Essentials of
Medical-Surgical Nursing

FOURTH EDITION

Susan C. deWit, MSN, RNCS

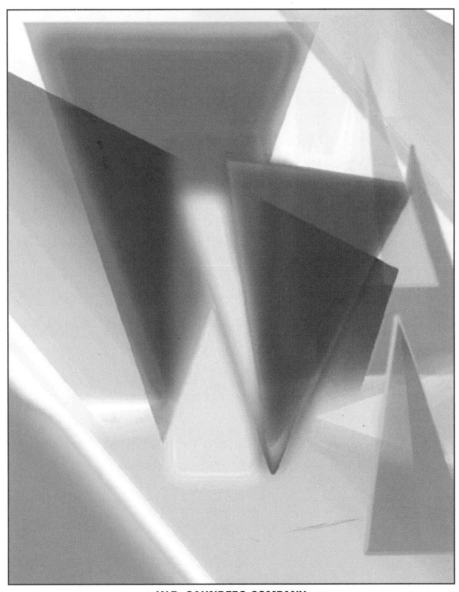

W.B. SAUNDERS COMPANY
A Division of Harcourt Brace & Company
Philadelphia London Toronto Montreal Sydney Tokyo

W.B. SAUNDERS COMPANY
A Division of Harcourt Brace & Company
The Curtis Center
Independence Square West
Philadelphia, Pennsylvania 19106

Library of Congress Cataloging-in-Publication Data

deWit, Susan C.
Essentials of medical-surgical nursing / Susan C. deWit. — 4th ed.

p.   cm.

Rev. ed. of: Keane's essentials of medical-surgical nursing. 3rd
ed. / Susan C. deWit. c1992.
Includes bibliographical references and index.

ISBN 0-7216-6920-4

1. Nursing.   2. Surgical nursing.   I. deWit, Susan C.   Keane's
    essentials of medical-surgical nursing.   II. Title.
    [DNLM: 1. Nursing.   2. Perioperative Nursing.   WY 150 D521e 1998]

RT41.D44 1998   610.73—dc21

DNLM/DLC   97-36860

Essentials of Medical-Surgical Nursing   ISBN 0-7216-6920-4

Printed in the United States of America

Last digit is the print number: 9   8   7   6   5   4   3   2   1

❖   ❖   ❖   ❖   ❖   ❖

In memory of:
"Bogie"
My deeply loved aunt, who departed for a better
place this year and is sorely missed

❖   ❖   ❖   ❖   ❖   ❖

To my cousins:
John and Georgia Wiester
and
Patty Sims
Who have been so supportive and generous in helping me
permanently locate close to them in beautiful central
coast California

❖   ❖   ❖   ❖   ❖   ❖

Contributors

Thomas Emanuele, BSN, RN, C, ACRN
Parkland Health and Hospital System
Amelia Court Clinic
Dallas, TX

Care of the Patient with AIDS

Barbara Wray Wayland, RN
Weekend Care Manager and Supervisor
Staff Builders Home Health
San Luis Obispo, CA

Care of Patients with Pain
Care of Patients with Disorders of the Female Reproductive System
Care of Patients with Sexually Transmitted Diseases

Barbara J. Michaels, RN, MS, EdD
Psychiatric Registered Nurse
The Holiner Psychiatric Group
Dallas, TX

Care of Patients with Anxiety and Mood Disorders
Care of Patients with Substance Use Disorders
Care of Patients with Cognitive Disorders
Care of Patients with Thought and Personality Disorders

Reviewers

Jan Marie Anderson, RN, MSN
Santa Barbara City College
School of Nursing
Santa Barbara, California

Roxanne Aubol Batterden, MS, RN, CCRN
The Johns Hopkins Hospital
Baltimore, Maryland

Jimmie C. Borum, RN, BSN
Medical Case Manager
Presbyterian Hospital of Dallas
Dallas, Texas

Mary Rose Chasler, RN, MSN
Jamestown Community College
School of Nursing
Jamestown, New York

Rebecca Coffey, RN, MSN
Ohio State University Hospitals
Columbus, Ohio

Carrie Dowdy, MSN, RN, C
Piedmont Virginia Community College
School of Nursing
Charlottesville, Virginia

Catherine A. Eddy, RN, MSN, CCRN
University of South Dakota
Department of Nursing
Rapid City, South Dakota
Rapid City Outreach
Rapid City, South Dakota

Frances Anne Freitas, MSN, RNC
Kent State University
School of Nursing
Ashtabula, Ohio

Karolyn R. Hanna, RN, MSN, PhD
Santa Barbara City College
School of Nursing
Santa Barbara, California

Sandra K. Harting, RN, CEN
Presbyterian Hospital of Dallas
Dallas, Texas

Shaula Hijazi, RN, MSN, FNP
Santa Barbara OB/GYN Associates
Santa Barbara, California

Renee S. Hyde, RN, MSN, CNRN
CMHA School of Nursing
Charlotte, North Carolina

Kathleen J. Jones, RN, MS, ANP
Walter Reed Army Medical Center
Washington, District of Columbia

Deitra Leonard Lowdermilk, RNC, PhD
University of North Carolina
School of Nursing
Chapel Hill, South Carolina

Lisa J. Massarweh, RN, MSN, CCRN
Kent State University
School of Nursing
Ashtabula, Ohio

Martha Megginson, RN, BSN, AD
Presbyterian Hospital of Dallas
Dallas, Texas

Kay Bowers O'Neal, MSN, RN
El Centro Community College
School of Nursing
Dallas, Texas

Patricia A. O'Neill, RN, MSN, CCRN
De Anza College
School of Nursing
Cupertino, California
O'Connor Hospital
San Jose, California

Arlene M. Polaski, MEd, MSN, RN
York Technical College
School of Nursing
Rock Hill, South Carolina

Dianna Lee Reding, RN, BS, MS, ACLS
Dallas County Community College District
El Centro College
Dallas, Texas
Parkland Hospital, Burn Unit
Dallas, Texas

Margaret Spath, RN, C, MSN
Kent State University
School of Nursing
Ashtabula, Ohio

Ruth A. Stocklas, MSN, RN, CS
Kent State University
School of Nursing
Ashtabula, Ohio

Kay I. Swiger, RNC, MN
York Technical College
School of Nursing
Rock Hill, South Carolina

Suzanne E. Tatro, BSN, MS, RN, CS
York Technical College
School of Nursing
Rock Hill, South Carolina

Linda M. Tunks, RN, BSN
Aetna Health Plans
Dallas, Texas

Judith P. Warner, BSN, RN
Vivra Renal Care
Erie, Pennsylvania
Forestview Nursing Center
Erie, Pennsylvania

Preface

As the health care environment is undergoing radical change, so is nursing. This fourth edition of *Essentials of Medical-Surgical Nursing* retains the basic elements that Claire Keane introduced in the first edition: clarity and conciseness of language and current data on disease processes and medical treatment. But it has been redesigned into a cohesive learning system constructed around the evolving role of the medical-surgical nurse today.

New chapters on issues and trends, community care and rehabilitation, leadership and management, and professional issues have been added to this edition, along with an entire unit on mental health nursing of the adult.

Costs effectiveness is the yardstick by which all aspects of care are presently measured. For this reason, registered nurses (RNs) and vocational practical nurses (LPNs, LVNs) are finding that the duties and skills required to perform their jobs are expanding. This new edition addresses expanded roles through four interwoven threads: (1) the use of the nursing process to organize and deliver appropriate care; (2) a focus on the patient as a consumer of health care and a person with psychosocial as well as physical needs; (3) an emphasis on wellness and preventive health care; and (4) collaboration with other health care professionals to provide coordinated, cost-effective patient care and promote rehabilitation.

Today more than ever, the practical nurse needs a thorough knowledge of the nursing process. This text teaches students the **application** of the nursing process and its five components. Use of the nursing process is illustrated throughout the chapters as a **tool,** while patients' needs are the focus of nursing care. Competence in skills is essential, but the knowledge of how and when to use those skills is what clinical medical-surgical nursing is all about.

There is a heavy emphasis on practical assessment: assessment to determine problems, assessment to monitor for the onset of complications, and assessment to determine the effectiveness of care (evaluation). As nurses function more and more in settings outside of the hospital where nursing practice is more autonomous, the ability to properly assess the patient, and to determine the effectiveness of treatment and care, become major factors in the return to optimum wellness for the patient.

Planning holistic care must include consideration of the patient's cultural orientation and its impact on perception of health and illness and health practices, and the ability of the patient to accomplish activities of daily living. Tables and boxes stressing specific areas of patient education are interspersed throughout the discussions of nursing care and encompass discharge planning.

Implementation of nursing actions is the heart of patient care. Nursing actions in this edition have been expanded and are specific and comprehensive. They are organized by common care problems to decrease repetition of information within a chapter and help students learn by mastering concepts rather than by memorizing facts.

Evaluation of nursing actions requires re-assessment of the patient and analysis of data. Thus, increasing student awareness of ways to specifically evaluate is a focus in each chapter.

Because our population is aging at a rapid rate, this edition includes expanded content on the geriatric patient. Assessment of the geriatric patient requires greater ability to elicit pertinent information from the patient or family as well as a knowledge of normal physiologic changes. Each chapter includes specific Elder Care Points. Suggestions for assessment and particular interventions for the long-term care and the home care patient are included.

A wellness focus requires more attention to **preventive health teaching.** Each "clinical" content chapter contains a section pointing out ways in which nurses can teach the public how to prevent many of the problems discussed.

Rehabilitation guides the patient toward wellness. Toward this end, a special chapter, "Extended Care within the Community: Chronic Illness and Rehabilitation," has been added to this edition. This chapter is concerned with rehabilitation of patients with burns and major disorders of the cardiac, respiratory, musculoskeletal, and neurologic systems for which rehabilitation is pertinent.

Clear, on-going, communication among health care professionals is essential for collaborative care to be effective. The ability to effectively communicate with and delegate tasks to ancillary personnel is essential when caring for multiple patients in any care setting. Chapter 36, "Leadership in Medical-Surgical Nursing," covers this as well as beginning management skills. Chapter 37, "Professional Issues," assists the student in obtaining a job, becoming a valued employee, contributing to the profession and community, and maintaining professional competence.

Student Learning Focus

This edition has been designed with student learning in mind. Illustrations and tables use visual appeal to pique students' interest, enhance content, illustrate a particular point, or summarize essential content. Important points throughout each chapter stand out in bold print. Essential-to-know information is inset and highlighted in red.

The language has been kept to a level consistent with today's students' reading ability without compromising the need to impart scientific and medical information. An English-as-a-Second Language (ESL) consultant has provided ideas to make the text more "user friendly" and understandable for the student with limited English proficiency (LEP). A section in each chapter of the *Student Learning Guide* has been designed to assist LEP students to more easily master the chapter content and to enhance English skills.

Potentially unfamiliar terms are printed in bold the first time they are introduced in the body of the text and a brief definition is given. All vocabulary terms are defined in the glossary. Chapter objectives are written to assist the student in focusing on what is most important in the chapter and to assist with the application of knowledge gained from the chapter. Exercises in the *Student Learning Guide* are geared to assist the student in achieving the objectives.

A brief review of the anatomy and physiology relevant to the content discussion is presented at the beginning of each "clinical" chapter. Normal function of the body system is reviewed. Correlation of how pathologic conditions interrupt normal function is included with the discussion of each disorder so that the student can visualize how illness or injury disrupts homeostasis.

"Think About" questions to check reading comprehension and promote critical thinking are interspersed throughout each chapter. Clinical Case Problems with questions are provided for integration of content into the student's overall knowledge base. A study outline provided at the chapter's end helps the student review the content, thereby enhancing retention. Questions are included in the *Student Learning Guide* for each chapter to test assimilation of content.

Pharmacology information and nutritional concerns are addressed along with the relevant nursing care for the most common disorders. Tables of the drugs most frequently utilized for treatment of the major disorders in the chapter have been added. A table of diagnostic tests and nursing implications is included for each chapter concerning medical-surgical problems.

Nursing Care Plans, Critical Pathway examples, and a table of nursing diagnoses and expected outcomes paired with specific nursing interventions are included for the most common disorders in each chapter dealing with "clinical" problems. Specific points to consider for evaluation of the effectiveness of care have been added. A chapter section of exercises in the *Student Learning Guide* is aimed at increasing comprehension and application of the nursing process for specific problems or disorders.

Since there are both male and female nurses, physicians, and patients, the use of "he" and "she" for patient, physician, and nurse varies from chapter to chapter.

The *Instructor's Curriculum Guide* presents a lecture outline for each chapter with suggestions for presentation of material and questions to involve students in discussion. Ideas for short answer quizzes for each chapter, suggestions for small group learning activities, suggestions for assisting limited English proficient students, clinical activities, and ways to integrate theory into the clinical setting are presented. Numerous transparency "masters" can be photocopied to overhead transparencies for lecture use.

The test bank has been revised and expanded to assist in preparing students for NCLEX CAT-type questions. Although many multiple-choice questions are free-standing for this reason, situations with several related questions and short-answer questions are included for the purpose of stimulating critical thinking. Answers with rationale are included with the test bank.

Although the text is designed so that it can be used free-standing, it is hoped that the learning system comprising the text, the *Student Learning Guide,* the *Instructor's Curriculum Guide,* and the test bank will be utilized to achieve the goals of mastery of content, synthesis of knowledge, development of critical thinking skills, and an increased ability to make sound clinical judgments for each student.

Susan C. deWit, MSN, RNCS

Acknowledgments

I am very appreciative of the work done by Claire Keane on the early editions of this text. She provided a fine foundation on which to work. Many thanks to my contributors Barbara Michaels, Barbara Wayland, and Tom Emanuele who helped build upon that foundation by doing a fine job on their chapters for this book.

Thanks to my colleagues in Santa Barbara, Santa Maria, and Dallas who have been so available with advice and answers to questions and to all those who reviewed chapters. Particular thanks to Ellen White at Alan Hancock College, Frances Warrick, Kathy Pritchett, Kay O'Neal, Barbara Michaels, and Jimmie Borum at El Centro College, Jackie Huth, Jan Anderson, Karolyn Hanna, and Janie Guillermo at Santa Barbara City College, and Faye Gregory at Long Beach City College for informal reviews, specific information, and helpful suggestions. Thanks to Mary Helen Madrid and Sandra Harting for supplying EKG rhythm strips and sharing ideas for teaching materials and to Rosa Babcock for supplying initial suggestions on how to make learning easier for students with limited English proficiency. Gail Boehme, the ESL/LEP consultant diligently reviewed every chapter, submitted suggestions for making reading easier for LEP students, and suggested types of learning activities for the Student Learning Guide and the Instructor's Curriculum Guide that could facilitate the learning process for these students.

Thanks to my steadfast friend, Dawn Vallendar, who has helped me through the difficult times and who has been my walking companion. I am very grateful to Linda Yankie, my secretary and friend, who took care of a lot of the correspondence and attention to detail that a project like this requires.

Special thanks to our photographer, Glenn Derbyshire, TC, and the rest of his crew who worked so hard to offer the flexibility needed to work with real patients and who created magnificent photos to grace the pages of the book. Kathie Morgan did a fine job of juggling people and places in coordinating the photo shots. I'm very grateful to the staff at Goleta Valley Cottage Hospital, the Santa Barbara City College VN students, and patients, who provided us with subjects, supplies, and opportunities to photograph nursing in action in their lovely facility. Thanks also go to Carol Cachelin and Debbie McCoy the Visiting Nurse Association of Santa Barbara, The Cancer Foundation in Santa Barbara, and the Leigh Block Hospice for allowing us to photograph patients undergoing nursing care and therapy. I extend special thanks to Margarite Wordel, the staff, and patients, at The Rehabilitation Institute at Santa Barbara for allowing us to photograph in the Institute and for working so hard to fit our photo shoots into their routine.

Special thanks also to Ilze Rader, who helped me begin this project before she left Saunders; to Kevin Law, my editor; and to Tony and Maria Caruso, who coordinated production of this text. I am very thankful to have had Marie Thomas again as Editorial Assistant. Marie always attends to the smallest detail efficiently and cheerfully. The quick, professional attention from all those at Saunders who worked on the text is deeply appreciated. Thanks go to all those involved in the project: Thomas Eoyang, Robin Richman, Lee Henderson, Joan Sinclair, Elizabeth Byrd, Marie-Josee Anne Schorp, and Julie Lawley.

Susan C. deWit, MSN, RNCS

Brief Contents

Unit Four ◆ Mental Health Nursing of the Adult   995

Unit Five ◆ Managing Medical-Surgical Issues   1049

Contents

8 Care of the Patient with AIDS   183

Thomas Emanuele, BSN, RN, C, ACRN

9 Care of Patients with Cancer   206

10 Care of Patients with Pain   241

Barbara Wray Wayland, RN

11 Care of the Immobile Patient: Preventing Complications   255

Unit Three ◆ Nursing Care for Specific Medical-Surgical Disorders   321

23   Care of Patients with Urological Disorders   715

24   Care of Patients with Endocrine Disorders: Pituitary, Thyroid, Parathyroid, and Adrenal Glands   765

25   Care of Patients with Endocrine Disorders: Diabetes Mellitus and Hypoglycemia   793

26 Care of Patients with Disorders of the Female Reproductive System   825

Barbara Wray Wayland, RN

27 Care of Patients with Disorders of the Male Reproductive System   857

Unit Four • Mental Health Nursing of the Adult   995

32   Care of Patients with Anxiety and Mood Disorders   997

Barbara J. Michaels, RN, Ed D, MS

33   Care of Patients with Substance Use Disorders   1009

Barbara J. Michaels, RN, Ed D, MS

34   Care of Patients with Cognitive Disorders   1023

Barbara J. Michaels, RN, Ed D, MS

35   Care of Patients with Thought and Personality Disorders   1036

Barbara J. Michaels, RN, Ed D, MS

Unit Five • Managing Medical-Surgical Issues   1049

36   Leadership in Medical-Surgical Nursing   1051

Medical–Surgical Nursing

The evolving health care system with its focus on cost-effectiveness is changing the ways in which medical–surgical nurses work. The first chapter in this unit addresses the issues and trends that are affecting the medical–surgical nurse. The role of the licensed practical/vocational nurse (LPN/VN) in various medical–surgical settings is explored. The basic economics of health care, health maintenance organizations, preferred provider organizations, and the disbursement system of Medicare are explained.

Chapter 2 focuses on assessment skills and the application of the nursing process in clinical practice. It is increasingly important that LPN/VNs develop good assessment skills as they venture out of the hospital into community care settings. The nurse uses the nursing process in every phase of daily work; it is essential that it become "second nature." Clinical pathways are presented as a cost-effective tool for tracking patient progress.

Chapter 3 discusses the psychosocial aspects that affect a patient's reaction to illness. Specific factors to be considered when planning nursing care are described. Nursing in the community requires that nurses give even more attention to psychosocial factors as they work with patients and families.

CHAPTER 1

Caring for Medical–Surgical Patients: Issues and Trends

OBJECTIVES

Upon completing this chapter, the student should be able to:
1. Give an example of each of the five functions of the medical–surgical nurse.
2. Describe three specific practice settings in which it would be desirable to work.
3. Explain the difference between a Health Maintenance Organization (HMO) and a Preferred Provider Organization (PPO).
4. List three disadvantages of allowing unlicensed personnel to perform nursing functions.
5. Identify four factors that have contributed to rising health care costs.
6. Describe how a hospital is reimbursed under the diagnostic-related group (DRG) payment system of Medicare.
7. Give two examples that illustrate how a focus on health promotion and prevention of illness could decrease health care costs.

CARING FOR MEDICAL–SURGICAL PATIENTS

The role of the licensed practical/vocational nurse, along with other health care team members, is to promote and maintain health, prevent disease and disability, care for individuals during rehabilitation and assist the dying patient to maintain the best quality of life possible. She or he uses the nursing process to plan and deliver safe, competent care to patients (or clients). Practical nurses carry out prescribed protocols and therapeutic regimens by acting in various capacities.

◆ Caregiver

Practical nurses perform treatments, give medications, and provide care to meet patients' basic needs. They gather data to assist in planning and evaluating care. They give baths and comb hair, insert catheters, administer medications, and perform various treatments. They assist patients with exercise and help them to obtain sufficient rest. They see to it that the patients' immediate environment is neat, clean, and orderly. They interact with the patients in a therapeutic manner, using effective communication skills, and maintain appropriate documentation of the care given and the status of their patients.

Think about . . . When delivering care, what can you do to treat the patient as a "valued customer"?

◆ Educator

Practical nurses provide health teaching to patients and significant others to maintain wellness or promote healing. They teach how to treat a wound and change a dressing, how to take prescribed medications, what side effects to report, and the self-care activities necessary to promote rehabilitation. They also provide information about community resources and self-help groups that could be beneficial to patients and their families.

◆ Collaborator

Collaborating with the other members of the health care team to provide the patient with an integrated, comprehensive, plan of care is another function of practical nurses. They work closely with nursing aides and registered nurses to ensure that all aspects of the patients' basic needs are met. They share information and uses the experience and expertise of others. They recognize the patient in crisis, intervene to maintain patient safety, and make appropriate referrals as needed. They contribute to the discharge plan of the patient and deliver discharge instructions.

Think about . . . Discuss with a classmate, what other health care providers you might collaborate with when caring for a patient with a breathing disorder such as pneumonia.

◆ Delegator

Knowing when and which tasks to delegate to nursing assistants or others is a function of the practical nurse that becomes easier and more effective with experience. Working with others in this supervisory capacity requires tact and effective communication skills. **Nurses are responsible for the care given by others that they have delegated. They must verify that the tasks have been accomplished properly and must document the care given. They must be knowledgeable about the skills and judgment capabilities of those to whom they delegate.**

Think about . . . Name three tasks you might assign to a nursing assistant when you are caring for three patients yourself. How would you verify that the work has been done satisfactorily?

◆ Upholder of Clinical Practice Standards

Practical nurses are accountable for the nursing care they administer. They know and apply the ethical principles of the profession. They adhere to state laws and continue their education to maintain a current knowledge base and skills in their area of practice. They serve as patient advocates, protecting patients' rights and consulting with others when necessary.

The roles of the registered nurse and the practical/ vocational nurse (LPN/VN) often overlap and in many settings are blurred. The practical nurse is more likely to give direct, basic, patient care, whereas the registered nurse supervises and coordinates care and performs the more complex procedures some patients require. The registered nurse is responsible for more in-depth assessment of the patient, although the practical nurse also performs assessment. The practical nurse often performs basic supervisory functions when working in an extended care facility or a clinic, but she functions under the supervision of a registered nurse who is ultimately responsible for the care of patients in that facility.

The role of the LPN/VN continues to evolve. Money constraints in the health care system are causing greater demands to expand the functions of practical nurses. With added education and training, LPN/VNs will probably continue to increase their capabilities and take on tasks that were formerly performed only by registered nurses (RNs).

Think about . . . Describe two ways in which you might continue your learning after graduation from the practical nurse program.

PRACTICE SETTINGS FOR THE MEDICAL–SURGICAL NURSE

Table 1-1 shows the many places the medical–surgical nurse can find employment today:

LPNs/VNs in many states make up the majority of the nursing staff in long-term care facilities, Health Maintenance Organization (HMO) clinics, rehabilitation centers, and physicians' offices. More opportunities also are becoming available in the field of home health care (Figure 1-1).

ISSUES AND TRENDS

The health care delivery system is undergoing many changes. People are living much longer, and improved health care is doing much to keep them alive. There is a continuously growing elderly population, many of whom have extensive and expensive health care needs. Hospitalized patients who are acutely ill and require much more nursing skill, time, and expertise than ever

TABLE 1-1 ◆ *Employment Settings for the Medical–Surgical Nurse*
Hospitals
Same-day surgery facilities
Intermediate or subacute care facilities
Long-term or extended-care facilities
Home health care agencies
Physicians' offices
Ambulatory clinics
Health maintenance organization clinics
Emergency centers
Neighborhood emergency clinics
Rehabilitation programs
Renal dialysis centers
Hospices

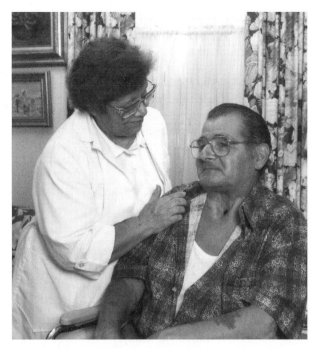

FIGURE 1-1   Licensed vocational nurse caring for the patient in a home care setting. (Photo by Glen Derbyshire. Courtesy of Santa Barbara Visiting Nurse Association.)

before. Less acutely ill patients are cared for outside the hospital, in subacute or extended care facilities, in the home, or at community clinics.

◆ The Changing Face of Health Care Delivery

To decrease costs, health care providers are grouping together to provide services. *Health Maintenance Organizations (HMOs)* operate by enrolling patients for a set fee per month. They then provide care for the patient by a team of doctors and other professionals that they employ. The monthly fee stays the same regardless of the number of visits or the type of treatment. Because they do not have to pay, or pay only a small fee for each visit, patients usually seek earlier treatment that helps them to avoid serious illness. The goal of an HMO is to keep its subscribers healthy and out of the hospital by means of regular health screening, health education, and preventive services such as immunizations.

An HMO patient must have prior approval to seek care from someone other than an assigned primary physician. If they do not have that approval, they are individually responsible for the costs involved.

Preferred Provider Organizations (PPOs) contract with businesses and insured groups to provide a group of physicians who will discount their fees in return for a steady supply of clients. Using PPOs allows insurance companies to keep their premium rates down, and in turn low rates appeal to employers who provide health

insurance as a benefit to employees. Policyholders associated with a PPO keep their health care costs down by using physicians and providers from the PPO list. They may select other physicians and service providers not on the list, but there will be an out-of-pocket cost for those services.

It is becoming increasingly difficult for physicians to work on a fee-for-services basis with individual patients. Employers in search of ways to stop the increases in health care premiums for their employees are more and more contracting with HMOs or PPOs.

There is considerable controversy as to whether the trend improves health care or causes it to deteriorate. Certainly more emphasis on health education and the promotion of wellness should bring positive effects. However, patients enrolled in HMOs and PPOs may find that they no longer have one physician over a long period. Employers switch the group with whom they contract, and physicians leave the employ of the HMO or disassociate with the PPO. Continuity of care by a physician who knows the patient well is disrupted. Time will tell whether this will decrease the quality of health care the patient receives.

Think about . . . Which would you rather your family be covered by, an HMO or a PPO? Give three reasons for your choice.

◆ Licensure Issues

Presently, nurses are licensed to practice by state boards of nursing and their practice is tightly controlled. To contain costs, a movement has been initiated to use less trained personnel to perform many of the tasks that are in the realm of nursing and other health professions. These people are "cross-trained" to perform a variety of functions in the hospital or are specifically trained in a specialty area to be "nurse extenders." They function under the *jurisdiction* (control) of the hospital or the physician and are not regulated by practice laws. There is considerable resistance on the part of nurses to allow this practice to continue. Professional nursing organizations are trying to educate the public about the dangers of allowing minimally trained people to perform duties that require considerable skill and judgment.

On the other hand, professional nurses are pushing to expand the scope of their practice to incorporate many of the health maintenance services that have traditionally been performed by physicians. Nurse practitioners are heavily utilized by HMOs and are sought as primary care providers in many rural areas where physicians won't locate. Licensing laws are changing fslowly to allow expanded practice for properly trained people.

THE ECONOMICS OF HEALTH CARE DELIVERY: COST CONTAINMENT

◆ Factors Contributing to Rising Costs

The increase in lawsuits against physicians has made malpractice insurance costs sky-rocket. The trend has been for physicians to practice "defensive medicine," ordering costly diagnostic tests to back up their diagnoses. This practice has contributed considerably to the rising cost of health care.

The increase in the elderly population who are living much longer lives is draining the Medicare system. Although many elderly are relatively healthy, a large percentage have chronic illnesses that require frequent health care treatments. The advances in technology have made diagnosis and treatment better, but these technologies are very expensive. The expense of diagnostic tests such as CT scans and magnetic resonance imaging (MRI) is another factor in rising costs.

Many elderly are taking multiple prescription drugs, and many drugs cost $1.00 or more a dose. Whether insurance covers a portion of these costs or not, they add to the total cost of health care.

◆ Attempts to Decrease Costs

Diagnostic-Related Groups   The number of elderly receiving Medicare benefits has mushroomed, straining the Social Security System. *Diagnostic Related Groups (DRGs)* were designed to cut the costs of Medicare expenses. The government has made a list of some 467 DRGs and figured the average cost of hospital care for each of them. An admitting diagnosis such as "pneumonia" is allotted so many days of hospitalization, so much money for diagnostic tests, medication, nursing care, and so on, in one lump sum paid by the government Medicare division. Hospitals are now reimbursed by this set amount for each DRG. If a patient's treatment requires more days than are designated or more tests than are included, the hospital bears the extra cost. It is very common for a percentage of patients to need extra hospital days. Many times this is because the patient has one or more chronic illnesses besides the one for which he or she is hospitalized. This system began in 1983, and the trend is for private insurance companies to adopt similar payment plans.

Because a majority of hospital patients are elderly and are covered by Medicare, hospitals are absorbing a great deal of the expense of care. Small hospitals cannot sustain such expense, and many have become bankrupt and have closed. All hospitals continue to cut staff in an effort to decrease expenses so that they can stay open. This has led to much heavier workloads for the remaining staff. Many physicians and nurses feel that the DRG system and consequent staff cuts have decreased the quality of care and directly threaten the safety of patients.

However, DRGs have forced hospitals to evaluate their operating procedures, evaluate costs, improve efficiency, and become more effective in the use of resources to provide effective health care. Hospitals have switched from a "health" to a "business" focus to survive. Nurses must learn to function with a cost-containment perspective, constantly questioning which is the most cost-effective way to do a treatment or provide care.

Managed Care   The trend toward a *managed care* system is a result of the focus on cost containment. Managed care is a term applied to a way of organizing health care delivery that centers on coordinating the care by various health team members in a timely manner for cost-effectiveness purposes. **The end goal of managed care is to facilitate the patient's recovery and discharge from the facility or agency.**

Clinical pathways are tools used to track a patient's progress along a set path in a managed care system (Clinical Pathway 1-1). The path is a carefully devised grid of activities to be accomplished by each member of the health care team involved in the patient's care for each day of hospitalization. A care manager is assigned to follow the progress of the patient and solve problems if expected progress along the path is not occurring. Clinical pathways standardize basic care for patients with each diagnosis. Each pathway is individualized for the particular patient by adding activities to the path as needed. Documentation is done on the pages of the pathway, on the back of the pathway pages, or in the progress notes, depending on hospital policy. In any event, documentation is simplified and takes less of the nurse's time. This system is evolving and is continually being refined. When a clinical pathway is used, a separate nursing care plan is unnecessary.

Access to Care   Another issue brought about by the steps toward cost containment is whether all persons should be entitled to health care whether they can pay for it or not. The costs to federal and state governments have risen beyond the taxpayers' willingness, and ability, to pay for them. To reduce expenditures, political and philosophical decisions must be made. How shall we decide who is entitled to free health care services? How long should the public pay for services to any one individual? Should people continue to be allowed to neglect their health, indulge in harmful life-styles, and then be given free health services when serious illness occurs?

Ethical considerations also raise questions. For example, should the person beyond eighty years be allowed to have open-heart surgery at Medicare (public) expense? Should the elderly person who has suffered a stroke and is long-term comatose be cared for in an extended care facility paid for by Medicare? What are our alternatives?

Think about... Consider your feelings about the following situation: an active 80-year-old man is told he needs cardiac bypass surgery, or he will most likely die of a coronary occlusion. He is used to gardening daily and still plays golf. Should Medicare pay the cost of a surgery that is in excess of $100,000? Think about how you would feel if this man was your father or favorite uncle.

Alternative Treatments   The quest for cost containment and research on the body–mind connection and its relevance to health and healing have caused health care providers to look anew at alternative treatments and methods of healing. Natural substance remedies are gaining favor, and much research is being conducted on the effectiveness of various herbs and treatments to determine whether there is a scientifically based reason for using them.

Acupuncture (technique to relieve pain or problem by inserting thin needles into specific points in the body) is becoming more accepted as an alternative treatment for many ailments. Many physicians are seeking training in acupuncture. Nurses are beginning to learn *acupressure* (technique to relieve pain by applying pressure to specific points on the body) to ease a patient's distress more readily, and *therapeutic touch* is being used in more creative ways. *Yoga* has been found to greatly decrease the symptoms of menopause, and *daily meditation* can decrease blood pressure and relieve anxiety. *Homeopathic medicine* is emerging as a treatment option. *Homeopathy* techniques involve administering minute, diluted quantities of a substance or a drug that in large amounts produces symptoms of disease in healthy individuals. It is similar to the desensitization techniques used in treating allergies. As more research studies are published showing their effectiveness, various alternative treatment methods will more readily be used to enhance, supplement, or lessen the need for more expensive medical therapies.

Focus on Health Promotion   *Healthy People 2000* objectives speak directly to National health promotion and disease prevention. These objectives were published by the U.S. Department of Health and Human Services in 1990, with an update published in 1996. The objectives cover areas of health promotion, health protection, preventive services, surveillance, and data systems.

They provide measurable guidelines for reducing death and disability.

A shift to a focus on health promotion should help decrease health care costs. The role of the practical nurse can be major in promoting and accomplishing these objectives. Contact with each patient is an opportunity to teach illness prevention, safe practices, and health promotion. The question is, *how do we make people accountable for taking care of their health?* Many insurance companies offer lower premiums to nonsmokers. Is it possible to structure health insurance costs according to the way people attempt to maintain good health in other ways?

People today spend the largest part of their extra income on dining out. Although information has been available regarding the advantage of a low-fat diet for many years, restaurants have been slow to convert their menus and food preparation to provide low-fat food. It is possible to eat lower fat meals when dining out now, but the majority of items offered are not low fat and are very high in calories. In the abundance of our country and our competitive market place, servings have become larger and larger over the years. Obesity and heart disease are two of our major health problems. Public pressure on food providers to adjust portion sizes, fat, and calorie content could do much to promote healthier lifestyles and decrease health care costs across the country. Our collective love of "junk food" has certainly been a factor in the development of both obesity and heart disease. Can we develop the self-discipline to change our eating habits? As you can see, society wide health-promoting changes are not easy to accomplish.

Think about... In what ways could you change your life-style to promote good health? Which of the ways would be easy for you to accomplish? Which would be most difficult?

Continuing to educate people about exercise, nutrition, ways to decrease stress, the use of sunscreen when outside, safe sexual practices, information on when screenings for cancer should be done, and the avoidance of harmful substances can promote a healthier society. It is each nurse's responsibility to educate each patient about these topics. **Nurses can be instrumental in educating the community about health promotion through membership in both professional and community organizations.** Medical–surgical nursing does not stop when nurses leave their workplace, it continues as they function in other roles in the community.

CRITICAL THINKING EXERCISES

1. Describe to your best friend outside of your nursing class, the various roles and functions you will perform when you are an LPN/VN.

CLINICAL PATHWAY 1-1 ◆ *Gastrointestinal Bleeding (Nonvariceal)*

Nursing Diagnosis/Collaborative Problem	Expected Outcome (The Patient Is Expected to . . .)	Met/Not Met	Reason	Date/Initials
Fluid volume deficit (hypovolemia)	Have stable VS and no evidence of active bleeding			
Electrolyte imbalance	Have lytes WNL and no S/S of electrolyte imbalance			
Potential for recurrent GI bleed	Follow discharge instructions regarding meds, diet, lifestyle changes, early detection			

Aspect of Care	Date ___ Day 1	Date ___ Day 2	Date ___ Day 3	Date ___ Day 4
Assessment	VS q 1→4 h, depending on stability; Monitor vomitus and stool for gross and occult blood; Systems assessment	VS q 2→4 h, depending on stability; Monitor vomitus and stool; Systems assessment; Assess for weakness, postural hypotension	VS QID; Monitor vomitus and stool; Systems assessment; Assess for weakness, postural hypotension	VS QID; Systems assessment; Monitor stools for OB
Teaching	Orient to hospital and unit; Review clinical pathway/plan of care with patient and family; Reinforce importance of NPO, meds, IVs, and diagnostic studies	Teach pre- and post-test care for endoscopic examination	Begin discharge teaching including ◆ Meds ◆ Diet ◆ Lifestyle changes ◆ When to call MD ◆ Monitoring stools	Reinforce/review discharge instructions
Consults	Gastroenterology/surgery; Social worker	N/A	Dietician	N/A
Lab tests	CBC with diff. SMA-6 (6/60). INR(PT)/APTT, type and crossmatch, stools for OB	Hgb and Hct stools for OB	Hgb and Hct stools for OB	Hgb and Hct
Other tests	Chest X-ray if >40 years old or if history of cardiac disease	Endoscopy	N/A	N/A
Meds	Zantac or other H₂ blocker continuous IV or IVPB; Blood transfusions until Hgb and Hct increase to baseline range; D/C all other nonessential meds	Same as Day 1 (blood if indicated for low Hgb and Hct)	PO antacids, carafate, and/or H₂ blocker; D/C IV meds	PO antacids, Carafate, and/or H₂ blocker

	Day 1	Day 2	Day 3	Day 4
Treatments/interventions	I & O q 8 h HOB elevated at least 30° unless severely hypotensive If severely hypotensive, may need shock blocks Provide emotional support	Same as Day 1	D/C I & O	N/A
Nutrition	NPO	NPO or clear liquids	Clear → full liquids; advance DAT (may need special diet if peptic ulcer disease, diverticulitis, or inflammatory bowel disease	DAT (or special diet for peptic ulcer disease, diverticulitis, inflammatory bowel disease)
Lines/tubes/monitors	Continuous IV fluids with KCl for volume, lyte replacement (18g) If upper GI bleeding, may use NGT to low suction	Continue with IV fluids May clamp or D/C NGT if bleeding subsides	D/C NGT if still present D/C IV and convert to saline loc	D/C saline loc, if present
Mobility/self-care	Bed rest Assist with ADLs as needed	Bed rest Assist with ADLs as needed	BSC or BRPs with supervision Assist with ADLs as needed	Up ad lib
Discharge planning	Assess support systems and financial needs; assess need for home health services or NH placement	Same as Day 1	Complete arrangements for home health or NH placement Arrange for follow-up appointment with MD as specified	Discharge to home or NH Follow-up appointment with MD or clinic

Source: Ignativicius, D. D., Hausman, K. A. (1995). *Clinical Pathways for Collaborative Practice.* Philadelphia: Saunders, pp 168–170.

2. Choose three practice settings that might appeal to you after graduation.

3. Explain to a family member what the differences are between an HMO and a PPO.

4. Make a list of your own health-promotion practices.

BIBLIOGRAPHY

AJN Newsline. (1995). Layoffs loom as Kaiser turns to "multiskilled caregivers." *American Journal of Nursing.* 95(5):77, 82.

Benefield, L. E. (1996) Making the transition to home care nursing. *American Journal of Nursing.* 96(10):47–49.

Chapman, A. H., Sebastian, W. (1996). Selected issues in quality improvement and risk management. *Seminars in Oncology Nursing.* 12(3):231–237.

Harris, M. D. (1996). Medicare coverage of medical supplies. *Home Healthcare Nurse.* 14(7):513–515.

Ignatavicius, D. D., Hausman, K. A. (1995). *Clinical Pathways for Collaborative Practice.* Philadelphia: Saunders.

Ignatavicius, D. D., Workman, M. L., Mishler, M. A. (1995). *Medical-Surgical Nursing: A Nursing Process Approach,* 2nd ed. Philadelphia: Saunders.

Katz, J. R., Clemons, P. (1996). Surviving a merger. *Nursing 96 Career Directory.* Springhouse, PA: Springhouse.

Kurzon, C. R. (1993). *Contemporary Practical/Vocational Nursing,* 2nd ed. Philadelphia: Lippincott.

Lessner, M. W., et al. (1994). Orienting nursing students to cost effective clinical practice. *Nursing & Health Care.* 15(9):458–462.

Nornhold, P. (1996). What networks mean to you. *Nursing 96 Career Directory.* Springhouse, PA: Springhouse.

Seeber, S., Baird, S. B. (1996). The impact of health care changes on home health. *Seminars in Oncology Nursing.* 12(3):179–187.

Swackhamer, A. H. (1995). It's time to broaden our practice. *RN.* 58(1):49–51.

Tabone, S. (1994). Unlicensed assistive personnel: dilemmas for RNs? Is quality care compromised? *Texas Nursing.* September, p. 8–10.

Thompson, D. G. (1994). Critical pathways: good idea, right reason? *Critical Care Nurse.* 15(6):112.

U.S. Department of Health and Human Services (1990). *Healthy People 2000: national health promotion and disease prevention objectives. Summary report.* Washington, DC: Government Printing Office.

Walsh, G. G. (1996). How subacute care fills the gap. *Nursing 96 Career Directory.* Springhouse, PA: Springhouse.

Weston, M. A. (1996). Case management in acute care. *MEDSURG Nursing.* 5(5):378–379.

Zerwekh, J., Claborn, J. C. (1997). *Nursing Today: Transition and Trends,* 2nd ed. Philadelphia: Saunders.

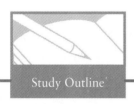

Study Outline

I. Caring for Medical–Surgical Patients: Roles of the Practical Nurse

A. Caregiver

1. Provides care to assist patients to meet their basic needs.

2. Competently performs basic nursing procedures.

3. Uses the nursing process to plan, deliver, and evaluate nursing care.

4. Interacts in a therapeutic manner using effective communication skills.

5. Maintains appropriate documentation of care given and patient status.

B. Educator

1. Teaches self-care practices to promote healing and rehabilitation or maintain wellness.

2. Includes the family or significant others in teaching.

3. Provides information about community resources.

C. Collaborator

1. Collaborates with other health team members in planning and delivering integrated, comprehensive care to patients.

2. Shares information and utilizes the expertise of other health professionals.

3. Recognizes the need for and makes referrals as needed.

D. Delegator

1. Is responsible for the nursing care delegated to others.

2. Uses good judgment in delegating tasks to others.

E. Upholder of standards of clinical practice

1. Is accountable for care given.

2. Applies ethical principles of the profession.

3. Adheres to state laws and the legal parameters of practice.
4. Updates skill and knowledge base through continued education.
5. Serves as a patient advocate.

II. **Practice Settings for the Medical–Surgical Nurse (Table 1-1)**

III. **Issues and Trends**
   A. The changing face of health care delivery
      1. From fee-for-service to managed care.
      2. Health Maintenance Organizations (HMOs).
      3. Preferred Provider Organizations (PPOs).
      4. Licensure issues: increase in unlicensed assistive personnel.
      5. Expanding practice of professional nurses.
   B. The economics of health care delivery: cost containment
      1. Factors contributing to rising costs.
         a. Lawsuits and expense of malpractice insurance.
         b. Practice of "defensive" medicine.
         c. Rapidly increasing elderly population entitled to Medicare benefits.
      2. Attempts to decrease the cost of health care.
         a. Diagnostic-related groups (DRGs).
         b. Shift in hospital administration from a "health" focus to a "business" focus.
         c. Attempts to limit access to care: decreasing welfare and rationing care.
         d. Managed care practices using clinical pathways.
         e. Focus on health promotion
            (1) Health education for health maintenance.
            (2) Avoidance of harmful substances and practices.

CHAPTER 2

Performing Assessment and Applying the Nursing Process

O B J E C T I V E S

Upon completing this chapter the student should be able to:
1. Define the nursing process and its goals.
2. Describe the role of the licensed practical nurse (LPN) in applying the nursing process.
3. Consider the underlying beliefs, give an example for each of them, and show how they are interwoven.
4. Perform a nursing assessment on a peer or a family member.
5. Discuss the types of data that might be obtained from a chart review.
6. Cite the areas to be included in a psychosocial assessment.
7. State how a spiritual assessment might help the nurse better to meet the health care needs of a patient.
8. Apply techniques of physical assessment to assess a peer, family member, or patient.
9. Describe how properly to formulate a nursing care plan.
10. Compare and contrast a nursing care plan and a clinical pathway.

Nursing greatly depends on good problem-solving abilities and should be approached and carried out in a scientific and orderly manner. Thinking of nursing as a problem-solving process provides nurses with a framework for identifying and dealing with the actual or potential problems presented by their patients. The components of the nursing process give organization and direction to the activities that are in the area of nursing care. Nurses enter into the process when they accept responsibility for the care of each patient, recognize him or her as a unique individual, and plan the care they will give according to the patient's specific health care needs at any given moment. In addition, the orderly approach inherent in the nursing process provides the means by which **outcomes** (results of actions) can be predicted and the results of nursing activities evaluated.

Communication is an essential part of any effective interaction among people. Documentation of the nursing process is the method by which vital information is communicated to all who provide health care to a patient. Written records provide continuity of care. Accurate and complete written records tell others on the health care team what is planned, what has been done, and how the patient has responded to whatever was done.

CHARACTERISTICS OF THE NURSING PROCESS

A *process* can be defined as a series of actions that move forward from one point to another on the way to achieving a goal.

In a process there is continuous progress through stages, each stage being dependent on the other and leading to a specific result, outcome, or product. In every process there is a moving force that controls and systematically directs activities so that the goal is achieved and the desired result reached. The actions taking place in a process are carefully carried out in a logical way. If a process is without a goal or there are no deliberate efforts to achieve it, the process will sooner or later break down. The *nursing process* is a goal-directed series of activities whereby the practice of nursing is approached in a systematic and orderly way.

The goal of the nursing process is to alleviate, minimize, or prevent real or potential health problems.

The problems that are identified in the nursing process are those that nurses are qualified to treat by virtue of their education, experience, and commitment to the goals of nursing.

The nursing process is deliberate. It is not haphazard, routine, or unmindful of the needs of the patient. It demands careful thought about what is happening to patients and how they are responding to actions intended to improve their health and well-being. It is, therefore, a rational and logical approach to the task of helping patients meet their health needs.

The nursing process demands knowledge, skills, and a belief in the worth of every person.

The actions of nurses are based on their knowledge of nursing theory, competence in performing the techniques of nursing practice, and understanding of and commitment to the basic philosophical beliefs and scientific principles derived from theories of nursing and other disciplines.

Each step of the nursing process builds on the preceding step. Data obtained by assessment are analyzed to determine what the patient's most pressing problems are and nursing diagnoses are chosen to address those problems. Goals are set to solve the problems and specific expected outcomes are written. Interventions are planned to assist the patient to meet the goals. **The plan is implemented, and then the nurse evaluates whether or not the actions performed are assisting the patient to meet the goals.**

The American Nurses' Association (ANA) provides standards to judge the competency of nurses and to evaluate the quality of services nurses give. These measures are the Standards of Medical–Surgical Nursing Practice, which were written to ensure that high-quality services will be provided by nurses. These standards are continually revised to reflect the emerging scope of practice for nurses. The ANA Standards for Medical–Surgical Nursing Practice in an acute care setting are presented in the discussion of each phase of the nursing process.

◆ Differences in Roles in the Nursing Process

Because of differences in their educational preparation for nursing practice, graduates of 1-, 2-, 3-, and 4-year programs are expected to perform at different levels. In actual practice these role differences are not nearly so clearly defined as they might be; there remain some questions about who is qualified—and therefore expected—to perform at what level. The National League of Nursing (NLN) is continuing work to clarify the roles and expectations for the graduates of these programs.

In addition to differences in formal educational preparation for the practice of nursing, there are differences in the amount of experience each nurse has obtained and in the setting in which he or she practices. In general, graduates of 1- and 2-year programs begin work in acute health care settings, long-term care facilities, or clinics, where they use the nursing process to achieve goals related to recovery from sickness and injury. Graduates of baccalaureate programs are more likely to practice in community-oriented settings where they deliver primary health care and practice independently and without direct supervision.

◆ Applying the Nursing Process in Medical–Surgical Nursing

The essential tasks of the beginning nurse are: (1) to establish a data base for the patient by collecting information using a standardized form, performing basic psychosocial assessment, and taking objective measurements of body functions; (2) to develop nursing care plans and then implement the established plan of care by; (3) performing basic therapeutic and preventive nursing measures; and (4) evaluating the care given by reporting observed outcomes and making necessary changes according to the results of the evaluation.

The information presented in this chapter and the remainder of this text is intended to help to prepare the beginning nurse to perform these tasks competently. The relatively complex tasks within the nursing process demand a sound knowledge of nursing principles and a commitment to the basic assumptions and beliefs presented.

The nursing process is based on some fundamental beliefs about human life, the role of nursing, and the delivery of health care:

◆ Every person is endowed with worth and dignity.

◆ Every person has basic needs common to all humans, and these needs must be met to some degree if a person is to survive and enjoy an acceptable level of wellness.

◆ Meeting one's basic human needs may require assistance from someone else until one is able to resume responsibility for oneself.

◆ Every person has the right to high-quality service regardless of his or her socioeconomic status, cultural background, race, or religious beliefs.

◆ Patients and their families prefer a patient-centered approach that actively seeks their input and respects their thoughts, feelings, and needs.

◆ The focus of nursing should be on maintaining health, preventing disease, and helping the sick and injured.

◆ The nurse who engages in the nursing process will continue to work toward her own self-fulfillment by studying, learning, and improving competence.

To give competent, cost-effective care the nurse today must develop good assessment skills, identify the patient's most pressing problems, work with nursing diagnoses, carefully plan care to achieve goals in a minimum of time, draw on a broad knowledge base to choose appropriate actions to achieve the set goals, skillfully implement the care, and evaluate the success of the plan.

ASSESSMENT (DATA COLLECTION)

ANA Standard: Assessment: The nurse collects client health data

The purpose of a nursing assessment is to collect a complete, relevant data base from which the patient's problems can be identified using a nursing diagnosis. Information for the data base is gathered in a purposeful way. In general, the more relevant information one has about a problem, the more likely one is to identify the problem correctly and arrive at a satisfactory resolution. However, in a life-threatening situation requiring immediate intervention, the nurse quickly assesses the patient's needs and determines the appropriate action to take.

Careful assessment is essential to providing good care and is the key to detecting signs of complications before serious problems occur.

During the nursing process, assessment and reassessment are ongoing tasks. An **initial** (first) assessment is made at the time of admission to the hospital or clinic. The information or data gathered at this time are used to establish a *data base* from which nursing diagnoses can be chosen. A data base is a collection of factual information. The data base also can be used later to determine whether the patient is progressing or not. For example, the nurse might learn through her initial assessment that the patient with heart disease is 100 lb overweight. This information is useful in setting a realistic goal for a return to normal weight and in deciding whether the goal has been reached. The Canadian Nurses Association Standards of Nursing covers the nursing process in Standard II:

Nursing practice requires the effective use of the nursing process. Nurses are required in any practice setting to do the following: (1) collection of data; (2) analysis of data; (3) planning of the intervention; (4) implementation of the intervention; and (5) evaluation.

◆ Sources and Techniques for Assessment

Several sources of assessment data are available to the nurse. If nursing care is to be patient-centered, the most obvious source is the patients, their family members, and other persons significant in the life of the patient (significant others). Information-gathering techniques include (1) review of records; (2) the interview; (3) psychosocial assessment; (4) spiritual assessment; (5) observation; (6) physical examination (including objective measurement of vital signs and other bodily functions); (7) review of laboratory and diagnostic test data and consultation with other health team members.

Review of Records   At the time of admission to an in-patient facility, some information about the patient will be available on an admission form. This will tell the admitting nurse such things as the patient's name, age, religious affiliation, and medical diagnosis; the reason for admission; and other pertinent information. If the patient has had previous admissions, medical records and documentation of care received will be available for the nurse making an initial assessment. Numerous previous admissions usually give an idea of the chronic nature of the illness or illnesses suffered by a patient and his or her long-term needs for nursing intervention. The physician's history and physical examination report will contain valuable information about the overall health of the patient.

Interviewing   An interview is conducted with the patient and, whenever possible, one or more family members. At this time a nursing history is obtained. This is sometimes referred to as an *admissions interview, health appraisal,* or *assessment questionnaire.* The interview is conducted in a systematic and orderly manner, using a printed format so that the nursing data base will be as complete as possible. The printed form might be organized according to body systems, a "head-to-foot" approach, or by patterns of health-related behaviors such as nutrition, elimination, activity and exercise, sleep and rest, and so on. A nursing history and assessment form that is organized under nine health-related categories and that assists with nursing diagnosis is shown in Figure 2-1. In addition, information regarding health problems in relatives is recorded.

Before starting the interview, nurses should gather as much information about patients as they can from

DATE:	NIGHTS TIME _____	DAYS TIME _____	EVENINGS TIME _____
DIET TYPE OF DIET	NONE☐ TYPE_____	NONE☐ TYPE_____	NONE☐ TYPE_____
AMOUNT TAKEN	_____	BREAKFAST _____LUNCH _____	_____
DIETARY SUPPLEMENT AND SNACK	NONE☐ TYPE_____	NONE☐ TYPE_____	NONE☐ TYPE_____
CALORIE COUNT (SPECIFY)	YES☐ NO☐	YES☐ NO☐	YES☐ NO☐
FOOD TAKEN PER	SELF☐ ASSIST☐ FED☐	SELF☐ ASSIST☐ FED☐	SELF☐ ASSIST☐ FED☐
TUBE FEEDING (INDICATE SOLUTION & RATE)	NA☐ SOLUTION_____ RATE _____	NA☐ SOLUTION_____ RATE _____	NA☐ SOLUTION_____ RATE _____
FLUIDS	NA☐ ☐ENCOURAGED ☐RESTRICTED	NA☐ ☐ENCOURAGED ☐RESTRICTED	NA☐ ☐ENCOURAGED ☐RESTRICTED
SKIN HYGIENE BED BATH, SPONGE BATH, TUB BATH **(CIRCLE)** SHOWER BATH, SITZ BATH	SELF☐ ASSIST☐ COMPLETE☐	SELF☐ ASSIST☐ COMPLETE☐	SELF☐ ASSIST☐ COMPLETE☐
SHIFT CARE	AM☐ SHAVE☐	AM☐ SHAVE☐	PM☐ HS☐ SHAVE☐
ORAL CARE	NA☐ SELF☐ ASSIST☐ COMPLETE☐	NA☐ SELF☐ ASSIST☐ COMPLETE☐	NA☐ SELF☐ ASSIST☐ COMPLETE☐
PERI CARE	NA☐ SELF☐ ASSIST☐ COMPLETE☐	NA☐ SELF☐ ASSIST☐ COMPLETE☐	NA☐ SELF☐ ASSIST☐ COMPLETE☐
SKIN CARE	NA☐ SELF☐ ASSIST☐ COMPLETE☐	NA☐ SELF☐ ASSIST☐ COMPLETE☐	NA☐ SELF☐ ASSIST☐ COMPLETE☐
CONDITION	WARM☐ COLD☐ DIAPHORETIC☐ DRY☐ CLAMMY☐	WARM☐ COLD☐ DIAPHORETIC☐ DRY☐ CLAMMY☐	WARM☐ COLD☐ DIAPHORETIC☐ DRY☐ CLAMMY☐
ABRASIONS/RASH/SKIN TEAR	NA☐ LOCATION_____	NA☐ LOCATION_____	NA☐ LOCATION_____
EDEMA (LOCATION, EXTENT)	YES☐ NO☐	YES☐ NO☐	YES☐ NO☐
DECUBITUS (CIRCLE)	Y/N FLOW SHEET IN USE: Y/N TURN SHEET IN USE: Y/N	Y/N FLOW SHEET IN USE: Y/N TURN SHEET IN USE: Y/N	Y/N FLOW SHEET IN USE: Y/N TURN SHEET IN USE: Y/N
ACTIVITY EQUIPMENT	NA☐ EGGCRATE☐ OTHER _____	NA☐ EGGCRATE☐ OTHER _____	NA☐ EGGCRATE☐ OTHER _____
TYPE OF ACTIVITY	BED☐ CHAIR☐ AMB☐ BSC☐ DANGLE☐ BRP☐ ROM☐	BED☐ CHAIR☐ AMB☐ BSC☐ DANGLE☐ BRP☐ ROM☐	BED☐ CHAIR☐ AMB☐ BSC☐ DANGLE☐ BRP☐ ROM☐
HOW ACCOMPLISHED	SELF☐ ASSIST☐ P.T.☐	SELF☐ ASSIST☐ P.T.☐	SELF☐ ASSIST☐ P.T.☐
LENGTH OF TIME, DISTANCE TOLERANCE	_____	_____	_____
DEEP BREATHE AND COUGH	NA☐ Q2H ASSISTED☐ Q2H SELF☐	NA☐ Q2H ASSISTED☐ Q2H SELF☐	NA☐ Q2H ASSISTED☐ Q2H SELF☐
REPOSITION	NA☐ Q2H ASSISTED☐ Q2H SELF☐	NA☐ Q2H ASSISTED☐ Q2H SELF☐	NA☐ Q2H ASSISTED☐ Q2H SELF☐
SAFETY UNIVERSAL PRECAUTIONS	IN USE_____ INITIAL _____	IN USE_____ INITIAL _____	IN USE_____ INITIAL _____
EQUIPMENT	NA☐ K-PAD☐ IVAC☐ TEDS☐ TIME ON ____ TIME OFF ____	NA☐ K-PAD☐ IVAC☐ TEDS☐ TIME ON ____ TIME OFF ____	NA☐ K-PAD☐ IVAC☐ TEDS☐ TIME ON ____ TIME OFF ____
SIDERAILS (UP/DOWN)	HEAD ↑ ↓ ☐ FOOT ↑ ↓ ☐	HEAD ↑ ☐ ↓ ☐ FOOT ↑ ☐ ↓ ☐	HEAD ↑ ↓ ☐ FOOT ↑ ↓ ☐
BED IN LOW POSITION	YES☐ NO☐	YES☐ NO☐	YES☐ NO☐
CALL BUTTON WITHIN REACH	YES☐ NO☐ OTHER _____	YES☐ NO☐ OTHER _____	YES☐ NO☐ OTHER _____
SEIZURE PRECAUTIONS	NA☐ YES☐ NO☐	NA☐ YES☐ NO☐	NA☐ YES☐ NO☐
RESTRAINTS (ON/OFF)	NA☐ POSEY☐ WRIST☐ ANKLE☐ TIME ON: _____ TIME OFF: _____	NA☐ POSEY☐ WRIST☐ ANKLE☐ TIME ON: _____ TIME OFF: _____	NA☐ POSEY☐ WRIST☐ ANKLE☐ TIME ON: _____ TIME OFF: _____
ISOLATION	NA☐ TYPE_____	NA☐ TYPE_____	NA☐ TYPE_____
PAIN LOCATION & INTENSITY/DESCRIBE	NA☐ _____	NA☐ _____	NA☐ _____
MEDICATION GIVEN	NA☐ YES☐	NA☐ YES☐	NA☐ YES☐
RESULTS	NO RELIEF☐ RELIEF: MILD☐	NO RELIEF☐ RELIEF: MILD☐	NO RELIEF☐ RELIEF: MILD☐
NOTE ACTION TAKEN IN NRS DOC.	MOD☐ COMPLETE☐	MOD☐ COMPLETE☐	MOD☐ COMPLETE☐
MD. CALL PHYSICIAN CALLED NAME:	_____	_____	_____
REASON FOR CALL:	_____	_____	_____
RESPONSE:	_____	_____	_____
SIGNATURES	11-7 _____	7-3 _____	3-11 _____
	11-7 _____	7-3 _____	3-11 _____

FIGURE 2-1 Portion of activity flowsheet and assessment record used to document routine nursing care for each patient. (Courtesy of Santa Ynez Valley Hospital, Inc., Solvang, California.)

their admission forms, agency file, physician's orders accompanying the patient (if any), and previous hospitalization records (if available). **This is done to avoid repetition of data gathering. Having to answer the same kinds of questions posed by several different people can be exasperating to the patient and can give the impression that members of the health care team do not communicate with one another.**

Elder Care Point... Plan extra time for an interview with a patient who is elderly. The elderly person who is ill may think and speak more slowly and often has a longer health history to relate than a younger person.

The nurse begins the interview by introducing himself and explaining why he is going to be asking the questions. The patient should be told that her responses will be recorded and the information used to help her nurses get to know her better and plan her care more effectively. She is assured that she is free to answer or not answer any of the questions asked and that she may add any pertinent information at any time she thinks it would be helpful. **The interview should be conducted in a place in which there will be some privacy and freedom from distraction and should take no more than 20 to 30 minutes to complete.**

It is important to obtain a list of the medications the patient is taking, both prescription and over-the-counter drugs. The patient should be asked what she sees as her most important problems, or "chief complaint." At the end of the interview the nurse briefly summarizes the data he has gathered and clarifies with the patient any important points or questions she might have.

Summarizing the information with the patient shows her that the nurse has been an interested and attentive listener and is concerned about her. Maybe at this point the patient begins to trust the nurse and is able to express her feelings more openly and ask questions more freely. As a final gesture the nurse might ask if there is anything that has been missed during the interview that the patient thinks is important to her care or her problem. Table 2-1 provides a guide for an abbreviated general patient interview. More detailed interview questions are provided in the focused assessments in the chapters concerning medical–surgical disorders.

Think about . . . How many sources can you identify that would provide information for a nursing data base on a patient who has been admitted to a long-term care facility?

A mini-interview is more casually conducted each day to determine patient progress and the status of body systems. Questions are asked about previously described symptoms to determine present status, level of pain, if a bowel movement has occurred, whether there are any problems with urination or sleep, how the patient's appetite is, and whether there are any new complaints. These questions are usually asked while the nurse is measuring vital signs, providing care, giving a treatment, or performing an assessment.

◆ Psychosocial Assessment

To care for the "whole" patient, the nurse must gather sufficient data on the psychological and sociological areas of the patient's life. *Sociological* data include the patient's educational level; employment status; marital status; number of children, their ages, and whether they are living at home; whether the patient has health insurance; where she lives and what the household is like; whether she has a pet; what her hobbies or leisure activities are; with whom she has significant relationships; and any significant problems she might presently have other than her state of health.

Cultural Factors   Cultural beliefs and values, especially in relation to illness and health care, need to be assessed. The nurse must question the patient to obtain data about individual beliefs the patient has about illness, pain, bathing practices, foods during illness, medication, and other aspects of treatment as they apply. **The nurse should not assume that, just because the patient is a member of a particular ethnic group, she adheres to all the cultural health beliefs of that group.** Basic knowledge about the cultural beliefs and health practices of a particular ethnic group should be used as a guideline for questions about the individual patient's beliefs. Does this particular Hispanic patient believe in "hot" and "cold" forces that may be thrown out of balance in illness? Does the southern African-American patient believe that illness is a punishment sent by God? Does the Asian woman have particular dietary needs after her hysterectomy?

Cultural assessment is a matter of asking the patient and the family about preferences, what they think, and who should be consulted about decisions. Family decision-making patterns and lines of authority are important, and they do vary from one culture to another. It is important that the nurse phrase questions in a positive, nonthreatening way. For example, ask the patient what she believes regarding a particular topic rather than what superstitions she practices.

Psychological Factors   *Psychological* assessment focuses on how the patient sees her state of health, her coping abilities, her past pattern of reacting to stress, her level of self-esteem, her roles, and the dynamics of family relationships. Are there signs of extreme nervousness, anxiety, or depression? Each of these states can interfere with the patient's ability to take in information and quickly return to wellness.

Many times, home or work problems affect the patient just as much as or more than her current health problem. An effective care plan can be devised only if the entirety of the patient's life is considered.

Educational level can be assessed by determining how well the patient reads, paying attention to the vocabulary she uses, determining her occupation or profession, or asking about her school years. Level of education plays a key part in determining how the patient can best be taught what she needs to know to take care of herself.

When seeking information about past response to stress and usual coping patterns, find out what stresses she has experienced in the past, and then ask her how

TABLE 2-1 ◆ *Abbreviated General Patient Interview Guide*

Social Data

What is your marital status? Who lives with you?

What is your occupation?

Are you an active church member or belong to any organizations?

Do you have health insurance?

How are things at home with you here?

Are there any medical problems that run in the family?

Have you had previous surgeries or serious injuries?

Who do you have in your life that is supportive to you?

What prescription drugs do you take? What over-the-counter medicines?

Do you smoke? How much?

Do you enjoy wine or alcohol? When and about how much do you drink?

Are you allergic to any medication? Foods? Other substances?

What do you like to eat? Describe yesterday's meals and snacks.

Physical Data

What brought about your admission here?

What health problems do you have?

Do you routinely see other doctors? For what?

Review of Systems

Ask questions about the presence of the following:

Head and neck

Do you have frequent headaches; dizziness, ringing of the ears, problems hearing; visual problems, glaucoma, cataracts, do you wear wear glasses or contact lenses; surgery of the brain, eyes, or ears; frequent colds; nasal allergies; sinus infections; frequent sore throats; hoarseness; trouble swallowing; swollen glands; mouth sores; When was your last dental exam; Do you have a history of thyroid problems; Do you use a hearing aid; Do you have any difficulty sleeping; Do you take naps

Chest

Cough, sputum production; asthma, wheezing, frequent bronchitis; history of pneumonia; tuberculosis; exposure to tuberculosis; exposure to occupational respiratory hazards; (female: frequency of breast exams; When was your last mammogram; nipple discharge; breast lumps); palpitations, chest pain; shortness of breath; history of heart problems, murmurs, hypertension; anemia; surgery

Abdomen (GI)

Indigestion; pain; nausea; vomiting; excessive thirst or hunger; frequency of bowel movements; change in bowel movements; rectal bleeding; black or tarry stools; constipation; diarrhea; excessive gas; hemorrhoids; history of gallbladder or liver problems

Genitourinary

Problems with urination; up at night to urinate; dribbling of urine; history of urinary tract infection; stones; (female: sexually active; problems; menstrual cycle and any problems; last menstrual period; bleeding between periods or after menopause; vaginal discharge; date of last Pap smear; history of herpes or other vaginal disorders); (male: sexually active; genital problems or penile discharge; history of herpes or other sexually transmitted diseases)

Extremities and musculoskeletal

Joint pain or stiffness; back problems; muscle pain; limited range of motion; vascular problems in legs or arms; easy bruising; skin lesions; history of phlebitis, thrombophlebitis; gout, arthritis, fractures, injury

Psychological Data

Are you experiencing anxiety? Depression?

Do you have unusual memory problems?

Do you have difficulty thinking?

Are you ever confused?

---

she reacted and made decisions. Does she gather data, withdraw, and carefully consider the facts before making a decision and taking action? Or does she quickly assess the situation and make a snap decision? Does she lose her temper and yell? Or is she cool and calm? Does she adapt to almost any situation and make the best out of it? Whom does she rely on for support in difficult times? It is essential to determine whether the patient has a solid support system.

Spiritual Beliefs

Regardless of whether one agrees that spiritual care is within the realm of nursing care, commitment to meeting the needs of the whole person must take into account the spiritual aspect of human nature.

Assessing spiritual needs and planning to meet those needs are not emphasized in the nursing literature. One reason usually given for this reluctance to deal with spiritual concerns and distress in a patient is that religion and matters of spirituality are personal and private. It is feared that patients and their families might resent having a nurse inquire into their beliefs and practices. Many nurses assume that they and their patients would be uncomfortable dealing with the subject. However, as has been pointed out by several authors, nurses usually have no difficulty asking the most intimate questions about their patients' bodily functions and sexual feelings and practices.

Another reason frequently given for failure to help a patient spiritually is that nurses are not qualified to handle problems of this kind. However, of all health care personnel, it is nurses who spend the most time with their patients, are most readily available in times of spiritual and emotional crises, and are presumably the most committed to holistic health care. Moreover, it is reasonable to expect a competent nurse to be able to use his "self" as a source of strength and hope when his patient is trying to cope with questions about the meaning of life and death and of sickness and suffering. Such competence is gained only by actively seeking answers for oneself and by sharing one's insights and beliefs with others.

During the assessment phase of the nursing process, most often spiritual assessment is limited to finding out from the admission sheet whether the patient is affiliated with some religion. This is obviously not enough information to do any more than pay lip service to nursing the whole patient. At the time of the initial interview, the nurse might more thoroughly assess a patient's spiritual needs once he has gained her trust and confidence. It is best if questions about values and beliefs are asked toward the end of the interview. It is important to respect the patient's religious beliefs and her right to remain silent if she does not wish to talk about the spiritual dimension of her life.

Another approach is to question the patient about whether spirituality is important to her. What does she do to nurture her spiritual self? Does she pray or meditate? What sources of spirituality does she feel give her strength? Does she have a spiritual adviser?

Table 2-2 lists questions that are helpful for a spiritual assessment. These questions can be asked at admission or at any point during nurse–patient interaction when it seems appropriate to help a patient to deal with her spiritual needs.

Once a patient's spiritual needs have been identified, the nurse can draw on a number of sources of help

TABLE 2-2 ◆ *Spiritual Assessment Guide*
◆ Has your illness affected your religious practices?
◆ Is spirituality important to you?
◆ Do you have a minister, priest, rabbi, or other spiritual adviser?
◆ What sorts of things do you do to nurture your spirituality?
◆ Does prayer help in your life?
◆ Do you meditate regularly?
◆ What helps you most when you are afraid or need special help?

for the patient. He can, as stated, draw on his own inner strengths and resources. Other sources include praying with the patient, reading religious passages, providing quiet time for meditation, and referring to and consulting with clergy or a spiritual adviser.

◆ Chart Review

When the nurse is assigned to a patient he did not admit himself, he must quickly gather information that will assist him to establish priorities of care for that patient. A quick, orderly chart review is a good way to begin the shift. The face sheet provides information on marital status, age, insurance coverage, occupation, significant others, and location of home. The most current set of physician's orders provides a clue as to the plan for that day (i.e., tests or treatments). The physician's history and physical examination give an overview of the patient's total health status and provide a summary of her current health problems. This part of the chart can provide a great deal of information, including allergies. The admission nursing assessment form also can provide additional helpful data.

Skimming through current lab data can give an idea of any abnormal values and areas that need to be monitored closely. Other test data can provide information on what might be in store for the patient and areas where teaching might be needed. The medication profile sheets tell what is currently ordered for the patient and what PRN (as needed) medications he has actually needed. Consultation sheets and dietitian's or respiratory therapist's notes also are helpful. Nurses' notes from the previous 24 hours should be read, and all of the flow sheets should be skimmed (Figure 2-1). The nurse who regularly skims all of these data will have a much better knowledge of the patient's needs and will be more comfortable and proficient in caring for her.

◆ Techniques of Physical Examination

Inspection and Observation   Inspection or observation is done by using the eyes to pick up clues about the physical and mental condition of the patient. Much can be learned simply by observing a patient's general appearance. Many an experienced nurse has sensed that something was wrong with a patient by noticing her facial expression, posture in bed, bodily movements, and ability or inability to cooperate or respond appropriately.

Observation might be considered the most important of all assessment activities

During assessment, the nurse inspects skin, hair, nails, and mucous membranes. He notices the patient's mood, whether there are signs of self-care such as combed hair, and evidence in the room of support for the patient by relatives and friends, such as cards, gifts, or flowers. The chart also is inspected for helpful information. Visual inspection is a vital assessment tool.

Olfaction (Smelling)   The nose is used to identify particular smells. In some instances, specific odors can be helpful in diagnosing certain disorders. For example, the sweetish, fruity odor of acetone can indicate diabetic acidosis; the smell of newly mown clover can accompany hepatic coma. The odor of alcohol is usually detected rather easily in acute alcoholism, unless the person has been drinking vodka, which is relatively odorless. A patient who is suffering from acute alcoholism also might smell of Sterno, lighter fluid, after-shave lotion, or other sources of alcohol.

Mouth odors that are foul or metallic usually indicate poor oral hygiene and periodontal disease (disease of the tissues around the teeth). A nasal odor can be caused by chronic sinusitis with postnasal drip or an obstruction in the nasal passages. In children, one might suspect a foreign object such as a bean or pea in the nose when there is a distinctly foul nasal odor.

The patient who wears excessive amounts of perfume or cologne may be hiding a serious body odor problem that is symptomatic of anemia, endocrine dysfunction, or an abnormality of the central nervous system. If the nurse suspects that the patient is trying to hide an embarrassing odor, he should seek to gain the patient's confidence and trust so that she can talk freely about her problem and receive help in coping with it.

The female with a foul odor about the genital area most likely has a vaginal infection. A genital odor in the bedridden elderly, frail female may indicate an inability to carry out proper bathing of this area.

Palpation   The sense of touch is used to gather information about the patient by the "laying on of hands." By touching the patient, nurses can distinguish between normal, healthy skin and skin that is coarse, dry, dehydrated, **edematous** (swollen with fluid), or cold and clammy. They can feel the extremities and other body parts to determine if they are cold because of poor circulation or hot because of a localized inflammation. The fingertips are used to palpate the pulses. The flat of the hand is used to palpate the abdomen to determine whether it is soft or hard and to find any tender spots. Breasts are palpated to detect abnormal growths. Lymph nodes are palpated to detect swelling or tenderness.

Auscultation   The ears are used to gather further information about a patient's condition. The nurse listens for normal breathing and distinguishes between a cough that is dry and hacking and one that is moist and "bubbly." He hears the wheezing of an asthmatic patient or the crowing sound produced by an obstruction of the air passages. The stethoscope amplifies sound so that the nurse can determine whether sounds in the lungs are normal or not. Applied to the area of the heart, the stethoscope provides a way to count the **apical** (at apex of heart) pulse and to determine whether there are any abnormal heart sounds (Figure 2-2). A stethoscope is used after surgery to listen for the return of bowel sounds that tell the nurse that the patient is now able to have fluids or food. The ears are vital to obtaining a thorough patient history and in picking up subtle clues about the patient's state of mind from what is said during all aspects of care.

Percussion   Percussion is a technique used more often by physicians and nurse practitioners than by staff nurses. It involves light, quick tapping on the body surface to produce sounds. Variations in the sounds reflect the characteristics of the organs or structures below the surface. Percussion is used primarily over the chest, abdomen, and kidney area to determine the size, location, and density of organs that lie within. The nurse sometimes uses percussion on the abdomen. This is done by striking the middle finger of one hand with the tip of the index or middle finger of the other hand. When tapping, the wrist rests on the patient's body and the forearm is not moved; the movement is done with a quick snap of the wrist. The tapping finger makes a quick contact with the other hand, and after two or three taps in one location, the hands are moved to another area. Different sounds occur as the nurse moves from a resonant area to a less resonant area, indicating air-filled structures or denser tissue beneath.

Think about . . . Can you identify four types of data that can be obtained by using a stethoscope?

Taking and Interpreting Vital Signs and Measurements   Height, weight, body temperature, pulse, respiration, and blood pressure measurements and values are included in the physical examination. Familiarity with these routine procedures can cause the nurse to overlook their importance to the overall assessment of a

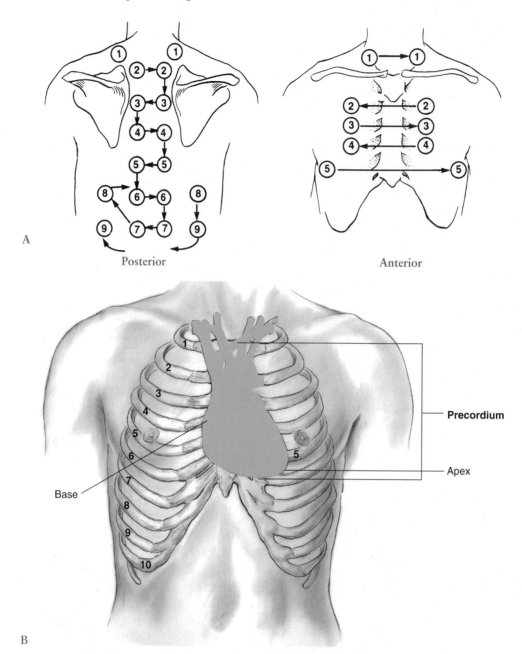

Posterior

Anterior

A

Precordium

Apex

Base

B

FIGURE 2-2 **(A) Place the stethoscope on the bare skin at these locations to hear the lung sounds.** (*Source:* deWit, S. (1994). *Rambo's Nursing Skills for Clinical Practice,* 4th ed. Philadelphia: Saunders, p. 309.) **(B) Place the stethoscope at the apex of the heart to listen to the apical pulse.** (*Source:* Jarvis, C. (1996). *Physical Examination and Health Assessment.* Philadelphia: Saunders, p. 515.)

patient's condition, but they are truly "vital signs" that are significant indicators of what is happening to a patient at any given moment. Rather than just measuring the vital signs, the nurse must correlate the present readings with the baseline data and the trend of past readings. Is the blood pressure still high, or is the antihypertensive medication the patient is receiving doing its job? Is the temperature rising slightly every afternoon? Does the pulse rate vary significantly from morning to afternoon? Do variations in weight reflect edema or fluid retention? Such data provide significant information about the patient's condition and her response to medication.

◆ Practical Physical Assessment

Most staff nurses do not have the luxury of sufficient time to perform a thorough head-to-toe physical assessment on each patient. Judgment about what must be assessed for a particular patient is developed over time. **Generally, an overall abbreviated general physical assessment is done on each assigned patient, and** then a more focused assessment is performed for systems in which the patient is experiencing health problems.

Beginning at the head, check the patient's skin color, eye appearance, condition of the hair, and general **affect** (emotional reaction). Determine **level of consciousness (LOC)** and ability to **mentate** (think) by talking with the patient and asking questions as you assess. Measure the vital signs, and auscultate the lungs, applying the stethoscope to the chest as in Figure 2-2. Turn off the TV or radio so that you can hear adequately. Listen to the heart at the apex, checking the rhythm for regularity, and determine whether there are any extra heart sounds. Check the skin **turgor** (elasticity) by gently lifting the skin between thumb and forefinger and seeing whether it quickly lies back down when you let go. With the patient lying down, listen for bowel sounds in all four quadrants (Figure 2-3). Gently palpate the abdomen with the palm side of the fingers to determine whether there are areas of tenderness. Check on bowel and bladder status and intake and output for the previous 24 hours. Determine whether the patient can move all extremities purposefully as you assess her.

The extent to which physical examination is performed by a particular nurse depends on the agency in which he or she works and his or her experience and expertise in the techniques. Many nurses have become quite proficient in this area.

Assessment is a very complex task, and beginning nurses might not be as proficient at some aspects of the physical examination and the interview as more experienced nurses or nurses with more advanced clinical skills. They should, however, be aware of the importance of this phase of the nursing process and the valuable contribution they can make toward determining the nursing needs of the patient. Because they frequently are at the patient's bedside and communicate personally with the family, nurses can use their knowledge and interpersonal, observation, and communication skills to collect additional information about the patient. In many occasions when nurses are in an excellent position to clarify a patient's statement and verify data already obtained, making sure that the information used for the patient's care plan is indeed accurate and not misunderstood.

It is extremely important that nurses who work in the home care setting refine their assessment skills. Many times those nurses are the only health professional to see the patient for weeks at a time. Skillful assessment by the nurse can catch signs of problems early and often prevent the need for hospitalization or extensive treatment.

Think about . . . How would you obtain a nursing data base on an elderly client who is very hearing impaired?

A guide for areas to be covered when assessing each assigned patient is provided in Table 2-3. Information obtained is entered on a chart form similar to the one in Figure 2-4. Focused assessments are carried out for various body systems once initial problems are identified. More in-depth techniques for focused assessment are included in each of the chapters dealing with medical–surgical disorders.

◆ Laboratory Data

Information about laboratory test results and other diagnostic procedures performed by other departments within the hospital or clinic can be helpful to nurses, who continually assess the status of patients. They can use the information to identify general areas in which a patient might have a health care problem or to validate a nursing diagnosis. For example, below-normal red blood cell (RBC), hematocrit, and hemoglobin counts provide data to validate the patient's fatigue and lack of energy. Checking the values of the blood count as test results are available allows the nurse to verify whether bleeding has stopped and whether the chosen therapy to correct the anemia is effective.

◆ Consultation

While assessing patients' needs, nurses use a variety of information sources, including nursing textbooks, professional journals, and other forms of nursing literature that provide information about the patient's condition and probable needs. Members of the health team who might be consulted include pharmacists, social workers, dietitians, occupational therapists, clinical specialists,

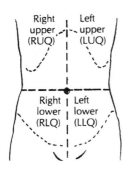

Quadrants of the abdomen

FIGURE 2-3   Listen for bowel sounds in all four quadrants of the abdomen. (Modified from Bolander, V. (1994). *Sorenson and Luckmann's Basic Nursing: A Psychophysiologic Approach,* 3rd ed. Philadelphia: Saunders, p. 686.)

TABLE 2-3 ◆ *Beginning-of-Shift General Assessment*	
Initial observation	Skin turgor and temperature
Ease of respiration	Peripheral pulses; compare bilaterally
Skin color	Presence of edema
Appearance	**Tubes and equipment**
Affect	Intravenous catheter: condition of site, fluid in progress, rate, additives; time next fluid is to be hung
How the patient is feeling	Nasogastric tube: suction setting; amount and character of drainage; patency of tube, security of tube
Head	Urinary catheter: character and quantity of drainage; not under patient
Level of consciousness	Dressings: location, drains in place, wound suction devices, amount and character of wound drainage
Ability to respond to questions	Oxygen cannula: liter flow rate
Appearance of eyes	Pulse oximeter: intact probe; readings
Ability to communicate	Traction: correct weight, body alignment, weights hanging free
Vital signs	Other equipment: applied properly, functioning as ordered
Temperature	**Pain**
Pulse rate, rhythm	Level of pain
Respiration rate, pattern, and depth	Frequency of use of medication
Blood pressure; compare with previous readings	Present status; need for medication
Chest: General heart and lung assessment	Patient-controlled analgesia (PCA) pump functioning; medication left
Auscultate lung fields	**Assessment of needs**
Listen to heart rate at apex	Call bell in reach
Inspect for equal bilateral movement of chest wall	Tissues and waste container in reach
Abdomen	TV control in reach
Shape	Water and personal items positioned conveniently
Soft or hard	Determine what supplies will be needed in room for remainder of shift
Auscultate bowel sounds	
Appetite	
Time of last bowel movement	
Voiding status	
Extremities	
Normal movement bilaterally	

Note: Focused in-depth assessment of systems in which the patient has a problem are added to the general assessment (i.e., respiratory assessment, cardiac assessment, neurological assessment).

physical therapists, respiratory therapists, physicians, and pastoral counselors or chaplains.

ANALYSIS AND NURSING DIAGNOSIS

Standard: Diagnosis: The nurse analyzes the assessment data to determine diagnoses.

In the analysis phase of the nursing process, the data base is **synthesized** (put together in a new meaningful whole) and analyzed to determine where problems exist. There is ongoing controversy concerning the role of the LPN in this step of the nursing process. Certainly, the LPN is expected to survey the data and determine what the patient's major problems are in basic terms, such as "difficulty breathing," "infection," or "anxiety." In some agencies it is up to the registered (RN) to choose or formulate nursing diagnoses for the plan of care. In some long-term care facilities, the LPN charge nurse, being the highest trained nurse present at the time of a patient's admission, will be expected to translate the identified problems by choosing nursing diagnoses from the approved (NANDA) list to initiate the patient's plan of care. An RN may review and finalize the care plan at a later time. So, LPNs must become familiar with nursing diagnoses.

A nursing diagnosis is a concise statement of a patient's actual or potential health problem based on a nurse's judgment of a patient's condition and clinical status, response to treatment, and nursing care needs.

A nursing diagnosis is chosen based on a cluster of information indicating an actual or potential health problem. The diagnoses express the patient's ability—or inability—to meet basic needs, cope with illness, and develop to his or her full potential.

The categories of nursing diagnoses shown in Table 2-4 are general statements, or stems, concerning a patient's problem. In this form they are *not* statements of an individual patient's problems; this cannot be determined without assessing the patient's health status. Information about the individual patient's problem

NURSING ASSESSMENT

Chief complaint as stated by patient: _____ Patient's understanding of condition _____
Secondary health problems: _____

PHYSICAL ASSESSMENT   TIME _____ T _____ P _____ R _____ BP: L. Arm _____ R. Arm _____ Ht. _____ Wt. _____

Neurological: No known problem ____ Oriented ____ Lethargic ____ Comatose ____ Muscular weakness ____ Paralysis ____
Headaches: _____ Seizures _____ Vertigo _____ Syncope _____
COMMENTS: _____

Sensory Deficit: No known problem ____ Speech ____ Tactile ____ Pain ____ Hearing ____ Vision _____
COMMENTS: _____

Integumentary: No known problem ____ Intact ____ Color _____ Diaphoretic ____ Dry ____ Temperature _____ Drainage ____
COMMENTS: _____

Muscuolskeletal: No known problem ____ COMMENTS: _____

Respiratory: No known problem ____ Dyspnea ____ Productive Cough ____ Non-productive cough ____ Char. of Resp. ____
Breath Sounds _____ COMMENTS: _____

Cardiac: No known problem ____ Angina ____ Irregular Rhythm ____ Palpitations ____ COMMENTS: _____

Circulatory: No known problem ____ Cyanotic ____ Pain· ____ Varicosities ____ Bleeding ____ Edema ____ Pulses ____
COMMENTS: _____

Endocrine: No known problem ____ Diabetes ____ Thyroid Dysfunctions ____ COMMENTS: _____

G.I.:   No known problem ____ Abd: Soft ____ Tender ____ Firm ____ Distended ____ Nausea ____ Vomiting ____
Present Diet (cultural considerations): _____ Food Allergies _____
Diarrhea ____ Normal Bowel Pattern: _____ Aids: _____
Bowel Sounds: _____ COMMENTS: _____

G.U.:   No known problem ____ Freq. ____ Dysuria ____ Hematuria ____ Nocturia ____ COMMENTS: _____
Reproductive/Genital: Do you do monthly: self breast exam? Yes ____ No ____ Testicular exam? Yes ____ No ____ Changes Noted ____
Date of last breast exam by physician: _____ Date of last pap smear _____
Breasts: No change ____ Lumps ____ Discharge ____ COMMENTS: _____
LMP _____ Contraception _____ Grav ____ Living ____ Para ____
No known problem ____ Rash ____ Tenderness ____ Swelling ____ Discharge ____ Itching ____ Sores ____
COMMENTS: _____

CONDITION OF SKIN
Abrasions/Bruises   •
Lacerations/Scars   —
Decubiti   O
Reddened Areas   □
Burns   ★
Rash   △

COMMENTS:

Locomotion: Independent? YES _____ NO _____
Dependent due to: _____
Aids used: _____

PREVIOUS MEDICAL/SURGICAL HISTORY AND COMPLICATIONS		PREVIOUS MEDICAL/SURGICAL HISTORY AND COMPLICATIONS	
DATE	Chronic illnesses or diseases and surgeries	DATE	CONTINUED

CURRENT MEDICATIONS				
NAME	DOSE	FREQ.	HOW LONG?	LAST DOSE

Brought to Hospital? Yes ____ No ____ Sent to Pharmacy Yes ____ No ____
ALLERGIES (what and type of reaction) _____

Tobacco Use: (#PPD, # Years, Type) _____   Alcohol:(Type, Amt., Freq.) _____
ENVIRONMENTAL EXPOSURE: Toxic Chemicals: _____   Infections: _____
Environmental Allergies _____

FAMILY HEALTH HISTORY: Diabetes: _____ Heart: _____ Hypertension: _____ Epilepsy: _____
Cancer: _____ Respiratory: _____ Kidney: _____ Mental Health Problems: _____ Other: _____

Psychological Data: Are you worried about anything now? _____ Behavior observed: _____
How do you handle stress/worries? _____ What do you do to relax? _____
What can we do to help you feel more comfortable during this hospital stay? _____
Name of Physician Notified: _____ Date/Time _____ Family Physician _____
Nurse's Signature and Title _____ Date/Time _____

ADDRESSOGRAPH

PATIENT'S STRENGTHS	SIGNIFICANT SOCIOCULTURAL DATA		DISCHARGE PLANS	
	MARITAL STATUS:	SIGNIFICANT OTHER:	Projected Date:	Discharge To:
	OCCUPATION:		Potential Problems	Projected Needs
	INSURANCE:			
CARE PLAN REVIEWED/UPDATED	SPIRITUAL DATA: (Sources of Strength)	LIVING ARRANGEMENTS:		
Date and Initial Appropriate Box When Updated				
	DATE	SIGNIFICANT CLINICAL EVENTS		
			Referrals/Date ( ) Social Service _____ ( ) Clergy _____ ( ) Home Health Care _____ ( ) _____ ( )	

ADM. DATE	DIAGNOSIS	HOSPITAL #	SURGERY/DATE	PT. CLASSIFICATION	
				INITIAL	DISCHARGE
RCOM	NAME	AGE	DOCTOR	DRUG ALLERGIES	

FIGURE 2-4   Sample form for recording data from nursing history and initial assessment. (Courtesy St. Mary's Hospital, Athens, GA.)

is linked to the "stem" of the nursing diagnosis taken from the list to formulate the entire nursing diagnosis. For example, "Ineffective airway clearance related to excessive, thick, secretions" is a complete nursing diagnosis for a particular patient.

Arriving at a nursing diagnosis requires thorough assessment and a sound knowledge of nursing theory and practice. Identifying patient care problems and establishing nursing diagnoses are the responsibility of the nurse assigned to admit or care for the patient and are derived from data collected by all health team members. From these data an informal list is constructed that describes the patient's problems or needs. The problems on the list are **prioritized** (listed in order of importance), and then the nursing diagnoses are developed.

TABLE 2-4 ◆ *Approved Nursing Diagnoses*	
Activity intolerance	Health maintenance, altered
Activity intolerance, risk for	Health-seeking behaviors (specify)
Adaptive capacity: intracranial, decreased	Home maintenance management, impaired
Adjustment, impaired	Hopelessness
Airway clearance, ineffective	Hyperthemia
Anxiety	Hypothermia
Aspiration, risk for	Incontinence, bowel
Body image disturbance	Incontinence, functional
Body temperature, risk for altered	Incontinence, reflex
Breastfeeding, effective	Incontinence, stress
Breastfeeding, ineffective	Incontinence, total
Breastfeeding, interrupted	Incontinence, urge
Breathing pattern, ineffective	Infant behavior, disorganized
Cardiac output, decreased	Infant behavior or, disorganized, risk for
Communication, impaired verbal	Infant behavior, potential for enhanced organized
Conflict, decisional (specify)	Infant feeding pattern, ineffective
Conflict, parental role	Infection, risk for
Confusion, acute	Injury, risk for
Confusion, chronic	Knowledge deficit (specify)
Constipation	Loneliness, risk for
Constipation, colonic	Management of therapeutic regimen: community, ineffective
Constipation, perceived	Management of therapeutic regimen: families, ineffective
Coping, community, ineffective	Management of therapeutic regimen: individual, effective
Coping, community, potential for enhanced	Memory, impaired
Coping, defensive	Mobility, impaired physical
Coping, family, ineffective: compromised	Noncompliance (specify)
Coping, family, ineffective: disabling	Nutrition, altered: less than body requirements
Coping, ineffective individual	Nutrition, altered: more than body requirements
Coping, family, potential for growth	Nutrition, altered: potential for more than body requirements
Denial, ineffective	Oral mucous membrane, altered
Diarrhea	Pain
Disuse syndrome, risk for	Pain, chronic
Diversional activity deficit	Parental role conflict
Dysreflexia	Parent–child attachment, risk for altered
Energy field disturbance	Parenting, altered
Environmental interpretation syndrome, impaired	Parenting, altered: risk for
Family coping, compromised, ineffective	Perioperative positioning injury, risk for
Family coping, disabling, ineffective	Peripheral neurovascular dysfunction, risk for
Family coping, potential for growth	Personal identity disturbance
Family processes, altered	Poisoning, risk for
Family process, altered: alcoholism	Posttrauma response
Fatigue	Powerlessness
Fear	Protection, altered
Fluid volume deficit	Rape-trauma syndrome
Fluid volume deficit, risk for	Rape-trauma syndrome: compound reaction
Fluid volume excess	Rape-trauma syndrome: silent reaction
Gas exchange, impaired	Relocation stress syndrome
Grieving, anticipatory	Role performance, altered
Grieving, dysfunctional	Self-care deficit: bathing/hygiene, dressing/grooming, feeding,
Growth and development, altered	toileting

The nursing diagnosis states psychosocial factors, risks of suboptimal wellness, or the patient's response to the pathological condition. Nursing diagnoses and interventions are primarily concerned with (1) physical, psychosocial, and spiritual comfort and well-being; (2) prevention of complications; and (3) patient education. Nursing diagnoses do not include health problems that are treatable by surgery, medications, or other forms of

TABLE 2-4 ◆ *Approved Nursing Diagnoses* (Continued)	
Self-esteem, chronic low	Suffocation, risk for
Self-esteem disturbance	Swallowing, impaired
Self-esteem, situational low	Thermoregulation, ineffective
Self-mutilation, risk for	Thought processes, altered
Sensory/perceptual alterations (specify: visual, auditory, kinesthetic, gustatory, tactile, olfactory)	Tissue integrity, impaired
	Tissue perfusion, altered (specify: cardiopulmonary, cerebral, gastrointestinal, peripheral, renal)
Sexual dysfunction	
Sexuality patterns, altered	Trauma, risk for
Skin integrity, impaired	Unilateral neglect
Skin integrity, risk for impaired	Urinary elimination, altered patterns of
Sleep pattern disturbance	Urinary retention
Social interaction, impaired	Ventilation, spontaneous, inability to sustain
Social isolation	Ventilatory weaning response, dysfunctional (DVWR)
Spiritual well-being, potential for enhanced	Violence, risk for: self-directed or directed at others
Spiritual distress	

Source: North American Nursing Diagnosis Association, 1994.

Note: The term *risk for* may be added to any nursing diagnosis to indicate an identified potential problem that actions need to be instituted to prevent its occurrence.

therapy that have been legally defined as the practice of medicine. An example of how the medical and nursing diagnoses complement one another follows:

◆ Medical diagnosis: chronic obstructive pulmonary disease
◆ Assessment data: shortness of breath; cough; thick, tenacious, yellow sputum; pursed-lip breathing; respirations at 24 per minute; unable to walk for more than a short distance without stopping to rest and catch his breath; sleeps with three pillows behind his back
◆ Appropriate nursing diagnoses:
  1. Ineffective breathing pattern related to dyspnea and copious sputum
  2. Risk of infection related to retained secretions
  3. Activity intolerance related to shortness of breath upon exertion
  4. Self-care deficit related to inability to perform activities of daily living (ADLs) without shortness of breath

Nursing diagnoses provide the basis for planning nursing interventions that will help prevent, minimize, or **alleviate** (reduce the severity) specific health problems. In the example, physical well-being is the major focus of the interventions.

The concept of nursing diagnosis is not totally accepted and used by all health care professionals because it pertains only to "nursing." Collaborative plans of care (clinical pathways or care paths) involving all the health team members concerned with a patient's treatment are being used in many agencies rather than a formal nursing care plan that speaks only to nursing care.

Think about . . . Your patient is very weak from the vomiting and diarrhea of intestinal flu. She is unable to navigate to the bathroom safely by herself. What would be an actual nursing diagnosis that relates to her weakness? (Choose from the list of approved nursing diagnoses.)

PLANNING

Standard: Outcome Identification: The nurse identifies expected outcomes individualized to the client.

Standard: Planning: The nurse develops a plan of care that prescribes interventions to attain expected outcomes.

The planning phase of the nursing process provides a blueprint for nursing interventions to achieve designated goals. If no problems have been identified during assessment (as with a client in a community health care clinic), together the nurse and client discuss goals for maintaining wellness. In a hospital, nursing home, or home care setting the patient will most certainly have some health-deficit problems that are responsive to nursing care. After all, one of the main reasons for hospitalization is to make 24-hour nursing care available to patients who need such care. Home care is provided for patients with specific health problems who most often do not need constant nursing attention. Planning for the patient at the ambulatory clinic may involve setting goals to maintain health rather than to alleviate illness.

During the planning phase the nurse collaborates with the physician and other members of the health care team, such as the physical therapist, respiratory therapist, pharmacist, speech therapist, or social worker, to consider every aspect of care and treatment necessary. The nurse works to coordinate the diagnostic tests, treatments, necessary rest periods, and teaching for the patient.

The steps included in the planning phase of the nursing process are: (1) prioritizing the patient's nursing diagnoses; (2) setting short-term and long-term goals for dealing with problems associated with each diagnosis; (3) developing expected outcomes by which success of the interventions can be measured; and (4) writing nursing orders.

◆ Priority Setting

Priorities are set according to what is most important for the well-being of the patient and are determined according to (1) a hierarchy of needs; and (2) what is perceived as important to the patient. For example, although elimination of infection (physiological need) might be seen as most important by the nurse, the patient might feel that obtaining a good night's sleep after several sleepless nights is more important right now.

◆ Goals and Expected Outcomes

Goals should be stated in terms of observable outcomes. They are set by the patient and the nurse and are in line with the patient's ability to achieve them. Goals are achievable within a specifically stated time frame and relate to one of three aspects of care: (1) restoration to health when there is a health problem; (2) maintenance of health when the patient needs to continue using his or her resources to stay healthy; and (3) promotion of health when the patient's resources can and should be so directed. **Goals may be long term or short term, meaning that some are achievable in the near future and others will take considerably more time for the patient to reach.** For example, a long-term goal for a stroke patient who has right-sided weakness might be: "Patient will feed himself without assistance." A short-term goal might be: "Patient will feed herself finger foods at lunch time before discharge."

Objectives are steps toward accomplishing major goals and are placed on the care plan in the form of expected outcomes. They should be stated in behavioral terms; that is, they should describe what the patient should be able to do or how he has improved as a result of nursing actions. They relate directly to the goal that is derived from the nursing diagnosis. For example, if the nursing diagnosis is "Potential for infection related to surgical incision," the goal is to prevent infection. The outcome criteria might be:

- White blood cell (WBC) count within normal limits (WNL) at discharge
- Temperature within normal limits by third postoperative day
- Incision clean, dry, and without signs of infection such as redness or swelling at time of discharge

Expected outcomes are written with a subject, a verb, conditions or modifiers, and the *criterion* for desired performance. (A *criterion* is a standard against which judgments are made.) They should include the following elements: (1) patient activity that can be observed by the nurse or patient knowledge that can be assessed (e.g., side effects of a medication); and (2) a description of how the patient's behavior will be measured, such as the time by which the objective is to be met and the accuracy or quality of performance. Two examples of expected outcomes are: (1) "The patient will walk to the end of the hall 3 times a day by 9/7/98"; and (2) "The patient will demonstrate each step of self-administration of insulin correctly by 10/2/98." By writing expected outcomes that are very specific, it is easy to determine whether the planned nursing interventions have worked to achieve the goal. If so, the expected outcomes will occur.

Nursing Orders   *Nursing orders* are the nursing actions and patient activities chosen by the nurse to help achieve the stated goals and expected outcomes. They are written on the nursing care plan to be carried out by all nurses caring for the patient and by assistants to whom tasks are assigned or delegated.

Think about . . . Can you write expected outcomes for the patient who meets the nursing diagnosis of "ineffective breathing pattern related to copious secretions?"

◆ Daily Planning

Planning the day-to-day delivery of care requires that the nurse collaborate with the patient and other health team members to coordinate nursing care, ordered treatments and tests, and adequate rest.

Computerized Care Plans   Many hospitals now have available for each nurse a printed sheet of current data about the patient. This sheet usually contains a demographics line listing the room, name, date of admission, age, doctor, and admitting diagnosis. A list of nursing diagnoses is given. A list of nursing orders is included that tells when vital signs should be taken; flow of oxygen, if in use; need for safety devices; type of diet; schedule for turning, coughing and deep breathing; or

IV information. A medication schedule should soon be incorporated into this data sheet.

This sheet can be used as a worksheet during the shift, and if notations are made on it about assessment and treatments completed, it provides an excellent guide for charting. Before relying on a computerized care plan, the nurse must be certain that the data it contains are up-to-date and correct. Each computerized care plan must be reviewed by a nurse and updated at least once every 24 hours.

Kardex Care Plans   Many agencies use a Kardex-type care plan (Figure 2-5). The information on the Kardex is recorded in pencil so that the plan can be easily updated as orders and patient condition change. Notations are included for all physician orders related to treatments, tests ordered, medications, activity allowed, and diet. **Patient allergies are highlighted in red ink.** Each time the physician writes new orders, the unit secretary changes the pertinent information on the patient's Kardex. The charge nurse checks that the information is entered accurately. **It is vitally important that each nurse review the Kardex information for each assigned patient at the beginning of the shift.** As care needs change, the nurse primarily responsible for the patient alters the care plan on the Kardex.

◆ Organization and Prioritization of Tasks

After the patient assignment is received for the shift, the nurse must sit down and organize all data to plan the day's work efficiently. Each patient's care plan is reviewed, current orders are noted, and priorities of care for each patient are set. **When setting priorities, the patient's most pressing problems are considered first, along with the physician's orders. Then, as time permits, less pressing problems may be attended to.**

Priorities often are set by using a hierarchy of needs. Physiological needs are considered first, and respiration has the highest priority. Circulation is considered next. Then the other physiological needs follow. Figure 2-6 presents both Maslow's hierarchy of needs and an adapted hierarchy used by nurses to prioritize care. Which needs come first at a particular time greatly depends on the individual patient's view of his or her situation. Most of the time the physiological needs should come first, but sometimes higher needs are of greater importance to the patient. Priorities should be set according to the patient's view of his needs, in addition to the physician's orders and the nurse's assessment.

The nurse then organizes the workday depending on the order of priority of tasks to be accomplished (e.g., obtaining weights before breakfast takes priority over morning treatments). Preparing preoperative patients for surgery is a high priority and would come before performing morning assessments on stable patients.

Think about . . . Your patient is admitted with pneumonia and weakness. The following nursing diagnoses are appropriate:

◆ Fatigue related to decreased oxygenation
◆ Ineffective airway clearance related to excessive secretions

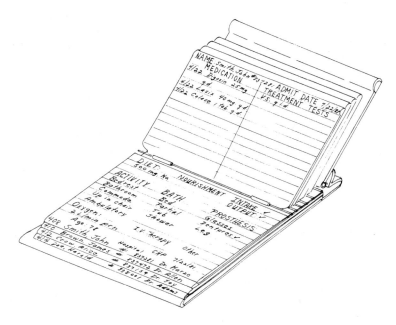

FIGURE 2-5   Kardex nursing care plan.
(*Source:* deWit, S. (1994). *Rambo's Nursing Skills for Clinical Practice,* 4th ed. Philadelphia: Saunders, p. 72.)

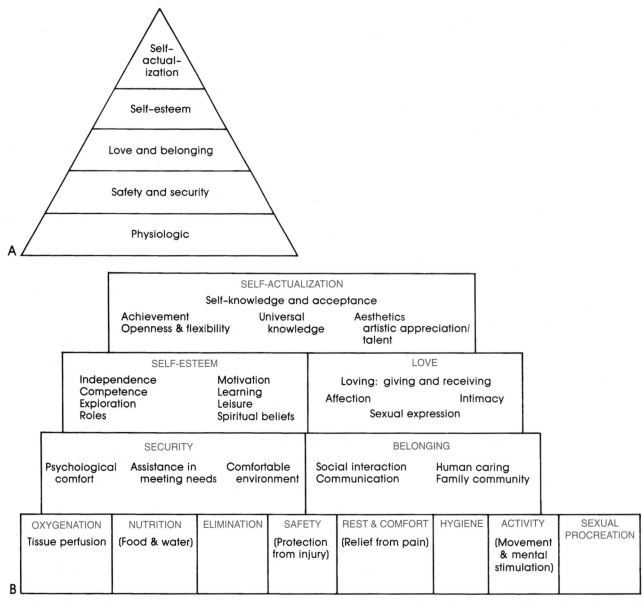

FIGURE 2-6   (A) Maslow's hierarchy of needs. (B) Evolving hierarchy of needs adapted by nursing to help to determine priorities of care.

- Activity intolerance related to weakness
- Self-care deficit related to weakness and shortness of breath
- Constipation related to inactivity
- Knowledge deficit related to possible side effects of medication

Can you place the diagnoses in order of priority according to the hierarchy of needs in Figure 2-6?

The shift report also gives clues about high-priority tasks and times for certain tasks to be accomplished. It is best to use a work organization sheet and lay out what needs to be done and at what time particular treatments are due (Figure 2-7). Time-flexible tasks are entered onto the worksheet between time-set tasks. When planning times for tasks, consider whether the patient has scheduled treatments by another health team professional, such as the respiratory therapist or physical therapist. Will the patient be off the unit for a diagnostic test today? What time does the patient's physician usually make rounds? Not considering these possibilities can destroy the time lines of the most carefully made work plan.

After initial shift assessment is done on each patient, the work schedule may need to be revised if data obtained suggest a need for a shift in the priority of care for a patient. This is particularly true if a patient's condition has become more acute.

SHIFT WORK ORGANIZATION SHEET

	8:00	9:00	10:00	11:00	12:00	13:00	14:00	15:00
PATIENT/ROOM J.D. 521	V.S. Quick Assess	9³⁰ Shower 9⁴⁵ Δdressing		Full Assess Chart	V.S. Glucometer	Pre-op teaching Chart	I + O Tape report	Close chart
PATIENT/ROOM R.S. 523'	V.S. 8²⁰ Quick Assess	Feed Full Assess	Bathe + Bed	Chart	Feed	Let Nap	Empty Foley I+O	Close chart
PATIENT/ROOM B.W. 523²	V.S. Quick Assess √ IV	Full Assess √ IV	Shower + Bed √ IV	Chart √ IV	V.S. √ IV	√ IV	I + O √ IV	Close chart √ IV
PATIENT/ROOM								

FIGURE 2-7   Shift work organization sheet. (*Source:* deWit, S. (1995). *Saunder's Student Nurse Planner.* Philadelphia: Saunders, p. 172.)

IMPLEMENTATION (INTERVENTION)

Standard: Implementation: The nurse implements the interventions identified in the plan of care.

During the implementation phase the plan of action is put into effect. The nurse coordinates her activities with other members of the health care team directly concerned with the patient. Procedures and activities involving the patient should be carefully timed to allow sufficient rest so that natural healing and body energies can do their work to restore a higher level of wellness.

In some instances implementation will include ordered medical treatments such as medications, irrigations, and oxygen therapy. At times, nursing care involves unplanned and prompt intervention, as when a crisis arises that demands immediate and decisive action on the part of the nurse.

During implementation the effectiveness and accuracy of the nursing care plan are tested. Nursing interventions may not have the intended effect, or a change in the patient's condition may present more crucial problems. **The implementation phase concludes with the documentation of nursing care.** The written note includes the nursing action performed, the outcome of the activity, and the patient's response.

◆ Documentation and Interstaff Communication

Nursing process includes communicating what has been done for the patient, pertinent observations, data on physical parameters, such as vital signs and input and output, how the patient is reacting to medication and other treatments and his or her psychological and emotional state and present needs. Good communication between health team members is vital to good patient care. Two to three different sets of staff on a unit are in charge of the care of each patient during a 24-hour period. Rarely does a patient have the same nurse for each shift for several consecutive days. **If communication is inadequate, patient care will be very fragmented and the nursing process breaks down.**

Good, thorough documentation is one way in which continuity of care can be achieved. The other way is through adequate verbal communication among staff members. Usually, each type of communication complements the other, and it is only by being thorough in each area—written and verbal—that high-quality, holistic care can be given to the patient.

◆ Giving or Taking a Report on Patients

Oral communication on patient care is conveyed during report. A report on each patient is given by the departing staff to the staff arriving for the next shift. There are many methods of giving and receiving report. A tape-recorded report is probably the most efficient method because only one nurse is involved at a time. When the arriving staff is getting the report from the tape, the departing staff can be on the floor addressing patient needs. The problem with a taped report is that often it is not clearly audible or well organized, and the listener cannot ask any questions about the patients. However, if the departing staff remain on the unit until the arriving staff have finished listening to the report, questions can be asked and answered.

Oral report from one staff member to others is usually given by the charge nurse to all of the arriving staff members. The entire arriving staff may listen to the report on all patients; in this way staff members are more knowledgeable about all patients and can assist each other by answering call lights, filling in during meal breaks, and so on. This method is time-consuming, as each arriving nurse stays for the entire report for every patient on the unit.

A *focused report* is a method whereby the department nurse gives a report on specific patients assigned to the arriving nurses and only to them. Thus each nurse is occupied only for the time it takes to listen to the reports on his or her 4 to 10 patients. However, with this method, the other nurses do not know much about other patients on the unit.

Walking rounds are another way of giving and receiving report. The departing and arriving nurses caring for specific patients go to the various patient rooms, and the departing nurse, along with the patient, describes what has happened during the previous shift and what the patient and nurse see as current needs and priorities for the present shift. This method allows patients a greater feeling of input and control over their care. It is more-time consuming than other methods, as patients usually are not as concise as the nurse in communicating needs.

Traditionally, a format such as the one shown in Table 2-5 has been used to organize and give report. Table 2-6 provides an example of a report on each patient. With the need to conserve the nurse's time and the extensive documentation systems currently in use, perhaps a modified report format might be more workable and efficient. Certainly with computerized care plans in hand, the nurse does not need to repeat, or listen to, a lot of the same data orally.

EVALUATION

Standard: Evaluation: The nurse evaluates the client's progress toward attainment of outcomes.

TABLE 2-5 ◆ *Shift Report Data*
1. Room number and bed designation, patient name, age, sex, date of admission, medical diagnoses, primary physician
2. Tests and treatments/therapies performed in past 24 hours and patient response to them (i.e., blood transfusion, blood gas analyses, surgery, arteriogram); intake and output
3. Significant changes in patient condition (use nursing process to organize the data in systematic fashion—assessment data, nursing diagnosis [if appropriate], planning, intervention, and evaluation)
4. Scheduled tests; consults or surgery; current IV solution, flow rate, and amount remaining or when next bag is due to be hung; oxygen flow rate; equipment in use and current settings (gastric suction, ventilator, CPM, PCA pump, etc.)
5. Current problems (i.e., fever, draining wound, severe pain, depression, anxiety, insufficient rest, abnormal lab values or test results) and amount of assistance needed
6. Scheduled treatments, status on PRN medications with times and amounts given, response to medications and treatments
7. Concerns, need for order changes, teaching, pertinent family dynamics, emotional status

Abbreviations: CPM, continuous passive motion; PCA, patient-controlled analgesia.

Evaluation is the process of judging or appraising the effectiveness of what has been done. In the nursing process, to evaluate means to identify to what degree the patient's goals and expected outcomes have been met. Nurses continually evaluate as they go about giving patient care and performing nursing interventions. They should continually ask, "Is this action effective? Is the outcome of the action performed expected or unexpected? Does the plan of care need to be revised and the nursing orders rewritten?" If the expected outcomes have been met, the nursing diagnoses and nursing orders for that problem can be noted "achieved," and that portion of the care plan can be closed or deleted.

Each nursing intervention under a nursing diagnosis should be evaluated to see whether it is effective and is still needed. Once daily the data obtained regarding the patient's response to the nursing interventions are examined, and a decision is made as to whether the various interventions should be continued, stopped, or changed.

Consider, for example, a nursing diagnosis of "fluid deficit related to nausea and vomiting" and an expected outcome of "takes in 3,000 mL of fluid each 24 hours." During evaluation the nurse would note how much fluid the patient took in during the previous 24 hours and also assess whether the patient was able to keep the fluid down. If the patient could take in only 2,200 mL but managed to keep the fluid down, the nursing intervention is appropriate and should be continued until the patient is taking 3,000 mL per day for several days without difficulty.

TABLE 2-6 ◆ *Example of Report*

Room 728, bed A, Mr. Harold Donald, 48-year-old male patient of Dr. Hopwitz admitted on the 2nd with abdominal pain; had an appendectomy yesterday with the wound left open because the appendix was ruptured.

No problems during surgery; continuous IVs and IVPB antibiotics, NPO with NG tube to Gomco with low suction, no bowel sounds, wound irrigations with antibiotic solution tid. Intake 2,550 mL, output 1,730 mL.

Temperature has risen to 100.8°F, skin flushed, given Tylenol suppository at 8:00 and 12:00; decreased temperature to 99.6°F, but it went right back up. Some purulent drainage noted on wound irrigation; Dr. Hopwitz notified.

Wound culture ordered before next irrigation; IV D5 ½ NS with 20 mEq KCl at 125 mL/h, count 675 mL remaining, PCA pump with Demerol; he's using it appropriately, and pain appears to be well controlled.

Vital signs q 4 h, but take temperature q 2 h until stable again; observe for changes in secretions in wound drainage or signs of abdominal abcess; watch his electrolyte values—they were within normal limits this morning. WBC count was 14,200. Needs help to stand to urinate and with turning, coughing, and deep breathing. He smokes, so encourage coughing and deep breathing; with that open wound, he doesn't like to cough.

The irrigation solution is in the medication refrigerator and needs to be allowed to warm up before you use it. The equipment is in his room. Irrigations are done at 10:00, 2:00, and 8:00. He has Montgomery straps to ease dressing changes. Dressing has needed changing every 2 hours. He's on Unasyn and Mefoxin piggybacks; we are waiting for culture results.

He is very worried about the wound being left open and just how long he will be off work. He works as a carpenter and doesn't get paid when he is off. He will need to be taught proper wound care before discharge. His wife visits, but they have three small children at home and she can't stay long.

If the patient has been drinking 3,000 mL of fluid but is vomiting most of it, the nursing care plan must be revised to assist the patient with this problem. Perhaps the nurse will need to obtain a different order for an antiemetic or give it more frequently than twice a day.

A good way to evaluate treatment and care collaboratively is to make rounds with the physician and obtain an overall perspective on the result of treatment. In this way a change of orders can readily be obtained if needed.

◆ Quality Management

Another broader aspect of evaluation in nursing practice is the overall evaluation done to determine whether the hospital unit is performing as well and as efficiently as possible. *Continuous quality management (CQM)* audits are a form of evaluation in which various nursing and hospital services are scrutinized to see whether they are meeting standards. The structure of the unit and its physical facilities, equipment, staffing, and other characteristics that affect the quality of nursing care are evaluated periodically. The Joint Commission on Accreditation of Hospitals is a governing body that reviews care given by hospitals. Within this procedure is a series of **retrospective** audits. (*Retrospective* means dealing with the past.) An *audit* is an examination of a record or chart. Objective criteria are applied to patients' chart after discharge to see whether the care received met set standards for the type of problem. Every hospital must perform both medical and nursing audits to achieve and maintain accreditation.

Each hospital has a quality management board or committee that coordinates audit activities. Generally each nursing unit must do a number of chart audits of data to see whether a particular standard of practice is being met. An example would be an audit to see how often intravenous (IV) tubing is being changed. The procedure manual may state that all IV tubing is to be changed every 48 hours. A review of charts for a specific period of time will identify how often this "standard" or criterion is being met. One nursing unit may be meeting it 98% of the time, whereas another that has a nurse shortage for that time may have met the criteria only 78% of the time.

Process evaluations center on the activities of the nurses and what they have done to assess, plan, implement, and evaluate nursing care. The criteria used in process evaluation are the Standards of Nursing Practice developed by the ANA.

An important question in evaluating nursing care is, "What can be done to improve the care?" Evaluation is not done so that someone can be blamed for inefficiency, carelessness, or incompetence. It is done to achieve continuous quality improvement (CQI) by identifying specific areas that need change for the better. Some weaknesses that might be found include vague or inaccurate statements of the problem because of poor assessment or inability to analyze data correctly, unrealistic goal setting caused by overestimating what a patient is capable of doing, and well-intentioned, but ineffective, nursing interventions that simply do not accomplish the desired goal. Whatever the results of an evaluation, they should be seen as a means of improving the quality of nursing care.

Nursing Care Plan 2-1 shows how the components of the nursing process can be used to provide a systematic plan of care for an individual patient. Sample care plans are provided throughout this text to familiarize the reader with the manner in which each phase of the process is recorded to document and communicate to others the planned care of patients with specific problems and the nursing diagnoses related to their health status.

Nursing Care Plan 2-1

Selected nursing diagnoses, goals/expected outcomes, nursing interventions, and evaluations for a patient with hypertension

Situation: 53-year-old male with a blood pressure of 170/100 found during routine screening of all employees at a local plant. A visit to the hypertension clinic reveals that he is hypertensive, is 75 pounds overweight, smokes two packs of cigarettes a day, and eats snacks during the day and in the evening while watching television. The physician prescribes a low-sodium diet and a mild antihypertensive. During her interview with the patient the nurse notes that he does not understand the nature of his illness, how his lifestyle is related to hypertension, and the purpose of the low-sodium diet and the expected action of the diuretic.

Nursing Diagnosis	Goals/Expected Outcome	Nursing Interventions	Evaluation
Altered systemic tissue perfusion related to increased peripheral vascular resistance. SUPPORTING DATA BP, 172/102; P, 96; feet cool and pale; pedal pulses, 1+; capillary refill >4 s.	Patient will maintain adequate tissue perfusion as evidenced by: 1. BP within normal limits at end of 2 weeks. 2. Pulse returns to normal range by discharge. 3. Skin of feet warm and dry within 4 weeks. 4. Capillary refill time less than 3 s within 4 weeks. Patient will quit smoking within 1 month.	Teach to take antihypertensive as ordered; and monitor BP b.i.d. Assess skin and peripheral pulses each visit. Discourage smoking; encourage him to quit smoking. Discourage intake of foods high in caffeine. Maintain sodium restrictions. Have patient weigh himself daily and keep record.	BP, 156/96; P, 86; skin on feet pale and cool; smoked only five cigarettes today; weight down 2 lb. Continue plan.
Altered nutrition, exceeding body requirements; related to overeating and lack of exercise. SUPPORTING DATA Weight, 285 lbs; height, 6 ft; consumes lots of junk food between meals; no daily exercise program; watches television a lot.	Patient will lose 2 lbs within 2 months. Consultation with dietician within 2 weeks. Patient will maintain 2-lb/wk weight loss until normal weight of 210 lbs is attained. Patient will have developed daily exercise plan within 2 weeks.	Explain need to lose excess weight; encourage him to participate in weight loss plan. Assist with development of daily exercise plan.	Weight, 283 lb; is considering options for daily exercise plan.
Knowledge deficit related to self-care aspects of hypertension: how to take blood pressure, medication rationale and side effects, low-sodium diet, need for exercise, need for continued medical follow-up. SUPPORTING DATA Does not know how to take blood pressure; has never taken antihypertensive medication; unaware of sodium content of foods and sodium's relationship to hypertension; unaware of the benefits of exercise on the cardiovascular system; complains of cost of going to doctor for a check-up.	Patient will demonstrate correct technique for taking own blood pressure within 1 week of teaching. Patient will explain action of antihypertensive medication and possible side effects 1 week after teaching session. Patient will describe effects of exercise on cardiovascular system after teaching session. Patient will state which foods are high in sodium when given a list from which to choose foods after teaching session. Before discharge patient will give three reasons why continued follow-up is necessary for patients with hypertension.	Develop teaching plan covering the following points: 1. How to take own blood pressure. 2. Action and side effects of antihypertensive medication. 3. Beneficial effects of exercise program on cardiovascular system. 4. How sodium increases water retention and elevates blood pressure. 5. Foods to avoid that contain excess sodium. 6. Potential complications of uncontrolled blood pressure and reason for physician examination to detect beginning complications.	First teaching session completed; verbalizes action and three side effects of antihypertensive medication; can pick foods high in sodium from a list. Continue teaching and plan.

COLLABORATIVE CARE PLANS

The nursing process is a framework for delivering nursing care. Sequential thought processes are necessary to identify patient needs and to plan and deliver comprehensive care. For the student and the beginning nurse in particular, studying prepared care plans and writing care plans for assigned patients are effective ways to develop the habit of thinking in a logical, orderly way. In practice settings, many institutions use standardized care plans that are either printed or available on computer. The nurse uses the standardized care plan as a guide and individualizes it for the patient. In addition, care plans may eventually take a form that is usable by all health team members for collaborative care.

It is logical that having one plan of care is preferable to having several plans, each devised by a member of the team, such as respiratory therapist, physical therapist, physician, or nurse. Such collaborative care plans may be named *clinical pathways, care paths,* or *multidisciplinary action plans (MAPs)* and are being developed for the most common patient problems and medical diagnoses. They are an attempt to coordinate all aspects of treatment and care into one clearly defined plan of care. **Clinical pathways are a tool used for *case management*** in a hospital or health care agency. The case manager coordinates services provided by the interdisciplinary health care team. Many varieties of case management are used today. Some are clinically oriented and others are business oriented. The one thing that seems clear is that well-structured case management models do decrease the length of stay in the hospital and thus provide significant cost savings. Many third-party payors such as health insurance companies are offering discounts or other incentives to hospitals who use a case management system. Other advantages of case management include improved quality of care and improved communication among the members of the health care team.

Clinical pathways have four major features: patient outcomes, a timeline, collaboration among members of the health care team, and directions for comprehensive aspects of care. Expected outcomes are listed for the projected date of discharge. Timelines for sequencing interventions to meet the expected outcomes are listed. The pathway is developed by all members of the health care team who will be involved in the treatment and care of the patient. Interventions are listed on the timeline for various aspects of care, such as diagnostic tests, nutrition, treatments, medications, mobility and activity, patient teaching, and discharge planning. The case manager oversees and coordinates the patient's care and documents deviations (called variances) from the pathway.

Case management methods will continue to evolve and be refined, as many aspects of clinical pathways and case management still need to be developed, researched, and evaluated.

CRITICAL THINKING EXERCISES

Clinical Case Problems

Read each clinical situation and discuss the questions with your classmates.

1. Mrs. Farmer, age 48, is admitted to the outpatient surgery unit with abnormal menstrual bleeding. She is scheduled for a dilatation and curettage (D&C) for diagnostic purposes.
   a. During the interview what kinds of nursing assessment questions would you expect to ask when Mrs. Farmer is admitted?
   b. How could you contribute to the collection of data for assessing and identifying the patient care problems Mrs. Farmer is likely to have?

2. Outline exactly what you would do for your physical assessment of Mrs. Farmer.

3. Mr. Johanssen has just been told by his physician that he has a chronic and incurable illness. He will be able to manage the illness if he is willing to learn about it and follow his physician's orders. Mr. Johanssen alternates between being very angry and very depressed and bewildered. Discuss with your classmates how a nurse might assess Mr. Johanssen's spiritual needs and what might be done to help him cope with his illness.

4. You have been caring for Mrs. Wolonski this shift. She is recovering from a fractured femur that is being treated with balanced traction. When you examine her pin sites, you notice a slight amount of bloody drainage around the pin on the left. Her pain is controlled for only 2 hours on the ordered oral analgesics, and she is complaining of stuffy head and sinuses. Give a report to the incoming nurse at the end of your shift.

BIBLIOGRAPHY

American Nurses' Association. (1991). *Standards: Medical-Surgical Nursing Practice*. Kansas City: American Nurses' Association.

Bonczek, M. E., and Ryan, L. A. (1993). Beyond QA, the easy way. RN. 56(8):19–23.

Canadian Nurses Association (1987). *A Definition of Nursing Practice: Standards for Nursing Practice*. Ottawa, Canada: Author.

Carson, V. B. (1989). *Spiritual Dimensions of Nursing Practice*. Philadelphia: Saunders.

Cox, S. S. (1994). Taping report: tips to record by. *RN*. 57(3):64.

Dawson, M. J. (1994). Not documented, not done. *Nursing 94.* 24(8):63–64.

deWit, S. C. (1994). *Rambo's Nursing Skills for Clinical Practice,* 4th ed. Philadelphia: Saunders.

Diaz-Gilbert, M. (1993). Caring for culturally diverse patients. *Nursing 93.* 23(10):44–45.

Doenges, M., Moorhouse, M. F. (1992). *Application of Nursing Process and Nursing Diagnosis: An Interactive Text.* Philadelphia: F. A. Davis.

Esler, R., Bentz, P., Sorensen, M., Van Orsow, T. (1994). A case management success story. *American Journal of Nursing.* 94(11):34–38.

Frawley, K. A. (1994). Confidentiality in the computer age. *RN.* 57(7):59–60.

Gordon, M. (1979). The concept of nursing diagnosis. *Nursing Clinics of North America.* 14(3):487.

Harrington, A. M. (1989). Eight steps for evaluating a new long-term care patient. *Nursing 89.* 19(5):74.

Ignatavicius, D. D., Hausman, K. A. (1995). *Clinical Pathways for Collaborative Practice.* Philadelphia: Saunders.

Ignatavicius, D. D., Workman, M. L., Mishler, M. A. (1995). *Medical–Surgical Nursing: A Nursing Process Approach,* 2nd ed. Philadelphia: Saunders.

Iyer, P. W., Taptich, B. J., Bernocchi-Losey, D. (1991). *Nursing Process and Nursing Diagnosis,* 2nd ed. Philadelphia: Saunders.

Jarvis, C. (1992). *Physical Examination and Health Assessment.* Philadelphia: Saunders.

Luquire, R., Hurley, M. L., et al. (1994). Focusing on outcomes. *RN.* 57(5):57–59.

Predd, C. S. (1989). Great tips for setting priorities. *Nursing 89.* 19(10):120.

Ramdayal, I. (1990). For smoother shift changes, try walking rounds. *RN.* 53(9):19.

Simpson, R. L. (1994). Case-managed care in tomorrow's information network. *Nursing Management.* 24(7): 14–15.

Sparks, S. M., Taylor, C. M. (1994). Formulating a nursing diagnosis. *Nursing 94.* 24(3):32H–32J.

Tripp-Reimer, T. (1994). Crossing over the boundaries. *Critical Care Nurse.* 94(6):134–141.

Ulrich, S. P., Canale, S. W., Wendell, S. A. (1994). *Medical–Surgical Nursing Care Planning Guides,* 3rd ed. Philadelphia; Saunders.

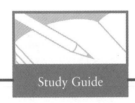

Study Guide

I. Characteristics of the Nursing Process

A. Process: a series of actions toward achieving a goal.

B. Actions are carried out carefully and systematically.

C. Nursing process: series of actions directed toward the delivery of high-quality nursing care.

D. Goal is to alleviate, minimize, or prevent real or potential health problems that a nurse is qualified to treat.

E. Specific expected outcomes are written for each goal.

F. Nursing process is a deliberate, rational, and logical approach to helping the patient deal with health problems.

G. Demands knowledge, skills, and belief in the worth of every person.

II. Differences in Nursing Roles

A. Based on differences in educational preparation and experience.

B. Minimal expectation for new graduates of various nursing programs have been defined by the NLN.

C. Essential tasks of beginning nurses are:

1. Collecting specific kinds of information.

2. Contributing to the development of nursing care plans.

3. Performing basic therapeutic and preventive nursing measures.

4. Participating in evaluating outcomes of care.

III. Underlying Assumptions or Beliefs

A. Fundamental beliefs about human life, role of nursing, and the delivery of health care

1. Respect the worth, dignity, and individuality of each person.

2. Recognize common human needs and the fact that people require help to meet those needs.

3. Emphasize the right to patient-centered, high-quality health care and the importance of patient input.

4. Focus on the role of nursing in health maintenance and care of the sick and injured.

5. Encourage self-fulfillment and continued learning and effort to increase competence.

IV. Applying the Nursing Process in Medical–Surgical Nursing

A. All five parts of the nursing process are systematically used to care for patients.

B. Assessment (data gathering).

1. Purpose is to collect data about patient's health status to establish nursing diagnoses.

2. Information should be relevant to the problem and of sufficient quantity to allow valid conclusions to be drawn.

3. Assessment is continuous; therefore, a plan of care can be revised when there is new information.

4. Initial assessment is made at the time of a nurses's first encounter with the patient to provide a data base. Baseline information is useful for later comparisons of patient's status.

5. Sources of data include patients or clients, their family members or significant others, and findings of other health team members.

6. Techniques for gathering information about the patient include:

   a. Records: new admission records and old records from previous admissions.

   b. Interview: to obtain nursing history.

      (1) Purpose is explained to the patient.

      (2) Conversational tone using direct and indirect open-ended questions.

      (3) Summarizing at end of interview helps to clarify and validate information.

      (4) A mini-interview is conducted with each patient each day in a casual manner.

      (5) Psychosocial assessment.

         (a) Educational level, employment status, marital status, number of children, health insurance, type of household, hobbies, leisure activities, pets.

         (b) Significant relationships and support system.

         (c) Other problems that might affect patients' health.

         (d) Cultural beliefs and values, especially regarding illness and health care.

         (e) How patients perceive their state of health.

         (f) Coping patterns (How the patient deals with difficulties).

         (g) Level of self-esteem, perceived roles, dynamics of family relationships.

         (h) Signs of anxiety or depression.

      (6) Spiritual assessment:

         (a) Necessary for holistic care of the patient.

         (b) Can be done during initial assessment interview or at any time that seems appropriate.

         (c) Guidelines for pertinent questions (see Table 2-2).

         (d) Sources of spiritual help include the nurse's own belief system, prayer, meditation, Scriptures, and referral to or consultation with clergy.

   c. Chart review is performed to gather data.

   d. Physical examination includes vital signs, inspection, auscultation, and palpation.

   e. Laboratory data.

   f. Consultation with people and review of written records.

C. Assessment: techniques of physical examination

1. Visual inspection is a vital assessment tool.

2. Smelling (olfaction) provides information about disease conditions, presence of infection, degree of cleanliness, and ingestion of alcohol.

3. Palpation of the skin, abdomen, and other areas of the body provides information about temperature, firmness, tenderness, swellings, and the rate and character of pulses.

4. Percussion is used to outline body organs and their characteristics.

D. Physical examination

1. Measurement of height, weight, respiration, pulse, and blood pressure.

2. Comparison of results with prior data to determine trends.

3. Practical physical assessment; an abbreviated physical assessment done on each assigned patient.

   a. Check skin color, eye appearance, condition of the hair, and general affect.

   b. Measure vital signs, auscultate the lungs, and listen to the heart at the apex.

   c. Check skin turgor and color.

   d. Assess abdomen, listening for bowel sounds and checking for tenderness; determine bowel and bladder status.

   e. Assess extremity movement.

   f. Determine ability to perform activities of daily living.

4. Check diagnostic test and laboratory data for current status and problems.

5. Consult with other health team members and survey the chart; consult texts and journals about the disease process as needed.

E. Analysis and nursing diagnosis.

1. A nursing diagnosis is a short statement of a patient's actual or potential health problem based on a nurse's judgment of a patient's condition and clinical status, response to treatment, and nursing care needs.

2. Categories of nursing diagnoses are continuously being refined, (first proposed in 1972 at the National Conference on Classification of Nursing Diagnoses).

a. Goal is to standardize nursing diagnoses to facilitate communication among nurses and identify specific outcome criteria and nursing interventions to solve patient care problems.

3. Nursing diagnoses are primarily concerned with:

a. Patient's comfort and sense of well-being.

b. Prevention of complications.

c. Patient education.

4. Medical diagnosis and nursing diagnosis complement one another.

5. Nursing diagnoses give direction to nursing care plan.

F. Planning

1. Provides a blueprint for nursing interventions.

2. Requires input from patient and family.

3. The nurse collaborates with the patient, physician, and health care team to construct a holistic plan of care.

4. Steps include:

a. Determining priorities from problem list.

b. Setting goals. Goals are broad statements that describe how to restore, maintain, or promote health.

c. Developing expected outcomes to reach goals. Expected outcomes are measurable and attainable steps toward accomplishing overall goals. Elements include patient activity that can be observed or tested, conditions provided to help patient to reach objective, time by which objective will be met, and quality of performance.

d. Writing nursing orders. Nursing orders include actions of nurse and patient activities prescribed to help reach outcomes and goals.

5. Plan is revised as problems are resolved and others arise or when nursing intervention is changed.

6. The computerized care plan or the Kardex care plan is consulted before completing a daily work plan.

7. Data about the current needs and priorities of care for the patient are obtained during report.

G. Implementation

1. Implementation is the phase during which the plan is put into action.

2. Nursing actions are coordinated with other forms of therapy so that the total care given is beneficial to the patient.

3. Implementation concludes with documentation of care given and the patient's response to that care.

4. Communication to other staff about the patient's condition, what has been done during a shift, and outcome of treatment are done by documenting in the patient's chart and reporting to oncoming staff.

H. Evaluation.

1. The evaluation step of the nursing process is continuous and ongoing.

a. Nursing interventions are evaluated to see whether they have been effective.

b. Interventions are judged effective if outcome criteria are met.

c. If intervention seems ineffective, the plan needs to be revised.

2. Quality management is aimed at evaluating the hospital, unit, nursing care, and other aspects of hospital function.

a. Quality management audits look closely at various aspects of hospital care to see whether they are meeting standards.

b. The Joint Commission on Accreditation of Hospitals reviews care given by hospitals.

c. A chart audit is done after patients are discharged to see whether the care they received meets set standards for the type of problem they had.

d. Each hospital has a quality management committee or board that coordinates audit activities.

e. The ANA Standards of Nursing Practice are used as criteria for process evaluation of nursing care.

3. The ultimate goal of all evaluation activities is to improve nursing care.

4. Evaluation is *not* done to find someone to blame. It is done to *improve* nursing care.

V. **Future Trends**

A. More emphasis on collaborative care.

B. Case management is a model of practice that is gaining favor in hospitals, home care agencies, and other types of health care facilities.

C. Clinical pathways are used in case management and present a collaborative approach to patient care along a clearly defined timeline.

CHAPTER 3

Psychosocial Aspects of Medical–Surgical Nursing

O B J E C T I V E S

Upon completing this chapter, the student should be able to:
1. List three ways in which the nurse promotes a therapeutic relationship with a patient.
2. Explain why it is important for the nurse to have some knowledge of the patient's cultural attitudes and beliefs.
3. Identify ways in which the nurse obtains information about patients' cultural values and preferences.
4. List three expectations that patients have of nurses.
5. Discuss specific ways to implement the strategies for pleasing patients.
6. Discuss examples of ways in which a nurse might help a patient to meet the three overall goals of patient teaching.
7. Identify two ways in which delivering nursing care in the home care setting is different from providing care in the hospital.
8. Give three examples of ways to meet the psychosocial needs of an elderly patient in an extended-care facility.
9. Identify the relationship of unmet needs to withdrawn, dependent, and hostile behaviors.
10. Describe two nursing interventions to meet needs of patients exhibiting each of the following types of behavior: dependent, withdrawn, depressed, hostile, manipulative.

To provide nursing care for the whole person, nurses consider both the physical and emotional needs of patients. Often patients cannot direct their energies toward healing because they are so involved with emotional concerns such as finances, who is caring for the children, or what is going to happen to their job. Anxiety interferes with learning and can interfere with normal coping mechanisms. Anxiety can be decreased through a trusting patient–nurse relationship. For the patient to develop trust in the nurse, the nurse must be knowledgeable and respectful of the patient's cultural beliefs and value system. Hope comes from the patient's spiritual or philosophical view. The nurse must provide for the patient's spiritual activities to promote hope and inner strength.

Patients today are consumers of health care, and they are aware that there is competition. They expect to be treated with the respect and dignity that a valued customer receives in the business world.

A very important aspect of nursing care is to teach patients what they need to know to care for themselves, prevent complications, restore health, or prevent illness. Learning relieves some fear and anxiety and psychologically prepares patients to attend to their own health care needs.

Providing psychosocial care includes attending to all of these needs. As the focus of nursing moves from the hospital setting to the community, attention to the psychosocial aspects of care become even more important because the family and other support persons will provide much of the daily personal care and treatments that nurses give in the hospital.

PSYCHOSOCIAL ASSESSMENT

To plan appropriate psychosocial care, the nurse must have a data base from which to identify the psychosocial needs of the patient. Table 3-1 is a guide for psychosocial assessment. This assessment can be done along with

TABLE 3-1   ◆ *Guide for Psychosocial Assessment*

Spiritual

Is there a pastor or church member you would like notified of your admission (or your illness)?

Do you use a quiet time each day for meditation, prayer, or spiritual reading?

Social

With whom do you live?

How will your illness/hospitalization affect your family?

Who will care for your children? (if appropriate)

Do you have sick leave at work? (if employed)

How will your illness affect your job? (if employed)

Do you have health insurance?

Who are the people in your life that can be of help at this time?

Will you be able to manage at home? Do you need assistance with bathing, meals, cleaning, errands, etc. (whichever is appropriate).

Are you able to obtain your medications, treatments, and/or needed equipment for your treatment?

Cultural

Do you have any dietary or food requirements that I can help you with?

Would you share with me any beliefs about your illness and treatment that are particular to your family or culture? (home remedies, aids toward wellness).

Psychological

What do you see as most stressful for you right now?

What are your biggest concerns/worries right now?

Are there other concerns that will affect your ability to recover/improve?

Do you ever have a problem with depression?

When you have a problem or face a difficult situation, how do you usually cope with it? Does this method of dealing with it usually help?

the admission interview. Nurses often learn more about patients and the family as they work with them over a period of time.

ESTABLISHING THERAPEUTIC RELATIONSHIPS

The nurse–patient relationship focuses on the patient, has goals, and is defined by the patient's needs and the nurse's role in promoting healing and wellness. A therapeutic relationship is one that promotes healing.

Characteristics that help to build a therapeutic relationship include effective communication skills, the quality of empathy, a desire to help, honesty, a nonjudgmental attitude, genuineness, acceptance, and respect for the individual.

The nurse focuses on the patient's feelings and problems without being judgmental. She expresses warmth, tact, respect, and caring. The nurse is someone the patient can rely on to do what she says she will do. If she tells the patient or family that she will get a cup of coffee or a pain medication, that need is attended to promptly; the therapeutic nurse is dependable (Figure 3-1).

By being nonjudgmental and accepting the patient's right to his own values, the nurse can refrain from taking a patient's anger, insult, or ungrateful behavior personally. She can allow the patient to own his own problems while sturdily being there to help him to choose alternatives and to make decisions.

What each of us brings to nursing is slightly different. Each one of us is a unique individual—the

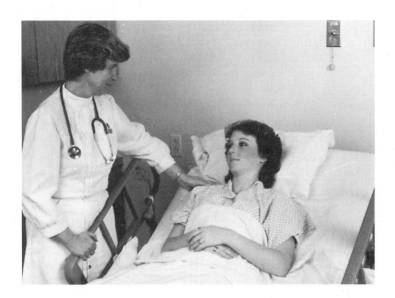

FIGURE 3-1   The nurse enters into a special kind of therapeutic relationship with her patient by being there when needed and showing care and concern. (Photo by Ken Kasper.)

total of our physical, psychological, social, and spiritual dimensions. Each patient is also unique in the same ways and must be considered as an individual.

> In personalized nursing care the patient's feelings, values, and expectations for his own care are of primary concern to the nurse.

The patient can make a significant contribution to planning, implementing, and evaluating his treatment and nursing care and must have the opportunity to do so insofar as he is able to. Time has proven that the ideal nurse–patient relationship is that of a partnership: a collaborative effort between the nurse and patient results in more effective health care.

In general, the nurse gives of herself in three broad areas: (1) in the knowledge she has acquired through study and experience; (2) in the hands-on skills she possesses; and (3) in the values and beliefs she feels are important and that she expresses in her behavior. Nurses use their knowledge of the physical, biological, social, and behavioral sciences to promote health, prevent disease, and give the best care of which they are capable to those who are unable to meet their own health needs. Throughout their professional life nurses are obligated to continue studying and expanding their store of knowledge. Psychomotor (hands-on) skills are used when performing procedures and giving treatments to meet patients' needs efficiently, safely, gently, and expertly. Nurses continually learn how to perform new procedures and develop expertise in using new equipment and supplies. Nurses are expected to be able to handle sophisticated monitoring devices and complex instruments that provide information about the physiological status of patients and to use machines that give life-sustaining support to those who cannot maintain vital functions on their own. The patient's confidence in the nurse's ability has a major psychological effect on his well-being.

Think about . . . Can you describe three ways in which you could consciously attempt to interact therapeutically with a patient? What personal values help you to interact therapeutically?

CULTURE, VALUES, BELIEFS, AND ATTITUDES

The nurses' Code of Ethics recognizes a person as a whole being with needs other than the purely physical (Table 3-2).

The culture in which each person was raised has a direct influence on the development of that person's attitudes, values, and beliefs. The Asian woman may

TABLE 3-2 ◆ *Code for Nurses*
1. The nurse provides services with respect for human dignity and the uniqueness of the client, unrestricted by considerations of social or economic status, personal attributes, or the nature of health problems.
2. The nurse safeguards the client's rights to privacy by judiciously protecting information of a confidential nature.
3. The nurse acts to safeguard the client and the public when health care and safety are affected by the incompetent, unethical, or illegal practice of any person.
4. The nurse assumes responsibility and accountability for individual nursing judgments and actions.
5. The nurse maintains competence in nursing.
6. The nurse exercises informed judgment and uses individual competence and qualifications as criteria in seeking consultation, accepting responsibilities, and delegating nursing activities to others.
7. The nurse participates in activities that contribute to the ongoing development of the profession's body of knowledge.
8. The nurse participates in the profession's efforts to implement and improve standards of nursing.
9. The nurse participates in the profession's efforts to establish and maintain conditions of employment conducive to high-quality nursing care.
10. The nurse participates in the profession's effort to protect the public from misinformation and misrepresentation and to maintain the integrity of nursing.
11. The nurse collaborates with members of the health professions and other citizens in promoting community and national efforts to meet the health needs of the public.

Source: American Nurses' Association (1985). *Code for Nurses with Interpretive Statements.* Kansas City, MO: Author.

have a much greater degree of modesty about revealing her body than the average American woman. The Hispanic man grows up with a much greater emphasis on the man being the decision maker in the family than does the Anglo male in America.

Cultural attitudes and beliefs extend to ideas about health care and practices to cure illness. When a patient's cultural beliefs and practices are different from those of the medical community, problems with following treatment plans occur. The nurse must first gain understanding of the patient's culture and belief system to establish a trusting relationship (Figure 3-2). Respect for patients includes accepting their cultural attitudes and beliefs. Allowing cultural health practices in which patients believe, as long as they are not harmful, meets the patients' psychosocial needs and assists them to regain health more quickly. Once trust is established, the nurse can begin to educate the patient about any cultural practices that are harmful to health.

Cultural beliefs are entwined in each person's entire being and need to be considered by nurses as they work with each individual. They need to review what effect

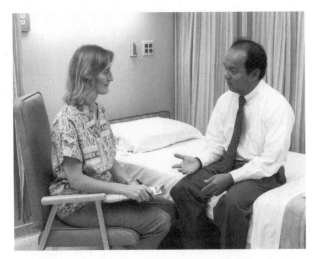

FIGURE 3-2   Obtaining cultural information for planning patient care. (Photo by Glen Derbyshire; Courtesy of Goleta Valley Cottage Hospital, Goleta, CA.)

their own culture has on their perspective of patients and their problems, as well as consider the effect of the patients' cultural background and beliefs on their view of their illness and recommended treatment. There is not room in this book to present all of the particular cultural beliefs and values that exist among the populations of the United States today. Each nurse must work at obtaining a knowledge of the cultures of the patient population in her area. Some examples of cultural beliefs and practices are interwoven in chapters of this book. Cultural considerations should be a part of holistic care and should be viewed in the context of the individual rather than a group.

Nurses must be careful not to assume that, because a patient is part of a particular ethnic group, his beliefs and preferences are the same as those attributed to that group.

The nurse obtains information about cultural values and preferences by interacting with patients and their families, asking appropriate questions about preferences, and seeking the patients' point of view about their illness and treatment.

A person's values, beliefs, and attitudes are outwardly expressed in his or her behavior. Although nurses must learn to be as "judgment free" as possible, their values do affect their professional judgment. The many ways in which a nurse might share her values and personal beliefs are not easily defined and measured.

The sensitive nurse will try to place herself in the patient's position, try to see things from the patient's point of view, and not try to impose her beliefs and values on the patient.

Think about . . . Can you identify a cultural belief or practice related to your own health practices that came from your childhood home?

It is most often the nurse who is called upon when the patients and their families and loved ones must cope with the sadder aspects of human existence. To give strength and support in times of pain and human suffering, nurses must have some inner resources of faith and hope to draw on. One cannot give to others what one does not have. It is important that each nurse have a clear idea of what his or her inner resources of strength are and how to draw on them. Each person must attempt to interpret the meaning of illness, or death, for himself or herself, drawing on spiritual beliefs and philosophy of life. The nurse can only assist the patient to seek his own answers.

Helping the patient to maintain hope is a vital part of the nurse–patient relationship. There can always be hope of some sort. Even when in pain, a patient can hope for a cheerful moment, a good laugh, or a loved visitor. The nurse helps to establish realistic hopes, but does not deny the patient his unrealistic hopes. Hope is what helps patients to cope with difficult situations.

SELF-ESTEEM: THE NURSE AND THE PATIENT

Self-concept, self-esteem, or self-image are integral parts of each person's personality and greatly influences a person's mental and physical health.

People who have a positive self-image are more capable of developing and maintaining warm interpersonal relationships. They also can resist psychological and physical illness better than those who have poor self-esteem.

It is the responsibility of the nurse to assess patients' level of self-esteem and, if it is low, to assist the person to develop a more positive self-image. The nurse's self-concept also is very important. The nurse who has a positive self-image is better equipped to help patients to meet their needs because he or she can respond to them in a healthy and positive manner.

Essentially, *self-concept* and *self-image* mean how a person sees her- or himself. *Self-esteem* indicates how people feel overall about themselves. Table 3-3 lists some behaviors that are associated with low self-esteem.

People with low self-esteem tend to be critical of themselves and their ideas and actions. The nurse can assist them to develop more positive thoughts and images about themselves by providing a model for them with positive statements about herself, such as, "I did a really good job redecorating the family room last

TABLE 3-3 ◆ *Behaviors Associated with Poor Self-Esteem*
◆ Avoids direct eye contact
◆ Poor grooming; appears unkempt
◆ Stooped posture
◆ Makes statements critical of self
◆ Has difficulty accepting compliments
◆ Apologizes frequently
◆ Avoids interacting with others
◆ Fails to complete or follow through with projects
◆ Is indecisive; has difficulty making up mind about things
◆ Overly dependent
◆ Verbalizes inability to cope
◆ Displays lack of energy
◆ Poor problem-solving ability
◆ Verbalizes feelings of guilt

weekend," or "I finally cooked a pie with a really good crust yesterday" and then asking what the patient has done lately that he feels good about—no matter how small the example. She also can give the patient honest, positive feedback such as "You managed more of your bath by yourself today!" Talking with the patient and getting him to express things he feels good about in his life can help him to focus on positive, rather than negative, aspects of himself.

PATIENTS' EXPECTATIONS

Hospitals and other health care facilities are concerned about how the people they serve view the quality of care they receive in their institutions. Administrators and staff members are genuinely concerned about the quality of care they give and are interested in having satisfied consumers. There are, of course, many reasons for their concern; one important reason is to minimize or eliminate altogether the possibility of lawsuits against them. In the days of the family doctor, who often was a friend of the family, knew each patient intimately, and was a respected and well-known member of the community, malpractice suits against physicians were rare. As medical and nursing care have become more depersonalized, legal action against physicians and nurses has increased greatly.

> People are less likely to take legal action against an individual or institution if they see the nurses caring for them as friendly, helpful, and striving to do their best.

The two major components of nursing are *competence* and *compassion*. Patients want to be tended by caring individuals who are fully competent in the skills of nursing. They want nurses to know what they are doing and to act as if they know what to do. They expect

them to have the necessary equipment at hand before beginning a procedure, to be skillful and adept in using it, and to perform repeated procedures in the same manner and sequence as much as possible. Performing nursing procedures with consistency can reduce the patients' anxiety and build their confidence in the competence of the nurses.

There are several strategies for pleasing patients. The first is to *keep patients informed* of what is happening and of anything relevant to their time in your care. This means that they need information about hospital routine, how to work the TV, the call light, the room lights, shower controls, and other aspects of their patient environment. They should be told what to expect regarding a procedure, when meals will be served, and when they might see you at the bedside again. If their doctor does not make rounds until after dinner, they would appreciate having that piece of information. Giving sufficient information and answering questions decrease patients' anxiety.

Give good service. Treat patients with common courtesy. Treat them like real persons, not "diseases." Ask them what they think. Actively listen to their answers, as well as concerns and fears. Respect and protect their privacy. Answer call lights promptly; try to anticipate toileting needs. Check on IV lines frequently, and prevent problems. See that the patient environment is kept clean and orderly and that meal trays do not sit around when the meal is over. Share that you will be busy for 10 minutes down the hall, but that you want to know whether anything is needed before you leave. Remind the patient that there is someone available at the desk to see that he or she gets needed assistance even when you are not available.

Take ownership of problems, even if you have nothing to do with the situation. Patients expect nurses to see to it that problems are handled. If the last shift left things undone, make sure that they are accomplished quickly, and try to troubleshoot so that the same situation doesn't happen again. Don't blame, just take care of it. This attitude promotes patient–consumer satisfaction.

Continually reassess your patient's needs. If you can anticipate a need before it is expressed, so much the better. Patient satisfaction multiplies when needs are met time and time again. Assess the need for further pain medication before the next dose is due; determine whether the medication is effective. If it is not doing the job, speak to the physician and get the order changed.

Do your best to exceed patient expectations. Straighten the bed when the patient is up to the bathroom; give a back rub along with pain medication when appropriate; volunteer information to the patient or family about progress or when test results can be expected. Focus on the patient and speak to him before attending to equipment in the room. Be an advocate for the patient's rights (Table 3-4), protecting confidentiality and privacy, respecting his or her right to informed consent and to refuse treatment. Show that you are concerned for your patient's total well-being.

Think about... Can you name three ways in which these strategies can be carried out in a home care setting? How would they differ in an outpatient clinic setting?

A major consideration of all health care workers should be the human rights of the patient (Table 3-4). Make sure that the patient is treated as a person. Hospitals are working on becoming more flexible, allowing patients to wear their own clothes if they are ambulatory, extending visiting hours, and improving dietary menus. Hospitals and other health agencies are required to have some rules and regulations that provide a safe and therapeutic environment for their clients. But strict following of rules for the sake of legality, rather than for the welfare of the patients, can lead to violating patient rights. An example of such a rule is that in many hospitals patients who have been ambulatory about the halls must be discharged in a wheelchair—in spite of their protests or feelings of loss of dignity.

When patients are consulted as partners, they are being told that they are worthwhile individuals whose thoughts and ideas count. The partnership recognizes our human need to have some control over what happens to us and some voice in the decisions that

---

TABLE 3-4 ♦ *Patients' Bill of Rights*

We consider you a partner in your hospital care. When you are well-informed, participate in treatment decisions, and communicate openly with your doctor and other health professionals, you help make your care as effective as possible. This hospital encourages respect for the personal preferences and values of each individual.

While you are a patient in the hospital, your rights include the following:

♦ You have the right to considerate and respectful care.

♦ You have the right to be well-informed about your illness, possible treatments, and likely outcome and to discuss this information with your doctor. You have the right to know the names and roles of people treating you.

♦ You have the right to consent to or refuse a treatment, as permitted by law, throughout your hospital stay. If you refuse a recommended treatment, you will receive other needed and available care.

♦ You have the right to have an advance directive, such as a living will or health care proxy. These documents express your choices about your future care or name someone to decide if you cannot speak for yourself. If you have a written advance directive, you should provide a copy to the hospital, your family, and your doctor.

♦ You have the right to privacy. The hospital, your doctor, and others caring for you will protect your privacy as much as possible.

♦ You have the right to expect that treatment records are confidential unless you have given permission to release information or reporting is required or permitted by law. When the hospital releases records to others, such as insurers, it emphasizes that the records are confidential.

♦ You have the right to review your medical records and to have the information explained, except when restricted by law.

♦ You have the right to expect that the hospital will give you necessary health services to the best of its ability. Treatment, referral, or transfer may be recommended. If transfer is recommended or requested, you will be informed of risks, benefits, and alternatives. You will not be transferred until the other institution agrees to accept you.

♦ You have the right to know if the hospital has relationships with outside parties that may influence your treatment and care. These relationships may be with educational institutions, other health care providers, or insurers.

♦ You have the right to consent or decline to take part in research affecting your care. If you choose not to take part, you will receive the most effective care the hospital otherwise provides.

♦ You have the right to be told of realistic care alternatives when hospital care is no longer appropriate.

♦ You have the right to know about hospital rules that affect you and your treatment and about charges and payment methods. You have the right to know about hospital resources, such as patient representatives or ethics committees, that can help you resolve problems and questions about your hospital stay and care.

♦ You have responsibilities as a patient. You are responsible for providing information about your health, including past illnesses, hospital stays, and use of medicine. You are responsible for asking questions when you do not understand information or instructions. If you believe you can't follow through with your treatment, you are responsible for telling your doctor.

This hospital works to provide care efficiently and fairly to all patients and the community. You and your visitors are responsible for being considerate of the needs of other patients, staff, and the hospital. You are responsible for providing information for insurance and for working with the hospital to arrange payment, when needed.

Your health is dependent not just on your hospital care but, in the long term, on the decisions you make in your daily life. You are responsible for recognizing the effect of life-style on your personal health.

A hospital serves many purposes. Hospitals work to improve people's health; treat people with injury and disease; educate doctors, health professionals, patients, and community members; and improve understanding of health and disease. In carrying out these activities, this institution works to respect your values and dignity.

directly affect us. It implies a cooperative effort and a mutual thought that the therapy being employed can and will have a desirable effect.

INTEGRATING HEALTH TEACHING

One way in which nurses can help patients to maintain their "rights" is to communicate effectively and to integrate teaching into every aspect of their care. To be most effective, patient teaching must begin with admission and continue until discharge. The nursing diagnosis "Knowledge deficit" should always be considered for the nursing care plan of each patient. Teaching should not be left for a 5- to 15-minute segment on the day of discharge.

The overall goals of patient teaching are that the patient learn (1) necessary self-care; (2) ways to promote better health; and (3) ways to prevent complications or illness. The teaching-learning process is similar to the nursing process in that both are flexible and dynamic—that is, subject to change whenever the patient's needs and problems require attention. The components of the teaching-learning process are (1) assessment, (2) planning, (3) instruction, and (4) evaluation.

During her initial admission assessment, the nurse should begin thinking about the various topics of health teaching that will be appropriate for this patient. Providing some general information is a start: how the television works, how to call the nurse, what the mealtime schedule is, and so on.

A review of the initial physician's orders gives clues about other topics. Teaching what to expect for scheduled diagnostic tests or upcoming surgery and about each prescribed medication should come next. After a diagnosis is finalized, determine the patient's understanding of what the physician has told him, and reinforce teaching about his disorder and its effect on his life-style. Assess what he needs to know to perform self-care.

Evaluating patients' educational level, cultural beliefs, and personality type is necessary to determine what methods of teaching will be most effective with them. Some patients will need simple, concrete explanations; others do better with an audiovisual presentation or written materials.

A plan is based on the evaluation findings. Before writing a plan, an assessment of what patients already know and what they feel they need to learn is done. An outline of what patients need to learn and a time frame for learning it are the starting points. Specific expected outcomes are written for each aspect of what patients are to be taught.

Teaching is implemented for each of the points to be covered. Discharge teaching regarding diet, level of activity, continued medications, signs and symptoms to

report, and the importance of follow-up care is begun as soon as the patient is well enough to retain the information.

Evaluating the plan's effectiveness is performed together with the patient. A major part of patient teaching is to take the time to obtain feedback about what you have taught. What he has learned must be validated, errors in understanding corrected, and reinforcement given for him to incorporate what you have taught into his daily living. Return demonstration of a motor skill is essential and will make the patient more confident in his ability to carry out the procedure correctly once he is home. Table 3-5 provides a guide for general topics that should be covered for every patient before discharge.

PSYCHOSOCIAL ASPECTS OF DELIVERING HOME CARE

Leaving an in-patient facility and entering into the world of home care requires a change in perspective on the part of nurses. In the home, you are on the patient's turf, whereas in the hospital he was on your turf. It is even more important to listen to the patient's point of view, acknowledge his wishes about his care, and be respectful of his property and home environment. If the home is messy, full of obstacles that could contribute to a fall, or is dirty, the nurse must work with the patient to bring about changes that are more beneficial to his health. The patient must first trust the nurse; building trust takes time. Being respectful of the person the patient is now is necessary before the nurse can expect to bring about changes in the way a patient lives or does things.

The family or significant other is a major factor in the care and treatment of the home patient. The home care nurse spends a lot of time communicating with family members, teaching them, listening to them, and being supportive. It is the entire family that is really the "patient," not the lone individual.

Psychosocial care is of vital importance in the home care setting. The nurse must collaborate with the social worker, other health team members, friends, and family to provide the emotional support and take care of the social needs of the patient. Ordering a special mattress to prevent pressure sores will not work unless provision for payment for the device is in place and someone can pick up the equipment. Considerable attention is paid to referral of the patient and the family members to various community agencies and support groups. Home care nurses and social workers collaborate to provide homemaking and bathing or personal care services for the patient. For some patients, the visit by the nurse is the only human contact he has for days at a time.

TABLE 3-5 ◆ *Topics for Discharge Teaching*	
Wound care	Cleansing of wound, types of dressings to use, frequency of dressing changes. How to assess the wound; what to report to the doctor.
Diet	Type of diet; food restrictions; expected fluid intake or restriction. Need for protein, Vitamin C. iron, or added postasium. Sodium restriction.
Treatments	How to perform wound irrigations, handle wound suction devices, rate of oxygen flow and how to correctly apply the cannula; catheter and tube care; how to empty drainage containers; heat or cold applications; how to perform other treatments. Use of incentive spirometer or other breathing and coughing regimens. Need to weigh and record weight and how often. Measuring and recording intake and output. Need to wear elastic stockings—when and how to apply.
Medications	What each medication is for and how to take it; side effects to report; expected action of each medication; importance of compliance.
Pain control	When to treat pain; use of pain medication; measures to avoid constipation from narcotic analgesics; alternative methods of reducing pain. What to do if pain is not relieved or worsens.
Activity	Positioning desired; how to perform range of motion or other specific exercises and how often to do them. Frequency and distance for ambulation. Restrictions on lifting, weight bearing, and other strenuous activity; when might be allowed to drive; when might be allowed to resume intercourse and other usual activities. Amount of sleep and rest desirable. What to do if unable to sleep well.
Bathing	Whether allowed to shower or bathe in tub; how to cover wound if necessary; precautions.
Support	Who to call and at what telephone number with questions or if a problem arises. Date of next doctor appointment or when to call for an appointment. When to expect contact from a Home Health Agency if such care is expected. Names and phone numbers of community agencies or support groups that might be helpful to the patient.

CONSIDERATIONS FOR LONG-TERM CARE

Most long-term care residents are elderly. There are a few basic principles for psychosocial care of these patients. The elderly will adjust better if they are allowed to do things for themselves and if they can help to take care of others. This participation gives them a sense of purpose. They need some control over their environment and should be consulted about care decisions.

Surrounding the patient with items from home such as pictures, books, a quilt, or whatever is most important to him will help him to adjust and feel less displaced. The patient should direct the placement of his personal articles. Once they are placed, they should not be moved to another location without permission.

Last, interactions with others are very important. Light exercise, crafts, music, special guest speaker programs, and such can make a definite difference in the quality of life of the residents. Even if the activity is not in itself meaningful to the individual, the socialization and contact with others is important to his well-being.

◆ Psychosocial Aspects of Caring for the Elderly

It should be remembered that, when the elderly patient is out of his normal home setting, it is likely that he will feel out of balance with his surroundings. Routine and familiarity are more important to the older person.

When an elderly person is removed from his home, he feels the loss of familiar surroundings, may miss a pet, does not have contact with his usual neighbors, friends, and so on. It is important to try to increase the patient's feelings of self-worth and give him some control over his life and surroundings. Psychosocial care includes trying to provide familiar objects around the patient, learning his usual routines, and trying to adapt agency routine to fit.

When interacting with the elderly patient, give information slowly and carefully. Wait for one piece of information to be processed before supplying another. Ask for feedback to see that information or instructions have been understood. Leave printed instructions so that the patient has something he can refer to for clarification. Printed instructions must be in print large enough for the elderly person to read and should be on nonglare paper. Ask the patient whether he can read the print easily and if there is anything he does not understand.

Address the elderly patient by his formal name and inquire if that is what he wishes to be called. Face the patient when speaking as he may be hearing impaired. Speak at a normal volume and use a medium to low pitch. Enunciate clearly. Approach each patient contact with patience. It takes more time for the elderly to rise from a bed or chair, walk to the bathroom, locate items, and formulate responses. Wait for an answer to your question. Be tactful. If you are trying to obtain specific information and your patient is rambling on about something else, you might say, "I'd like to hear about that, but I believe we'd better get back to . . . at the moment." If possible, state a specific time when you can continue the patient's topic of conversation. "I'd like to hear more about . . . when I come to help you with your bath" lets the patient know that he is a person of interest.

Speak directly to the elderly patient when discussing his care; it is disrespectful to speak to a family member over his head when he is present. Think about how you would want your mother or father treated if they were in the patient's place. Let the patient speak for himself as much as possible so that he feels in control of his own life. Be a good patient advocate by helping him to assert his right to be included in the decision making and planning for his care.

Touch of a therapeutic nature is a major means of communicating caring and warmth to your elderly patient. It is best to ask whether the patient minds being touched or hugged before doing so. In some cultures, touching by a stranger is very threatening. Taking a hand in yours, placing an arm around the shoulders, giving a hug, all say to the patient that he is a person worthy of your caring. However, do not use patting on the shoulder with phrases of "It will be all right"; that is treating him like a child.

As the end of life nears, people have a need to go through a life review, talking about past events and people. Assist your patient to do this by listening to his tales attentively and patiently. You may always express the need to break away to perform some task, just express the desire to continue the story later and then return to do so. The elderly have a wealth of experience and a different perspective from the young; one can learn much from them and be very enriched by the experience.

Think about . . . How could you assist the elderly home-bound patient to be less lonely?

COPING WITH PATIENTS WHO DISPLAY DIFFICULT BEHAVIORS

Being hospitalized for any illness or injury can create emotional problems and unacceptable behaviors in patients, who, under less trying circumstances, are mentally sound and emotionally mature. A holistic and personalized approach to nursing care certainly must respect a patient's need for both emotional and physiological support and provide planned nursing intervention to meet each patient's emotional needs. Identifying and meeting a patient's emotional needs are part of the responsibility of the nurse in all care settings, from acute care to home care.

Patients' emotional needs and resulting behaviors may be temporary and related to the stresses of the illness, or they may be related to underlying disorders that will benefit from a psychiatric consultation or treatment. Psychiatric disorders and nursing care to promote mental health are discussed in Chapters 32 through 35.

Even patients whose primary illness is a physiological rather than psychological disorder can sometimes express emotional discomfort through dependent, withdrawn, hostile, or manipulative behavior. They may behave in ways that are uncomfortable for the nurse who is not prepared to intervene effectively.

The nurse who is able to provide effective planned intervention to meet a patient's emotional needs has learned to respond in an appropriate and therapeutic manner when a patient's extreme behavior is uncomfortable for her.

There are techniques and interventions that nurses can effectively use to deal with patients who exhibit dependent, withdrawn, hostile, or manipulative behaviors, but first and foremost the nurse must remember that the patient needs to have his behavior accepted. The nurse should look for what emotion is underlying the behavior. If the patient is extremely dependent, often he is extremely frightened. If he is withdrawn and depressed, he frequently needs help in increasing his coping techniques. Hostility is sometimes an expression of anger toward the illness or oneself. Manipulation just might be a grasping for some control over a part of life when everything else seems out of control.

♦ Dependency Behavior

Patients exhibiting extreme dependency behavior are attempting to satisfy an unmet need to depend on someone other than themselves.

In an extreme form of dependency the patient may refuse to do anything for himself. He might be unreasonably demanding of the nurse's time and attention, show little or no initiative in performing the simplest of self-care activities, or exhibit flirtatious behavior to attract attention to himself. This is the patient who is constantly ringing for the nurse and can't seem to do anything for himself.

Attempts to force the patient to do things for himself and develop some independence usually have the opposite effect, causing further regression into an even more dependent state and an escalation of unacceptable attention-getting behaviors.

Nursing interventions for dependent behavior are first directed toward meeting the patient's dependency needs and then gradually fostering independence once the dependency needs are met and the patient feels secure. Nursing actions initially include increasing the amount of time spent with the patient, establishing trust, anticipating his needs and wants, utilizing therapeutic touch, and assuring him that his needs will be met. Next, the nurse should encourage him to do one small task of daily care on his own, such as wash his own face or put on his own gown. When this is accomplished, lavish praise should be given. It also is helpful to focus on the patient's abilities and to praise each and every thing he does for himself. If constant ringing for the nurse is a problem, sometimes this can be cured by setting limits. Meet all of the patient's current requests and then tell him that you will check on him in 30 minutes if he does not use the call bell. Be sure that you check on him in exactly 30 minutes. By returning as promised, you help him feel secure that his needs will be met, and the time period between checks can be lengthened to 45 minutes and then to 1 hour.

◆ Withdrawn Behavior

Withdrawn behavior is a withdrawal from contact with others.

> Extreme withdrawn behavior reflects a need to feel safe and secure and can indicate feelings of anxiety, fear, or sometimes anger. However, depression can also cause this type of behavior.

Although some degree of caution in establishing close contact with a stranger is natural when a relationship is new, continued withdrawal from the nursing staff can interfere with effective care and prevent a therapeutic nurse–patient relationship from being formed.

Withdrawn behavior is characterized by silence, failure to make eye contact, recoiling from touch, superficial conversation without any self-disclosure or sharing of feelings, and denial of feelings. The patient also may deny a reality, such as his own illness and its effects on his life.

Nursing interventions to meet a patient's need to feel safe and secure include providing a consistent routine of care so the patient knows what to expect; reducing environmental stress, confusion, and disorder; and limiting the number of health care providers the patient must interact with. Primary nursing as a mode of care is ideal for this kind of behavior problem.

Because these patients have a need for structure and trust, it is important that their nurses develop a reliable and trusting relationship with them. Whispering and secretive behavior on the part of the nurse can destroy trust. Teasing, joking, and otherwise failing to establish a bond of real friendship with the patient also can damage a trusting relationship and destroy the patient's confidence in the nurse.

◆ The Depressed Patient

Depression can range from occasionally feeling "blue" and sad to unrelenting despair and suicidal tendencies. Although some degree of depression might be expected in hospitalized patients, symptoms of depression should not be ignored.

> A person's frame of mind can directly affect his rate of recovery and will to live.

Depression often is expressed in withdrawn behavior. Signs and symptoms of depression are not always readily recognized. Loss of appetite, fatigue, vague aches and pains, insomnia, poor posture, gazing into space, and difficulty making decisions are all possible signs of depression. Sometimes the patient will make statements such as, "Nobody cares about me," "I don't feel like eating or going anywhere," or "I don't care whether I get better or not."

One helpful nursing action is just to spend silent time with the patient. This assures him that someone cares and is there for him, yet respects his desire to be withdrawn and silent.

Several other nursing interventions are sometimes helpful in relieving a patient's depression:

- Encourage and help the patient to engage in activities of daily living.
- Work at a slower pace and be patient and gentle.
- Emphasize the patient's good qualities, and point out his accomplishments and strengths.
- Do not overdo being bright and cheerful in his presence or admonish him to "cheer up and look at the bright side of things."
- Show that you care by being with the patient and interacting with him.
- Encourage exercise and social interaction with others.

Many times a depressed patient becomes more and more withdrawn and silent. Physical appearance and personal hygiene begin to deteriorate, and the patient has no interest in what is going on around him. Statements such as "I don't have anything to live for any more" warrant psychiatric consultation or referral.

All caregivers should be alert for signs of self-destruction and the potential for suicide. Depression is a treatable medical/psychiatric problem and should be dealt with as such (see Chapter 32).

◆ Hostile Behavior

> Hostile behavior is an expression of the patient's need to have control over what is happening to him.

It can arise from fear, desperation, anger, and frustration. Illness inevitably represents some degree of loss. For some patients it is a loss of independence, loss of control over some body functions, or loss of the means to care for and financially support themselves or their family members. Others suffer a loss of self-esteem or a disturbance in self-image because of body changes brought about by illness, disability, or surgery.

Losses of any kind can intensify the need to regain power and control over one's life. Behaviors that indicate a need to gain power or control include shouting, criticism, threats to "report" the nurse, and constant complaints about the care provided. Under a barrage of this kind of behavior, it sometimes is extremely difficult for the nurse to be compassionate toward and concerned about the abusive patient. Planned and consistent nursing intervention often can change the patient's behavior to a more acceptable and comfortable level and make his hostile behavior less uncomfortable for the nurse.

Sometimes it is not the patient who exhibits this kind of behavior, but a family member who is upset over a serious, rapidly progressing, or perhaps fatal illness of a loved one. In either case, no matter who is the aggressor, the natural reaction is either to become defensive or to counterattack and wage a power struggle. Neither of these reactions is an appropriate response to the patient's or family member's need for control.

Nursing interventions to deal with expressions of anger that represent hostile behavior should begin with letting the person know you are aware of his anger and allowing him to express his feelings freely. The person could be asked what is upsetting him and what can be done to help him feel less angry and frustrated.

It is important to listen actively to the person who is exhibiting hostile behavior.

Usually the opportunity to release some of his pent-up anger provides some relief and permits a calmer and more logical approach to his problem.

Other interventions include allowing the patient to make suggestions about his care and meeting his demands when they are not unreasonable and will not threaten his recovery. Physical activity can help release the pent-up energy associated with frustration and anger. Providing the patient with opportunities to participate in decisions and make choices in regard to his care can give the patient a sense of power and control.

Patients or family members who have a need for power and control sometimes feel better when they can talk to a supervisor or other person in a position of higher authority. This is not to say that the nurses caring for the patient are not providing the best of care, but rather that the patient or family member has a need to exercise some power and control and they see summoning an authority figure as a way to satisfy that need.

◆ The Manipulative Patient

Manipulative patients may use charm or flattery, seductiveness, lies, or threats to get what they want from the nurse. Sometimes they play one staff member against another ("splitting"). Examples of these various behaviors include: "Gee Paula, you do such a good job! They ought to promote you. Couldn't I have an extra dessert tonight?" "A hug would make me feel so much better." (Tomorrow he wants a full body clinch.) "The doctor said I only have to walk to the door." "If I don't get more pain medicine I'll kill myself." "I'm so glad you are here! Sally didn't come into my room all night. You are the only one who understands me."

This type of behavior has various causes. It may be a learned behavior that the patient uses as a way of communicating and responding to stress, or it may be a manifestation of a psychiatric disorder. However, many times it is based on fear of losing control.

The manipulative person fears losing total control of himself or his environment.

Suggested ways of dealing with the manipulative patient include: (1) helping to reduce the need for control by decreasing anxiety; (2) helping the patient use alternate ways of coping; and (3) maintaining an environment in which he feels safe, regardless of his behavior.

Specific interventions include the following:

◆ *Set limits.* Respond to the undesirable behavior as calmly as possible. Indicate that you will not tolerate the behavior. Tell him "Don't swear at me" or "Your screaming is inappropriate and disturbing to other patients and is making it impossible for me to help you; please stop and then tell me how I can help you."

◆ *Be consistent and firm.* Tell him when someone can help him and how often someone can check on him, and remind him of that when he demands attention between scheduled times.

◆ *Don't take insults personally or become defensive.* Take any threat of suicide seriously. Explore the situation by saying something such as, "That threat sounds like you are experiencing a lot of feelings you are not talking about. Can you tell me about them?" This lets him know you care.

◆ *Be aware of your own feelings.* This patient may remind you of a family member or friend who has used such tactics on you before.

If all of these strategies fail, rather than get into a shouting match or promote further hostility, tell the patient you are leaving the room because of his behavior and that you will be back when he has calmed down. State when you will be back, and be sure you arrive on time. Of course, this can be done only if the patient is not in need of some immediate care.

> Accept a patient's less than desirable behavior as part of his illness and not necessarily typical of the way he might react under more normal circumstances.

If we understand that a person's response to a particular situation is the best he is capable of at that particular time, it is easier to accept his or her behavior, even though we might not like it. The task of the nurse is to recognize the patient's behavior as resulting from the demands being placed on him or her at the moment. This requires kindness, understanding, and often firmness on the part of the nurse. People tend to become childlike and fearful when they are ill, and they appreciate having someone with them who can guide them through their ordeal gently and kindly.

CRITICAL THINKING EXERCISES

Clinical Case Problems

Read each clinical case problem and discuss the questions and complete the exercise with your classmates.

1. Mary is a 16-year-old who dove into the shallow end of a swimming pool and sustained a cervical fracture and paralysis. She is almost totally dependent on others for the most basic of self-care activities.

   a. What might you expect in the way of psychosocial problems for Mary and her family? Choose three appropriate psychosocial nursing diagnoses for Mary from the Approved Nursing Diagnoses List (Table 2-4, pgs. 24-25).

   b. Considering Mary's physical limitations and extremely poor prognosis for recovery, how can her life have meaning? How can she focus on her strengths and find activities that will be both meaningful and satisfying?

2. Mr. Porter has been hospitalized many times in the past few years and has earned the label "difficult patient" because of his abrasive and demanding personality.

   a. What do you think Mr. Porter's expectations of nurses might be?

   b. Conduct a survey among yourselves in the classroom to determine what each person thinks a patient should reasonably expect of nurses. Ask each person to list five expectations. After the survey, compare these expectations with those you listed for Mr. Porter and those listed in this chapter.

3. Sally is a 10-year-old Korean girl who is hospitalized with a fracture of the right tibia that she sustained in a bicycle accident. She also has a weeping wound of the left knee. She is to be discharged home on Friday.

   a. How would you assess what teaching will need to be done before discharge?

   b. Who will need to be included in the teaching sessions?

   c. How can you determine whether learning about cast care, medications, and wound care has taken place?

   d. What cultural implications related to the care of this patient might need to be considered in your teaching?

BIBLIOGRAPHY

Advice PRN. (1995). Difficult patient: master of manipulation. *Nursing 95.* 25(7):9–10.

Angelucci P. (1995). Notes from the field. Cultural diversity: health belief systems. *Nursing Management.* 26(8):72.

Antai-Otong, D. (1988). What you should and shouldn't do when your patient is angry. *Nursing 88,* 18(2):44.

American Hospital Association. (1976). *Statement on a Patient's Bill of Rights.* Chicago: American Hospital Association.

Badger, J. M. (1994). Calming the anxious patient. *American Journal of Nursing.* 94(5):46–50.

Baker, L. J. (1995). Communicating across cultures. *Nursing 95.* 25(1):79.

Boyle, J. S., Andrews, M. M. (1989). *Transcultural Concepts in Nursing Care.* Boston: Scott, Foresman.

Brady, J. (1995). Branching out into home health care. *American Journal of Nursing.* 95(6):34–36.

Buchwald, D., et al. (1994). Caring for patients in a multicultural society. *Patient Care.* 20(11):105–109, 113–114, 116.

Carson, V. B. (1989). *Spiritual Dimensions of Nursing Care.* Philadelphia: Saunders.

Corso, M. T. (ed.). (1984). *Practices.* Springhouse, PA: Springhouse.

Diaz-Gilbert, M. (1993). Caring for culturally diverse patients. *Nursing 93.* 23(10):44–45.

Fascione, J. (1995). Healing power of touch. *Elderly Care.* 7(1):19–21.

Franklin, K. (1995). The final rule . . . residents in extended-care facilities . . . right to be fully informed about own care and treatment. *Nursing 95.* 25(7):4, 6.

Giger, J. N., Davidhizar, R. E. (1991). *Transcultural Nursing:* Assessment and Intervention. St. Louis, MO: Mosby.

Grossman, D. (1994). Enhancing your "cultural competence." *American Journal of Nursing*. 94(7):58–62.

Hall, P. (1996). Providing psychosocial support. *American Journal of Nursing*. 96(10), 16N–16O.

Kozier, B., Erb, G., Olivieri, R. (1994). *Fundamentals of Nursing Concepts and Procedures,* 5th ed. Menlo Park, CA: Addison-Wesley.

Lewis, S., Blumenreich, P. (1993). Defusing the violent patient. *RN.* 56(12):24–29.

Long, C. O., Greeneich, D. S. (1994). Four strategies for keeping patients satisfied. *American Journal of Nursing.* 94(6):26–27.

Marion, P. S., et al. (1995). Relocation stress syndrome: a comprehensive plan for long-term care admissions. *Geriatric Nursing.* 16(3):100–112.

Messner, R. L. (1993). What patients really want from their nurses. *American Journal of Nursing.* 93(8):38–39.

Murray, R. B., Zentner, J. P. (1988). *Nursing Concepts for Health Promotion,* 5th ed. Englewood Cliffs, NJ: Prentice-Hall.

Neff, L. (1995). Positive responses to difficult behavior. *Journal of Post Anesthesia Nursing.* 10(6), 332–335.

Norris, J., Kunes-Connell, M. (1985). Self-esteem disturbance. *Nursing Clinics of North America.* 20(4):745.

Pelletier, L. R., Kane, J. J. (1989). Strategies for handling manipulative patients. *Nursing 89.* 19(5):81.

Robinson, L. (1990). Stress and anxiety. *Nursing Clinics of North America.* 25(4):935.

Rogers, C. (1961). *On Becoming a Person.* Boston: Houghton Mifflin.

Rosenbaum, J. N. (1991). A cultural assessment guide. *The Canadian Nurse.* 87(4):32.

Ruscitti, C. (1992). Caring for a combative patient. *Nursing 92.* 22(9):50–51.

Simms, C. (1995). How to unmask the angry patient. *American Journal of Nursing.* 95(4):37–40.

Smith, J., et al. (1995). The resident: the heart of it. *Geriatric Nursing.* 16(3):113–116.

Spector, R. E. (1991). *Cultural Diversity in Health and Illness,* 3rd ed. New York: Appleton & Lange.

Timm, P. (1994). Improving your self-esteem. *Nursing 94.* 24(11):92–93.

Tripp-Reimer, T. (1994). Crossing over the boundaries. *Critical Care Nurse.* 14(6):134–136.

Ufema, J. (1994). Defusing Will's anger. *Nursing 94.* 24(7):60–61.

Valente, S. M., Saunders, J. M. (1989). Dealing with serious depression in cancer patients. *Nursing 89.* 19(2):44.

Zook, R. (1996). Take action before anger builds. *RN.* 59(4):46–49.

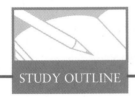

STUDY OUTLINE

I. Introduction

A. Holistic care involves assisting patients to meet both psychosocial and physical needs.

  1. Meeting psychological needs involves helping the patient to cope.

  2. Spiritual activities promote hope and inner strength.

  3. Respecting cultural beliefs and considering them in the plan of care enhance patient trust and compliance.

  4. The patient is a "consumer" of health care—a valued customer.

  5. Teaching is an important aspect of nursing care.

B. Establishing therapeutic relationships.

  1. Effective communication skills, empathy, a desire to help, honesty, a nonjudgmental attitude, genuineness, acceptance, and respect for the individual help to build a therapeutic relationship.

  2. The nurse focuses on the patient's feelings and problems without being judgmental.

  3. By being nonjudgmental and accepting the patient's right to his own values, the nurse can avoid taking the patient's undesirable behavior personally.

  4. The patient's feelings, values, and expectations for his own care are of primary concern to the nurse delivering personalized nursing care.

  5. The ideal nurse–patient relationship is that of a partnership.

  6. The nurse gives of herself in three broad areas: knowledge, hands-on skills, and her values and beliefs.

  7. The nurse is obligated to continue her education and expand her store of knowledge.

  8. The nurse must learn how to perform new procedures and develop facility in using new equipment and supplies.

C. Culture, values, beliefs, and attitudes.

1. One's culture has a direct influence on the development of the person's attitudes, values, and beliefs.

2. Cultural considerations should be a part of holistic care.

3. Obtain information about cultural values and preferences by interacting with the patient and his family, asking appropriate questions about preferences, and seeking the patient's point of view about his illness and treatment.

4. Be nonjudgmental; try to see things from the patient's point of view; do not impose your own beliefs and values on the patient.

5. To give strength and support, the nurse must have some inner resources of faith and hope to draw on.

6. Helping the patient to maintain hope is a vital part of the nurse–patient relationship.

II. Self-Esteem: The Nurse and the Patient

A. Self-esteem influences mental and physical health.

B. Certain behaviors may indicate low self-esteem (Table 3-3).

C. Methods for assisting patient to increase self-esteem include:

1. Modeling with positive statements and behaviors.

2. Giving honest, positive feedback.

III. Patients' Expectations

A. There is concern about how patients view the quality of care they receive.

B. People are less likely to take legal action if they perceive the nurse caring for them as friendly, helpful, and working to do her best.

C. There are several strategies for pleasing patients:

1. Keep patient's informed of what is happening; give adequate information.

2. Give good service.

3. Take ownership of problems.

4. Continually reassess the patient's needs.

5. Try to exceed expectations.

6. Protect the patient's rights (Table 3-4).

IV. Integrating Health Teaching

1. Goals of patient teaching include the patient's need to learn necessary self-care; ways to promote better health; ways to prevent complications or illness.

2. Assess teaching-learning needs on initial assessment; use patient interview and chart information to identify needs.

3. Assessment of educational level, own cultural biases, and personality type is needed to determine most effective teaching methods.

4. Before creating a plan, assess what the patient already knows and what he feels he needs to learn.

5. Areas to be covered in discharge teaching include diet, level of activity, medications, treatments, signs and symptoms to report, and follow-up care.

6. Obtaining feedback about material taught is essential; return demonstrations of motor skills aids confidence when at home.

V. Psychosocial Aspects of Delivering Home Care

A. Home care requires recognition by the nurse that this is the patient's territory.

B. Building trust is essential to help the patient to change unhealthy patterns of living.

C. Home health care means interacting with the family and including them in planning the patient's care.

D. Psychosocial care is even more important to successful nursing in the home setting.

E. Home health care involves collaboration with many other health care workers.

VI. Considerations for Long-Term Care Facilities

A. The patient displaced from his home needs a sense of control and a sense of purpose.

B. Allowing patients to do as much for themselves as possible and to help others with tasks helps them to meet part of their psychosocial needs.

C. Familiar personal items provide a sense of individuality.

D. Interaction with others in activities provides the social contact necessary to mental well-being.

VII. Psychosocial Aspects of Caring for the Elderly

A. Routine and familiarity are more important to the older person.

B. Separation from friends and neighbors decreases the sense of belonging.

C. Work with the patient to integrate his lifelong habits and preferences for bathing, sleeping, and other activities of daily living into the facility routine.

D. Treat the elderly person with respect, warmth, tact, and caring.

E. Go slower; do not give too much information too rapidly.

F. Be patient; the elderly person may take longer to do things.

G. Reinforce teaching with large-print instructions on nonglare paper.

H. Seek feedback to verify that you are being understood.

I. Touch used therapeutically can convey warmth and caring to the elderly patient.

J. Assist with the patient's life review by listening actively.

VIII. Coping With Patients Who Exhibit Difficult Behaviors

A. Illness and injury make unmet emotional needs more intense; which can be identified through nursing assessment and handled by planned nursing interventions.

B. Effective nursing intervention for undesirable behaviors resulting from unmet emotional needs are needed in all care settings.

C. The patient needs to have his behavior accepted by the staff.

D. Dependency behavior is used to satisfy an unmet need.

1. The patient's needs must be consistently met by the nurse; establishing trust is vital.

2. Behavior modification is then used to alter the dependent behavior.

3. Praise for self-care actions is important.

E. Withdrawn behavior.

1. Withdrawal can be an expression of anxiety, fear, anger, or depression and reflects a need to be safe and secure.

2. Characterized by silence, failure to make eye contact, recoiling from touch, superficial conversation, denial of reality.

3. Nursing interventions include providing structure and developing trust.

a. Provide consistent routine of care.

b. Reduce environmental stress, disorder, and confusion.

c. Assign primary nurse for patient care.

d. Avoid secretive behavior, teasing, and joking with patient.

F. The Depressed Patient: Symptoms Should Not Be Ignored.

1. Depression affects recovery from illness.

2. Symptoms of depression include loss of appetite, fatigue, vague aches and pains, insomnia, poor posture, difficulty making decisions, withdrawal, and poor hygiene.

3. Spending time just in silence with patient can be helpful.

4. Prolonged depression requires psychiatric intervention. Suicide assessment should be done if patient is deeply depressed.

5. Nursing interventions can be helpful in alleviating patient's depression.

a. Encourage engagement in activities of daily living and exercise.

b. Do not rush patient.

c. Emphasize his good qualities and point out accomplishments and strengths.

d. Do not be too cheerful and bright.

e. Encourage social interaction.

f. Be alert for signs of self-destruction and suicidal tendencies.

G. Hostile behavior: an expression of a need for control over what is happening.

1. Hostile behavior can arise from fear, desperation, frustration, and anger. Patient experiences sense of loss and powerlessness as a result of illness or injury.

2. Characterized by shouting, criticism, threats, and constant complaints. Family members also can exhibit hostile behavior because of concern for patient.

3. Nursing interventions are aimed at allowing person to ventilate pent-up feelings. Constructive help includes giving patient choices and opportunities for exercising control.

a. Actively and nonjudgmentally listen to person.

b. Allow person to make decisions and give in to demands that will not jeopardize his welfare.

c. Encourage physical activity.

d. Respect person's need to speak with authority figure.

e. Do not take anger or hostility personally.

f. Assist to find source of anger.

g. Set limits on patient's expressions of anger and hostility when necessary.

h. Seek help when unable to deal effectively with another person's anger or hostility.

i. If anger is getting out of control and harm may ensue, get help immediately.

H. Manipulative patients may use charm, flattery, seductiveness, lies, or threats to get what they want.

1. Manipulative behavior has various causes; it may be a learned behavior and used as a method of communication.

2. It may be a manifestation of a psychiatric disorder.

3. It may be based on fear of losing control.

4. Suggestions for dealing with the manipulative patient include:

a. Helping to decrease the need for control.

b. Assisting with alternate ways of coping.

c. Maintaining a safe environment regardless of the behavior.

d. Setting limits; responding to undesirable behavior calmly.

e. Being consistent and firm.

f. Not taking insults personally or becoming defensive.

g. Being aware of one's own feelings.

Medical–Surgical Patient Care Problems

Chapters 4 through 13 deal with general problems that the medical–surgical nurse encounters regularly. Chapter 4 discusses all aspects of care of the surgical patient. Chapter 5 talks about correcting fluid, electrolyte, and acid–base imbalances. Chapter 6 presents ways to prevent infection in all patients and the nursing care involved in treating the patient who does experience an infection. Chapter 7 presents major problems of immune response. Chapter 8, a new chapter, relates information necessary for the care of the HIV/AIDS patient. Chapter 9 discusses the specifics of care for the cancer patient. Chapter 10 builds on information about pain learned in introductory or fundamentals courses and focuses on pain identification and control. Chapter 11 reviews the problems that result from immobility and discusses the assessment and nursing care needed to prevent or alleviate such problems. Chapter 12, a new chapter, discusses care within the community for patients with chronic illness and includes nursing in an extended-care facility. This chapter also presents the concepts of rehabilitation nursing. Chapter 13 covers the dying patient and hospice care, focusing on care of the terminal patient in the home or hospice setting.

These chapters are building blocks for the care of patients with disorders of the various body systems, which are discussed in Unit Three.

CHAPTER 4

Care of Surgical Patients

OBJECTIVES

Upon completing this chapter, the student should be able to:

1. Discuss three technological changes that have made surgery less invasive and have lessened recovery time.
2. Identify the types of patients most at risk for surgical complications, and state why each type is at risk.
3. Perform a thorough nursing assessment for a preoperative patient.
4. Prepare patients physically, emotionally, and psychologically for surgical procedures.
5. Plan and implement patient and family teaching to prevent postoperative complications.
6. Compare and contrast various types of anesthesia and the nursing care that is unique to each type.
7. Assess the status of patients during the immediate postoperative period while they are in the recovery area.
8. Discuss the steps in assessing and taking care of a surgical wound.
9. Prepare a general teaching plan for the patient being discharged from the ambulatory or same-day surgery unit.
10. Identify signs and symptoms of common postoperative complications.
11. Provide routine postoperative care for patients who have had various types of surgery.

Surgical procedures are performed to repair tissue or correct defects, remove undesirable growths, remove damaged tissue or organs, alleviate pain, and to treat certain diseases. Since the invention of anesthesia, surgical techniques have continued to be improved, granting greater quality and quantity of life to many.

Not as many patients are hospitalized for surgery today as in the past. To avoid the expense of an overnight stay, many common surgeries are done on an outpatient basis, (e.g., cataract extraction, simple hernia repair, arthroscopy, cholecystectomy, hemorrhoidectomy). Independent day surgery centers have increased in numbers to fill this need. However, most large hospitals have an outpatient surgery unit where the patient is admitted the morning of surgery, prepared for surgery, and given postrecovery room care before discharge that afternoon. Diagnostic testing is done the 2 days before surgery. The nurse cares for these patients before and after the surgical procedure, and assists in determining that the patient is stable and may be discharged.

For patients who are hospitalized for planned surgery, the preparation also is often begun before admission. Because the patient comes to the hospital very early the morning of surgery, there is little time for the nurse to perform preoperative teaching. The patient is given printed materials by the surgeon on topics such as what to expect and exercises to prevent postoperative complications. The day surgery or staff nurse is the one who ensures that the patient leaves for home confident that he can manage with the help of his family or significant others.

TECHNOLOGICAL ADVANCES IN SURGERY

Since the mid-1980s, an array of lasers and endoscopes have enhanced the practice of surgery. Operating microscopes combined with these instruments have promoted a surge in microsurgical procedures. Body parts are now often successfully reattached, smaller surgical incisions are required for many procedures, and operations can be performed successfully that were only dreamed of a couple of decades ago. **Laser** is an acronym for Light Amplification by the Stimulated Emission of Radiation. This radiation is not ionizing radiation but is light energy. A laser is a tube containing a medium, such as carbon dioxide or other active gas, that is energized by electricity. The energized molecules reflect back and forth between mirrors and a bright light is generated that forms the laser beam. The light beam is converted to heat as it is absorbed by tissue. The carbon dioxide laser emits an invisible light that is absorbed by the water in tissue. It turns the water into steam, destroying tissue and sterilizing at the same time. It has a shallow penetration. These lasers are used in various types of surgery. Other types of lasers are used for specialized procedures. Lasers are used extensively in eye surgery and to remove growths on the vocal cords. They also are used in gynecological and genitourinary surgery and to some degree in most other surgical areas.

The use of fiberoptics in the operating room (OR) is the other innovation that has made surgery less invasive. By using an endoscope through a very small incision, the surgeon can remove growths and small organs without making a traditional surgical incision. The endoscope may be hooked up to an operating microscope to provide a magnified visual field for the surgeon, or it may be equipped with a video camera. The picture of the area is then viewed on a screen, and the surgeon can see the anatomy more clearly. Laparoscopic surgery, in which an endoscope is introduced through the abdominal wall, has been used to remove the appendix and the gallbladder. Three other puncture holes are made for the video camera and the instruments needed to perform the surgery. Laparoscopic cholecystectomy has reduced time off work for gallbladder removal from 6 weeks down to approximately 1 week. Experimental laparoscopic surgery is being conducted for surgery on the bowel, and endoscopic surgery will probably be used in place of other traditional surgical techniques in the future.

◆ Autologous Blood for Transfusion

Since the mid-1980s, patients undergoing elective surgery have had the option of donating their own blood so that it is available in the event that a transfusion is needed during or after surgery. The blood is withdrawn at the blood bank several weeks before the surgery, prepared, and stored for future transfusion to the patient. This is called an **autologous** *(related to self)* transfusion. The ability to do this has greatly decreased the anxiety of many patients who feared

transfusion with blood that might possibly be contaminated with a bloodborne virus, such as HIV or hepatitis B or C.

THE PREOPERATIVE PERIOD

◆ General Assessment

Before surgery is undertaken, the patient should be in the best possible physical condition. In emergencies, of course, this cannot be controlled, but planned surgery might be postponed for days or weeks until the patient is physically able to withstand the stress of anesthesia and major surgery. To determine the patient's readiness for surgery, a thorough assessment of his health status and risk factors is conducted.

Elder Care Point . . . Patients over the age of 75 have surgical complication rates three times higher than other adults. The elderly individual's body is less able to adjust and compensate for the stress of surgery as physiological reserves have declined.

Laboratory Data   Required tests before surgery include a complete blood cell (CBC) count and urinalysis. A chest radiograph is usually performed, and an electrocardiogram (EKG) is ordered for many patients over 40 years of age. Other tests commonly ordered include tests to determine electrolyte and blood glucose levels, prothrombin time (PT), and partial thromboplastin time (PTT) (which indicate blood clotting ability), blood type, and cross-match for transfusion, and a profile that gives data about liver and kidney function. If the laboratory reports indicate any abnormal values, measures will be taken by the physician to improve the general health of the patient before surgery is scheduled. Most surgeons prefer to postpone surgery if a patient's hemoglobin level is below 10 gm/mL. To contain health care costs, not as many laboratory tests are performed before surgery as in the past. This makes it even more important for the nurse to be a good interviewer and history taker.

Think about . . . Why would anemia make a patient a poor surgical risk?

Surgery puts a strain on the cardiovascular, urinary, and respiratory systems. Liver function is also important because the liver is involved in synthesizing clotting factors, producing albumin, and metabolizing and detoxifying drugs.

Requesting preoperative diagnostic tests is the responsibility of the physician, but the nurse will need to explain to the patient why these tests have been ordered.

The elderly patient is more likely to have impaired renal, hepatic, respiratory, and cardiac function and chronic diseases that cause vulnerability to fluid and electrolyte imbalances during and after surgery.

◆ Nursing Assessment

The nurse's assessment of the patient's health status prior to surgery facilitates planning of his care during and after surgery. During assessment the nurse will check the patient's temperature, pulse, respiratory rate, and blood pressure. **Any significant deviations from normal range should be brought to the attention of the surgeon.** For example, an elevated temperature might indicate an infection that would need to be brought under control before surgery could be done. Knowing the patient's usual blood pressure reading is necessary for comparison later when postoperative shock is a concern. Height and weight are measured and charted so the anesthesiologist can accurately calculate anesthetic dosages.

Think about... Why would infection be a contraindication for surgery in some instances?

Allergies must be identified and noted on the front of the patient's chart. *All* allergies should be documented. Because the surgical patient is frequently exposed to iodine antiseptics used preoperatively to cleanse the skin (e.g., povidone-iodine [Betadine]), it is especially important to note any allergy to iodine or shellfish (which contain iodine) on the front of the chart, in the chart, and on the preoperative checklist. An allergy to adhesive or paper tape also must be noted.

It is very important to obtain a list of all prescription and over-the-counter medications the patient has been taking. Of particular importance is whether or not the patient is taking a corticosteroid. Patients should be questioned about allergy medicines and eye drops that may contain a corticosteroid. Corticosteroids may delay wound healing, can alter fluid and electrolyte balance, and affect several metabolic functions in the body.

Nutritional status and *body weight* are significant factors in healing and repair of the surgical site. Obesity presents problems related to such routine procedures as venipuncture, intubation for general anesthesia, and prolonged uptake of anesthetic drugs. Obese patients have difficulty breathing as deeply and effectively as they should to avoid respiratory complications. Preoperative instruction must be tailored to meet the obese person's special needs, because there is more danger of strain on the surgical wound and greater demand for oxygen in these patients.

Obesity often prolongs surgery and increases tissue trauma, especially when the surgical site is the abdominal or thoracic cavity. **Healing is slower and infection more of a threat, because fat contains fewer blood vessels.** This limits the availability of nutritional elements for repair and defensive elements to fight infection. Obese patients also dehydrate more easily, because there is less body fluid in adipose tissue than in other tissues.

The malnourished or emaciated patient also is at risk because of the need for protein to replace blood cells and serum lost during surgery. Protein also is needed to form antibodies and defensive cells and to repair damaged cells. After surgery there is a metabolic change in which the **catabolic** (destructive) phase predominates. This results in a *negative protein balance,* which the emaciated patient can ill afford. Vitamins and other food elements necessary for tissue healing and repair are discussed in the section on wound healing.

Nursing History   An assessment of factors that place the patient at risk for complications of surgery should be carefully completed. Elderly patients are at greater risk because they often have chronic illnesses. People with respiratory, cardiac, or liver disorders or diabetes likewise have an increased risk.

Smoking has a negative effect on wound healing and on pulmonary function. It alters platelet function so that there is greater risk for abnormal clot formation and obstruction of blood vessels, particularly the small vessels that nourish tissue cells. Respiratory problems during the postoperative period are related to the reduced level of functional hemoglobin for the transport of oxygen, decreased lung expansion, inadequate oxygenation of the blood, and possible acid–base imbalance.

The *diabetic* person is more at risk during and after surgical procedures. Stress and other factors can upset the blood glucose level and predispose the patient to either hypo- or hyperglycemic reactions. In the poorly controlled diabetic person there is greater chance for delayed healing, because high blood sugar levels impede the release of oxygen to the cells. Infection also is a potential problem because poorly controlled diabetes inhibits the action of phagocytes, which are necessary to defend the body against infectious agents.

Liver disease patients are at added risk, as impaired liver function interferes with normal clotting of blood and the liver cannot properly detoxify anesthetics and other drugs.

Respiratory disease is an important risk factor both during the surgery and in the postoperative period. **Many anesthetics are given by inhalation, and some of these irritate the respiratory mucosa, creating more secretions. In addition, the immobility imposed by** surgery increases the possibility of accumulated secretions and inflammation of the lungs and bronchial tree. Impaired respiration slows down oxygen and carbon dioxide exchange and predisposes the patient to delayed wound healing and possibly acid–base imbalance. Table 4-1 summarizes a variety of factors that impose an added risk during surgery or for postoperative complications.

Think about . . . What points would you make when explaining to a patient that smoking affects the body in ways that are harmful to the surgery patient?

Psychological Assessment   The news that surgery is needed usually comes as an emotional shock to patients and their families. The changes it brings about in the routine of their lives will naturally place some personal and financial burdens on them. For some patients the surgery will alter their lives permanently and possibly leave them physically impaired in some way. Others might expect to be greatly helped by the surgical procedure. In any event, there will be some fears and misgivings about the prospect of undergoing anesthesia and surgery.

During their assessment of the patient's level of anxiety and emotional readiness for surgery nurses might seek answers to the following questions:

◆ What does the patient know about the surgical procedure to be done? What questions does she have about the procedure? What misinformation might she have that could cause needless worry?

TABLE 4-1 ◆ *Factors That Increase the Risk of Complications During Surgery or in the Postoperative Period*

◆ Age over 65, especially if over 75
◆ Bedridden patient prior to surgery
◆ Concurrent disorder: diabetes mellitus; immune deficiency; autoimmune disorder; cardiac disease; hypertension; pulmonary disease; liver disease; renal impairment; anemia; coagulation disorder; infection; other chronic disease
◆ Malnutrition
◆ Obesity
◆ Arthritis of the rib cage
◆ Tobacco use
◆ Excessive alcohol use
◆ Illicit substance use or medication abuse
◆ Currently taking: antidepressants; antihypertensives; anticoagulants; corticosteroids; nonsteroidal antiinflammatory drugs (NSAIDs)
◆ History of: reaction to anesthesia; previous postoperative complications; malignant hyperthermia (self or family member); bleeding disorder; allergies

---

◆ Has she ever had surgery before? What was done then? What experiences does she remember, and were they good or unpleasant?
◆ Does she have any particular concerns or fears now?
◆ Is she especially fearful of any medical problems that might affect her recovery from surgery? What can be done to help allay her fears?

Elder Care Point . . . Older patients who are experiencing serious depression are at high risk for complications of surgery because their motivation for recovery often is very low.

Spiritual Assessment   Most people are concerned about whether they will "wake up" or survive the anesthesia and surgical procedure. Some patients have the strong spiritual beliefs that they need to cope with sickness, suffering, and death. Others may need help in finding the spiritual support they need. Still others do not want to discuss this particular facet of their lives.

If a patient does not seem to have spiritual support, the nurse should help him to find and use the available resources. The resource could be himself or another person, such as a special friend, family member, minister, or hospital chaplain. Table 2-2 on p. 18 summarizes the kinds of questions the nurse might ask during his assessment of the patient's spiritual needs.

Assessment of Learning Needs   There is some general information the surgical patient should have about what will be happening to him immediately before, during, and after surgery. There also are specific preventive measures he might need to learn to perform. Instruction in these and other pre- and postoperative procedures are discussed later in the Intervention section.

If it is expected that members of the family or supportive friends will assist the patient during the postoperative period, they need to be included in teaching sessions (Figures 4-1 and 4-2).

◆ Nursing Diagnoses

Nursing diagnoses commonly used for the preoperative patient include "Knowledge deficit," "Fear," "Spiritual distress," and "Ineffective coping" as appropriate. Each diagnosis is supported by data obtained during nursing assessment.

Expected outcomes include:

◆ Verbalizes understanding of operative procedure and consequences, pre-, intra-, and postoperative routine.
◆ Preoperative anxiety and fear is lessened.

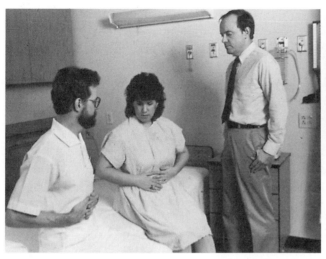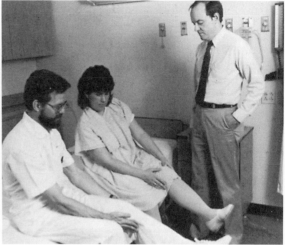

FIGURE 4-1   Deep-breathing and leg exercises demonstrated by nurse and practiced by patient. Spouse will help in post-operative care. (Photos by Ken Kasper.)

◆ Spiritual support is obtained.
◆ Effectively coping with surgery.

◆ Planning

The nurse who is assigned preoperative patients must carefully plan the work for the shift to have surgical patients ready without neglecting the needs of other assigned patients. Checking at the beginning of the shift to see that all preoperative medications ordered for the patient are on the unit saves time later. The surgery schedule is usually posted, and some estimate as to what time the OR will call for the patient to be "pre-oped" can be made. The efficient nurse can anticipate the call and have the preoperative medications drawn up and ready to give. This is done by carefully calculating the ordered dose, drawing up the medications, and taping them to a

med tray with a label stating the patient's name, room number, and the name and dosage of each medication. Then when the OR calls for the patient, the nurse can immediately give the medications. Checking at the beginning of the shift to see that the surgical consent form has been signed also decreases problems later in the shift. A quick look at the pre-op checklist (Figure 4-3) to see what is still to be done also is a good idea.

◆ Intervention

Patient Teaching   In most hospitals it is the nurse's job to provide the patient the information needed to help feel less anxious and better prepared to undergo surgery. Explanation of what can be expected before, during, and after surgery begins when the operation is scheduled. This can be valuable reinforcement for the

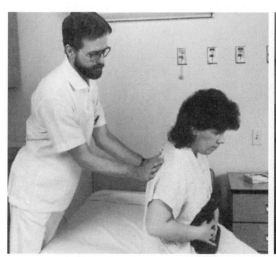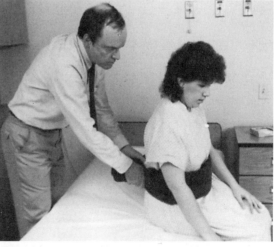

FIGURE 4-2   Coughing is more effective and less painful when the patient splints the operative site with a towel or pillow and the nurse gives firm support to the patient's back. Bracing with a towel pulled snug on the side opposite the operative site during coughing is another way to provide support. (Photos by Ken Kasper.)

anxious patient who can't take in all the information at one time. Some hospitals also make available pamphlets, filmstrips, and other teaching aids to instruct preoperative patients.

General information about surgery.   General

information that almost all surgical patients should receive includes information related to:

♦ *Preoperative procedures.* Enemas, skin preparation, care of belongings, restriction of food and liquid

ALLERGIES:

FLOOR CHECK LIST	OPERATING ROOM CHECK LIST

	CHECK	COMMENT

1. Consent for surgery form signed __Yes __No

2. Special Consent form signed __Yes __No

   Sterilization___Abortion___Disposal___

3. History & Physical   ___Yes ___No

4. Doctors orders __Yes ___No

**5. Consultation   ___Yes ___No

6. Urinalysis   ___Yes ___No

*7. C.B.C.   ___Yes ___No

8. Type & Cross match __Yes __No __Number

***9. Preoperative profile   ___Yes ___No

10. Prep done by_____

11. Patient dressed   ___Yes ___No

12. T.P.R._____Time_____

13. B/P _____Time_____

14. Oral Hygiene done ___Yes ___No

15. Voided_____Time_____

16. Retention Catheter ___Yes ___No

17. PROSTHESES:| NONE |REMOVED|DISPOSITION.|LEFT IN|

	NONE	REMOVED	DISPOSITION.	LEFT IN
Bridges				
Partials				
Plates				
Artifical Limbs				
Artifical Eyes				
Contact Lenses				
Hearing Aid				
Wig				

18. VALUABLES:| REMOVED |

	YES	NO	DISPOSITION, IF REMOVED
Rings			
Watch			
Medal & Chains			
Glasses			

19. Identification band checked with chart
    ___Yes ___No

20. Pre-op medications and times _____

_____

_____

By_____

_____
Signature of Charge Nurse

_____
           Date

Operating room checklist numbered 1. through 20.

POSTOPERATIVE

Sponge Count Correct   ___Yes ___No

Specimen to Lab   ___Yes ___No

Culture Done   ___Yes ___No

Packing in Place   ___Yes ___No

Procedure Done _____

_____

_____

_____
Signature of Circulating Nurse

Drains Left In_____

Catheter In_____

*NOTIFY DR. AND O.R. IF HEMOGLOBIN BELOW
 11 Grams
** CONSULTATION ON ALL FIRST CAESAREAN
   SECTIONS
   CONSULTATION ON ALL HYSTERECTOMIES 35
   YEARS OLD AND YOUNGER
*** FOR ALL PATIENTS 35 YEARS OLD OR OLDER

   CBC AND URINALYSIS MUST BE REPEATED
   IF OVER 48 HOURS.

FIGURE 4-3   Sample preoperative checklist.

intake, and administration of bedtime sedatives and preoperative medication; time to report to hospital.

♦ *Technical information.* Anticipated surgical procedure; location of incisions; and dressings, tubes, drains, or catheters that are expected.

♦ *Day of surgery.* Time surgery is scheduled, time to report to hospital or the time patient is to leave his room, probable length of procedure, effects of preoperative medications, where family will wait, when and where they can see the patient after surgery, pain control, and postoperative routine.

♦ *Postanesthesia care unit (PACU).* General environment (noise, lights, equipment), frequent taking of vital signs, and administration of oxygen.

♦ *Intensive care unit (surgical ICU)* (if patient is to go there from PACU). Location of the unit, expected length of stay, and visiting privileges.

Elder Care Point... It is particularly important to reinforce instruction and information given to the elderly patient. The anxiety of surgery, unfamiliar surroundings, and forgetfulness may decrease retention of information. Seek specific feedback periodically of points that are important for the patient to remember. Treat the elderly person with respect and dignity.

Special information. The specific kinds of information a surgical patient needs will depend on the surgical procedure planned and anticipated length of recovery. There are distinct advantages to teaching the patient certain procedures and practices that will be of benefit postoperatively. Such instruction gives the patient an opportunity to participate in care as much as possible, enlists cooperation in preventing postoperative complications, and reduces anxiety.

Specific preoperative instruction varies from one institution to another but usually includes deep-breathing and coughing techniques, use of an incentive spirometer, leg exercises, and practice in moving about in bed and getting in and out of bed. Figure 4-4 shows the kind of sheet that can be used to teach the patient during the preoperative period.

Now that admission to the hospital no longer occurs days ahead of surgery, the office nurse may be the person who will be doing most of the preoperative teaching and information giving.

Instruction techniques. The *how* of teaching might include (1) giving the patient a pamphlet to read or a filmstrip to view and returning later to answer questions and clarify what has been read or seen; (2) demonstrating the use of special equipment (e.g., an incentive spirometer) that will be used after surgery; (3) having the patient read about specific exercises to perform after surgery, demonstrating them, and then having the patient practice them with guidance; and (4) calling in such resource personnel as the physical therapist to teach specific exercises, the respiratory therapist, recovery room nurse, and any others who are in a better position to explain certain aspects of the patient's surgery and recovery period.

Informing the surgical patient is a continuous process during the preoperative period. The purpose is to allow information to be absorbed and to provide an atmosphere in which questions can be freely asked.

The family of the in-patient should be advised to come to the hospital 1 to $1\frac{1}{2}$ hours before surgery. They should be told about the usual routines, the approximate time the patient may be expected to return, and what to anticipate in the way of tubes, equipment, and patient appearance after surgery. This knowledge keeps them from thinking the patient has "taken a turn for the worse" when they see the extra equipment for suction, oxygen, or intravenous therapy in use after surgery. A warning about the occasional delays in starting surgery can keep the family from becoming excessively anxious if the patient is not back at the expected time.

♦ Preparation for Surgery

Preparation of the Skin   Scrubbing and shaving the operative site is most often done just before surgery. Hair may be shaved, clipped, or removed with a depilatory cream according to the surgeon's preference. For some types of surgery (i.e., bone and heart surgery and some plastic reconstructions), preoperative skin preparation may be started 24 to 72 hours beforehand. The patient is given a bacteriostatic cleansing solution (e.g., Hibiclens or pHisoHex) to use in the shower or on a designated body part.

Restriction of Oral Intake   The surgeon will leave written orders regarding restriction of food and drink intake before surgery. **It may be necessary for the nurse to explain to the patient that nothing is allowed by mouth because of the danger of vomiting with subsequent aspiration of the vomitus into the air passages during or immediately after surgery.** Patients who smoke are asked to stop 24 hours before surgery. In some cases, a nasogastric tube may be inserted into the stomach and gastric suction started the evening or morning before surgery. This tube is to be clamped off and left in place just before the patient is taken to the operating room. It may reassure the patient if she understands that gastric suction eliminates much unnecessary distention, nausea and vomiting, and consequent pain postoperatively. The nurse should clarify with the surgeon which, if any, routine medications should be administered (e.g., glaucoma, heart, or diabetic medications). Medications can be given with just a sip of water.

Elder Care Point... The elderly patient who has been NPO for diagnostic tests or who has had preoperative enemas must be watched for dehydration. This patient may need an intravenous infusion during the NPO period prior to surgery to maintain fluid balance.

Elimination **Surgery involving the abdominal cavity, rectum, or perineum usually requires a cleansing of the lower intestinal tract by catharsis and/or enemas.** This preparation will reduce the possibility of contamination of the operative area during surgery, when the sphincter muscles are relaxed and will also help to eliminate distention following surgery. "Enemas until clear" may be ordered for patients having rectal surgery or other operative procedures in which the surgeon does not wish the patient to have a bowel movement for several days after surgery. These can be exhausting and should be given slowly and with care, allowing the patient to rest between enemas.

Rest and Sedation The body needs all its strength and physical resources when coping with surgical procedures. Thus the patient should have adequate sleep

After your surgery, it is extremely important to breathe deeply, cough, change positions, and exercise your legs every 2 hours. These exercises may be uncomfortable but they are necessary to prevent complications.

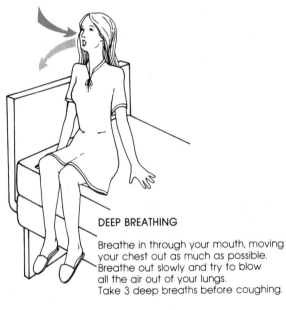

DEEP BREATHING

Breathe in through your mouth, moving your chest out as much as possible. Breathe out slowly and try to blow all the air out of your lungs. Take 3 deep breaths before coughing.

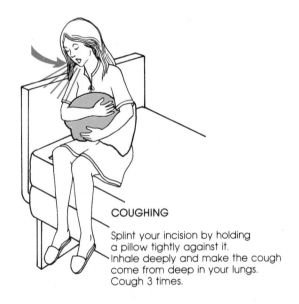

COUGHING

Splint your incision by holding a pillow tightly against it. Inhale deeply and make the cough come from deep in your lungs. Cough 3 times.

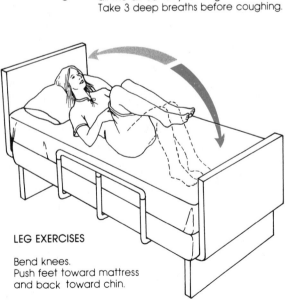

LEG EXERCISES

Bend knees. Push feet toward mattress and back toward chin.

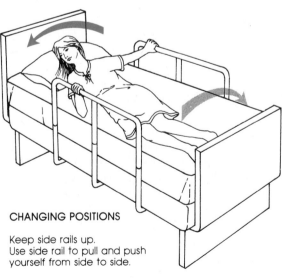

CHANGING POSITIONS

Keep side rails up. Use side rail to pull and push yourself from side to side.

FIGURE 4-4   Postoperative exercises.

the night before surgery. A sedative is usually ordered, but this does not always guarantee that the patient will sleep well. He should be checked on frequently. If he is awake and restless, the nurse should take time to talk with him, dispel fears, offer a soothing backrub, and repeat the sedation if necessary. If the patient is sleeping well, disturbance for routine procedures during the night and morning of surgery should not be necessary. The patient who is to report to the hospital early the morning of surgery should retire early, taking a sedative if needed, to obtain a good night's sleep.

Consent for Surgery **Before the surgeon can perform an operation, she must have written permission signed by either the patient or his guardian.** This written consent protects the surgeon against claims of unauthorized surgery and provides the patient an opportunity to exercise his right of informed consent. In most hospitals, the "contract" is a printed form that the patient signs before surgery. The consent form is then attached to the patient's chart and is sent to the OR with the patient. The patient has the right to change his mind and revoke his consent up until the time of surgery. **The nurse must always check to see that a consent form has been signed before giving the preoperative medication.** Figure 4-5 shows an example of a standard consent form.

Think about . . . What happens if a patient has been given his preoperative medication and then it is discovered that the surgical consent form has not been signed?

CONSENT TO OPERATION

Date _____ Time $\begin{array}{l}\text{a.m.}\\\text{p.m.}\end{array}$

1. I hereby authorize Dr. _____ and whomever he may

designate as his assistants, to perform upon _____
Name of Patient or "Myself"

the following operation: _____
Nature of Procedure(s) to be Performed

and if any unforeseen condition arises in the course of the operation in his judgement for procedures in addition to or different from those now contemplated, I further request and authorize him to do whatever he deems advisable.

2. The nature and purpose of the operation, possible alternative methods of treatment, the risks involved, and the possibility of complications have been fully explained to me. I acknowledge that no guarantee or assurance has been made as to the results that may be obtained.

3. I consent to the administration of anesthesia to be applied by or under the direction

of _____

_____ or _____, and to the use of such anesthetics as may be deemed by any of them advisable with the

exception of _____
("None", "Spinal Anesthesia", etc.)

4. I am aware that sterility may result from this operation although such result has not been guaranteed. I know that a sterile person is incapable of parenthood.

5. I consent to the disposal by authorities of the _____ Hospital of any tissues or parts which may be removed.

I CERTIFY THAT I HAVE READ AND FULLY UNDERSTAND THE ABOVE CONSENT TO OPERATION, THAT THE EXPLANATIONS THEREIN REFERRED TO WERE MADE, AND THAT ALL BLANKS OR STATEMENTS REQUIRING INSERTION OR COMPLETION WERE FILLED IN AND INAPPLICABLE PARAGRAPHS IF ANY, WERE STRICKEN BEFORE I SIGNED.

Signature of patient _____

Signature of patient's husband or wife _____

Signature of person authorized to consent for patient
when a patient is a minor or incompetent to give consent _____

Witness: _____ Relationship to patient _____

FIGURE 4-5   Sample consent form for surgery.

Immediate Preoperative Care The patient must wear only a hospital gown to the operating room. Hair should be covered with a surgical paper cap or towel. People with very long hair should have it combed and plaited into braids, and all hairpins must be removed from the hair. If the patient wishes to wear a wedding ring, it should be secured in place with tape. Watches and other valuables must be removed from the bedside table and placed under lock and key according to hospital policy. Dentures are often removed, placed in a labeled denture cup, and kept in a designated place according to hospital policy. Sometimes the anesthesiologist will request that the dentures be left in place, because they help maintain the contour of the face and facilitate the administration of inhalation anesthesia. **Unless there is a urinary catheter in place, preoperative patients are asked to empty their bladder before the preoperative medication is administered.**

> The patient's identification bracelet or tag is checked with the chart for accuracy to avoid any error or mixup of patients in the operating room.

A delay in giving the preoperative medication may cause difficulties for the patient and a great inconvenience to the person administering the anesthesia. All preliminary preparations should be done before the medication is given so that it will have maximum effect.

> The preoperative medication must be administered at exactly the time ordered by the surgeon or anesthesiologist. This is essential because the amount of anesthesia and time of induction have been calculated according to the hour the premedication was expected to be given.

Preoperative medications are given to (1) reduce anxiety and promote rest; (2) decrease secretion of mucus and other body fluids; (3) counteract nausea and reduce emesis; and (4) enhance the effects of the anesthetic. The sedatives usually given include secobarbital (Seconal) and pentobarbital (Nembutal). Drying agents include atropine and scopolamine. Narcotics such as morphine and meperidine hydrochloride (Demerol) are given to supplement the anesthetic (Table 4-2).

Elder Care Point . . . Because of decreasing liver and kidney function that occurs with age, the elderly patient, especially those over 75, will need reduced dosages of preoperative narcotics and sedatives.

Other agents commonly administered immediately prior to surgery are promethazine hydrochloride (Phenergan), hydroxyzine hydrochloride (Vistaril), or chlorpromazine hydrochloride (Thorazine), all of which produce sedative, antihistaminic, and antiemetic effects; and diazepam (Valium) or midazolam hydrochloride (Versed), which calm the patient. To decrease stomach acid production during surgery, cimetidine (Tagamet), rantidine hydrochloride (Zantac), or famotidine (Pepcid) are often administered IV. An antacid or simethicone may be given to reduce stomach acidity and gas production.

It is important to attend to all the items on the checklist that can be handled ahead of time early in the morning. This avoids last-minute haste, prevents mistakes, and makes it easier to give the preoperative medication on time. **After the preoperative medication is given, the patient is told not to get out of bed without assistance, siderails are raised, and the call bell is placed within reach.**

When the transport person comes to take the patient to surgery, the nurse assists with transferring the patient to the stretcher. The patient's identification band is compared with the request to transport. If the patient has great difficulty seeing without her glasses or cannot hear without a hearing aide, these should be sent to the OR with the patient so that they are available when arousal from anesthesia occurs. A notation is made on the preop checklist about the device and the reason for sending it. A notice is taped to the front of the chart and the glasses or hearing aide may also be attached to the chart. The nurse checks the chart to make certain everything is in order and that the preoperative checklist is complete. An entry is made in the nurse's notes, such as that presented in Figure 4-6.

Think about . . . How would you handle a situation where a patient is insisting on wearing underwear to surgery?

INTRAOPERATIVE CARE

When the patient arrives in the anesthesia holding area he is checked in by the nurse. The operative permit is checked with the patient's identification band, and the nurse verbally checks that the patient is the right person and that the surgical procedure scheduled is the correct one. The chart is checked again to see that all preparations are complete and the nurse rechecks for allergies.

All personnel who will be entering the OR don scrub outfits, hair cover, shoe covers, and mask, and perform a surgical scrub prior to entering. Strict surgical asepsis is observed throughout the operating room area. The circulating nurse and the scrub nurse, or scrub technician, are preparing the operating room by opening and laying out instruments and needed sterile supplies (Figure 4-7).

The anesthesiologist or nurse anesthetist inserts an

TABLE 4-2 ◆ *Commonly Prescribed Preoperative Medications*			
Drugs	**Average Doses**	**Purposes**	**Nursing Implications**
Sedatives			
Nembutal sodium Seconal sodium	100 mg IM 90 minutes before surgery	Decrease anxiety; lower blood pressure and pulse; enhance action of anesthetic.	Be alert for opposite effect in certain patients, particularly the elderly, who may become restless and confused. Must be given at precise time ordered.
Tranquilizers			
Thorazine Phenergan	12.5 to 25 mg IM up to 2 hours before surgery	Reduce anxiety; promote relaxation. *Note:* Can cause severe hypotension.	Patient should be confined to bed after injection because of danger of fainting. Sensitive children and adults may exhibit motor restlessness and opisthotonos. Check blood pressure for signs of extreme hypotension.
Hydroxyzine pamoate (Vistaril)	25 to 50 mg IM	Reduce anxiety and tension; promote relaxation.	Raise side rails. Give IM Z-track.
Diazepam (Valium)	5 to 10 mg IM	Reduce tension and anxiety; promote relaxation; decrease muscle spasm.	Reduce dosage of narcotics. Monitor respirations.
Midazolam hydrochloride (Versed)	0.07 to 0.08 mg/kg IM	Induce drowsiness and relieve apprehension.	Conscious sedation; sedation before short-term diagnostic or endoscopic procedures; amnesic effect.
Drying agents			
Atropine sulfate Scopolamine (Hyoscine)	0.03 to 0.6 mg IM 0.03 to 0.6 mg SC	Inhibit secretions from mucous membranes of mouth and respiratory tract.	Do not give to patients with glaucoma. Observe for rash, flushing of skin, and elevated temperature, which are common side effects, particularly in children. Bed rails and close supervision of patient who has received scopolamine; may become very drowsy or restless and injure self.
Glycopyrrolate (Robinul)	0.004 mg/kg IM	Diminish secretions; block cardiac vagal reflexes.	Contraindicated in glaucoma. Check dosage carefully. Use smaller doses in elderly. Watch for adverse reaction in elderly patients. Monitor for urinary heistancy.
Analgesics			
Morphine sulfate Meperidine (Demerol)	8 to 15 mg SC 50 to 100 mg IM	Reduce anxiety; promote relaxation; not necessarily to relieve pain when given preoperatively.	Check respiratory rate before giving. Nausea, vomiting, and constipation may result. Observe patient for increased restlessness, tremors, and delirium, which may occur as side effects.
Hydromorphone hydrochloride (Dilaudid)		Reduce anxiety; promote relaxation.	Check vital signs before giving. Raise side rails.

intravenous line, and when the operating room is ready the patient is transferred to the table. **The circulating nurse again checks the patient's identification and the surgical consent form to verify both that they have the correct patient and that the patient is being prepared for the correct surgery. The patient is carefully positioned on the table with padding to prevent injury to nerves and to minimize pressure over bony prominences.**

Safety straps hold the patient in position. As the patient is being draped, the anesthesiologist or certified registered nurse anesthetist (CRNA) begins to anesthetize the patient. If the skin prep was not done in the patient's room, it is done at this time. When the patient has been prepped, the surgical team is scrubbed and ready, and when the anesthesiologist says the patient is ready, surgery begins.

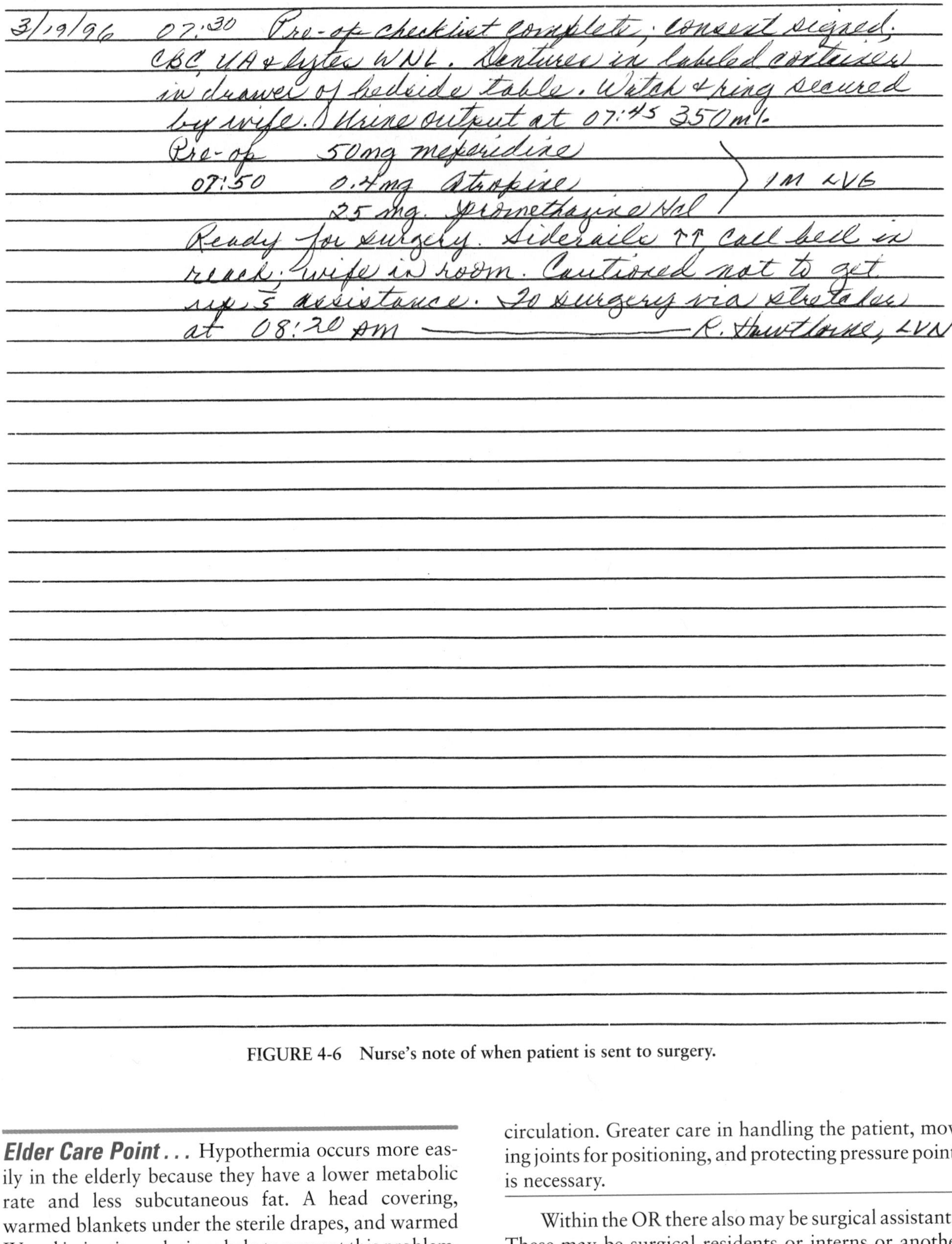

> 3/19/96   07:30   Pre-op checklist complete; consent signed.
> CBC, UA & lytes WNL. Dentures in labeled container
> in drawer of bedside table. Watch & ring secured
> by wife. Urine output at 07:45 350 ml.
> Pre-op   50 mg meperidine
> 07:50   0.4 mg atropine   ) IM LVG
>   25 mg. promethazine HCl   /
> Ready for surgery. Siderails ↑↑ call bell in
> reach; wife in room. Cautioned not to get
> up, c̄ assistance. To surgery via stretcher
> at 08:20 AM ——————— R. Hawthorne, LVN

FIGURE 4-6 Nurse's note of when patient is sent to surgery.

Elder Care Point . . . Hypothermia occurs more easily in the elderly because they have a lower metabolic rate and less subcutaneous fat. A head covering, warmed blankets under the sterile drapes, and warmed IV and irrigating solutions help to prevent this problem.

Tissue ischemia also is a greater risk as the elderly have thinner skin, stiffer joints with less tissue protecting them, and some degree of decreased peripheral circulation. Greater care in handling the patient, moving joints for positioning, and protecting pressure points is necessary.

Within the OR there also may be surgical assistants. These may be surgical residents or interns or another physician. Although the surgeon is "captain of the ship" and is in charge, each participant is responsible for his or her own actions in the OR.

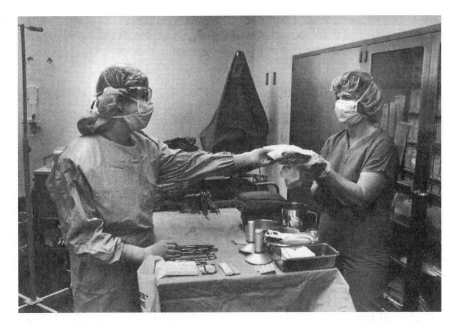

FIGURE 4-7 **Setting up the sterile field.** (Source: Ignatavicius, D. D., Workman, M. L., Mishler, M. A. (1995). *Medical-Surgical Nursing: A Nursing Process Approach,* 2nd ed. Philadelphia: Saunders, p. 385.)

◆ Role of the Circulating Nurse

The circulating nurse observes for breaks in sterile technique from his place outside the sterile field and protects the safety of the patient. He also supervises the activities of the scrub person. It is the circulating nurse who gives care to the patient during the preparation period for the procedure. He provides instruments and supplies to the scrub person as needed. He assists other members of the surgical team to gown and glove after their surgical scrub and positions platforms or stools for the surgeon, scrub person, and assistants as needed. He checks the function of each piece of equipment to be used during the surgery, makes certain the patient is properly grounded if electrocautery is to be used, and hooks up suction and O$_2$ tubing. He performs a sponge count with the scrub nurse before the surgery begins and another closing sponge count when the surgery ends. Interim sponge counts may be done as the two nurses desire. The circulating nurse positions the kick buckets for waste, furnishes sterile solutions to the scrub nurse and surgical team during the operation, and turns on equipment as it is needed. He also is the one who mops the perspiration from the brows of the OR team. The circulating nurse also assists with sharps and instrument counts at the close of surgery and may care for tissue specimens. He obtains blood from the blood bank and fetches IV solutions, sutures, and other supplies as needed.

The circulating nurse is the communication link between the surgical team and those outside the OR. Although this role was formerly almost always filled by a registered nurse (RN), lack of sufficient trained RNs for the OR is causing these positions to be filled by technically trained personnel. It is still required that an RN be available in case of emergency.

◆ Role of the Scrub Person

The scrub nurse may be a surgical technician or a specially trained LPN/VN. This person prepares the sterile Mayo tray with drape and instruments and arranges instruments, drapes, and supplies on a sterile supply table. Instruments are checked for proper function, suture packets are opened, and ligatures (ties) and sutures are placed in the sequence in which the surgeon usually uses them. The scrub person counts all sponges, needles, sharps, and instruments with the circulating nurse and gowns and gloves the surgeon. The scrub person hands the instruments and supplies to the surgeon as needed and receives them back again, anticipating needs and maintaining sterile technique at all times. This person performs several other tasks as well. **Any member of the OR team who notices a break in sterile technique should immediately point it out so that sterility can be reestablished.**

◆ Anesthesia

Anesthesia (the loss of sensory perception) came into use as an accepted part of surgical procedure in the 1840s. With the advent of drugs that safely produced anesthesia, the performance of surgical operations became a more widely accepted and successful means of treating disease and injury. Few of us would accept surgery without the advantage of being insensible to pain during the operation, and modern surgical procedures requiring several hours would be impossible without adequate anesthesia.

The first anesthetics used were ether and nitrous oxide. It is interesting to note that these drugs were used as a source of entertainment and amusement before anyone considered using them in medical practice. Nitrous oxide, commonly called "laughing gas," was sometimes administered to a volunteer from the audience of a side show for the purpose of watching the antics of the victim as he was transported into a state of euphoria and became hysterical with laughter. Today ether is rarely used because it is highly explosive; however, nitrous oxide remains a frequently administered anesthetic.

There are three main objectives when administering an anesthetic: (1) to prevent pain; (2) to achieve adequate muscle relaxation; and (3) to calm fear, allay anxiety, and induce forgetfulness.

To achieve these objectives, anesthetics can be administered in a number of ways. The choice of anesthesia and route of administration rest with the anesthesiologist and depend on the type of surgery to be performed, the age and physical condition of the patient, and the patient's ability to tolerate the anesthetic and the surgical procedure.

Inhalants   Inhalation is the oldest, most easily controlled, and most frequently used method of administering anesthesia. Halothane (Fluothane) may be administered by the nonrebreathing, partial rebreathing, or closed technique. It often is given in combination with nitrous oxide. Because of its potential for damage to the liver, it is not given to patients with hepatic or biliary disease. Adverse reactions, in addition to liver toxicity, include hyperpyrexia, shivering, nausea, and emesis.

Methoxyflurane (Penthrane) is a form of ether that has been altered chemically so that it is not highly volatile. Analgesia and drowsiness from the effects of Penthrane may persist after the patient has regained consciousness and thus minimize the need for narcotics immediately after surgery. Renal toxicity associated with Penthrane seems to be related to the total amount given and the length of time it is administered. It is not recommended for diabetic patients and others with existing or potential kidney disease.

Intravenous Anesthesia   The major advantages of administering an anesthetic by vein are (1) a rapid induction in which the patient quickly goes to sleep; and (2) the absence of nausea and vomiting during the postoperative period. However, drugs administered intravenously are usually barbiturates, which are comparatively poor anesthetics and present a risk of asphyxiation, from laryngospasm and bronchospasm. The drug most commonly used as an IV anesthetic is thiopental sodium (Pentothal).

Thiopental sodium used in combination with fentanyl-droperidol (Innovar) is another popular anesthetic. It may also be used with fentanyl (Sublimaze). In recent years, morphine has been considered the agent of choice for open-heart and vascular surgery.

Another drug, ketamine (Ketalar), also may be administered alone or in combination with nitrous oxide. The patient who has been given ketamine may be delirious, have disturbed dreams, or possibly hallucinate. The nurse should provide a quiet, nonstimulating environment while the patient is emerging from the effects of the anesthetic.

Regional Nerve Block   In this type of anesthesia, only one area of the body is deadened to pain; the patient remains conscious. Because the patient is awake and immobile for less time, there are fewer respiratory difficulties due to pooling of mucus in the air passages.

Regional anesthetics may be administered topically (directly on the surface of the area to be treated) and by injection either into the skin and subcutaneous tissues or into the spinal column. Drugs commonly used for regional anesthesia include butacaine, tetracaine (Pontocaine), lidocaine (Xylocaine), and cocaine.

Whenever a local anesthetic is administered, there is the potential for anaphylaxis due to hypersensitivity to the drug if it accidentally enters the blood stream. Precautions are the same as for any highly allergenic drug, and emergency equipment should be readily available.

Spinal anesthesia, which is a form of regional anesthesia, can be used only for surgery below the diaphragm, but it is very effective and produces complete muscular relaxation, even though the patient remains awake during the operation.

The postoperative care of the patient receiving spinal anesthesia is basically the same as for general anesthesia, although there are usually fewer gastrointestinal and respiratory complications to be guarded against following spinal anesthesia. On the other hand, the nurse must realize that respiratory difficulties and cardiovascular complications can develop when spinal anesthesia is given. If the anesthesia ascends beyond the point of injection, innervation of the respiratory muscles and blood vessels is affected. This produces depression of respiration and lowers blood pressure.

As the anesthesia wears off, the patient may complain that she cannot move her legs and that they feel numb and heavy. This is to be expected at first and will gradually subside. Patients used to be kept flat in bed for 6 to 12 hours to prevent headache, but this practice has fallen out of favor. They now may be turned from side to side unless there are specific orders to the contrary.

The patient may experience spinal headache. Nursing intervention includes restricting her to bed rest; maintaining a quiet, darkened room; maintaining hydration orally or with IV fluids; and administering analgesics as needed.

Epidural or caudal anesthesia is used primarily in obstetric procedures. The anesthetic is injected into the epidural space rather than the subarachnoid space.

Conscious Sedation   Conscious sedation is used in combination with regional anesthesia or by itself for minor procedures, such as cardiac catheterization, endoscopy, D&C, vasectomy, or extensive suturing. It consists of the use of local anesthetic with intravenous opioids and sedatives. Often a registered nurse administers the IV drugs. It provides a minimally depressed level of consciousness where the patient retains the ability to respond appropriately to verbal commands. The patient can cooperate during the procedure, but has partial amnesia afterward. The technique is safer than general anesthesia as it causes less change in vital signs and airway patency is maintained. The patient recovers very quickly from this type of sedation.

A comparative summary of the types of anesthesia, their uses, advantages and disadvantages, and nursing implications can be found in Table 4-3.

◆ Hypothermia

The term **hypothermia** refers to a reduction of body temperature. Its purpose in surgery is to lower metabolism and thereby decrease the need for oxygen. In many types of surgery involving the heart, blood vessels, or brain, it is necessary to interrupt the flow of blood through the body. Lowering the body temperature to between 32°C (89.6°F) and 26°C (78.8°F) reduces the metabolic needs of the vital organs so that they are less likely to be damaged by a decreased supply of blood and oxygen.

There are several ways in which hypothermia can be achieved. In *external hypothermia*, the patient's body is wrapped in a cooling blanket, packed in ice, or submerged in a tub of ice water. This is done after the patient has been anesthetized and immediately before the surgical procedure is performed.

In *extracorporeal* cooling, the patient's blood is cooled outside the body. It is removed from a major vessel, circulated through a refrigerant unit for cooling, and returned to the body by the way of another large blood vessel. This is the quickest way to achieve hypothermia, and it is usually the method used for patients undergoing open-heart surgery.

During the rewarming process, the patient's temperature is raised gradually. Care must be taken to avoid burns if warm baths or heating blankets are used. The rewarming procedure is discontinued when the body temperature is within 1 or 2 of normal.

> Observations during the rewarming include checking the pulse, blood pressure, and respiration, as well as the temperature. Any sudden change must be reported immediately.

Because research is showing that maintaining normal body temperature during surgery markedly reduces postop wound infection rates and reduces blood loss, hypothermia may not be used as much as in the past.

◆ After Surgery

When the surgical procedure is complete, a final count of the sponges, sharps, and instruments is performed before the wound is closed. Wound closure is achieved by suturing or securing with surgical staples. When the count is verified as correct, the wound is closed and the dressing applied. The anesthesiologist tapers the anesthesia, allowing the patient to reemerge slowly to a conscious state. The patient is transferred to a stretcher or bed and taken to the postanesthesia care unit (PACU) for observation. She is not discharged back to her unit until she is adequately aroused and her vital signs are relatively stable.

IMMEDIATE POSTOPERATIVE CARE

The period immediately following surgery is a critical one for the patient and involves constant observation by specially trained nurses. The *recovery room*, or *postanesthesia care unit (PACU)*, care plan includes interventions to meet all basic needs. An example of routine immediate PACU observations and care is given in Figure 4-8. While recovering from anesthesia the patient is totally helpless. Caring aspects of nursing become vitally important. The nurse positions the patient so that comfort will be maintained while preventing complications such as aspiration. The patient's lips are moistened, lights adjusted so they don't shine directly in the eyes, and the patient is covered with warmed blankets to prevent chills. The nurse must use her knowledge and skills to help to maintain the patient's oxygenation and circulation, to provide safety and comfort, to meet basic needs, and to prevent complications.

◆ Postanesthesia Care Unit

Following surgery, most patients are taken to the postanesthesia recovery room (PAR), located near the ORs. This unit is staffed with specially trained nurses and equipped with all items needed to handle postop-

TABLE 4-3 ◆ *Types of Anesthesia: Uses, Advantages, and Disadvantages*

Route of Administration	Agents Commonly Used	Advantages and Disadvantages	Nursing Implications
General anesthesia			
Inhalation	Methoxyflurane (Penthrane)	Renal toxicity: related to total dose.	Contraindicated in patients with actual or potential kidney disease. Rarely used now. Can reduce need for narcotics during immediate postoperative period.
	Halothane	Possible liver damage.	Monitor respiratory rate and pulse for signs of respiratory and circulatory depression.
	Nitrous oxide (laughing gas)	Relatively nontoxic; can cause hallucinations and dreams.	None
	Ethrane	Rapid induction, possible respiratory depression and cardiac arrhythmia; similar to halothane, but does not cause kidney or liver damage.	Monitor for possible seizure activity.
	Isoflurane (Forane)	Rapid induction and recovery; enhances muscle relaxants; does not depress myocardium; causes respiratory depression.	Monitor respiration and blood pressure.
Intravenous	Combination of fentanyl and droperidol (Innovar), and thiopental Fentanyl (Sublimaze)	Not as easily controlled as inhalation anesthesia.	Do not give in combination with other sedatives, hypnotics, or other strong analgesics because of possible additive effects, chiefly hypotension and respiratory depression.
		Major dangers are laryngospasm and bronchospasm.	Monitor closely for signs of laryngospasm.
	Morphine sulfate	Increases cardiac output. Agent of choice for open-heart surgery and vascular surgery.	Observe for respiratory depression.
	Ketamine (Ketalar) used alone or with nitrous oxide	Onset brief, suitable for short procedures.	Given with caution to elderly patients with atherosclerosis and contraindicated in patients with hypertension because of increased cardiac output and elevation of blood pressure.
		Postoperative hallucinations in adults.	Protective safety measures to prevent injury during irrational behavior, excitement, and confusion.
		Airway obstruction and vomiting may occur.	Provide quiet environment; avoid visual, auditory, and tactile stimulation.
	Methohexital sodium (Brevital)	Very short acting; five times stronger than sodium pentothal; less likely to cause bronchospasm.	Monitor respiration closely.
	Proprofol (Diprivan)	Short-acting; quickly responsive postoperatively; minimal nausea, vomiting or sedation postoperatively. May cause allergic skin reaction; quicker awareness of postoperative pain.	Monitor for need of analgesia early in the postoperative period; use alternative pain relief methods along with analgesia.
	Bupivacaine (Marcaine)	Available with epinephrine to decrease bleeding. May cause tremors, twitching, shivering; respiratory arrest can occur if absorbed systemically.	Mixed with epinephrine may cause ischemia of area, so monitor for adequate blood flow postoperatively; protect area until full sensation has returned.

TABLE 4-3 ◆ *Types of Anesthesia: Uses, Advantages, and Disadvantages* (Continued)

Route of Administration	Agents Commonly Used	Advantages and Disadvantages	Nursing Implications
Regional anesthesia			
Topical anesthesia	Cocaine Tetracaine (Pontocaine)	Immediate effect, generally nontoxic.	Check for history of drug sensitivity or other allergies.
	Lidocaine (Xylocaine)	Major disadvantage is possibility of drug sensitivity and anaphylactic shock.	Have emergency equipment and drugs for treatment of anaphylactic shock readily available.
Local block	Procaine hydrochloride (Novocain)	Danger of anaphylactic shock if drug is accidentally injected into a vein.	Same as for topical anesthesia. Protect involved part from injury during period of insensitivity after local anesthesia. Do not allow patient to rub eyes, caution about biting inside of mouth, withhold food and fluids until return of tissue sensitivity.
	Mepivacaine (Carbocaine)	Absorbs into blood stream; can cause cardiac depression.	Contraindicated if patient has been taking monoamine oxidase inhibitors. Monitors blood pressure.
	Bupivacaine (Marcaine)	Available with epinephrine to decrease bleeding. May cause tremors, twitching, shivering; respiratory arrest can occur if absorbed systemically.	Mixed with epinephrine may cause ischemia of area, so monitor for adequate blood flow postoperatively; protect area until full sensation has returned.
Spinal anesthesia	Procaine hydrochloride Tetracaine (Pontocaine)	Relatively safe method. May produce nausea, vomiting, pain during surgery.	Position patient only as directed during administration of anesthetic.
		Headache not uncommon, may last for days after surgery.	Assess neurological status of patient during recovery period.
		Respiratory paralysis can occur if drug reaches upper levels of spinal column.	Keep patient lying down to decrease possibility of headache and auditory and visual problems related to increased intracranial pressure.
		Neurological complications include muscle weakness and paraplegia	Patient allowed to sit up when spinal fluid pressure returns to normal. Numbing and tingling are expected, will abate after short period of time; reassure patient.

erative emergencies. Doctors and anesthetists check on their patients frequently and are close at hand when needed.

Postoperative patients remain in the PACU until they have recovered from anesthesia and are able to respond to the stimuli around them; this generally takes 2 to 6 hours. Very critically ill patients, such as those recovering from open-heart surgery, are often taken directly to the intensive care unit (ICU) for anesthesia recovery. **Wherever patients are sent for recovery, they are always attended closely by a nurse at all times until their condition is stable.**

The PACU is equipped with specialized monitors and equipment, drugs, and fluids needed for postoper-

ative care, oxygen, suction, and devices for measuring vital signs for each patient. Equipment for emergency **resuscitation** (revival after apparent death) is close at hand.

When the patient is transferred from the OR, the anesthesiologist or nurse anesthetist gives a report to the nurse who will care for the fresh postoperative patient. The usual ratio of staff is one nurse per 1 or 2 patients. Information relayed includes the patient's name and age; the surgical procedure performed and any complications that occurred; pertinent medical history; the type of anesthesia administered; drug allergies; the preoperative medications given; the drugs used during surgery; the solution infusing; the oxygen flow rate; vital

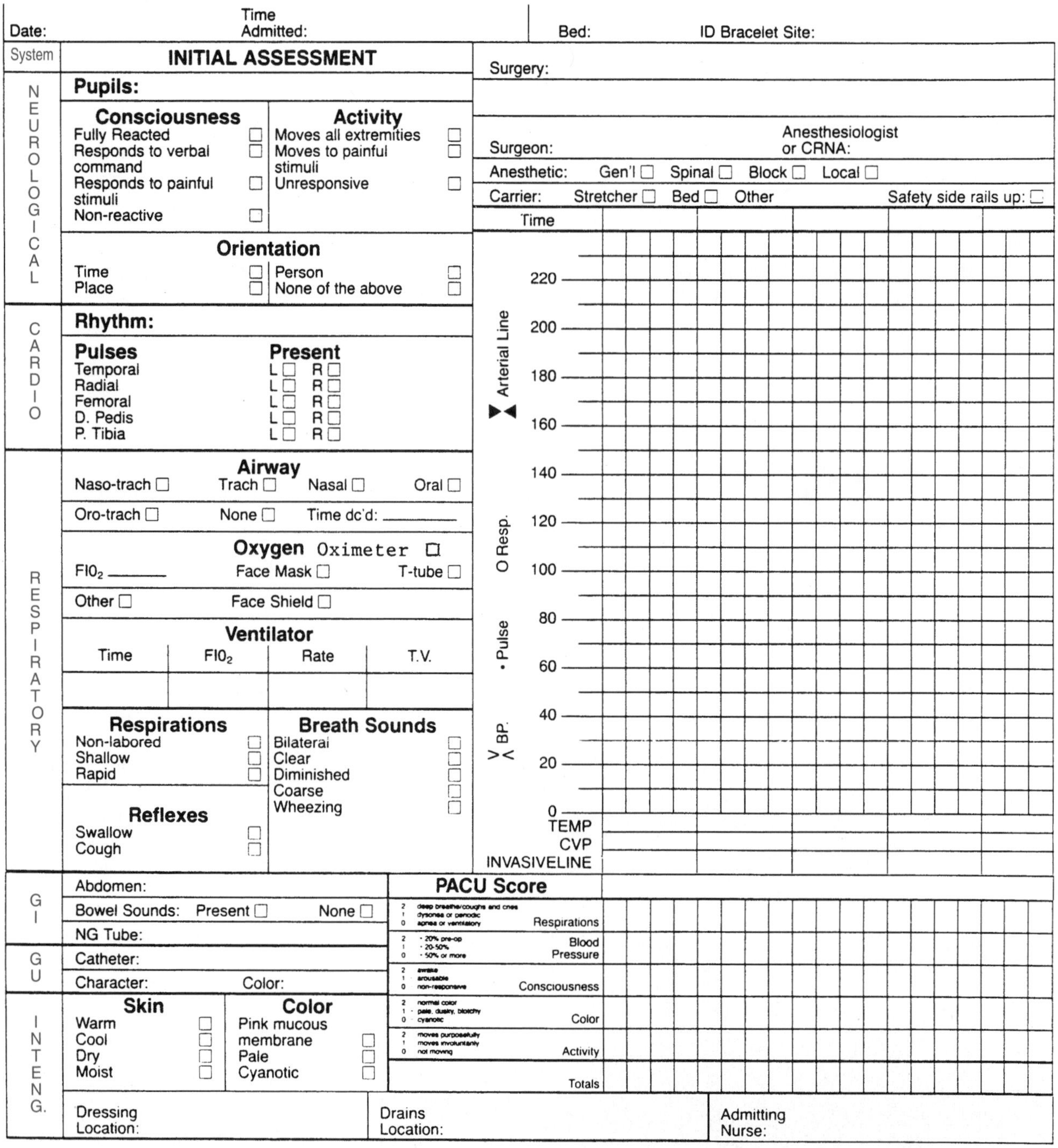

Date: _____ Time Admitted: _____   Bed: _____   ID Bracelet Site: _____

System	INITIAL ASSESSMENT

Surgery: _____

Surgeon: _____   Anesthesiologist or CRNA: _____

Anesthetic: Gen'l ☐ Spinal ☐ Block ☐ Local ☐

Carrier: Stretcher ☐ Bed ☐ Other   Safety side rails up: ☐

NEUROLOGICAL

Pupils:

Consciousness
Fully Reacted ☐
Responds to verbal command ☐
Responds to painful stimuli ☐
Non-reactive ☐

Activity
Moves all extremities ☐
Moves to painful stimuli ☐
Unresponsive ☐

Orientation
Time ☐   Person ☐
Place ☐   None of the above ☐

CARDIO

Rhythm:

Pulses   Present
Temporal   L ☐ R ☐
Radial   L ☐ R ☐
Femoral   L ☐ R ☐
D. Pedis   L ☐ R ☐
P. Tibia   L ☐ R ☐

RESPIRATORY

Airway
Naso-trach ☐   Trach ☐   Nasal ☐   Oral ☐
Oro-trach ☐   None ☐   Time dc'd: _____

Oxygen Oximeter ☐
FIO$_2$ _____   Face Mask ☐   T-tube ☐
Other ☐   Face Shield ☐

Ventilator

Time	FIO$_2$	Rate	T.V.

Respirations
Non-labored ☐
Shallow ☐
Rapid ☐

Breath Sounds
Bilateral ☐
Clear ☐
Diminished ☐
Coarse ☐
Wheezing ☐

Reflexes
Swallow ☐
Cough ☐

GI
Abdomen: _____
Bowel Sounds: Present ☐   None ☐
NG Tube: _____

GU
Catheter: _____
Character: _____   Color: _____

INTEG.
Skin
Warm ☐
Cool ☐
Dry ☐
Moist ☐

Color
Pink mucous membrane ☐
Pale ☐
Cyanotic ☐

Dressing Location: _____   Drains Location: _____   Admitting Nurse: _____

Arterial Line ►◄ ◄◄
O Resp.
• Pulse
> BP. <

220
200
180
160
140
120
100
80
60
40
20
0
TEMP
CVP
INVASIVELINE

PACU Score

Respirations
2 deep breathe/coughs and cries
1 dyspnea or periodic
0 apnea or ventilatory

Blood Pressure
2 ± 20% pre-op
1 ± 20-50%
0 ± 50% or more

Consciousness
2 awake
1 arousable
0 non-responsive

Color
2 normal color
1 pale, dusky, blotchy
0 cyanotic

Activity
2 moves purposefully
1 moves involuntarily
0 not moving

Totals

FIGURE 4-8   Flowsheet used for charting nurses' observations in the postanesthesia care unit.

sign trends; intake and output during surgery; the estimated blood loss; allergies; placement of drains, tubes, and suction devices; and any orders for analgesia during recovery.

Nursing care of the postoperative patient includes maintaining a patent airway; positioning the patient on his side or with the head turned to the side or supine using a chin lift jaw thrust maneuver to keep the airway open; taking vital signs at least every 15 minutes; administering supplemental oxygen by nasal cannula or face mask at 3 to 5 L/minute; suctioning secretions as needed; monitoring dressings, tubes, and drains; regulating the flow of IV fluids; and encouraging the patient to wake up, breathe deeply, and cough. The nurse also provides warmth and comfort, assuring the patient that the surgery is over. All observations and interventions are documented on the PACU flowsheet (Figure 4-8).

While the patient is still under anesthesia, the recovery room staff should keep conversation to a minimum. The patient is repeatedly told where he is and that the surgery is over. Communication with staff members should be done in a low voice.

`Discharge Criteria Met ☐`

TIME

Discharge Assessment

NEUROLOGICAL

Pupils:

Consciousness		Activity	
Fully Reacted	☐	Moves all	☐
Responds to verbal command	☐	extremities Moves to painful stimuli	☐
Responds to painful stimuli	☐	Unreactive	☐
Non-reactive	☐		

Orientation			
Time	☐	Person	☐
Place	☐	None of the above	☐

CARDIO

Rhythm:

Pulses	Present	
Temporal	L ☐	R ☐
Radial	L ☐	R ☐
Femoral	L ☐	R ☐
D. Pedis	L ☐	R ☐
P. Tibia	L ☐	R ☐

RESPIRATORY

Airway

Naso-trach ☐   Trach ☐   Nasal ☐   Oral ☐

Oro-trach ☐   None ☐   Time dc'd: _____

Oxygen Oximeter ☐

FI O₂ _____   Face Mask ☐   T-tube ☐

Other   Face Shield ☐

Ventilator

Time	FI O₂	Rate	T.V.

Respirations		Breath Sounds	
Non-labored	☐	Bilateral	☐
Shallow	☐	Clear	☐
Rapid	☐	Diminished	☐
		Coarse	☐
Reflexes		Wheezing	☐
Swallow	☐		
Cough	☐		

GI

Abdomen:

Bowel Sounds: Present ☐   None ☐

NG Tube:

GU

Catheter:

Character: Color:

INTENG.

Skin		Color	
Warm	☐	Pink mucous	
Cool	☐	membrane	☐
Dry	☐	Pale	☐
Moist	☐	Cyanotic	☐

Dressing Location:

Drains Location:

Date:

Allergies:

Time	Medication	Route	Site	Signature

Time	System	Assessment

Diagnostic Tests

Time	Tests	Results

	Intake					Output				
	Time	Fluids	I.V.	Blood	Other	Total	Time	Urine	NG	EBL	Total
OR							OR				
PACU		Fluids	I.V.	Blood	Other	Total	PACU	Urine	NG	Other	Total
I & O											
		PACU Total					Output				

Disposition: I.C.U. ☐   D.S.U. ☐   NSG Unit ☐   ☐

Discharged By:

Discharge Nurse: Report To:

	PACU	B.P.	P.	R.	on unit

Released By:

Received		B.P.	P.	R.	on unit

FIGURE 4-8   *Continued*

During the time that the patient is recovering from the effects of anesthesia, the nurse must provide simple nursing measures to relieve some of his discomfort. Because the patient has had nothing by mouth for 8 hours or more, he may experience severe thirst. After the gag reflex has returned, and if not contraindicated, a few ice chips may be offered; otherwise his lips and mouth can be moistened with a washcloth or gauze square dipped in ice water. If he is receiving intravenous fluids, the rate is checked, and the site is inspected and positioned so that the cannula will not be dislodged.

Many surgical procedures extend over hours, which means that the patient has been lying motionless, in a fixed position, on a hard table for that length of time. The nurse should check pressure points for the position that the patient was in during surgery and provide padding and appropriate positioning for areas that are uncomfortable.

Think about... Your postoperative patient was placed in a right side lying position during surgery. Which specific places should you check for signs of pressure problems? How would you position the patient who is complaining of pain in the right hip as well as pain in the left flank where the surgery occurred?

Pain is an important factor in the care of the patient who is recovering from anesthesia. Before resorting to analgesic medications, the nurse should try to determine the cause of the pain. Dressings should be checked to see whether they are too tight and the bladder and abdomen should be assessed for distention. If the patient complains of chest pain, or pain either on inhaling or exhaling, this should be reported to the anesthesiologist.

Operating rooms are kept very cool so that the staff members working under the bright lights do not become overheated and so that the patient's metabolism will slow, decreasing oxygen needs. The patient's temperature in this environment often decreases, especially during prolonged abdominal surgery where the peritoneal cavity has been open for hours. His temperature should be checked frequently, and if there is an indication that hypothermia (temperature below 97.5°F [36.4°C]) is present or developing, warm blankets should be used to help to maintain normal body temperature. The shivering that accompanies hypothermia produces an early need for analgesics, as these patients experience additional pain caused by uncontrollable shivering.

Nausea and vomiting following anesthesia are not uncommon. Supportive measures such as holding the patient's head or turning it to the side to prevent aspiration of the vomitus are most helpful. Suction is used to clear the mouth and throat. An alert patient may have a few sips of water to rinse his mouth after the siege of vomiting is over. If nausea continues, the patient is given antinausea medication as ordered.

Once aroused, the patient should be asked whether he needs to empty his bladder, particularly if several liters of IV fluid were infused during surgery or it has been 6 to 8 hours since the last voiding.

A family member or two may be allowed a brief visit once the patient is awake. This offers reassurance that loved ones are near and allows the family or significant others to see that the patient has made it safely through surgery. Both the patient and family are kept informed of what is happening and when transfer back to the nursing unit or discharge from the same-day surgery unit is likely.

Discharge from the PACU occurs when the patient is sufficiently recovered from anesthesia, that is, is arousable and *lucid* (has a clear mind), can move all unrestrained extremities, demonstrates the ability to deep-breathe and cough, and has near-normal skin color and vital signs that are within acceptable limits and stable. A scoring system is usually used to determine whether the patient is sufficiently recovered or not; such systems vary from one facility to another. When the patient is about ready to transfer back to the original nursing unit, the PACU nurse calls the unit, advises of the coming transfer, and notifies the staff of any special equipment that will be needed to care for the patient.

The patient is accompanied back to the nursing unit by a nurse who gives a report to the staff nurse who will be caring for the patient in that unit. If someone else is transporting the patient, the PACU nurse phones the report to the staff nurse. Table 4-4 presents the data to be relayed to the staff nurse assigned to the patient.

The first 72 hours after surgery require frequent observations to detect signs of postoperative complications. The patient will need extra assistance with personal needs and help with activities of daily living (ADLs) during this period.

TABLE 4-4 ◆ *Outline for a Report by the PACU Nurse to the Staff Nurse*

- Patient's name, age, and sex
- Surgery performed
- Pertinent past medical or surgical history
- Type of anesthesia administered
- Known allergies
- Amount of blood loss
- Location of tubes, drains, and dressings
- IV fluids infused and currently hanging
- Urine and other output
- Medications given during surgery or recovery
- Any problems the patient experienced
- Current vital signs
- General condition and degree of arousal
- Special equipment in use and the settings ordered

CARE AND DISCHARGE FROM AN AMBULATORY OR SAME-DAY SURGERY UNIT

Many surgery patients are in the hospital for only a few hours. The ambulatory or day surgery unit, or a surgical center that is freestanding and not attached to any hospital, handles the preoperative and postoperative care for these patients. For minor procedures, the patient may bypass the PACU and be transferred from the OR to the ambulatory or day surgery general unit for brief monitoring before discharge. This occurs most commonly when the patient has had only conscious or intravenous sedation rather than general anesthesia or has had local or regional anesthesia. Other patients go to the PACU and then are transferred to the ambulatory unit for further observation before discharge.

The nurse monitors the patient's airway, circulation, vital signs, neurological status, fluid intake and output, wound drainage and dressings, and comfort level. When the vital signs are stable, the patient is allowed to sit up. Early ambulation is encouraged, and when the patient can ambulate without assistance, he may be discharged if the vital signs are stable. Oral fluids are started when the gag reflex has returned fully. Swallowing motions indicate that the patient is swallowing saliva and then small sips of water may be given. Recovery time in the ambulatory unit is generally 1 to 3 hours.

Discharge teaching is begun before surgery and continues when the patient is again alert and able to concentrate on instructions. Written instructions are sent home to reinforce the teaching. If the patient has had more than a local anesthetic, another adult driver must provide transportation home. Surgery patients are advised not to resume normal activities or make important decisions for at least 24 hours after surgery. The phone number of the surgeon is written on the postoperative instruction sheet in case of complications. Table 4-5 presents a discharge teaching checklist. A skillful assessment of the patient's postoperative status is essential to establish that he can be safely discharged.

Think about . . . How would you assess a patient to determine whether or not the gag reflex has returned sufficiently to allow him to have a few ice chips?

GENERAL POSTOPERATIVE NURSING CARE

◆ Preparation of the Postoperative Patient Unit

While the patient is in surgery, the unit is prepared for her return. The bed is made and the covers are either

TABLE 4-5 ◆ *Discharge Teaching Checklist for Same-Day Surgery Patients*

The following points should be covered for the postoperative patient before discharge:

Diet
  Type of diet and importance of proper nutrition for healing
  Dietary restrictions, if any
  Avoiding alcohol for first 24 hours after anesthesia
  Special dietary recommendations
  Recommended fluid intake

Activity
  Recommended exercise and frequency
  Instructions for special equipment: crutches, walker, cane, splint, etc.
  Schedule for deep breathing, coughing, and leg exercises; how long to continue these activities; remember to splint the incision when coughing and getting out of bed
  Recommended rest periods
  Activity restrictions, i.e., driving, intercourse, and lifting
  Application, use, and care of antiembolism stockings

Wound care
  Dressing changes and frequency
  Cleansing of wound; irrigations
  Drainage observations
  Signs to report
  Use of heat or cold packs
  Supplies and where to obtain them

Temperature monitoring
  Record time and temperature
  Report temperature >100°F

Type of bath and frequency

Medications
  Analgesics
  Antibiotics
  Sedatives
  Vitamin supplements
  Other medications

Precautions related to anesthesia or side effects of medication
  Caution regarding using machinery
  Caution regarding making decisions for 24 hours
  Drug interactions
  Potential for constipation
  Potential for urinary retention

Next scheduled appointment with the doctor

Signs and symptoms to report
  Elevated temperature
  Increasing malaise
  Severe pain or swelling
  Bleeding through bandage
  Decreased sensation below surgical site
  Severe nausea and vomiting

Expectation for return to usual activities
Expectation for return to feeling normal

---

folded to the side or the bottom of the bed. A protective pad is placed at the head of the bed and at the torso area. A drawsheet is positioned at shoulder height on the bed for the use in turning the patient. The bed is left at the height of the transfer stretcher, and the near side rail is left down so that the stretcher can be put against the bed. The furniture is arranged so that the stretcher can be easily positioned to transfer the patient.

The emesis basin, tissues, frequent vital signs sheet, intake and output sheet, paper, and a pencil are placed on the bedside table or over-bed table. A thermometer, sphygmomanometer, and stethoscope also are placed in the room or are readily available. An IV pole is placed at the head of the bed, on the side that corresponds with the IV site, if known. Oxygen and suction setups are put into place if they are needed and any other equipment is placed in the room as soon as the PACU notifies the unit of such needs.

◆ Nursing Assessment

After receiving a report on the patient from the PACU nurse, checking his identity, and settling him in bed, the nurse performs her initial postoperative assessment. Frequent assessment can detect the signs and symptoms of postoperative complications. The earlier a complication is detected, the quicker it can usually be remedied, and the less harm the patient experiences.

Initial assessment of the postoperative patient when she returns to the nursing unit is presented in Table 4-6. **Ongoing assessment of dressings, drains, tubes, comfort, safety, and equipment function is performed whenever vital signs are taken.**

◆ Nursing Diagnosis

Common nursing diagnoses for postoperative patients who had general anesthesia include:

- ◆ Pain related to the surgical procedure
- ◆ Risk of infection related to surgical wound
- ◆ Impaired gas exchange related to the effect of anesthesia on the lungs
- ◆ Risk of ineffective airway clearance related to inability to breathe deeply and cough without discomfort
- ◆ Self-care deficit related to decreased mobility, tubes, and dressings
- ◆ Risk of injury related to sedation, decreased level of consciousness, and excessive blood loss
- ◆ Altered tissue perfusion related to surgery, anesthesia, and positioning on the operating table
- ◆ Risk of ineffective coping related to loss of body part or change in body image

Nursing diagnoses for patients who underwent spinal anesthesia include the first two items in the list plus:

TABLE 4-6 ◆ *Initial Postoperative Assessment upon Return to Unit*

Respiratory status
Airway: patent
Respirations: rate, depth, character
Breath sounds: character, presence bilateral

Circulatory status
Pulses: apical, brachial, and those distal to surgical site
Skin: color, temperature
Capillary refill
Body temperature

Neurological status
Level of consciousness
Orientation
Ability to move all extremities to command
Gag reflex fully returned

Dressing
Location
Presence of drainage
Drainage tubes: where located; not kinked
Wound suction functioning

Comfort
Level of pain
Presence of nausea or vomiting
Positioning: as ordered; in correct body alignment; facilitates respiration
Bladder: nondistended; Foley bag below bladder level with tubing free of kinks; amount of urine output
Nasogastric tube: attached to suction; correct setting; functioning

Safety
Bed in low position
Side rails up
Call bell in reach
Extra blankets as needed for warmth
Emesis basin and tissue at hand
Need for restraint to preserve function of tubes
Monitors attached and functioning correctly
IV: site patent and secure; correct solution, correct additives and dosage; correct flow rate; amount left in container
Orders checked; special positioning performed

- ◆ Impaired mobility related to effects of spinal anesthesia
- ◆ Risk of injury related to decreased sensation and movement in lower extremities

◆ Planning

The goals of nursing care depend on the individual patient and the specific nursing diagnoses chosen. General goals include:

- ◆ Maintaining patent airway and adequate respiratory function
- ◆ Maintaining adequate tissue perfusion

- Promoting comfort and rest
- Promoting wound healing
- Preventing complications
- Promoting psychological adjustment to lifestyle or body image changes

When planning her daily work, the nurse must remember that frequent assessments of fresh postoperative patients is a high priority. Careful planning is essential to fit in these assessments every 15 to 60 minutes without getting behind in meeting needs of other patients.

◆ Implementation

After Spinal Anesthesia   The patient is helpless while his legs are paralyzed by spinal anesthesia, and the side rails must be kept raised for safety. The patient may be groggy from preoperative sedation or other drugs given during surgery. Reassure the patient that a sensation of numbness and heaviness in the legs is usual and that feeling will soon return to normal. Function returns in the reverse order in which it was depressed. Position sense returns first, then sensation to deep pressure, voluntary movement, and finally the ability to feel superficial pain and temperature. Continue to observe for hypotension even after movement and sensation have returned.

The patient used to be kept flat for 12 hours after surgery to prevent headache. However, this practice has not proven effective and has been largely abandoned. If the patient develops a spinal headache, keeping him flat tends to decrease the pain. Encourage spinal anesthesia patients to drink fluids, particularly those containing caffeine. The fluids replace lost body fluids and the caffeine raises vascular pressure at the spinal puncture site, helping to seal the hole. Caffeine also is a vasoconstrictor and acts to decrease cerebral volume and lower intracranial pressure. As the spinal anesthesia wears off, the patient experiences a feeling of "pins and needles" in the legs and may have pain in the operative area.

Think about . . . How would your care for the patient who has had spinal anesthesia differ from that of the patient who has had general anesthesia?

Monitoring Vital Signs   Vital signs are monitored as frequently as indicated by the physician's orders. By the time the patient has returned to his room his vital signs should have stabilized. The purpose of continued monitoring is to note and report any significant changes that could indicate such complications as hypovolemic shock from bleeding and fluid loss, in-

fection, **hyperthermia** (high temperature), and cardiac and respiratory problems. A temperature below 97.5°F (36.4°C) indicates hypothermia and the patient should be warmed.

Think about . . . The initial vital sign readings for your patient at return from surgery were blood pressure (BP) 138/86, pulse 76, respirations 14, temperature 97.8°F. An hour later they were BP 126/74, pulse 80, respirations 14, temperature 98.0°F. What action, if any, should you take?

Promoting Respiratory Function   The postoperative patient is at risk for respiratory problems because of anesthesia and immobility. All postoperative patients have some degree of **atelectasis** (collapse of alveoli in the lungs). Mild **hypoxemia** (insufficient oxygen supply in the blood) is common for about 48 hours after surgery. One fourth to one half of all patients who had either abdominal or thoracic surgery suffer from such pulmonary complications as increasing **atelectasis** and pneumonitis. If any area of the lung remains atelectic for more than 72 hours, hypostatic pneumonia from retained secretions is likely to occur.

Assessment of the patient for adequate respiratory function requires auscultating the lungs, observing the patient's rate and depth of breathing, and noting any cough and whether it is productive and wheezing or moist "bubbling" sounds when the patient breathes. **Subjective data include complaints of shortness of breath, pain on inspiration, and extreme fatigue due to hypoxemia.**

Turning, coughing, and deep-breathing. Preventive measures include helping the patient to turn, cough, and deep-breath. Turning changes the distribution of gas and blood flow in the lungs and moves secretions. Because moving about and turning in the bed can put a strain on healing wounds, the patient should be assisted in turning when he is still drowsy from anesthesia or physically weak and unable to move himself without great effort. Overhead trapeze bars should *not* be used by patients who have had abdominal surgery because this causes an increase in intraabdominal pressure. When the surgical patient is able to get up on his own, he should be taught to roll to one side, flex his legs, and push himself up on his elbow when getting out of bed.

The purpose of *deep-breathing* is to expand and aerate the lungs. To accomplish this the patient should concentrate on inhaling deeply and holding the inhaled breath as long as comfortably possible. This is called *sustained maximal inspiration (SMI).* Another procedure for SMI involves using an *incentive spirometer,* which some authorities feel is the most effective way to

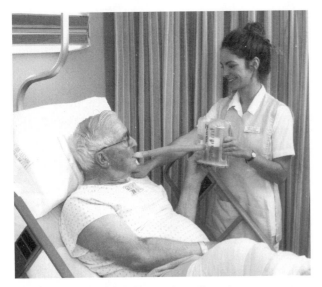

FIGURE 4-9 Patient using an incentive spirometer postoperatively. (Photo by Glen Derbyshire; Courtesy of Goleta Valley Cottage Hospital, Goleta, CA.)

avoid postoperative pulmonary problems (Figure 4-9). Maximum benefit from this instrument is obtained if the patient has been taught to use it before surgery.

Incentive spirometers are named "incentive" because the patient is encouraged to inhale deeply by watching the movement of one or more balls or lights in response to his efforts. As the patient inhales, these balls move upward in a cylinder. The spirometer must be held upright to obtain maximum therapeutic value. The nurse should monitor the patient's use of the incentive spirometer at first (Table 4-7 presents guidelines for use of an incentive spirometer.)

Coughing is encouraged for the purpose of removing secretions that have accumulated in the air passages. Although it is a forced expiratory movement that causes discomfort in abdominal and thoracic surgical wounds, it can help to prevent pulmonary complications. When it is appropriate and done properly, coughing usually is

---

TABLE 4-7 ◆ *Patient Teaching: Using the Incentive Spirometer*

Instruct the patient to:
- Insert the mouthpiece, covering it completely with the lips.
- Take a slow deep breath and hold it for at least 3 s.
- Exhale slowly keeping the lips puckered.
- Breathe normally for a few breaths.
- Try to increase the inspired volume by at least 100 mL with each breath on the spirometer.
- Once maximal volume is achieved, attempt to inspire this volume 10 times, resting a few breaths in between each attempt.
- Clean the mouthpiece of the spirometer when finished.

---

effective in removing these secretions, thereby minimizing or eliminating the need for suctioning. The area of the surgical incision should be splinted with a small pillow or with the nurse's or the patient's hands to decrease discomfort.

The patient is taught to take a deep breath and forcibly exhale with the mouth open. She is asked to do this "huff" maneuver again; then she is told to take a deep breath and cough strongly enough as she exhales to move the secretions out of the airways. Little coughs that just clear the throat do not do the job. Several successive huff coughs will then bring up secretions so they can be **expectorated** (spat out).

Coughing is contraindicated in some kinds of abdominal surgery (e.g., hernia repair), following eye surgery, ear surgery, and after most types of brain surgery when it is dangerous to increase intracranial pressure.

Elder Care Point . . . The elderly patient is at greater risk for respiratory problems because of the effects of aging on the lungs, such as decreased compliance and tidal volume, and also because arthritis frequently affects the rib cage, inhibiting inspiration. It is important for the nurse to encourage and supervise deep-breathing and coughing in these patients to prevent complications.

A pulse oximeter may be used to determine how well the patient is oxygenating his blood. Obtain pulse oximetry readings as ordered. Check the machine and the probe frequently if the patient is being monitored continuously. Report SaO_2 readings below 90% to the physician (Figure 4-10). The procedure for attaching the patient to a pulse oximeter is covered in Chapter 16.

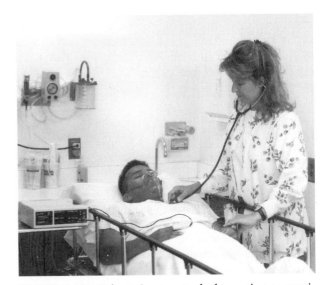

FIGURE 4-10 Pulse oximeter attached to patient to monitor his oxygenation status in recovery area. (Photo by Glen Derbyshire; Courtesy of Goleta Valley Cottage Hospital, Goleta, CA.)

Promoting Circulatory Function If considerable blood is lost during surgery, the patient may receive blood transfusions. If the surgery is elective, the patient may donate some of his blood several weeks before surgery and have it held for him. This decreases the risk of AIDS, hepatitis B or C, and transfusion reaction. Autologous transfusion of the patient's blood collected through loss during surgery also may be done.

Movement of the extremities and leg exercises encourage venous return to the heart and help to prevent thrombus formation. Elastic stockings, TEDS® or Jobst hose, are sometimes also ordered. They should be checked frequently to see that they fit smoothly. They may be removed for 15 to 30 minutes per shift for bathing and to allow air circulation to the skin. Pneumatic compression devices that alternately inflate and deflate, putting pressure intermittently on the legs to encourage venous return often are used postoperatively. Low-dose subcutaneous heparin injections are commonly ordered for any patient who has a history of **thrombophlebitis** (clot and inflammation in a blood vessel). Thrombophlebitis does not usually occur until after the fifth day of bed rest. The vigilant nurse will question the patient about pain or tenderness in the legs. She should assess for **Homan's sign** (pain in the calf when the leg is raised with knee bent and then straightened while dorsiflexing the foot).

If the patient complains of leg pain, the area should be gently felt for increased warmth, and the physician must be notified. **The leg should *never* be massaged, as this might dislodge a blood clot and cause an embolus that could lodge in the lungs.**

Promoting Comfort, Rest, and Activity

Pain. After the stress of surgery, the patient needs all her resources to recover. Pain and discomfort interfere with rest and inhibit the processes of healing and repair. Although analgesic drugs are almost always prescribed for the postoperative patient, comfort measures also should be used. **NSAIDs and non-narcotic analgesics may be used to augment opioids, as they work on both the peripheral and the central nervous system to control pain.** Opioids tend to depress respirations and the cough reflex and therefore may contribute to the development of pulmonary problems. They also can increase the possibility of nausea and vomiting. Using other drugs in combination with opioids helps to control pain with the least amount of side effects. Pain must be reduced so that the patient will rest, turn, cough, and deep-breathe frequently. **Pain medication should be given consistently for the first 24 to 48 hours postoperatively.** The nurse should assess the pain level and effectiveness of analgesia at least every 3 hours. **Consistent pain relief is achieved by giving analgesics regularly before pain builds.**

Before administering any analgesic drug, it is best to try to determine whether a distended bladder, abdominal distention, tight dressings or cast, or some other condition is interfering with the patient's comfort. A change of position, soothing backrub, quiet environment, or soothing music may be all that is needed to relieve discomfort. If an analgesic medication is given, comfort measures used before the drug is administered, or along with the drug, will serve to increase and prolong its effect.

> If the patient is hypotensive or bradycardic, the physician should be consulted before pain medication is administered.

Comfort measures and prompt attention to expressions of pain and discomfort can be reassuring to the patient. Be certain that the patient is warm enough; feeling chilled contributes to discomfort. Operating rooms are kept cool, and patients who become cold have a difficult time getting warm again while they are so inactive. Applying socks to the feet may help the patient to rewarm more quickly.

Relaxation techniques also can help to decrease the patient's discomfort. Teach him to use jaw relaxation and slow breathing techniques. For jaw relaxation, tell him to allow the lower jaw to drop slightly, just like at the start of a yawn. Relax the tongue and let it lie on the bottom of the mouth; keep it still. Relax the lips; feel them becoming soft. Breathe slowly and in a steady rhythm; inhale, exhale, rest; inhale, exhale, rest. Continue to relax and breathe slowly.

Pain medication may be administered by subcutaneous (SC) or intramuscular (IM) injection, intravenously (IV), epidurally, or by intermittent administration of local anesthetic into the pleural space via an intrapleural catheter. Two methods very commonly used for pain control are the epidural catheter and the patient-controlled analgesia (PCA) pump. The problem of pain, methods of pain control, pain medications, and their administration are discussed in greater detail in Chapter 10.

Elder Care Point... The elderly feel pain just as they did when they were younger, but they tend to report less pain. Many older individuals have become stoic and do not wish to complain or "bother" the nurse. Moreover, the postoperative elderly patient may experience joint pain from positioning on the operating table.

The effects of aging predispose the elderly patient to constipation. **When narcotic analgesics are used postoperatively, the nurse must vigilantly monitor and take action to prevent this side effect.**

The knowledge that something is being done and the belief that it will be effective can have a placebo effect and thereby relieve discomfort and promote relaxation. Once the patient's needs have been attended to and she is resting comfortably, every effort should be made not to disturb her any more than is absolutely necessary to monitor her status and carry out prescribed treatments.

Nursing interventions for pain and for other selected problems in a patient undergoing surgery are summarized in Nursing Care Plan 4-1. It is the nurse's responsibility to evaluate the effectiveness of the pain relief methods ordered for the patient and to get the orders changed if pain is not being properly controlled.

Therapeutic Communication Interaction 4-1

Mrs Wilson is a 76-year-old who is recovering from abdominal surgery. Although her body language tells her nurse she is experiencing pain, she has denied any need for pain medication since she administered her PCA dose 3 hours before.

"Mrs. Wilson, I would like to see you able to cough more vigorously, move about in bed more, and ambulate more frequently. I think that if you would use your pain pump more often you would be more comfortable doing your exercises and coughing."

"I'm not that uncomfortable and those medications always cause problems for me."

"Problems?"

"Yes, I get really constipated."

"The doctor has a stool softener ordered for you to help to prevent constipation, and by increasing fluids, we should be able to control that. Do you have other problems with the pain medication?"

Nursing Care Plan 4-1

Selected nursing diagnoses, goals/expected outcomes, nursing interventions, and evaluations for a patient undergoing a mastectomy

Situation: Patient is a married 38-year-old female and the mother of two children ages 16 and 14. She is scheduled for simple mastectomy as treatment for a localized malignant tumor, detected by self-examination of her breasts.

Nursing Diagnosis	Goals/Expected Outcome	Nursing Interventions	Evaluation
Fear related to cancer, disfigurement, death. SUPPORTING DATA Malignant tumor by biopsy; grandmother died of breast cancer; is crying at intervals and is worried about husband's reaction to loss of breast.	Patient will discuss fears openly. Patient will look at incisional area before discharge. Patient will talk about having cancer. Patient will join support group for cancer patients. Patient will identify spiritual support. Patient will utilize community resources.	Establish rapport and trust. Encourage her to discuss fears with nurse and family. Help her to identify specific fears and deal with each one separately. Encourage her to think of cancer as a challenge. Teach relaxation exercises to decrease anxiety. Do preoperative teaching for patient and family: routine procedures, NPO, expected tubes and drains, equipment to expect in room, probable length of surgery, where family will wait, pain relief measures, handling of arm on operative side, coughing, deep breathing and leg exercises, ambulation, diet, daily postoperative routine. Call pastor/chaplain if patient desires a visit. Provide private time for patient and husband and patient and family. Seek physician's order for Reach to Recovery program.	Preop teaching done; states she is "afraid to die of cancer"; minister visited; relaxation exercise taught and practiced; continue plan. Outcomes partially met.

Nursing Care Plan 4-1 *(Continued)*

Nursing Diagnosis	Goals/Expected Outcome	Nursing Interventions	Evaluation
Impaired skin integrity related to surgical wound. SUPPORTING DATA Right mastectomy 5/10/97	Wound will be free of signs of infection. Wound will heal completely.	Keep Jackson-Pratt suction functioning properly. Note character and amount of drainage; document. Reinforce dressing as needed. Assess for excessive bleeding q h for 4 h, then q 2 h for first 24 h. Assess pulses in arm q 2 h to detect excessive swelling in arm. Monitor temperature and WBCs. Assess wound for signs of infection with each dressing change. Change dressing q 8 to 24 h as needed.	Serosanguinous drainage in J-P; dressing dry and intact; brachial and radial pulses equal at 3+; Temp, 99.8°F; WBCs, 10,800; no signs of infection; continue plan. Meeting outcomes.
Pain related to surgical incision SUPPORTING DATA Right mastectomy Rigid in bed Complains of incisional pain	Pain is controlled by analgesia as noted by patient. Patient appears relaxed. Pain is controlled by oral analgesia by discharge.	Assess need for pain measures q 3 to 4 h. Provide comfort measures. Administer analgesics as ordered; note response and assess for side effects. Refrain from giving injections in right arm (side of surgery.)	Demerol per PCA pump—dosage adequate for control; repositioned q 2 h; states she is reasonably comfortable; pain controlled. Outcomes met.
Impaired gas exchange related to residual effects of anesthesia, immobility, and incisional pain. SUPPORTING DATA Inhalation anesthesia Right mastectomy Bed rest with BRP only	No atelectasis Lung sounds clear	Have patient deep-breathe and cough q 2 h. Auscultate lungs q 8 h. Encourage ambulation when ordered. Monitor temperature and respirations.	Deep-breathed and coughed at 8, 10, 12, and 2 o'clock; lungs clear to auscultation bilaterally; resp 22; continue plan. Outcomes being met.
Risk for grieving related to loss of body part and perception of feminity. SUPPORTING DATA Right mastectomy Concern about husband's reaction to surgery and loss of breast.	Patient will verbalize feelings of self-worth and confidence. Patient will discuss sadness over loss of breast. Patient will discuss ways to develop new positive body image.	Have patient list her strengths and positive attributes. Encourage sharing of sad feelings and fears with husband. Talk with husband privately about his feelings. Involve husband in patient's care. Encourage daughters to discuss their feelings and fears with patient. Encourage independence in patient.	Husband appears supportive but scared: "I don't want to talk about it until the final report is in." Will wait 2 days postop before speaking to daughters about their fears. Patient assisted with own bath this AM.

"Yes, it makes me light-headed and unsteady on my feet."

"If the medication makes you light-headed, we can switch you to a different medication. One of us will stay with you when you are out of bed to see that you do not fall."

"I'm very afraid of falling, breaking a hip, and adding to my troubles."

"By taking the medication and being more comfortable, you'll feel more like doing your exercises. That's how you can help prevent postoperative complications such as pneumonia or blood clots."

"I certainly don't want pneumonia or a blood clot!"

"*Moving about more will also increase circulation and help your wound to heal faster.*"

"O.K., I'll take the pain medication if it will help me prevent complications."

Rest and sleep.   Planning care so that the patient has undisturbed rest periods is equally important. **Insufficient sleep slows the healing process and causes undue fatigue.** Try to coordinate changing out IV fluid containers, giving other medications, and taking vital signs at the same time, especially during the night, so that the patient is not repeatedly disturbed every hour. If the patient has considerable difficulty sleeping, a sedative may be ordered to ensure a good night's sleep. Foam ear plugs can dampen noise and allow patients to sleep more easily despite the activity inherent in a hospital environment.

Nutrition and fluids.   A healthy surgical patient may be kept on nothing but IV fluids for up to 5 days without developing a serious nutritional problem. If extensive tissue repair is required for healing, supplemental nutrition by enteral or parenteral feeding may be started. A patient who is kept on intravenous fluids only will lose some weight as there are insufficient calories in the IV fluids to meet total daily requirements. **A liter of 5% Dextrose (D5W) in water contains only 200 calories.** The surgeon will calculate the correct amount of fluid and electrolyte replacement that the patient needs to restore balance in the body. It is an important function of the nurse to see to it that the IV site remains patent and the fluids are given at the correct rate.

When bowel sounds have returned and the patient is passing gas per rectum, peristalsis has resumed and the patient may safely begin taking liquids by mouth. Usually the diet progresses from clear liquids to full liquids, to a soft diet, and then to a regular diet. The nurse must judge whether or not the patient is tolerating each type of diet before allowing progression to the next type. **If the patient is consuming the meal, has no complaints of nausea, diarrhea, distention, or pain, and bowel sounds are still present, it is usually safe to progress to the next type of diet.** Food choices containing lots of vitamin C, zinc, and protein will provide the nutrients needed for healing (Table 4-8).

Nausea and vomiting.   Nausea and vomiting caused by anesthesia are common in the early postoperative period but generally last only 12 to 24 hours after surgery. An emesis basin should be placed close to the patient. Medication is usually ordered for nausea, and the nurse should administer it *before* the patient starts vomiting. Mouth care may eliminate any unpleasant taste from anesthesia and help decrease nausea. **Applying a cool cloth to the forehead and back of the neck, rinsing the mouth, ridding the room of odors, and providing a quiet environment also help to reduce nausea.**

TABLE 4-8   ◆   *Foods High in Vitamin C and Protein*

Patients undergoing surgery need a diet high in vitamin C and protein. When counseling patients about their diet, encourage the following food choices:

Foods high in vitamin C

Citrus fruits and juices	Turnip or collard greens
Strawberries	Broccoli
Cantaloupe	Mangos
Tomatoes	Peaches
Bell pepper	Pineapple
Cabbage	Potatoes

Foods high in protein

Meats: chicken, beef, pork*	Beans
Cottage cheese	Eggs
Milk*	Ice cream
Cheese	Grain products: breads, pasta
Peanut butter	Tofu; soy products

*Meats and milk products contain the highest amounts of protein.

If vomiting continues in spite of medication, a nasogastric (NG) tube may have to be inserted to solve the problem and prevent both aspiration and continued stress on the incision.

Hiccups.   This condition usually is a minor discomfort that disappears in a few minutes or, at the most, several hours. Sometimes, however, the spasms of the diaphragm persist for days or weeks, causing serious problems of discomfort, stress on the suture line, and interference with eating and rest.

Treatment usually involves administering carbon dioxide by having the patient rebreathe exhaled air in a paper bag or by inhaling the carbon dioxide gas through a mask. Sedatives and tranquilizers are sometimes prescribed to promote relaxation and reduce irritation of the phrenic nerve. Severe, persistent cases may require surgical interruption of impulses along the nerve pathways so as to remove the cause of the spasms of the diaphragm.

An alternate treatment for hiccups is to massage the ear lobes. Massage activates the accupressure points interrupting the hiccup reflex. Many "folk" remedies for hiccups often are effective for patients (Table 4-9).

TABLE 4-9   ◆   *"Folk" Remedies for Hiccups*

- Fill a glass with at least 4 oz of water. Lean over a sink and drink water from the backside of a glass. Drink continuously until the glass is empty.
- Stick a finger in each ear, and hold your breath; drink from a glass that someone else is holding for you.
- Place a paper bag over the head and breathe deeply 20 times.
- Place a teaspoon of sugar or peanut butter on the tongue and let it slowly melt; the hiccups will be gone when the sugar or peanut butter has dissolved.

Distention (gas). Patients who have had general anesthesia or who have had abdominal organs manipulated during surgery tend to develop considerable gas postoperatively. Antacids formulated to reduce gas may be given to decrease this problem. These patients should refrain from drinking through a straw as more air tends to be swallowed in this manner and they should drink fluids that are neither really hot or ice-cold. Ambulation helps the gas to move along the intestines so that it can be expelled. Gentle massage over the large intestine in the path of normal evacuation may help the gas to move out. If such a position is not contraindicated, lying with the body at a slant with the feet, legs, and lower abdomen above the level of the chest helps gas move out (gas will rise).

Thirst. The patient who must remain on NPO status after surgery will complain of thirst and dry mouth. Moistening the mouth with a slightly wet washcloth can be soothing. Cleansing the mouth frequently with a toothette also helps. Sometimes ice chips are allowed. If so, instruct the patient to take them a teaspoon at a time and to let them dissolve completely in their mouth before swallowing.

Constipation. A sluggish bowel after general anesthesia, the effects of narcotic analgesics, lack of usual activity, and an altered diet status often lead to constipation in the postoperative patient. Encouraging adequate fluid intake in those who are allowed fluids may help. A stool softener may be ordered as soon as the patient is allowed something by mouth. When the diet is resumed, adding extra fiber quickly resolves the problem. In the meantime **it is important for the nurse to judge, based on the time the patient has been NPO and the resumption of food by mouth, when the patient should be having a normal bowel movement.** If the patient has been eating a normal diet for 3 days, but has not had a bowel movement and is complaining of feeling constipated, an order should be sought for a suppository or a laxative.

Think about . . . Can you name four specific interventions you might try to prevent constipation in your postoperative patient who is receiving narcotic analgesics for pain?

Activity. Activity is necessary to prevent venous **stasis** (stagnation of normal flow) and thrombophlebitis. After the patient recovers from anesthesia, she should be asked to perform leg exercises at least every 2 hours while awake until she is up and about normally. She should rotate the ankles, bend the leg at the knee, and dorsiflex the foot, repeating these movements at least five times on each side. If possible, the patient is ambulated within 12 hours of surgery. This promotes better circulation and expansion of the lungs. After allowing the patient to sit on the side of the bed for a bit,

with slippers or shoes in place, the nurse assists the patient to stand and stabilize. Then, **with a firm hold on the patient,** the nurse assists her to walk about the patient unit. Progressive ambulation will involve walking to the bathroom, down the hall a short way, and then the full length of the hall. The nurse assists until it is judged that the patient can walk safely on her own. Resuming more and more self-care activities increases the patient's activity.

If the patient cannot be up out of bed, the nurse supervises active range of motion exercises on unaffected extremities and performs passive range of motion on the affected extremities as ordered.

Clinical Pathway 4-1 presents a collaborative care plan for a patient undergoing an abdominal hysterectomy.

◆ Promoting Wound Healing

Pathophysiology of Wound Healing   When it has been injured the body responds by initiating the inflammatory and repair process. There are three possible outcomes of the attempt toward healing: *recovery, regeneration,* and *replacement.*

If the cells are not damaged beyond recovery, they will restore themselves, and there will be no permanent evidence of injury. If an infection is present and is localized, the **exudate** (fluid accumulation) is removed, and the tissues return to normal. This is called *localization* and *resolution.* The outcome is recovery, that is, restoration of the tissue to its former state.

A second possibility is that some of the cells may be fatally injured (**necrosis**). The affected area then must heal by *regeneration,* which means that new cells similar in structure and function to the dead ones are produced as replacements. This is not possible in all types of tissue. The epithelial, fibrous, bony, and lymphoid tissues regenerate well, but the nervous, muscular, and elastic tissues do not.

The third possible outcome is replacement of the damaged tissue with fibrous scar tissue (**scarring**). The exudate associated with the inflammatory process contains fibrin, which forms a network of strands on which granulation tissue forms. As the debris from the inflammatory site is removed by the leukocytes, the capillaries and immature fiber cells begin to move into the remaining spaces. These small blood vessels and fiber cells give the granulation tissue a soft, reddish appearance.

Scar formation is a natural result of the process of repair. The capillaries and connective tissue cells in the wound shrink and become taut, appearing as hard reddish tissue and gradually becoming white and glossy to form the typical scar tissue with which we are all familiar. Collagen overgrowth results in a "keloid"-type scar, which occurs mostly in dark pigmented skin. Internally, the formation of scar tissue can create some

CLINICAL PATHWAY 4-1* ◆ *Total Abdominal Hysterectomy*

Nursing Diagnosis/ Collaborative Problem	Expected Outcome (The Patient is Expected to . . .)	Met/Not Met	Reason	Date/Initials
Pain.	State that pain is relieved following appropriate interventions.			
Potential for postoperative complications (hemorrhage, infection).	Have Hgb and Hct WNL, stable VS, and WBC WNL; incision clean and dry.			
Potential for ineffective coping/ body image disturbance.	Participate in self-care, ventilate feelings about effects of surgery, and identify support systems.			

Aspect of Care	Date ___ Pre-admission/Pre-op	Date ___ Day 1 (DOS)	Date ___ Day 2 (POD #1)	Date ___ Day 3 (POD #2)
Assessment	Systems assessment. Preop checklist. Psychosocial assessment.	*PACU* Systems assessment. Pain assessment. VS q 15 min × 4, q 30 min × 4. Check abdominal dressing for drainage. Assess vaginal discharge with VS checks. *Postop* Pain assessment. VS q 1 h × 4, then q 4 h. Check abdominal dressing and vaginal discharge with VS checks. Systems assessment.	VS QID. Monitor abdominal dressing. Breath sounds and bowel sounds q 8 h. Check for spontaneous voiding after Foley removal.	VS q 8 h. Assess incision for S/S of infection. Assess for BM.
Teaching	Preop teaching regarding surgical procedure, incision, pain management, and postop expectations. Review plan of care/clinical pathway with patient and family.	Orient to hospital and unit. Teach/demonstrate procedure of DB & C and incentive spirometer. Remind patient to report excessive bleeding or severe pain. Reinforce basic understanding of surgical procedure.	Teach additional pain relief measures, such as muscle relaxation and visual imagery. Teach perineal care procedure.	Review discharge instructions regarding: Wound care. Pain management. Physical activity. Sexual activity. Complications. Physical changes. Meds.
Consults	N/A	Social worker.	N/A	N/A

Lab tests	Admission labs. INR(PT)/APTT.	Hgb and Hct in PM or next AM.	N/A	N/A
Other tests	Chest x-ray and ECG if >40 years old or history of cardiac disease.	N/A	N/A	N/A
Meds	Prophylactic antibiotic at least 1 h before OR. Preanesthesia meds.	PCA with meperidine or morphine until POD #1 AM. Antiemetic PRN. Toradol IM PRN for breakthrough pain. Antibiotic IVPB q 6–8 h ×3–4 doses.	D/C PCA; switch to Percocet (Tylox) PO or other opioid q 3–4 h PRN.	Percocet or other opioid q 3–4 h PRN. Fleet's enema or suppository if no BM before discharge.
Treatments/interventions	N/A	I & O ×24 h. Perineal care q 4 h W/A. DB & C q 2 h with incentive spirometer. Reinforce abdominal dressing PRN. Emotional support; encourage ventilation of feelings about surgery and body image effects.	Perineal care q 8 h (patient may do own). DB & C q 2 h with incentive spirometer. Reinforce abdominal dressing PRN.	Same as Day 2 (POD #1). MD to change or remove dressing.
Nutrition	NPO after 12 midnight.	NPO except ice chips or sips of H_2O sparingly.	Clear → full liquids; progress as tolerated if bowel sounds present.	DAT
Lines/tubes/monitors	N/A	Continuous IV fluids. Foley catheter. Monitor Foley output and measure q 8 h.	D/C Foley if urine clear and output adequate. D/C IV fluids when patient voids and takes adequate PO fluids without nausea.	N/A
Mobility/self-care	Activity ad lib.	Dangle at bedside; up in chair with assistance in PM if early AM surgery. Thigh-high antiembolism stockings; ankle pumps and LE ROM q 2 h.	Progressive ambulation. May shower (per MD's order). Thigh-high antiembolism stockings.	Same as Day 2.
Discharge planning	N/A	Assess home situation for support systems and financial status.	Reassess home needs and support.	Arrange for follow-up appointment as MD specified. Home health referral if patient is unstable to provide self-care.

*Abbreviations
WNL   Within normal limits
s/s   Signs and symptoms
DB&C   Deep breathe and cough
POD   Postop day
LE   Lower extremities

difficulties. **Adhesions** (fibrous bands that hold parts together that are normally separated) may form and become troublesome when tough fibrous tissues interfere with the normal functions of the internal organs around which they form. If the scar tissue is very large, it may interfere with normal function; for example, a large area of scar tissue in the heart muscle after recovery from a myocardial infarction inhibits the heart's pumping action.

There are two general types of wound healing: (1) healing by primary union, called *first intention;* and (2) healing by secondary union, called *second intention.* In the first type, the two edges of the wound are close together and a crust forms between them to seal the wound. A thin scar results (Figure 4-11). A clean surgical incision where the edges are held close together is an example of healing by first intention.

In healing by second intention, the edges of the wound are far apart and cannot be brought together (Figure 4-12). Usually a large amount of tissue is lost because of **necrosis** (tissue death) or severe physical trauma. The area in the middle fills with granulation tissue, and the wound heals from the edges inward. A pressure ulcer is an example of a wound that must heal by second intention.

Factors Promoting Wound Healing   Adequate rest, sufficient blood supply, and proper nutrition all promote wound healing. Resting or immobilizing the area in which the wound is located prevents disruption of the healing tissues. This is especially true of wounds that heal slowly, such as a broken bone. Rest decreases the metabolic rate and allows nutrients to be available for healing rather than being used for the energy of activity.

Blood contains the amino acids and other elements needed for rebuilding tissue and is essential to healing. Good circulation ensures that the blood reaches the wound. Blood flow also is necessary to remove the waste products of metabolism and the inflammatory process from the wound site. **A lack of exercise during bed rest**

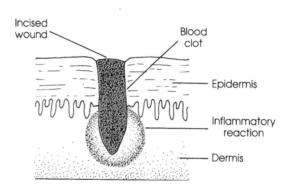

A. Incised wound is held together by a blood clot and possibly by sutures or surgical clamps. An inflammatory process begins in adjacent tissue at the moment of injury.

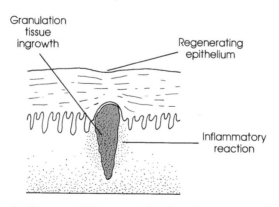

B. After several days, granulation tissue forms as a result of migration of fibroblasts to the area of injury and formation of new capillaries. Epithelial cells at the wound margin migrate to the clot and seal the wound. Regenerating epithelium covers the wound.

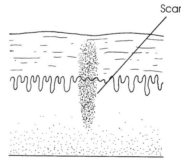

C. Scarring occurs as granulation tissue matures and injured tissue is replaced with connective tissue.

FIGURE 4-11   Wound healing by primary, or first, intention. In primary wound healing there is no tissue loss.

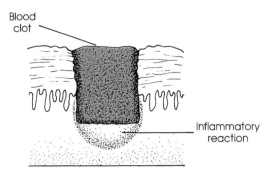

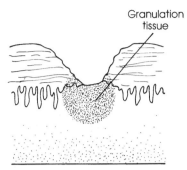

A. Open area is more extensive; inflammatory reaction is more widespread and tends to become chronic.

C. Fibroblasts and capillary buds migrate toward the center of the wound to form granulation tissue, which becomes a translucent red color as the capillary network develops. Granulation tissue is fragile and bleeds easily.

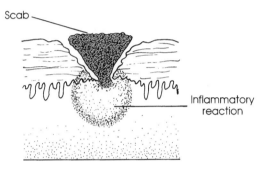

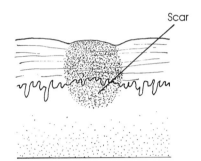

B. Healing may occur under a scab formed of dried exudate or dried plasma proteins and dead cells (eschar).

D. As granulation tissue matures, marginal epithelial cells migrate and proliferate over connective tissue base to form a scar. Contraction of skin around the scar is a result of movement of epithelial cells toward the center of the wound in an attempt to close the defect. The surrounding skin also moves toward the center of the wound in an effort to close the defect.

FIGURE 4-12 Healing by second intention occurs when there is tissue loss, as in extensive burns and deep ulcers. The healing process is more prolonged than in healing by primary intention, because large amounts of dead tissue must be removed and replaced with viable cells.

slows blood flow to healing tissues. Active or passive range of motion exercise promotes good circulation as should be encouraged every 2 hours while the patient is awake.

Vitamins, minerals, and trace elements are essential for adequate wound healing. *Vitamin A* is needed for the creation of collagen for scar formation and for the growth of epithelial cells over **denuded** (without protective covering) surfaces. The *B vitamin complex* is necessary for proper functioning of the enzyme system. *Vitamin C* is necessary for collagen production, the formation of capillaries that bring blood to the healing tissues, and resistance to infection. *Vitamin K* plays an important role in normal clotting. The minerals zinc,

copper, and iron assist in the formation of collagen. *Proteins* provide the amino acids that are the building blocks of tissue and are vital to the healing process.

Factors Interfering with Wound Healing **Smoking produces a decrease in the amount of hemoglobin available to carry oxygen to the healing tissues. Healing time in cigarette smokers is prolonged.** Mechanical injury from friction, pressure, or abrasion, such as can occur when tape is removed, disrupts the healing tissue and prolongs wound healing. Physical injury destroys granulation tissue, which is the framework on which new cells grow and mature to form a covering for the wound. All healing wounds should be handled gently and shielded from injury. When dressings are removed from a wound, care must be taken not to dislodge the granulation tissue.

Corticosteroid drugs that depress the immune system also suppress inflammation and delay healing. Many drugs used to treat cancer have the same effect.

The presence of pathogenic organisms in a wound prolongs the inflammatory process and delays healing. **Sterile technique is used in the care of the wound so that no infectious agents are introduced.** Antiinfective drugs are sometimes given postoperatively to prevent wound infection, and they should be administered at the times ordered to maintain appropriate blood levels of the drug.

Excessive stress, apprehension, and emotional disturbances seem to make the body more vulnerable to invasion by foreign organisms by depressing the immune system. When it is under excessive stress, the body also is less able to mobilize the elements and cells that promote healing.

The manner in which a person is physically handled, the tone of voice used in speaking to him, and the availability of others to listen to him can have profound effects on his physical condition. We must not forget that nursing is a healing profession. Much of what is done to, for, and with a patient reflects a willingness to use one's self to heal another.

During her studies on "therapeutic touch," which attempted to measure in a scientific manner the effects of "laying-on of hands with the intent to heal," Dr. Dolores Krieger became convinced the *intent to heal* another is a critical factor. Noting that even the most basic of nursing skills cannot be performed without the act of touching the patient, Dr. Krieger contends that touch can be therapeutic when used appropriately.

Elder Care Point... The elderly patient's wounds heal more slowly than the young adult's. The elderly person often has chronic diseases that interfere with oxygenation and transport of nutrients to the cells and removal of wastes from the cells. Vitamin and mineral deficiencies are common in the elderly, contributing to poor wound healing. Regeneration of tissue takes more time, partially because of the slower metabolic rate that occurs with age.

Interventions for Wound Care   The surgical wound should be inspected at least daily and more often if dressings are changed more than once a day. Assessment includes observing the incision line for signs of excessive swelling, formation of a **hematoma** (blood-filled swelling), **seroma** (serum-filled swelling), redness, and tearing of the skin or other signs of separation of the edges of the skin that have been sutured together. Normally, a surgical wound is sealed within hours and little drainage

is expected. If there is evidence of bleeding, **purulence** (pus), or any other sign that the wound is not healing as it should, this should be reported and documented.

The best way to prevent *nosocomial* (hospital acquired) infection of a surgical wound is always to wash your hands before doing wound care or touching the patient, use aseptic technique and standard precautions for dressing changes, and change the dressings as frequently as ordered.

Additional factors that may slow wound healing in a postoperative patient include vomiting, abdominal distention, and strenuous respiratory efforts, such as coughing and forcefully exhaling breaths of air without proper splinting of the incision. Nursing interventions for the patient with nausea and vomiting are covered in Chapter 6. Abdominal distention usually is relieved by inserting a NG tube attached to a suction device. Care of a patient with a tube of this kind is discussed in Chapter 20. The wound should be properly splinted for coughing (Figure 4-2 on p. 60).

Tubes and drains.   Tubes and drains are used to remove fluid and air from around the operative site or from a body structure such as the stomach, intestine, or urinary bladder. Each tube must be kept **patent** (open), and there should be some evidence of the expected drainage—urine, bile, stomach contents, serosanguinous fluid—coming through it.

Although the purpose of a specific tube inserted during surgery will be discussed in more detail in appropriate chapters throughout this text, **the importance of monitoring tubes and drains cannot be emphasized enough.** In general, tubes are inserted into the stomach (NG tubes) to remove gastric fluids and air, chest cavity (thoracotomy or chest tube) to remove air thereby reinflating the lung or to remove blood or fluid, and the bladder (urinary catheters) to empty urine. *Drains* are used to (1) prevent accumulation of fluids or air at the operative site; (2) protect suture lines; and (3) remove specific fluids, such as bile, cerebrospinal fluid, or drainage from an abscess. Some drains require continuous suction and are therefore connected to some type of apparatus that creates suction to facilitate removal of drainage. If a drain is kinked, the accumulated fluid and gas can cause pain, create dead air space (which delays healing), damage the healing tissue at the suture lines, and delay healing by compressing surrounding capillaries and cutting off oxygen supply to the cells.

Another kind of drain system is the closed-wound suction device (e.g., Hemovac). The drainage catheter is connected to a spring-loaded drum, collapsed periodically to create the desired suction, that pulls fluid into a collection area of the device. *Jackson-Pratt* suction devices are about the size of the bulb on a blood pressure

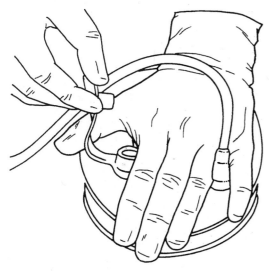

A. Hemovac.

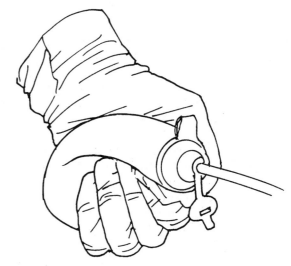

B. Jackson-Pratt bulb.

FIGURE 4-13   Reactivating surgical wound suction devices. (*Source:* deWit, S. C. (1994). *Rambo's Nursing Skills for Clinical Practice,* 4th ed. Philadelphia: Saunders, p. 850.)

cuff. They have a valve on top that is opened to allow removal of fluid and collapse of the bulb and then is closed to create negative pressure, which provides the suction. As drainage accumulates in the bulb, it is emptied and recompressed (Figure 4-13).

Nursing responsibilities for drains include the following:

◆ Frequent monitoring to ensure that the drain is open and working as it should.

◆ Keeping the suction device functioning by checking it frequently and recollapsing it as necessary.

◆ **Using strict aseptic technique and standard precautions when changing dressings or emptying the drainage.**

◆ Changing the dressings around the drain site at least every 8 hours or more often if so ordered by the physician.

◆ Measuring amount of drainage in the collection device and recording it as output. Sometimes, when there is a significant amount of drainage oozing from around the drain and onto the dressings, it is important to estimate the amount, especially if it is bright red from blood.

◆ Assessing the skin around the area where the drain exits from the body and documenting the status of the skin and cleansing the area.

Drains that do not attach to a suction device either are attached to a drainage bag or have dressings placed to catch the fluid. An example of a drain is the *Penrose,* which is inserted into the abdominal cavity or any other area where an abscess, fistula, or other condition requires drainage.

Dressings. Surgical dressings should be checked each time vital signs are taken for the first 24 hours after surgery, every 4 hours during the next 24 hours, and then at least every 8 hours as long as the surgical wound is covered with a dressing. If drainage is outlined and the time and date noted, the nurse can tell if the wound is draining more than it should be over a period of hours. The surgeon usually does the first dressing change. If the dressing becomes saturated before this, it should be reinforced. The outer dressings are removed, leaving those in direct contact with the wound, and new dressings are secured in place. When there is excessive drainage, the dressing probably will require reinforcing or changing every 4 hours. Changing the dressing more often than this is not recommended because of the danger of introducing infectious agents, traumatizing the wound, and interfering with the regeneration of tissue.

Each time the dressing is changed, the amount and characteristics of drainage on it should be noted and documented. If the wound is infected, the odor of the drainage can give a clue as to the kind of organism causing the infection. A musty odor is characteristic of aerobic organisms. An acrid or putrid odor is characteristic of anaerobes. Anaerobic infections are frequently seen in colorectal and vaginal surgery.

Removing sutures and staples. When an order is written to remove sutures or staples, the nurse checks the order, gathers the proper equipment, informs the patient about the procedure, correctly identifies the patient, washes her hands, gloves, and inspects the incision carefully. For a long incision or an incision over a joint, remove every other suture or staple first. If the edges of the incision do not pull apart, remove the rest of the sutures or staples. Often *steri-strips* (small, reinforced strips of adhesive) are applied to hold the incision together until healing is complete.

◆ Complications of Surgical Wounds

Wound Infection   Infection of a wound can occur in any surgical procedure, but it is more common in old wounds caused by accidental injury and in those that were infected at the time of surgery. A few doses of antibiotics may be ordered to prevent the occurrence of postoperative wound infection. If a wound infection is not caused by organisms that were introduced prior to hospitalization or surgery, the infection is considered **nosocomial** (hospital acquired).

> Improper sterilization (i.e., improper handling of sterilized equipment and supplies), poor handwashing, and incorrect aseptic techniques are responsible for the nosocomial infections caused by doctors, nurses, and other health care workers.

In patients with an intact immune system, infection causes inflammation. See Table 4-10 for a review of the inflammatory process. The nurse should assess for signs and symptoms of wound infection by looking for pain, redness, swelling and hardness in the area, purulent drainage, fever, increased pulse rate, an elevated white blood cell (WBC) count, or swollen lymph nodes in adjacent areas. **If an infection is going to develop, it usually becomes apparent 2 to 7 days postoperatively.** For most patients this means that they will already be at home when postoperative infection becomes evident. **Subjective complaints that may indicate infection include fatigue, loss of appetite, headache, nausea, or general malaise or pain.**

> Any patient with a surgical incision is at risk of developing a nosocomial infection, and "Risk for infection" should be a nursing diagnosis on the care plan.

Should an infection occur, cultures are obtained and appropriate antibiotics are given for a specific time. Wound irrigations may be ordered for an open, infected wound. The physician orders the appropriate irrigating solution. Fluids that are often used include sterile normal saline, hydrogen peroxide diluted with sterile water, providone-iodine solution, or acetic acid. The wound may be packed with dressings moistened with one of these solutions.

> A noninfected wound should not be cleaned or irrigated with anything but sterile normal saline as other substances irritate the tissue and slow healing.

Category-specific isolation precautions or body substance precautions are instituted when a wound is

---

TABLE 4-10 ◆ *Review of the Inflammatory Process*

- Inflammation is an immediate response of the body to any kind of injury to its cells and tissues.
- The inflammatory process can be induced by mechanical, chemical, and infectious microorganisms.
- The terms *infection* and *inflammation* do not mean the same thing. *Inflammation* is a localized protective response brought on by injury or destruction of tissues. *Infection* means that the inflamed area has been invaded by infectious agents.
- Changes due to the inflammatory process occur at the site of injury and may occur systemically.
- Changes involve
  Cells of the damaged tissues and adjacent connective tissues release histamine and serotonins, triggering the inflammatory response.
  Blood vessels in and near the site of injury constrict and then dilate, bringing more blood to the damaged cells.
  Blood cells, particularly the leukocytes (neutrophils in particular) are released from the bone marrow and transported to the injury site.
  Monocytes from the mononuclear phagocyte system become macrophages and migrate to the inflammatory site; here they ingest foreign particles and dead tissue.
  The immune system produces specific antibodies and antitoxins in response to the infectious agent or harmful substance; transported to the inflammation site, these substances attack foreign cells and neutralize the poisons these cells produce.
  The hormonal system releases aldosterone, which stimulates the inflammatory process; or cortisone may be released, which has an antiinflammatory action.
- The basic purposes of the inflammatory response are to:
  Neutralize and destroy harmful agents.
  Limit their spread to other tissues in the body.
  Prepare the damaged tissues for repair (Figure 5-6).
- Increased blood flow to the affected area produces heat and redness.
- Increased permeability of the capillaries and leakage of fluid from the blood into the tissue spaces around the cells result in swelling.
- The chemicals released by the defensive cells and the accumulation of fluid in the area irritate the nerve endings and produce pain.
- Movement is inhibited to lessen pain, causing a loss of motion in the affected part.
- Laboratory tests will show an elevated white blood cell (WBC) count if inflammation is systemic.

---

infected. Gowns, as well as gloves, are worn when performing dressing changes or wound irrigations on infected wounds. If splattering is likely, protective eye wear and masks are also worn. **Dirty dressings and supplies are bagged in plastic barrier bags and deposited in a biohazard trash receptacle. Dressings from an infected wound should never be placed in the patient's room trash container.**

Dehiscence and Evisceration   Throughout the period following abdominal surgery, the nurse must be alert for possible disruption or separation of some or all the layers of the surgical wound. This is called **dehiscence**. If the wound completely separates and the contents of the abdominal cavity (viscera) protrude through the incision, the condition is called **evisceration**.

Dehiscence can occur at any time during the postoperative period, but it most commonly occurs between the 5th and 12th postoperative day. The separation or disruption usually is brought on by a sudden strain or stress on the suture lines, as for example when the patient sneezes, coughs, or has an episode of retching and vomiting.

Patients who are most at risk for dehiscence and evisceration are those who are obese, malnourished, or dehydrated, have a malignancy, have experienced multiple trauma to the abdomen, or have an infected wound. Abdominal distention, strenuous coughing, and broken sutures also are factors in wound disruption.

When the nurse checks an abdominal surgical wound, she should be particularly aware of any drainage on the dressing. In about half the cases of dehiscence, there is a noticeable increase in the amount of **serosanguinous** (i.e., composed of serum and blood) drainage on the wound dressing before the separation of the wound layers becomes apparent. Subjectively, the patient may not notice any symptoms until he feels something "give way" in the wound.

Needless to say, wound dehiscence and evisceration can be upsetting events for the patient and his nurse. They create an emergency that requires immediate surgery and are very serious complications. Between the time the dehiscence and exposure of the intestines occur and surgery is done, the wound should be covered with either a sterile towel or dressing moistened with sterile normal saline. For the home care patient, a sterile gauze moistened with sterile water, or if that is unavailable, fresh water, should be placed over the exposed bowel. The object is to keep the bowel membrane moist. The patient should notify the home care agency or the doctor immediately, call someone to help, and lie down with the moistened dressings in place.

Think about . . . Can you identify seven assessment findings that together would indicate that the patient most likely has a wound infection?

COMPLICATIONS OF SURGERY

◆ Hemorrhage and Shock

The two most common complications of anesthesia and surgery are shock and infection. Of these, shock presents the most immediate danger to the patient, as it can quickly develop into a life-threatening emergency condition. The person in shock is suffering from a disruption of blood flow. This disruption can result from (1) failure of the heart to function as a pump *(cardiogenic shock),* as in cardiac arrest (see Chapter 19); (2) a low volume of blood *(hypovolemia),* as in hemorrhage; (3) collapse of the blood vessels as a result of faulty nervous system regulation *(neurogenic shock)* (see Chapter 14); (4) **anaphylaxis** (severe, allergic reaction), as in hypersensitivity to a drug or other allergen (see Chapter 7); and (5) sepsis, occurring when the toxins from bacteria bring about a relaxation and dilation of blood vessels with a resultant drop in blood pressure (see Chapter 6).

In the immediate postoperative period the patient is most likely to suffer from cardiogenic, hypovolemic, or neurogenic shock. However, any of the five kinds of shock are a possibility after anesthesia and surgery. The symptoms of shock depend to some degree on the cause of circulatory failure.

With hypovolemic shock from hemorrhage the patient may complain of thirst, restlessness, and blurred vision.

Patients with neurogenic and cardiac shock may not present any warning signs of impending shock other than changes in the vital signs.

As the shock progresses, the blood pressure begins to drop. The pulse rate increases and may be bounding at first, but becomes thready and indistinct as circulatory collapse occurs. The skin becomes cold and clammy, and pallor becomes evident. There may be air hunger, with cyanosis of the lips and nail beds as a result of tissue hypoxia. As shock deepens, the blood pressure continues to fall, and the patient loses consciousness, eventually becoming comatose. Unrelieved shock ultimately is fatal.

Assessment of the postoperative patient must include frequent monitoring for the signs and symptoms of shock. Vital signs must be monitored frequently regardless of the type of anesthesia used during the operation. Urine output should be more than 30 mL per hour. Less than this amount may indicate inadequate blood circulation to the kidneys and can be a sign of beginning shock. Both general and local anesthesia can bring about circulatory collapse. If there is evidence that the patient is in the early stage of shock, he should be placed in the supine position with the lower extremities elevated to add blood volume to the vital organs. **Patients in cardiogenic shock are placed in a Fowler's position to lower the diaphragm** and increase oxygenation as long as they do not become too hypotensive. Pain contributes to the progression of shock, but large doses of narcotics can add to low blood pressure.

Intravenous fluids and medications are important to prevent and treat shock. They must be given as ordered, and the patient's response to them must be observed and recorded. Supplemental oxygen also is usually given to combat tissue hypoxia and cardiac response. Table 17-8 presents care guidelines for the patient experiencing hypovolemic shock.

Think about . . . After consulting Table 17-8, describe the measures you would take if you suspected that your patient was experiencing hemorrhagic shock.

◆ Pneumonia

Hypostatic or bacterial pneumonia occurs most frequently after surgery in the elderly, the immobile patient, and in those who have had abdominal or chest surgery. Aspiration pneumonia can occur in any patient who experiences regurgitation and aspiration of stomach secretions into the airway and lungs. **Careful positioning, certainty that the gag reflex has returned before giving the patient anything by mouth, and medicating for nausea before vomiting begins can help to prevent aspiration pneumonia.**

Elder Care Point . . . Vital capacity, forced expiratory volumes, and maximum breathing capacity decrease with age. Muscle tone and sensitivity to stimuli decrease, making laryngeal, pharyngeal, and other airway reflexes less effective. This increases the risk of aspiration in the elderly patient.

Other types of pneumonia can be prevented by diligent deep-breathing and coughing, use of an incentive spirometer, and early, frequent, ambulation. Signs of pneumonia include fever, malaise, increased sputum, purulent sputum, cough, flushed skin, dyspnea, pain on inspiration, and abnormal breath sounds, such as crackles and rhonchi. The treatment of the pneumonia depends on the cause. Sputum cultures are performed, and if a microorganism is responsible, an antimicrobial agent is ordered.

◆ Thrombophlebitis

Signs and symptoms of thrombophlebitis include pain or warmth in the calf, warmth to the touch over the area, swelling, and temperature elevation. Treatment includes keeping the patient well hydrated and administration of heparin by SC injection or IV infusion.

◆ Pulmonary Embolus

Although pulmonary embolus is not a common complication of surgery, it can and does occur. It is seen most frequently 2 to 14 days postoperatively and mostly occurs in those who have thrombophlebitis or preexisting irregular heart beats, particularly *atrial fibrillation*. **Signs and symptoms include sudden onset of shortness of breath, anxiety, chest pain, rapid pulse and respirations, cough, bloody sputum, and cyanosis.** Treatment is directed at dissolving the clot or removing it if it is large and at preventing further clots. After diagnostic lung scans and other tests, continuous heparin infusion often is ordered.

◆ Malignant Hyperthermia

Malignant hyperthermia (MH) is a complication of general anesthesia that is life-threatening. It occurs in genetically predisposed people. Agents that may trigger MH include halothane, isoflurane, enflurane, and succinylcholine. It occurs from a biochemical reaction. Signs of MH include high temperature, cardiac dysrhythmia, muscle rigidity of the jaw or other muscles, hypotension, tachypnea, and dark cola-colored urine. The temperature may rise up to 111.2°F (44°C). The extremely high temperature is a late sign. The anesthesiologist and surgeon should be notified immediately if any of these signs occur. If it is not treated swiftly and effectively, MH kills the patient. Treatment is the medication dantrolene. The patient is immediately placed on a hypothermia blanket, ice bags are applied, and iced saline may be administered.

◆ Fluid Imbalance

Because of the stress on the body induced by surgery and anesthesia, fluid shifts occur within the body. Intravenous fluids are administered while the patient is NPO. The most frequent fluid imbalance is overhydration. **Signs and symptoms include crackles in the lungs, edema, weight gain, restlessness, and confusion.** Output should be greater than input during the first 72 hours after surgery and anesthesia.

Dehydration also can occur at times with signs and symptoms such as weight loss, diminished pulse, dry mucous membranes, decreased tissue turgor, and feelings of thirst. The nurse can monitor for these imbalances by auscultating the lungs each shift, monitoring the intake and output, weight, and skin turgor, and checking for edema.

Hydration status must be carefully assessed, as elderly patients can become quickly dehydrated from vomiting. Circulatory overload from too much or too rapid administration of IV fluid also can occur. Mild to moderate confusion from fluid and electrolyte shifts is not uncommon in the early postoperative period. Family members need to be assured that this is most likely a temporary state.

Treatment is aimed at identifying the reason for the imbalance, giving fluids for dehydration, restricting fluids for excess, and administering a diuretic if ordered.

◆ Ileus

Patients who have had trauma to the abdomen, experience shock, have respiratory problems, or have a metabolic disturbance are at great risk for intestinal problems related to inadequate peristalsis. Such a condition is termed *adynamic ileus, paralytic ileus,* or simply **ileus.** This is not a common postoperative problem.

Because there is little or no peristaltic action when ileus occurs, fluids and gas accumulate in the intestine and cause distention. If the condition continues unchecked, the enlarged abdomen causes difficulty in breathing, while the intestinal fluids press against blood vessels and impede venous return of blood. The patient is in danger of developing atelectasis, pneumonia, hypovolemia due to escape of fluids from the blood into the intestinal tract, and metabolic alkalosis.

Subjective signs of ileus include complaints of abdominal pain and tenderness and nausea. Objective signs include increasing expansion of the abdominal girth due to abdominal distention, the absence of bowel sounds, no passage of either feces or gas rectally, and vomiting. Because of upward pressure against the diaphragm, the patient has increasing difficulty breathing and is subject to atelectasis and pneumonia. Impairment of venous return can lead to decreased cardiac output, diminished flow of urine (**oliguria**), and a decrease in blood pressure. If the buildup of gas and fluid in the intestine is not relieved, there is a potential for wound dehiscence and evisceration. Regular ambulation and light abdominal massage are helpful in encouraging the passage of gas.

Any and all symptoms of adynamic ileus should be reported and well documented. The diagnosis is confirmed by x-ray, which shows a dilated bowel with accumulations of gas throughout the intestine.

The condition is usually relieved by inserting an NG tube or Miller-Abbott tube attached to suction for decompression. This removes the accumulated fluids and gas and often allows the bowel to return to its normal position and function. The passage of flatus and fecal material and the return of bowel sounds indicate that peristalsis has returned. If intubation and decompression do not relieve the distention, surgery may be necessary to relieve an intestinal obstruction.

◆ Urinary Retention

Patients need to void within 8 to 10 hours of surgery. A common problem following surgery is retention of urine in the bladder. It can occur as a result of anesthetic medication, narcotics, trauma to the bladder or urethra during the operation, or anxiety and fear of pain.

Subjective data for urinary retention include complaints of fullness and pressure in the bladder region. Objective signs include distention of the bladder, which can be noted by palpation and observation, and either total absence of urinary output or dribbling of small amounts of urine (not more than 50 mL), which indicates retention with overflow. **When a patient has difficulty voiding after surgery, this information should be shared in the change-of-shift report.**

The nurse can use any of a number of methods to induce voiding; catheterization is used only when other measures fail. Some nursing actions that do not require a physician's order include providing privacy for the patient, warming the bedpan before placing it in position, helping the patient to stand or sit to void, and applying gentle, but firm, pressure over the bladder. Hearing the sound of running water or placing hands in water also help some patients, as does pouring warm water over the perineum, which has the effect of relaxing the muscles, thereby encouraging urination. Blowing through a straw into a glass of water while on the commode or bedpan is sometimes effective for female patients.

◆ Urinary Tract Infection

Urinary tract infection may occur as a result of surgery on the urinary system, bedrest, inadequate fluids, preexisting low-grade infection, and poor aseptic technique during urinary catheterization or from an indwelling urinary catheter. **Signs and symptoms include pain on urination, frequent need to urinate, foul-smelling urine, or cloudy urine.** Treatment is to force fluids, unless contraindicated, obtain a urine culture and sensitivity, and treat the responsible microorganism with an antimicrobial agent.

The postoperative complication of renal failure is not nearly so common as urinary retention. It is, however, a very serious condition that requires extensive treatment. Renal failure is discussed in more detail in Chapter 23. Signs of renal failure include decreasing urine output or lack of urination.

Think about . . . Can you identify four types of patients or situations where the patient would be at risk for a urinary tract infection?

PROMOTING PSYCHOLOGICAL ADJUSTMENT

The patient may experience anxiety postoperatively over the outcome of the surgery of life-style changes that the surgery will cause. They may be concerned about the ability to perform self-care or acceptance of an altered body or health status by family and friends.

Depending on the type of surgery performed, the patient may experience considerable change in body image. If there is extensive scarring, a body image change is likely. If part of an extremity an organ, or part of a breast has been lost, the necessary psychological adjustment is considerable. Such adjustment takes a lot of time. The patient should be assessed for signs of ineffective coping, such as withdrawn, depressed behavior, less attention to grooming than before, and poor communication efforts. If these signs occur, the nurse should work with the patient to identify areas of concern and then collaborate with the other health team members to develop a plan of assistance.

The nurse can help the patient by encouraging talking about feelings regarding what has been lost and the effect it might have on the patient's life. Being an active listener and gradually having the patient focus on the positives in life rather than on the loss incurred, is helpful. Referral to an appropriate community support group with people who have undergone a similar loss and are learning to cope can be very helpful. The nurse cannot solve the patient's problem, but he can listen. He can help the patient to draw on her own strengths to overcome this loss.

DISCHARGE PLANNING

With same-day surgery and early release from the hospital after in-patient surgery, it is vital that discharge planning be started at admission or several days before the surgery. Needs for home care must be assessed. Will the patient need assistance with bathing? Meals? Dressing changes? It may be necessary to arrange home health care with an aide to assist with bathing and a nurse to assess the patient's condition and attend to his wound. Equipment, such as oxygen, suction, or an IV pump, may need to be ordered before discharge so that the transition to home goes smoothly.

The family or significant others must be included in discharge planning and teaching. Often it is a family member who will do the dressing changes, monitor for side effects of medication, alert the physician to signs of complications, and be generally supportive to the patient during recovery.

When the patient is discharged, the nurse reviews specific instructions regarding care at home, including care of incision or wound, diet, activity level, medications, and signs and symptoms of complications to report. The nurse makes certain the patient understands when he is next to see the doctor. Sufficient supplies of items needed for dressing changes are sent home with the patient, and he is told where such items can be obtained. The nurse makes every attempt to see to it that the patient does not go home with unanswered questions concerning his care.

COMMUNITY CARE

The patient may be given follow-up care at an outpatient clinic, doctor's office, subacute care unit, extended-care unit, or the home. The home care nurse may be a "private duty" nurse staying with one patient for a full shift or may be visiting several patients per day. The nurse assesses the patient's condition and progress and performs treatments and procedures such as wound care. The nurse case manager will coordinate the care of the whole team, collaborating with the social worker, the physical therapist, respiratory therapist, nurse aide, dietitian, pharmacist, physician, and other health professionals. The quality of nursing care delivered often is the factor that prevents complications and rehospitalization of the patient.

The home care, office, or outpatient clinic nurse must reinforce teaching about the signs and symptoms of complications, such as infection, dehiscence, or thrombophlebitis, and verify that the patient can adequately perform his own self-care. Some physicians discharge patients who are ambulatory and normally self-sufficient thinking that they can do complicated wound care. This is often not the case; most patients need assistance with anything more than a simple dressing change. This is particularly true if the patient lives alone. The nurse collaborates with the patient, physician, social worker, and community agencies to secure the assistance the patient needs.

Think about . . . Which health care professionals would it be necessary to collaborate with to plan appropriate continuing care for the elderly patient who has had a hip replacement (and also has chronic lung disease) and is being discharged home to the care of her 76-year-old husband?

CRITICAL THINKING EXERCISES

Clinical Case Problems

Read each clinical case problem and discuss the questions with your classmates.

1. You are assigned to care for a 37-year-old male who just had a surgical repair of a ventral hernia with spinal anesthesia. He is a same-day surgery patient.

   a. How does the care of this patient differ from that of a patient who had inhalation anesthesia?

   b. If this patient has difficulty voiding after surgery, how could you assist him?

   c. If he develops a spinal headache, what measures could be taken to decrease his discomfort?

2. This is your first day on a surgical unit. You are assigned a patient who is scheduled for surgery at 10:00 AM. He has preoperative medication ordered: "Demerol 50 mg, Phenergan 35 mg, and atropine 0.04 mg IM on call." You also are assigned two other patients who are ambulatory.

   a. List what you would check in the surgery patient's chart as part of his preoperative preparation.

   b. Describe the steps you would take to complete the preoperative checklist and charting for this surgical patient in your assigned hospital.

   c. What steps are necessary in preparing and administering the preoperative medication?

3. Mrs. Johnson just had a colon resection for a tumor. You are assisting with her care in the PACU. She is waking up, but is still groggy. Her breathing is somewhat shallow.

   a. What would you do to improve her respiratory status?

   b. Describe the method used to manually open the airway.

4. Mrs. Hanson, a 78-year-old female, returned to the nursing unit from surgery 1 hour ago. She underwent an abdominal hysterectomy and exploration for cancer of the uterus. She has an IV infusion running into the right forearm. Her blood pressure has gradually fallen from 138/88 to 102/62. She is restless, complains of thirst, and is anxious.

   a. What assessments would you make?

   b. What actions would you take? In what order would you perform these actions?

BIBLIOGRAPHY

Agency for Health Care Policy and Research. (1992). *Acute pain management in adults: operative procedures.* (AHCPR Pub. No. 92-0019). Rockville, MD: U.S. Department of Health and Human Services.

Ball, K. A. (1990). The basics of laser technology. *Nursing Clinics of North America.* 25(3):619–634.

Barret, J. B., Deehan, R. M. (1992). Preoperative patient teaching: A video approach. *Nursing 92.* 22(2):32F, 32H.

Bove, L. A. (1994). How fluids and electrolytes shift after surgery. *Nursing 94.* 24(8):34–39.

Brockopp, D. Y., et al. (1994). Postoperative pain: getting a grip on the facts. *Nursing 94.* 24(6):49.

Burden, N. (1992). Telephone follow-up of ambulatory surgery patients following discharge is a nursing responsibility. *Journal of Post Anesthesia Nursing.* 7(4):256–261.

Campbell, A., Johnston, C. A. (1991). OR-PACU reports: what they should tell you about your postoperative patient. *Nursing 91.* 21(10):49.

Carroll, P. (1992). Using cuffs to prevent clots. *RN.* 55(4):57–59.

Cassidy, J., Marley, R. A. (1996). Preoperative assessment of the ambulatory patient. *Journal of PeriAnesthesia Nursing.* 11(5):334–343.

Chiarella, M. (1991). The role of the nurse in today's operating room. *AORN Journal.* 4(4):15–16.

Dellasega, C., Burgunder, C. (1991). Perioperative nursing care for the elderly surgical patient. *Today's OR Nurse.* 13(6):12–17, 30–32.

deWit, S. C. (1994). *Rambo's Nursing Skills for Clinical Practice,* 4th ed. Philadelphia: Saunders.

Drago, S. S. (1992). Banking on your own blood. *American Journal of Nursing.* 92(3):61–66.

Eddy, M. E., Coslow, B. L. (1991). Preparation for ambulatory surgery: a patient education program. *Journal of Post Anesthesia Nursing.* 7(4):243–250.

Ehrlichman, R. J., et al. (1991). Common complications of wound healing. *Surgical Clinics of North America.* 71(6):1323–1351.

Evans, C., Kenny, P. (1993). Postoperative confusion in the elderly. *NURSEweek.* 6(14):30–31.

Fraulini, K. E., Borchardt, K. C. (1988). Guide to solving postanesthesia problems. *Nursing 88.* May:66.

Gallagher, M. T., Kahn, C. (1990). Lasers: scalpels of light. *RN.* May:46–52.

George, S., Bugwadia, N. (1996). Nutrition and wound healing. *MEDSURG Nursing.* 5(4):272–275.

Good, M. (1995). Relaxation techniques for surgical patients. *American Journal of Nursing.* 95(5):38–43.

Grennan, A. J. (1987). Helping your patient get his strength back . . . first few days at home. *RN.* March:70.

Hinojosa, R. J. (1992). Nursing interventions to prevent or relieve postoperative nausea and vomiting. *Journal of Post Anesthesia Nursing.* 7(1):3–14.

Ignatavicius, D. D., Workman, M. L., Mishler, M. A. (1995). *Medical–Surgical Nursing: A Nursing Process Approach,* 2nd ed. Philadelphia: Saunders.

Johnson, G. M., Bowman, R. J. (1992). Autologous blood transfusion: current trends, nursing implications. *AORN Journal.* 56(2):281–285, 288–293, 296–298.

Jones, P. L., Millman, A. (1990). Wound healing and the aged patient. *Nursing Clinics of North America.* 25(1): 263–277.

Jurf, J. B., Nirschl, A. L. (1993). Acute postoperative pain management: a comprehensive review and update. *Critical Care Nursing Quarterly.* 16(1):8–25.

Kaempf, G., Goralski, V. (1996). Monitoring postop patients.

Kane, A. M., Kurlowicz, L. H. (1994). Improving the postoperative care of acutely-confused older adults. *Medical–Surgical Nursing.* 3(6):453–458.

Krasner, D. (1992). The twelve commandments of wound care. *Nursing 92.* 22(12):34.

Lambert, D. H. (1992). Continuous spinal anesthesia. *Anesthesiology Clinics of North America.* 10(1):87–102.

Lawler, M. (1991). Preventing postop complications: managing other complications. *Nursing 91.* 21(11):33, 40–48.

Leckrone, L. (1991). Preparing your patient for surgery. *Nursing 91.* 21(7):47–49.

Litwack, K. (1991). What you need to know about administering preoperative medications. *Nursing 91.* 21(8): 44–47.

Litwack, K. (1992). Managing postanesthetic emergencies. *Nursing 92.* 21(10):49.

Longinow, L. T., Rzeszewski, L. B. (1993). The holding room: A perioperative advantage. *AORN Journal.* 57(4): 914–924.

Marley, R. A., Moline, B. M. (1996). Patient discharge from the ambulatory setting. *Journal of Post Anesthesia Nursing.* 11(1):39-49. *RN.* 59(7):31–34.

Marley, R. A (1996). Postoperative nausea and vomiting: The outpatient enigma. *Journal of PeriAnesthesia Nursing.* 11(6):147–161.

Marshall, M. (1993). Postoperative confusion: helping your patient emerge from the shadows. *Nursing 93.* 28(1): 44–47.

McConnell, E. A. (1991). Preventing postop complications: minimizing respiratory problems. *Nursing 91.* 21(11): 33–39.

McConnell, E. A. (1992). Assessing postoperative chills and tremors. *Nursing 92.* 22(4):110–114.

McConnell, E. A. (1992). Assessing wound drainage . . . wound dehiscence. *Nursing 92.* 22(7):66.

Meeker, B. J., Rothrock, J. C. (1991). *Alexander's Care of the Patient in Surgery,* 9th ed. St. Louis, MO: Mosby Year Book.

Metzler, D. J., Fromm, C. G. (1993). Laying out a care plan for the elderly postoperative patient. *Nursing 93.* 23(4): 67–74.

Moore, J. L., Rice, E. L. (1992). Malignant hyperthermia. *American Family Physician.* 45(5):2245–2251.

Neal, J. M. (1992). Management of postural puncture headache. *Anesthesiology Clinics of North America.* 10(1): 163–178.

Reichenbach, S. L. (1995). Neuromuscular blockade: when paralysis is intentional. *RN.* 58(6):43–48.

Rowland, M. A. (1990). Myths and facts about postop discomfort. *American Journal of Nursing.* 90 (5):60.

Saleh, K. L. (1993). The elderly patient in the post anesthesia care unit. *Nursing Clinics of North America.* 28(3): 507–518.

Schaefer, A., et al. (1990). Are they ready? Discharge planning for older surgical patients. *Journal of Gerontologic Nursing.* October:16.

Shaw, C., Weaver, C. S., Schneider, L. (1996). *Journal of Post Anesthesia Nursing.* 11(1):13–19.

Somerson, S. J., Husted, C. W., Sicilia, M. R. (1995). Insights into conscious sedation. *American Journal of Nursing.* 95(6):26–32.

Spearing, C., Cornell, D. J. (1988). Incentive spirometry: inspiring your patients to breathe deeply. *Nursing 88.* 18(6):50.

Strong, N. S. (1993). Assessing the postanesthesia patient. *Critical Care Nursing Quarterly.* 16(1):1–7.

Sutherland, E. (1991). Day surgery: all in a day's work. *Nursing Times.* 87(March 13–19):26.

Unkle, D. W. (1990). Postoperative care after the patient's had a spinal. *RN.* September:93.

Walhout, M. F. (1992). Treat for hypothermia. *RN.* 55(4): 50–55.

Walker, J. R. (1996). What is new with inhaled anesthetics: Part 1. *Journal of PeriAnesthesia Nursing, 11(5): 330–333.*

Walsh, J. (1993). Postop effects of OR positioning. *RN.* 56(2):50–58.

Watson, D. S. (1991). Safe nursing practices involving the patient receiving local anesthesia. *AORN Journal.* 53(4): 24–27.

Woodin, L. M. (1993). Cutting postop pain. *RN.* 56(8): 26–34.

Woodin, L. M. (1996). Resting easy: How to care for patients receiving I. V. conscious sedation. *Nursing 96.* 26(6):33–40.

Young, M. S., Kindred, D. (1993). Malignant hyperthermia: not just an operating room emergency. *Medical Surgical Nursing.* 2(1):41–43, 46.

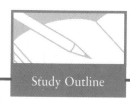

I. Introduction

A. Outpatient surgery is common today.

B. There is limited time in hospitals for preoperative teaching.

II. Changes in Operative Techniques

A. New technology, such as operating microscopes, surgical lasers, and fiberoptic endoscopes, have made less invasive surgery possible.

B. Autologous blood is gathered before surgery so that the patient may receive his or her own blood if a transfusion is needed during or after surgery.

III. Preoperative Period

A. Assessment.

1. Determine the patient's readiness for surgery and identify those most at risk.

2. Chest radiograph; EKG is common if patient is over 40.

3. Laboratory data: blood profile, urinalysis.

4. Nursing assessment.

   a. Vital signs to establish baseline. Report abnormalities.

   b. Allergies and drug idiosyncrasies; current drug history.

   c. Body weight; obesity increases risk: anesthesia, respiratory function, fluid balance, wound healing.

   d. State of nutrition; malnutrition carries greater risk for slow healing.

5. Nursing history.

   a. Smoking: harmful effect on wound healing, clot formation, and pulmonary function.

   b. Diabetes mellitus: risk for variations in blood glucose level, delayed healing, and infection.

   c. Liver disease: jeopardy for excessive bleeding, poor wound healing, and poor detoxification of drugs.

   d. Respiratory disease: patient at greater risk for atelectasis, hypoxemia, and pneumonia.

6. Psychological assessment.

   a. Different expectations for outcome of surgery.

   b. Determine cause of fear and anxiety if possible.

7. Spiritual assessment:

   a. Determine whether patient needs and wants support.

   b. Ask about usual ways of expressing spirituality and finding comfort.

8. Assessment of learning needs.

   a. What do patient and family want to know about?

   b. What do they need to know to reduce anxiety?

B. Planning

1. Be certain preoperative medications are on the unit ahead of time.

2. Verify that the surgical consent form has been signed at the beginning of your shift.

3. Verify what remains to done for the preop checklist; coordinate preop patient care with care for other patients.

C. Intervention—preoperative period

1. General information: preparation for surgery, preoperative routine, recovery room routine, postoperative routine.

2. Assess learning needs and do preoperative teaching for patient and family.

   a. Deep-breathing, coughing, and incentive spirometry techniques.

   b. Leg exercises, how to turn and get in and out of bed.

   c. Measures for pain control.

   d. Diet restrictions and progression postoperatively.

3. Reinforce teaching with available hospital audiovisual materials.

4. Complete preoperative checklist.

5. Preparation for surgery.

   a. Signed consent form.

   b. Diagnostic tests completed.

   c. NPO 8 to 12 hours before surgery.

   d. Cleansing of intestinal tract; use of nasogastric (NG) tube and suction.

   e. Sedation on the night before surgery.

   f. Indwelling urinary catheter.

   g. Intravenous infusion started.

6. Preoperative routine.

   a. Preoperative medication and purpose.

     (1) Reduce anxiety and promote rest.

     (2) Decrease secretions.

(3) Prevent nausea and vomiting.

(4) Enhance anesthesia effect.

b. Removal of jewelry, underwear, hairpins, dentures.

c. ID bracelet checked with chart, verifying name and patient number.

d. Bladder emptied.

e. Preoperative medication given.

f. Side rails up, bed placed in low position, and call bell placed within reach.

g. Documentation completed.

IV. Intraoperative Care

A. Patient taken to anesthesia holding area and checked in.

B. All personnel entering the OR must perform a surgical scrub and wear clean scrub clothes.

C. An intravenous line is inserted.

D. The patient is carefully positioned and padded on the OR table.

E. The skin prep is completed.

F. When the surgical team is ready, the patient is anesthetized.

G. Role of the circulating nurse: monitors for breaks in sterile technique, protects patient safety, supervises and assists scrub person, provides instruments and supplies as needed; assists others to gown and glove; cares for room and equipment; assists with sponge, sharps, and instrument counts; documents all care given.

H. Role of the scrub person: prepares the sterile field and checks instruments; prepares ligatures and sutures; passes instruments and supplies to the surgeon; anticipates needs; performs sponge, sharps, and instrument counts.

V. Anesthesia: Loss of Sensory Perception

A. Types include inhalants, IV anesthetics, regional and topical anesthetics, and hypothermia (see Table 4-3).

B. Objectives of anesthesia: prevent pain, achieve adequate muscle relaxation, calm fear, allay anxiety, and induce forgetfulness.

C. Local anesthetic agents may cause anaphylaxis; precautions must be taken when they are administered.

D. Spinal anesthesia produces complete muscular relaxation, even though the patient remains awake.

E. Conscious sedation with IV opioids and sedatives in conjunction with regional or local anesthesia is used for many minor procedures and for endoscopic procedures.

VI. Hypothermia: Reduction of Body Temperature

A. Used in some types of surgery to lower metabolism and decrease oxygen needs.

B. Methods.

1. External hypothermia: ice packs or other forms of external cold.

2. Extracorporeal hypothermia: rerouting the blood outside the body, through a cooling unit, and back into the body.

3. The patient is rewarmed slowly after surgery.

4. Use of hypothermia being questioned now.

VII. The Elderly Patient in Surgery

A. Patients over age 75 have surgical complication rates three times higher than other adults; body has less physiological reserves.

B. Elderly more likely to have impaired renal, hepatic, respiratory, and cardiac function and more chronic diseases, causing greater vulnerability to fluid and electrolyte imbalances during and after surgery.

C. Older patients with serious depression are at high risk for complications of surgery due to lack of motivation for recovery.

D. Reinforce instruction for elderly patient frequently to enhance retention of information.

E. Elderly patients are at risk for dehydration from preparation for surgery and NPO status.

VIII. Immediate Postoperative Care

A. The patient is totally helpless while recovering from anesthesia.

B. Recovery from general anesthesia generally takes 2 to 6 hours.

C. The postanesthesia care unit (PACU) receives the patient from surgery.

1. The nurse receives a report on the patient from the OR personnel.

2. The patient is closely monitored: vital signs, respiration, circulation, wounds, tubes, drainage, level of consciousness.

3. The PACU nurse meets basic needs of patients; provides comfort and reassurance.

4. Patient is positioned to prevent aspiration and promote respiration; either turned on side or with head turned to the side.

5. The chin-lift, jaw-thrust maneuver is used to keep the tongue from occluding the airway.

6. The recovery area is kept quiet to prevent complications as patients emerge from anesthesia.

7. Pressure points from the operating table are checked and treated.

8. The patient is kept warm.

9. The nurse checks for bladder distention.

10. Suction is turned on and kept close in case the patient vomits.

11. When the patient has awakened, family members often are allowed to visit for a few minutes.

12. Discharge from the PACU is based on a scoring system determining that vital signs, respiration, and circulation are stable.

13. The PACU nurse gives a report on the patient to the staff nurse who will be caring for him.

IX. Care and Discharge From an Ambulatory or Same-Day Surgery Unit

A. Same-day surgery units may be in the hospital or be freestanding.

B. Nurses prepare patients for surgery and monitor them after surgery.

  1. The nurse monitors respiration, circulation, vital signs, neurological status, fluid intake and output, wound drainage and dressings, and comfort level.

  2. Recovery in an ambulatory unit is generally 1 to 3 hours.

  3. When the patient is stable, can ambulate on his own, has emptied his bladder, and is drinking fluids, he is discharged home.

  4. Discharge teaching begins before surgery and is continued when the patient is alert again.

  5. Written discharge instructions are sent home with the patient.

  6. Someone must drive the patient home if he has had general anesthesia.

X. General Postoperative Care

A. Preparation of the postoperative unit is done when the patient is sent to surgery.

  1. The bed is made, "opened," and positioned to receive the patient.

  2. An emesis basin, tissues, frequent vital signs sheet, intake and output sheet, and a pencil are placed by the bed.

  3. Vital signs equipment and any special equipment the patient will need is obtained and connected.

  4. An IV pole is set up.

B. After receiving a report on the patient, the nurse performs her own initial assessment (Table 4-6).

C. The nurse incorporates appropriate nursing diagnoses into the nursing care plan.

D. Specific expected outcomes are written for the goals of postoperative care.

E. The nurse constructs her work plan to include taking frequent vital signs and doing frequent assessments on her fresh postoperative patients.

F. Implementation.

  1. After spinal anesthesia, the side rails are raised even, even though the patient is alert.

  2. Function returns in the reverse order in which it was depressed.

  3. Encouraging fluids containing caffeine may prevent a spinal headache.

  4. Vital signs are assessed q 15 minutes × 4; q 30 minutes × 4; q 1 × 2; then q 4 h.

  5. Interventions are performed to meet the goals of postoperative care.

    a. Promote respiratory function: repositioning q 2 h; turn, cough and deep-breathe q 2 h; auscultate lungs each shift.

    b. Using an incentive spirometer decreases atelectasis and helps to prevent hypostatic pneumonia.

    c. Turning prevents any one portion of the lung from remaining dependent too long, preventing pooling of secretions.

    d. Coughing removes secretions from the lungs and helps to prevent pneumonia.

    e. Abdominal and chest incisions must be splinted while the patient coughs.

    f. A pulse oximeter is used to measure the oxygen saturation in the blood.

    g. Turning, ambulating, and performing range of motion activities promotes circulation.

    h. Performing foot and leg exercises decreases the risk of thrombus formation.

    i. Elastic hose, sequential pneumatic compression devices, or low-dose heparin may be used to prevent thrombophlebitis and pulmonary embolus.

    j. Blood loss may be replaced by autologous transfusion or by donor blood transfusion.

    k. The nurse checks for a positive Homan's sign.

    l. The legs of a patient at risk for thrombus formation are never massaged.

    m. Adequate treatment is necessary to control postoperative pain.

      (1) Continuous, regular doses of pain medication should be given for the first 48 to 72 hours postoperatively.

      (2) A PCA pump or epidural catheter infusion may be used to control pain.

      (3) Patients should be assessed every 3 hours for pain status.

      (4) Alternative comfort measures can do much to relieve pain and increase the effectiveness of pain medication.

      (5) The physician is consulted before giving pain medication if the patient is hypotensive or bradycardic.

(6) Elderly patients often need encouragement to take sufficient pain medication.

(7) Patients taking narcotic analgesics must be monitored for constipation.

n. Adequate sleep is essential for healing.

o. NPO status is maintained until bowel sounds have returned.

p. Protein, vitamins, and trace minerals are all needed to promote healing.

q. The diet progresses from clear liquids, to full liquids, to regular.

r. Patients should be medicated for nausea before they begin to vomit.

s. Providing mouth care after anesthesia may reduce nausea.

t. Discomforts of anesthesia and surgery include thirst, hiccups, and gaseous distention.

u. Constipation may occur from lack of activity, lack of normal diet, and pain medications.

v. Physical activity, particularly ambulation, is the best method of decreasing postoperative discomforts and complications.

w. Patients should be assisted the first few times they are out of bed after surgery in case they become faint or unsteady.

XI. Promoting Wound Healing

A. Pathophysiology of wound healing.

1. The inflammatory response initiates wound healing.

2. Healing occurs by recovery, regeneration, or replacement.

3. Replacement healing causes a scar.

4. Most surgical incisions heal by primary or first intention.

5. Wounds from trauma often heal by secondary intention.

B. Factors that promote wound healing.

1. Adequate rest, sufficient blood supply, and proper nutrition all promote wound healing.

2. Immobilization and rest of the area of the wound prevents disruption of the healing tissue.

C. Factors that interfere with wound healing.

1. Smoking decreases the oxygen carried to the cells.

2. Mechanical injury from friction, pressure, or abrasion disrupts healing tissue.

3. Corticosteroids depress the immune response and slow wound healing.

4. Presence of infection interferes with wound healing.

5. Excessive stress seems to make the body more vulnerable to invasion by foreign organisms by depressing the immune system.

6. A nurse's gentle, caring attitude and attention promote healing.

7. The wounds of the elderly heal more slowly.

D. Interventions for wound care.

1. Observe for bleeding and signs of infection: swelling, redness, pain, pulling of sutures, purulent drainage; document findings.

2. Frequent hand washing and aseptic technique for wound care should be followed to prevent infection.

3. A dressing should be checked with each set of vital signs for the first 24 hours.

4. Dressing reinforced as needed until changed by surgeon; then changed at least q 24 h or q 4 h as needed.

5. Suction device; maintain suction.

a. Amount and characteristics of drainage.

b. Skin care around drain.

c. Dressing; all care with aseptic technique.

6. Removing sutures and staples.

a. Remove every other suture or staple; observe for separation of wound; apply steri-strips; then remove remaining sutures or staples.

E. Complications of surgical wounds.

1. Wound infection.

a. Preventive antiinfectives often prescribed. increased pulse rate, elevated WBC, swollen adjacent lymph nodes.

b. A culture is obtained if infection is suspected.

c. Pain, redness, swelling, purulent drainage, fever, increased pulse rate, elevated WBC, and swollen adjacent lymph nodes are signs of infection.

d. Body substance precautions are used when caring for an infected wound.

2. Dehiscence and evisceration: 5th to 12th day.

a. Risk factors: obesity, malnourishment, wound infection, abdominal distention, multiple trauma, strenuous coughing.

b. Signs and symptoms: increased serosanguinous drainage; feel that wound "gave way."

c. Cover with sterile towel; if viscera are protruding, moisten towel with sterile saline.

XII. Complications of Surgery

A. Hemorrhage and shock.

1. Various types of shock may occur: hypovolemic, cardiogenic, neurogenic, anaphylactic, or septic.

2. With hypovolemic shock from hemorrhage the patient may complain of thirst, restlessness, and blurred vision.

3. Vital sign changes are hallmarks of shock.

4. The blood pressure falls, pulse rate increases and becomes thready, the skin becomes cold and clammy, and pallor becomes evident; respirations increase as air hunger occurs; as shock progresses, urine output falls, and the patient loses consciousness.

5. Unrelieved shock is fatal.

6. Table 17-8 presents the nursing care for the patient experiencing hypovolemic shock.

7. Hypostatic pneumonia occurs after surgery in the elderly, the immobile patient, and in those who had abdominal or chest surgery.

8. Turning, coughing, and deep-breathing every 2 hours and ambulation are the best measures to prevent pneumonia.

9. Signs of pneumonia include fever, malaise, increased sputum, purulent or rusty sputum, cough, flushed skin, dyspnea, pain on inspiration, and abnormal breath sounds, such as crackles and rhonchi.

10. Thrombophlebitis is caused by inflammation of the vein by a thrombus.

11. Signs of pulmonary embolus include sudden onset of shortness of breath, anxiety, chest pain, rapid pulse and respirations, cough, bloody sputum, and cyanosis.

12. Treatment is directed at dissolving the clot and at preventing the formation of further clots; continuous IV heparin is given.

13. Malignant hyperthermia is a complication of anesthesia and occurs in genetically predisposed people.

14. Signs of malignant hyperthermia (MH) include high temperature, cardiac dysrhythmia, muscle rigidity of the jaw or other muscles, hypotension, tachypnea, and dark cola-colored urine.

15. MH may kill if not treated immediately with dantrolene.

16. Fluid imbalance is due to the stress of surgery and anesthesia.

17. Signs of overhydration include crackles in the lungs, edema, weight gain, restlessness, and confusion.

18. The elderly are especially prone to fluid imbalances.

19. Output should be greater than input in the first 72 hours after surgery and anesthesia.

20. Monitor for fluid imbalance by auscultating the lungs each shift, monitoring the intake and output, checking weight, testing skin turgor, and assessing for edema.

21. Adynamic ileus occurs when peristaltic action does not return to normal after surgery and anesthesia.

22. Fluids and gas accumulate in the intestine during ileus, causing distention and pain and interfering with respiration and circulation.

23. Ileus is treated with intestinal intubation if it does not resolve quickly.

24. Urinary retention may occur after surgery and anesthesia and is most common in males.

25. The patient should void within 8 to 10 hours of surgery.

26. If the patient cannot empty his bladder, catheterization is necessary.

27. Urinary tract infection may occur postoperatively when the urinary tract has been entered surgically or by catheterization.

28. Elderly patients who do not empty their bladder completely, are inactive, and are not drinking fluids are at risk for urinary tract infection.

29. Signs and symptoms include burning, urgency, discomfort, and foul-smelling urine.

XIII. **Promoting Psychological Adjustment**

A. When there is a considerable change in body image from loss of a body part, body function, or scarring, the patient may need assistance with adjustment.

B. Allowing the patient to talk about his concerns and grief is beneficial.

C. Active listening and focusing on the patient's strengths and the positives of life help.

D. Referral to a support group may be beneficial.

XIV. **Discharge Planning Begins at the Time of Admission or the Time the Surgery is Scheduled**

A. Collaboration with many health team professionals is essential to provide continuous care through recovery.

B. The patient and family are central to the discharge planning process.

C. Discharge teaching is begun at admission.

D. Written discharge instructions are sent home with the patient. (See Table 3-5)

E. The nurse must check that the patient understands the discharge instructions and measures for self-care.

F. Supplies for dressing changes are sent home with the patient, along with information on where to replenish the supplies.

XV. **Community Care**

A. Follow-up care may be given at home, a subacute or extended-care facility, or an outpatient clinic.

B. The home care nurse, through good assessment and intervention, may prevent the complications of surgery and keep the patient from having to be rehospitalized.

C. The community nurse reinforces the discharge teaching regarding self-care, the prevention of complications, and symptoms to report.

XVI. Elder Care

A. Elder patient at greater risk for respiratory problems: decreased compliance and tidal volume. Arthritis may inhibit inspiration; supervise deep breathing and coughing.

B. Pain sensation is not diminished in the elderly; may be more stoic.

C. Take measures to combat constipation in the elderly when administering narcotic analgesics.

D. Wounds heal more slowly in the elderly; chronic disease may interfere with oxygenation and transport of nutrients to the cells.

E. The elderly person is at greater risk for aspiration due to decreased muscle tone causing decreased airway reflexes.

F. The elderly patient may become quickly dehydrated from vomiting; circulatory overload can occur from too rapid or too much IV fluid; fluid imbalances may cause confusion.

CHAPTER 5

Correcting Fluid, Electrolyte, and Acid–Base Imbalances

OBJECTIVES

Upon completing this chapter the student should be able to:
1. List the various functions fluid performs in the body.
2. Describe three ways in which body fluids are continually being distributed among the fluid compartments.
3. Compare the signs and symptoms of various electrolyte imbalances.
4. Describe the signs and symptoms of fluid volume deficit and its consequences.
5. Identify three types of patients who might experience a fluid volume excess.
6. State the major causes of acid–base imbalances.
7. Identify intravenous fluids that are isotonic.
8. Discuss the steps in managing an IV infusion.
9. Describe the measures used to prevent the complications of IV therapy.
10. Identify the symptoms of a transfusion reaction and the appropriate measures to be taken when this occurs.
11. Compare interventions for the care of a patient receiving total parenteral nutrition with one undergoing intravenous therapy.
12. Discuss why the elderly have more problems with fluid and electrolyte imbalances.

The fluid portion of the body accounts for about 56% of its total weight. The actual percentage depends on a number of factors: age, sex, nutritional status, and state of wellness. Throughout life there is a gradual decline in the amount of body water and the elderly person's body is about 45% water. **The elderly and the very young are more likely to experience severe consequences with even minor changes in their fluid balance.** The greater the amount of fat in the body, the less the percentage of body water as fatty tissue does not contain as much water as other tissue. Persons of all ages and states of wellness need a normal fluid balance to survive.

Keeping body fluids within a normal range is necessary because the life processes of each cell of every organ take place within fluid. The nutrients needed for life, reproduction, and the normal functioning of a cell must be dissolved or suspended in water. Moreover, the largest part of each cell is fluid. For all of the cell's life processes to take place there must be a continuous

exchange of water, glucose, oxygen, nutrients, electrolytes, and waste products.

When a person becomes ill or suffers an injury, the symptoms he experiences are manifestations of changes within the cells and in the fluid that surrounds them. Just as the whole body cannot survive in an unhealthy and static environment, so, too, each cell requires a constant or stable and healthy environment to function normally.

PHYSIOLOGY

The fluid outside each cell makes up its environment and is often called the body's *internal environment*. The term *homeostasis* is used by physiologists to refer to the maintenance of a constant or stable environment for the body's cells. **Virtually every organ in the body is involved in the task of maintaining homeostasis so that** the environment of every cell is essentially the same. In the healthy person, there is an equilibrium of water loss and water gain.

DISTRIBUTION OF BODY FLUIDS

◆ Fluid Compartments

Even though the body fluids are continually in motion (moving in and out of the blood and lymph vessels, the spaces surrounding the cells, and the bodies of the cells themselves), physiologists identify body fluid according to its location. That is, fluid within the cell is considered to be in one *compartment* (**intracellular**) and fluid outside the cell in another (**extracellular**).

The extracellular fluid is further divided into three types (Fig. 5-1). When fluid leaves a cell by passing through its outer membranes, it enters the spaces surrounding the cell. These spaces are called *interstitial spaces*, and the fluid in them is called *interstitial fluid*. When the fluid moves from these spaces into the blood and lymph vessels, it is called *intravascular fluid*.

A third type of body fluids is the so-called **transcellular fluid**. This fluid is composed of the secretions and excretions that move through the cell membranes (hence the prefix *trans-*) and eventually leave the body. Examples of transcellular fluid include gastrointestinal secretions, saliva, aqueous humor, urine, pericardial,

EXTRACELLULAR COMPARTMENT =
Intravascular (plasma) fluid
  +
Interstitial (lymph) fluid
  +
Transcellular fluid
(e.g., cerebrospinal fluid, pleural fluid,
peritoneal fluid, pericardial fluid,
gastrointestinal secretions,
aqueous humor, saliva)

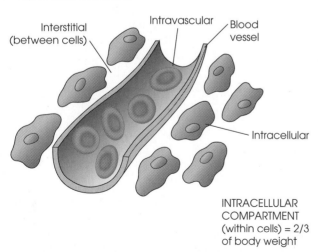

INTRACELLULAR
COMPARTMENT
(within cells) = 2/3
of body weight

FIGURE 5-1 Fluid compartments.

TABLE 5-1 ◆ *Distribution of Body Fluids*	
Intracellular fluid	That which is within the cell walls. Constitutes the internal environment of the body. Transports water, nutrients, oxygen, waste, etc., to and from the cell. Regulated by renal, metabolic, and neurological factors. Cell walls are permeable to water.
	Accounts for about 2/3 of total body weight.
	Most of the cell body is fluid.
	High in potassium (K^+).
Extracellular fluids	Accounts for about 1/3 of total body weight.
	High in sodium (Na^+).
Intravascular fluid	Extracellular fluid that is within the blood vessels. Blood cells do not normally pass in and out of the vascular compartment, and so the fluid is made up of plasma and the substances it transports.
	Contains electrolytes and large amounts of protein.
Interstitial fluid	Extracellular fluid that is in the spaces surrounding the cell. High in sodium (na^+).
Transcellular fluid	Secreted by epithelial cells.
	Passes through the permeable cellular membrane.
	Includes aqueous humor, saliva, cerebrospinal, pleural, peritoneal, synovial, and pericardial fluids and gastrointestinal secretions.

pleural, synovial, and cerebrospinal fluid. Table 5-1 summarizes information about the fluids that are in the various compartments.

When fluid shifts from the vascular space (from the plasma) to the interstitial space, dehydration and **hypovolemia** (too little blood volume) can occur. This occurrence often is termed "third spacing." It may occur with extensive trauma, burns, peritonitis, intestinal obstruction, nephrosis, sepsis, and cirrhosis of the liver where there is an increase in *capillary hydrostatic pressure* or increased capillary membrane *permeability*. (Permeable means that substances can pass through). Capillary hydrostatic pressure is the push of the water contained in blood against the vascular walls. **Leakage from the intravascular space also occurs when there is decreased protein content of the blood. When the red blood count is low or there is a decrease in albumin levels, the osmotic pressure within the vascular space decreases, and the fluid "pulling" pressure is lessened.** (Osmotic pressure occurs when there is a greater number of particles on one side of a permeable membrane than on the other side.) This is why people with severe protein deficiency anemia become edematous. The fluid that has escaped from the vascular compartment collects in the intestine, pleural cavity (pleural effusion), the peritoneal cavity (ascites), or between the cells, causing massive edema. The danger is that with a decreased circulating blood volume, the blood pressure drops, blood flow to the kidneys is greatly decreased, and acute kidney failure may occur.

◆ Transport of Fluids and Their Constituents

The distribution and composition of body fluids depends on a dynamic movement of the fluids and the substances in them. Water and the molecules of the elements dissolved and suspended in it must move freely from one compartment to another so that they are uniformly distributed throughout the body. Many factors contribute to the continuous motion of body fluids. Among the more important are (1) the pumping action of the heart (hydrostatic pressure); (2) the spontaneous exchange of molecules, ions, cellular waste, and other substances *(diffusion);* and (3) the movement of molecules of water across a semipermeable membrane *(osmosis).*

Heart Action The heart actually works as a two-phase pump. First the blood is pumped from the right side of the heart through the pulmonary circulation to discard carbon dioxide and pick up a fresh supply of oxygen. The oxygenated blood is emptied into the left side of the heart where the second phase pumping action moves blood through the general circulation to the rest of the body. As the blood moves through the large blood vessels and on to smaller ones, it eventually passes through the capillaries. These extremely small blood vessels are so abundantly scattered throughout the body tissues that there is not one cell that is more than 50 microns (μ, mu) away from a capillary. (A micron is one-thousandth of a millimeter.) Thus each cell in the body has access to the plasma once it moves out of the capillary and into the interstitial spaces.

Diffusion As the plasma moves along a capillary, large amounts of fluid filter through pores in the capillary walls. The fluid moves into and out of the capillaries. It does this by filtering through the permeable capillary wall or cell membrane walls. There is a capillary hydrostatic pressure inside the capillary that pushes against the wall of the capillary. When the solution on one side of the membrane is more concentrated than the solution on the other side of the membrane, the particles in the more concentrated solution "pull" water toward them in an attempt to equalize the concentration of the two solutions. The direction of water flow depends on which side of the membrane has the greatest concentration of solutes.

Once fluid moves from one compartment to another, diffusion occurs. Diffusion is possible because of *kinetic* motion, which diffuses the molecules in the intracellular fluid and the plasma. These molecules literally bounce off one another, mixing and stirring the body fluids. Diffusion, then, is a spontaneous mixing and moving that allows the exchange of molecules, **ions** (electrically charged particles), cellular nutrients, wastes, and other substances dissolved or suspended in body water. With diffusion, molecules and ions move from an area containing more particles (**solute**) or ions to an area where there are less. It is a process of equalization.

Think about… Can you explain to a classmate the difference between osmosis and diffusion?

Osmosis The principle of *osmosis* is related to the movement of molecules of water. The body does not tolerate differences in the concentrations of fluids in the various compartments. **It tends to equalize the concentrations by moving water from the less concentrated solution to the more concentrated until the solutions are of equal concentration.**

For osmosis to occur, there must be a semipermeable membrane, that is, one that allows water and some other substances to pass through it and prohibits the passage of other particles. Figure 5-2 shows the factors that influence body fluid distribution.

When there is a higher concentration of particles (solute) on one side of a semipermeable membrane than on the other side, **osmotic pressure** occurs. This pressure draws water from the compartment outside of the membrane that has the lower concentration of particles (solute). Osmotic pressure is "water-pulling pressure." Osmotic pressure in the interstitial fluid helps "pull" fluid from the capillary into the interstitial fluid. Likewise there is capillary osmotic pressure within the capillaries and hydrostatic pressure in the interstitial fluid. When the concentration of solute is equal for the amount of water on each side of the membrane, equilibrium occurs and there is no osmotic pressure. **Osmotic pressure is what holds fluid in the vascular space.**

COMPOSITION OF BODY FLUIDS

◆ Body Water

There is far more water than electrolytes in the body fluids. It is essential to normal functioning of the body because it is the medium in which all physiological and

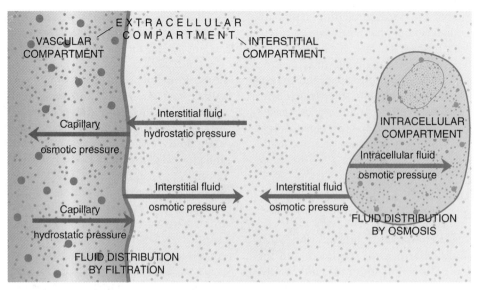

FIGURE 5-2   **Factors that influence body fluid distribution.** (From Copstead, L. C. (1995). *Perspectives on Pathophysiology*. Philadelphia: W. B. Saunders, p 526.)

chemical activities of the cells take place. Water transports substances to and from the cells. These include oxygen and carbon dioxide, as well as the chemicals and nutrients that are used immediately by the cells and those that are stored for future use. **The end products of cellular metabolism are diluted by water so that they are less injurious to the cells;** they are excreted in water by the kidney.

> The body water (1) serves to transport substances to and from the cells; (2) assists the body to regulate its temperature by the evaporation of perspiration; (3) helps maintain the delicate $H^{\pm}$ balance in the body; and (4) provides water to aid the enzymes of digestion.

Think about... Why does increasing fluid intake for the patient with fever lower the body temperature?

◆ Electrolytes

Body fluid has been compared with sea water because both contain many of the same chemical compounds. Some of these substances remain intact and do not break up into atomic particles. Other molecules, when placed in solution, undergo a separation of their atoms into electrically charged *ions.* The molecules of electrolytes break up into atomic particles that are either negatively charged *(anions)* or positively charged *(cations).* For example, when sodium chloride (table salt) is dissolved in body water, its molecules separate into sodium ions, which are positively charged (Na^+), and chloride ions, which are negatively charged (Cl^-).

The electrolytes derive their name from the fact that their atomic particles are capable of conducting an electric current. And because some are positively charged and some are negatively charged, they are chemically active. **This chemical activity allows for the creation of an electrical impulse across the cell membrane, making possible the transmission of nerve impulses, contraction of muscles, and excretion of hormones and other substances from glandular cells.** It is thus apparent that electrolytes are essential to the normal functioning of the body.

> Although all of the electrolytes perform important functions, those of major significance to the nurse who is caring for patients with fluid and electrolyte imbalances are sodium, calcium, potassium, magnesium, and phosphorus. Almost every illness is in some way affected by fluid and electrolyte balance.

Sodium   Sodium is the most abundant electrolyte in extracellular fluid. Sodium influences the irritability of nerves and muscles and is an important factor in nerve conduction. Sodium helps initiate heart contractions. It plays an important role in the movement of fluid back and forth between the intracellular and extracellular compartments. Sodium also promotes acid-base balance by renal exchange for hydrogen ions. The average intake from the diet is 6 to 12 g per day. Serum sodium level is regulated by the kidney in response to levels of aldosterone, antidiuretic hormone (ADH), and atrial natriuretic peptide (ANP). Aldosterone signals the renal tubules to reabsorb sodium. ADH tells the kidney to reabsorb water. As the extracellular fluid levels of sodium increase, the secretion of aldosterone decreases. **Water imbalance, whether too much or too little, is always associated with sodium gain or loss.**

Whenever sodium is retained in the body, there will be a retention of water and an increase in the extracellular volume.

That is why the intake of sodium is restricted in patients who have a heart condition, kidney disease, or liver disease in which there is retention of water in the spaces between the body cells (interstitial fluid). This condition is called *edema*, which is discussed in more detail later in this chapter. **The normal serum range in the adult for sodium is 135 to 145 mEq/liter.** Table 5-2 presents sodium imbalances. When sodium levels are low, the first measure is usually to restrict fluid intake. When sodium levels are elevated, dietary sodium is restricted. See Appendix II for low sodium diets.

Think about . . . Can you explain why some Chinese food causes fluid retention?

Calcium   About 99% of the calcium in the body is found in the bones. The other 1% in the blood is crucial to the normal functioning of the nerves and muscles. **Calcium regulates neuromuscular activity, including that of the heart and skeletal muscle. It also plays a role in blood coagulation.**

Normal serum levels in the adult are 8.4 to 10.6 mg/dL. Excess amounts of calcium (hypercalcemia) can cause cardiac arrest.

Table 5-3 presents calcium imbalances. When the calcium level is low, increases in dietary intake of yellow cheese, milk products, and dark green vegetables may help to raise it.

When assessing for hypocalcemia, the nurse tests for Trousseau's sign by placing a blood pressure cuff around the upper arm, inflating the cuff above the patient's normal systolic pressure, and keeping it inflated for 1 to 4 minutes. This causes hypoxia in the hand, and, if hypocalcemia is present, muscle spasms occur (Figure 5-3). Chvostek's sign also is checked by tapping on the patient's face just below and in front of the ear over the facial nerve. If hypocalcemia is present, muscle twitching affecting one side of the mouth, nose, and cheek will occur (see Figure 5-4).

Elder Care Point . . . Elderly patients may decrease their intake of calcium because of an intolerance to milk products (lactose intolerance). Encourage the intake of green leafy vegetables for these patients.

TABLE 5-2 ◆ *Sodium Imbalances*			
	Potential Causes	**Signs and Symptoms**	**Nursing Interventions and Treatment**
Hypernatremia (>145 mEq/L)	**Increased water loss:** fever, watery diarrhea, dehydration, hyperventilation, excessive sweating, infection with increased metabolic rate. **Decreased water intake** (NPO) **Decreased sodium excretion:** renal failure, corticosteroid therapy, Cushing's syndrome, diabetes insipidus. Administration of hyperosmotic tube feedings.	Dry mucous membranes, loss of skin turgor, intense thirst, flushed skin, decreased urine output with increased specific gravity, elevated temperature, muscle twitching, fatigue; late: confusion, seizures, diminished deep tendon reflexes.	Correct underlying cause. **Restrict sodium intake.** **Increase fluid intake.** Give water between tube feedings. Monitor vital signs.
Hyponatremia (<135 mEq/L)	**Inadequate sodium intake** (NPO), very low sodium diet. **Increased sodium loss:** diuretic therapy, heavy sweating, excessive wound drainage, gastrointestinal suction, extensive burns, nausea and vomiting, diabetic ketoacidosis, syndrome of inappropriate antidiuretic hormone. **Retention of fluid:** kidney failure, heart failure. **Excessive intake of water:** IV fluids without electrolytes, irrigation with hypotonic fluids.	Mental confusion, altered levels of consciousness, anxiety, coma; rapid pulse, weakness, abdominal cramping, muscle twitching, and eventual convulsions.	**Restrict water intake.** **Increase sodium intake if permitted.** Give sodium solution IV slowly, 2 mEq/hour to prevent cerebral edema, seizures, and death. Treat underlying cause.

TABLE 5-3 ◆ Calcium Imbalances

	Potential Causes	Signs and Symptoms	Nursing Interventions and Treatment
Hypercalcemia (>10.6 mg/dL)	Excess intake of calcium from calcium-containing antacids or supplements. Excess intake of vitamin D. Conditions that cause calcium to move from bones into extracellular fluid: bone tumor, multiple fractures, osteoporosis, immobility. Tumors of the lung, stomach, and kidney. Decreased excretion of calcium: **renal failure,** use of thiazide diuretics; hyperparathyroidism, hyperthryoidism, use of glucocorticoids, lithium therapy; adrenal insufficiency.	Increased heart rate and blood pressure; full bounding pulses, widened T wave, bradycardia, cardiac arrest; decreased clotting time, muscle weakness, diminished deep tendon reflexes, nausea, anorexia, constipation, abdominal distention, confusion, lethargy, coma.	**Continuous cardiac monitoring. Restrict calcium intake.** Stop thiazide diuretics, switch to furosemide, which enhances calcium excretion. Give IV normal saline if kidney function is normal and fluid not restricted. Give calcium chelator mithramycin or penicillamine. Give calcitonin, phosphorus, biphosphonates, or nonsteroidal antiinflammatory drugs to inhibit calcium resorption from bone. Dialysis may be necessary.
Hypocalcemia (<8.4 mg/dL)	**Inadequate intake of calcium. Impaired absorption of calcium from intestinal tract,** diarrhea, inadequate intake of vitamin D, **end-stage renal disease,** overuse of phosphate laxatives and enemas, decreased secretion of parathyroid hormone. Crohn's disease, sprue, acute pancreatitis, massive blood transfusions.	Tachycardia, hypotension, cardiac dysrhythmias, paresthesias, twitching, cramps, tetany, seizures, positive Trousseau's sign, positive Chvostek's sign; diarrhea, hyperactive bowel sounds; bronchospasm.	**Calcium supplementation** 1–2 hours after meals to increase absorption. Give drug to decrease neuromuscular irritability. May give magnesium sulfate. Increase dietary calcium and vitamin D. **Decrease environmental stimuli and sensory input. Institute seizure precautions.** Teach correct use of laxatives, phosphate enemas, and antacids.

Potassium   Potassium is the most abundant electrolyte in *intracellular fluid* and is important for the maintenance of normal fluid volume within each cell and for cell growth. Like calcium, **potassium is involved with regulating neuromuscular activity of heart, skeletal, and smooth muscle.** A drastic change in the level of potassium, either too much or too little, can have an impact on the heart and bring about cardiac arrest. Potassium also affects the hydrogen ion concentration in the blood, which is the determining factor in maintaining acid–base balance and is necessary for transport of glucose into the cell. **Normal serum range in adults for potassium is 3.5 to 5.0 mEq/L.** When potassium levels are low, potassium is increased in the diet (Table 5-4) or is given as an oral or intravenous (IV) supplement. **Potassium chloride is never given IV as a "push" or undiluted medication.**

One of the most common causes of potassium depletion is diuretic therapy. Patients taking a potassium-sparing diuretic should be watched for increases in potassium levels. Diarrhea is another common cause of potassium depletion. Other drugs that

may cause potassium deficit include amphotericin B, Carbenicillin, and corticosteroids. Table 5-5 presents potassium imbalances.

Elder Care Point... Patients taking both digitalis and a potassium-wasting diuretic must be closely watched for digitalis toxicity. Hypokalemia predisposes to digitalis toxicity. Always check potassium lab values and for signs of hypokalemia before administering digitalis.

TABLE 5-4 ◆ Nutrition Point: Common Foods High in Potassium

Counsel the patient taking a potassium-wasting diuretic to add these foods to the daily diet:*

◆ Avocado	◆ Cod fish	◆ Raisins
◆ Baked potato	◆ Meats	◆ Salmon
◆ Bananas	◆ Milk	◆ Tuna
◆ Cantaloupe	◆ Orange	

*Patients in renal failure may need to restrict their intake of these foods.

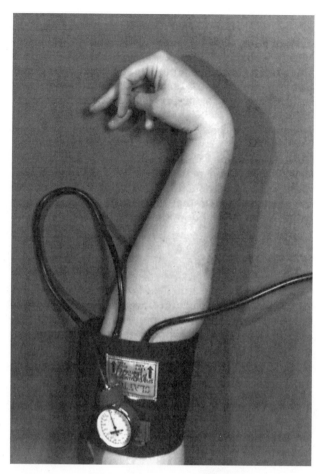

FIGURE 5-3   Palmar flexion (positive Trousseau's Sign in hypocalcemia). (From Ignatavicius, D. D., Workman, M. L., and Mishler, M. A. (1995). *Medical-Surgical Nursing: A Nursing Process Approach,* 2nd ed. Philadelphia: W. B. Saunders, p 307.)

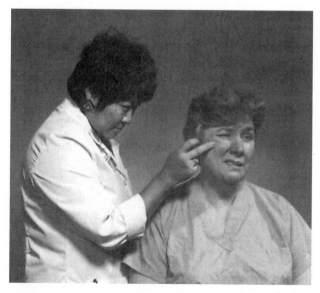

FIGURE 5-4   Facial muscle response (positive Chvostek's sign in hypocalcemia). (From Ignatavicius, D. D., Workman, M. L., and Mishler, M. A. (1995). *Medical-Surgical Nursing: A Nursing Process Approach,* 2nd ed. Philadelphia: W. B. Saunders, p 308.)

Magnesium   Magnesium, the second most abundant intracellular cation, in the intracellular fluid acts as a catalyst for many chemical reactions involving enzymes. It is particularly important in those reactions related to carbohydrate metabolism. In the extracellular fluid, **magnesium is required for the transmission of nerve impulses, dilatation of peripheral blood vessels, and normal contractions of the heart muscle.** Normal adult serum levels are 1.3 to 2.1 mg/dL. See Table 5-6 for magnesium imbalances. Good food sources of magnesium include raw spinach, rolled oats, avocado, and tuna fish.

Phosphorus   Phosphorus is necessary to metabolize nutrients and is essential for bone formation. Intracellularly it acts as a cofactor in many enzyme systems active within the cells. Extracellularly it has a major effect on the regulation of calcium and phosphorus, and **acts as a buffer to promote acid–base balance.** Normal adult serum levels, measured as phosphate, are 3.0 to 4.5 mg/dL. Imbalances are presented in Table 5-7. Food sources high in phosphorus include tuna fish, cod, pork, beef, liver, milk products, and peanuts.

Chloride   Chloride is the major anion in the extracellular fluid and works with sodium to maintain osmotic pressure. It is important in the formation of hydrochloric acid in the stomach and necessary for digestion. Normal adult serum levels are 96 to 106 mEq/L. A chloride deficit most often results from gastric fluid loss related to vomiting or gastric suction. Most diets contain adequate chloride to meet the needs of the body. Chloride imbalances are not common.

♦ Electrolyte Imbalances

Assessment and nursing interventions related to fluid and electrolyte imbalances are summarized in Tables 5-2–5-7.

Nursing Diagnosis   Nursing diagnoses for problems of electrolyte imbalance are written to reflect the actual problem the imbalance is causing. For example, hypokalemia might cause muscle weakness or cardiac arrhythmias. Therefore appropriate nursing diagnoses might be:

♦ Impaired physical mobility related to muscle weakness.

♦ Decreased cardiac output related to arrhythmias.

TABLE 5-5 ◆ *Potassium Imbalances*

	Potential Causes	Signs and Symptoms	Nursing Interventions and Treatment
Hyperkalemia (>5.0 mEq/L)	Conditions that alter kidney function or decrease its ability to excrete potassium (**kidney failure**). Intestinal obstruction that prevents elimination of potassium in feces. Addison's disease, potassium-sparing diuretics, **massive tissue damage** that releases potassium from the cells, **metabolic acidosis**. **Excessive potassium intake:** potassium supplements, potassium-rich foods, salt substitutes, too much potassium in IV fluids. Increased potassium intake in conjunction with renal insufficiency.	Muscle weakness, paresthesias, hypotension, increasing and ascending paralysis leading to respiratory problems. Irregular heart rate, wide QRS, prolonged PR interval. Diarrhea, hyperactive bowel sounds.	**Decrease potassium intake,** stop IV with potassium and potassium supplements. Restrict intake of potassium-containing foods. **Increase fluid intake.** Restrict use of salt substitute containing potassium. Provide adequate carbohydrate intake to prevent use of proteins for energy. May treat with glucose and insulin to move K^+ into the cells, potassium-excreting diuretics, **cation exchange resins** by mouth or enema (Kayexalate). Dialysis may be necessary.
Hypokalemia (<3.5 mEq/L)	Potassium-wasting **diuretic therapy, diarrhea,** vomiting, inadequate intake of potassium-rich foods, excessive gastric suction, excessive fistula drainage, Cushing's syndrome, **corticosteroid therapy,** too much IV fluid without potassium added, renal disease preventing reabsorption of potassium, total parenteral nutrition, diabetic ketoacidosis, alkalosis.	Leg and abdominal cramps, lethargy, weakness, confusion, gaseous distention, hypoactive bowel sounds, ileus, weak, thready pulse, postural hypotension, shallow respirations, decreased or absent reflexes, flat or inverted T waves.	**Give potassium supplements** orally or IV. Increase potassium in diet and instruct to eat foods high in potassium. **Watch for digitalis toxicity** if on digitalis. Teach signs of hypokalemia.

TABLE 5-6 ◆ *Magnesium Imbalances*

	Potential Causes	Signs and Symptoms	Nursing Interventions and Treatment
Hypermagnesemia (>2.1 mEq/L)	Overuse of antacids and laxatives containing magnesium. **Renal insufficiency and kidney failure.**	Hypotension, bradycardia, weak pulse, heart block; sweating and flushing; respiratory depression.	**Restrict magnesium intake.** Teach to avoid abuse of antacids and laxatives. Give extra fluids if permitted; may give loop diuretics; administer calcium for severe cardiac symptoms.
Hypomagnesemia (<1.3 mEq/L)	Malnutrition, diarrhea, celiac disease, Crohn's disease, **alcoholism,** prolonged gastric suction, **ileostomy or colostomy,** acute pancreatitis, biliary or intestinal fistula, diabetic ketoacidosis, eclampsia, **chemotherapy,** sepsis.	Twitching, paresthesias, hyperactive reflexes, irritability, confusion, hallucinations, positive Trousseau's sign, positive Chvostek's sign, seizures, tetany, shallow respirations, tachycardia.	Correct underlying cause. Discontinue drugs that contribute to hypomagnesemia. **Give magnesium supplements,** monitor infusions closely; increase magnesium in diet with milk and cereals.

TABLE 5-7 ◆ *Phosphate Imbalances*

	Potential Causes	Signs and Symptoms	Nursing Interventions and Treatment
Hyperphosphatemia (4.5 mg/dL)	Phosphate laxative and enema abuse. Renal insufficiency. Chemotherapy treatment for leukemia, lymphoma, and small cell lung cancer. Tumor lysis syndrome. Hypoparathyroidism.	Mainly those caused by accompanying hypocalcemia: neuromuscular irritability, muscle weakness, hyperactive reflexes, tetany. Soft tissue calcification.	**Monitor calcium levels. Treat hypocalcemia. Monitor kidney function.**
Hypophosphatemia (<3.0 mg/dL)	Malnutrition, **use of magnesium-based or aluminum-hydroxide–based antacids.** Renal failure, malignancy, hyperparathyroidism, hypercalcemia, alcohol withdrawal, diabetic ketoacidosis, respiratory alkalosis.	Confusion, seizures, weakness, decreased deep tendon reflexes, shallow respirations, increased bleeding tendency, cardiomyopathy, immunosuppression, bone pain.	**Oral supplement** with vitamin D. Decrease intake of calcium-rich foods and increase intake of meats and whole grains that contain phosphorus. Give phosphate if imbalance is severe.

◆ Self-care deficit related to muscle weakness and fatigue.

Nursing diagnoses for other electrolyte imbalances are determined in the same way. The nurse looks at the problems the imbalance causes and then formulates the nursing diagnosis.

Expected Outcomes   Expected outcomes are written specifically to the appropriate nursing diagnosis. The overall goal is that electrolytes will be within normal range within a specified time.

Evaluation   Evaluation is performed by checking the laboratory values of the electrolytes and assessing patients for signs of continuing imbalances.

FLUID IMBALANCES

The main source of water intake is the water that we drink. However, solid foods contain up to 85% water and water is also produced in the body as a by-product of metabolism. The average amount of fluid taken in each day is about 1,500 mL as plain water or in liquids such as milk, juice, coffee, etc.; 700 mL of water are obtained from foods and about 250 mL is produced from metabolism. Body secretions are partially excreted, but a lot are reabsorbed.

When it is not possible for a person to obtain an adequate intake of water through the gastrointestinal tract, fluids usually are given intravenously or by feeding tube. Fluids are lost from the body through urine, feces, expired air, and perspiration (Figure 5-5). The total 24-hour output of fluid in urine and feces and through the lungs and skin is about 2,500 mL. Extra fluid is lost when the metabolic rate is accelerated, such as occurs in thyroid crisis, burns, severe trauma, states of extreme stress, and fever. Perspiration can account for a fluid loss of a maximum of 2 L/hr. For every degree of fever on the Celsius scale, an **insensible** (not aware of) water loss of 10% may occur. When the weather is hot and dry, water loss from the body is greater. Patients on mechanical ventilators, those with rapid respirations, and those with severe diarrhea or excessive wound or fistula drainage also lose greater quantities of water.

In a healthy person, balance between intake and output is maintained by drinking a sufficient amount of water each day and by having a diet that contains the essential substances needed to replace water and electrolytes lost through normal excretory functions. **The major organ involved in maintaining fluid and electrolyte balance is the kidney, which regulates both the volume and the composition of extracellular fluid.**

Illness can affect the fluid and electrolyte balance in many different ways. There may be an inability to ingest liquids or an impairment of absorption of liquids that enter the gastrointestinal tract. A kidney disorder that affects either secretion or tubular reabsorption greatly affects both fluid and electrolyte balance. Because circulation of fluids is important to maintaining balance, any disease that affects circulation (e.g., congestive heart failure) will ultimately affect the distribution and composition of body fluids. Burns, in which large amounts of body fluid may be lost through the open wounds, also present problems of fluid balance. In fact, virtually every patient who is seriously ill is at risk for a fluid and electrolyte imbalance.

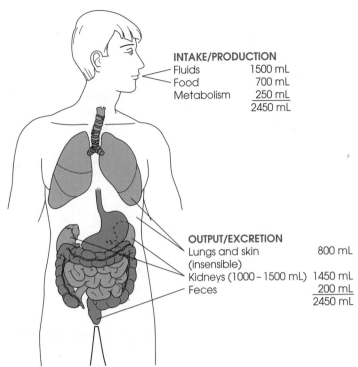

INTAKE/PRODUCTION
Fluids   1500 mL
Food   700 mL
Metabolism   250 mL
                2450 mL

OUTPUT/EXCRETION
Lungs and skin   800 mL
(insensible)
Kidneys (1000 – 1500 mL) 1450 mL
Feces   200 mL
                              2450 mL

FIGURE 5-5   Sources of fluid intake and production and fluid output and excretion.

Fluid intake and output are balanced in the healthy person

PATHOPHYSIOLOGY

A fluid imbalance exists when there is either a **deficit** (too little) or an **excess** (too much) of body water and one or more of the substances dissolved in it. Although it is possible for a person to suffer from an imbalance involving only one component of body fluids, it is more often the case that several substances are out of balance. Body water does not exist as pure water. It always has substances dissolved in it, and the concentration of these substances affects the shifting of fluid from one compartment to another and the eventual loss or retention of fluid. **When water is lost, sodium usually is also lost. When sodium is lost, potassium is often retained.**

Fluid Volume Deficit   A fluid volume deficit occurs when there is either too little fluid taken into the body or too much lost without replacement. It is not always possible to prevent fluid deficit and dehydration, particularly in patients who are acutely ill or have undergone surgery. However, many patients can be spared the harmful effects of a fluid deficit if the nurse is alert to its threat, especially for those who are most at risk. Assessment of the patient, identification of early signs of dehydration, and appropriate nursing intervention often can prevent more serious problems of fluid imbalance.

Elder Care Point . . . Fluid volume deficit is a very common problem in the elderly. There is an age-related decline in total body water and a decrease in thirst sensation and taste that causes elderly people to skimp on fluids and they easily become dehydrated.

Nursing Responsibilities in the Prevention and Treatment of Fluid Deficit

Assessment.   Patients most likely to suffer from fluid volume deficit that can be prevented or corrected relatively easily are (1) those who are unable to take in sufficient quantities of fluids because of difficulty in swallowing, extreme weakness, unavailability of water, confusion and disorientation, and coma; and (2) those who lose excessive amounts of fluid through prolonged vomiting, diarrhea, and copious drainage through operative wounds, burns, and fistulas.

Other factors that may contribute to fluid deficit are related to treatments for an underlying disorder, such as, the administration of diuretics or continuous gastrointestinal irrigation and suctioning of gastric contents.

The symptoms of fluid deficit are essentially those of cellular dehydration. When there is not enough water in the plasma, it becomes too concentrated, and so water is drawn out of the body cells to equalize the concentrations. This causes the cells to shrivel from dehydration.

Subjective symptoms include thirst, complaints of dizziness and of feeling faint upon standing up (postural hypotension), rapid weight loss (1–2 lb in a day or two), and weakness. Objective symptoms of fluid deficit are production of less than 30 mL of urine per hour over several hours; dark and concentrated urine with an increased specific gravity; dry, cracked lips; additional furrows in the tongue; dryness in the mouth where the cheek and gum meet; dry skin that lacks **turgor** (elasticity or fullness); flat neck veins or collapse of neck veins with each inspiration of air; increased pulse rate and weak, thready pulse; and elevated temperature in the absence of infection. **The most accurate measure of fluid gain or loss for any age group is weight change.**

Elder Care Point... Skin turgor is altered in the elderly. As a result, when assessing for dehydration, the nurse should assess the skin on the forehead or the sternum to check turgor. However, because pinching the skin may cause bruising, gentle palpation and visual inspection are used. The condition of the tongue and oral mucosa is a more useful indicator of fluid status in this age group. A furrowed, dry tongue that is not the result of drug therapy indicates a fluid deficit.

Fluid volume deficit contributes to constipation and orthostatic hypotension with related dizziness and falls and makes the person more susceptible to infection.

Many elderly people rely on laxatives and enemas to clear the bowel. This practice can cause fluid volume deficit along with sodium and potassium loss. Depending on the type of laxative or enema, this practice also can cause other electrolyte imbalances.

Medical treatment and nursing intervention. Many times a fluid volume deficit occurs because the patient is unable to get a sufficient supply of water on his own, is too nauseated to keep it down, or is too confused and disoriented to recognize the need for fluids. The responsibility of the nurse in these instances simply is to provide an adequate intake for those who are unable to do this for themselves. An accurate record of intake and output must be maintained, and techniques must be employed to ensure that the patient drinks or receives sufficient fluids. Insertion of a nasogastric tube may be necessary if the patient is unable to swallow and will need continuous care over a long period. The newer small-bore feeding tubes, such as the Dobhoff, have allowed longer periods of **enteral feeding** (i.e., feeding via the gastrointestinal tract) with fewer complications, such as esophageal-tracheal fistula. Many of the small-bore tubes are placed into the duodenum. Correct placement of these tubes is confirmed by radiograph. There are formulas of various combinations of nutrients to meet the particular patient's nutritional needs (see Chapter 20).

Nursing interventions particular to these nasogastric tubes include verifying that the tube is in the proper position before beginning a feeding either by radiograph or by aspirating stomach contents and checking the pH of the secretions. Other interventions include checking for residual before the next feeding, irrigating the tube with 30 to 50 mL of tap water after the feeding to prevent clogging, and placing the patient in a semi-Fowler's position before beginning the feeding and for 30 to 60 minutes afterward.

For those patients who require only short-term supplementation feeding, IV therapy may be prescribed to ensure adequate fluid intake. However, conscientious nursing care to combat fluid volume deficit may prevent the need for IV administration of fluids.

> It is essential to measure, rather than estimate, fluid intake and output.

The patient's preferences for type, temperature, and taste of the liquids he is to drink should be included in the plan of care. Water alone will not restore a fluid deficit. The patient also needs electrolytes and therefore should receive fruit juices, bouillon, and any other nutritious liquid he is able to tolerate.

The plan must take into account the physical strength of the patient and his mental and emotional state. He may be totally dependent on the nurse to assist him in drinking the fluids he needs to avoid dehydration, or he may not fully understand the importance of an adequate fluid intake. (See Nursing Care Plan 5-1.)

If the patient's problem is not inadequate intake, but rather excessive loss of fluids, the nursing care is directed toward helping him cope with the specific condition that is contributing to a fluid imbalance. A frequent cause of excessive loss of fluids is abnormally rapid excretion of intestinal fluids, such as that which occurs in vomiting and diarrhea.

The Patient with Nausea and Vomiting Nausea is a feeling of discomfort or an unpleasant sensation vaguely felt in the epigastrium and abdomen. It is accompanied by a tendency to vomit. Nausea usually is experienced when nerve endings in the stomach and other parts of the body are irritated. Usually the irritated nerve endings in the stomach send messages to the part of the brain that controls the vomiting reflex, but nerve cells in other parts of the body can trigger the same response. An example is intense pain in any part of the body. Pain can trigger the nausea-vomiting mechanism. Nausea and vomiting are an automatic response of the involuntary autonomic nervous system to unpleasant stimuli.

The *causes* of nausea and vomiting are many and varied. They include gastrointestinal irritation from foods, viruses, radiation, and some drugs and other chemicals; certain types of anesthetics; and pregnancy.

Nursing Care Plan 5-1

Selected nursing diagnoses, goals/expected outcomes, nursing interventions, and evaluations for a patient with fluid volume deficit

Situation: A 79-year-old female is admitted to the hospital with a fractured femur. She is confused, disoriented, unable to feed herself, and extremely weak.

Nursing Diagnosis	Goals/Expected Outcomes	Nursing Intervention	Evaluation
Fluid volume deficit related to weakness, confusion, and lack of fluid intake. SUPPORTING DATA Found on floor at home 7 hours after injury; no oral intake for 11 hours. Too weak to drink by herself; 200-mL intake last shift.	The patient will have a normal fluid balance as evidenced by: 1. Normal skin turgor. 2. Moist mucous membranes. 3. Blood pressure and pulse in normal range, stable with position change. 4. Balanced intake and output. 5. Urine-specific gravity between 1.010 and 1.030.	Assess skin turgor and mucous membranes q shift. Measure specific gravity q 24 h. Record accurate intake and output. Offer fruit juices in small quantities totaling 8 oz. q 1h. Offer sips of tap water in between juice. Give mouth care q 2 h. Apply lubricant to lips prn. Offer hard candy q 2 to 3 h while awake to stimulate flow of saliva; stay with patient while candy is in mouth.	Taking 6 oz. of fluid per hour. Mucous membranes not as dry. Intake this shift, 495 mL; output, 320 mL. Urine-specific gravity, 1.030. Patient improved; continue plan. Outcomes are being met.

Prolonged vomiting can lead to sodium and potassium deficits and metabolic alkalosis.

Assessment. Subjective data indicating nausea and vomiting include complaints of nausea or feeling "sick to my stomach," queasiness, abdominal pain, epigastric discomfort or burning, and a history of vomiting. Objective data include pallor; mild diaphoresis; cold, clammy skin; excessive salivation; and attempts to remain quiet and motionless. **If vomiting occurs, the vomitus should be observed for odor, color, contents (e.g., undigested food), and amount.** Noting and recording vomiting patterns, conditions that trigger vomiting, and quality of nausea as described by the patient can be helpful in planning treatment.

Medical treatment. Medical treatment most often consists of administering one of the antiemetic drugs. These drugs usually are given to depress the vomiting reflex. Many also have a tranquilizing effect. Some must be used with caution, however, because they can produce oversedation, respiratory depression, and a lowering of blood pressure. Antihistamines, sedatives and hypnotics, anticholinergics, phenothiazines, and other drugs are used to control nausea and vomiting.

Nursing intervention. During an episode of vomiting intervention includes having the patient lie down and turn his head to one side or sit and lower the head between the legs so that vomitus is not aspirated into the respiratory tract. An emesis basin is held close to the side of the face. A cool, damp wash cloth can be used to wipe the patient's face and back of neck. Breathing through the mouth may also help. After the episode is over, the patient may appreciate a mouthwash or cold water to rinse the mouth. Sucking on ice chips helps reduce nausea in some patients.

Patients who are nauseated should be in a quiet, cool, odor-free environment. Physical activity and ingestion of food can trigger further attacks of vomiting. When a patient is able to resume eating and drinking, small meals of cool drinks and foods can be gradually added to his intake. Sips of carbonated drinks are usually tolerated well at first. Foods and drinks that do not have a strong odor are less likely to bring on nausea and another episode of vomiting. Frequent, gentle, oral hygiene is a must for patients who have prolonged periods of nausea.

If nausea and vomiting persist, the patient must be observed for early signs of dehydration. Intravenous therapy may be indicated to replace fluids and nutrients that have been lost because of vomiting and cannot be replaced because of nausea.

Elder Care Point... Older patients must be rehydrated cautiously. Elderly patients who have cardiac problems are at risk for fluid overload from IV infusions. Allowing a liter of fluid to infuse too fast can sometimes cause the patient to go into congestive heart failure. **If an IV infusion falls behind, it should not be regulated to make up for lost time by infusing fluid at a rate faster than ordered.**

The Patient with Diarrhea Diarrhea is defined as the rapid movement of fecal matter through the intestine. It results in the loss of water and electrolytes and poor absorption of nutrients. These substances, especially the potassium needed by the body to prevent alkalosis, are lost in large amounts.

Major *causes* of diarrhea are related to local irritation of the intestinal mucosa, especially that caused by infectious agents, such as *Salmonella Clostridium difficile,* and *Escherichia coli, C. difficile,* gastrointestinal flu, and chemicals. Chronic and prolonged diarrhea is typical of such disorders as ulcerative colitis, irritable bowel syndrome, allergies, and nontropical sprue. Obstruction to the flow of intestinal contents, as from a tumor or a fecal impaction, also can produce diarrhea.

Assessment. The most outstanding subjective symptoms of diarrhea are a history of frequent watery bowel movements, abdominal cramping, and general weakness. Objective signs include numerous watery stools that often contain mucus and are blood-streaked. It is the consistency rather than the number of stools per day that is the hallmark of diarrhea. In some cases the number can be as high as 15 to 20 liquid stools. If the condition is chronic, the patient can suffer from dehydration, malnutrition, and anemia. Diarrhea usually is the result of increased peristaltic activity; hence bowel sounds heard through a stethoscope are likely to be loud gurgling and tinkling sounds that come in waves (**borborygmi**) and are hyperactive.

When assessing diarrhea the nurse should clarify what the patient and family mean by diarrhea when they report this during an interview. For some people more than one stool a day constitutes diarrhea. When a nurse is directly responsible for the care of a patient with diarrhea, she must note and record the number of stools during her shift and the characteristics of each stool, i.e., color, consistency, unusual contents, such as blood, or mucus, any peculiar odor, and associated pain.

Elder Care Point . . . Any time an elderly patient has a change in mental status from alert to confused that cannot be linked to obvious physical problems, the nurse should carefully look for indications of fluid and electrolyte problems. Even slight alterations in electrolytes can cause confusion in this age group.

Medical treatment and nursing intervention. The strength of the patient with diarrhea diminishes rapidly. Nursing measures should be aimed at providing physical and mental rest, preventing unnecessary loss of water and nutrients, protecting the rectal mucosa, and eventually replacing fluids. Diarrhea is a symptom, rather than a disease, and it sometimes requires extensive testing to determine its cause. The nurse will need to explain the purpose of these tests to the patient, enlist his cooperation, and give him the support he needs to endure what could be trying and exhausting procedures.

In acute diarrhea the stomach and intestines are rested by limiting the intake of foods. Once oral feedings are allowed, they usually start with clear liquids and progress to bland liquids and then solid foods with increased calories and high-protein, high-carbohydrate content. Rehydrating solutions containing glucose and electrolytes are given first. These solutions may be purchased at the pharmacy or are ordered by the physician. The patient should avoid iced fluids, carbonated drinks, whole milk, roughage, raw fruits, and highly seasoned foods.

Diarrhea can be and often is associated with nervous tension and anxiety. The patient often is embarrassed by his condition and inconvenienced by frequent trips to the bathroom or the need to request a bedpan. This emotional stress only serves to aggravate the condition and make it worse. The nurse can help break the vicious cycle by maintaining a calm and dignified manner, accepting and understanding the patient's behavior, and providing privacy and a restful environment for him.

An important goal in a plan of care for a patient with diarrhea is a return to normal patterns of bowel elimination. Other goals might be (1) reporting less abdominal cramping; (2) maintaining the integrity of the skin around the anus; (3) having adequate nutrition; (4) restoring and maintaining fluid and electrolyte balance; (5) reducing stress and tension through relaxation techniques; and (6) getting sufficient rest. If diet therapy is used to treat, minimize, or prevent a problem of chronic diarrhea, a major goal would be that the patient follow the prescribed dietary regimen.

Medications prescribed for diarrhea depend on the cause of the disorder and the length of time the condition has been present. Mild cases usually respond well to kaolin and bismuth preparations, (e.g., Kaopectate), which coat the intestinal tract and make the stools more firm. Antispasmodic drugs such as belladonna or paregoric reduce the number of stools by decreasing the peristaltic rate and relaxing the intestinal musculature. Bismuth subsalicylate (Pepto-Bismol) is helpful in that it soothes the mucosa and binds water. It is the recommended treatment for "traveler's diarrhea" and can also be used for prevention of this type of diarrhea. Codeine, diphenoxylate (Lomotil), or loperamide (Imodium) are useful to decrease the peristaltic action that causes the frequency of stools. If the patient with diarrhea shows signs of nervous tension and anxiety, sedatives or tranquilizers may be prescribed. Diarrhea caused by infections may be treated with drugs that are specific for the causative organism. If metabolic acidosis occurs, it is treated by giving buffer solutions.

Think about . . . How would you assess the patient with diarrhea for signs of dehydration?

Patients with Fluid Volume Deficits from Other Causes   The improper use of gastric suction can rapidly deplete the level of body fluids. It is estimated that as much as 2,500 mL of gastric fluid and 1,500 mL of saliva can be removed from the body in a 24-hour period when there is continuous gastric suction.

> It is essential, then, that an accurate record be kept of the amount of drainage removed by suction so that these fluids can be replaced and dehydration avoided.

Drainage fistulas and abscesses can also produce fluid volume deficit. These conditions require careful observation of the patient for signs of a fluid and electrolyte imbalance. An accurate recording of intake and output is essential, even though the amount of fluid lost by drainage on to dressings can only be estimated. One way in which estimates can be made with greater accuracy is to record *every* dressing change that is needed to keep the patient dry and comfortable.

Burn patients lose body fluids through the open wounds in the skin. To compensate for this loss, there is a shifting of fluids from one compartment to another. First the fluid leaves the plasma and moves into the interstitial spaces. Later the fluid moves in the opposite direction. These patients require careful monitoring of their fluid and electrolyte levels to avoid the serious consequences of fluid shift and fluid volume deficit. Burns are discussed more fully in Chapter 29. Patients with fluid deficits from any cause are taught carefully to observe for signs of dehydration and those at risk are asked to weigh daily.

Nursing Diagnosis   Nursing diagnoses for patients with fluid volume deficit could be:

- Fluid volume deficit related to loss of body fluids or electrolytes.
- Risk of fluid volume deficit related to diarrhea.
- Risk of fluid volume deficit related to nausea and vomiting.

Expected Outcomes   Expected outcomes for patients with fluid volume deficits are based on the specific nursing diagnoses and usually relate to the correction of the underlying cause. Overall goals would include: (1) Fluid balance is restored as evidenced by intake and output within normal limits; (2) Absence of signs of dehydration; and (3) Electrolytes within normal range.

◆ Fluid Volume Excess

An excessive amount of *body water* usually occurs first in the extracellular compartment because the water enters and leaves the body from this compartment. When it is ingested or inhaled, water quickly moves into the circulatory system or intravascular compartment. When it is administered intravenously, it goes directly into the intravascular compartment.

Normally, an excess of water alone is not a problem. Healthy persons do not ordinarily drink too much water. When they become ill, however, they may take in more water than they excrete. This can happen if they receive too rapid an infusion of IV fluids, are given tap water enemas, or are persuaded to drink more fluids than they eliminate. The last situation can occur when there is inaccurate and inconsistent measurement of intake and output. When any of these conditions is present, the patient is likely to suffer from *water intoxication*.

A more common fluid imbalance is associated with the retention of water, sodium, and chloride, which produces **edema**. Edema is defined as an accumulation of freely moving interstitial fluid, that is, fluid in the spaces surrounding the cell. Edema also can occur in body cavities, as in the peritoneal cavity (**ascites**) and the cranial cavity. The accumulation of body fluids can affect almost all of the tissue spaces, in which case it is known as *generalized edema,* or it can affect a limited area, in which case it is called *localized edema*. **Whenever sodium is retained in the body, there also is water retention.** *Generalized edema* occurs when the body's mechanisms for eliminating excess sodium fail. The sodium, along with water, accumulates in the body. It becomes life-threatening when it overloads the circulatory system, as in congestive heart failure, and when it involves the lungs, as in pulmonary edema.

Generalized edema can occur as a result of (1) kidney failure and a resulting retention of sodium and water; (2) inadequate circulation of blood through the general circulation (heart failure) or through the portal circulation (liver failure); and (3) hormonal disorders, which involve the overproduction of aldosterone and antidiuretic hormone (ADH). Thus the administration of large doses of hormones from the adrenal cortex (i.e., the corticosteroids) may have a similar effect. Malnutrition, decreased serum albumin, and anemia also can produce a generalized nonspecific edema. This occurs because, with the decrease of proteins in the blood, vascular osmotic pressure drops and fluid is pulled into the interstitial spaces.

Localized edema can be a sign of inflammation and increased permeability of the capillaries. This allows for the flow of unusual amounts of fluid out of the capillaries and into the tissue spaces. Localized edema usually is nonpitting, does not come and go, and is characterized by tight, shiny skin that is stretched over a hard and red area. Causes of localized edema include trauma, allergies, burns, obstruction of lymph flow, and liver failure.

Dependent edema is noted in the feet, ankles, and lower legs or in the sacral region of patients confined to bed or chair. It is an effect of gravity and therefore can be somewhat relieved by elevating the affected part 18″ or above heart level when possible and repositioning the patient frequently.

Nursing Responsibilities for Patients with Fluid Excess

Assessment. Subjective and objective symptoms of fluid excess will depend on the kind of edema present, its location, its severity, and the extent of fluid shift from the plasma into the tissue spaces. The history given by the patient can be very significant. For example, the patient who states that he must sleep on several pillows or sitting up in a chair to breathe comfortably may be experiencing excess fluid trapped within a body cavity (for example, the abdominal or pleural cavity) and suffering from the effects of pressure against the abdominal and thoracic organs, especially when lying down. **Listening for crackles in the lung bases is one way to assess for fluid excess.** Assessing patients with specific kinds of edema is discussed in more detail in appropriate chapters.

If there is a possibility that fluid is seeping into the abdominal cavity forming *ascites*, the nurse should measure abdominal girth. Once every 24 hours, measure the abdomen at the level of the umbilicus. Mark where the tape is centered at the sides of the patient so that the next person will measure in exactly the same place. Chart the measurement.

An objective measure of water excess and circulatory overload is the hematocrit. This is a measurement of the volume percentage of red blood cells in whole blood. **Normal hematocrit values range from 35 to 54 mL of red blood cells per 100 mL of whole blood, depending on age and sex. If there is an excess of water, the proportion of red blood cells to milliliters of blood will be lower, and the hematocrit will be below the normal values.**

"Pitting edema" is common in patients with dependent edema. The name is derived from the fact that a pit or depression can be created by pressing a fingertip against the swollen tissue. **To check for pitting edema the thumb is pressed into the patient's skin at a bony prominence, such as the tibia or malleolus, and held for 5 seconds.** If the depression, or "pit," remains for a while after the pressure is released, the patient has pitting edema. Assessing the severity and progress of pitting edema in the feet and ankles *(pedal edema)* can be made more accurately by rating the findings and comparing assessments from one shift to another (Figure 5-6).

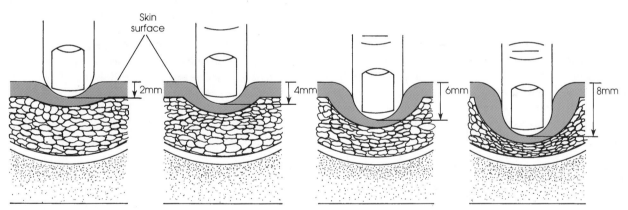

Skin surface

2mm   4mm   6mm   8mm

A. One method for a relatively accurate measurement of the progress of a patient with pedal edema is gently pressing the tissue and estimating the depth of tissue depression in millimeters.

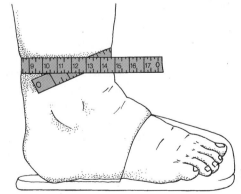

B. The progress of edema in the lower extremities can be assessed by using a measuring tape to measure in inches the circumference of the ankle or calf.

FIGURE 5-6   Measuring pedal edema.

Another scale rating system that is often used by physicians and nurses is:

1+   Mild pitting. Slight indentation with no swelling of the leg.

2+   Moderate pitting. Indentation subsides quickly.

3+   Deep pitting. Indentation remains for a short time, leg looks swollen.

4+   Very deep pitting. Indentation lasts a long time and leg is very swollen.

Ambulatory patients may say that their edema of the feet and ankles gets worse during the day but goes down at night. However, they also report an increasing need to get up during the night to urinate. This nocturia occurs because the fluid in the lower extremities is mobilized during the night when the patient is lying down as the kidneys function more efficiently when the body is supine. The fluid is then excreted as urine.

> A common sign of edema, other than obvious swelling, is weight gain. A liter of water weighs 2 lb, and therefore an accumulation of water in the tissues causes a gain in body weight.

Medical Treatment and Nursing Intervention   The sacral region and buttocks of bedridden patients should be checked frequently for signs of edema. Frequent changes of position can help prevent accumulations in one area. For the patient who is able to sit up, exercises of the legs increase circulation, and periodic elevation of the feet and legs promotes removal of the excess fluid by the blood and lymph vessels. Lightweight elastic stockings, available from the hospital central supply department or a surgical supply house, can be used to counteract edema formation. Sequential compression devices (SCD) may assist venous return in the bedridden patient.

The physician usually requests that the patient be weighed daily when edema is present so that he or she can determine the amount of body fluid being lost or retained. When daily weight measurement is ordered, the nurse must be careful to obtain as accurate a reading on the scales as possible. Ideally, the patient is weighed before breakfast and at exactly the same time every day. The same scales are used at each weighing, and the patient should be wearing the same type of clothing. **The loss or gain of 1 or 2 pounds of body weight can be quite significant in the course of a fluid volume excess. Each pint (500 mL) of excess fluid retained equals 1 lb of added body weight.**

Another symptom of fluid retention can be decreased urinary output. Accurate measurement is vitally important for fluid intake and output. The intake reflects all fluids taken into the body, whether orally, intravenously, or any other way. Output includes all urine, vomitus, watery stools, wound drainage, and unusual sweating. Recording these measurements is a nursing responsibility and does not require a physician's order.

Think about . . . Can you describe the assessments you would make to determine whether your 68-year-old patient is experiencing edema?

Strange as it may seem, edematous patients can suffer from dehydration. The fluid that has accumulated in one of the body cavities is trapped there and is therefore not available to other parts of the body. If the patient develops signs of dehydration, this should be reported immediately. The physician will assess the need for additional fluids and the method by which they are to be provided.

Sometimes the patient's fluid intake is *restricted* to a certain amount within a 24-hour period. The nursing care plan must then include a schedule of fluid intake arranged so that liquids are spaced evenly and the patient *does not* receive all of the allowed liquids in a short time, leaving many hours before he can again have something to drink. If they are not prohibited, hard candies and chewing gum can help relieve thirst. Frequent mouth care is essential.

Skin care is especially important in preventing a breakdown over the area of edema. The skin covering the edematous areas is extremely fragile. It has a decreased blood supply and is stretched beyond its normal limits so that it is no longer flexible. Care must be taken to preserve the skin as much as possible. Bed linens are kept dry and smooth, and the patient is turned frequently to relieve the pressure of the body's weight on susceptible areas. In turning and moving the patient, it is necessary to be as gentle as possible and to avoid friction against the skin. A break or abrasion of edematous skin can very rapidly develop into a pressure ulcer. The use of a turning sheet for repositioning helps prevent abrasions from the sheets.

> Because sodium retention is invariably accompanied by water retention, the patient with edema is placed on a low-sodium diet.

Table salt is not allowed, and special attention must be paid to all foods and liquids consumed by the patient. There are many hidden sources of sodium in foods in their natural state as well as in those that are commercially prepared. Patients should avoid high-sodium foods such as those listed in Table 5-8.

Occasionally it is necessary for patients with edema to receive IV fluids. The administration of these fluids must be carefully monitored, particularly if the patient has or is likely to develop pulmonary edema. An infusion pump is used to prevent too much fluid from accidentally being infused over any one period. The nurse must still check on the IV frequently to see that it

---

TABLE 5-8 ◆ Nutrition Point: Foods High in Sodium

The patient experiencing a fluid volume excess or who is to decrease sodium intake should avoid the following foods:

- buttermilk
- canned meats or fish
- canned soups
- canned vegetables
- casserole and pasta mixes
- catsup
- cheese (all kinds)
- delicatessen meats
- dried fruits
- dried soup mixes
- foods containing MSG
- frozen vegetables with sauces
- gravy mixes
- ham
- hot dogs
- olives
- pickles
- prepared mustard
- preserved meats
- processed foods
- salted nuts
- salted popcorn
- salted snack foods
- softened water
- soy sauce
- tomato or vegetable juice

Note: Check all packaged food for sodium content.

---

is patent and that the pump is functioning properly. Diuretics also are commonly prescribed to control generalized edema, especially when it is a manifestation of congestive heart failure (see Chapter 19).

When a patient with edema is to be discharged from the hospital, he should be instructed in the ways in which he can participate to manage his illness, control his symptoms, and prevent complications.

Some expected outcomes that might be used for a patient with water and sodium retention related to congestive heart failure and those suitable for a patient with ascites are shown in Table 5-9.

Nursing Diagnosis   Some nursing diagnoses that may be appropriate for patients with fluid volume excess are:

TABLE 5-9 ◆ Goals/Expected Outcomes for Evaluating Nursing Interventions to Manage Different Types of Edema

Nursing Diagnosis	Goals/Expected Outcomes
Fluid volume excess related to inadequate heart action and resultant edema.	Heart rate returned to baseline. No significant dependent edema. Blood pressure within baseline. Lungs clear on radiograph and auscultation. Intake is balanced with output. Body weight returned to normal and maintained with no more than ½ lb. fluctuation.
Fluid volume excess (ascites) related to liver failure.	Decreased abdominal girth. Decreased peripheral edema.

- Fluid volume excess related to excessive fluid or sodium intake.
- Fluid volume excess related to compromised regulatory mechanisms.
- Fluid volume excess related to low protein intake or low serum protein levels.
- Risk of fluid volume excess related to decreased heart function.
- Risk of fluid volume excess related to decreased excretion by failing kidneys.

Expected Outcomes   Expected outcomes are written based on the specific nursing diagnosis and usually relate to correcting the underlying cause of the fluid excess. Overall goals would include: (1) Fluid balance as evidenced by correct ratio of intake and output, lungs clear to auscultation, and absence of signs of edema; and (2) Electrolytes within normal ranges.

Patient Education   Patients should be taught to seek treatment quickly when a fluid or electrolyte deficit occurs. The elderly could prevent hospitalization and extended illness if they replaced lost fluids with an appropriate electrolyte solution right away rather than waiting several days to seek medical care.

Patients who are taking diuretics and eating bananas or other high-potassium foods to replace the lost electrolyte should consult their physician when nausea or vomiting interferes with their ability to take daily medications or to eat. If diarrhea is severe or lasts more than a day, the physician should be notified as there may be considerable fluid and electrolyte loss. The home care nurse frequently obtains blood samples for serum electrolyte tests.

ACID–BASE BALANCE (HYDROGEN ION CONCENTRATION)

To understand the concept of acid–base balance and how it is maintained in the body fluids, one should be familiar with some basic facts about biochemistry and the terms commonly used in discussions of hydrogen ion concentration. Some of the more important facts about acid–base balance are:

- An acid is defined as a substance capable of giving up a hydrogen ion during chemical exchange.
- A base is a substance capable of accepting a hydrogen ion.
- Acids react with bases to form water and a salt.
- **A reaction of an acid and a base to form water and a salt is a *neutralization* reaction because both the acid and the base are neutralized.**

◆ Acids react with carbonates and bicarbonates to form carbon dioxide gas.

◆ The term *pH* refers to the concentration of hydrogen (H) in a solution. The *p* represents a *negative* logarithm, which is an inverse proportion. Thus **the higher the concentration of hydrogen ions in a solution, the lower the pH.** A higher pH indicates the opposite, that is, a lower concentration of hydrogen ions.

◆ A chemically neutral solution has a pH of 7.00.

◆ **The pH of the body's fluids is normally somewhat alkaline (between 7.35 and 7.45).**

◆ A pH above 7.8 (*alkalosis*) or a pH below 6.9 (*acidosis*) usually is fatal.

◆ A blood pH of 7.4 indicates a ratio of 1 part carbonic acid to 20 parts base bicarbonate.

◆ *Acidosis* is the result of either a loss of base or an accumulation of acid.

◆ *Alkalosis* is the result of either a loss of acid or an accumulation of base. (See Figure 5-7 for an easy way to interpret blood gases.)

◆ Pathophysiology

Most of the body's metabolic activities produce carbon dioxide gas, which moves from the tissues into the

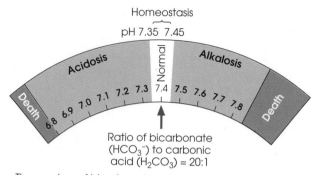

Homeostasis
pH 7.35 7.45

The number of bicarbonate ions in proportion to carbonic acid diminishes with acidosis and increases with alkalosis. A pH below 6.9 or above 7.8 is incompatible with life.

FIGURE 5-8   Acid–base balance: pH 7.35–7.45.

blood, where it combines with water to form carbonic acid. The body deals with this constant manufacture of acid in a number of ways so that the ratio of carbonic acid to bicarbonate can be maintained and an alkaline environment provided for normal cellular activities. If the ratio is not maintained, the acid–base balance is upset. The pH will either fall below the normal range and acidosis will occur, or it will rise above normal range and alkalosis will be present (Figure 5-8).

In general, there are two main types of mechanisms by which the pH is controlled: those concerned with respiration and those concerned with metabolism. As long as the ratio of carbonic acid to bicarbonate is maintained at 1:20, the pH remains within normal limits.

There are, therefore, four possible states of an acid–base imbalance: (1) respiratory acidosis; (2) respiratory alkalosis; (3) metabolic acidosis; and (4) metabolic alkalosis.

The progression of each of the four types of acid–base problems is depicted in Figure 5-9. The role played by the lungs in a respiratory imbalance is concerned with the retention or "blowing off" (excretion) of carbon dioxide (CO_2). In *hypoventilation*, the lungs do not eliminate enough CO_2, and it remains in the body, unites with water, and forms carbonic acid. The opposite is *hyperventilation*, in which too much CO_2 may be excreted.

The kidneys are the principal organs of control in maintaining a normal pH during *metabolic* **activities** because they either reabsorb or excrete bicarbonate. If they eliminate too much bicarbonate, acidosis will develop. Conversely, if they fail to eliminate enough bicarbonate and allow it to be reabsorbed into the bloodstream, alkalosis will develop.

The bottom boxes of Figure 5-9 provides a brief summary of the body's attempts to compensate for an acid–base imbalance. **In the presence of respiratory**

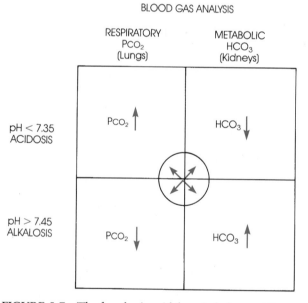

BLOOD GAS ANALYSIS

	RESPIRATORY PCO₂ (Lungs)	METABOLIC HCO₃ (Kidneys)
pH < 7.35 ACIDOSIS	PCO₂ ↑	HCO₃ ↓
pH > 7.45 ALKALOSIS	PCO₂ ↓	HCO₃ ↑

FIGURE 5-7   The four basic acid–base imbalances. The boxes illustrate the four basic acid-base imbalances. The top left is respiratory acidosis, and the top right is metabolic acidosis; the bottom left is respiratory alkalosis, and the bottom right is metabolic alkalosis. The arrows show in which direction the components deviate from normal. The inner circle represents how the other system compensates for the primary abnormality. (Courtesy of Kathleen M. White, RN, MS, CCRN.)

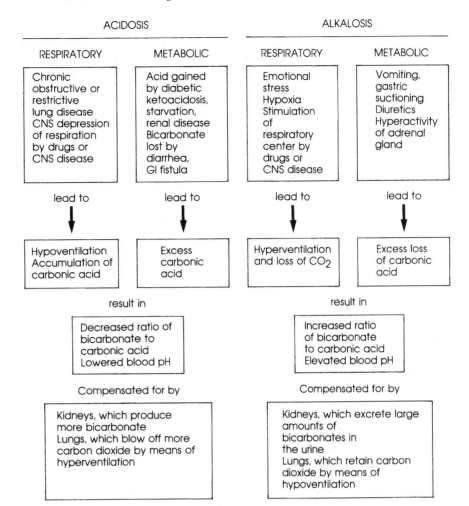

FIGURE 5-9 Comparison of causes, physiological effects, and compensatory mechanisms for acidosis and alkalosis.

acidosis, the kidneys will retain and manufacture more bicarbonate than normal so that it is available to neutralize the excess acid. However, this is a slow process that takes from a few hours to several days. In the presence of respiratory alkalosis, the kidneys will increase their excretion of bicarbonate. In response to metabolic acidosis, the patient will involuntarily hyperventilate to remove carbon dioxide so that it is not available to produce carbonic acid. Should metabolic alkalosis develop, the patient will hypoventilate to retain the supply of carbon dioxide.

The foregoing information on acid–base balance, hydrogen ion concentration, and the carbon dioxide-bicarbonate ratio does not represent an in-depth explanation. Many complex chemical activities are involved in the maintenance of an internal environment that must be slightly alkaline for normal body function. For a more thorough study of the subject, the reader is referred to the Bibliography.

It is important, however, that the nurse have some appreciation of the reasons for various metabolic and respiratory illnesses that are related to either acidosis or alkalosis. With an understanding of the rationale of medical management, the nurse will be better able to plan nursing care that is coordinated with and supportive of medical care. In the following pages, we describe the kinds of acid–base problems patients are likely to encounter and discuss ways in which the nurse might help patients cope with these problems. Because acidosis and alkalosis are common to a great variety of medical and surgical conditions of illness, the chapters on specific illnesses will frequently refer to problems of this kind.

◆ Arterial Blood Gas Analysis

Studies of the percentages of gases (oxygen and carbon dioxide) in the blood and the hydrogen ion concentration (pH) are useful in assessing the status of both respiratory and metabolic acid–base imbalances. They do not detect disease or distinguish the specific cause of the imbalance, but blood gas studies are valuable indicators of a patient's progress toward recovery or lack of it. They reflect the ability of the lungs to exchange oxygen and carbon dioxide, the effectiveness of the kidneys in balancing retention and elimination of bicarbonate, and the effectiveness of the heart as a pump.

The results of analyses of arterial blood gases (ABGs) are reported as follows:

- *PaO$_2$*. Partial pressure (P) exerted by oxygen (O$_2$) in the arterial blood (a). **Normal value is 80 to 100 mm Hg.**

- *PaCO$_2$*. Partial pressure of carbon dioxide in the arterial blood. **Normal value is 35 to 45 mm Hg.**

- *pH*. An expression of the extent to which the blood is alkaline or acid. **Normal value is 7.35 to 7.45.**

- *SaO$_2$* (also abbreviated O$_2$Sat). Percentage of available hemoglobin that is saturated with oxygen, that is, combined to the total amount of oxygen the hemoglobin can carry. **Normal value is 94% to 100%.**

- *HCO$_3$*. The level of plasma bicarbonate; an indicator of the metabolic acid-base status. **Normal value is 22 to 26 mEq/L.**

- *Base excess or deficit.* Indicates the amount of blood buffer present. Alkalosis is present when this value is abnormally high. Abnormally low values indicate acidosis. Measured in "+" or "–".

◆ Acid–Base Imbalances

Respiratory Acidosis

Assessment. Patients most likely to suffer from respiratory acidosis are, of course, those whose respiratory functions are impaired so that the lungs are unable to remove sufficient amounts of carbon dioxide. *Acute* respiratory acidosis develops suddenly and occurs when an airway obstruction, acute respiratory infection with retained secretions, or acute pulmonary edema interferes with the normal exchange of oxygen and carbon dioxide, with a resulting accumulation of carbon dioxide in the blood.

Think about . . . What could you do to help your home care patient who has pneumonia prevent respiratory acidosis?

Chronic respiratory acidosis is a slower process that accompanies the gradual loss of pulmonary function. The most common condition in which this is likely to occur is chronic obstructive pulmonary disease (COPD). This condition is explained in more detail in Chapter 16. A patient with COPD is most likely to develop acute acidosis when an infection of the respiratory tract further impairs his breathing capacity and the removal of carbon dioxide.

Subjective symptoms of respiratory acidosis include complaints of increasing difficulty in breathing, a history of respiratory obstruction (acute or chronic),

weakness, dizziness, restlessness, sleepiness, and change in mental alertness. Objective data include increased levels of carbon dioxide in the blood, dyspnea, and obvious respiratory problems.

Respiratory Acidosis
pH   < 7.35
pCO$_2$ > 45 mm Hg

Nursing diagnosis. Nursing diagnoses appropriate for the patient experiencing respiratory acidosis are:

- Impaired gas exchange related to airway obstruction, bronchoconstriction, acute respiratory infection, or pulmonary edema.

- Impaired gas exchange related to carbon dioxide retention secondary to COPD.

Expected outcomes. Expected outcomes for acid–base imbalances are written for each specific nursing diagnosis and often relate to correcting the underlying cause of the imbalance. The overall goal for any acid–base imbalance is "Acid–base balance is restored with pH 7.35 to 7.45." It should be noted that patients with longstanding lung disease may never reach a pH of 7.35 and will remain slightly acidotic.

Medical treatment and nursing intervention. The initial treatment for respiratory acidosis is immediate establishment of an airway if airway obstruction is at fault. This may involve a tracheostomy or the insertion of an endotracheal tube. Adequate ventilation is maintained by administering oxygen and possibly assisted ventilation using a mechanical ventilator. Conservative treatment in other patients is by postural drainage, deep-breathing exercises, bronchodilators, and antibiotics if indicated.

Care must be taken when administering certain drugs that depress the respiratory center. These include narcotics, hypnotics, and tranquilizers.

In patients with COPD, the respiratory drive mechanism is altered, and oxygen can act as a respiratory depressant. Oxygen should be administered with great care to these patients (no more than 2 to 3 L/min) because it can cause respiratory arrest.

If a patient's history is unknown, oxygen is begun at a rate of 2 to 3 L per minute until it is determined that he can tolerate a higher flow rate.

The patient must be watched closely for respiratory and cardiac arrest. Should either occur, it will be necessary to maintain respiration and circulation artificially through cardiopulmonary resuscitation.

Respiratory Alkalosis

Assessment. Respiratory alkalosis arises when hyperventilation results in excessive loss of carbon dioxide from the lungs. Patients hyperventilate for a variety of reasons; these include **hypoxemia** (insufficiency of oxygen, which triggers an automatic increase in respiration), fever, early stages of salicylate poisoning, reactions to certain drugs, pain, anxiety, and hysteria. The overzealous use of mechanical ventilation also can cause hyperventilation when too much CO_2 is blown off.

Symptoms of respiratory alkalosis include deep, rapid breathing, tingling of the fingers, pallor around the mouth, dizziness, and spasms of the muscles of the hands.

Respiratory Alkalosis
pH > 7.45
pCO_2 < 35 mm Hg

Nursing diagnosis. A nursing diagnosis appropriate for the patient experiencing respiratory alkalosis is:

◆ Ineffective breathing pattern related to hypoxemia or fever (hyperventilation). Expected outcomes would be: Normal breathing patterns and normal pH and pCO_2.

Medical treatment and nursing intervention. If the underlying cause of respiratory alkalosis is hysteria, treatment is aimed at preventing further hyperventilation and helping the patient reestablish a normal level of carbon dioxide in his blood. Sedatives may be given to calm the patient. To aid in the retention of carbon dioxide, the patient may be instructed to hold his breath or to breathe into a paper sack and rebreathe the carbon dioxide he has just exhaled. This recycling of the carbon dioxide can eventually restore normal carbonic acid levels in the blood.

Patients who develop respiratory alkalosis from causes other than hysteria or overzealous use of a ventilator will require treatment of the primary illness. If the cause is anxiety, a sedative or tranquilizer may be given.

Metabolic Acidosis

Assessment. The usual causes of metabolic acidosis are (1) excessive burning of fats, such as occurs (a) when a diabetic patient does not metabolize carbohydrates because of insulin insufficiency and instead burns fat, the end products of which are fatty acids; and (b) in persons who are on low-carbohydrate, high-protein diets to lose weight; (2) abnormal carbohydrate metabolism in which, in the absence of oxygen, lactic acid accumulates in the blood; (3) failure of the kidneys to reabsorb bicarbonate; and (4) loss of bicarbonate through diarrhea or a gastrointestinal fistula.

The symptoms of metabolic acidosis include weakness, malaise, and headache. If the acidosis is not relieved, these symptoms progress to stupor, unconsciousness, coma, and death. The breath of the patient may have a fruity odor owing to the presence of ketone bodies (**ketoacidosis**). Vomiting and diarrhea may occur and aggravate the problem because of the loss of fluids and electrolytes, which are essential to restoring the acid–base balance.

Metabolic Acidosis
pH   < 7.35
HCO_3 < 22 mEq/L

Medical treatment and nursing intervention. Prevention of acidosis is by far more desirable than treating the condition once it has developed. If the underlying cause is diabetic acidosis, it may be that the patient does not understand his role in managing the illness (Chapter 25).

One way in which metabolic acidosis can be prevented is by carefully observing patients receiving IV fluids that could upset the acid–base balance. Others who should be watched for early signs of acidosis are patients in shock, patients with hyperthyroidism, liver disease, and fluid volume deficiency, and patients with continuous gastric or intestinal suction.

Treatment of metabolic acidosis is aimed at the underlying cause. Insulin is administered if the patient is in diabetic ketoacidosis. Dialysis may be necessary to correct the problem in the patient with kidney failure.

Immediate treatment of severe metabolic acidosis requires administration of IV bicarbonate or lactate. When either of these drugs is administered, the patient should be watched closely, and vital signs should be recorded frequently. Careful measuring of intake and output helps determine how well the kidneys are able to regulate the acid–base balance.

As with any patient likely to develop disorientation or convulsions, safety precautions are taken to avoid injury. Mouth care using an alkaline mouthwash such as baking soda (sodium bicarbonate) will help reduce discomfort from acids in the mouth. Because these patients often breathe rapidly through their mouths, frequent mouth care is necessary.

Metabolic Alkalosis

Assessment. There are three major causes of a shift toward the alkaline range of body fluids. These are (1) excessive loss of acid; (2) either excessive intake or retention of base; and (3) a low level of potassium in the blood (**hypokalemia**).

Loss of fluid from the gastrointestinal tract by gastric suction or emesis is the main cause of metabolic alkalosis. Other causes include drainage from intestinal fistula, diuresis resulting from potent diuretics that increase potassium loss in the urine, and steroid therapy, which causes retention of sodium and chloride and loss of potassium and hydrogen.

Symptoms of metabolic alkalosis include such neurological signs as irritability, disorientation, lethargy, and convulsions; and respiratory manifestations such as slow, shallow respirations, decreased chest movements, and cyanosis. In addition, there may be symptoms of potassium and calcium depletion.

Metabolic Alkalosis

pH   > 7.45
HCO_3 > 45 mEq/L

Medical treatment and nursing intervention.

Because metabolic alkalosis often is associated with some form of medical treatment, the nurse usually is able to detect it in its early stages and prevent more serious developments. However, once the condition is well established, the treatment is directed at correcting the underlying cause and attempting to restore the body fluids to a less alkaline state. Drug therapy is aimed at correcting the underlying cause of the alkalosis. Fluids and electrolytes are replaced orally and parenterally as needed. Emergency measures include the administration of an acidifying solution such as ammonium chloride. Patients receiving this form of therapy must be watched carefully for signs of overcompensation and a resulting acidosis.

Again, it is necessary to take and record vital signs frequently. If the pulse rate increases sharply and the blood pressure drops, the patient may be suffering from potassium depletion (see Table 5-5 for symptoms.) A record of intake and output is necessary so that replacement of lost fluids and electrolytes can be planned. Safety precautions are necessary because the patient may experience mental confusion. If there are muscle spasms, they may be symptomatic of hypocalcemia.

Think about . . . Your patient has a pO$_2$ of 94, pH 7.32, pCO$_2$ of 48, and HCO$_3$ of 26. What type of acid–base imbalance does he have?

It must be noted that blood gas interpretation is somewhat more complicated than presented here because, as changes are taking place, the body is compensating by getting rid of H$^+$ ions or by retaining HCO$_3$. With practice in interpreting ABGs, the nurse can determine how the body is compensating for the imbalances that are occurring.

THERAPY FOR FLUID/ELECTROLYTE IMBALANCES

♦ Intravenous Therapy

The administration of fluids through the veins is the most common means by which water, electrolytes, nutrients, and some drugs may be given when oral intake is not possible or must be supplemented. Medications may be administered in an IV solution when rapid action is required. A form of therapy called *total parenteral nutrition* (TNP) also is used for the parenteral administration of all nutrients for patients with gastrointestinal problems. This form of therapy will be discussed in more detail at the end of the chapter and in Chapter 20.

Some terms related to the concentration of an IV fluid and the effect this has on cells are:

- *Isotonic.* A solution that has the same osmotic pressure as intracellular fluid. Body cells can be bathed in an isotonic solution without net flow of water across the cell membrane.
- *Hypotonic.* A solution that has a lower osmotic pressure (is less concentrated) than that of body fluids. Cells bathed in a hypotonic solution will swell as water passes from the less concentrated solution across the cell membrane and into the cell. *Note:* Sterile distilled water is hypotonic and is never added to an IV solution.
- *Hypertonic.* A solution that has a higher osmotic pressure than that of body fluids. Cells bathed in a hypertonic solution will shrink as water passes out of the cell into the fluid surrounding it.

An example of an isotonic solution is 0.9% normal saline. Hypotonic solutions are those with less than 5% glucose or with anions less than 150 mEq/L.

Some fluids commonly used in IV therapy include:

- *Normal saline* (0.9%), which contains sodium and chloride ions in water.
- *Dextrose or glucose* solution, which contains water and carbohydrate for calories.
- *Lactated Ringer's solution*, which contains water, sodium, potassium, chloride, calcium, and lactate.

Table 5-10 shows commonly ordered IV solutions.

Blood-related fluids that are given IV include whole blood, packed cells from which the plasma has been removed, and plasma. Whole blood is given to replace that which has been lost through hemorrhage. Packed cells may be administered to patients with anemia or some other blood disorder or to patients who cannot tolerate a large volume of fluid very well, such as those with renal disease or congestive heart failure. Plasma is

TABLE 5-10 ◆ *Commonly Ordered Intravenous Solutions*		
Isotonic Solutions	**Hypotonic Solutions**	**Hypertonic Solutions**
Fluid stays in intravascular compartment.	Fluid shifts out of intravascular compartment into intracellular and interstitial compartments.	Fluid shifts out into intravascular compartment from intracellular and interstitial compartments.
0.9% saline (normal saline, NS)	0.45% saline (½ NS).	5% dextrose in normal saline (D2NS).
Lactated Ringer's solution (RL).	2.5% dextrose in water.	5% dextrose in 0.45% saline (D51/2NS).
D5W (5% dextrose in water).	0.33% saline.	10% dextrose in water (D10W), 5% dextrose in 0.33% saline

given to increase blood volume (as in shock), to provide protein and to treat disorders of coagulation.

In the treatment of shock, fluids called *plasma expanders* are administered to increase the volume of plasma. Examples of plasma expanders are low-molecular-weight dextran, albumin, Hespan, and plasmanate.

Nursing Responsibilities in Administering IV Fluids   Responsibility for the safe and effective administration of IV fluids rests with every member of the nursing staff. As with any therapeutic measure, IV therapy is not without its hazards to the patient. Many complications can be avoided through careful handling of equipment and meticulous monitoring of the patient's reaction to the fluids he is receiving.

> The four goals of nursing care for a patient receiving an IV infusion are (1) preventing infection; (2) minimizing physical injury to the veins and surrounding tissues; (3) administering the correct fluid at the prescribed time and at a safe rate of flow; and (4) observing the patient's reaction to the fluid and medications being administered.

All equipment and fluids used for IV therapy must be sterile and safe for administration. Before any bottle or plastic bag of solution is added to an IV set, it must be checked for leaks and possible contamination. A plastic bag of solution may be squeezed to check for leaks. Any solution that is discolored or has small particles, a white cloud, or film in it should not be used. If there is no vacuum in the bottle when it is opened, the solution may be contaminated.

When a new bottle of fluid or additional medication is added to an IV already in progress, strict surgical asepsis must be observed. Each time a new unit of solution or medication is added to an IV setup, there is a danger of introducing bacteria into the patient's blood system. Because of the danger of incompatibility, it is essential that the nurse check each drug and each solution to be certain they can be mixed.

The site of venipuncture should be watched closely for signs of inflammation. Redness, swelling, and heat in the area should be reported as they are possible signs of phlebitis. Chills and an elevation of body temperature may indicate a bacterial infection.

When an IV is discontinued, the tubing is clamped, all tape is removed, and the needle or catheter is gently, but quickly, withdrawn using *standard precautions*. A dry sterile gauze is held on the site with enough pressure to control the leakage of blood and to avoid the formation of a hematoma. If possible, raising the patient's limb for a minute or two to drain blood from the site of insertion will help prevent leakage of blood from the punctured vein.

The IV administration of fluids requires the same safety precautions as any other medication does. The label must be read several times to ensure that the correct solution is being given to the correct patient. The patient's ID band must be checked each time.

Rate of Flow   *Rate of flow* is an important factor in safe and effective IV therapy. IV setups should be checked once an hour to be certain that the fluid is running correctly and there are no problems. When possible, an IV pump that is set for the specific rate of flow is used to administer IV fluids. IV pumps, although not infallible, keep IV fluids flowing at the desired rate and act as safeguards should a problem arise.

Principles that affect the rate of flow for IVs not administered by a pump are:

◆ The higher the container is placed above the level of the patient's heart, the faster the rate of flow.

◆ The fuller the container, the faster the rate of flow.

◆ The more viscous the fluid, the slower the flow; for example, whole blood will flow more slowly than 5% dextrose in water.

◆ The larger the diameter of the needle and tubing, the faster the flow. IV sets usually indicate the number of drops per milliliter delivered by the set.

◆ The higher the pressure within the vein, the slower the flow. As an infusion progresses and the veins become fuller, the IV solution may drip more slowly.

◆ Fluid will pass through a straight tube faster than through one that is coiled or hanging below the level of the cannula.

There usually is a chart available to the nurse who needs to determine the number of drops that should be given per minute to administer a given amount of fluid in a specified time. The IV tubing package will contain information about the number of drops the set will deliver per milliliter. If a chart is not available, the number of *drops per minute* can be calculated using a simple proportion and solving for *x*. Bear in mind that the set gives information about drops per *milliliter*. To check the rate of flow, the nurse must know how many drops should pass through the drip chamber in *1 minute*.

For example, the patient is to receive 1,000 mL (1 L) of fluid in 8 hours (480 minutes). The IV set states that the equipment will deliver 10 drops per milliliter. This would be a total of 10,000 drops because the bottle contains 1,000 mL. The ratio of drops to minutes is 10,000 drops in 480 minutes. The problem is written as:

$$\text{Total time of infusion in minutes} = \frac{\text{Total infusion volume} \times \text{drops/mL}}{} = 1{,}000 \text{ mL} \times 10 \text{ drops/mL}$$

$$480 \text{ minutes} = 10{,}000 \text{ drops}$$
$$480 \text{ minutes} = 20.8 \text{ drops/minute or } 21 \text{ drops/minute.}$$

An alternative method for the equation is to use the following chart based on the number of drops the administration set delivers:

gtt factor	divide the quantity of mL per hour by
60	1
20	3
15	4
10	6

For example if 1,000 mL are ordered to be given over 8 hours and the drop factor is 10 gtt/mL, then:

$$\frac{1000 \text{ mL}}{8} = 125 \text{ mL/hr}$$

$$\frac{125 \text{ mL/hour}}{6} = 20.8 \text{ or } 21 \text{ gtt/min}$$

Once the number of drops per minute has been determined, the IV set must be checked at 30- to 60-minute intervals to be sure that it continues to flow at the prescribed rate. As explained in the list of principles that affect the rate of flow, any number of factors can speed up or slow down the infusion.

If the IV slows down and has not been checked and readjusted for some time, **no attempt should be made to "catch up"** a large volume of fluid by speeding up the rate of flow beyond that ordered. This can lead to circulatory overload and a volume excess that may produce pulmonary edema in susceptible persons. Remember that elderly persons and those with either renal

or cardiac conditions cannot tolerate rapid administration of fluids. The symptoms of circulatory overload and other possible complications of IV therapy are shown in Table 5-11.

Think about . . . How would you calculate the rate of flow for the following order: "1,000 mL of D5W over 8 hours" using a drip set that delivers 15 gtt/mL? How would the rate differ if the drip set delivers 20 gtt/mL? How would you calculate the flow rate for this order? "250 mL NS at 50 mL/per hour" using a microdrip set (60 gtt/mL)?

Intravenous Intake   The total amount of IV fluid infused during the shift is calculated at the end of the shift. For example, if the beginning count was 350 mL (amount in container at beginning of shift) and a new solution of 1000 mL was added after the 350 mL was infused, then the 350 mL infused is added to whatever amount of the 1,000 mL that was added has infused by the end of the shift:

	Count	Infused
Count at beginning of shift	350 mL	
New solution added at 11:30	1,000 mL	350 mL
Count left at end of shift	525 mL	475 mL
Total amount of IV intake for shift		825 mL

Intravenous therapy may become such a commonplace procedure to nurses that they are tempted to be complacent about it. However, it should never be thought of as a routine procedure that requires little attention. **Any fluid or medication that enters a vein has an immediate effect.** There is no margin for error in its administration. Nursing Procedure 5-1 presents information on managing IV infusions.

TRANSFUSION OF BLOOD COMPONENTS

A transfusion is the IV administration of whole blood or one or more of its components. Among the components frequently transfused are plasma, packed red blood cells, granulocytes, platelets, and leukocytes. Table 5-12 shows some commonly used blood products, the usual amount given per transfusion, and reasons why each is used.

Special precautions are always taken when whole blood or any of its components are given. Blood banks have written procedures and policies for withdrawing and dispensing blood for transfusion. These procedures must be followed to minimize the possibility of an adverse reaction or administration of the wrong blood

TABLE 5-11 ◆ *Problems, Assessment, and Nursing Interventions for IV Therapy*

Problem	Assessment Data	Nursing Interventions
Infiltration caused by needle or catheter displacement or leakage of blood from vein.	Pain, redness, swelling around site, absence of backflow of blood, diminished rate or complete cessation of flow.	Stop flow of fluid and remove needle or catheter. Splint arm to stabilize it when site is over a joint. If noticed within 30 minutes of onset, apply ice to swelling. If noted later than 30 minutes, apply warm compresses to encourage absorption.
Air embolism caused by air in tubing, allowing container to run dry.	Cyanosis, drop in blood pressure, weak and rapid pulse.	Make sure all connections are airtight. Clear air from tubing before attaching the needle. Monitor and change containers promptly. If embolism occurs, place in Trendelenburg position and turn to left side.
Circulatory overload caused by inability of cardiovascular system to handle fluids at current rate of flow and volume.	Rise in blood pressure, headache, dyspnea, flushed skin, discrepancy between fluid intake and urinary output. Increased jugular venous distention.	Know patient's cardiovascular status. Monitor urinary output. Slow infusion rate to keep vein open. Elevate head of bed. Monitor vital signs. Adminsiter oxygen as prescribed.
Thrombophlebitis caused by injury to vein from movement, irritating additive, overuse of vein; too-slow flow rate that allows clot to form at end of needle.	Pain, redness, hardness along vein site. Sluggish flow rate. Swelling of limb.	Stabilize needle or catheter to minimize trauma to vein. Select large vein to help dilute additive. Alternate sites. Maintain desired flow rate.
Infected venipuncture site.	Swelling and soreness, yellow and foul-smelling discharge.	Use aseptic technique during venipuncture. Discontinue IV. Notify infection control officer so culture can be taken. Notify physician; apply antimicrobial ointment and dressing as prescribed.
Pyrogenic reaction caused by inadequate sterile technique, improper handling of tubing.	Rapid rise in temperature; severe chill 30 minutes after infusion started.	Check sterile technique when doing venipuncture. Avoid contamination of system when it is accidentally disconnected. Notify physician and administer prescribed therapy for infection.
Allergic reaction caused by hypersensitivity to additive.	Itching, rash, dyspnea.	Stop flow immediately; keep IV open with normal saline. Notify physician.

type to a recipient. Although many reactions and complications cannot be anticipated, carelessness in handling transfusion products cannot be excused.

Nursing Intervention   The staff nurse checks to see that a consent form allowing blood administration has been signed by the patient. Next, she determines whether the patient has an IV site already established and what size catheter is in place. It is best to give blood through an 18-gauge or larger catheter.

Blood is given with a blood administration set with a filter, preferably a Y-set. This allows one arm of the Y

to be used for the blood and the other to be used for normal saline. If a reaction to the blood occurs, the blood can be quickly shut off and the normal saline opened to maintain patency of the IV site.

Before the blood is started, two nurses (most hospitals require registered nurses) verify the patient's name and identification number, the number on the blood bag label, and the ABO group and RH type on the blood bag label with the corresponding information on the patient's identification band and blood bank band on his wrist. Both nurses sign the blood bank form if everything is correct. The blood must be started within

Nursing Procedure 5-1

Managing an intravenous therapy infusion All nurses are expected to monitor IV sites and ensure that intravenous fluids are administered as ordered. Any nurse may discontinue an IV infusion once such an order has been written.

Steps	Rationale
1. Verify that the solution hanging is the correct solution by checking the physician's order.	All IV solutions are ordered by the physician.
2. Check the IV site for redness, swelling, edema, blanching of the skin, coolness, or moisture, and question the patient about discomfort at the site.	Redness or swelling may indicate vein irritation; moisture indicates that the tubing is loose from the cannula or that the site is leaking and needs to be changed.
3. Verify that the tubing is unkinked and hanging free. Note when it was last changed.	For the solution to flow at the correct rate, the tubing must be unobstructed. If the patient is lying on the tubing, it will slow the rate; if the tubing is caught in the bedding, it may pull loose from the cannula. Tubing is changed every 24–48 hours.
4. Assess for signs of fluid volume excess by checking for edema, shortness of breath, or confusion and by auscultating the lungs. Verify that the patient's urine output is adequate.	Crackles in the lungs and edema may indicate fluid volume excess when accompanied by shortness of breath and confusion. If findings are positive, slow the infusion to a keep open rate and notify the nurse in charge and the physician. Urine output should be at least 30 mL/hour.
5. Calculate the correct flow rate, and adjust the flow accordingly; or check the IV pump for the correct settings. Be certain the alarm is "on" if using an IV pump.	The flow rate must be accurate so that the solution is infused as ordered.
6. If the solution does not flow properly, assess patency of the site by: kinking the tubing a few inches from the cannula and then pinching the tubing between the kink and the cannula. If resistance is felt, a clot may have formed at the tip of the cannula. Determine whether the cannula is lying against the side wall of the vessel; readjust it slightly. Raise the container slightly to increase the pull of gravity.	These actions will correct flow problems if the site is patent. If not, the IV should be discontinued and restarted in another location by someone certified to do so.
7. Look at the dressing to see that it is clean and dry and to check when it was last changed.	A dry dressing prevents the entrance of microorganisms at the site. Dressings are changed every 48 hours.
8. When there is 100 mL left in the container, notify the person responsible for hanging the next solution. Ascertain that the next solution ordered is available on the unit.	The new solution may be hung when there is 50 mL still remaining in the container. Making certain that the next solution is on the unit prevents the IV from running dry.
9. At the end of the shift, calculate the amount of solution left in the container. Calculate the amount of IV fluid that infused for the shift.	Calculating the amount "left to count" gives the oncoming shift a status report on the patient's IV. The amount of IV fluid infused must be added to the shift intake record.

To discontinue the IV infusion:

10. Check the physician's order. Gather the needed supplies, wash hands, don gloves, and explain the procedure to the patient.	An order is necessary to discontinue an IV. 2 × 2 gauze, alcohol swab, adhesive bandage, and near-by biohazard container are needed. *Standard precautions* must be used to prevent blood contamination.
11. Turn off the IV pump or shut the clamp on the IV tubing to stop the infusion. Remove the dressing. Place the gauze lightly over the site, and gently withdraw the cannula. Apply pressure to the site with the gauze. Place the cannula/needle and tubing where it will not stick anyone. Clean any blood off the skin around the site with the alcohol swab, and apply the adhesive bandage.	The IV will continue to flow after the cannula is removed if it is not shut off. Dry gauze and pressure will stop the bleeding at the site. Care must be taken not to allow the cannula/needle to stick anyone. An adhesive bandage will protect the site from microorganisms.

Nursing Procedure 5-1 *(Continued)*

Steps	Rationale
12. Place the cannula in a biohazard container, remove the gloves, wash the hands, and discard the remaining IV solution per agency policy.	The cannula is contaminated with blood. *Standard precautions* are necessary.
13. Document all IV care, including site condition, tubing change, dressing change, and discontinuation of the IV.	Most documentation is done on the IV flow sheet. Some documentation may be required on the daily activity and assessment sheet. Problems should be documented in the nurse's notes.

30 minutes of arrival on the unit and should never be left at room temperature for more than 4 hours; it takes from 1½ to 4 hours for a unit to run into the patient.

A set of baseline vital signs is taken just before the blood is administered to the patient. **For the first 15 minutes of the transfusion, the blood is run at 10 drops per minute and the patient is observed for signs of reaction such as chills, nausea, vomiting, skin rash, back pain, or tachycardia. Vital signs are taken every 5 minutes for the first 15 minutes. If any of these signs occur, the transfusion is stopped immediately and the charge nurse is notified at once.** If no signs of reaction occur during the first 15 minutes, vital signs are retaken. If they are within normal limits, the infusion may be set to run at the ordered rate. Assess the patient again 15 minutes after the rate has been increased and retake the vital signs. As long as there are no signs of adverse reaction, the patient is assessed and vital signs are taken every 30 to 60 minutes until the transfusion is completed depending on agency policy. The procedure for a blood transfusion is included in Chapter 17.

Elder Care Point . . . Vessels in the elderly are fragile. A 19-gauge cannula may be used rather than an 18-gauge for transfusion. Blood products should be transfused more slowly to allow the body time to adjust to the added fluid. Careful assessment for fluid overload during and after the transfusion is essential. A lag period of 2 hours should be observed between each unit transfused.

The word *reaction*, when used in reference to the transfusion of blood or the infusion of fluids, means a sensitivity to the blood itself or to the preservatives or other substances that have been added to a solution. Reactions to red blood cells are the result of incompatibility between blood types. There are antigens on the surfaces of red blood cells that can bring about a reaction if exposed to blood that is not the same type and is incompatible. The antigen–antibody reaction causes the cells to clump together and obstruct the flow of blood through the capillaries.

TABLE 5-12 ◆ *Blood Products and Their Use*

Product	Volume	Use
Whole blood	450–500 mL	Massive acute blood loss such as occurs with accidental injury and hemorrhage during surgery; infrequently administered.
Packed red blood cells	250–350 mL	Acute or chronic blood loss with tachycardia, shortness of breath, and low hemoglobin, and hematocrit.
Platelets	200–400 mL	Control or prevent bleeding from platelet deficiencies; for bleeding with platelet count <50,000/mm^3.
Fresh frozen plasma	200–250 mL	Clotting deficiencies; hypovolemia.
Granulocytes	100–400 mL	Granulocytopenia, especially in conjunction with infection.
Cryoprecipitate	5–10 mL (10 units tranfused at a time)	Factor VIII deficiency; Hemophilia A; von Willebrand's factor XIII, and fibrinogen.
Coagulation factor concentrates: Factor VIII, Factor XI	Dosage calculated individually	Treat congenital factor deficiencies.
Plasma derivatives: albumin, plasma protein fraction	200–500 mL 50–100 mL	Blood volume expansion; decreased plasma proteins; shock, massive hemorrhage, acute liver failure, burns, hemolytic disease of the newborn.

The symptoms of a reaction may be so mild as to go unnoticed or so severe that death is the eventual outcome. In milder cases the patient may develop a rash, hives, itching, or facial flushing. In more severe reactions the patient may experience dyspnea, sudden chills and fever, chest pains or tightness, low back pain, and shock. A delayed reaction due to hepatitis, syphilis, malaria, or other infectious agents might not be evident until 4 to 6 weeks or more after the blood has been given.

Treatment of a reaction depends on its cause and severity. If it is a mild allergic reaction, the physician may order an antihistamine (diphenhydramine hydrochloride, Benadryl) to relieve the symptoms. In severe anaphylactic reactions the treatment is the same as for anaphylaxis due to any extreme hypersensitivity.

Hospitals and other health care facilities in which blood transfusions are administered have written policies and procedures to guide the nursing staff when a patient shows signs of an adverse reaction. It is common practice to stop a transfusion immediately and notify the physician when early signs and symptoms of a reaction appear. The intravenous line usually is kept open with normal saline until further orders are obtained from the physician.

Think about... Your patient is receiving a unit of packed RBCs. When you assess him after the first hour of the transfusion, his pulse rate has increased from 78 to 84, he is slightly restless, and he is complaining of discomfort in his back. His temperature has risen from 98.4°F. to 99°F. He has no skin rash and denies nausea. What would you do?

PARTIAL OR TOTAL PARENTERAL NUTRITION

Many patients with fluid and electrolyte imbalances are nutritionally depleted. Partial parenteral nutrition (PPN) is given when a patient cannot maintain an adequate nutritional status with oral intake. PPN is given through a large peripheral vein in the arm. If sufficient nutrition cannot be delivered by oral intake and PPN, or by enteral feedings, total parental nutrition (TPN) is begun.

TPN solution is made up of a nitrogen (protein) source, hypertonic dextrose, and supplementary vitamins and minerals. The solution is hypertonic and contains 1 calorie/mL or 1,000 calories/liter. Some solutions also contain lipids. Because of its degree of concentration, it must be infused to a central vein, usually the subclavian, where the high rate of blood flow quickly dilutes it. The Hickman, Broviac, and Groshong and are the most frequently used central line catheters

and can be used for long-term therapy. TPN solution is administered with a pump or an infusion controller device so that the rate is constant. **The flow rate is never changed to "catch up" on the amount of fluid that should have been infused if the flow has slowed for some reason.**

TPN solutions and catheters must be handled with strict asepsis, as the solution is an ideal medium for bacterial growth. Infection is a major complication of total parenteral nutrition. The TPN solution is mixed in the pharmacy under sterile conditions. There are many complications of TPN in addition to infection, including glucose intolerance, electrolyte imbalance, phlebitis, allergic reaction, and fluid overload. The port through which TPN is administered is not used for any other solution. The patient must be carefully monitored. When TPN is begun, the flow rate is slowly started, at about 60 to 80 mL/hour, and gradually increased at 25 mL per hour until the maintenance rate is reached. This allows the body to adjust to the glucose load. Blood sugar determinations are performed frequently during the stabilization period, which is usually the first week. If the patient's body has difficulty with glucose tolerance, insulin may be ordered and is added to the TPN solution. At the end of therapy, the flow rate is tapered down for 1 to 2 hours before stopping the fluid to allow the body to adjust.

Peripheral parenteral nutrition is used for patients in whom central venous access is not possible and who will need IV nutritional support for only 7 to 10 days. The concentration of the solution given is less because it does not flow into a vessel with a large blood flow, which would dilute it. Table 5-13 summarizes the principles for administering TPN.

TABLE 5-13 ◆ *Principles for Administration of Total Parenteral Nutrition (TPN)*

- Placement of a central venous catheter must be verified by radiograph before beginning the infusion of the TPN solution.
- Use an infusion pump to administer TPN solution; start infusion slowly at first and increase to desired rate over a 24-hour period.
- If solution is administered cyclically (at night only), taper to the desired flow over 1 to 2 hours and taper flow down to 1 to 2 hours before completion.
- Check the amount actually infusing every 30 to 60 minutes; do not rely solely on the pump functioning accurately.
- Before administering other solutions or drugs through another lumen of the central line, check compatibility with the TPN solution.
- Monitor continuously for signs of complications such as glucose intolerance, infection, fluid volume excess, phlebitis, and sepsis.
- Record the intake and output accurately.
- Never speed up the solution flow rate beyond that ordered if it falls behind for some reason.

COMMUNITY CARE

Nurses in long-term care facilities deal every day with the problems of delicate fluid balance in their elderly patients. These patients often are taking multiple drugs that can affect their fluid and electrolyte status. Diuretics in particular can upset fluid and electrolyte status. It is especially important that the long-term care and home care nurse be vigilant for the signs of hypokalemia (Table 5-5). Potassium imbalances are particularly dangerous for the heart patient. Hypokalemia alters the way digitalis is metabolized in the body and predisposes to digitalis toxicity. Signs of digitalis toxicity are fatigue, anorexia, headache, blurred vision, yellow-green halos around lights, nausea, diarrhea, and cardiac dysrhythmias.

Any patient in a long-term care facility or at home who is taking digitalis and is experiencing nausea, vomiting, diarrhea, or fluid and electrolyte alterations should be questioned daily about symptoms of hypokalemia and digitalis toxicity.

Elder Care Point... Dehydration and hyponatremia secondary to infection or treatment of congestive heart failure account for the majority of hospital admissions of patients from long-term care facilities and home situations. It takes a caring, skillful nurse to see that long-term and home care patients take in enough fluids without interfering with their nutritional intake.

The home care nurse must collaborate with the infusion company nurse when the patient is receiving fluids at home or is on total parenteral nutrition. It is especially important that both nurses be consistent in teaching the patient and the family the procedures.

The elderly patient who has a fluid volume excess from congestive heart failure may already have a diminished appetite. In this instance, restricting sodium in the diet may do more harm than good. The nurse, along with the physician, must make individual judgments about the patient's priority needs.

Home care nurses must do considerable teaching to patients and family members when IV therapy is needed. Topics for teaching include purpose, precautions in rate of flow, aseptic techniques, potential complications, signs and symptoms to report, and whom to call if problems arise. Table 5-14 is a teaching guide that can be left with the patient.

CRITICAL THINKING EXERCISES

Clinical Case Problems

Read each clinical situation and discuss the questions with your classmates.

1. Mrs. Carlson, age 61, is admitted to the hospital with a diagnosis of congestive heart failure. She is extremely edematous and obese. Mrs. Carlson is slightly confused upon admission, and, although she is not on absolute bedrest, she tells you that she cannot get out of bed. She continues to refuse to get up or move about in bed the next morning when you are assigned to care for her.

   a. What type of diet would you expect Mrs. Carlson's physician to prescribe for her? How would you explain to her the restrictions of her diet and the need for her to follow it?

   b. How might you encourage Mrs. Carlson to get out of bed for her daily weighing?

   c. If Mrs. Carlson's fluid intake is restricted, how would you schedule her fluid intake?

   d. What problems might Mrs. Carlson's obesity and inactivity present?

2. Mr. Woo is a 35-year-old patient who has suffered a severe gastrointestinal upset producing nausea, vomiting, and diarrhea. He is admitted for rehydration, and his physician has written orders for IV fluids.

   a. List the observations you should make while caring for Mr. Woo.

   b. What nursing measures might be taken to relieve his symptoms? What medications might you expect him to receive?

   c. What are your responsibilities regarding Mr. Woo's IV therapy? Why is it necessary to check the infusion frequently? Would you measure his intake and output? In what electrolytes might he be deficient?

TABLE 5-14 ◆ *Patient Education: Home Care IV Therapy*

When should I call the home care nurse?

Call the nurse when:

- Swelling, redness, or pain occurs at the IV site or along the vessel.
- The solution will not flow even after you have checked that the clamps are open.
- The solution leaks at the catheter site and you have checked to see that the tubing is firmly attached to the catheter.
- The patient's temperature rises above 100° F (38° C).

Telephone number _____

BIBLIOGRAPHY

Andreoli, T. E., et al. (1993). *Cecil Essentials of Medicine*, 3rd ed. Philadelphia: Saunders.

Angeles, T., Barbone, M. (1994). Infiltration and phlebitis: assessment, management, and documentation. *Journal of Home Health Care Practice.* 7(1):16–21.

Angelucci, D., Todaro, A. (1993). Action stat! Reversing acute dehydration. *Nursing 93.* 23(6):33.

Batcheller, J. (1992). Disorders of antidiuretic hormone secretion. *AACN Clinical Issues in Critical Care Nursing.* 3(2):370–378.

Black, J. M., Matassarin-Jacobs, E. (1997). *Medical-Surgical Nursing: Clinical Management for Continuity of Care,* 5th ed. Philadelphia: Saunders.

Bove, L. A. (1994). How fluids and electrolytes shift. *Nursing 94.* 24(8):34–39.

Bove, L. A. (1996). Restoring electrolyte balance: sodium and Chloride. *RN.* 59(1):25–28.

Cirolian, B. (1996). Understanding Edema. *Nursing 96.* 26(2):66–69.

Copstead, L. C. (1995). *Perspectives on Pathophysiology.* Philadelphia: Saunders.

Coulter, K. (1992). Intravenous therapy for the elder patient: implications for the intravenous nurse. *Journal of Intravenous Nursing.* 15(suppl):S18–S23.

Cullen, L. (1992). Interventions related to fluid and electrolyte balance. *Nursing Clinics of North America.* 27(2):569–597.

Dennison, R. D., Blevins, B. N. (1992). Myths and facts . . . about acid–base imbalance. *Nursing 92.* 22(3):69.

deWit, S. C. (1994). *Rambo's Nursing Skills for Clinical Practice,* 4th ed. Philadelphia: Saunders.

Guyton, A. C. (1991). *Textbook of Medical Physiology,* 8th ed. Philadelphia: Saunders.

Harovas, J., Anthony, H. (1993). Your guide to trouble-free transfusions. *RN.* 56(11):26–35.

Hastings-Tolsma, M., Yucha, C. B. (1994). IV infiltration: no clear signs, no clear treatment? *RN.* 57(12):34–9.

Held, J. L. (1995). Cancer care: correcting fluid and electrolyte imbalances. *Nursing 95.* 25(4):71.

Ignatavicius, D. D., Workman, M. L., Mishler, M. A. (1995). *Medical-Surgical Nursing: A Nursing Process Approach,* 2nd ed. Philadelphia: Saunders.

Janusek, L. W. (1990). Metabolic acidosis. *Nursing 90.* 20(7):52.

Janusek, L. W. (1990). Metabolic alkalosis. *Nursing 90.* 20(6):52.

Kirton, C. A. (1996). Assessing edema. *Nursing 96.* 26(7):54.

Markel, S. (1994). PIC/PICC and extended peripheral catheters: five years' experience in home care. *Journal of Home Health Care Practice.* 7(1):35–40.

Martin, J. H., Larsen, P. D. (1994). Elder care: Dehydration in the elderly surgical patient. *AORN Journal.* 60(4):666–668.

Masoorli, S. (1995). Legally speaking. When IV practice spells malpractice. *RN.* 58(8):53–55.

Mays, D. (1995). Turning ABGs into child's play. *RN.* 58(1):36–40.

Mendyka, B. E. (1992). Fluid and electrolyte disorders caused by diuretic therapy. *AACN Clinical Issues in Critical Care Nursing.* 3(3):672–680.

Meyers, S., Texidor, M. S. (1994). Establishing a home health intravenous therapy program. *Journal of Home Health Care Practice.* 7(1):1–5.

Millam, D. A. (1992). Starting I.V.s: how to develop your venipuncture expertise. *Nursing 92.* 22(9):33–48.

Norris, M. K. (1994). Lab test tips: checking chloride levels. *Nursing 94.* 24(3):76.

O'donnell, M. E. (1995). Assessing fluid and electrolyte balance in elders. *American Journal of Nursing.* 95(11):41–45.

Owens, M. W. (1993). Keeping an eye on magnesium. *American Journal of Nursing.* 93(2):66–67.

Pals, J. K., et al. (1995). Clinical triggers for detection of fever and dehydration: implications for long-term care nursing. *Journal of Gerontological Nursing.* 21(4):13–19.

Perez, A. (1995). Hyperkalemia. *RN.* 58(11):33–36.

Perez, A. (1995). Restoring electrolyte balance: hypokalemia. *RN.* 58(12):33–36.

Perucca, R., Micek, J. (1993). Treatment of infusion-related phlebitis: review and nursing protocol. *Journal of Intravenous Nursing.* 16(5):282–286.

Ramer, F. (1994). How to identify electrolyte imbalances on your patient's E.C.G. *Nursing 94.* 24(6):54–58.

Roth, D. (1993). Integrating the licensed practical nurse and the licensed vocational nurse into the specialty of intravenous nursing. *Journal of Intravenous Nursing.* 16(3):156–166.

Sheldon, P., Bender, M. (1994). High-technology in home care: an overview of intravenous therapy. *Nursing Clinics of North America.* 29(3):507–519.

Sommers, J. (1990). Rapid fluid resuscitation—how to correct dangerous deficits. *Nursing 90.* 20(1):52–54.

Stringfield, Y. N. (1993). Acidosis, Alkalosis, and ABGs. *American Journal of Nursing.* 93(11):43–44.

Tasota, F. J., Wesmiller, S. W. (1994). Assessing A.B.G.s: maintaining the delicate balance. *Nursing 94.* 24(5):34–46.

Terry, J. (1994). The major electrolytes: sodium, potassium, and chloride. *Journal of Intravenous Nursing.* 19(5):240.

Toto, K. H., Yucha, C. B. (1994). Magnesium: homeostasis, imbalances, and therapeutic uses. *Critical Care Nursing Clinics of North America.* 6(4):767–783.

Vonfrolio, L. G. (1995). Would you hang these IV solutions? *American Journal of Nursing.* 95(6):37–39.

Ward, L. (1990). Home care: patient teaching for home IV therapy. *RN.* April:86.

Weinstein, S. M. (1993). *Plumer's Principles and Practice of Intravenous Therapy.* Philadelphia: Lippincott.

Wise, G. (1995). Intravenous therapy: are physicians asking the wrong nurses to do the task? *Journal of Practical Nursing.* 45(2):18–22.

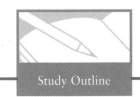

I. Physiology

A. Fluids account for about 56% of total body weight.

B. Differences depend on age, sex, and state of hydration.

C. There is a gradual decline of body fluids with age.

D. Maintenance of normal fluid balance is necessary in all ages, because all cell processes take place in a fluid medium.

E. When a person becomes ill or injured, his or her symptoms are manifestations of changes on a cellular level.

F. The internal environment of the body is the fluid that surrounds and bathes each cell.

G. Homeostasis is the maintenance of a constant, stable environment for the cells.

H. Every organ in the body is involved in the task of maintaining homeostasis so that the environment of every cell is essentially the same.

II. Distribution of Body Fluids

A. Factors that influence body fluids distribution are summarized in Figure 5-2; fluids and their compartments are summarized in Table 5-1.

  1. Intracellular fluid is contained within the body's cells.

  2. Extracellular fluid is fluid that is outside of the body's cells.

    a. Interstitial fluid is the fluid in the spaces between the cells.

    b. Intravascular fluid is the fluid contained in the blood and lymph vessels.

     (1) When fluid shifts from the intravascular space to the interstitial space, hypovolemia may occur. (Hypovolemia is low blood volume.)

     (2) This shift may occur with severe trauma, burns, intestinal obstruction, sepsis, cirrhosis of the liver, peritonitis, nephrosis—and is called "third spacing."

    c. Transcellular fluids are those that are secreted and excreted by the body: gastrointestinal secretions, saliva, aqueous humor in the eye, urine, pericardial, pleural, synovial, and cerebrospinal fluid.

B. Transport: movement of fluids to ensure normal distribution of fluids.

  1. Heart action necessary to pump intravascular fluid.

  2. *Diffusion:* the spontaneous mixing and moving of molecules.

  3. *Osmosis:* the passage of water molecules across a semipermeable membrane. Movement is from the less concentrated solution to the more concentrated, so that solutions on both sides of the membrane are made equally concentrated.

III. Fluid and Electrolytes

A. Water is in greatest proportion.

  1. Serves as the medium in which physiological and chemical activities occur.

  2. Transports essential nutrients.

  3. Dilutes toxins of waste.

  4. Allows electrolytes to become active by being in solution.

B. Electrolytes.

  1. Break into small atomic particles when placed in solution.

  2. Some particles are negatively charged (anions), and some are positively charged (cations).

  3. Difference in electric charge creates an electrical impulse across membranes.

  4. Important to contraction of muscles, nerve activity, and glandular secretions.

  5. Important electrolytes and their functions are summarized in Tables 5-2 to 5-7.

  6. Most illnesses affect fluid and electrolyte balance in some way.

  7. Whenever sodium is retained in the body, there will be water retention and an increase in the extracellular volume.

  8. Normal serum sodium range for the adult is 135 to 145 mEq/L.

  9. Calcium regulates neuromuscular activity and plays a role in the coagulation of blood.

  10. Normal serum calcium in the adult is 8.4 to 10.6 mEq/L.

  11. Excess amounts of calcium can cause cardiac arrest.

  12. Potassium helps regulate neuromuscular activity of heart, skeletal, and smooth muscle.

  13. Normal potassium levels in the adult are 3.5 to 5.0 mEq/L.

  14. Potassium chloride is never given IV as a "push" or undiluted medication.

15. Magnesium is required for the transmission of nerve impulses, dilatation of peripheral blood vessels, and normal contractions of the heart muscle.

16. Phosphorus is necessary for the metabolism of nutrients and is essential for the formation of bone; it acts as a buffer to promote acid–base balance.

17. Chloride is the major anion in the extracellular fluid; it is important in the formation of hydrochloric acid in the stomach and necessary for digestion.

18. Assessment and nursing interventions related to fluid and electrolyte imbalances are summarized in Tables 5-1 to 5-7.

IV. Fluid Imbalances

A. Main source of gain of body fluids is by ingestion and absorption from the digestive tract.

B. Average amount of water taken each day is 2,500 mL. Source is water, liquids, fruits, vegetables, and meat. 250 mL is produced during metabolism.

C. Normal output for a 24-hour period is about 2,500 mL.

D. Pathophysiology: fluid imbalance exists when there is either a deficit or excess of body water and the solutes it contains.

E. Fluid deficit.

1. Too little fluid taken in or too much lost without replacement.

2. Many patients can be spared the effects of fluid deficit if they receive planned and effective nursing care.

3. Nursing responsibilities in the prevention of fluid deficit.

   a. Assessment.

      (1) Patients at risk: those who are unable to drink sufficient quantities and those with excessive loss through prolonged vomiting, diarrhea, draining fistulas and operative wounds, and burns.

      (2) Treatments such as gastric suction, diuretic therapy, and tap water enemas predispose patients to fluid deficit.

      (3) Subjective symptoms: thirst, dizziness, feeling faint upon standing up (postural hypotension), weakness, and weight loss.

      (4) Objective symptoms: oliguria, dry mucous membranes, dry skin with poor turgor, and flat neck veins.

      (5) The most accurate measure of fluid gain or loss for any age group is weight change.

   b. Medical treatment and nursing intervention.

      (1) Measures to ensure adequate oral intake if at all possible.

      (2) Help control underlying disorder.

      (3) It is essential to measure, rather than estimate, fluid intake and output.

   c. Evaluation: see Nursing Care Plan 5-1.

4. The patient with nausea and vomiting.

   a. *Nausea:* feeling of discomfort in epigastrium and abdomen with tendency to vomit.

   b. Assessment:

      (1) Subjective symptoms: complaint of feeling nauseated or "sick to my stomach," queasiness, abdominal pain, epigastric discomfort or burning, history of vomiting.

      (2) Objective symptoms: pallor; mild diaphoresis; cold, clammy skin; attempts to remain motionless. Vomitus observed for amount, odor, color, and contents. Note and record patterns of vomiting and conditions that trigger it.

   c. Medical treatment and nursing intervention:

      (1) Administer medication ordered, position patient to prevent aspiration of vomitus, and wipe patient's face with cool, damp cloth during vomiting episodes.

      (2) Give ice chips and provide frequent oral hygiene.

      (3) Provide quiet and odor-free environment.

      (4) Reinstate diet slowly, beginning with clear liquids and gradually adding foods.

      (5) Goals usually appropriate for a nursing care plan for a patient with nausea and vomiting include:

         (a) Patient is able to renew intake of fluids and food; no episodes of vomiting.

         (b) Fluid intake and output balanced.

         (c) Electrolytes restored to normal values.

      (6) Prolonged vomiting can lead to sodium and potassium deficits and metabolic alkalosis.

      (7) Vomitus is observed for odor, color, contents, and amount.

5. The patient with diarrhea.

   a. Diarrhea: the frequent passage of watery stools; results in rapid loss of water, nutritive elements, and electrolytes.

b. Assessment:

(1) Patients at risk: likely to be those with intestinal infections, colitis, irritable bowel syndrome, and allergies. Also can occur with obstruction of bowel due to tumor or fecal impaction.

(2) Subjective symptoms: history of frequent, watery stools, abdominal cramping, general weakness.

(3) Objective symptoms: loose, watery stools; active bowel sounds. Stools observed for number and characteristics (e.g., color, consistency, unusual contents, and peculiar odor).

c. Nursing intervention and medical treatment.

(1) Provide rest and privacy.

(2) Explain diagnostic procedures and give patient support and encouragement.

(3) Limit intake of foods at first, then gradually add clear liquids and then more solid foods.

(4) Assist patient by maintaining calm, understanding approach.

(5) Administer antidiarrheic drugs as ordered.

d. Goals in a plan of care might include:

(1) Return to normal pattern of bowel elimination.

(2) Reduction in complaints of discomfort.

(3) Maintenance of integrity of perianal skin.

(4) Adequate nutrition; cessation of weight loss.

(5) Being able to get sufficient rest.

6. Fluid deficits from other causes.

a. Improper use of gastric and intestinal suction. As much as 2,500 mL of gastric fluid and 1,500 mL of saliva can be removed in a 24-hour period by continuous suction.

b. Observe and note fluid loss from draining fistulas.

c. Measure fluid intake and output of surgical patient.

d. Be especially alert to fluid loss in severely burned patients.

F. Fluid volume excess.

1. Excessive amount of body *water* alone is rare. It can occur, however, if patient drinks more water than needed, if IV fluids are administered too rapidly or in excess, or if tap water enemas are given.

2. Edema is a more common problem. Edema: the excessive accumulation of freely moving interstitial fluid. Can be either generalized or localized.

a. Generalized edema occurs when body fails to eliminate sodium and water. Can be result of:

(1) Kidney failure.

(2) Heart failure.

(3) Hormonal disorder with excess of aldosterone and ADH.

(4) Malnutrition.

b. Localized edema can occur as a result of trauma, allergies, burns, obstruction of lymph flow, and liver failure.

c. Dependent edema is an effect of gravity. Especially noticeable in feet and ankles and in sacral region of bedridden patients.

d. Whenever sodium is retained in the body, water is retained also.

e. Nursing responsibilities.

(1) Assessment.

(a) Subjective symptoms: history can be very significant (e.g., whether patient needs more than one pillow to sleep, gets up frequently during the night to urinate, has shortness of breath from pressure of fluid in abdominal cavity). History of weight gain.

(b) Objective symptoms: obvious edema of feet and ankles, sacral region, etc. Crackles in lungs upon auscultation. Lab analysis of blood usually shows a low hematocrit. Patient may have pitting edema of body parts that are below the level of the heart.

(2) Medical treatment and nursing intervention.

(a) Weigh patient daily.

(b) Measure intake and output; restrict fluid intake as ordered.

(c) Exercise legs; periodically elevate feet and legs.

(d) Give meticulous skin care to avoid breakdown of fragile edematous tissue.

(e) Limit sodium and fluid intake as prescribed.

(f) Carefully monitor IV fluids.

(g) Prepare patient for discharge by teaching self-care.

(h) Suggested outcome criteria for management of generalized edema and case of localized edema presented in Table 5-9.

(3) Patient education.

   (a) Teach elderly to pay attention to fluid loss immediately and seek replacement of fluids.

   (b) Patients taking potassium-wasting diuretics need to replace potassium daily: eat bananas or drink orange juice; report vomiting or diarrhea to the doctor promptly.

V. Acid-Base Balance (Hydrogen Ion Concentration)

A. Pathophysiology.

1. Body fluids normally are slightly alkaline, even though metabolic activities produce acids.

2. Two types of activities maintain normal pH.

   a. Respiratory activities in which carbon dioxide is exchanged for oxygen.

   b. Metabolic activities involving retention and excretion of bicarbonate by the kidney.

3. The higher the concentration of hydrogen ions in a solution, the lower the pH.

4. The pH of the body's fluids is normally somewhat alkaline (between 7.35 and 7.45).

5. The kidneys maintain pH during metabolic activities by either reabsorbing or excreting bicarbonate.

6. The lungs help maintain pH by slowing respiration to retain carbon dioxide (acid) or by speeding up to rid the body of more carbon dioxide.

B. Arterial blood gas analysis: useful in assessing status of imbalances related to both respiration and metabolism (See Figure 5-7).

1. In respiratory acidosis the kidneys will retain and manufacture more bicarbonate to neutralize the excess acid; this is a slow process and takes time.

2. In response to metabolic acidosis, the patient will hyperventilate to get rid of carbon dioxide so that it is not available for the production of carbonic acid.

C. Respiratory acidosis.

1. Assessment.

   a. Patients at risk are those with acute or chronic impairment of respiration that causes accumulation of carbon dioxide in the blood.

   b. Subjective symptoms: complaints of increasing difficulty breathing, history of respiratory obstruction, weakness, dizzi-

ness, sleepiness, change in mental alertness, and restlessness.

   c. Objective symptoms: increased levels of carbon dioxide in the blood (noted in blood gas analysis), dyspnea, and obvious respiratory problems. pH < 7.35, pCO_2 > 45 mm Hg.

2. Intervention.

   a. For acute respiratory acidosis, establish airway, administer oxygen with great caution; 2 to 3 L/min for patients with COPD.

   b. Inhalation treatments, postural drainage, bronchodilators, or antibiotics if indicated.

   c. Prevention includes cautious administration of drugs that depress respiration.

D. Respiratory alkalosis.

1. Assessment: common in those who hyperventilate.

   a. Subjective symptoms: complaints of dizziness and tingling of fingers.

   b. Objective symptoms: pallor around mouth, rapid and deep breathing, spasms of hands and feet. pH > 7.35, pCO_2 < 35 mmHg.

2. Intervention.

   a. Treat hysteria, if present; may require sedation.

   b. Have patient rebreathe exhaled air.

   c. Avoid overzealous use of ventilator.

E. Metabolic acidosis.

1. Likely to occur in those who have poor carbohydrate metabolism and burn fats for energy (e.g., those with uncontrolled diabetes, persons on low-carbohydrate, high-protein diet to lose weight, and those with kidney failure, diarrhea, and gastrointestinal fistula).

2. Assessment.

   a. Subjective symptoms: history of inadequate carbohydrate metabolism or intake (fad diets); weakness, malaise, headache.

   b. Objective symptoms: fruity odor to breath, vomiting and diarrhea, stupor, loss of consciousness. pH < 7.35, HCO_3 < 22 mEq/L.

3. Intervention.

   a. Help diabetic patients maintain control of their illness.

   b. Teach public about hazards of fad diets.

   c. Carefully monitor patients receiving IV fluid therapy.

   d. Administer bicarbonate or lactate as ordered.

e. Measure intake and output.

f. Implement safety precautions for disoriented and those subject to altered levels of consciousness.

g. Frequent mouth care.

F. Metabolic alkalosis.

1. Assessment: patients at risk include those with severe vomiting, gastric suction, intestinal fistulas, diuresis, steroid therapy. pH > 7.45, HCO_3 > 45 mEq/L.

2. Intervention.

a. Observe for signs of potassium depletion.

b. Measure and record intake and output.

c. Institute safety precautions.

d. Monitor vital signs.

e. Watch for signs of calcium depletion.

VI. **Therapy for Fluid/Electrolyte Imbalances**

A. IV therapy.

1. Purpose: administration of electrolytes, nutrients, water, etc.; rapid administration of drugs.

2. Concentration (osmotic pressure) of IV fluid has direct influence on hydration of cells.

3. Isotonic solution has same osmotic pressure as intracellular fluid.

4. Hypotonic solution has a lower osmotic pressure than that of body fluids.

5. Hypertonic solution has a higher osmotic pressure than that of body fluids; Will pull excess interstitial fluid into the vascular compartment.

6. Common IV solutions are normal saline, dextrose solution, and lactated Ringer's solution.

7. Nursing responsibilities.

a. Goals of care.

(1) Preventing infection.

(2) Minimizing trauma to veins and adjacent tissue.

(3) Administering correct fluid at prescribed rate of flow.

(4) Observing patient response.

b. Calculate the rate of flow

c. Calculate the IV intake at the end of shift.

B. Transfusion of whole blood and blood components.

1. Special precautions always are indicated.

2. Transfusion reaction can be mild or fatal. Signs and symptoms: rash, hives, itching, or facial flushing; dyspnea, sudden chills and fever, chest pains or tightness, low back pain, and shock.

3. Usual procedure is to stop transfusion, start saline and notify physician when signs of reaction occur.

4. Nursing interventions.

a. Patient data checked with data on blood bank slips by two nurses.

b. Baseline vital signs taken before blood is started.

c. Blood administration set used with filter and Y lines with normal saline and blood bag.

d. Begin blood at 20 drops per minute for first 15 minutes.

e. If no signs of reaction, increase flow to ordered rate.

C. Total parenteral nutrition

1. Provides long-term nutritional therapy for patients with fluid and electrolyte imbalances who cannot be fed orally or enterally.

2. Usually given by central line, usually in the subclavian vein, so that it will be immediately diluted by high blood flow. Types of central line catheters include the Hickman, Broviac, and Groshong.

3. Solution provides protein, glucose, vitamins, and minerals.

4. TPN can cause many complications such as infection, fluid overload, phlebitis, dehydration, and hyperglycemia.

5. Patients receiving TPN must be monitored closely.

6. For principles guiding administration of TPN, see Table 5–13.

VII. **Community Care**

A. Long-term care nurses deal with delicate fluid balance in their elderly patients daily.

B. Long-term care and home care nurses must be especially vigilant for signs of hypokalemia in patients taking diuretics.

C. Hypokalemia may cause digitalis toxicity: fatigue, anorexia, headache, blurred vision, yellow-green halos around lights, nausea, diarrhea, and cardiac dysrhythmias.

D. Dehydration and hyponatremia secondary to infection or treatment of congestive heart failure accounts for the majority of hospital admissions of elderly patients from long-term care facilities and home care.

E. If appetite is suppressed, sodium restriction may not be wise for the elderly patient with heart failure.

F. Home care nurses must collaborate with infusion company nurses on teaching patients receiving TPN or long-term IV therapy. (Table 5–14).

VIII. Elderly Care Points

    A. Fluid volume deficit is a very common problem in the elderly.

    B. The elderly become dehydrated easily.

    C. Fluid volume deficit causes constipation, orthostatic hypotension, and dizziness, which can contribute to falls.

    D. Mucous membrane and tongue condition are more reliable for assessment of fluid status in the elderly than skin turgor.

    E. If skin is assessed, use the skin of the forehead or sternum.

    F. Elderly with cardiac conditions are at risk for heart failure if they become overloaded with fluid; IV fluids must be very carefully regulated.

    G. Laxative and enema use among the elderly often lead to fluid, potassium, and sodium loss.

    H. If an elderly patient becomes confused for no obvious reason, suspect fluid and electrolyte imbalance.

    I. Fluid and electrolyte imbalances often lead to need for hospitalization among long-term care facility residents.

CHAPTER 6

Problems of Infection: Prevention and Nursing Care

The invasion of the body by microorganisms is what causes infection. An infection can be **communicable** (transmitted to another) or **noncommunicable** (not usually transmitted to another). Although vaccines and antibiotics have made the treatment of infectious disease more effective, new microorganisms as well as drug-resistant strains continue to arise and the incidence of infectious disease has been increasing. The greater use of invasive diagnostic procedures, the treatment of cancer, and transplant rejection with immunosuppressive agents are related to the increase in incidence of infectious diseases. The rise in the number of patients with AIDS who are highly susceptible to infection is another factor.

The emergence of the Ebola virus in Africa and the rise of antibiotic-resistant strains of *Enterococcus* species and *Stapholococcus aureus* in the United States make infection-control measures more important than ever. Between 1980 and 1992, deaths from infectious disease rose by 58%. Understanding the infection cycle, the body's protective mechanisms, and how to prevent transmission of pathogens can help prevent infection, decrease its spread, or minimize its severity.

OVERVIEW OF THE INFECTIOUS PROCESS

Infection is a process by which a pathogenic organism invades the body of a host and establishes itself to reproduce (colonization). If the body environment is favorable to the growth and reproduction of the pathogenic organism (**incubation**), infection occurs. If the body environment is hostile to the invader and kills or expels it, infection does not occur. When the pathogenic organism has reproduced in sufficient numbers to cause symptoms, the incubation period is complete. This period of incubation is the *latent period* where the patient shows no symptoms but the infectious organism can be shed from the body and transmitted to another person.

Infectious disease, and its symptoms, is the result of an invasion of a pathogen, the response

139

of the host to the destructive action of the pathogen or to the toxic substances the pathogen produces, and the immune responses that the body uses to fight the pathogen.

The period of communicability extends until the organism is no longer shedding from the body. This period varies with different pathogens and different diseases. **Pathogens that can cause infection include bacteria, viruses, rickettsiae, mycoplasmas, chlamydiae, protozoa, fungi, helminths, and prions.** Figure 6-1 shows some of the most common forms of pathogens.

PATHOGENIC ORGANISMS

◆ Bacteria

Bacteria are microscopically small organisms belonging to the plant kingdom. They can be classified into three major categories, according to their Gram-staining

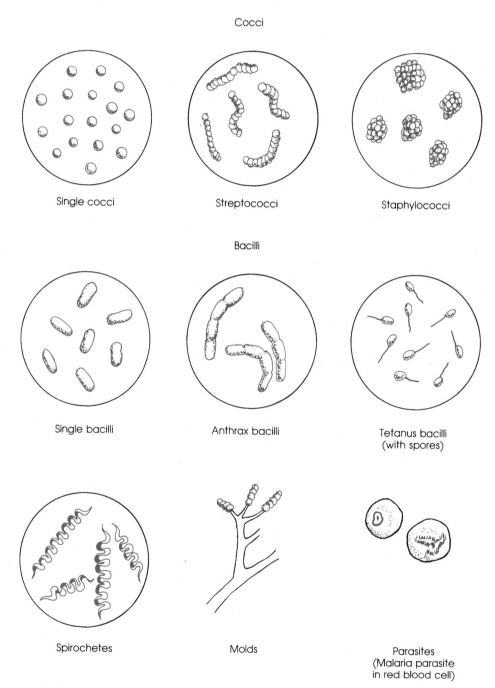

FIGURE 6-1   **Various pathogenic microorganisms as they appear under the microscope. Their shape and groupings determine classification.**

properties, their shape, and their requirements for oxygen. Bacteria that take up the gram stain (a dye) are gram-positive; those that will not take up a gram stain are gram-negative. *Cocci* are round, *Bacilli* are rod-shaped, and *Spirochetes* are spiral or corkscrew shaped. Some bacteria grow in chains *(Streptococci)*, some grow in pairs *(Diplococci)*, and some grow in clusters *(Staphylococci)*. Bacteria that require oxygen to live and reproduce are **aerobic**; those that cannot tolerate the presence of oxygen are **anaerobic**. When bacteria enter the body, they trigger the immune system to produce **antibodies** (proteins that fight and destroy antigens). Some bacteria produce poisonous substances called **endotoxins** (within the bacteria), others produce **exotoxins** (excreted by the bacteria).

Different bacteria thrive under different environmental conditions. Some form **spores** (reproductive cells with a thick membrane) to protect themselves against destruction from heat, cold, lack of water, toxic chemicals, and radiation. Others thrive best in water. The bacterium that causes tuberculosis can survive for years in dust. Some bacteria, such as *S. aureus* can survive very high temperatures. Different methods are necessary to rid the body and inanimate objects of these disease-producing agents.

♦ Viruses

Viruses have characteristics that make them particularly dangerous to humans. They are extremely small (visible only with an electron microscope); are composed of particles of nucleic acids, either DNA or RNA (the "stuff" of which genes are made), with a coat of protein and, in some cases, carbohydrate and fatty material; and they can grow and replicate only in a living cell. Viruses can camouflage themselves and take up residence in the body's cells without calling attention to themselves. Once there, they can trigger an immune response that is harmful to the body's cells or they can damage cells in other ways. In some acute viral infections, such as measles and chickenpox, the viruses reproduce within the cells, causing them to burst. In more chronic viral infections the viruses change the cells' membranes so that they are not recognized by the body as part of its "self." Thinking, then, that these altered cells are foreign, the body's immune system attacks and injures or destroys them. Many of the so-called slow viruses can reside in the body for years without producing symptoms and then suddenly cause an acute flareup of symptoms. Herpes viruses are examples of this type.

Viruses, like bacteria, vary in their resistance to destruction by chemical disinfectants. Most are easily inactivated by heat, but the hepatitis viruses can resist boiling for at least 30 minutes.

♦ Protozoa

Protozoa are microscopic one-celled organisms belonging to the animal kingdom. Protozoa that are pathogenic to man include the *Plasmodium* species that cause human malaria; *Enamoeba histolytica,* which causes amoebic dysentery; and other strains capable of causing diarrhea. **Protozoa are often transmitted via contaminated water or food.**

♦ Rickettsiae

Rickettsiae are small round or rod-shaped microorganisms that are transmitted by the bites of lice, ticks, fleas, and mites. Diseases of this kind are most likely to develop wherever sanitation standards are low and there is poor control of rodents and insects.

♦ Fungi

Fungi are very small, primitive organisms of the plant kingdom; yeasts and molds also are members of this group. They feed on living plants and animals and decaying organic material and thrive in warm, moist environments. Fungal infections in humans are called *mycoses* and are classified into three main types: (1) systemic or deep mycoses involving internal organs, especially the lungs; (2) subcutaneous mycoses, which involve the deeper layers of the skin, subcutaneous tissues, and sometimes bone; and (3) superficial or cutaneous mycoses, which grow in the outer layer of the skin, hair, and nails.

Fungal infections are difficult to eradicate once they have invaded a human host, mainly because fungi tend to form spores that are resistant to ordinary antiseptics and disinfectants. The course of treatment must be carried out conscientiously and over a long period. Athlete's foot and ringworm are two typical fungal infections. Fungi are very difficult to eliminate in the environment completely. Control is achieved by changing the environment so that their numbers are decreased, causing them to be too sparse to produce symptoms.

Systemic mycoses have become more frequent because of the increased incidence of people with AIDS who are more susceptible and because of the use of toxic drugs to fight cancer. These also upset the normal balance of body flora. *Histoplasmosis*, which affects the lungs, is transmitted by the inhalation of spores. Both systemic and topical drugs are used to treat fungal infections.

♦ Mycoplasmas

Mycoplasmas are very small organisms that no longer have the ability to form a cell wall. They cause infections of the genital tract or the respiratory tract such as mycoplasma pneumonia.

◆ Other Infectious Agents

Helminths are worms or flukes and belong to the animal kingdom. Pinworms are the most common in this country and mostly affect children. *Chlamydia* is the organism responsible for trachoma and is more prevalent in tropical and unindustrialized countries. Prions are rare; they cause Creutzfeldt-Jakob disease (Table 6-1).

The most effective means for destroying viruses and all other kinds of microorganisms is to expose them to moist heat at a temperature of 250°F (121°C) for 15 to 20 minutes.

Think about . . . Why do you think it has been more difficult to find ways to treat viral illnesses than it has been to find ways to treat bacterial illnesses?

THE INFECTION CHAIN

Infection occurs as a cyclical process, as shown in Figure 6-2. Each part of the cycle, or chain, is interrelated with the other parts. Disruption at any point in the chain will

TABLE 6-1 ◆ *Organisms That Produce Infection in People**

Organism Class	Common Examples	Common Disease Manifestations
Prions		◆ Creutzfeldt-Jakob disease
Viruses	◆ Poliovirus ◆ Hepatitis A virus ◆ Rhinovirus ◆ Influenza A virus ◆ Mumps virus	◆ Poliomyelitis ◆ Hepatitis ◆ Common cold ◆ Influenza ◆ Mumps
Chlamydiae	◆ *Chlamydia trachomatis* ◆ *C. psittaci*	◆ Trachoma, lymphogranuloma venereum, conjuncitivitis ◆ Psittacosis (parrot fever)
Mycoplasmas	◆ *Mycoplasma pneumoniae* ◆ *Ureaplasma urealyticum* ◆ *Mycoplasma hominis*	◆ Pneumonia ◆ Urethritis ◆ Pyelonephritis, pelvic inflammatory disease
Rickettsiae	◆ *Rickettsia rickettsii* ◆ *R. prowazekii* ◆ *Coxiella burnetii*	◆ Rocky Mountain spotted fever ◆ Typhus ◆ Q fever
Bacteria	◆ *Staphylococcus* sp. ◆ *Streptococcus* sp. ◆ *Neisseria meningitidis* ◆ *Escherichia coli* ◆ *Pseudomonas aeruginosa*	◆ Superficial skin infections, osteomyelitis, pneumonia, uremia ◆ Pharyngitis, skin infections, pneumonia ◆ Meningitis ◆ Urinary tract infection ◆ Skin infection, otitis, urinary tract infection
Fungi	◆ *Candida albicans* ◆ *Aspergillus* sp. ◆ *Cryptococcus neoformans* ◆ *Hisotoplasma capsulatum* ◆ *Coccidioides immitis*	◆ Thrush, vaginitis ◆ Sinusitis, brain abscess ◆ Meningitis, pneumonia ◆ Pneumonia ◆ Pneumonia
Protozoa	◆ *Entamoeba histolytica* ◆ *Plasmodium* sp. ◆ *Leishmania* sp. ◆ *Toxoplasma gondii* ◆ *Pneumocystis carinii*	◆ Diarrhea, colitis ◆ Malaria ◆ Fever, weight loss, cutaneous lesions ◆ Chorioretinitis, encephalitis ◆ Pneumonia
Helminths	◆ *Ancylostoma duodenale* (hookworm) ◆ *Ascaris lumbricoides* (roundworm) ◆ *Enterobius vermicularis* (pinworm) ◆ *Schistosoma* sp. (blood flukes) ◆ *Taenia solium* (pork tapeworm)	◆ Anemia ◆ Intestinal obstruction ◆ Anal pruritus ◆ Hydronephrosis ◆ Epilepsy from cysticercosis

*Organsism are presented in order of increasing complexity.
Source: Ignatavicius, D.D., Workman, M.L., Mishler, M.A. (1995). *Medical-Surgical Nursing: A Nursing Process Approach,* 2nd ed. Philadelphia: Saunders, p. 590.

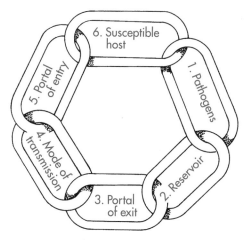

FIGURE 6-2 The cyclical process of infection. Each link of the infection cycle must be present and in proper sequence to produce disease.

prevent infection. Control of infection is aimed at interrupting the cycle. The **reservoir** is any place the pathogen is found; it can be **animate** (living) or **inanimate** (nonliving). People, animals, and insects are animate reservoirs. Inanimate reservoirs can be soil, water, surfaces of objects, contaminated solutions, or anything on which pathogens are located. The body can be a reservoir as pathogens can grow and multiply (**colonize**) in the skin and in body substances such as urine, feces, wound drainage, saliva, and respiratory secretions. **Even a person who does not have symptoms of disease, but harbors pathogens, can be a reservoir** *(a carrier)*. Out in the community, improperly cooked, contaminated food, stagnant water, or sewage can be reservoirs.

Think about . . . If you look around your home, what three "reservoirs" for microorganisms could you probably find?

The *portals of exit* and *portals of entry* **provide the means by which pathogens move in and out of the body.** A cut in the skin can let pathogens out via the bleeding that occurs or pathogens can come in through the cut; pathogens can enter or exit the respiratory tract via air inhaled that contains someone else's respiratory secretions from a sneeze or a cough or by the air exhaled when coughing or sneezing. Table 6-2 gives examples of organisms and the point at which they enter the body.

The *mode of transmission* **can be by direct or indirect contact.** Contact with a reservoir, such as the infected secretions of a wound or a contaminated vehicle (i.e., a contaminated needle, thermometer, cup or eating utensil, dressing, or piece of hospital equipment) can transmit pathogens. Organisms can be introduced any time a body is entered for a medical test or treatment if the equipment used is not sterile or the person performing the test or treatment does not use

strict asepsis. *Vectors* (carriers), **such as mosquitoes, fleas, ticks, flies, and other insects, can transmit pathogens by their bites or stings.**

Think about . . . Can you name three "modes of transmission" of infection you might encounter during an outing to a movie theater?

The *host* becomes *susceptible* **to infection when the body's own protective mechanisms fail to function efficiently.** When any of the body's defense mechanisms break down, the body is more susceptible to infection. Whenever a patient undergoes surgery or experiences physical trauma, the first line of defense against infection, the skin, is penetrated. The stress of the surgery and anesthesia on the body also make it more susceptible to infection. **Immune status plays the largest role in determining risk for infection.** It is because the human immunodeficiency virus (HIV) attacks the immune system and drastically damages it that AIDs patients die from other infectious diseases, such as *Pneumocystis carinii*, a form of pneumonia.

Some people are more susceptible to disease than others. Personal characteristics and actions increase or decrease the likelihood of an infection occurring. Heredity plays a role in natural resistance to disease; **the very young (especially under age 3) and the elderly have a less efficient immune system.** Certain ethnic groups are more susceptible to particular types of pathogens. For example, native Americans are more susceptible to tuberculosis than Caucasians. Nutritional state, general health, hormone balance, and the presence of a concurrent disease such as diabetes mellitus also are factors in susceptibility. **A state of malnutrition predisposes to contracting an infection.** Elderly people may have a decreased nutritional state for many reasons. Excessive stress is another factor. Students often contract colds or flu toward the end of a stressful exam week. Widowed people often develop an illness soon after losing their loved one. Keeping the body's protective mechanisms intact and in good working order decreases susceptibility to infection.

◆ Protective Mechanisms

The largest organ of the body, the skin, serves as a first line of defense against harmful agents in the environment. It functions as a protective covering for the more delicate and vulnerable underlying tissues. It also excretes, through sweat and sebaceous glands, lactic acid and fatty acids that inhibit the growth of bacteria.

Secretions from the mucous membranes lining the respiratory, gastrointestinal, and reproductive tracts contain an abundance of the enzyme *lysozyme*, which is bactericidal. The same enzyme is also found in tears and

TABLE 6-2 ◆ *Portals of Entry of Selected Disease-Producing Organisms*

Portal of Entry	Infecting Organisms	Resultant Diseases
Respiratory tract	◆ *Neisseria meningitidis*	◆ Meningococcal pneumonia, meningococcal meningitis, meningococcemia
	◆ *Cryptococcus neoformans*	◆ Cryptococcal meningitis, cryptococcal pneumonia
	◆ *Mycobacterium tuberculosis*	◆ Tuberculosis
	◆ Influenza A virus	◆ Influenza
	◆ *Streptococcus pneumoniae*	◆ Pneumococcal pneumonia
	◆ Measles virus (rubeola)	◆ Measles
	◆ *Legionella pneumophila*	◆ Legionnaires' disease
	◆ Varicella-zoster virus	◆ Chickenpox
Gastrointestinal tract	◆ *Salmonella enteritidis*	◆ Gastroenteritis
	◆ *Salmonella typhi*	◆ Typhoid fever
	◆ *Giardia lamblia*	◆ Diarrhea
	◆ *Clostridium botulinum*	◆ Botulism
	◆ Poliovirus	◆ Poliomyelitis
	◆ Hepatitis A virus	◆ Hepatitis A
Genitourinary tract	◆ *Neisseria gonorrhoeae*	◆ Gonorrhea
	◆ *Chlamydia trachomatis*	◆ Lymphogranuloma venereum, cervicitis, urethritis, endometritis
	◆ Enterobacteriaceae (*Escherichia coli*, *Klebsiella* sp., *Serratia* sp., *Proteus* sp.)	◆ Urinary tract infections
Intact skin or mucous membranes	◆ Rhinovirus	◆ Common cold
	◆ Respiratory syncytial virus	◆ Pneumonia, bronchiolitis, tracheobronchitis
	◆ *Schistosoma* sp.	◆ Schistososome dermatitis (swimmer's disease)
	◆ Herpes simplex virus	◆ Oral or genital herpes
Bloodstream	◆ Hepatitis B virus	◆ Hepatitis B
	◆ *Plasmodium*	◆ Malaria
	◆ *Clostridium tetani*	◆ Tetanus
	◆ Human immunodeficiency virus (HIV)	◆ AIDS

Source: Ignatavicius, D.D., Workman, M.L., Mishler, M.A. (1995). *Medical-Surgical Nursing: A Nursing Process Approach*, 2nd ed. Philadelphia: Saunders, p. 591.

saliva. Cilia, which line the respiratory tract, trap organisms and debris and propel them up and out of the body with a wavelike action.

The bone marrow and the liver are major components in the body's defense system. Infection spurs the bone marrow to produce more leukocytes and **leukocytosis** occurs. The bone marrow plays an important role in the production of defensive blood cells, neutrophils, macrophages, and lymphocytes. The liver's Kupffer's cells destroy bacteria that have found their way into the blood circulating through the portal system. No more than 1% of the bacteria that pass into the bloodstream from the intestines and enter into the liver escape destruction and pass into the general circulation. The body's defense mechanisms against pathogens are summarized in Table 6-3. These act either to prevent the invasion of the body by pathogens or to neutralize the pathogen chemically. The pH of body secretions and their chemical content act to inactivate pathogens. The **flora** (bacterial plant life) that is normally present on the skin, in the mucous membranes of the oral cavity, gastrointestinal tract,

and the vagina coexist with the body and control the growth of harmful pathogens. When the amount of the normal flora is diminished, other pathogens may cause infection. **When the body's immune system is suppressed from chemotherapy or AIDS, normal flora may grow out of control and cause infection.** *Candida albicans*, the yeast infection called thrush that frequently occurs during or after treatment with antibiotics, is an example of this process. Table 6-4 shows changes in the natural defense mechanisms that occur with age and cause the elderly to become more susceptible to infection.

The process of phagocytosis assists the body in destroying pathogens. Phagocytes ingest solid particles that may be microorganisms, their parts, foreign particles, or dead or damaged body cells. **The two types of phagocytic cells are the neutrophils and the macrophages.** Neutrophils are leukocytes (white blood cells) that leave the blood and migrate to the site of an infection where they engulf and digest the microorganisms. They then die. The accumulation of dead pathogens, neutrophils, and cellular debris is **pus**. Macrophages are

TABLE 6-3 ◆ *The Body's Mechanism of Defense Against Infection*

Mechanism	Factors Involved in Protection
Natural immunity	Determined by age, ethnicity, and genetics. Greater resistance to disease.
Intact skin	Skin is the first defense; slightly acid pH and normal flora present unfavorable environment for colonization of pathogens.
Mucous membranes	Mucous membranes with their mucocilliary action provide mechanical protection against invasion of pathogens. Mucous secretions contain enzymes that inhibit many microorganisms. Respiratory system clears about 90% of introduced pathogens.
Gastrointestinal tract	Peristaltic action empties the gastrointestinal tract of pathogenic organisms. Acid pH of stomach secretions, bile, pancreatic enzymes, and mucous protect against invasion by harmful pathogens.
Normal flora	Present on skin and in mucous membranes of oral cavity, gastrointestinal tract, and vagina. Helps prevent excessive growth of pathogens.
Genitourinary tract	Flushing of urine through the system washes out microorganisms. The acid pH of urine helps maintain a sterile environment in the system.
Phagocytosis by white blood cells	Leukocytes, neutrophils, and macrophages (large monocytes) engulf, ingest, kill, and dispose of invading microorganisms.
Inflammation	Cells damaged by pathogens release enzymes, and leukocytes are attracted to the area; the damaged area is "walled off" and phagocytosis disposes of the microorganisms and dead tissue.
Humoral immune response (antigen-antibody; B lymphocytes)	Antibodies are produced against invading pathogens and inactivate or destroy them.
Cellular immune response (T lymphocytes)	Sensitized T-cells kill or inactivate antigens by chemical release or secretion of substances that destroy the antigen.

monocytes (large leukocytes) that have left the bloodstream and migrated into the tissues. They both ingest and destroy pathogens and clear away the cellular debris and dead neutrophils in the latter stages of an infection. Macrophages cleanse the lymph as it passes through the lymph nodes and perform a similar action on the blood as it journeys through the liver and the spleen. The second line of defense is the inflammatory response.

THE INFLAMMATORY RESPONSE

Inflammation is an immediate, localized, protective response of the body to any kind of injury to its cells and tissues.

Inflammation occurs at the cellular level where the injury has taken place and is the most common kind of

TABLE 6-4 ◆ *Changes in Natural Defense Mechanisms That Occur With Age*

Change	Consequence
Decreased skin turgor and greater skin friability	Skin is more susceptible to friction damage and tearing.
Decreased elasticity and atherosclerosis of peripheral vessels	Decreased blood flow to extremities produces slower wound healing.
Calcification of heart valves	Provides a location for bacteria to attach and cause endocarditis.
Stiffness of thorax from arthritis or aging changes, weakened respiratory muscles, decreased ciliary action from smoking or exposure to air pollution	Decreased ability to maintain good oxygenation leads to less respiratory reserve; greater tendency to retain secretions as cilia cannot move foreign substances and secretions as easily and cough reflex and effort are diminished.
Gastrointestinal tract motility is decreased as muscles weaken; acid production is decreased	Insufficient acid to inhibit growth of pathogens; decreased motility allows organisms to remain in GI tract and multiply.
Prostate changes, bladder prolapse, and urethral strictures.	Bladder is not completely emptied at each voiding allowing stagnation; provides medium for growth of pathogens.
Immune response decreases as bone marrow does not produce new blood cells as rapidly	Wound healing is slower, mobilization of body defenses to fight infection is slower.

response to cell damage. **Almost all tissues of the body respond to injury by initiating the inflammatory process (Figure 6-3).**

The injury can be caused by infectious agents, mechanical or chemical trauma, or any other abnormal condition affecting the tissues. The basic purposes of the inflammatory response are to (1) neutralize and destroy harmful agents; (2) limit their spread to other tissues in the body; and (3) prepare the damaged tissues for repair.

◆ Inflammatory Changes

Changes that are part of the inflammatory process can occur locally at the site of injury and also systemically. These changes involve (1) the cells of the damaged

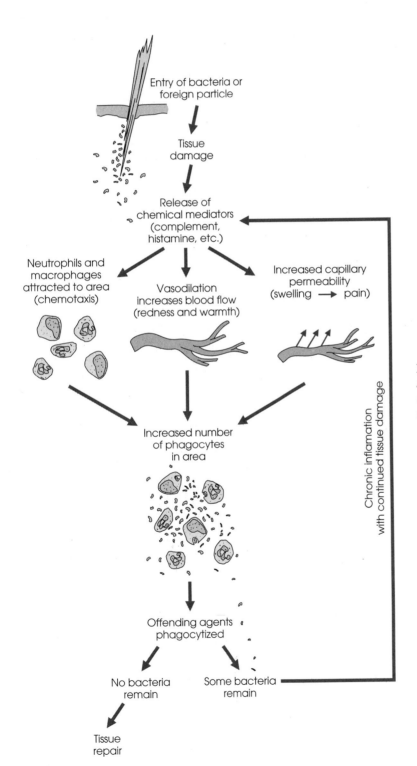

FIGURE 6-3   Steps in Inflammation. (*Source:* Applegate, E. J. 1995. *The Anatomy and Physiology Learning System: Textbook.* Philadelphia: Saunders, p. 294.)

tissues and adjacent connective tissues; (2) the blood vessels in and near the site of injury; (3) the blood cells, particularly the leukocytes; (4) the macrophages of the mononuclear phagocyte system; (5) the immune system; and (6) the hormonal system.

Chemical Release and Vascular Changes Encounter of a foreign substance by plasma cells may cause the activation of the complement system. The activation of these proteins enhances phagocytosis and the inflammatory process. If microbial invasion has occurred, interferon is released that acts to protect cells against viruses. As soon as injury occurs, the blood vessels in the injured area momentarily constrict and, as histamine and serotonin are released, they dilate so that more blood is brought to the damaged cells. The walls of the capillaries become more *permeable* (i.e., their pores enlarge) so that water, proteins, and defensive cells can pass out of the blood and into the fluid surrounding the damaged cells. **This leakage of fluid into the spaces around the cells produces a localized swelling, or edema, which is one of the classic outward signs of inflammation.**

When the fluid and fibrinogen brought by the blood leak through the walls of the capillaries, they fill the tissue spaces and block the lymphatic vessels with fibrinogen clots. This results in a "walling off" of the area and delays the spread of bacteria, toxins, and other harmful agents to other parts of the body.

Leukocytosis Another substance that is believed to be liberated from damaged cells is the *leukocytosis-promoting factor.* It acts on the bone marrow, which is stimulated to release granulocytes—especially neutrophils—that have been stored there. **These defensive cells then enter the bloodstream and are transported to the site of injury where they engage in phagocytosis.** The factor also increases the rate of production of granulocytes so that a supply of them is available as long as needed to inactivate and destroy harmful agents.

Phagocytosis Within the first few hours of the onset of the inflammatory process, the monocytes swell, becoming very large cells (macrophages), and migrate to the inflammatory site. There they ingest foreign particles and **necrotic** (dead) tissue.

After the neutrophils and macrophages engulf and destroy bacteria and foreign matter, they themselves die, producing debris that is composed of tissue fluid, dead cells, and their products. This exudate is commonly known as **pus.** A yellow or greenish purulent drainage is a sign of infection.

Immune Response **The third line of defense is the immune response, by which the body attempts to defend and protect itself.** The immune response is a remarkable series of complex chemical and mechanical activities that take place within the body. These activities involve (1) constant surveillance to detect the entry of foreign agents as soon as they gain access to the body's cells; (2) immediate recognition of the agents as "nonself" (that is, foreign or alien); and (3) the ability to distinguish one kind of foreign agent from another and to "remember" that particular agent if it appears again at a later time.

While the phagocytes are engulfing and destroying bacteria and other harmful agents, **the specific antibodies and antitoxins produced by the immune response are transported by the blood to the tissue spaces at the site of inflammation.** Here they attack foreign cells and neutralize the poisons these cells produce. The immune response is discussed fully in the next chapter.

Hormonal Response Some hormones, such as cortisone, have an *antiinflammatory* action that limits inflammation to the locally damaged tissues where it is most needed. Other hormones, such as aldosterone, are *proinflammatory* corticoids, which means that they stimulate the body's protective inflammatory response. Thus the hormones have a regulatory effect on the inflammatory process so that it is well balanced and provides maximum benefit. In some cases of severe inflammation, the physician may prescribe an antiinflammatory drug to relieve the symptoms of inflammation. However, hormones, such as the corticosteroids, can interfere with healing.

◆ Signs and Symptoms of Inflammation

Local Reactions

The five local signs and symptoms of inflammation are heat, redness, swelling, pain, and limitation or loss of function.

The increased blood flow to the affected area produces heat and redness. Swelling is the result of the increased permeability of the capillaries and the leakage of fluid from the blood into the tissue spaces around the cells. Blockage of lymphatic drainage from the site also contributes to the local swelling. **The chemicals released by the defensive cells and the accumulation of fluid in the area irritate the nerve endings and produce pain.** To lessen pain, the patient avoids moving the area, holding it immobile and thereby causing loss of motion in the affected part.

If there is an inadequate inflammatory response, which sometimes occurs in patients receiving certain drugs or suffering from chronic illness, the pathogens may cause active, systemic infection in the patient. Tissue repair is discussed along with wound healing in Chapter 4, Care of Surgical Patients.

Systemic reactions. Systemic reactions to inflammation are familiar to any of us who have had the flu or some other kind of generalized infection. Headache, muscle aches, and fever are common symptoms. Sweating and chills are sometimes experienced, as are anorexia and a sensation of "just feeling sick" and depressed. Laboratory tests will show that the white cell count is elevated; the leukocyte count can be as high as 30,000/mL of blood.

Patient care problems associated with systemic inflammatory responses include those related to inadequate nutrition and fluid intake, discomfort, need for rest, and need for maintenance of normal body temperature and fluid balance. If there is an inadequate inflammatory response, which sometimes occurs in patients receiving certain drugs or suffering from chronic illness, susceptibility to bacterial infections elsewhere in the body and delayed tissue repair and wound healing may occur.

CONTROLLING INFECTIOUS DISEASE

Infectious disease is controlled by breaking the transmission cycle. This is done by interrupting the chain at any one link. **Pathogens can be inactivated by disinfection, sterilization, or use of antiinfective drugs.** Eliminating the *reservoir* for the pathogen is another way of preventing transmission. Environmental sanitation, such as water and sewage treatment and rodent control, eliminates reservoirs for pathogens.

Interruption of transmission at the portal of exit is accomplished by detecting and treating clients who are infected by a pathogen. Barrier precautions and isolation techniques that include the proper handling and disposal of secretions, excretions, and exudates can prevent portal of exit transmission. Specific precautions and isolation techniques have been recommended by the Centers for Disease Control and Prevention (CDC) and are based on knowledge of how particular pathogens are transmitted.

The *mode of transmission* can be interrupted by proper disinfection and sterilization of medical equipment, aseptic technique in performing procedures and diagnostic tests, effective handwashing, and use of barrier and isolation precautions to prevent contamination. Teaching people to cover the mouth when sneezing or coughing, to dispose of soiled tissues correctly, to wash the hands after contact with potentially contaminated items, and to avoid contact with people who have an infection all prevent transmission of microorganisms. Controlling insects with programs such as spraying for mosquitoes and filtering the air in health care facilities also can prevent transmission of pathogens.

Transmission can be interrupted at the *portal of entry* by using only sterile and clean items when caring for patients. Barrier precautions (gloves, masks, condoms), safe handling of food and water, good personal hygiene, protection from insect bites and stings, and avoidance of high-risk behaviors all prevent entry of microorganisms.

> Effective handwashing technique by health care workers and by patients is a very important way to prevent the transmission of microorganisms.

Table 6-5 presents high risk behaviors that predispose toward the transmission of pathogens via a portal of entry.

Think about . . . How can an insect or rodent infestation in a restaurant kitchen and premises cause infections in customers?

Protecting *susceptible hosts* (patients who are more susceptible to infection) by using aseptic techniques, barrier precautions, and protective isolation can reduce disease transmission. Immunization and measures to boost immunity through proper nutrition and healthy lifestyle also increase resistance to infection. Table 6-6 lists factors that can make a host more susceptible to pathogens.

TABLE 6-5　◆　*Risk Factors for the Entry of Pathogens*	
Risk Factor	**Consequence**
Smoking or inhalation of toxic chemicals	Inhibits ciliary action of mucosa of respiratory tract that normally rids the body of inspired pathogens. Toxic chemicals may damage the bone marrow, inhibiting the production of leukocytes.
Intravenous drug abuse	Allows introduction of microorganisms into the bloodstream from contaminated needles or from lack of aseptic technique.
Unsafe sexual practices (not knowing history or health status of sexual partner, not using comdoms)	Allows entry of pathogenic organisms through the genital mucosa.
Unsafe handling of needles and sharps	Potential for breaks in the skin through which pathogens may enter.

TABLE 6-6 ◆ *Risk Factors for Increased Susceptibility to Infection*

Risk Factor	Consequence
Altered defense mechanisms	Body damage from trauma, breaks in the skin or mucous membranes; fractures.
Below normal leukocyte (WBC) count	Bone marrow suppression from chemotherapy or toxic agents; genetic or acquired agranulocytosis.
Age	Elderly patients and the very young are more susceptible to infection, probably because of declining or immature immune function.
Excessive stress or fatigue	These states seem to interfere with the body's normal defense mechanisms.
Malnutrition	Poor nutrition interferes with cell growth and replacement, which contributes to decreased immune function.
Alcoholism	Inhibits the immune system.
Preexisting chronic illnesses, such as diabetes mellitus, adrenal insufficiency, renal failure, or liver disease; serious illness such as pneumonia, peritonitis, etc.	These disease states upset the normal homeostatic balance within the body, impairing the normal defense mechanisms. Serious illness taxes the immune system, causing greater susceptibility to other pathogens.
Immunosuppressive treatment, chemotherapy, or corticosteroid treatment	Depresses the immune system or harms the bone marrow decreasing the number of leukocytes. Corticosteroids depress the inflammatory response, inhibiting one of the body's defense mechanisms.
Invasive equipment or indwelling tubes	Fracture pins, endotracheal or tracheostomy tubes, IV cannulas, feeding tubes, and urinary catheters provide a potential route for entry of pathogens.

◆ Hospital-Acquired (Nosocomial) Infections

The word *nosocomial* literally means hospital-acquired. A nosocomial infection occurs when a patient is infected while in a hospital. The term currently is used in a broader sense to include infections resulting from health services provided in all types of health care facilities.

There is a disturbing increase in the number of infections patients acquire during their stay in a hospital. Although inanimate objects such as needles, contaminated surgical instruments, and linen are major sources of infection in health care facilities, every patient is directly and indirectly in contact with untold numbers of persons, each of whom could be responsible for infecting the patient.

There is strong evidence that carelessness on the part of doctors, nurses, and other people in the patient's environment is primarily responsible for the unbelievably high incidence of hospital-acquired infections.

The cost of nosocomial infections is high in terms of treatment, human suffering, and time lost from work because of an extended recovery time. A small percentage of patients who contract nosocomial infections do not recover from them. The major sites of nosocomial infections, the infectious agent most often responsible, and some actions nurses may take to prevent infection at each site are presented in Table 6-7.

◆ Nursing Interventions to Prevent Nosocomial Infection

Infection is prevented by breaking the infection chain.

Careful attention to handwashing before and after any direct patient contact, before any invasive or sterile procedure, after invasive or sterile procedure, after contact with infectious materials (e.g., wound drainage, feces, urine, or sputum), and before contact with immunocompromised patients is the primary method by which infection can be prevented.

Changing soiled dressings promptly and replacing soiled linens quickly prevents spread of infectious organisms. Disposing of infectious materials, such as tissues, used dressings, and contaminated equipment, in covered, moisture-resistant biohazard containers helps contain organisms. Such items should not be left to sit in uncovered trash baskets in the patient's room. Insisting on maintaining strict aseptic technique for all invasive procedures (e.g., insertion of intravenous needles or bladder catheterization) also can greatly reduce the incidence of nosocomial infection.

Encouraging patients to move, cough, and deep-breathe on a regular basis will decrease the chance of respiratory infection. Protecting patients from others with respiratory infections and from visitors with other communicable diseases also is appropriate.

Along with preventive interventions, **the nurse must continuously assess the patient to detect early signs of**

TABLE 6-7 ◆ *Prevention of Nosocomial Infections*		
Most Common Sites	**Most Frequent Causative Organism**	**Nursing Actions to Prevent Infection**
Urinary tract	*Escherichia coli, Enterococcus, Klebsiella,* and *Proteus,* all from patient's own normal bowel flora. *Pseudomonas* and *Serratia* from other sources occur less frequently but often are resistant to antimicrobial drugs.	Observe sterile technique when catheterizing patients. Keep drainage system for indwelling catheter closed. Keep drainage bag below bladder level at all times to avoid reflux. Separate patients with known urinary tract infections. Catheterize only when absolutely necessary and follow faithfully the procedure for catheter care. Empty urine drainage bag into clean container without contaminating spout. Wipe spout with alcohol sponge before securing it.
Surgical wounds	*Staphylococcus aureus, Escherichia coli, Proteus,* and *Klebsiella.*	Administer prophylactic antibiotics as ordered. Follow strict aseptic technique during surgical procedures, whether minor or major and in whatever setting. Be sure patient's skin is correctly prepared for surgery. Use care in dressing and cleaning postoperative wounds. Ensure that patient has adequate nutrition and sufficient fluid intake, if he is able to eat and drink after surgery.
Respiratory tract	*Pseudomonas aeruginosa* and *Klebsiella.*	Adequately decontaminate respiratory therapy equipment. Perform suctioning, tracheostomy care, and other procedures under aseptic technique. Protect patient from others with colds or influenza.
Blood stream (bacteremia)	Secondary to infection elsewhere in the body or can be a primary infection caused by contamination of IV fluids, in which cases *Klebsiella, Enterobacter,* and *Serratia* are most common causative agents.	Scrupulous technique in the administration of IV fluids. Follow recommended procedure for daily care of insertion site and IV tubing, needles, and catheters.

infection so that treatment can begin immediately. The nurse also assesses every patient for appropriate immunization against infectious diseases, such as tetanus, pertussis, diphtheria, polio, influenza, hepatitis B, pneumococcal pneumonia, or measles.

Surveillance and Reporting   Surveillance demands that every nurse keep a watchful eye for signs of infection in every patient who is receiving health care. **Each patient should be routinely assessed for unexpected elevation of temperature; malaise; loss of appetite; purulent, or foul-smelling discharge; foul-smelling urine; cough; diarrhea; and sores and skin lesions that are red, swollen, and painful and contain pus.** The color of the purulent drainage is helpful in identifying the kind of organism causing an infection. For example, *S. aureus* produces a golden color and *Pseudomonas* organisms a bluish-green color.

The nurse particularly monitors those patients who are more susceptible to infection. Patients at greater risk are those who (1) are weakened by severe illness or injury; (2) have catheters IV cannulas, tubes, or other invasive devices for monitoring or treatment; (3) are very young or very old; (4) have had recent surgery; or (5) are immunocompromised from chemotherapy or immunosuppression. If an infection is suspected, the nurse takes extra precautions to prevent the possible spread of microorganisms. When an infection is discovered, it is reported to the infection control nurse of the institution and the patient's physician.

Destroying and Containing Infectious Agents The goals of destroying and containing infectious microorganisms are achieved by techniques and methods that (1) either kill the organisms or render them harmless by sterilization and disinfection; and (2) separate the sources of infection, so that they are isolated or "contained" within a specific area and therefore cannot spread to others.

Surgical and Medical Asepsis   Two important kinds of techniques and procedures used to destroy and contain infectious agents are surgical and medical asepsis. *Surgical asepsis* is concerned with destroying infectious agents *before* they enter the body. Medical *asepsis* is concerned with destroying the infectious agents *after* they *leave* the body of a patient who is infected and containing or isolating them within an area that is already contaminated.

Surgical asepsis involves sterilizing instruments, linens, and other articles used to treat the patient whenever surgery compromises the first line of defense. This compromise of defense occurs with surgical incisions, catheterization, the puncture of blood vessels for intravenous therapy and placement of monitoring devices, and other invasive procedures. Handwashing for surgical asepsis is more vigorous and must be done according to procedure. In a surgically aseptic environment, surgical gowns, masks, and gloves are necessary and must be put on and removed strictly according to surgical procedure. Surgical asepsis at the bedside requires sterile gloves, draping the patient with sterile drapes, and using sterile equipment and supplies; barrier precautions, such as mask and gown, may also be needed depending on the treatment to be given.

Medical asepsis includes hand washing, separation or isolation of the patient, precautions for handling and disposing of contaminated articles, and other techniques devised to destroy and contain infectious agents such as cleansing and sterilization.

> Handwashing, when done correctly, is the most effective of all the procedures recommended for prevention of the spread of infectious agents. Handwashing should be done with an approved soap or detergent under running water, using friction, for at least 20 seconds.

Standard Precautions   In the 1980s the spread of acquired immunodeficiency syndrome (AIDS) prompted the CDC to recommend the use of universal blood and body fluid precautions, or "universal precautions" (now called *standard precautions*), for every patient to prevent the spread of this lethal disease. **The purpose of these precautions is to protect hospital personnel from exposure to the human immunodeficiency virus (HIV), hepatitis B, and other bloodborne diseases.** In 1996 these precautions were revised to include all body fluids, except sweat, by the National Infection Control Practices Advisory Committee, the CDC, and the Public Health Service. These *standard precautions* are listed in Table 6-8 and are recommended for use with *all* patients.

Isolation Precautions   *Isolation precautions are designed to prevent the transmission of microorganisms from one patient to another as well as to protect the health care worker caring for the patient.* Table 6-9 describes the various category-specific isolation precautions, the disease for which each is used, and the equipment necessary. A colored card is placed on the patient's unit door or at the foot of the bed designating the precautions to be used by everyone entering the unit.

TABLE 6-8 ◆ *Standard Precautions*

1. Use barrier precautions, such as gloves, mask, gown, and protective eyewear to prevent exposure of skin or mucous membranes to patient's blood and body fluid.
   a. Use gloves when likely to come in contact with blood, body fluids, mucous membranes, or broken skin or when handling items or surfaces that are soiled with blood or body fluids.
   b. Change gloves between contact with each patient.
   c. Wash hands immediately after removing gloves.
   d. Discard used gloves; do not wash and reuse them.
   e. Wear a gown, mask, and protective eyewear during any procedure that might generate droplets of blood or body fluid.
2. Prevent injury by needle-stick or cut from sharp instruments.
   a. Be cautious and attentive any time a needle is handled.
   b. Do not recap a used needle by hand; scoop the cap onto the needle on a flat surface.
   c. Immediately dispose of a contaminated needle or other sharp instrument in the puncture-resistant container provided for that purpose in the room.
   d. Replace full puncture-resistant containers as needed; do not attempt to push needles bulging from the container down into it.
3. Prevent possible self-contamination through broken skin.
   a. If you have open lesions or weeping dermatitis on the skin, do not give direct patient care or handle patient care equipment until the condition is corrected.
4. Prevent possible self-contamination during cardiopulmonary resuscitation.
   a. Use disposable mouthpiece or resuscitation bag for emergency mouth-to-mouth breathing.
5. Prevent transmission of HIV or other bloodborne disease to the fetus.
   a. If pregnant, be especially diligent in maintaining standard precautions at all times.

Because of the broad groupings of diseases within a category, unnecessary techniques are used for some infections with this system.

Many hospitals today are switching to a disease-specific isolation procedure. This involves the use of a general instruction card (transmission precautions) for all patients with a transmissible infection. The card lists all possible specifications that might be needed to prevent transmission of the infection and the nurse checks which are to be used depending on the microorganism involved. The categories include Standard Precautions, Airborne Precautions, Droplet Precautions, and Contact Precautions. Check with your employing institution to see which isolation precaution system applies.

This individualized type of isolation saves money by eliminating unnecessary precautions. Its effectiveness depends on the nurse's knowledge of the microorganism involved and the ways in which it can be transmitted.

TABLE 6-9 ◆ Category-Specific Isolation Precautions (Transmission Based)

Isolation Category	Private Room*	Masks	Gowns	Gloves	Common Diseases Placed into Isolation Category
Strict isolation	◆ Always	◆ Always	◆ Always	◆ Always	◆ Varicella-zoster (chickenpox); pharyngeal diphtheria; shingles (zoster), localized in an immuno-compromised client or disseminated.
Contact isolation	◆ Always	◆ For close contact	◆ If soiling with infective material is likely	◆ If contact with infective material is likely	◆ Acute respiratory tract infection in infants and young children; disseminated herpes simplex; methicillin-resistant *Staphylococcus aureus*; pediculosis; scabies.
Respiratory isolation	◆ Always	◆ For close contact	◆ No	◆ No	◆ Measles; meningococcal meningitis, pneumonia, or meningococcemia; mumps; pertussis.
Acid-fast bacteria isolation	◆ Always	◆ Yes; special filter	◆ Only to prevent gross contamination	◆ No	◆ Tuberculosis (primary pulmonary or pharyngeal).
Enteric precautions	◆ Only if the client's hygiene is poor	◆ No	◆ If soiling with infective material is likely	◆ If contact with infective material is likely	◆ Enteroviral infection, including meningitis; infectious gastroenteritis (e.g., giardiasis, salmonellosis, shigellosis); hepatitis A, *Clostridium difficile* enterocolitis.
Drainage and secretion precautions	◆ No	◆ No	◆ If soiling with infective material is likely	◆ If contact with infective material is likely	◆ Minor or limited abscess, wound, burn, or skin infection; conjunctivitis.
Blood and body fluid precautions	◆ Only if the client's hygiene is poor	◆ If contact with blood or body fluids is likely	◆ If contact with splashes of blood or body fluids is likely	◆ If contact with blood or body fluids likely	◆ AIDS; hepatitis B; non-A, non-B hepatitis; malaria.

*In most cases when a private room is required, clients infected with the same organism may share a room.
Source: Ignatavicius, D.D., Workman, M.L., Mishler, M.A. (1995). *Medical-Surgical Nursing: A Nursing Process Approach*, 2nd ed. Philadelphia: Saunders, p. 595.

SEPSIS AND SEPTIC SHOCK

If a patient's infection is not adequately treated, the pathogen may enter the bloodstream causing a systemic infection, *septicemia* or *sepsis*. When microorganisms enter the bloodstream they are carried throughout the body and may invade any tissue. Sepsis is most commonly associated with bacterial invasion, particularly from gram-negative bacteria such as *P. aeruginosa, Escherichia coli,* and *Klebsiella pneumoniae,* and **gram-positive bacteria such as *Staphylococcus* and *Streptococcus*. The toxins secreted into the blood react with the blood vessels and cell membranes, stimulating a massive inflammatory and immune response.** Increased capillary permeability with resultant loss of fluid from the vascular space, cellular injury, and greatly increased cellular metabolic rate occurs. There is thrombus formation in the capillaries and poor oxygen uptake by cells. **Patients with sepsis may progress to *septic shock,* a condition in which there is decreased cardiac output, tissue damage, and hypovolemia leading to hypoxia throughout the body that can result in death.**

Each nurse must consider which patients are at greatest risk for sepsis. Postsurgical infections and peritonitis are two problems that can lead to sepsis. Patients who have delayed seeking treatment for an infection of any kind also are at risk. When a patient has been identified as being at risk for sepsis, monitor for slight changes in condition such as warm, dry, flushed skin; full, bounding pulse; normal to high blood pressure; and elevated urine output. The temperature may be normal or slightly elevated, although some patients do experience a high temperature with sepsis. Some patients, often the elderly, experience hypothermia when septic.

Sepsis is diagnosed from the results of serial blood cultures that show growth of the offending organism. Sensitivities are done to determine appropriate treatment. When the patient is known to have sepsis, the nurse must be vigilant for signs of septic shock. **Watch the urine output. If it begins to decrease hourly, notify the physician.** Monitor breath sounds for crackles, check for an increasing heart rate and decreasing blood pressure. Assess for increased fatigue, feelings of anxiety, and changes in mental status. Watch for dependent edema. If shock becomes established, the skin will become cool and clammy and the peripheral pulses will be weak and thready. Urine output will drop, and blood pressure will fall as hypovolemia becomes more pronounced. Septic shock often is accompanied by massive clot formation throughout the body called *disseminated intravascular coagulation* which can be life-threatening by itself. **Treatment involves controlling and eliminating the infection and supporting the patient with fluids, blood pressure control, oxygen, and preventing compli-** cations. If sepsis is discovered early, the chance of recovery is good. If septic shock progresses to the stage of tissue damage from microthrombus formation, death may occur.

NURSING CARE OF THE PATIENT WITH AN INFECTION

◆ Assessment

Detecting infection in a patient requires a thorough nursing assessment. Subjective data can be obtained by asking the following questions:

- When did your symptoms begin? What are you experiencing as symptoms?
- Have you had fever or chills?
- Do you have any back pain? a stiff neck? headache? pain anywhere?
- Do you have any urgency or burning when you empty your bladder?
- Have you had any diarrhea? stomach cramps? nausea or vomiting?
- Do you have a cough? What does your sputum look like?
- Do you have sores or broken spots on your skin?
- Have you had any discharge from the vagina/penis?
- Do you have allergies? sinus problems? frequent lung infections?
- Have you traveled outside the country recently?
- Have you been bitten by any insects or been out in the country or the woods? Do you have contact with animals?
- Do you have any chronic diseases, such as diabetes or kidney disease?
- What drugs do you take? (Look for immunosuppressive drugs.)
- Do you drink alcohol? Use recreational drugs? (Both may depress the immune system.)
- Have you been around anyone who has an infection lately?

Subjective complaints that may indicate infection include fatigue, loss of appetite, headache, nausea, or general malaise or pain.

Physical assessment includes checking the throat for redness, palpating the cervical lymph nodes or superficial lymph nodes close to an area of pain; listening to the lungs to check for abnormal breath sounds; inspecting the skin for lesions and rash; checking the urine for cloudiness, discoloration, and abnormal smell. Vital signs are taken and compared with previous readings, if available. Bowel sounds are auscultated and then the abdomen is gently palpated for signs of tenderness. Objective data often point to the specific body system affected by the infection, but may include systemic signs such as fever and increased pulse and respiratory rate.

> Signs of local infection are redness, swelling, pain or tenderness on palpation or movement, heat in the affected area, and possibly loss of function of the body part affected.

Elder Care Point . . . Many elderly people, especially over the age of 80, have a normally low body temperature. Because of decreased inflammatory and immune response, there may be very little rise in temperature in the presence of infection. Small increases in temperature in these patients may be quite significant. Signs of inflammation may not be present or may be less than the infection would produce in a younger person. **Clues that an infection is present may be a decrease in mental alertness, increased fatigue, or sudden onset of confusion, irritability, or apathy.**

Diagnostic Tests   Laboratory data that may indicate infection include an elevated white blood cell (WBC) count, changes in the distribution and number of the types of leukocytes on the differential WBC count, an elevated erythrocyte sedimentation rate (ESR), and cultures that test positive for microorganisms. Other serum tests for agglutination, precipitation, complement-fixation, or immunofluorescence may be performed to determine the causative agent.

Bacteriologic tests are done by culturing body fluids or wastes. *Cultures* are grown from specimens collected at the site of infection. When obtaining a culture, the nurse must be careful to (1) collect fresh material from the site only, avoiding contamination by microbes from nearby tissues and fluids; (2) use sterile equipment and the appropriate container for the sample; and (3) be sure the container is tightly covered to avoid spilling and contamination during transport to the laboratory.

Sensitivity tests are done in conjunction with cultures to determine which drug or drugs a particular microbe is sensitive to, that is, which antimicrobials can most effectively destroy or inhibit the multiplication and growth of the infecting microbe. Once this has been determined, the drug of choice must be administered exactly as prescribed. As explained, inadequate dosage or delay in administration can lead to genetic mutation and the development of a strain of microbe that is resistant to the drug.

Intradermal skin tests are done to determine the presence of certain active or inactive diseases, such as tuberculosis, histoplasmosis, diphtheria, coccidioidomycosis, and mumps. Radiography, computed tomography, or magnetic resonance imaging may be used to inspect the lung fields, locate abscesses, and detect changes in tissues.

Think about . . . Your lab partner is complaining of fatigue, headache, and malaise. What would you do to assess him or her for signs of infection?

◆ Nursing Diagnosis

Appropriate nursing diagnoses for patients with problems of infection include risk for infection and risk for injury.

The specific type of infection and the problem it presents determine the correct nursing diagnosis. For example, if the patient has a urinary tract infection, the nursing diagnosis would be "Alteration in urinary elimination"; if there is a wound infection, the nursing diagnosis would be "Impaired skin integrity." Collaboration with other health team members helps establish the correct nursing diagnosis. Secondary nursing diagnoses may include "Fatigue," "Fear," "Pain," "Activity Intolerance," and many others. The nursing diagnosis of "Knowledge deficit" related to lack of knowledge about the disease, prevention of infection, or self-care should always be considered.

Any patient entering the hospital for surgery or an invasive procedure is at risk for a nosocomial infection, and "Risk for Infection" should be listed as a nursing diagnosis on his care plan.

◆ Planning

The goals for recovery from infection include measures to help the patient use the body's defensive and healing processes; adequate rest; freedom from physical discomfort and mental anxiety or depression; adequate nutrition and hydration; and sufficient oxygen and blood supply to the infected tissues.

Expected outcomes may include:

- ◆ Temperature, pulse, and respirations are within normal range.
- ◆ The patient is able to rest comfortably and reports absence of or decrease in severity of pain or discomfort.
- ◆ Total fluid intake is at least 2,000 mL every 24 hours.
- ◆ Nutritional needs are met, weight loss gradually regained (if this is desired, depending on patient's weight status), and normal body weight maintained.
- ◆ The patient verbalizes the purposes of diagnostic tests, treatments, and special precautions.
- ◆ The patient and family maintain medical asepsis at all times and prevent the spread of infection.

- The patient is free from infection as evidenced by normal WBC, ESR, vital signs, and negative culture.
- The patient will experience decreased incidences of infection.

The planning phase of the nursing process should take into account the physical strength of the patient, his need for rest, and the psychological impact of isolation precautions. He may feel "dirty" and that people are avoiding him if he has a serious infection with a contagious organism.

Every effort should be made to maintain the integrity of the skin and mucous membranes so that they continue to serve as effective barriers to infectious agents. This means planning and implementing good skin care, oral hygiene, and personal cleanliness.

◆ Intervention

Providing a quiet environment with nursing care planned to provide expanses of uninterrupted rest time is important in the recovery period. Relieving the discomforts of fever and muscle aches is accomplished by tepid sponge baths, ice bags, use of antipyretics, and massage. Warm compresses and the application of heat, as appropriate, promote healing.

Mild physical exercise promotes circulation and helps the patient relax. **Good circulation of the blood to an infected area is necessary to remove waste products from metabolism and the inflammatory process.**

A diet high in protein, vitamins, minerals, and trace elements helps promote quicker healing by providing the nutrients necessary for cell growth. *Vitamin A* is needed for the **synthesis** (creation) of collagen for scar formation and for the growth of epithelial cells over denuded surfaces. The *vitamin B complex* is necessary for proper functioning of the enzyme system. *Vitamin C* is necessary for collagen synthesis, the formation of capillaries that bring blood to the healing tissues, and resistance to infection. *Vitamin K* plays an important role in normal clotting. The minerals zinc, copper, and iron assist in collagen synthesis.

Cultural Care Point . . . Asian patients believe that a balance of hot and cold foods should be eaten. When infection and fever are present, they may believe that cold foods such as watermelon or white radish soup are desirable.

Many Hispanic patients also believe in "hot" and "cold" forces that are thrown out of balance when illness strikes. They may want cold foods such as dairy products, honey, or fresh vegetables when they are suffering from infection.

For patients of both these cultures it is advisable to assess what their beliefs are and then to work with the family to provide the foods that they believe will assist in their recovery.

Accurate intake and output records are necessary to determine whether the patient is taking sufficient fluids. Good hydration helps the body expel the waste products of the fight against infection. The patient should drink at least 2,000 mL of fluid each 24 hours.

Think about . . . Your Hispanic patient is recovering from an auto accident. He has a large wound on his thigh. How would you specifically counsel him about eating a diet that would assist in healing of the wound?

Psychosocial care helps the patient deal with the unpleasant features of his illness and the discomfort of tests and treatments. **Stress seems to make the body more vulnerable to invasion by foreign organisms by depressing the immune system.** When under excessive stress, the body also is less able to mobilize the elements and cells that promote healing. The nurse should realize that her attitude toward a patient and the ways in which she strives to meet his needs can reduce stress and promote healing in ways that are not yet completely understood.

The manner in which a person is physically handled, the tone of voice used in speaking to him, and the availability of others to listen to him can have profound effects on his physical condition. We must not forget that nursing is a healing profession. Much of what is done to, for, and with a patient reflects a willingness (or a lack of it) to use oneself to heal another. If those who care for a patient share with him a strong desire for his recovery, his will to be healed is strengthened. If the illness is lengthy, concerns about work and home responsibilities may cause anxiety. Collaboration with the social worker for solutions to such problems may be needed.

The administration of antiinfective drugs is an important nursing responsibility. **The nurse must give the drugs on time to maintain effective blood levels.** She must monitor the patient for side effects of the drug and also evaluate to determine whether the drug is effective in eradicating the infection. Antiinfective drugs are far too numerous to list here, but Table 6-10 presents the general classification of antimicrobial drugs and the organisms for which they are effective. General nursing actions for the administration of an antimicrobial medications are shown in Table 6-11.

Patient Education   Nurses have an obligation to teach the patient how to care for himself and how to avoid infection by good personal hygiene and sanitation. **If a patient already has an infection, he and his family will need to know (1) the ways in which the**

**TABLE 6-10 ◆ *Classification of Antimicrobial Drugs by Susceptible Organisms* **

ANTIBACTERIAL
   Narrow Spectrum
      Gram-positive cocci and gram-positive bacilli
         Penicillin G and V
         Penicillinase-resistant penicillins: methicillin, nafcillin
         Vancomycin
         Erythromycin
         Clindamycin
      Gram-negative aerobes
         Aminoglycosides: gentamicin, others
         Cephalosporins (first and second generations)
      Mycobacterium tuberculosis
         Isoniazid
         Rifampin
         Ethambutol
         Pyrazinamide
   Broad Spectrum
      Gram-positive cocci and gram-negative bacilli
         Broad-spectrum penicillins: ampicillin, others
         Extended-spectrum penicillins: carbenicillin, others
         Cephalosporins (third generation)
         Tetracyclines
         Imipenem
         Trimethoprim
         Sulfonamides: sulfisoxazole, sulfamethoxazole, others
         Fluoroquinolones: ciprofloxacin, norfloxacin, others
ANTIVIRAL
   Acyclovir
   Azidothymidine
   Amantadine
ANTIFUNGAL
   Amphotericin B
   Ketoconazole
   Itraconazole

*The classification in this table is simplified.
Source: Lehne, R.A. (1994). *Pharmacology for Nursing Care,* 2nd ed. Philadelphia: Saunders, p. 915.

infection is transmitted; (2) **proper handwashing techniques; (3) the approved method of disinfection by boiling, steaming, using bleach solutions, alcohol, sunlight, or other bactericidal cleansers; (4) methods for proper handling and disposal of contaminated articles; and (5) other precautions indicated for the kind of infectious disease the patient has.**

Adequate teaching is essential so that the patient and his family will understand why precautions are necessary. Instruction should be given on how the infection is spread and how spread is prevented. **Before beginning teaching, the nurse needs to find out how much the patient and his family know about his condition and the problems it can present.**

If a patient is to take medications at home to control his infection, he must be taught how to take them. He must also be cautioned not to discontinue taking any antimicrobial medication even when he begins to feel better. **All antimicrobial drugs should be continued for as long as they are prescribed.** To stop before the full amount has been taken can lead to a second outbreak of the infection and possibly a return to the hospital.

Other aspects of teaching will depend on each patient's learning needs. A patient may need to learn how to change dressings or handle secretions without spreading infection to others or reinfecting himself. Nurses may also need to teach patients how to dispose of contaminated articles and maintain a clean and sanitary environment, how to plan nutritious meals that provide adequate protein and vitamin intake, and how to ensure the rest and activity necessary to promote healing.

◆ Evaluation

Periodic evaluation of the effectiveness of nursing actions is performed by **assessing vital signs and determining the trends, checking WBC lab values to see if they are moving toward normal, monitoring wounds for signs of improvement, and inquiring as to how the patient feels.** Evaluation is determined by how well the goals of care and expected outcomes have been met. **Lab values showing the absence of infection and a greater sense of well-being are other criteria that determine the effectiveness of care.** Nursing Care Plan 6-1 presents a plan drawn up for a 28-year-old patient with an *S. aureus* infection. Evaluating the effects of the medications the patient is receiving is a prime nursing responsibility.

COMMUNITY CARE

Controlling the spread of infectious diseases is a worldwide effort of public health officials. **Their major goals and those of nurses who work with them are to (1) promote sanitary standards in communities; (2) identify persons who are highly susceptible to infection and reducing their chances of developing an infectious disease; and (3) implementing immunization programs to protect people against certain infectious diseases.**

Nurses share the responsibility for educating the public and promoting sanitary living conditions in the communities in which they live and work. Each nurse also must be aware of what she is doing when working with her patients. She might be helping to contain and prevent the spread of infection, or she could actually be contributing to it. As more nurses work in the community, opportunities to educate the public about infection

TABLE 6-11 ◆ *General Nursing Implications for the Administration of Antimicrobial Drugs*

When giving an antimicrobial drug, the nurse should:

- ◆ Check the ID band of the patient before administering each dose to ensure that the right patient receives the drug.
- ◆ Follow the five rights of medication administration to prevent errors and injury to the patient.
- ◆ Verify allergies with the patient before administering a dose of an antimicrobial drug to prevent allergic reaction.
- ◆ Know the reason the patient is to receive an antimicrobial drug; this helps prevent drug administration errors. Question the order if the drug does not seem appropriate for the patient.
- ◆ If culture and sensitivity studies have been done, verify that the drug to be given is one to which the organism is sensitive.
- ◆ Give each dose of an antimicrobial drug as close to the scheduled time as possible to maintain a consistent blood level of the drug.
- ◆ Monitor the patient for effectiveness of the antimicrobial drug (i.e., check WBC levels, temperature trends).

Regarding possible side/adverse effects of the drug, the nurse should:

- ◆ Monitor the patient for side effects of the antimicrobial drug. The most common general side effects are: gastrointestinal upset, anorexia, nausea, diarrhea, rash, and photosensitivity. **Consult pharmacology book or drug insert for specific side effects for each particular drug.**
- ◆ Monitor patient for signs of allergic reaction, such as rash, hives, itching, drug fever, swelling of the oral mucous membranes, difficulty breathing, or anaphylaxis, to institute treatment quickly and prevent death.
- ◆ Monitor blood urea nitrogen, creatinine, liver functions and complete blood count (CBC) for abnormalities that might be drug induced (i.e., blood disorders, kidney damage, liver damage).
- ◆ Determine renal and liver function status of patients before administering an antimicrobial drug to prevent toxic circulating levels of the drug; most drugs are metabolized in the liver and excreted by the kidneys.
- ◆ Check for signs of superinfection in patients taking high doses of the antimicrobial drug for a long time (oral thrush, vaginal itching or discharge, diarrhea).
- ◆ Check precautions for administration of the antimicrobial drug when the patient is pregnant or lactating.

The nurse should teach the patient taking an antimicrobial drug to:

- ◆ Take the medication with a full glass of water to promote absorption.
- ◆ Refrain from drinking alcohol when taking an antimicrobial drug that can cause alcohol intolerance.
- ◆ Take all of an antimicrobial drug prescription to prevent drug-resistant microorganisms.
- ◆ Take the medication in appropriate relationship to meals for best absorption of the drug with minimal gastrointestinal side effects. (Different drugs vary in this respect; some need to be taken with food and some should be taken on an empty stomach; check pharmacology book or drug insert.)
- ◆ Eat yogurt and/or drink buttermilk to reestablish normal intestinal flora when taking an antimicrobial drug.
- ◆ Discontinue the drug and notify the physician if an allergic reaction occurs.
- ◆ Use a sunblock and protective clothing when sun exposure is unavoidable when taking an antimicrobial that causes photosensitivity.
- ◆ Increase fluid intake to 2,500 to 3,000 mL per day, especially when patient is taking a sulfa-type drug to prevent crystalization in the kidney and promote drug excretion.
- ◆ Check all drugs patient is receiving for drug interactions with the antimicrobial drug to prevent toxicity or lack of absorption.
- ◆ Check that dosage of an antimicrobial drug is appropriate for the elderly patient who may have decreased kidney function that could cause drug levels to build up to a toxic level.

transmission and the prevention of disease occur more frequently.

◆ Home Care

The home care nurse must work with family members to prevent the transmission of pathogens from the environment outside the house to the patient. Each person should thoroughly wash hands as soon as returning home from being out in a public place. Microorganisms are picked up on the hands from shopping basket cart handles, elevator buttons, telephone receivers, library books, soap dispensers, items in department stores, and every other place one goes to do errands and interact with others. The incidence of colds and flu might be decreased if during the heavy respiratory illness season people who are at risk for infection would stay away from crowded places and situations where pathogens are likely to be airborne, such as crowded stores and theaters.

Within the home the patient and family are taught how to contain infectious wastes such as dressings and soiled tissues in impermeable plastic bags—double bagged and sealed. Handwashing is stressed, and family members are taught not to share personal items, especially toothbrushes or razors that might be contaminated by blood. Dishes and eating utensils are washed in the dishwasher on the "sani" cycle or scalded with boiling water. The patient's linens, clothing, and towels should be stored in sealed plastic bags until washed.

Nursing Care Plan 6-1

Selected nursing diagnoses, goals/expected outcomes, nursing interventions, and evaluations for a patient with wound infection

Situation: Patient is a 28-year-old male with *Staphylococcus aureus* infection of a wound sustained during an automobile accident.

Nursing Diagnosis	Goals/Expected Outcomes	Nursing Interventions	Evaluation
Impaired skin integrity related to infected wound. SUPPORTING DATA Draining wound on right leg; positive culture for *Staphylococcus aureus.*	Staphylococcal infection will not be spread to others or other parts of patient's body.	Follow CDC's drainage/secretion precautions. Explain purpose of precautions to patient and visitors. Change wound dressing A.M. and P.M.; assist patient with bath to ensure skin has been cleaned and dressing does not become wet.	In drainage/secretion isolation; explanations given; dressings changed A.M. and P.M. using sterile technique; dressing remains dry. No evidence of spread of infection. Outcomes met.
Knowledge deficit related to proper wound care at home. SUPPORTING DATA "I don't know how to change a dressing properly."	Patient will state reasons for using special precautions for dressing change. Patient and family member will demonstrate proper handwashing technique before discharge. Patient and one family member will demonstrate dressing change, maintaining medical asepsis before discharge. Patient will list signs and symptoms that should be reported to physician. Patient will take full prescription of antibiotics exactly as directed.	Explain purpose of special precautions for dressing change and handling of soiled dressings. Demonstrate proper handwashing technique; observe patient and family member perform handwashing. Demonstrate proper dressing change and wound cleansing procedure; obtain return demonstration from patient and family member before discharge. Instruct patient to watch for elevated temperature; increased redness, swelling, or pain; or purulent discharge from wound and to report such findings to the physician should they occur. Explain importance of taking medication exactly as prescribed and of finishing entire prescription.	Patient verbalizes reasons for special precautions; patient and family member demonstrate proper handwashing, wound cleansing, and dressing change using medical asepsis; patient verbalizes signs and symptoms to report to physician and states that he understands how to take medication and why he must finish the prescription. Outcomes being met.

They should be washed separately in hot water, detergent, and a cup of chlorine bleach. Surfaces contaminated with traces of blood, urine, feces, or vomitus should be cleaned with a clean cloth and soap and hot water, and then recleaned with a 1:10 solution of chlorine bleach and hot water. Meats and poultry are handled properly during cooking preparation and stored in the refrigerator. Kitchen surfaces such as countertops and cutting boards are disinfected after poultry, meat, and fresh vegetables are prepared for cooking. They should be scrubbed thoroughly with hot soapy water, rinsed, and dried. Exposing cutting boards to direct sunlight for a couple of hours also helps. Phone receivers and other items that might become contaminated by contact with an infectious patient can be wiped with alcohol, a 1:10 chlorine bleach solution, or exposed to direct sunlight for at least an hour.

Maintaining a lifestyle that promotes increased resistance to infection is very helpful. Obtaining adequate sleep, eating properly, and exercising regularly all contribute to increased resistance. Adopting stress-reduction techniques that work and using them regularly also is beneficial. Nurses can help patients and family members plan and implement a program to increase resistance to infection.

The home care nurse must teach the techniques of asepsis to patients and family members to prevent cross infection from one person to another or the spread of infection in the patient.

◆ Long-Term Care

Infection control in long-term care facilities focuses on both residents and caregivers. Nurses and other health care workers must use medical aseptic techniques consistently to prevent the spread of microorganisms from one resident to another. Again, handwashing is the primary means of preventing the spread of microorganisms. Each health care worker needs to develop an aseptic "conscience" and remember to wash hands after every contact with a resident or items in the resident's unit. The elderly are more susceptible to infection because of age; those in long-term care facilities often have chronic illnesses that add to their susceptibility. Many elderly have low-grade infections of the urinary, respiratory, or gastrointestinal tract that can be passed on to others.

Patience in assisting residents to wash their hands before meals and after toileting, after being in community rooms such as the dining room or social activities lounge, and any time their hands become soiled will greatly reduce the incidence of nosocomial infection. Cleaning up incontinent patients promptly and securing soiled linens in plastic sealed bags is essential. The nurse is the key to preventing the spread of microorganisms in the long-term care environment.

CRITICAL THINKING EXERCISES

Clinical Case Problems

Read each clinical situation and discuss the questions with your classmates.

1. You have been asked to speak to a group of sixth-grade students about disease prevention and health promotion. The children are especially interested in "how people get sick" and how disease can be avoided.

   a. What kinds of disease-producing factors should you include in your discussion?

   b. Considering the age of your audience, what safety precautions might you stress?

2. Mrs. Compton, age 44, is admitted to the hospital for a hysterectomy. During the admission procedure, you notice a large, draining boil in her axillary region. She also has a temperature of 100°F, and she tells you that she has not felt well for the past few days.

   a. What would be your course of action following this discovery?

   b. What specific nursing actions could be taken to eliminate links in the chain of the infectious process so that Mrs. Compton's infection is not spread to others?

3. Conduct a survey in the clinical area in which you are practicing as a student nurse, observing ways in which infectious agents can be spread from one person to another through carelessness and poor sanitation practices. These might include failure to wash hands as often as needed, improper disposal of contaminated dressings and equipment, careless handling of soiled linens, and taking objects into a patient's room that are contaminated with infectious agents.

4. Ms. Maria Lopez 18 years of age, is admitted to the orthopedic unit following an automobile accident. She has sustained an open fracture of the femur and chest injuries. Her fractured leg has been placed in traction; the open wound is covered with a bandage.

   a. What protective body structures have been damaged in her injuries?

   b. What would be some expected signs and symptoms of inflammation that she might experience?

   c. What process would produce each of those signs and symptoms?

   d. What are some possible outcomes for each of her injuries?

   e. What specific problems might her care present for the nurse?

   f. How would you determine whether these problems were present?

   g. What nursing actions should be planned and implemented to deal with each of the problems you have identified?

5. Mrs. Dunn is a young mother who has recently moved into your neighborhood. She has not had her children immunized against any diseases because she fears that "the shots will only make my healthy children sick." One of her children, aged 5, will need immunization before he can enter school. Mrs. Dunn does not know whether her children received immunizations during infancy because she has moved from one community to another fairly often and has not taken them regularly to a pediatrician or to well-baby clinics.

   Mrs. Dunn is concerned about her children's health; she resists immunization only because she does not understand what these "shots" will do to the children and why they are necessary. She also has told you that she is worried about her children having tuberculosis because an aunt that once lived with them was diagnosed as having that disease.

   a. What would you say to try to convince her that her children should be immunized?

   b. How would you explain tuberculin testing to Mrs. Dunn?

   c. How would you describe the benefits of skin testing for the members of her family?

BIBLIOGRAPHY

American Hospital Association. (1989). *Infection Control in Hospitals*, 4th ed. Chicago, American Hospital Association.

Anastasi, J. K., Rivera, J. (1994). Understanding prophylactic therapy for infections. *American Journal of Nursing.* 94(2):36–41.

Applegate, E. J. (1995). *The Anatomy and Physiology Learning System: Textbook.* Philadelphia: Saunders.

Beam, T. R. (1994). Anti-infective drugs in the prevention and treatment of sepsis syndrome. *Critical Care Nursing Clinics of North America.* 6(2):275–293.

Borton, D. (1995). Combating infection: keeping your patient safe from VRE. *Nursing 95.* 25(5):28.

Borton, D. (1997). Isolation precautions: Clearing up the confusion. *Nursing 97.* 27(1):49–52.

Brown, K. K. (1994). Critical interventions in septic shock. *American Journal of Nursing.* 24(10):20–26.

Brown, K. K. (1994). Septic shock: how to stop the deadly cascade. *American Journal of Nursing.* 94(9):20–27.

Centers for Disease Control. (1989). Guidelines for the prevention of nosocomial infections. Atlanta: U.S. Department of Health and Human Services.

Centers for Disease Control. (1987). Recommendations for prevention of HIV transmission in health-care settings. *Morbidity and Mortality Weekly Report,* 36, no. 2S, August 21:3.

Centers for Disease Control. (1988). Update: universal precautions for prevention of transmission of human immunodeficiency virus, hepatitis B virus, and other blood-borne pathogens in health-care settings. *Morbidity and Mortality Weekly Report.* June 1988:377.

Copstead, L. C. (1995). *Perspectives on Pathophysiology.* Philadelphia: Saunders.

DeGroot-Kosolcharoen, J. (1996). Culture and sensitivity testing. *Nursing 96.* 26(9):33–38.

Eggleston, B. (1994). Infection-control update: choosing personal protective equipment. *Nursing 94.* 24(3):70–72.

Garb, J. R. (1996). Combating infection: managing body-substance exposure. *Nursing 96.* 26(1):26–27.

Garner, J. S., Simmons, B. P. (1989). CDC Guideline for Isolation Precautions in Hospitals. Atlanta: U.S. Department of Health and Human Services.

Gawlikowski, J. (1992). White cells at war. *American Journal of Nursing.* 92(3):44–51.

Gurevich, I. (1994). Your patients don't need diarrhea, too! *RN.* 57(4):52–53.

Guyton, A. C., Hall, J. E. (1996). *Textbook of Medical Physiology,* 9th ed. Philadelphia: Saunders.

Howland, W. A. (1995). Defending your patient against nosocomial pneumonia. *Nursing 95.* 25(8):62–63.

Ignatavicius, D. D., Hausman, K. A. (1995). *Clinical Pathways for Collaborative Practice.* Philadelphia: Saunders.

Ignatavicius, D. D., Workman, M. L., Mishler, M. A. (1995). *Medical-Surgical Nursing: A Nursing Process Approach,* 2nd ed. Philadelphia: Saunders.

King, M. (1994). Combating infection. How to stop the spread of M.R.S.A. *Nursing 94.* 24(11):23.

Lancaster, E. (1993). Tuberculosis comeback: impact on long-term care facilities. *Journal of Gerontological Nursing.* 19(7):16–21.

Lerner-Durjava, L. (1997). Combating infection: How to stop the pox. *Nursing 97.* 27(4):20.

Lerner-Durjava, L. (1996). Protecting against tetanus. *Nursing 96* 26(2):26–27.

Messner, R. L., Pinkerman, M. (1992). Preventing a peripheral I. V. infection. *Nursing 92.* 22(6):34–42.

Monahan, F. D., Drake, T., Neighbors, M. (1994). *Nursing Care of Adults.* Philadelphia: Saunders.

Morita, M. M. (1993). Methicillin-resistant staphylococcus aureus: past, present, and future. *Nursing Clinics of North America.* 28(3):625–637.

Reiss, P. J. (1996). Battling the super bugs. *RN.* 59(3):36–40.

Rodits, B., Meister, S. (1990). Home Care: Infection control takes top priority. *RN.* 53(12):59–62.

Russell, S. (1994). Septic Shock. *Nursing 94.* 24(4):40–52.

Wahl, S. C. (1995). Septic shock: How to detect it early. C. E. Test Handbook, Vol. 5: 17–23.

Warren, J. W. (1994). Catheter-associated bacteriuria in long-term care facilities. *Infection Control and Hospital Epidemiology.* 15(8):557–562.

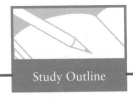

Study Outline

I. Introduction

A. Infections can be communicable or noncommunicable.

B. Increase in incidence of death from infectious disease.
1. More invasive procedures.
2. Treatment with immunosuppressive therapy.
3. Drug-resistant microorganisms.

C. Overview of the infectious process.
1. Process where body is invaded by pathogens.
2. Symptoms result from pathogen's destructive ability; toxic substances produced; body's immune response.

II. Pathogenic Organisms

A. Bacteria: microscopically small organisms belonging to the plant family.

1. Classification.
   a. Gram-positive: those that "take" Gram stain. All streptococci and staphylococci are gram-positive.
   b. Gram-negative: those that do not retain the stain. Tuberculosis bacillus and many hospital-acquired infectious agents are gram-negative.
   c. Morphology (shape).
      (1) Cocci: round.
      (2) Bacilli: rod-shaped.
      (3) Spirochetes: spiral.
   d. Arrangement in cultures:
      (1) Streptococci grow in chains.
      (2) Diplococci grow in pairs.
      (3) Staphylococci grow in clusters.
   e. Oxygen requirement.
      (1) Obligate aerobes must have oxygen to survive.
      (2) Obligate anaerobes cannot tolerate oxygen.
      (3) Facultative anaerobes can thrive with or without oxygen.
2. Control of bacteria: destruction of harmful microbes is not simply a matter of using one method of sterilization or disinfection. Microbes vary in their ability to resist heat, cold, water, and chemicals.

B. Viruses: extremely small, cannot be seen with ordinary microscope. Made up of a core of nucleic acids (of RNA or DNA), contained within a coating of protein, carbohydrate, or fatty material. Cannot live or replicate outside a living cell.
   1. Can camouflage themselves inside cells of the body. Once there, they can cause a cell to burst and die or to change its membrane so that it is attacked by the body's immune system.
   2. Many of the "slow" viruses can live in cells for years without causing symptoms and then suddenly cause an acute illness.
   3. Destruction of viruses.
      a. Most are easily inactivated by heat. However, some (for example, the hepatitis viruses) can resist boiling for at least 30 minutes.
      b. Most effective means of destroying viruses and all other microbes is by moist heat at 250°F (121 °C) for 15 to 20 minutes.
   4. Types of viruses: classified according to.
      a. Whether core is RNA or DNA.
      b. Size.
      c. Tissues they prefer.
      d. Types pathogenic to man.
   5. Response of host cell to virus.
      a. May allow it to live peaceably in dormant state.
      b. Host cell may die without reproducing.
      c. Host cell may divide and then die.
      d. Host cell may be changed and take on abnormal growth pattern.

C. Protozoa: microscopic, one-celled organisms belonging to the animal kingdom. Malaria is an example of a disease caused by protozoa.
D. Rickettsiae: small, round, rod-shaped, parasitic.
E. Fungi: members of a class of vegetable organisms, including yeasts and molds. Diseases caused by fungi include athlete's foot and systemic mycoses.
F. Mycoplasmas are small organisms causing infection of the genital and respiratory tracts.
G. Other infectious agents.
   1. Helminths.
   2. Chlamydiae.
   3. Prions.

III. The Infection Chain
   A. Each link in the circular chain must be present for the process to take place.
   B. Links.
      1. Pathogen.
      2. Reservoir.
      3. Portal of exit.
      4. Modes of transmission.
      5. Portal of entry.
      6. Susceptible host.
         a. Protective mechanisms.
            (1) Organs: skin, liver, bone marrow.
            (2) Natural flora.
            (3) Phagocytosis.
            (4) Inflammatory response.
               (a) Inflammatory changes: chemical release and vascular changes; leukocytosis; phagocytosis; immune response; hormonal response.
               (b) Signs and symptoms of inflammation: local reactions; systemic reactions.
   C. Preventing spread of infection is achieved by controlling the links of the process.

IV. Controlling Infectious Disease
   A. Major goals of public health officials and professionals.
      1. Promotion of sanitary living conditions.
      2. Identification of susceptible persons and reduction of their chances of developing an infectious disease.
      3. Immunization programs.
   B. Nosocomial infections.

1. Nosocomial literally translated means hospital-acquired. Now used to include all infections resulting from health care services in all kinds of agencies.
2. Nosocomial infections are becoming increasingly more costly in terms of dollars and human suffering and death.
3. Common features of nosocomial infections are summarized in Table 6-7.

V. **Signs and Symptoms of Infection**
   A. Detection of infection requires thorough nursing assessment.
   B. Subjective signs include fatigue, loss of appetite, headache, nausea, general malaise, or pain.
   C. Objective signs: fever, increased pulse and respiratory rate; vomiting; diarrhea; cough; decreased breath sounds; swollen lymph nodes; cloudy urine; purulent sputum—usually indicate the body system involved.
   D. Signs of local infection are redness, swelling, pain, or limitation of movement caused by discomfort.
   E. Laboratory data indicative of infection: elevated WBC count, changes in distribution of cells on differential count, elevated erythrocyte sedimentation rate, and positive culture result.
   F. Any patient admitted for surgery or other invasive procedure is at risk of infection.

VI. **Nursing Interventions to Prevent Nosocomial Infection**
   A. Close attention to handwashing is of primary importance.
   B. Changing soiled dressings and linens promptly removes growth medium for bacteria.
   C. Proper disposal of infectious materials and contaminated equipment decreases incidence of infection.
   D. Use strict aseptic technique for all invasive procedures.
   E. Encourage patients to move, cough, and deep-breathe to prevent respiratory infection.
   F. Protect patients from others with infections.
   G. Administer prophylactic antibiotics as ordered.
   H. Encourage adequate rest, nutrition, and fluid intake to increase resistance to infection.
   I. Vigilantly assess for beginning signs of infection.
   J. Surveillance and reporting.
      1. Every patient is assessed for signs and symptoms of infection.
      2. If signs are detected, the patient's physician and the infection control officer of the institution are notified.
   K. Destroying and containing infectious agents.
      1. Techniques and procedures used to destroy and contain infectious microbes include:

   a. Surgical asepsis: the destruction of organisms *before* they enter the body. Procedures include sterilization of instruments and linens, surgical masks, gowns, and gloves, and draping the patient.
   b. Medical asepsis: The destruction of microbes *after* they leave the body of an infected person and separation of the sources of infection from other people.
   c. Handwashing is the single most important procedure to prevent the spread of infection.
   d. Standard precautions are taken by all health care workers with every patient: barriers are used for contact with blood and body fluids or broken or weeping skin and when droplet contamination might occur (Table 6-8).
   e. Isolation and precautionary measures carried out according to type of infection presented by patient.
      (1) Category-specific isolation (Table 6-9).
      (2) Disease-specific isolation.

VII. **Sepsis and Septic Shock**
   A. Inadequately treated infection; pathogen enters bloodstream, causing a systemic infection.
   B. Septic shock: decreased cardiac output, tissue damage, and hypovolemia with hypoxia; may result in death.

VIII. **Nursing Care of the Patient with an Infection**
   A. Assessment.
      1. Obtain subjective data by interview. Complaints indicating infection include: fatigue, loss of appetite, headache, nausea, or general malaise or pain.
      2. Physical assessment: vital signs, check throat, palpate cervical nodes & superficial lymph nodes; auscultate lungs, inspect skin, check urine, assess abdomen.
         a. Local signs of infection: redness, swelling, pain or tenderness on palpation or movement, heat in affected area, loss of function of body part.
      3. Diagnostic tests: WBC, differential WBC, ESR, culture and sensitivity, agglutination, precipitation, complement-fixation, or immunofluorescence tests; intradermal skin tests.
   B. Nursing diagnosis.
      1. Risk of infection.
      2. Risk for injury.
      3. Specific nursing diagnoses for problems the infection presents.
   C. Planning.
      1. Goals include measures to use body's defense systems and healing processes.

2. Interventions designed to promote adequate rest, comfort, adequate nutrition and hydration, and sufficient oxygen and blood supply.

3. Maintain integrity of skin and other defenses.

D. Interventions.

1. Provide restful environment.

2. Insure adequate nutrition.

3. Provide psychosocial care.

4. Administer antiinfective drugs safely.

5. Patient teaching.

   a. How infection is transmitted.

   b. How to prevent spread.

   c. How to take medications; precautions.

E. Evaluation

1. Periodic evaluation of lab values and vital signs to determine effectiveness of treatment.

2. Monitor wounds for improvement.

IX. Community Care

A. Educate public about sanitation.

B. Educate about infection transmission and its prevention.

C. Educate about a healthy lifestyle that promotes resistance to infection.

D. Home care nurse teaches ways to prevent spread of infection, how to contain organisms, how to disinfect, and techniques of medical asepsis.

E. Long-term care nurses carefully monitor residents for signs of infection and practice good aseptic technique.

X. Elder Care Points

A. Many elderly have a normally low body temperature; there may be little rise in the presence of infection.

B. Clues that an infection is present may be a decrease in mental alertness, increased fatigue, or sudden onset of confusion, irritability, or apathy.

C. Elderly often are more susceptible to infection because of the presence of other chronic disease, malnutrition, diminished immune response, compromised defense mechanisms from changes of aging (Table 6-4).

Problems of Immune Response

Upon completing this chapter the student should be able to:
1. Contrast the characteristics of humoral and cellular immunity.
2. Identify the various ways in which immunity to disease occurs.
3. List the factors that interfere with normal immune response.
4. Explain why tissue matching is so important for organ and tissue transplants.
5. Describe the methods used to prevent transplant rejection.
6. Discuss ways in which immune deficiencies occur.
7. Explain how an allergic reaction occurs when a patient experiences an excessive immune response.
8. State measures to prevent and treat an anaphylactic reaction.
9. Explain how autoimmune disorders are thought to occur.
10. Formulate a nursing care plan for a patient who has systemic lupus erythematosus.

The immune response is a remarkable series of complex chemical and mechanical activities that take place in the body. These activities involve (1) constant surveillance to detect the entry of foreign agents (**antigens**) as soon as they gain access to the body's cells; (2) immediate recognition of the agents as nonself (that is foreign or alien); and (3) the ability to distinguish one kind of foreign agent from another and to remember that particular agent if it appears in the body again at a later time.

TYPES OF IMMUNE RESPONSE

Once a particular kind of foreign substance has been detected and identified, the body responds in two general ways. It immediately produces a protein (called an *antibody*) that is specifically designed to do battle with the *antigen*. This immediate response is called a *humoral response*. There also is a delayed response that involves the use of sensitized lymphocytes to attack whole cells, such as those of bacteria and viruses, and malignant cells. This second kind of response is called a *cellular*, or *cell-mediated*, response.

◆ T Lymphocytes and B Lymphocytes

Both humoral and cellular immunity originate in the lymphocytic stem cells found in the bone marrow of the developing fetus. Within a few months after birth those lymphocytes destined to provide cellular immunity have passed through the thymus and migrated to the lymph tissues throughout the body. **These are called the *T lymphocytes* (the *T* is for *thymus*) and they are further divided into helper T-cells, memory T-cells, suppressor T-cells, and sensitized T-cells (killer cells).** T-cells provide defense against viral infections. T-cells and macrophages secrete a variety of substances called lymphokines that help destroy antigens. Killer T-cells attach themselves to cells bearing antigen and secrete toxic substances that kill the antigen-bearing cells. This cell-to-cell contact response is called *cell-mediated immunity*.

The second group of lymphocytes, the B-cells, are involved in humoral immunity and the production of antibody. These cells are further divided into plasma cells and memory cells. These also arise from stem cells in the bone marrow. They are processed at an unknown place (maybe the fetal liver) in the body and then migrate to the lymph nodes. Because early research of the immune response showed that the preprocessing of these cells takes place in the bursa of Fabricius in birds, they were given the name B lymphocytes. When stimulated by an antigen, the B-cell becomes a plasma cell that can secrete antibody cells into the body fluids, or it becomes a memory cell capable of secreting this specific antibody. As shown in Figure 7-1, both T and B lym-

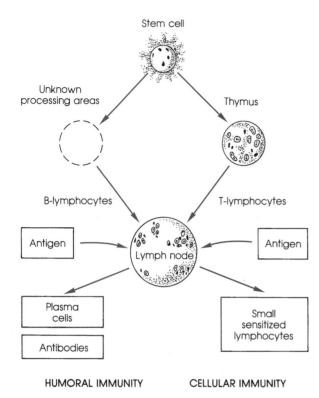

Stem cell

Unknown processing areas

Thymus

B-lymphocytes

T-lymphocytes

Antigen

Lymph node

Antigen

Plasma cells

Antibodies

Small sensitized lymphocytes

HUMORAL IMMUNITY   CELLULAR IMMUNITY

FIGURE 7-1   Origin of B and T lymphocytes responsible for cellular and humoral immunity. In response to antigens, B and T lymphocytes are sensitized by lymphoid tissue.

phocytes migrate to lymphoid tissue, where they wait in readiness to form either sensitized lymphocytes or antibodies.

B-cells secrete immunoglobulins called *antibodies* in response to the specific antigen they encounter. This is antibody-mediated, or **humoral immunity.** T-cells and B-cells interact with each other in complex ways. Helper T-cells must interact with B-cells before the B-cells can become plasma or memory cells. The suppressor T-cells regulate the amount of antibody that B-cells produce. **Both T-cells and B-cells are necessary for normal immune response to occur.**

The memory cells reactivate when the same antigen enters the body a second time. They rapidly respond by producing large quantities of the specific type of antibody needed to fight the particular type of antigen. It is an immediate and potent response, and antibodies continue to be produced for many months. Because of this secondary response, immunity from immunizations is usually achieved by administering the vaccine in divided doses over weeks or months. This sets in motion the more powerful, longer lasting secondary response. For example, infants are given immunizations at intervals during infancy and then periodically after that. To stimulate continued immunity, adults should have immunizations against tetanus and diphtheria every 10 years (Table 7-1).

Antigen   The word *antigen* is a combination of *anti-*, meaning against, and *-gen*, meaning generate or cause to be. Thus an antigen is any substance that can bring about or generate a substance that will fight it. The most common response to the antigen is the production of antibody.

Antibodies are produced to act against a specific antigen. The antibodies produced as a response to chickenpox do not provide immunity against mumps or any other kind of bacterial or viral infection.

Examples of antigens include the cells of bacteria, viruses, fungi, and other infectious organisms, as well as the toxins they produce. Nonliving matter such as pollen, dust, and the chemicals in detergent also can be antigens. For some people, foods are perceived as antigens. For example, the interpretation of the protein in milk as a harmful substance may trigger an allergic reaction to milk in some persons. The same is true of many other substances. Substances that have no harmful effect on some people may cause potentially fatal allergic reactions in others. This is discussed more fully in the section on allergies.

In instances in which transplanted organs are rejected by the recipient, the cells of the transplanted organs are seen by the body as foreign antigens. Red blood cells can become antigenic if they are mixed with cells of a different type, as in a transfusion of mismatched whole blood. The wrong type of red cells in the bloodstream of the recipient can stimulate the production of antibodies and result in the symptoms of a transfusion reaction.

TABLE 7-1 ◆ *Recommended Immunization Schedule*	
Birth	Hepatitis B
2 months of age	Hepatitis B; diptheria, tetanus, pertussis (DTP); *H. influenzae* type B; polio
4 months of age	Diptheria, tetanus, pertussis (DTP); *H. influenzae* type B; polio
6 months of age	Hepatitis B (between 6 and 15 months of age); diptheria, tetanus, pertussis (DTP); *H. influenzae* type B; polio (between 6 and 18 months)
12 months of age	Diptheria, tetanus, pertussis (DTP between 12 and 15 months of age); measles, mumps, rubella (MMR, between 12 and 15 months of age), Varicella (between 12–18 months of age)
4–6 years of age	Diptheria, tetanus, pertussis (DTP); polio; measles, mumps, rubella (MMR, now or at 11–12 years of age)
11–12 years of age	Tetanus, diptheria
Every 10 years	Tetanus

Antibody   Just as almost all antigens are proteins, so are the antibodies that are produced to fight them. Antibodies are a kind of protein synthesized by plasma cells. They are called **immunoglobulin. Globulins** are proteins that are soluble in moderately concentrated salt solutions. The prefix *immuno-* tells us that these kinds of globulins provide some kind of immunity.

There are five classes of immunoglobulins (Ig): IgA, IgD, IgE, IgG, and IgM. Each antibody is able to stick to the kind of antigen for which it is made. The number of sites at which an antibody can attach itself to its antigen depends on the class to which it belongs. This ability of an antibody to form a bond with its antigen is important to the destruction of the antigen, but it can sometimes result in damage to the body's own cells.

Antibodies are found in the serum of blood and in other body fluids and tissues, including the urine, saliva, tears, breast milk, interstitial fluid, spinal fluid, lymph nodes, and spleen. An antibody can either destroy or inactivate its particular antigen by (1) mechanically harming it; (2) activating a complement system; or (3) causing the release of chemicals that affect the environment of the antigen.

In some instances the antibody prepares the antigen for ingestion by phagocytes. It does this by a process called **lysis,** in which the antibody damages the membrane of the antigen's cell, causing it to rupture and making its contents accessible for digestion.

Another means by which antibody attacks antigen is through **agglutination.** This causes the antigens to lump together (agglutinate), forming a heavy, inactive mass. This is what sometimes happens in a transfusion reaction. When the mismatched red blood cells of the donor blood come into contact with the red cells of the recipient's blood, antibodies attach to the recipient's red cells. These antibodies stick to the antigens, causing the blood cells to clump together. The clumps of cells then obstruct small blood vessels and thereby produce some of the symptoms of a transfusion reaction.

Some antibodies cause their antigens to form a heavy mass that is insoluble. This causes them to settle into an inactive deposit of solid particles called a **precipitate.** The process is called *precipitation,* and the antibodies are called *precipitins.*

If the antigen is a **toxin** (poison) produced by a bacterial or viral cell, the antibody produced is called the **antitoxin** that is capable of neutralizing the poisonous chemical of the antigen by covering the toxic sites of the antigenic agent. An antitoxin is, therefore, a specific type of antibody that acts through the process of *neutralization.*

In the *complement* system, certain enzymes in the plasma that are normally inactive are stimulated by the antigen–antibody reaction. These enzymes not only attack the invading antigens, but also protect local body cells from damage by the foreign substances.

During the antigen–antibody reaction some of the antibodies attached to the tissue and blood cells cause these cells to rupture, bringing about the release of *histamine* and other substances that can be harmful to the body. If the reaction is extreme and widespread, the individual can die from circulatory shock and respiratory failure. This reaction is discussed more fully later in this chapter in the section on anaphylaxis.

◆ Humoral (Immediate) Response

When a bacterium or other antigen enters the body, it may encounter a B lymphocyte that is specific for that bacterium or antigen. The B lymphocyte becomes a plasma cell that secretes immunoglobulin, IgM (antibody) that attacks the bacterium or antigen. The first time this particular bacterium or antigen is encountered, it takes 4 to 8 days for the B lymphocyte to produce immunoglobulins that can attack. If the same bacterium or antigen enters the body a second time at a later date, the immunoglobin response by the memory cells is quicker, occurring in 1 to 2 days. The immunoglobulin produced is mostly IgG, and the response is stronger and longer lasting.

The major function of the humoral (antigen–antibody) response is to provide protection against acute, rapidly developing bacterial and viral diseases. The antigen–antibody response also is involved in allergies and transfusion reactions.

◆ Cellular (Delayed) Response

The second type of immunological response of the body involves various interactions with antigens by T lymphocytes. Unlike the humoral response, which takes place in cell-free plasma, the cellular response involves whole cells called *sensitized lymphocytes* and occurs out in the tissues. They are said to be *sensitized* because they have been made sensitive to a specific antigen after their first contact with it. They are special troops in the same sense that antibodies are special troops. Subsequent exposure to the antigen to which they are sensitive triggers a host of chemical and mechanical activities, all designed to either destroy or inactivate the offending antigen.

The T lymphocytes **mediate** (indirectly accomplish) the cellular response. When an antigen is complex (e.g., a bacterium or another type of living cell), T lymphocytes that are specifically reactive with the particular antigen mediate the cellular response in several ways. These specific T lymphocytes enter the circulating fluids of the body from the lymphoid tissues, migrate widely, and react anywhere in the body where they encounter the particular antigen. Destruction of the antigen may occur by release of chemicals into the membrane of the target cell, by secretion of lymphokines such as interleukin-2 or T-cell growth factor, or by other processes. This direct contact by the T lymphocytes with an antigen is called *killer activity,* and such lymphocytes are named *killer T cells.* Cellular immune response is often termed *delayed hypersensitivity.* The larger the amount of antigen present, the greater the response of sensitized T lymphocytes.

The T lymphocytes perform immune surveillance for the body by detecting cells that enter the host and have foreign antigens on their surface. They are defensive cells that patrol the blood and tissues. This is why transplanted tissue must have surface antigens that are very similar to those of the host tissue to be accepted by the host body. **Sensitized T lymphocytes are the cause of allergic reactions. T-cells are responsible for the inflammatory response present in people with a variety of** *autoimmune* **diseases.** *Autoimmune* means that there is a defective cellular immune response and that antibodies are produced against normal parts of the person's body. These T lymphocytes, along with migrating macrophages, are responsible for rejecting transplanted organs as well. Figure 7-2 depicts the humoral and cell-mediated immune responses.

Think about . . . Can you explain to a family member how the body reacts to protect itself against an invading virus?

IMMUNITY AGAINST DISEASE

There are two major types of immunity to specific diseases: natural (innate) immunity and acquired (adaptive) immunity. **Natural immunity is present at birth.**

Acquired immunity occurs by actively producing antibodies when the body has been invaded by pathogens or by receiving an immunization that causes antibodies to a specific pathogen to form.

◆ Innate (Natural) Immunity

Certain innate, or inborn, features of human cells make a person naturally immune to certain diseases. Some of us are immune simply because we belong to a certain species, race, or gender or because we have a particular kind of constitution. Humans are not susceptible to the same diseases as are animals of lower orders. Some people are able to resist disease more easily than others because they are physically and mentally healthier.

◆ Acquired Immunity

In acquired immunity a person can either actively produce his or her own antibody or passively receive antibodies that have been produced by another person or animal.

Naturally Acquired Passive Immunity   The fetus in the uterus can *passively* receive some natural immunity from its mother. Most antibodies in the mother's bloodstream can pass through the placenta and become mixed with the blood of the fetus, so that they are present in the infant's blood at birth. Thus an expectant mother who has a high level of immunity to diphtheria, tetanus, and whooping cough can be assured that her newborn baby will have some immunity to these diseases. Greater immunity can be passed to the infant through breast

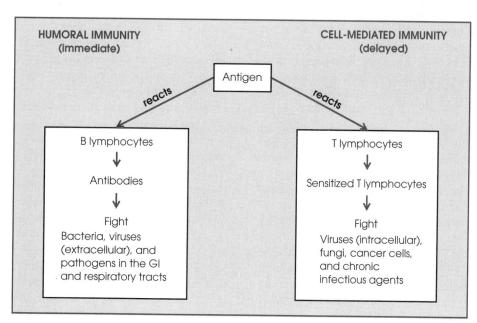

FIGURE 7-2   Humoral and cell-mediated immune responses.

milk. Breastfeeding is the best way to protect the newborn.

Naturally Acquired Active Immunity

Before immunization and inoculation became commonplace, the only way an individual could acquire immunity was to suffer an attack of the disease and, owing to a strong constitution and good fortune, manage to survive. Once he had survived this trial by fire, he was immune and no longer needed to fear that particular disease.

Artificially Acquired Active Immunity

The establishment of immunity by vaccination became widely accepted through the efforts of an English country doctor, Edward Jenner, who developed the smallpox vaccine. He knew that having had cowpox protected people against smallpox. He innoculated a boy with material from a sore on the hand of a milkmaid who had cowpox. Six weeks later he innoculated the boy with smallpox exudate. The boy proved to be immune to smallpox. To provide active immunity to diseases by artificial means, the actual pathogenic microorganisms are grown and cultured in the laboratory. They are divided into single doses under rigid controls and made into vaccines. These specially treated microorganisms are weakened or killed so that they will stimulate the production of antibodies but will not cause the disease itself. Vaccines from cowpox viruses, tetanus, and tubercle bacilli, and more recently the polio, influenza, measles, mumps, chickenpox, and hepatitis viruses, are all examples of agents used to produce an active immunity in humans.

This method of stimulating the production of immunizing substances in the body is successful in situations in which there is time to wait for the person to build up his own defenses. This immunity does not last indefinitely. The body must be reminded of the need to produce more antibodies. To achieve this a booster dose of an immunizing agent is given to jog the memory of the specific B-cells and cause them to actively produce more antibodies.

Artificially Acquired Passive Immunity

If a person has no immunity and contracts the disease, he needs antibodies that can go to work immediately to destroy the harmful antigens. This is achieved by providing passive immunity. As the name implies, passive immunity is acquired through the efforts of someone else. Usually the someone else is a horse or a rabbit, although it may be a human. The serum from the blood of one of these animals contains ready-made antibodies that include antitoxins. It is prepared in a laboratory by increasing the strength of injections of specific antigens given to the animals over a period of time so that they build up the necessary antibodies.

The most common diseases against which passive immunity is used effectively to bolster the patient's defenses are diphtheria, tetanus, scarlet fever, and gas gangrene. There also are *antivenins* containing antibodies against snake venoms and the poisons produced by the black widow spider. Injections that provide passive immunity should be given in the earliest stages of the disease because they can only help prevent damage to tissues; they cannot repair damage already done.

Sometimes passive immunity is established before the disease is contracted. In instances of known contact with a disease such as hepatitis, when the exposed person is considered too weak to withstand the rigors of a full-blown disease, human immune globulin is given to prepare the body in advance and to lessen the severity of the disease, should the person exposed actually contract it.

Human immune globulin, formerly called gamma globulin, contains antibodies against not just one, but many infectious diseases. It is used for some of the so-called childhood diseases because it is assumed that adults, from whom it has been taken, have been exposed to and developed antibodies against these diseases during their lifetime.

Think about . . . What type of immunity do you have after recovering from the chickenpox?

◆ Screening and Diagnostic Testing

The purpose of screening and testing is to identify persons who are in danger of contracting an infectious disease or who may have it without knowing it and therefore are likely to infect others. Persons at higher risk of contracting an infectious disease include all persons in an area in which there is an epidemic, where there is a polluted water supply, who live in substandard housing in crowded conditions, who are not well nourished, or who suffer from a chronic illness. Persons who come into close contact with the public frequently must be tested for tuberculosis. This includes all health care and food service workers.

Skin testing is one of the most commonly used techniques to measure immunity and to identify people who may have a dormant infectious disease. These tests include the *Schick test* to determine susceptibility to diphtheria and the *tuberculin test* to identify those who might need treatment for tuberculosis.

Testing for a reaction to tuberculin (a product of the organism that causes tuberculosis) can be done in several ways. These include the Mantoux test (intradermal injection), jet-gun injection, and multiple-puncture techniques. Interpretation of results will depend on the technique used. In general, a positive reaction means either that the person has had a tuberculosis infection somewhere in the body that has healed or that he has an infection that is currently active. It does not mean simply that the person has been exposed to someone who has active tuberculosis. **Tuberculin testing alone does not confirm a diagnosis of tuberculosis. It is a screening device to detect those who need a more thorough workup to establish or rule out a diagnosis of tuberculosis.**

◆ Immunization and Nursing Implications

The nurse has three major goals in regard to immunization against specific diseases: (1) to increase public participation in immunization programs recommended by health officials; (2) to contribute to identification of persons in need of immunization; and (3) to prevent or mitigate sensitivity reactions to immunizing agents.

Immunization Programs An important aspect of health teaching is to improve the general public's awareness of the importance of immunization as a means of avoiding certain diseases and their consequences. In spite of the availability of vaccines against poliomyelitis, measles, rubella, mumps, and other potentially dangerous diseases, there still are many children who have not been adequately immunized. Figure 7-3 shows the secondary response and longer lasting immunity provided by a second injection of an antigen. This is particularly true in areas that have a large, recent, immigrant population and in areas populated by the poor who do not have easy access to the health care system. **Nurses have a responsibility to inform the public of the purpose of immunization in terms the lay person can understand.**

Parents should be told why immunization is best for their children and be warned of the dangers faced by children who are not adequately immunized. This information must be presented in such a way that the

parents do not feel threatened or badgered by the nurse. Older adults and others who are particularly susceptible to influenza and pneumococcal pneumonia also should be immunized according to the recommendations of public health officials.

Circumstances that require postponing immunization include fevers, pregnancy, immune deficiency disease, immunosuppressive therapy, and administration of serum immune globulin, plasma, or whole blood transfusion 6 to 8 weeks before the immunization. Immunization also is contraindicated when a person is taking certain drugs. Brochures accompanying these drugs will state whether they prohibit the administration of an immunizing agent.

Think about . . . Describe two ways in which a person can obtain antibodies for the virus that causes measles.

Preventing or Decreasing Sensitivity Reactions
Whenever an immunizing agent is to be administered, precautions must be taken to ensure as far as possible that the patient is not hypersensitive to the components of the agent. Many times chick embryo, horse serum, and other substances are used to make the vaccine or immune serum. These substances can produce a serious allergic reaction in persons who are hypersensitive to them. Immunizing agents that are most often associated with anaphylaxis, a potentially fatal reaction, include tetanus antitoxin, diphtheria antitoxin, rabies antitoxin, and antilymphocytic globulin.

It is imperative that a history of allergies in the patient and his family be obtained before administering an immunizing agent. It also should be determined whether the patient has an immune deficiency disease of any kind that would prevent a normal immune response to the immunizing agent. If a patient does have a history of allergies or an immune deficiency, the physician should be made aware of this fact before the immunizing agent is given. If the patient has had an allergic reaction to the specific agent he is supposed to receive, the drug must not be given.

There are times when a skin sensitivity test is indicated before any serum is administered to a patient. Skin testing for sensitivity should not be confused with skin testing for diagnostic purposes. Testing for sensitivity is done to determine whether a minute amount of the immunizing agent will produce a local reaction. If it does, chances are the patient will have a severe reaction if the agent is given systemically.

In spite of these precautions it is possible that a patient will suffer from hypersensitivity to an immunizing agent. To avoid serious problems, the nurse should always be prepared to act quickly and effectively in such an emergency. In all patient care areas where immunizing agents are administered, emergency equipment

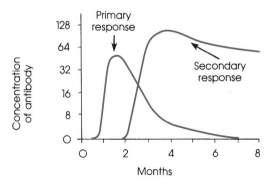

FIGURE 7-3   Time course of antibody responses to a primary immunization and to a secondary injection 2 months later.

should be readily available. This includes epinephrine, aminophyllines, and other drugs as indicated; syringes and other equipment for administration; a tourniquet; an airway; oxygen; and equipment for intravenous infusion. As an extra precaution to ensure prompt treatment of a hypersensitivity reaction if one occurs, it is advisable for persons receiving immunizing agents to remain in the clinic or office for 15 to 20 minutes after an injection.

Think about . . . What happens if a person does not get a tetanus booster every 10 years? Will he still have some immunity to tetanus?

DISORDERS OF THE IMMUNE SYSTEM

Abnormal responses of the immune system are divided into four basic categories: (1) *immune deficiency,* that is, insufficient production of either antibodies or immune cells or both; (2) *excessive response,* which involves increased growth of the plasma cells and the synthesis of abnormal antibodies; (3) *overreaction* or *hypersensitivity* to antigens from the external environment; and (4) *autoimmune disease,* in which the immune system reacts against the body's own cells or a substance arising in the body.

◆ Immune Deficiency

Inadequate function of the immune system can affect either the humoral or the cellular components of the system. Insufficient production of these components can be present at birth (congenital) or acquired during life. In some cases the acquired deficiency is a primary condition; in others it is secondary to some other disorder or treatment.

> In all cases, a deficiency of immune bodies leaves its victims unable to resist foreign agents and therefore susceptible to overwhelming infection.

Acquired immune deficiency can result from any of a number of factors. Contraction of the *human immunodeficiency virus (HIV)* and the subsequent development of *Acquired immunodeficiency syndrome (AIDS)* is the most serious of these disorders as it is eventually fatal. AIDS is covered in the next chapter. Secondary causes are cytotoxic drugs and chemicals that suppress or damage the bone marrow, long-term therapy with corticosteroid drugs, immunosuppressive drug therapy for autoimmune disease or to prevent transplant rejection, and radiation therapy. Cancer patients often have an imposed immune deficiency from chemotherapy and radiation therapy.

Elder Care Point . . . Aging does not affect the bone marrow to a significant degree. It does cause the thymus gland to become smaller and T-cells apparently diminish in the circulation. B-cell numbers remain the same. All the mechanisms involved in decreased immune function are not yet clear, but it is apparent that after age 70 there is a definite decline in the function of the immune system. This is evidenced by a marked increase in the numbers of cancerous tumors in the population over age 70 and in their decreased ability to fight infection.

Therapeutic Immunosuppression Sometimes it is beneficial to the patient to have his immune response deliberately suppressed. To illustrate, the patient who has received an organ transplant may suffer from total rejection of the organ by his own body cells if they react to the organ as if it were a harmful agent. **To avoid rejection of the transplanted organ, the patient may receive certain drugs that inhibit the action of his immune system.** As previously explained, certain cytotoxic drugs, as well as x-rays used to produce radiographs, can be immunosuppressive. Hence these agents can be used to benefit the patient when immunosuppression is desirable. The use of immunosuppressive agents requires the maintenance of a delicate balance between control of the immune response and control of infections that occur when the immune response is suppressed.

Three agents are generally used to prevent rejection after organ transplantation. They are azathioprine (Imuran), cyclosporine (Sandimmune), and a corticosteroid such as prednisone. The doses of these drugs are adjusted according to the immune response of each patient. This type of therapy increases the risk for bacterial and fungal infections in the patient. Cyclosporine acts as a selective immunosuppressant, leaving intact some of the body's defenses against infection. There is evidence that use of the drug increases the survival rate of patients with certain organ transplants, but it does not completely eliminate the danger of organ rejection. Another problem is that the immunosuppression tends to allow the growth of some cancers.

In addition to preventing the rejection of transplanted organs, immunosuppressive therapy also may be employed to manage multiple myeloma, rheumatoid arthritis, other kinds of neoplastic growths, and other autoimmune diseases.

Whatever the reason for the immune deficiency, the patient will require special nursing care so that the possibility of an overwhelming infection is kept at a minimum.

Treatment of Immune Deficiencies The management of immune deficiency depends on its degree of severity and its primary cause. Some patients have virtually no ability to synthesize antibodies or sensitized lymphocytes, whereas others experience only a temporary minor defect in humoral immune response and cell-mediated immunity.

Injections of immune globulin may be given on a regular basis to provide passive immunity for those who are unable to produce their own antibodies. Antibiotics are used in large doses as soon as an infection is evident, but these drugs are rarely used as a preventive measure because antibiotics themselves can be immunosuppressive.

In some types of immune deficiency, passive immunization can be accomplished by transfusing specifically sensitized lymphocytes to help the patient resist an infection. When function of the bone marrow is involved, as in leukemia, the patient may receive a bone marrow transplant to provide the stem cells that will eventually become immune bodies.

To help prevent or combat infection in immunosuppressed patients, granulocyte colony-stimulating factor (Neupogen) is used to promote the growth of neutrophils. This drug has been used for both AIDs patients and some types of cancer patients who have immunodeficiency.

Whenever possible, treatment is aimed at controlling the disease or eliminating the condition that is the primary cause of an inadequately functioning immune system. Sometimes, as in cases of nephrosis, liver disease, drug toxicity, and viral infections, this may be possible. In other instances, however, treatment consists of minimizing the effects of the immune deficiency.

Experimental drugs continue to be developed for use in the treatment of AIDS. Research also offers hope for infants with combined immune deficiencies through administration of specially treated bone marrow containing stem cells that mature into normally functioning T lymphocytes. Preventing and treating infection in patients with immune disorders is a nursing challenge.

Nursing Care of Patients with Immune Deficiency

Assessment. When an immune deficiency is suspected, the patient is questioned about frequent infections, exposure to HIV, immunosuppressive drug therapy, and family history of genetic immune disorders. Nutritional status is assessed by measuring weight and height, inspecting the skin and hair, general appearance of the patient, and inquiring about weight loss. Information is gathered about the current physical status of the patient, such as his general state of health, any infections he may have at the time, and how these infections are affecting him. Inquiring about occupational or environmental exposure to agents that might harm the bone marrow also is important. Excessive alcohol intake depresses the immune system, so gathering a drinking history is indicated. Determining whether or not the patient is on corticosteroid therapy is essential.

Physical assessment includes palpating the superficial lymph nodes to detect abnormalities and assessing of body systems involved in complaints. The abdomen is palpated to detect organ enlargement such as an enlarged liver or spleen.

Diagnostic tests. A complete blood count (CBC) with differential is obtained to determine the numbers of circulating lymphocytes. Other tests used to ascertain immune status include bone marrow studies, serum protein, protein electrophoresis, immunoelectrophoresis, T-cell and B-cell assays, and enzyme-linked immunosorbent assays (ELISA). Other tests specific to the type of disorder suspected may be performed.

Nursing diagnoses. Nursing diagnoses for patients with immune deficiency always include Risk for infection. Other nursing diagnoses are written according to the particular problems and complaints the patient has.

Planning. **The primary goals of the nurse caring for a patient who has an *immune deficiency* are to (1) protect the patient from infection; (2) improve health status; and (3) maintain as high a degree of wellness as possible so that the immune system can function at optimal level.**

Planning care for the patient with an immune deficiency focuses on preventing exposure to pathogens. If a patient's immune deficiency is severe, he will need to be placed in protective (reverse) isolation. Working with patients in this type of isolation requires more time because of the precautions involved. Integrating care of this patient with the rest of the assignment for the shift needs to be carefully planned. Nurses caring for immunodeficient patients should not be caring for patients with active infections at the same time.

Expected outcomes might include:

◆ Patient remains free from infection.
◆ B-cell and T-cell counts are within normal limits.

Intervention. Adequate nutrition is important as proteins are needed to synthesize antibodies. If the patient is on corticosteroid therapy, appetite control may be a problem and the patient must be watched for continuous weight gain.

When a severely immune deficient patient is hospitalized, ***protective (reverse) isolation* is implemented so that exposure of the patient to infectious agents is kept at a minimum (Table 7-2).** For any patient with immune deficiency, meticulous handwashing is essential before and after each contact with the patient or any object that may serve as a source of infection. Strict observance of surgical aseptic technique is essential during the performance of such nursing care procedures as catheterization, dressing changes, intravenous infusions, and all

TABLE 7-2 ◆ *Precautions for Protective (Reverse) Isolation*

◆ Patient is placed in a private room.
◆ No visitors are allowed to enter the room if they have a cold, influenza, or any other type of infection.
◆ Strict handwashing is performed before entering the room and before delivering patient care.
◆ Barriers of mask, protective garments such as clean scrub suits or gowns, hair coverings, and gloves are required.
◆ No fresh fruit or flowers are allowed in the room.
◆ Special linens may be used (sterilized).
◆ For extreme cases of immune deficiency, air purification filter systems are used.
◆ Invasive procedures are avoided as much as possible.
◆ Sterilized and disinfected equipment that is to be used on this patient only is kept in the room for taking vital signs, performing treatments, etc.

other activities that might lead to introducing pathogenic microorganisms into the body tissues.

Psychosocial care to assist the patient deal with the fear associated with the knowledge that he may contract a serious infection at any time is a nursing responsibility. The lives of patients with immune disorders often are disrupted by infections and by the therapy to control the disorder. They may have trouble remaining in school or at work because of frequent illness or malaise. Collaboration with the social worker is often indicated to assist with role changes and financial constraints.

The nurse can be instrumental in assisting the patient with techniques to reduce stress. **Excessive stress further depresses immune function.** Light exercise, meditation, relaxation techniques, or imagery are all appropriate.

Patient education. Patient education regarding the immune disorder and any therapy that the patient is to receive should be provided. The patient is taught continuously to assess for signs of infection and to report them immediately. Antimicrobial therapy should be started at the first signs of infection. Patients are encouraged to wash hands frequently and to refrain from mingling in crowds. Avoiding others who have an infection is essential. Foods should be well cooked and raw foods should not be eaten. Adequate rest is important to allow the body to function as well as possible.

Evaluation. Evaluation of nursing actions is performed to determine whether expected outcomes are being met. **Lab tests are checked to assess whether immune function is improving.** B-cell and T-cell assays are particularly important. The patient is evaluated for recovery from any infection that might have been present. Temperature is monitored for elevations, although immune deficient patients may not have a temperature elevation even in the presence of infection.

The patient also is evaluated for general well-being, appetite, weight maintenance, and for side effects of the medications he is taking.

◆ Excessive Immune Response

In an excessive response of the immune system, the plasma cells of the bone marrow begin to multiply very rapidly, forming a tumor within the bone marrow (myeloma) that causes bone destruction. Normal bone marrow functions are disrupted and the patient is more prone to infection. The abnormal plasma cells then invade the lymph nodes, liver, spleen, and kidneys; hence the term *multiple* myeloma. The disorder occurs in middle-aged and elderly people and in men more than women. More information on multiple myeloma is in Chapter 17.

Hypersensitivity and Allergy

Pathophysiology. An **allergy is an abnormal, individual response to certain substances that normally do not trigger such an exaggerated reaction.** Allergies are divided into three major groups: (1) delayed-reaction allergies involving sensitized lymphocytes; (2) antigen–antibody allergies caused by a reaction between IgG and antigen; and (3) atopic or inherited allergies, which are characterized by the presence of large amounts of IgE antibody.

Examples of *delayed-reaction, cell-mediated hypersensitivity* allergies include contact dermatitis resulting from exposure to certain drugs, chemicals such as those in cosmetics and household cleaners, and the toxins of plants such as poison ivy. On contact with the allergen the sensitized lymphocytes diffuse into the skin and bring about an immune response. During this reaction the lymphocytes release toxins and macrophages invade the tissues. If the process continues unchecked, **there can be extensive damage to the tissues as a result of inflammatory changes.**

Antigen–antibody allergies occur when a person **has a high titer of antibodies, especially the IgG type, circulating in his blood.** The reaction results in the formation of an antigen–antibody complex that precipitates and deposits small granules on the walls of blood vessels. Enzymes released during the reaction cause inflammation of the small blood vessels, which are subsequently badly damaged or destroyed. Examples of antigen–antibody reactions are transfusion reactions and drug reactions.

Atopic allergies affect about 10% of the population. **The hypersensitivity is inherited, and excessive amounts of IgE antibodies are produced.** Allergens that react specifically with IgE antibody include house dust, foods, and the venom of bees, wasps, and hornets. During this reaction histamine and other chemicals toxic to the body's cells are released. The chemicals cause dilation of blood vessels (which increases the transport of antibody and chemicals to the site of battle) and the contraction of smooth-muscle tissues in the bronchioles. These internal changes produce the symptoms of allergy, notably redness, swelling, increased exudate, and breathing difficulties such as wheezing and dyspnea.

As with all types of immune response, abnormal as well as normal, a full-blown reaction will not occur until an individual's immune cells have been sensitized to the specific substance that triggers the response. **This means that on first contact with the allergen, there will be very little specific antibody in the circulating blood or in the lymphoid tissues.** On second and subsequent contacts, however, the antibody specific to the allergen will be produced in large quantities and circulated in the body fluids, where it can be transported to the site of the allergic reaction.

Management of hypersensitivity and allergic reactions.

The major goals in managing hypersensitivity and allergic reactions are (1) to assist in the diagnosis of hypersensitivity; (2) to help the patient identify the particular substance or substances that trigger an allergic response; (3) to assist the patient in devising ways to avoid or at least limit exposure to these allergens; (4) to relieve the symptoms of an allergy; (5) to decrease the exaggerated response to the allergen(s); and (6) to provide health teaching.

Assessment.

Objective and subjective data suggestive of an allergy are summarized in Table 7-3. Identification of the specific allergen or allergens causing the allergic reaction may be fairly easy or extremely difficult. Reaction to stings, drug allergies, and other conditions that are not routine occurrences in the life of the patient are readily noticed because the cause-and-effect relationship is apparent, but vague symptoms, such as a stuffy nose from allergy to inhalants, may be less obvious.

Types of allergens.

To help the patient recognize less obvious allergic substances, you may want to put these substances in some kind of category. Four broad types of allergens may be distinguished according to the way in which they gain access to the body. **Inhalants** enter the body through the nose and mouth; they include dust, molds, pollen, animal dander, and some chemicals. **Contactants** come in direct contact with the skin. These include detergents and soaps, cosmetics, plants such as poison ivy, and dyes such as those used in shoe leather. **Ingestants** are swallowed. They usually are foods and drugs. Citrus fruits, tomatoes, cow's milk, wheat, seafoods, chocolate, and colas are common food offenders. Among the drugs, the most likely to cause an allergic reaction are aspirin, barbiturates, and antibiotics. **Injectables** enter the body through hypodermic, intramuscular, and intravenous injections; by snake and other animal bites; and by insect stings. Immunizing agents such as vaccines, animal saliva, and venoms are the allergens that most commonly enter the body by this route.

Identification of allergens.

Skin testing to identify specific allergens can be done in a number of ways. In the *scratch test*, the skin is slightly scratched so that only its upper layer is broken and no blood appears. A sampling of the suspected allergen is applied to the scratched area. In the *intracutaneous* or *intradermal*

TABLE 7-3 ◆ *Assessment Guide for Allergy*		
Location	**Objective Data**	**Subjective Data**
Skin	Dryness, scaling, irritations, inflammations, hives, rash (note symmetry and location), scratches, urticaria.	Itching, burning.
Eyes	Discoloration below eyes (allergic shiners); conjunctivitis; long, silky eyelashes; rubbing or excessive blinking.	Burning, itching, tearing; history of styes.
Nose	Allergic salute (pushing nose upward and backward with heel of hand), nasal polyps, nasal voice.	Nose twitching, "stuffiness," recurring nosebleeds, sudden episodes of sneezing, snorting.
Mouth and throat	Open-mouth breathing, continual throat clearing; shiny, bald patches on tongue with slightly elevated borders; mouth wrinkling with facial grimaces; redness of throat; swollen lips or tongue.	Ability to tolerate only moderate exertion without tiring, wheezing, or shortness of breath.
Ears	Drainage.	Hearing loss.
Neck	Palpable lymph nodes.	
General		History of food intolerances; colic; abdominal cramping; vomiting and diarrhea in absence of general illness; unusual reactions to drugs, insect stings, odors, or fumes; recurrent respiratory problems; seasonal flare-ups of any symptoms.

method, the sample of allergen is injected just below the epidermis. In the *patch test* a small amount of the allergen is simply placed on the surface of the skin and covered with an airtight dressing (patch). A positive reaction to these tests is indicated by the appearance of a small (dime-size) wheal at the site of contact with the allergen.

Another helpful tool for identifying suspected allergens in foods is the *elimination diet.* It usually starts with foods that are known to be frequent offenders. The patient is asked to eliminate one food at a time and to record in a food diary *all the foods eaten each day.* This includes additives and preservatives in processed foods that were eaten. If the patient's symptoms persist for a week to 10 days after eliminating one food (for example, milk and dairy products), he is allowed to resume his intake of that particular food, and another one is chosen for elimination.

Identification of allergens can be a tedious process. Many times more than one substance produces the symptoms of an allergy. The patient and family will need continued support and encouragement to keep looking for the offending substance or substances.

Nursing intervention. Goals for nursing intervention to assist the patient with an allergy are (1) to help the patient avoid exposure to known allergens; (2) to manage the symptoms of the allergy; (3) to participate in a program of hyposensitization or immunotherapy; and (4) to provide health teaching.

Avoiding exposure to allergens. Once the allergens are identified, the patient will need help in devising ways to avoid them or to limit exposure to them. In some cases, it may mean parting with a cherished family pet, overcoming the habit of smoking and asking others not to smoke in one's presence, or purchasing an air-conditioning unit that effectively filters out airborne allergens.

House dust and pollens are common allergens that are not easily eliminated from the environment. Overstuffed furniture, heavy draperies, and thick carpets serve as excellent reservoirs for these substances. Other common allergens found in the home include cleaning compounds, cosmetics, and dyes in fabrics and common materials. Some patients may need to wear rubber gloves each time they wash dishes, launder clothes, or perform other chores requiring contact with cleansing agents.

Nurses and others who handle certain drugs may develop allergies to these drugs. For example, penicillin and streptomycin can cause contact dermatitis in some persons who are regularly exposed to them.

As with the control of the spread of infectious agents, **avoiding exposure to allergens requires a knowledge of the nature of the allergen, how it is transmitted, its source or reservoir, and its portal of entry.** Once these have been established, the nurse and the patient work together to eliminate the allergen from the patient's environment insofar as this is feasible (see Nursing Care Plan 7-1).

Management of symptoms. As stated, symptoms of an allergic response vary widely depending on the severity of the attack and the site of the reaction. Relief from the potentially fatal symptoms of anaphylaxis is discussed later in this chapter. Other allergic symptoms, although less life-threatening, can certainly cause much discomfort and inconvenience.

Nursing Care Plan 7-1

Selected nursing diagnoses, goals/expected outcomes, nursing interventions, and evaluations for a patient with hypersensitivity to contactant—probably a dishwashing detergent

Situation: 34-year-old married female with a history of rash on both hands for several months that has become progressively worse. Improvement was noted during 1-week vacation when she did not do household chores. After returning to regular housework, symptoms worsened.

Nursing Diagnosis	Goals/Expected Outcomes	Nursing Intervention	Evaluation
Impaired skin integrity related to allergy to household cleaning products. SUPPORTING DATA Dry, scaling, cracking skin on hands and wrists with rash.	Skin on hands without rash, scaling, or cracking within 3 weeks.	Attempt to identify contact allergen by instructing how to record all activities in which hands are used for 3 days and noting each morning specific condition of hands. Have change brands of dishwashing detergent. Have wear rubber gloves for any activity using soap or cleaning solution beginning on day four.	Activity record kept; hands worse after mopping with cleaning solution. Rubber gloves worn starting day four; hands improving. Meeting goals.

Drug therapy. Drugs that play an important part in alleviating the systemic reactions to allergens include epinephrine, the antihistamines, bronchodilators, corticotropin (adrenocorticotropic hormone [ACTH]), and cortisone.

The antihistamines are particularly useful in controlling the symptoms of hay fever, serum sickness, and hives. These drugs are histamine-blocking agents, which means that they prevent the histamine released during an allergic reaction from coming in contact with its specific receptors in the body cells. Thus a reaction within the tissues is avoided or at least greatly reduced. The result of this blocking action is relief from itching, swelling of mucous membranes, increased secretions, and other symptoms of an allergic reaction.

Patients requiring antihistamines are warned of the side effects of drowsiness and impaired coordination, both of which contraindicate driving an automobile and operating machinery during the initial phase of therapy. Other side effects, such as dryness of the mouth, urinary retention, weakness, and blurred vision, are not uncommon.

Elder Care Point... Many elderly men experience hesitancy, urinary retention, and difficulty with ejaculation when they take antihistamines. Bladder distention must be monitored in these patients and the drug discontinued if the problem cannot be resolved.

Antiinflammatory agents such as corticotropin and cortisone are administered to reduce the inflammatory response that occurs in an allergic reaction. The bronchodilators help relieve the respiratory distress that may be a symptom of involvement of the respiratory tract. Tranquilizers and sedatives promote the rest needed for repair of body tissues and relieve the stress that aggravates an allergic reaction.

Local reactions involving widespread and deep skin lesions are treated with salves, wet compresses, and soothing baths. The patient also must be protected from a secondary bacterial infection.

The nurse should be aware that a warm environment and sweating increase the sensation of itching. The patient should be kept cool without chilling and warned not to take hot showers or hot baths. Another important aspect of care for these patients is prevention of scratching and excoriation of the skin.

Desensitization. When it is not possible for a patient to avoid exposure to allergens, or if the symptoms cannot be managed successfully, the physician may suggest desensitization. The purpose of this form of therapy is to render the patient less sensitive to the allergens. The program involves regular injections of minute quantities of selected antigens on a daily, weekly, or monthly schedule. The amount given is gradually increased until there is noticeable clinical improvement, and then a maintenance dose is given. The program may last for years, but improvement should be noted in about 6 to 24 weeks after it is begun.

Patient evaluation. Successful management of hypersensitivity depends in large measure on the ability of the patient to understand the allergy and to follow the prescribed regimen of treatment.

Patients who have a food allergy should be instructed to read the labels on all food products carefully before purchasing them. Monosodium glutamate, other preservatives, and artificial food coloring can be potent allergens for some people. Keeping the home and work environment as allergen free as possible is a daily challenge. Compliance is very difficult unless the person's allergy is severe, prompting every effort to control it. Rugs, overstuffed furniture, stuffed animals, drapes, and other household items that gather difficult-to-remove dust are best eliminated. Electrostatic filters and top-quality vacuum cleaners with filters are essential. Daily floor care and frequent dusting is essential. If there is an allergy to mold, house plants should be removed.

Anaphylactic Reaction and Anaphylactic Shock

Anaphylaxis is a serious, dramatic allergic reaction. When it occurs, there is swelling and rupture of the affected cells, with the release of histamine. This chemical substance causes dilation of small blood vessels, a pooling of blood, and release of fluid into tissues. These changes in turn may produce circulatory collapse and profound shock. The patient also suffers from difficult breathing as a result of the narrowing of the air passages and accumulation of mucus. Another manifestation of anaphylaxis is the appearance of hives (**urticaria**). These are sudden outbreaks of **wheals** (small areas of swelling) on the skin that itch and burn.

The patient with an anaphylactic reaction is in a very serious condition and requires immediate attention. Circulatory collapse can occur very rapidly leading to fatal *anaphylactic shock*. The heart muscle does not function as it should, causing decreased output of blood and a drop in blood pressure. The patient also experiences dyspnea of increasing severity, and convulsions may occur. If these conditions are not relieved immediately, the patient can die within 5 to 10 minutes.

Treatment of anaphylaxis includes (1) administration of antihistamine (diphenhydramine hydrochloride, Benadryl) to stop the effects of the histamine released by the body cells, thereby restoring the circulatory vessels and the bronchioles to a more normal state; (2) administration of aqueous epinephrine to counteract the effect of histamine, thereby causing relaxation of the bronchioles, an increase in cardiac output, and an elevation of the blood pressure; (3) establishment of a patent airway and administration of oxygen to relieve the symptoms of dyspnea and hypoxia; (4) measures to control shock; and (5) provision for psychological support.

Avoidance of anaphylaxis requires an awareness of previous allergic reactions in individuals and identification of those people who are likely to experience a serious reaction. **It is extremely important that anyone who is about to receive drugs that are likely to produce an allergic reaction be questioned about allergies before any medication is given.** An emergency tray should be readily available whenever vaccines, serum for passive immunization, and highly allergenic drugs are administered. Table 7-4 presents substances that are known to have caused anaphylaxis.

People who are aware of their extreme sensitivity to certain substances should wear an identification bracelet giving that information. In this way, any medical staff will be forewarned if the person requires emergency treatment and is unable to communicate with personnel. It also is advisable for individuals who are highly allergic to stings from bees, wasps, or other insects to carry with them a small kit containing diphenhydramine hydrochloride (Benadryl), epinephrine, syringe, needle, and tourniquet. These kits are available, by prescription, from a pharmacy and are recommended by allergists who realize the rapidity with which a bee sting or similar event can be fatal to someone who is highly sensitive.

It is extremely important that each nurse check the chart and question patients about allergies before (1) giving medications; (2) dispatching them for x-ray studies using contrast media; and (3) minor or major surgery. It is wise to check for allergies in several places, including the front of the chart, the physician's history, the nurse's admission history, and with the patient and the family. When people are ill or experiencing the stress of being hospitalized, they often forget about allergies or fail to mention an allergy that they do not think is significant.

Serum Sickness   *Serum sickness* is another type of generalized, widespread reaction to an antigenic substance. Usually the antigen is a drug or a foreign serum such as the immunizing sera that confer passive immunity.

Serum sickness develops more slowly than anaphylaxis, occurring over a period of 2 to 3 weeks after injection of the drug. It presents less serious symptoms and usually is self-limiting. Symptoms commonly associated with serum sickness include skin rash, edema, joint pain and swelling, renal vasculitis, swelling of lymph nodes, and sometimes high fever and prostration. Treatment most often involves administration of antihistamine and aspirin, the latter being helpful in reducing the inflammatory reaction that often affects the joints. More serious symptoms require treatment similar to that for anaphylaxis.

◆ Autoimmune Disease

Normally, the body is able to distinguish between substances that are part of itself and those that are foreign, but sometimes the body fails to recognize its own cells. When this happens, **the immune system attacks and attempts to reject substances that have been mistakenly identified as foreign agents. This reaction against the body's own cells is called an *autoimmune reaction*.**

There are many theories as to why there are cases of mistaken identity that result in the body's destruction of some of its own tissues. There also is much disagreement as to which diseases are actually autoimmune. Many of the diseases that are considered to be related to the mechanism of autoimmunity are those in which there is some involvement of collagenous connective tissue, a type of tissue that is found throughout the body. (These disorders are sometimes called collagen diseases.) Table 7-5 shows disorders that are considered autoimmune. Systemic lupus erythematosus (SLE) is presented here as an example. Other autoimmune diseases are discussed in later chapters under the heading of the specific disease. In general, treatment is aimed at managing the excessive inflammatory responses common to almost all autoimmune diseases and relieving the patient's symptoms. This includes (1) administering such antiinflam-

TABLE 7-4 ◆ *Substances Known to Cause Anaphylaxis*	
Drugs	
Aspirin	Nonsteroidal antiinflammatory
Cephalosporins	drugs (NSAIDs)
Chemotherapy agents	Penicillins
Insulins	Sulfonamides
Local anesthetics	Tetracyclines
Diagnostic and treatment agents	
Allergenic extracts for de-	Iodine-contrast media used
sensitization	for x-rays
Blood products	
Antitoxin serums	
Diptheria antitoxin	Snake venom antitoxin
Poisonous spider antitoxin	Tetanus antitoxin
Foods	
Chocolate	Nuts (especially peanuts)
Eggs	Shellfish
Fish	Strawberries
Milk	
Insect stings	
Ants (particularly fire ants)	Wasps
Bees	Yellow jackets
Hornets	

TABLE 7-5 ◆ *Autoimmune Disorders*	
Collagen Diseases	
Ankylosing spondylitis	Scleroderma
Polyarteritis nodosa*	Systemic lupus
Rheumatoid arthritis*	erythematosus*
Rheumatic fever*	
Organ-specific diseases	
Glomerulonephritis	Multiple sclerosis (MS)
Goodpasture's syndrome	Myasthenia gravis
Grave's disease	Pernicious anemia
Hashimoto's thyroiditis*	Progressive systemic sclerosis
Hemolytic anemia*	Thrombocytopenic purpura*
Idiopathic Addison's	Type I diabetes mellitus
disease	Ulcerative colitis
Mixed connective tissue	Uveitis
disease	Vasculitis

*Most authorities agree that these are autoimmune disorders.

matory agents as the corticosteroids or nonsteroidal antiinflammatory drugs (NSAIDs); (2) suppressing the immune response (therapeutic immunosuppression) through radiation by x-ray or radioactive substances or through immunosuppressive drugs; and (3) administering aspirin and other salicylates to provide pain relief.

Systemic Lupus Erythematosus   Lupus is a chronic inflammatory disease of the collagen contained in connective tissue. Systemic lupus is an immune complex disorder in which the inflammation and tissue damage occur from the formation of soluble immune complexes that are deposited in tissues and cells.

Signs and symptoms include joint inflammation and pain; skin rashes; fatigue; and involvement of the nervous, vascular, and renal systems. The skin rash characteristically forms a butterfly over the cheeks and nose or presents as a disc-like rash on the body. Vasculitis and Raynaud's phenomenon are vascular manifestations; nephritis may occur; and cardiac, pulmonary, and nervous system manifestations are common.

Diagnosis is made by history, physical examination, and results of multiple diagnostic tests, including lupus erythematosus (LE) cell reaction, ANA titer, anti-double standard DNA, anti-Sm, and by false-positive VDRL.

Treatment is based on the system involved and symptoms. Administration of salicylates, NSAIDs, and corticosteroids for arthritic symptoms are used, and immunosuppressants are added as needed. For some patients, antimalarial drugs are added. Patients who survive the first 2 years after diagnosis without extensive complications tend to live a normal life span.

Nursing care is aimed at helping patients deal with individual symptoms, assessing for complications, teaching about medications and their side effects, and providing psychosocial support. Patients who are photosensitive are taught to protect themselves against exposure to sunlight with sunblock, long sleeves and pants, and a brimmed hat. These patients also need to avoid skin exposure to certain types of fluorescent light in the same manner. Patients are taught stress-reduction techniques and to avoid fatigue. Frequent rest periods are helpful. Patients taking antimalarial drugs need regular eye examinations.

Community Care   Each nurse should be alert to pollution in the community that might cause damage to the bone marrow and immune system. Nurses must be active in teaching the public about healthy lifestyles and avoidance of activities and practices that might cause immune deficiency. The next chapter speaks to public education about the dangers of HIV and avoiding contact. Certainly refraining from drug abuse, including alcohol abuse and smoking, can help keep the immune system healthy.

Considering the many causes and varying degrees of immune deficiency, it is likely that the nurse will frequently encounter patients who are highly susceptible to infection because of abnormal function of the immune system. **It is the responsibility of the nurse to identify such patients and to plan their care so that the goals of preventing infection and strengthening resistance are accomplished in cooperation with the patient and his family.** Chapters nine and eleven provide further information on patient education to prevent the spread of infection in immunodeficient patients.

Nurses working in long-term care facilities or in home care may encounter patients who are being treated for other disorders but also have rheumatoid arthritis or another autoimmune disorder. In these instances, thorough assessment of all body systems is essential and careful coordination of care for both acute and chronic disorders can be a challenge to the nurse. Collaboration with many people on the health care team is necessary, including the dietitian, physical therapist, occupational therapist, physician, and social worker.

CRITICAL THINKING EXERCISES

Clinical Case Problems

Read each clinical situation and discuss the questions with your classmates.

1. Mr. Watson is a 45-year-old patient who is admitted to the hospital for an abdominal hernia operation. You notice that he has cold symptoms, and you ask him about them. Mr. Watson replies that he is allergic to something and often has these symptoms.

   a. How might you help Mr. Watson determine the airborne substances to which he is allergic?

b. What techniques are used to determine foods that may be allergens?

c. What role does histamine play in the symptoms of an allergic reaction?

d. Why are antihistamines helpful in managing allergy symptoms?

e. What measures should be taken to avoid a fatal allergic reaction to drugs that are administered in a hospital or clinic?

2. Ms. Marilyn Jost, aged 15, is a young friend of yours who is highly allergic to penicillin and bee stings. The last time she experienced a reaction to a bee sting on her leg, the entire limb became swollen. Marilyn is active in the teen church group and frequently goes on camping trips. Her physician has suggested that she wear an identification bracelet stating her allergies and that she carry an emergency kit when she is on a camping trip. Her mother sees no need for these precautions because Marilyn is a perfectly healthy girl. Marilyn says she wouldn't know what to do with the kit if she did get stung by a bee or wasp.

a. How would you explain to Marilyn and her mother the need for the identification bracelet and the kit?

b. How would you go about teaching Marilyn to use the diphenhydramine hydrochloride (Benadryl), epinephrine, syringe, needle, and tourniquet in the kit?

BIBLIOGRAPHY

Applegate, E. J. (1995). *The Anatomy and Physiology Learning System: Textbook.* Philadelphia: Saunders.

Carrol, P. (1994). Speed: the essential response to anaphylaxis. *RN.* 57(6):26–31.

Centers for Disease Control. (1987). Recommendations for prevention of HIV transmission in health-care settings. *Morbidity and Mortality Weekly Report.* 36(2S), August 21:3.

Centers for Disease Control. (1988). Update: universal precautions for prevention of transmission of human immunodeficiency virus, hepatitis B virus, and other blood-borne pathogens in health-care settings. *Morbidity and Mortality Weekly Report.* 37(24):377.

Copstead, L. C. (1995). *Perspectives on Pathophysiology.* Philadelphia: Saunders.

Dambro, M. R. (1996). *Griffith's 5-Minute Clinical Consult.* Baltimore: Williams & Wilkins.

Ferrante, C., Derivan, M. C. (1995). Caring for patients with systemic lupus erythematosus. *Nursing 95.* 25(11):67–68.

Giuliano, K. K. (1997). Organ Transplants. *Nursing 97.* 27(5):34–39.

Guyton, A. C., Hall, J. E. (1996). *Textbook of Medical Physiology,* 9th ed. Philadelphia: Saunders.

Harwood, S. (1997). Actionstat anaphylaxis. *Nursing 97.* 27(2):33.

Howard, B. A. (1994). Guiding allergy sufferers throughout the medication maze. *RN.* 56(4):26–30.

Ignatavicius, D. D., Workman, M. L., Mishler, M. A. (1995). *Medical-Surgical Nursing: A Nursing Process Approach,* 2nd ed. Philadelphia: Saunders.

Jackson, R. (1991). The immune system: basic concepts for understanding transplantation. *Critical Care Nursing Quarterly.* 13(4):83–88.

Kernich, C. A., Kaminski, H. J. (1996). Myths and facts about myasthenia gravis. *Nursing 96.* 26(7):22.

Kuper, B. C., Failla, S. (1994). Shedding new light on lupus. *American Journal of Nursing.* 94(11):26–32.

Lisanti, P. (1996). Anaphylaxis. *American Journal of Nursing.* 96(11):51.

Monahan, F. D., Drake, T., Neighbors, M. (1994). *Nursing Care of Adults.* Philadelphia: Saunders.

O'Neill, S. (1990). Critical difference: anaphylactic shock. *American Journal of Nursing.* 90(12):40.

Patton, B., Holt, J. (1992). When your patient is allergic. *American Journal of Nursing.* 92(9):58–61.

Pavel, J. N. (1989). Hemotalogic problems: blood cell abnormalities: leukocyte disorders. In *Nurse Review,* ed. K. Goldberg. Springhouse, PA: Springhouse Corporation.

Payne, J. (1992). Immune modification and complications of immunosuppression. *Critical Care Clinics of North America.* 4(1):43–61.

Price, S. A., Wilson, L. M. (1989). *Pathophysiology: Clinical Concepts of Disease Processes,* 3rd ed. New York: McGraw-Hill.

Roitt, I. (1991). *Essential Immunology,* 7th ed. London: Blackwell Scientific Publications.

Schenkein, D. (1992). Intravenous IgG for treatment of autoimmune disease. *Hospital Practice.* 27(10A):29–36, 39–40, 42.

Weinstein, R. (1992). Bone involvement in multiple myeloma. *American Journal of Medicine.* 93(6):591–594.

Workman, J., Ellerhorst-Ryan, J., Koertge, V. (1993). *Nursing Care of the Immunocompromised Patient.* Philadelphia: Saunders.

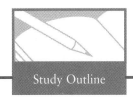

Study Outline

I. Introduction

A. Immune response is a series of complex mechanical activities involving:

1. Surveillance for and recognition of foreign agents (antigens).
2. Recognition of antigens as nonself.
3. Ability to distinguish foreign cells one from another.
4. Ability to remember the antigen if it appears in the body again at a later time.

II. Types of Immune Response

A. T lymphocytes and B lymphocytes.

1. Originate in the lymphocytic cells of the developing fetus. T-cells pass through the thymus gland. B-cells are preprocessed in an area not yet known but similar to the bursa of Fabricius in birds; hence the name B-cells.
2. Both T-cells and B-cells migrate to lymphoid tissue, where they wait to form either sensitized lymphocytes for cellular immunity or antibodies for humoral immunity.
3. Some young B-cells do not go on to form plasma cells for the production of antibody. Instead, they lie dormant as memory cells. When a specific antigen enters the body, the memory cells greatly increase the number of sensitized lymphocytes available for defense.
4. T lymphocytes are responsible for rejection of transplanted tissue.
5. Both T-cells and B-cells are necessary for normal immune response.

B. Humoral (immediate) response:

1. Takes place in body fluids (humor).
2. Is an antigen–antibody response.
3. Provides protection against acute, rapidly developing bacterial and viral organisms.
   a. Antigen: any substance capable of a specific immune response.
   b. Antibody: protein synthesized by plasma cells in response to a specific antigen.
      (1) There are five classes of antibodies (immunoglobulins). The number of sites where an antibody can attach itself to its antigen depends on the class to which it belongs.
      (2) Chemical and mechanical actions by which antibody can attack antigen include lysis, agglutination, precipitation, formation of antitoxin, and use of the complement system in which certain enzymes attack the foreign agents and protect body cells by neutralizing them.

C. Cellular (delayed) response:

1. Utilizes sensitized T lymphocytes.
2. Is active against slowly developing bacterial infections. It also is involved in autoimmune response, some allergic reactions, and rejection of foreign cells.
3. Sensitized lymphocytes have been sensitized to a specific antigen. Subsequent exposure triggers many chemical and mechanical activities.
   a. Some sensitized lymphocytes are transformed into killer cells.
   b. Chemicals involved include lymphokines and macrophage-activating factor.
4. Cellular immune response often is termed *delayed hypersensitivity.*
5. Sensitized T lymphocytes are the cause of allergic reactions.

III. Immunity Against Disease

A. Two major types: (1) natural or innate and (2) acquired or adaptive:

1. Natural (innate): present at birth; based on sex, age, race, constitutional makeup, and other individual traits.
2. Acquired: person can receive it passively from his mother's antibodies or animal serum or actively produce his own antibody in response to a disease or; immunization also produces active acquired immunity.

B. Screening and diagnostic testing:

1. Part of assessment is to identify persons in need of immunization or treatment.
2. Consideration of risk factors (e.g., inadequate housing, poor nutrition, age, chronic illness).
3. Skin testing for allergy to pollens or other inhalants.

IV. Immunization and Nursing Implications

A. Goals: (1) increase public participation; (2) identify people in need of immunization; (3) prevent or decrease sensitivity reactions to immunizing agents.

B. Immunization programs:

1. Nurse is responsible for encouraging public participation in programs to protect people from disease. (The recommended vaccination schedule is shown in Table 7-1.)

2. Contraindications to active immunization include fevers, pregnancy, immune deficiency disease, immunosuppressive therapy, administration of certain drugs, and a history of allergy or hypersensitivity to any drug, chemical, or natural antigen.

C. Preventing or mitigating sensitivity reactions to immunizing agents:

1. History must be taken before administration.

2. Findings of allergic reactions in the past must be reported to physician.

3. Patient with an allergy to a specific immunizing agent must not be given the agent.

4. If there is doubt about whether a reaction will occur, a minute amount of the agent can be given intradermally to determine whether there will be a local reaction.

5. In all areas where immunizing agents are given, there must be emergency equipment readily at hand in case a reaction occurs.

V. Disorders of the Immune System

A. Immune deficiency: absence or inadequate production of immune bodies. Can affect either humoral or cellular immunity or both.

1. Congenital, primary immune deficiency can range from a complete absence (agammaglobulinemia) to an inadequate level (hypogammaglobulinemia). Prognosis depends on the available immune bodies and the kind of infections the child develops.

2. Secondary acquired immune deficiency can result from a host of factors:

a. Age: infants and the elderly have less resistance.

b. Malnutrition, malignancy, stress, certain drugs, liver disease, and lymphatic disorders also are causative factors.

c. Therapeutic immunosuppression:

(1) To prevent rejection of organ transplant.

(2) To minimize autoimmune reaction.

(3) To treat cancer.

3. Treatment of immune deficiency disorders depends on the degree of inadequacy of immune bodies and its primary cause.

a. Passive immunization can provide some protection. This is accomplished through injections of human immune globulin and transfusion of sensitized lymphocytes.

b. Prevention of infection.

4. Nursing care of patients with immune deficiency

a. Assessment:

(1) History for factors that decrease immune function.

(2) History of frequent infections.

(3) Nutritional status and general state of health.

(4) History of alcohol and drug abuse.

(5) Taking corticosteroids or not.

(6) Physical assessment for abnormalities of lymph tissue.

(7) Diagnostic test: CBC and differential count; serum protein, protein electrophoresis, bone marrow studies, T- and B-cell assays, enzyme-linked immunosorbent assays (ELISA); other tests specific to the disorder suspected.

b. Nursing diagnoses: Risk for infection and Risk for injury; others for specific problems.

c. Planning:

(1) Goals: (1) protect from infection; (2) improve health status; (3) maintain high degree of wellness to promote optimal immune function.

(2) May need to plan for protective isolation.

(3) Expected outcomes: (1) Patient remains free from infection; (2) B-cell and T-cell counts are within normal limits.

d. Interventions

(1) Promote balanced, adequate nutrition.

(2) Protect from infection: protective isolation as needed (Table 7-2).

(3) Use of strict aseptic technique.

(4) Psychosocial care to decrease fear, help deal with lifestyle changes or role changes, and reduce stress.

(5) Patient teaching regarding disorder, therapy, signs of infection, and self-care.

e. Evaluation

(1) Determine whether expected outcomes are being met.

(2) Monitor lab test values for improvement.

(3) Monitor temperature and vital signs.

(4) General well-being and side effects of medication.

B. Excessive response: hypergammaglobulinemia, secondary to myeloma.

C. Hypersensitivity and allergy:

1. Three major groups of allergies:

a. Delayed reaction is a cell-mediated hypersensitivity. Examples include contact dermatitis associated with cosmetics, plants, chemicals.

b. Antigen–antibody allergy occurs when person has high amount of antibodies, particularly IgG. Examples are drug reactions and transfusion reactions.

  c. Atopic allergies affect about 10% of the population. Characterized by excessive amounts of IgE antibodies. Allergens include house dust, foods, and the venom of bees and wasps.

2. In all types of allergies a reaction occurs only on second and subsequent contacts with the allergen.

3. Management of hypersensitivity and allergic reactions:

  a. Assessment: objective and subjective data summarized in Table 7-3.

    (1) Identification of particular allergen-causing problem.

    (2) Types of allergens: Inhalants, contactants, ingestants, and injectables.

      (a) Skin testing to identify allergens.

      (b) Elimination diet to identify food allergens.

      (c) Identifying allergen is a slow and tedious process. Patient and family will need support and encouragement.

  b. Goals of intervention:

    (1) To help patient avoid exposure to known allergens.

      (a) Patient will need to know sources of allergens, how it comes into contact with body cells (inhalation, etc.).

      (b) Care must be taken not to make patient feel like an invalid or that his life must be completely disrupted.

    (2) To manage symptoms.

      (a) Antihistamines are useful. However, warn of side effects: drowsiness and impaired coordination, and less frequently dryness of mouth, urinary retention, weakness, blurred vision.

      (b) Antiinflammatory agents, cortisone, used to decrease allergic reaction.

      (c) Salves, wet compresses, and soothing baths used to treat local reactions.

    (3) To participate in desensitization.

    (4) To provide patient education.

      (a) Avoid exposure to allergens.

      (b) Minimize reactions.

4. Anaphylaxis: a serious and dramatic allergic reaction with release of histamine from damaged cells; profound shock and death may occur.

  a. Treatment: administering antihistamines (diphenhydramine hydrochloride, Benadryl) and epinephrine, establishing a patent airway, and providing measures to control shock; provision for psychological support.

  b. Prevention: teaching hypersensitive persons how to avoid allergens, recommending identification bracelet to be worn at all times, and having person carry a kit for immediate treatment of reaction.

  c. Questioning each patient about allergies before administering a drug.

  d. Check charts thoroughly for evidence of known allergies.

5. Serum sickness: delayed, generalized reaction to antigenic substances, often immunizing sera.

  a. Treatment often involves administration of antihistamines and aspirin.

D. Autoimmune disease:

1. Body is unable to recognize its own cells as part of itself.

2. Often affects collagenous tissue.

3. No agreement regarding many diseases considered by some to be autoimmune.

4. Treatment:

  a. Administration of antiinflammatory agents and nonsteroidal antiinflammatory drugs.

  b. Immunosuppression through drugs or radiation.

  c. Aspirin and other salicylates for pain.

E. Systemic lupus erythematosus (SLE)

1. Inflammatory disease of collagen contained in connective tissue.

2. Signs and symptoms include butterfly or disc-shaped rash, joint inflammation and pain, and involvement of the nervous, vascular, and renal systems.

3. Diagnosis made by diagnostic tests combined with clinical findings.

4. Treatment based on system involved and symptoms; antiinflammatories, corticosteroids, immunosuppressants.

5. Nursing care aimed at helping patient deal with individual symptoms, decrease stress, teach about disease and treatment; provide psychosocial support.

6. Photosensitive patients are taught to protect against exposure to sunlight.

VI. Community Care

A. Be alert to factors that can cause immune damage in community and environment.

B. Teach healthy lifestyle.

C. Identify patients with immune deficiency; plan care to prevent infection and strengthen resistance.

D. Long-term and home care nurses deal with patients with an acute disorder and accompanying chronic immune deficiency.

    1. Requires careful care planning.

    2. Requires collaboration with other health team members.

VII. Elder Care Points

A. Aging does not affect the bone marrow much.

B. The thymus gland shrinks and the number of T-cells diminishes.

C. After age 70, there is a definite decline in the function of the immune system.

D. There is an increase in the incidence of cancer in those over age 70.

E. The ability to fight infection is diminished in those over 70.

Care of the Patient with AIDS

As discussed in Chapter 7, the immune response is a remarkable series of complex activities that take place in the body. As a result of a disturbance in these activities, the continuous search within the body for foreign invaders is disrupted and the ability of the body to prevent infection is less than adequate, resulting in many problems.

Nurses are on the front lines in the fight against the **Human Immunodeficiency Virus and Acquired Immune Deficiency Syndrome (HIV/AIDS).** It must be remembered that it is not only the individual infected with this virus that is affected, but also the family of the individual, the significant other and friends, as well as the community at large. Another facet of care for the patient with HIV/AIDS is education provided for colleagues, family, friends, and community.

Caring for an individual with HIV/AIDS challenges all the skills, knowledge, and spirit of the nurse. This challenge will truly allow a synthesis of all previous experiences and an opportunity to combine the art and science of nursing.

More than half of the individuals diagnosed with AIDS have died. There are many areas of care to address, including physical, spiritual, and emotional aspects. Clients may have difficulties in all three of these areas at the same time.

AIDS is a multisystem process in which the patient may have multiple infective disorders concurrently. Patients may also have experienced multiple personal losses such as altered body image and lowered self-esteem, as well as the emotional trauma of being diagnosed with a disease for which there is currently no cure.

However, as challenging as this sounds, there will be great satisfaction in using the nursing process to deal effectively with this population and to achieve both personal and professional growth through caring for them.

NATURAL HISTORY AND EPIDEMIOLOGY

Acquired immune deficiency syndrome (AIDS) was first described in 1981 by the Centers for Disease Control and Prevention (CDC). Initially, young men who had no reason for becoming ill with certain cancers and other opportunistic infections were being diagnosed with these diseases. No one is certain where the disease came from. There are many theories, but none have been proven. In 1983 the cause was discovered to be a virus, eventually named human immunodeficiency virus (HIV), which is transmitted through blood and body fluids. Along with the many physical problems that develop as a result of immune deficiency, there are numerous psychosocial issues that arise for patients who are seropositive for HIV. One such problem is becoming ill with a life-threatening illness in the most productive years of life. The cumulative incidence of AIDS cases in adult and adolescent age groups, according to the CDC case definition, in December 1996 is estimated at 581,429 cases. Pediatric cases (defined as patients <13 years old), totaled 7,629. Approximately 65% of the people who have been diagnosed with AIDS have died. Reviewing these numbers shows that this disease is no minor problem.

The initial population affected by this virus seemed to be homosexual and bisexual men, later described as men who have sex with men. Other populations affected at this time were prostitutes, Haitians, people from Central African countries, and injectable drug users, as well as some recipients of tainted blood transfusions and blood products, such as Factor VIII. At this time the heterosexual population did not seem to think they would be affected. This proved to be a false and very dangerous assumption, and although the numbers in the heterosexual population are smaller in the United States, it is a different case in the rest of the world. For example, in Central and Western Africa, AIDS is predominantly a heterosexual disease. It is transmitted through sexual contact and from mother to baby.

The disease is caused by infection with HIV, a *retrovirus,* that integrates itself into the genetic material of the cell it infects, changing the DNA of the host cell. This causes the host cell to be unable to fulfill its normal functions in the immune system. The primary host cell for HIV is the CD_4 lymphocyte, the quarterback of the immune system. HIV seriously impairs the ability of the cell-mediated immune response from working as effectively as it would normally. *Cell-mediated immunity* is defined as a type of immunity mediated by cells, the CD_4 lymphocytes, rather than by antibodies. The disease presents many clinical problems and involves multiple systems. Although presently there is no cure for the underlying immune deficiency, some treatments are effective for opportunistic infections.

As with other types of immune deficiencies, there are periods of exacerbations interspersed with remissions. The current thought about HIV infection versus AIDS is that there is a period after the initial infection during which the virus appears to be latent. In fact, during this time, although there are very few outward signs of infection, the virus is very busy replicating and

infecting cells and organs. When the immune system is sufficiently depleted, as evidenced by a large decrease in CD_4 lymphocytes, infections the person had previously been exposed to and had an antigen to may manifest as opportunistic infections.

Some people infected with HIV have no symptoms for a long time. As the immune system is less and less functional, symptoms of sentinel infections (infections that may indicate an underlying immunosuppression), such as oral thrush, recurrent vaginal candidiasis, or seborrheic dermatitis, appear. Table 8-1 lists the chief signs and symptoms of AIDS.

More extensive information on the care of the pediatric patient with HIV/AIDS can be found in pediatric textbooks.

TABLE 8-1 ◆ *Chief Signs and Symptoms of AIDS*	
Hematological	Dry, flaky scalp
White blood cell	Psoriasis
CD_4 count <200	Poor wound healing
cells/mm^3	Drenching night sweats
Inverted CD_4/CD_8 ratio	Lesions of the skin
Neutropenia	
Red blood cell	**Malignancies**
Anemias	Kaposi's sarcoma (KS)
Thrombocytopenia	Invasive cervical cancer
Hypovolemia	B-cell lymphomas
	Hodgkin's lymphoma
Immunological	Non-Hodgkin's lymphoma
Fatigue	
Lymphadenopathy	**Opportunistic Infections**
Hypergammaglobulinemia	*Bacterial infections*
	Mycobacterium tuberculo-
Respiratory	sis (MTb.)
Cough	Atypical *Mycobacterium*
Dyspnea on exertion	infections
Shortness of breath	*M. avium* complex
	(MAC)
Gastrointestinal	*M. kansasii*
Nausea	*M. marinum*
Vomiting	*Protozoal*
Diarrhea	Pneumocytosis
Flatus	Giardiasis
Weight loss	Cryptosporidiosis
	Toxoplasmosis
Central Nervous System	*Viral*
Short-term memory loss	Cytomegalovirus (CMV)
Confusion	Herpes simplex (HSV-I,
Headache	HSV-II)
Fever	Varicella zoster (shingles;
Visual changes	VZV)
Dementia/HIV	*Fungal*
Encephalopathy	Candidiasis (thrush;
Alterations in comfort	vaginitis)
Chronic/acute pain	Histoplasmosis
Neuropathic pain	Cryptosporidiosis
Personality changes	Coccidiomycosis
Integumentary	
Dry skin (seborrheic	
dermatitis)	

TRANSMISSION AND PREVENTION

Gaining knowledge about HIV and educating others—patients, colleagues, and community—is an important part of the nurse's role. There must be an understanding of the pathophysiology of the virus to dispel fears associated with HIV/AIDS infectivity. The nurse must be able to assess the risk behaviors practiced by every patient to slow and eventually stop the transmission of this virus.

The first step in the prevention of HIV infection is knowledge, and teaching is the method available to us as health care providers. **Current medical research has shown that HIV cannot be transmitted by casual contact.** It has been proven that there are specific modes of transmission. These are as follows:

◆ Through unprotected sexual contact with an HIV-infected partner (sexual transmission).

◆ Through exposure to HIV-infected blood, body fluids and tissue, and breast milk (occupational and maternal transmission).

Health education agencies, as well as the gay community, have made a Herculean effort to educate people about the possibility of exposure through unprotected sex. There is a push to end the sexual promiscuity that evolved during the 1960s; a monogamous sexual relationship is the far safer option.

Safer sex prevents transmission by putting a barrier, a condom or other impermeable barrier, between the body fluids of one partner and the other. **This method of prevention is not called *safe* sex because the only guaranteed way to prevent transmission sexually is through abstinence.**

When we discuss *safer* sex, we are talking about methods to reduce the possibility of exposure. The use of latex condoms is recommended because they are more impermeable than other types of condoms that may allow penetration of the virus through the membrane of the material used. There are some other ways to further reduce the possibility of exposure sexually, such as participating in a **mutually monogamous** relationship, avoiding anal or vaginal intercourse with a partner who is seropositive with HIV, and if neither partner has a sensitivity to nonoxynol-9, using a spermicide that contains it. Nonoxynol-9 has been shown in studies to inactivate or kill HIV. If either partner has a sensitivity to nonoxynol-9, it may cause the tissue to become irritated and more prone to infection. Avoidance of anal intercourse prevents microscopic tears in the lining of the anus which is thinner than the walls of the vagina.

There is no reason for HIV-infected individuals to completely discontinue sexual activity. Touch and intimacy are important parts of any relationship. However

there is a need to reduce the risk of transmitting the virus to others and at the same time prevent exposure to any other **sexually transmitted diseases (STDs).** Sexually transmitted diseases are more difficult to treat when the immune system is suppressed.

Safer sex may make one become more inventive in sexual encounters. It gives an opportunity to talk about what is needed and wanted and also to listen to what the partner's needs and wants are. Remember to consider the whole person. Some safer methods are massage, cuddling, hugging, mutual masturbation, frottage (body-to-body rubbing), and the incorporation of fantasy into sexual activities.

Some **unsafe** practices include being the receptive partner in anal or vaginal intercourse without a latex condom, as well as being the insertive partner; orogenital (felatio or cunnilingus) or oroanal stimulation (rimming) without a barrier (dental dam). Contact with all body fluids, such as semen or vaginal secretions and blood, must be avoided.

> The key to being less prone to becoming infected with HIV, or other STD (e.g., syphilis, gonorrhea, cytomegalovirus, chlamydia, hepatitis B, herpes, and condyloma), is to know methods of protection and to use them consistently. Barrier sex must be practiced with *every* sexual encounter.

Think about . . . Can you list the ways in which HIV might be transmitted from one person to another? What is the first step in the prevention of spread of HIV virus? How can this be accomplished?

Should a person wish to know his or her HIV status, testing is available from a physician, local public health clinic, or by home test kit. Home test kits are not as reliable as a laboratory blood test. Be aware that if an HIV blood test is reported as positive, further testing is necessary to verify correctness of the result. A test done by taking a buccal scraping also is available to test for the presence of HIV. HIV tests search for antibodies to the virus; there is no test to detect the actual virus (Table 8-2). There may be a lag period after infection occurs before antibodies appear in the blood. Therefore, a negative HIV test is not considered accurate in the first 6 months after exposure.

MANAGEMENT OF EARLY HIV INFECTION

When an individual tests positive for HIV and the diagnosis is confirmed by repeated testing, a comprehensive examination of health status is conducted.

TABLE 8-2 ◆ *HIV Tests*

ELISA (enzyme-linked immunoabsorbent assay)
Normal value: negative
> HIV-antibody screening test (positives must be confirmed with a Western blot).
> Antibody assays do not detect HIV-antibody in the earliest stages of the infection. (HIV antibodies may be detected normally from 2 weeks to 6 months after the acute infection.)
> False-positive ELISA may be seen in the presence of maternal antibodies.
> Sensitivity: 98%

Western blot (WB)
Normal value: negative
> HIV-antibody test used to confirm a positive ELISA.
> False-positive WB may be seen in the presence of maternal antibodies.

Polymerase chain reaction (PCR)
Normal value: negative
> A qualitative measurement of cell-associated proviral DNA.
> Sensitivity: 100%

Immunofluorescent antibody assay (IFA)
Normal value: negative
> Sensitivity: 99.8%

Particular attention is paid to eye and mouth condition, neurological status, skin and lymph nodes, and any signs of opportunistic infection. A psychological assessment is added to help determine the patient's present and long-term needs. The assessment includes a sexual history and a substance use history. A CD_4 lymphocyte count is performed to establish the stage of HIV infection and to decide the timing of initiation of antiretroviral therapy and prophylaxis for opportunistic infections. CD_4 cell counts are performed every 3 to 6 months depending on CD_4 levels.

Selecting optimal therapy is based not only on clinical data but also on individual factors, such as past health status, medication history, quality of life issues, and patient expectations of therapy. Antiretroviral therapy is begun when CD_4 counts are less than 500 cells/μL or below 25% or when there are any symptoms of HIV disease (e.g., weight loss; chronic or unexplained fever; night sweats; recurrent thrush or vaginal yeast infections; or a viral load greater than 30,000 to 50,000 copies/mL).

◆ Antiretroviral Therapy

These classes of drugs are specifically used to fight the HIV infection and act directly on the virus itself. *Nucleoside analogs* act by incorporating themselves into the DNA of the virus, stopping the replication process. The resulting DNA is incomplete and cannot create new virus.

Nonnucleoside reverse transcriptase inhibitors stop HIV production by binding directly onto reverse transcriptase and preventing the conversion of RNA to DNA. Even though they work at the same site as nucleoside analogs, they act in a completely different way.

Protease inhibitors work at the last stage of the viral reproduction cycle. They prevent HIV from being successfully assembled and released from the infected CD_4 cell. Other drugs mentioned in this chapter are used to prevent or treat the causative agents for specific opportunistic infections. The dosing recommendations and information about certain nursing implications related to these drugs are found in Table 8-3.

Nucleoside reverse transcriptase inhibitors (NRTI's) are the first drugs used in treatment of HIV infection. If they are not effective or not tolerated a second class of drugs, non-nucleoside reverse transcriptase inhibitors (NNRTI's) may be added or substituted. A third class, protease inhibitors, (PI's) are showing great promise in reducing the HIV viral load and seemingly allowing the immune system to repair or rebuild itself as evidenced in the rise in the CD_4 lymphocyte count. Failure to follow strict medication administration schedule could make the virus resistant to treatment and cause a potential health risk by creating drug-resistant strains of the virus. *If the CD_4 lymphocyte count rises above 200 cells/m^3, prophylaxis therapy should continue according to new CDC guidelines.* Currently the most effective treatment seems to be a combination of drugs. New antiretroviral and protease inhibitor drugs are quickly becoming available. One drawback is that therapy may cost $16,000 a year or more and the patient must take many pills at fixed times throughout the day and night.

PATHOPHYSIOLOGY, CLASSIFICATION, AND CLINICAL SIGNS AND SYMPTOMS

The CDC definition of AIDS is based on a classification scheme for HIV disease that depends on the pathophysiology of the disease as immune deficits increase and function decreases (Table 8-4).

- *Stage I.* Acute infection (CDC Group I).
- *Stage II.* Asymptomatic infection (CDC Group II).
- *Stage III.* Symptomatic infection (CDC Group III) includes persistent generalized lymphadenopathy lasting longer than 3 months.
- *Group IV-A* includes the symptoms of fever or diarrhea lasting more than 1 month or a weight loss of more than 10% of the baseline body weight.
- *Group IV-B* contains all the previous symptoms in addition to neurological diseases, such as dementia, neuropathies, and myelopathy.

◆ *Groups IV-C and IV-D* include all the previous symptoms plus a CD_4 lymphocyte count lower than 200 mm³ and clinical conditions such as **opportunistic infections**, recurrent **community-acquired pneumonia**, cervical cancers in women, pulmonary tuberculosis (TB), and malignancies (Table 8-2).

The continuum of HIV infection may last from 18 months to longer than 10 years depending on the type of exposure, lifestyle, and strain of, or virulence, of the virus. Personal factors that may hasten the progression of HIV disease are stress, pregnancy, poor nutritional status, exposure to other strains of HIV, and infection with other STDs, such as syphilis, herpes, and cytomegalovirus (CMV).

Suppression of the immune response as a result of HIV infection is the cause of AIDS. Two types of HIV have been identified, HIV type-1 and HIV type-2 (HIV-1 and HIV-2, respectively). HIV-1 is the most common cause of HIV infection in the United States, Europe, and Asia. HIV-2 is widespread in western Africa.

HIV-1 and HIV-2 are both retroviruses. Retroviruses differ from other viruses because of an enzyme called reverse transcriptase, which helps with the viral replication process in the host cell. HIV types 1 and 2 have only ribonucleic acid (RNA) as their genetic material. When they replicate, their genetic material is placed in the deoxynucleic acid (DNA) of the host cell. The resulting new DNA continues the process of replication, and its RNA produces larger numbers of viral particles, as many as 50 million to 2 billion a day. These viral particles are released from the host cell into the circulatory system where they infect other cells, such as macrophages and lymphoid tissue.

The immune cells have a specific receptor site called a CD_4 receptor site. This is where HIV attaches and begins the process of infecting the CD_4 lymphocytes, the quarterback of the immune response. When these cells are infected, they do not function normally, and their malfunction can cause neutropenia, lymphocytopenia, and abnormally functioning macrophages and CD_4 cells.

TABLE 8-3 ◆ *HIV/AIDS Medications*

Popular Name	Trade Name	Generic Name	Usual Dose
Nucleoside reverse transcriptase inhibitors (NRTIs)			
AZT (100 mg capsules)	Retrovir	Zidovudine	200 mg tid PO Observe for signs of anemia.
ddI (25 mg; 50 mg; 100 mg; 150 mg tablets; 20 mg/ml suspension)	Videx	Didanosine	200 mg bid PO Observe for signs of pancreatitis.
DDC (0.375 mg; 0.75 mg tablets)	Hivid	Zalcitabine	0.75 mg tid PO Must take 1 hour AC or 2 hours PC.
d4T (15 mg; 20 mg; 30 mg; 40 mg capsules)	Zerit	Stavudine	20–40 mg bid PO Monitor liver function tests and level of peripheral neuropathy.
3TC (150 mg tablet)	Epivir	Lamivudine	150 mg bid PO None of these drugs should be used alone as resistance develops rapidly.
Non-nucleoside reverse transcriptase inhibitors (NNRTIs)			
None	Viramune	Nevirapine	200 mg qd × weeks; then increase dose to 400 mg qd Observe for rash as side effect.
100 mg tablets	Rescriptor	Delavirdine	400 mg tid
Protease inhibitors (PIs)			
200 mg tablets	Invirase	Saquinavir	600 mg tid PO Take within 2 hours of a full meal.
100 mg capsule	Norvir	Ritonavir	600 mg bid PO Keep refrigerated; Take with meals. Titrated lead-in dosing: Start with: day 1: 300 mg bid; days 2–3: 400 mg bid; day 4: 500 mg bid.
400 mg capsule	Crixivan	Indinavir	800 mg q 8 h PO Take on an empty stomach 1 hour AC or 2 hours PC. Drink at least 1.5 L of water a day to prevent crystals forming in the kidneys.
250 mg tablets	Viracept	Nelfinavir	750 mg tid PO

TABLE 8-4 ◆ *Centers for Disease Control and Prevention (CDC) Classification of HIV*	
Class	Criteria

Group I
Acute infection with HIV
Flu-like symptoms, resolve completely
HIV antibody negative

Group II (HIV asymptomatic)
HIV antibody positive
No laboratory or clinical indicators of immune deficiency

Group III (HIV symptomatic)
HIV antibody positive
Persistent generalized lymphadenopathy

Group IV-A
HIV antibody positive
Constitutional disease
    Persistent fever or diarrhea
    Weight loss >10% of normal body weight

Group IV-B
Same as group IV-A, *plus*
Neurological disease
Dementia
Neuropathy
Myelopathy

Group IV-C
Same as group IV-B, *plus*
CD_4 lymphocyte count <200 cells/mm^3
Opportunistic infections

Group IV-D
Same as group IV-C *plus*
Pulmonary tuberculosis, invasive cervical cancer, or other malignancy

Source: Adapted from Centers for Disease Control and Prevention, March 1993.

◆ Opportunistic Infections

Opportunistic infections are defined as diseases caused by microorganisms commonly present in the environment or the body; **the organisms cause disease only when a change in the normal, healthy condition of the body leads to a weakening or suppression of the immune system.**

The major OIs are *Pneumocystis carinii* pneumonia (PCP), *Mycobacterium avium* complex (MAC), cytomegalovirus (CMV), Kaposi's sarcoma (KS), toxoplasmosis (Toxo), histoplasmosis (Histo), *Cryptococcus neoformans* (Crypto), cryptosporidium, candidiasis, and the herpes family viruses.

A description of the most common bacterial, fungal, and protozoal infections seen in HIV-infected patients follows. The main neoplasms associated with HIV also are discussed. See Table 8-5 for information regarding signs and symptoms, diagnostic tests, nursing implications, and treatment for the major OIs.

Bacterial Infections

Mycobacterium *tuberculosis* (MTb). This infection may present as a pulmonary infection, but in approximately 50% of people infected with HIV, MTb is found in **extrapulmonary** sites, sites outside the respiratory tract, such as bone, skin, liver, central nervous system (CNS), spleen, and the gastrointestinal tract (GI).

Symptoms of pulmonary TB include dyspnea, cough, fever, chest pains, weight loss, night sweats, and anorexia. Symptoms of systemic infection are fever, chills, weight loss, night sweats, and anorexia. Extrapulmonary infection symptoms are site related.

Mycobacterium *avium* complex (MAC). The causative bacterium for MAC are *M. avium* and *M. intracellulare*. The sites generally infected by these bacteria are the respiratory system and GI tract. However, it may infect the bone marrow and thus the circulatory system as well. Symptoms may include fevers, night sweats, weight loss, lymphadenopathy, malaise, or organ disease. *MAC* becomes a threat when the immune system is seriously depleted, for example when the CD_4 count is generally 50 cells per mm^3. At this point many primary care providers will initiate prophylaxis for MAC and/or serial blood cultures to identify AFB in the blood. A bone marrow examination also may be performed if MAC is suspected and anemias of unknown etiology are present.

Fungal Infections

Cryptococcosis. Cryptococcosis often presents as a meningitis and is the fourth most common OI in HIV-infected individuals. The causative agent is *Cryptococcus neoformans*. In HIV-infected individuals with a low CD_4 count, generally about 100 cells per mm^3, cryptococcosis may manifest as a fungal meningitis or **disseminated** (widespread) disease. Usual sites of infection are the CNS and circulatory system. It also may appear in the lung, heart, GI tract, bone, prostate, lymphatic system, and skin. Symptoms are any or all of the following: fever, headache (H/A), visual changes, nausea, vomiting, nuchal rigidity, confusion, and altered mental status. Neurological changes and seizures may also occur. This fungus is found in pigeon droppings and in the soil.

The usual entry point is the lungs, where it causes an asymptomatic infection. Because of severe immune suppression, the cell-mediated immunity response does not destroy the fungi. It reactivates in immunosup-

This immune dysfunction makes the person infected more prone to reactivation of opportunistic infections (OIs). This infection does not kill the macrophages that are reservoirs of the viruses.

TABLE 8-5 ♦ Opportunistic Infections

Opportunistic Infection	Signs and Symptoms	Diagnostic Tests	Nursing Implications	Treatment/Medications
Pneumocystis carinii pneumonia (PCP)	Shortness of breath, dyspnea on exertion; fever, drenching night sweats; dry; nonproductive cough	Chest x-ray; bronchoscopy; induced sputum; pulse oximetry; pulmonary function tests	Auscultate lungs. Assess for distress or cyanosis. Reposition patient PRN. Assess night sweats. Assist with activities that increase dyspnea.	Trimethoprim-sulfamethoxazole (TMP/SMX) (PO, IV). Pentamidine (aerosolized, IV). Hypotension, cardiac arrhythmias; hypoglycemia, Dapsone (PO) O_2 as ordered
Cytomegalovirus (CMV) Eye: retinitis Lung: pneumonia GI: gastritis	Eye: loss of visual field; blurry vision; scarring of the retina. Lung: cough; shortness of breath, dyspnea on exertion. GI: diarrhea Neurological: personality changes; motor impairment.	Eye: ophthalmoscopic exam; Amsler Grid exam Lung: bronchoscopy GI: stool culture Neurological: lumbar puncture; biopsy	Precautions for neutropenia; anemia; thrombocytopenia. Assess renal function (serum creatinine). Assess patients for safe environment because of decreased vision; teach good handwashing; encourage good hygiene and skin care after stools. Instruct NOT to clean litter boxes without mask and NOT to dig in ground without rubber gloves.	Ganciclovir (Cytovene) (IV, PO, intraocular implant) Foscarnet (Foscavir) (IV) Cidofovir (Vistide) (IV) **Filgastrim** (GCSF, granulocyte colony stimulating factor) (Neupogen) is a drug that is used to treat the neutropenia caused by the drugs used to treat CMV. It stimulates the production of neutrophils by the bone marrow. It allows neutropenic patients to continue chemotherapy for CMV. Erythropoetin (Epogen; Procrit) is a drug used to treat anemia caused by the therapy for CMV. It is not used to treat the CMV, but allows the patient to continue chemotherapy for CMV. Both of these drugs may be given IV or SQ. Labs: CBC with differential for the hemoglobin and hematocrit and absolute neutrophil count (ANC); must be checked at least weekly to adjust the dose of these medications.
Mycobacterium tuberculosis (MTb)	Fever; wasting; moist, productive cough	Chest x-ray; sputum analysis, AFB smears	Respiratory isolation. Instruct in medication administration regimen. Instruct in infection-control procedures; provide masks for patient and visitors if needed.	Isoniazid (INH) (PO); ethambutol; rifampin; streptomycin

(Table 8-5 continued)

189

TABLE 8-5 ◆ Opportunistic Infections (Continued)

Opportunistic Infection	Signs and Symptoms	Diagnostic Tests	Nursing Implications	Treatment/Medications
Mycobacterium Avium Complex (MAC) disseminated	Blood/bone marrow: anemia; fever; drenching night sweats GI: watery diarrhea; wasting	Blood/bone marrow: blood cultures GI: stool cultures	Provide supportive care for fevers, weakness, and possible dyspnea. Teach infection-control measures. Offer nutritional counseling.	INH: Ethambutol; rifabutin; ciprofloxacin; azythromycin; clarythromycin
Kaposi's Sarcoma (KS)	Skin: purplish lesions (nonblanching) Lung: dyspnea GI: altered bowel pattern; diarrhea or constipation	Skin: biopsy Lung: chest x-ray; bronchoscopy; biopsy GI: upper gastrointestinal series; colonoscopy; biopsy	Symptomatic support: elevate testicles in males if swollen; elevate lower extremities if lymphedema is present. Teach infection-control measures if wounds are weeping Medicate for pain as ordered. Use comfort measure, reposition frequently; use good skin care.	Skin: intralesional injections Lung and GI: radiation; chemotherapy
Histoplasmosis	Fever; pneumonia; sepsis	Chest x-ray; sputum culture; biopsy; bronchoscopy	Treat fevers; provide symptomatic support.	Suppressive therapy only amphotericin B (IV); itraconazole (PO); ketoconazole (PO or IV)
Cryptococcus Lung GI	Lung: fever; malaise; pneumonia Neurological: altered mental status; headache; fever	Lung: chest x-ray; sputum culture Neurological: CT scan; MRI	Provide symptomatic support for fevers. Encourage periods of rest for malaise. Provide safe environment.	Amphotericin B (IV), Itraconazole (PO)
Cryptosporidiosis	Voluminous watery diarrhea; flatus; abdominal distention; pain; fever	Stool culture; bowel biopsy	Teach infection-control measures. Encourage to drink bottled or boiled water. Teach skin care.	Antispasmodics; paromomycin; antidiarrheals (esp. opiates)

Disease	Signs and symptoms	Diagnostic tests	Medications	Nursing interventions
Toxoplasmosis	Altered mental status; headache; cognitive impairment	CT; MRI; serum antibody for *Toxoplasma gondii*	Pyrimethamine (PO); sulfadiazine (PO) *or* pyrimethamine alone *or* in combination with clindamycin	Teach food and water safety. Provide safe environment. Teach importance of medication regimen.
Candidiasis (thrush)	Creamy, white, curd-like patches found on the buccal mucosa and tongue surfaces. These patches can be wiped or brushed off, leaving a red or bleeding surface. Dysphagia, odynophagia and altered taste may occur. Occasionally retrosternal pain will be present.	Gross examination, endoscopy or biopsy of the affected tissue, because culture is not reliable	Clotrimazole troches, nystatin suspension, ketoconazole, fluconazole, and itraconazole (all antifungal agents). Cutaneous Candida may be treated topically with creams or ointments, generally in conjunction with PO medications.	Establish routine oral hygiene regimen. Teach how to detect early signs of infections; infection-control measures; if placed on nystatin suspension, instruct in swish and swallow technique; if placed on mycelex troches instruct to suck on troche until it is dissolved, not to swallow or chew it.
Herpes viruses Herpes simplex 1 (HSV I) Herpes simplex 2 (HSV II) Herpes Zoster (HZV, VZV, shingles)	Painful vesicular lesions that rupture and cause ulcers on the tongue, lips, pharynx or buccal mucosa; fever; pharyngitis; cervical lymphadenopathy; labial lesions	Direct viral culture, gross examination	Acyclovir is the first line of treatment in most cases of HSV and HZV/VZV infections. It may be given PO, IV, or may be used topically on cutaneous lesions. It is used PO and topically in some cases. There is an acyclovir-resistant HSV that is treated somewhat effectively with foscarnet.	Teach infection-control measures and skin care. Offer symptomatic support. Instruct in medication regime. Teach about transmission/prevention methods. Teach comfort measures. Administer pain medications as ordered.

pressed individuals because the T lymphocytes and macrophages cannot destroy the organism. The fungi enters the circulatory system and are carried to the CNS by the macrophages and lymphocytes.

Treatment is generally with IV Amphotericin B, an antifungal drug. This drug can cause renal toxicity, which is generally reversible if the drug is stopped. The dosage is 0.3 to 1.0 mg/kg per day, until a total dose of 1 to 1.5 g is achieved. There are side effects with Amphotericin B, such as fevers and shakes (rigors). To prevent these, the primary care providers may premedicate the patient prior to the infusion with a combination of diphenhydramine hydrochloride (Benadryl) and acetaminophen (Tylenol). Meperidine (Demerol) may be given to prevent rigors. Initially the patient receives treatment daily. Treatments may be reduced to 3 to 5 days a week to decrease the incidence of renal toxicity.

The medication is best given via a central venous access device, as phlebitis may occur if the medication is given via a peripheral vein. The risk of phlebitis is lower if corticosteroids are mixed into the infusion.

Fluconazole (Diflucan) is used for long-term management. Fluconazole is an antifungal that may be given orally or IV. In the oral form it does not cause the renal toxicity and depletion of potassium, magnesium, or phosphate that occur commonly with Amphotericin B. The maintenance dosage is generally 100 to 200 mg per day.

Histoplasmosis. The causative agent is *Histoplasma capsulatum*. This infection is generally related to the environment or region of the country where the patient has lived. The northeastern region of the United States and along the Canadian border is called the "Histo belt" because of the higher incidence of histoplasmosis found there. Generally histoplasmosis presents as a pulmonary infection, but may become disseminated. Symptoms may include dyspnea, weight loss, fever, and cough. The affected sites of disseminated disease are commonly the liver, spleen, and other lymphoid tissue. This infection also has a cutaneous manifestation.

Candida albicans. *Candida albicans* is the fungus responsible for this OI. It can affect the skin, mucous membranes in the mouth, vagina, or GI and urinary tracts.

In HIV-infected individuals it usually presents as white patches on the surface of the tongue, buccal mucosa, or in the pharynx or esophagus, and hard palate, with complaints of sore throat and altered taste sensation. It is commonly referred to as **thrush**. Repeated outbreaks of vaginal candidiasis may be the initial presenting symptom of HIV infection in women. Esophageal candidiasis can be characterized by difficulty or pain when swallowing.

Pneumocystis carinii pneumonia (PCP). There are two schools of thought about the causative agent for pneumocystosis. The first contends that it is a protozoon; the second, a fungus. What is important is that the drugs used to treat this infection are used mainly to treat protozoal infections. The organism is transmitted by the respiratory route. This infection is usually encountered by healthy children, but remains latent until the immune system is sufficiently suppressed; when the CD_4 count is 200 cells per mm^3 or less, it activates. The presenting symptoms may be a dry, nonproductive cough, fever and night sweats, malaise, shortness of breath, dyspnea on exertion, and weight loss (see Table 8-4 on p. 188). This infection may become disseminated, and the symptoms will be site related. It may infect the kidneys, eyes, liver, spleen, and lymph nodes.

There are now multiple effective treatment regimens for pneumocystosis as well as mechanisms to prevent activation of the latent infection. This infection also is seen in both patients who have received chemotherapy for cancer as well and who have had organ transplants and have been therapeutically immune suppressed to prevent organ rejection.

Toxoplasma gondii. Toxoplasmosis (Toxo) is caused by a protozoon called *Toxoplasma gondii* and is ubiquitous around the world. It is the major cause of focal cerebral lesions in HIV infection. Cats carry oocysts in their urinary tract and excrete it in their urine. In approximately 24 hours the oocysts have become spores that remain in the environment for about 1 year. In initial Toxo infection there is a severe inflammatory response, and if the Toxo survives, it becomes cysts. When sufficient immune suppression exists the cysts break down and infect the patient's body. Most commonly toxoplasmosis infects the CNS, although it may also infect the lungs, heart, peritoneum, and GI tract, especially the colon, and skin.

The clinical manifestation may be nonspecific and include fever, headache, nausea and vomiting, and malaise. CNS symptoms predominate (focal neurological symptoms or seizures, fever, and headache). Altered mental status, confusion, lethargy, cognitive impairment, and coma may also be CNS manifestations of toxoplasmosis.

Cryptosporidium. This intestinal protozoon presents in HIV-infected individuals with severe, large volume, foul-smelling, watery diarrhea. The diarrhea is self-limiting in some cases to anywhere from 4 to 20 days. It can cause severe abdominal cramping, malaise, and electrolyte imbalance, especially of sodium, potassium and chloride from the loss of large volumes of intestinal fluids. It may cause weight loss, dehydration, malnutrition, skin breakdown, and debilitation. Psychosocially it may cause the individual to withdraw socially because of the fear of foul-smelling, involuntary bowel movements, the inconvenience of frequent trips to the restroom, an emotional reaction to the change in body image, and worry about what friends may think.

Viral Infections

Cytomegalovirus (CMV). Cytomegalovirus, a member of the herpes virus family, is common. It may be associated with crowded living conditions, lower economic status, and poor sanitation. This virus also is transmitted sexually and by intimate contact. Transmission in utero and during the birth process and breast-feeding can also occur. It is usually carried in the respiratory tract and the urinary tract.

Cytomegalovirus may infect the retina, lung, GI tract, liver, CNS, and circulatory system. Pulmonary infections produce shortness of breath, dyspnea on exertion, and nonproductive cough.

The two most common sites of infection are the retina (may cause blindness) and the GI tract (causing abdominal cramps and diarrhea, weight loss, and anorexia). These symptoms are severe and long-lasting. The CMV infection in the GI tract is more easily treated than in the eye, and may afford long periods of remission. This is not the case in the eye. If treatment for CMV retinitis is not continuous, there is a possibility that vision will be lost. The first sign in the eye is loss of peripheral vision, and the infection may be unilateral. There are ganciclovir-resistant strains of the virus isolated and the treatment for them is usually with foscarnet (Foscavir). It should be noted that it is given IV only and is nephrotoxic. Observe the patient's creatinine and blood urea nitrogen. Foscarnet is given IV at a dose of 40 mg/kg q 12 h for 21 days as an induction regimen. The maintenance dose is 90 mg/kg q 24 h.

Foscarnet is very irritating to the peripheral veins and therefore should be given via a central venous access. If given peripherally it must be given doubly dilute. Because of its nephrotoxicity, it requires preinfusion hydration with at least 500 to 1000 mL of 0.9% NaCl solution. Some patients require postinfusion hydration as well. One sign that the patient is receiving the drug too rapidly is tingling around the mouth. If this happens, the rate of infusion should be reduced, and if the tingling does not resolve, the physician must be notified. CNS symptoms may cause memory loss, muscle weakness, paralysis, lethargy, headache, parasthesias, and personality changes.

There is a third drug now available for treatment of CMV retinitis, cidofovir (Vistide). Its side effects are similar to those of foscarnet: renal impairment and damage. It also is given only IV. The benefits of cidofovir are (1) an induction period of one dose a week for 2 weeks; (2) a maintenance dose once every other week; (3) a total administration time of approximately 1 hour; and (4) the fact that it can be given through a peripheral venous access (IV). This reduces the cost and risk of infections resulting from central venous catheters that are left in place for a much longer time.

To reduce the risk of damage to the kidneys, the patient must take Probenecid 2 g PO 3 hours prior to beginning the cidofovir infusion. The patient is then prehydrated with 1 L 0.9% NaCl over 1 hour. The cidofovir is administered according to body weight at 5 mg/kg and diluted in 100 mL 0.9% NaCl. This infusion lasts for 1 hour. The physician may order a second liter of hydration with 0.9% NaCl during or after cidofovir administration. Two hours after the cidofovir infusion is completed, the patient must take Probenecid 1 g PO and a third dose of 1 g 8 hours after completing the infusion, for a total dose of 8 g of Probenecid.

Patient instructions must include recommendations to increase oral fluid intake, and any fluids lost through vomiting, diarrhea, or excessive perspiration must be replaced to prevent possibly irreversible damage to the kidneys.

The blood must be checked for neutropenia as well as anemia and elevated creatinine. The urine must be checked for proteinuria. These tests must be run within 24 hours of the scheduled infusion.

There are ways to adjust the dose if the creatinine increases or there is protein in the urine. It is imperative that the physician be made aware of any changes in renal function **prior** to infusing the medication.

Patients are much more compliant with this medication because of the improved quality of life resulting from an administration schedule that allows a more normal lifestyle.

Herpes viruses. The herpes family of viruses consists of many well-known members. Herpes simplex types I and II, herpes zoster (shingles), CMV, Epstein-Barr virus (EBV), and Varicella (chicken pox) are some of them. Discussion of most of these will follow because they cause many problems for the HIV-infected individual.

In HIV-infected individuals, herpes usually presents as outbreaks in the oral, genital, and perirectal areas. Patients experience a prodrome of itching and tingling 24 to 48 hours prior to the actual outbreak of vesicles at the site of infection. As with any of the herpes viruses, the clear liquid from the vesicles is highly infectious and the lesions are very painful. The pain decreases as the lesions get to the crusting stage. Chronic ulcerative lesions may form after the vesicles rupture. Symptoms of fever, pain, bleeding, lymph node enlargement, headache, myalgia, and malaise may occur if the infection becomes systemic.

Herpes simplex type I and type II (HSV I and HSV II, respectively) may be transmitted sexually. HSV I usually is isolated in the nose, mouth, pharynx, and esophagus. HSV II generally appears in the genital, perineal, and perirectal areas. Because of cross infection, HSV II may be cultured from the usual HSV I sites and vice versa.

The drug of choice is acyclovir (Zovirax). The initial oral treatment dose is 200 mg five times a day. More severe infections may be treated with intravenous acyclovir. There have been acyclovir-resistant strains of the virus isolated, and the treatment for them is usually with foscarnet (Foscavir). It should be noted that it is given IV only and is nephrotoxic. Observe the patient's creatinine and blood urea nitrogen. Foscarnet is given IV at a dose of 40 mg/kg every 8 hours for 7 to 10 days or until there is a resolution of the outbreak.

Foscarnet is very irritating to the peripheral veins and therefore is given via a central venous access or given doubly dilute. Because of its nephrotoxicity, it requires preinfusion hydration with at least 500 to 1000 mL 0.9% NaCl solution. Some patients require postinfusion hydration as well.

Therapy with this drug causes individuals to become socially withdrawn and may make them unable to continue gainful employment because of the time they must spend each day getting their infusion. This drug may be given with great success at home, so consider making a home care referral prior to discharge.

Herpes zoster/varicella zoster. This virus has two names because it is the same virus that causes chicken pox in children. After infection with chicken pox, the virus becomes dormant in the dorsal ganglion, and when immune suppression become severe enough, it reactivates. Sometimes called zoster and sometimes shingles, the virus manifests itself with a prodrome of itching or tingling, usually 24 to 48 hours prior to the appearance of vesicles. The vesicles usually appear along a **dermatome** (nerve tract). Varicella pneumonia and varicella encephalitis also have been reported. The vesicles fill with a clear liquid that is highly infectious. As they rupture they shed virus that can infect the individual in other areas of the body. It is especially important to instruct the patient not to inoculate the eyes, nose, or oral cavity with the virus. They can prevent this cross infection by using good handwashing and hygiene practices.

Recurrent HZV infections may occur because of immune suppression. It is usually at times of increased stress that the outbreaks occur. Reactivation of the infection in HIV-infected individuals may signal the onset of other OIs and may lead to disseminated disease in visceral and cutaneous sites.

Complications of HZV infection include scarring and postherpetic neuralgia that appear as prolonged pain at the site of the outbreak. Eruptions that occur on the face usually involve the seventh cranial nerve and may involve the eye. The symptoms of shingles are itching and tingling along the affected nerve, headache, and low-grade fever.

Neoplasms

Kaposi's sarcoma (KS). As of 1993, Kaposi's sarcoma (KS) was the most commonly seen neoplasm in HIV-infected individuals. That may be changing as an increase in the number of cases of non-Hodgkin's and CNS lymphoma are diagnosed. Kaposi's sarcoma is a tumor that involves the endothelial cells of the blood vessels. Some researchers believe it is a herpes family virus that causes the cells to proliferate. Kaposi's sarcoma usually appears as a cutaneous problem. Initially the lesions may appear to be a bruise. They then develop as plaques that may become very large. This may eventually cause restriction of movement such as inability to bend an arm or leg.

Another site where early KS may be identified is in the oral cavity. The tumors also may appear in the GI tract, eye, liver, lungs, and lymph nodes. The lesions are highly vascular, but do not bleed when cut or traumatized. Although KS is not usually the cause of death, it is a contributor to morbidity in the HIV-infected individual. If the tumors are located near a lymph node, pressure from increasing size may cause decreased lymph flow, causing lymphedema. This is especially true if the involved area is the inguinal lymph node, with resulting edema of the lower extremities as well as edema of the testicles and penis. This tumor generally affects males, although there have been a small number of females diagnosed with it as well.

Discussion of treatments for KS is brief because no treatment seems to be curative; rather palliation is achieved. The types of treatment available are either local or systemic. The systemic treatment is chemotherapy. One problem with the chemotherapy is that it worsens the immune suppressed state of the patient. Local treatments are somewhat effective in changing the appearance of the lesions, but not in curing them. Intralesional vinblastine injection can reduce the size and appearance of the lesions. Liquid nitrogen also is employed for the same outcome.

Radiation therapy is probably the most commonly used local therapy. Low-dose radiation is used for small skin lesions. Larger doses are required for internal organs and lymph node involvement. Radiation treatment has been effective in reducing the size of tumors near lymph nodes, thus allowing release of lymph that was trapped by the pressure on the node, resulting in a decrease in distal lymphedema.

Researchers at the University of Southern California are finding in preliminary trials that injections of human chorionic gonadotropin (hCG) into the tumors shrinks them. In 10 of the 12 patients receiving the highest dose of hCG, the tumors disappeared completely. These studies are promising.

Lymphomas Lymphomas are tumors of the immune system. There are four types seen in HIV-infected individuals. The four types are non-Hodgkin's lymphoma, B-cell lymphoma, Burkitt's lymphoma, and primary lymphoma of the CNS. Discussion of non-

Hodgkin's lymphoma follows, because it is the most commonly seen type of lymphoma in patients with AIDS.

Non-Hodgkin's lymphoma. This lymphoma may occur after the occurrence of other OIs, or it may be the primary manifestation in unsuspecting individuals who believe that they are at low risk for HIV infection. It is of unknown etiology.

This tumor usually presents as a unilateral, painless enlargement of a lymph node. Other symptoms are nonspecific but may include fever, night sweats or weight loss greater than 10% of baseline body weight. As the tumor enlarges, it spreads to adjacent lymph nodes or organs such as the liver, GI tract, spleen, respiratory system, and the CNS. Symptoms related to other organs are site specific and include nausea, vomiting, elevated liver enzymes, cough, shortness of breath, high fevers, chills, night sweats, and elevated intracranial pressure.

Treatment may be effective depending on which stage the tumor is diagnosed. Surgery may be employed if the tumor is localized. Radiation is used in conjunction with chemotherapy or surgery. Combination chemotherapy, described as the use of more than one agent, is the most common treatment.

AIDS Dementia/HIV Encephalopathy

AIDS dementia/HIV encephalopathy is a manifestation of HIV infection that may occur at any point on the HIV disease continuum. In some individuals it may be the presenting symptom. However, it usually is preceded by one of the OIs. Its etiology is unknown, but it is thought that infected macrophages are responsible for infecting the brain.

The presenting symptoms have a very subtle beginning and are difficult to differentiate from depression, Parkinson's, and Alzheimer's disease (Table 8-6). One clue that differentiates these symptoms as being related to HIV infection is that they are generally present in a younger individual.

There currently is no therapy or treatment for HIV encephalopathy, and because the CNS is involved, treatment of the underlying HIV infection appears to be the best course of action. Treatment with antiretrovirals appears to slow progression. The nursing intervention focuses on preventing the individual from doing harm to himself or others. Safety issues become paramount, and a referral to a home care agency for skilled nursing assessment of the patient, the home environment for safety, and of home maintenance status is needed. The skilled nurse should assess the individual's ability to perform personal care, activities of daily living (ADLs), food preparation, and ability to remember to eat and to take medications. Referrals to community-based AIDS organizations is appropriate with the patient's or responsible party's consent.

TABLE 8-6 ◆ *Chief Signs and Symptoms of AIDS Dementia/HIV Encephalopathy*

Early signs and symptoms
Cognitive impairment
   Short-term memory loss
   Slowed thinking
   Mental slowing/slowed reaction time
   Impaired concentration
   Forgetfulness

Behavioral impairment
   Apathy
   Withdrawal
   Agitation
   Hallucinations
   Depression
   Hyperactivity

Motor Impairment
   Tremor
   Leg weakness
   Loss of balance
   Impaired handwriting
   Slowed motor performance

Late signs and symptoms
Mental status
   Confusion
   Disorientation
   Organic psychosis
   Global dementia

Neurological
   Urinary and fecal incontinence
   Ataxia

NURSING MANAGEMENT

◆ Confidentiality and Disclosure Issues

Confidentiality is essential for all patients. In the case of a patient with HIV, it becomes very important to prevent discrimination and loss of respect and self-esteem.

There is no greater safety in knowing which patients are infected with HIV. The nurse has the skills and responsibility to protect the staff and patients from infection by utilizing standard precautions. The need to know exists only to provide appropriate, supportive, and safe care to HIV-infected patients.

Confidentiality is an ethical requirement for health care professionals. When interviewing patients, some very personal and sensitive information about themselves and their families or significant others is obtained. If this information is released inappropriately, there may be severe penalties such as legal or financial sanctions because of existing laws in most states. A lawsuit may be the consequence for the nurse who is indiscreet. For the patient, the consequences may be loss of job, loss of housing, as well as loss of insurance benefits, job and social discrimination, and rejection by families and friends.

> The right to disclose HIV status is regulated by the state in which you are working.

It is important for every licensed nurse to be aware of the state regulations and of the policies in the employing agency or institution. When a patient's family member asks what is wrong with the patient, if the patient has given permission for explanations to the family, explain the symptoms and what progress or lack thereof is occurring. Leave it to the patient to disclose diagnostic information and HIV status to the family.

When an incident arises that deals with the patient's right to confidentiality, consult the nurse manager, the hospital administrative staff plus a member of the hospital's Pastoral Care Department, such as a chaplain, minister or rabbi.

Occupational Exposure   The first question that comes to mind when caring for a individual with HIV infection has to be, "How can I protect myself from becoming infected and still provide care?" In response to this continually asked question, the CDC, the American Nurses' Association, the Occupational Safety and Health Administration (OSHA), and many health care agencies, private and governmental, have developed research-based guidelines to prevent exposure and infection with HIV and other bloodborne pathogens.

First, follow the CDC's *standard precautions* and the guidelines of the institution for the prevention of transmission of bloodborne pathogens. There are standard policies in all institutions. Second, review the personal protective equipment provided by the institution, where it is located, and how to use it properly. Know what your rights and responsibilities are according to the state and institutional policy, should there be an accidental occupational exposure. Report any exposure to your manager or supervisor immediately and to the employee health department, and follow through with the protocols that are in place.

Infection control is the key to safety anywhere you encounter a person with an injury. Health care workers need to review the CDC standards and take the following precautions:

- *Handwashing.* Use thorough handwashing practices according to your institution's policy, before gloving and after removing gloves, and wash vigorously after any contact with blood or body fluids.
- *Barrier equipment.* Also called PPE or personal protective equipment. Use **gloves, gowns, aprons, masks, glasses, goggles or face guards, and waterproof shoes** as the exposure potential indicates a need for them and per *standard precautions* and

agency guidelines. **Use the PPE *consistently*. The type of PPE used must be appropriate for the task at hand, and the risk of exposure to blood and/or body fluids present.**

- *Sharp object disposal.* Any sharp objects that are disposable, including needles, surgical staples, scalpels and scissors, must be disposed of in a hard-wall, puncture-resistant container. **These containers should be in close proximity to the area where the procedure is being performed to reduce the risk of exposure to other employees, patients, and visitors.** The recapping of nonsheathed needles has been shown to be a very high-risk behavior. Avoid it whenever possible. If there is no disposal unit available, you should utilize the "scoop" technique. This simply means using only the one hand holding the syringe to scoop up the needle cap from a flat surface onto the used needle. **Remember however, the correct procedure is to dispose of *uncapped* needles and sharps in a hard-wall, puncture-resistant container, immediately after use.**
- *Leakproof containers.* Liquid waste and lab and tissue samples should be placed in leakproof containers and should be labeled as hazardous materials. **This goes for every specimen, all tissues, and liquid waste; not just those from known HIV-infected patients.**
- *Skin integrity.* Health care workers with any open sores, lesions, or excoriated skin, should refrain from direct patient care.

Isolation   The only types of isolation that should be used institutionally are protective isolation for burn or neutropenic patients and respiratory precautions for suspected or identified pulmonary tuberculosis patients.

For more information about safety and prevention of occupational exposure, you may check with your institution's infection control department or call the federal OSHA office at (202) 523-8151.

Think about . . . What is the one occupational mistake some nurses make that can lead to contracting the HIV virus?

◆ The Nursing Process

The nursing process is the same for all patients. In patients with a diagnosis of asymptomatic HIV infection, or a patient with advanced disease, the *process* is the same.

Assessment.   Assessment in the adult with HIV infection, including symptomatic AIDS, is very important. It is during the assessment that a determination of the patient's physical, mental, and psychosocial status is made. This basic data-collection step becomes the basis for the plan of care for the each patient on the HIV infection continuum. A complete head-to-toe physical assessment should be performed and any deviations from normal findings should be documented and considered significant. The assessment should include an evaluation of signs and symptoms, physical status, functional level (ability to perform ADLs), self-care abilities, support systems, financial status, and living environment. The assessment of the functional level of the patient must be an ongoing assessment.

History. The history should include a general assessment of the patient's past and present status to help determine specific teaching needs as well as any risk behaviors the patient may practice. Obtain a sexual history to ascertain the risk of transmission and possible exposure to other sexually transmitted diseases. Current medications and treatments should also be included, as well as whether the patient is on any experimental or complementary therapies. If the patient was diagnosed HIV positive previously, ascertain if any OIs have been acquired. Also ask if any of the community-based AIDS service organizations have been accessed. If not, referral should be made prior to discharge.

Nutritional history. The nutritional history is very important. Obtain present weight. Note the patient's past and present weight and any recent weight loss or gain. Present nutritional status should be compared to the patient's past pattern to note any changes that exist and that the patient may not have noticed. Ask if the patient is experiencing nausea, vomiting, or diarrhea. These states not only can affect the patient's ability to take in sufficient calories, nutrients, and fluids, but also may lead to problems with electrolyte balance. If the patient is experiencing diarrhea, the volume and quality should be noted, and assessment for signs of dehydration and potassium depletion, such as leg cramps or cardiac arrhythmias should be done. If the patient is vomiting, hyponatremia may occur. Assess for pale mucous membranes and dry flaky skin. Wasting syndrome in HIV disease causes a loss of lean muscle mass and subcutaneous adipose tissue, so skin turgor is not a good sign of dehydration in this population.

Cardiovascular history. Obtain vital signs. Especially significant are pulse and blood pressure. Observe for signs of hypotension and **orthostatic hypotension.** Also assess for signs of peripheral and periorbital edema and lower-extremity **lymphedema.** In advanced HIV disease observe the patient for **anasarca** (generalized massive edema) resulting from severe depletion of albumin.

Neurological history. Assess cognition, concentration abilities, level of consciousness, and orientation to place and time. Assess for mood changes, irritability, and depression. **Situational depression** related to the HIV/AIDS diagnosis may be noted. However, it may be an appropriate response, considering the HIV seropositive status. Clinical depression and other behavioral changes also may be noted. The patient also may experience motor and sensory changes, such as gait changes, imbalance, and changes in vision, particularly in peripheral visual fields. The neurological history is the initial time to question the patient about any pain or numbness in the extremities, any changes in ability to walk, or any balance problems.

Respiratory history. Ask about the patient's history of respiratory illnesses that may put them at risk for current problems, such as pneumonia, chronic obstructive pulmonary disease, or asthma. Observe for any abnormal breath sounds. Cough is a very important symptom to assess in HIV disease. Question whether the patient smokes, how much, and for how long. If the patient is experiencing a cough, is it dry and nonproductive or moist and productive. Is the patient experiencing any drenching night sweats? Any shortness of breath or dyspnea on exertion? These questions may indicate the possibility of pulmonary tuberculosis or pneumonia. Table 8-1 lists the chief signs and symptoms of AIDS.

Psychosocial history. HIV infection causes stress in HIV-infected healthy persons and in those with clinical disease. It generates a unique series of stresses for the infected person, sexual partners, family members, and health care professionals. These stresses can predispose the patient to a variety of psychiatric symptoms, such as paranoia, anxiety, hallucinations, and mania. The symptoms identified require intervention and support from the primary care provider and the nurse. By collecting data during psychosocial assessment, the nurse is better able to anticipate the needs and vulnerabilities of the patient and is in a better position to plan and implement interventions.

This assessment should include a substance use history, a history of interpersonal relationships, educational level, and career information. Look at the past **coping skills** to see what coping techniques may be useful in the present situation. Learn about the social support system. Has the patient experienced multiple losses of friends? What is the living situation? Does someone live with the patient? Is there any community organization membership? Church or synagogue attendance? Identify the patient's social set. Is there support available within that community? The answers to these questions will provide information to enable development of a functional plan of interventions and referrals.

◆Nursing Diagnosis

As with any other disease process, the patient with HIV/AIDS can have nursing diagnoses formulated specifically for any of their problems. However, some of the NANDA nursing diagnoses occur in this population frequently. These diagnoses may be associated with systemic, psychosocial, or specific body system responses to HIV (See Table 8-7).

◆ Planning

Planning is a very important part of the nursing process. To develop a plan that will work, you must collaborate with other members of the health care team. These include the patient, other nurses, the physician, and the primary care giver at home. If the patient is to adhere to the plan, he must have ownership of it, and the way to get the patient to own the plan is to give him every chance to make the decisions that will affect the outcome of his nursing care. The patient also must believe that the plan will be evaluated and reassessed along the way, so changes can be made when necessary. The nurse should supply information, education, and support, as well as help the patient decide on goals and expected outcomes for the plan of care. When these steps are included in the planning stage, the implementation of the plan goes very smoothly. Expected outcomes are written individually for each nursing diagnosis chosen for the care plan.

◆ Implementation

Major goals associated with implementing the plan of care for all adults with HIV/AIDS are (1) preventing secondary bacterial, viral, and fungal infections; (2) preventing wasting due to malnutrition; (3) maintaining or improving the present level of immune function; (4) maintaining adequate social functioning; and (5) maintaining or improving current mental status. Table 8-7 lists common nursing diagnoses, expected outcomes, and interventions used for patients with AIDS.

Teaching the patient and significant other careful and consistent handwashing is very important. As stated in Chapter 7, meticulous handwashing by the care provider before and after each encounter with the patient is the single most important way to prevent infections. It also is very important to practice this same method of handwashing during meal preparation.

Wasting is a physiological problem associated with HIV infection. However, if the patient and caregiver are knowledgeable about methods to maintain adequate nutritional status, wasting may not become a problem. Referral to a nutritionist or dietician is one option. If this is not available, instruct the patient in the use of the food pyramid, and if possible provide them with handouts for future reference at home. Calorie intake can be boosted by encouraging plenty of butter, mayonnaise, sour cream, or other high-calorie condiments; recommending sweets and ice cream for snacks; adding honey to coffee or tea; adding more peanut butter and deviled eggs to the diet; and adding skim milk powder to milk and sauces. Suggestions for serving six small meals a day or for using food supplements may be needed.

Instruct the patient in the appropriate method of medication administration. By taking antibiotic and antiretroviral medications consistently as ordered, less resistance to the drugs occurs, and the effect of the drugs is prolonged.

Encourage social interaction and independence in activities as tolerated and refer to support groups to boost the patient's self-esteem and worth. This may reduce the effects of situational depression and empower the patient. Consistency in promoting a positive attitude also will reduce the powerlessness the patient experiences.

◆ Evaluation

The evaluation of nursing actions is performed to determine whether the expected outcomes have been met. Data indicating that the outcomes have been met must be collected and analyzed. The patient's ability to participate in the care must be factored into the plan. A regular time frame should be set to evaluate the outcomes as a team with input from the patient. The patient's expectations may not be the same as those of the health care team or the primary care giver's, and when you evaluate the outcomes, you must address unrealistic expectations.

Frequent laboratory testing to determine immune status, blood cell status, and effects of medications is a large part of the evaluation process.

ELDER CARE

Elder care is an area that often is forgotten when discussing HIV infection. This may be a result of the "youth fixation" in the United States. Age is no barrier to becoming infected with HIV, and in some cases may actually predispose people to infection. A myth that must be discarded is that elders, generally considered to be people over the age of 55, are no longer interested in a sexual relationship. This is simply not true. With many people becoming single as a result of death of a spouse or partner or divorce and life expectancy increasing well past 70, this is a population who is at very high risk. People in this age group often have had transfusions for surgery done some years ago; this puts them at greater risk of having contracted HIV from this source.

Times and values are changing, and older people may not have the comfort level to negotiate safer sex. Their self-esteem may be low, and their body image changed. They may not know how to protect themselves. Because pregnancy is not a consideration in this age group, condoms are not used as often as they should be. It is imperative to give older patients the appropriate

TABLE 8-7 ◆ Nursing Diagnosis and Interventions for the Patient with HIV/AIDS

Nursing Diagnosis	Expected Outcomes	Nursing Interventions
Risk of infection Elevated body temperature Depressed immune function	Patient will exhibit no signs of infection; normal temperature.	Monitor for outward signs of infections and for symptoms of opportunistic infection. Monitor body temperature daily. Assess for signs of dehydration and altered mental status.
Impaired gas exchange Excessive lung secretions Use of respiratory accessory muscles for breathing	Patient's oxygenation will improve to within normal levels within 3 weeks.	Monitor breath patterns and sounds q 4 h. Position to allow for maximum chest expansion. Provide supplemental oxygen as ordered. Encourage deep-breathing and coughing as need indicates. Conserve strength and oxygen by assisting with activities of daily living. Monitor blood gases as ordered. Suction airway as ordered PRN.
Impaired skin integrity Multiple areas of skin abrasion State of dehydration	No further areas of skin breakdown will occur. Areas of abrasion will heal within 2 weeks.	Assess skin status q 4 h; assess for areas of excoriation, lesions, rashes, and discoloration. Report changes from baseline findings. Keep skin clean and dry. Change linens as needed if diaphoresis or incontinence are present. Use elbow and heel protectors and special mattress while patient is immobilized. Apply lotion to dry skin. Assess for dehydration q 4 h. Encourage adequate fluid intake per physical status. Assess for signs of fluid overload/edema. Monitor input and output.
Alteration in oral mucous membranes Fungal infection Irritation from drug therapy	No evidence of fungal infection at the end of 3 weeks.	Assess and monitor the status of the mouth, tongue, and teeth. Refer for dental care. Teach proper dental hygiene. Refer for nutritional counseling as need indicates.
Alteration in nutrition; less than body requirements Weight loss Loss of appetite Impaired swallowing	Patient will not experience further weight loss. Patient will gain at least 0.5 lb per week.	Assess patient's ability to take in food, chew, and swallow. Assess for pain in throat; loss of taste sensation. Monitor weight twice a week. Record input and output. Administer antiemetics as ordered. Assess the availability of food within living situation. Assess ability of caregiver to meet patient's nutritional needs. Assist with planning for small frequent meals. Administer dietary supplements if required.

(Table 8-7 continued)

TABLE 8-7 ◆ Nursing Diagnosis and Interventions for the Patient with HIV/AIDS (Continued)

Nursing Diagnosis	Expected Outcomes	Nursing Interventions
Pain Pressure on nerves from Karposi's sarcoma lesions Discomfort from peripheral neuropathy	Pain will be controlled within tolerable levels within 4 days.	Assess levels of pain. Assess patient's methods to relieve it. Relieve causes of pain by correcting underlying condition if possible. Administer pain medications as ordered. Assess amount of relief provided by medication; if relief is not adequate, consult with physician for more effective protocol for pain relief. Explore use of NSAIDs and antidepressant medications for pain relief in conjunction with other analgesics. Implement adjunctive therapies to assist with pain relief: massage, cold or hot applications, repositioning, distraction, meditation, imagery, etc. Teach relaxation techniques.
Activity intolerance Weakness Central nervous system and peripheral nerve involvement Fatigue	Level of activity intolerance will improve within 1 month.	Encourage periods of rest alternated with periods of activity. Plan activities according to usual stamina levels. Change schedule of activities as degree of fatigue indicates need. Assist with activities of daily living as needed to conserve energy. Encourage self-care in small increments as condition improves.
Altered thought processes Drug side effects Impaired oxygenation Effects of disease process	Oxygenation will be improved, if possible, within 2 days. Electrolyte imbalances contributing to problem will be corrected within 3 days.	Assess mental and thought processes to establish a baseline. Monitor for causes of interference in thought processes: anemia, electrolye imbalances, drug side effects, impaired oxygenation or dementia. Orient patient to person, time, and place frequently. Utilize techniques to assist with memory lapses; calendar, clock, labels for things. Structure the environment per patient's wishes; do not move placement of belongings and frequently utilized items such as eye glasses, tissues, book, etc. Decrease outside stimuli when patient is trying to concentrate.
Alteration in self-concept Considerable weight loss Altered physical appearance Inability to maintain employment	Patient will verbalize personal strengths within 3 weeks. Patient will take action to find ways to increase feelings of worth within 2 months.	Encourage socialization to prevent withdrawal and social isolation. Refer to support group for strengthening of self-concept. Refer to nutritionist to improve nutrition and physical appearance. Encourage volunteer work to increase self-worth and feelings of accomplishment.
Altered sexuality pattern HIV status Decreased physical well-being Fatigue Presence of ano-genital lesions	Patient will develop methods of sexual expression and intimacy that will not endanger self or others.	Instruct patient to plan periods of rest around periods of sexual activity. Offer referral to support groups or therapy to deal with issues of altered body image. Instruct patient and significant other in the effective practice of abstinence, use of condoms, and barrier sex. Discuss alternative methods of intimacy until ano-genital lesions are healed.

Nursing diagnosis	Patient outcomes	Interventions
Ineffective individual coping Diagnosis of life-threatening illness Fatigue Anxiety	Patient will marshall usual effective coping techniques to meet challenges of the illness.	Establish rapport with the patient, significant other, and family. Assess past methods of effective coping. Assess patient's strengths. Schedule activities that may cause stress when the patient is most rested or has support person available. Review effective methods for problem solving.
Powerlessness Diagnosis of life-threatening disease Increasing fatigue	Patient will maintain control over treatment and lifestyle choices.	Show patient respect. Allow patient control of daily schedule, activity, and treatment choices. Foster independence in the patient by allowing to do as much self-care as possible. Reinforce behaviors that indicate the patient is planning for the future.
Anticipatory grieving HIV status Diagnosis of a life-threatening disease	Patient will express feelings within 3 weeks.	Encourage verbalization of feelings; provide nonthreatening, supportive environment; be an active listener. Refer to support group to facilitate grief process. Refer to social services and pastoral care to assist with directives to physicians, living will, and designation of power of attorney. Encourage positive thinking for increased energy level and constructive handling of grief.
Sensory perceptual alteration, visual Loss of visual fields HIV damage to CNS	Patient will develop methods of dealing with visual changes within 1 month.	Assess amount of visual deficit. Orient patient to the environment. Speak to and touch the patient frequently while in the room. Keep patient informed of what you are doing and what will be happening to decrease fear and anxiety. Instruct to report any further change in vision. Assist with methods to enhance remaining vision and to prevent injury.
Self-care deficit Fatigue Deterioration of physical condition Mental changes Neurological impairment	Patient will accomplish as many activities of daily living as possible without undue fatigue. Patient will accept assistance with activities of daily living within 2 weeks.	Assess ability to perform own activities of daily living. Provide assistance for activities the patient is unable to perform. Refer to occupational and physical therapy for assistive devices and home equipment needed. Instruct significant other and family members how to assist with activities of daily living.
Impaired home maintenance Fatigue Activity intolerance Inadequate finances	Patient will achieve adequate home maintenance within 1 week.	Assess availability of caregiver in the home to assist with shopping, cleaning, meal preparation, and transportation. Assess income for adequacy to support living and needed medical care. Refer to social services and community agencies for help and other resources.

information while respecting their feelings. Women, in general, are more vulnerable to HIV infection from sexual transmission because semen has far higher concentrations of the virus than infected vaginal secretions. A woman's male sex partner is statistically more likely to have had multiple other sexual contacts, increasing the likelihood of HIV infection. HIV testing for *both* partners, before entering into a new sexual relationship should be encouraged, along with recommendations to use barrier techniques.

There are normal aging processes that put older women and men at higher risk as well. Skin and mucous membranes are more fragile in the elderly person, possibly making transmission easier (e.g., atrophic vaginitis in elderly women). To a small degree, the bone marrow is affected by the aging process. After the age of 70 there is a definite decline in the functioning of the immune system as evidenced by the increase in neoplasms and the decreased ability to fight infections. Age-specific referrals to a geriatric nurse practitioner or counselor with experience working with older adults may be appropriate.

COMMUNITY CARE

Nurses are on the front lines of the AIDS epidemic. The skill and ability to educate and care for the patients and community are part of nursing responsibility. Each nurse should be alert to the possibility of transmission of HIV and the methods of prevention and take every opportunity to share this information with at-risk populations. This means not only the patients we treat and care for, but also their significant others, families, and friends, as well as professional colleagues.

Nurses provide care in many different places: the neighborhood school, churches, the nursing home, homeless shelters, or the patient's home. In each of these situations, take the opportunity to use the nursing process to assess and refer for care. Assessment should include evaluating the patient and family for risk of infection due to high-risk behaviors or reduced immune function. The need identified may be to educate about infection control, to preventing transmission of HIV, or to provide a referral to community agencies for further information. Nurses have the opportunity to meet the challenge of care for the person with HIV/AIDS. This disease presents many problems to the status quo in nursing and gives our profession an opportunity to provide improved, quality, and compassionate care to these individuals.

CRITICAL THINKING EXERCISES

Clinical Case Situations

1. Mary Ross is a 40-year-old white female who is admitted to the hospital with a dry, nonproductive cough, and a 10-lb weight loss. She has been treated for a week by her primary care provider for an upper-respiratory infection presenting as a fever and weight loss with night sweats. She has been very adherent to her medication schedule and has not missed any of her antibiotics. Her doctor has admitted her and counseled her about the possibility of being HIV infected. She believes that she cannot be infected and that she must be ill with something else, even though she had a short relationship with a man she met while she and her husband were separated last year. She knows that they did not have protected sex. She refuses to take an HIV antibody test. Her doctor is treating her **empirically** for PCP. He also ran a CD_4 lymphocyte count, which is in the low 200s. He feels that she is HIV seropositive and wants to talk to her husband about the type of treatment she needs and about the possibility of testing him for HIV. He knows that he needs Mary's permission to share the information that she may be HIV-infected with her husband. Yet because she is in denial, he feels he must make her husband aware of the risk in which he may be placing himself if they continue to practice unprotected sex.

   a. As the nurse assigned to Mary, what would you do to protect her confidentiality when her husband asks you what is wrong with her?

   b. What type of referrals would you plan for this patient?

2. Epimenio Costa is 48-year-old Hispanic man who has come to the employee health clinic at the hospital where you are working. You are taking his history before he sees the doctor. He complains of something growing in his mouth and a 15-lb weight loss over the last month. During that time he states that he hasn't been able to sleep one complete night because he is having terrible diarrhea. This is the second time this year he has experienced these symptoms. He is married with four children ages 16, 14, 13, and 10. His wife doesn't speak English and works as a domestic and is undocumented. He states they have no primary care provider. When any of them are sick, they just go to the emergency room at the hospital or to the *curandero,* a Latino natural/faith healer who may use prayer, herb, and home remedies. The last time he went to the ER, the doctor tested him for HIV, but he never went back for the results. He said that he wasn't a homosexual and didn't use injection drugs, so how could it be possible for him to HIV positive? He did not deny having sexual intercourse with prostitutes.

   a. As the nurse doing the initial assessment, what related physical symptoms would you look for?

   b. What type of referrals would you plan to make, if he agreed with the plan of care?

   c. What nutritional teaching would you make available to Mr. Costa?

BIBLIOGRAPHY

Agency for Health Care Policy and Research. (1994). *Evaluation and Management of Early HIV Infection*. Rockville, MD: U.S. Department of Health and Human Services.

American Journal of Nursing. (1996). New drugs: A new class of anti-HIV drugs debuts. *American Journal of Nursing*. 96(7):59–64.

Anastasi, J. K., Lee, V. S. (1994). HIV wasting: how to stop the cycle. *American Journal of Nursing*. 94(6):18–24.

Anastasi, J. K., Rivera, J. (1992). Identifying the skin manifestations of H.I.V. *Nursing 92*. 22(11):58–61.

Anastasi, J., Sun, V. (1996). Controlling diarrhea in the HIV patient. *American Journal of Nursing*. 96(8):35–41.

Anastasi, J. K., Thomas, F. (1994). Dealing with H.I.V.–Related pulmonary infections. *Nursing 94*. 24(11):60–64.

Brooke, P. S. (1997). HIV and the law: An update. *RN*. 60(5):59–64.

Centers for Disease Control. (1987). Human Immunodeficiency virus infections in health-care workers exposed to blood of infected patients. *MMWR*. 36:285–289.

Centers for Disease Control. (1987). Recommendations for prevention of HIV transmission in health-care settings. *MMWR*. 36(S2S):3S–12S.

Centers for Disease Control. (1987). Revision of case definition for AIDS for surveillance purposes. *MMWR*. 36(suppl.):1S–8S.

Centers for Disease Control. (1989). Guidelines for prophylaxis against *Pneumocystis carinii* pneumonia in persons infected with human immunodeficiency virus. *MMWR*. 38(S5):1–9.

Cerrato, P. L. (1996). HIV report: Always a death sentence? *RN*. 59(8):22–27.

Cerrato, P. L. (1993). Nutrition support: what diet can do to combat HIV infection. *RN*. 56(6):71–72.

Flaskerud, J., Ungvarski, P. (1995). *HIV/AIDS: A Guide to Nursing Care*, 3rd ed. Philadelphia: Saunders.

Geer, J., Heiman, J., Leitenberg, H. (1984). *Human Sexuality*. Englewood Cliffs, NJ: Prentice-Hall.

Grimes, D., Grimes, R. (1994). *AIDS and HIV Infection*. Mosby's Clinical Nursing Series. St. Louis, MO: Mosby.

Holzemer, W., Henry, S., Reilly, C., Portillo, C. (1995). Problems of persons with HIV/AIDS hospitalized for *Pneumocystis carinii* pneumonia. *Journal of the Association of Nurses in AIDS Care*. 6(3):23–30.

Kenny, P. (1996). HIV infection: how to bolster your patient's fragile health. *Nursing 96*. 26(8):26–35.

Lubkin, N. (1997). What to do if you're exposed to HIV. *Nursing 97*. 27(2):23.

Macalinao, M., Kirton, C. A. (1994). The AIDS patient with respiratory failure. *American Journal of Nursing*. 94(11):5–10.

Muma, R., Lyons, B., Borucki, M., Pollard, R. (1994). *HIV: Manual for Health Care Professionals*. Norwalk, CT: Appleton & Lange.

Nursing 92. (1992). Aids update: how H.I.V. affects the eye. *Nursing 92*. 22(6):26.

Sande, M. A., Volberding, P. (1993). *The Medical Management of AIDS*, 4th ed. Philadelphia: Saunders.

Schmidt, J., Crespo-Fierro, M. (1995). Who says there's nothing we can do? *RN*. 58(10):30–35.

Tannenbaum, I. (1993). Women and HIV. *RN*. 56(5):34–40.

Ungvarski, P. J. (1997). Update on HIV infection. *American Journal of Nursing*. 97(1):44–51.

Ungvarski, P. (1996). Waging war on HIV wasting. *RN*. 59(2):26–32.

Whipple, B., Scura, K. W. (1996). The overlooked epidemic: HIV in older adults. *American Journal of Nursing*. 96(2):23–28.

Wilson, B. A. (1997). Understanding strategies for treating HIV. *MEDSURG Nursing*. 6(2):109–111.

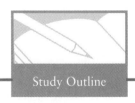

Study Outline

I. Introduction
A. Mortality rate for diagnosed AIDS patients is approximately 65%.
B. Aspects of care should address physical, spiritual, and mental needs.
C. AIDS is a multisystem disease process.
D. People diagnosed with AIDS experience multiple losses, physically, emotionally, and psychosocially.

II. Natural History and Epidemiology
A. Acquired immune deficiency syndrome (AIDS) was first described by the Centers for Disease Control and Prevention (CDC) in 1981.
B. In 1983 the cause of AIDS was identified to be a virus.
C. Pediatric AIDS cases are defined as patients younger than 13 years of age.
D. The primary host cell for HIV is the CD_4.

E. HIV impairs the cell-mediated immune response.

F. There is no period of latency in the infection, although, like in other immune deficiencies, there are periods of exacerbation and remissions.

G. Sentinel infections, such as recurrent *Candida* infections or seborrheic dermatitis, may indicate an underlying immunosuppression.

III. **Transmission and Prevention**

A. First step in prevention of transmission is knowledge.

B. HIV cannot be transmitted through casual contact.

C. Specific modes of transmission are as follows:

1. Unprotected sexual contact with an HIV-infected partner (sexual transmission).

2. Exposure to HIV-infected blood, body fluids, tissues, and breast milk (occupational and maternal transmission).

D. Safer sex is practiced by putting a barrier to prevent transmission of the virus between the partners via body fluids.

E. Latex condoms are recommended because they are more impermeable than other types of materials.

F. Spermicides containing nonoxynol-9 are recommended because they have been shown to inactivate the virus.

G. An allergy to nonoxynol-9 may actually increase the risk of viral transmission because it inflames the tissues and makes it easier for the virus to penetrate them.

H. Sexually transmitted diseases are more difficult to treat in HIV-infected individuals.

I. The key to reducing the possibility of infection with HIV sexually is knowledge of transmission modes and consistency in practicing either abstinence or barrier sex methods.

IV. **Management of Early HIV Infection**

A. A complete physical and psychological examination is performed when an individual tests HIV positive.

B. CD$_4$ lymphocyte counts are performed every 3 to 6 months to determine the progression of the infection.

C. CD$_4$ cell counts are used to determine when to begin therapy with antiretroviral medication and prophylaxis against opportunistic infections.

D. Antiretroviral medications include Zidovudine (ZDV), didanosine (Videx), and Zalcitabine (ddC); others are becoming available.

V. **Pathophysiology**

A. The CDC has developed a classification system for AIDS. This system is described in Table 8-4.

B. Suppression of the immune response as a result of infection with HIV is the cause of AIDS.

C. The continuum of HIV infection may last from 18 months to more than 10 years depending on the type of exposure, lifestyle (healthy vs. unhealthy, sexual orientation), and strain or virulence of the virus.

D. There are two types of HIV infection: HIV-1 and HIV-2. The type found in the United States is HIV-1.

E. There are different types of test to determine HIV serostatus. The ELISA and the IFA are the most commonly performed HIV screening tests. Descriptions of these tests and others can be found in Table 8-2.

F. Pretest and posttest counseling should be provided to the client to ensure an understanding of the methods of HIV transmission.

VI. **Clinical Manifestations and Opportunistic Infections**

A. Opportunistic infections (OIs) are diseases caused by microorganisms commonly present in the environment or the body that cause disease only when a change in the normal, healthy condition of the body leads to a weakening or suppression of the immune system.

B. The opportunistic infections are classified as either bacterial, fungal, viral, or protozoal. These infections can be reviewed in Table 8-5.

C. AIDS dementia/HIV encephalopathy may occur anywhere on the HIV continuum.

D. The symptoms are subtle and are difficult to differentiate from depression, Parkinson's, and Alzheimer's disease. The age of the HIV-infected individual is one clue that may make diagnosis easier in that these disease processes usually occur in adults older than the general HIV-infected population.

E. Safety issues are important to assess in order to protect the patient from doing harm to himself or others.

F. A description of manifestations of AIDS dementia/HIV encephalopathy is found in Table 8-6.

VII. **Nursing Management**

A. Patient confidentiality and disclosure issues.

1. Prevention of inappropriate disclosure of HIV status is important to prevent discrimination and loss of respect and self-esteem.

2. For the health care worker there is no greater safety in knowing a patient's HIV status. The responsibility of prevention of occupational exposure is that of the practicing nurse, utilizing CDC *standard precautions*.

3. Confidentiality is an ethical requirement of health care workers. There may be legal recourse against the nurse who inappropriately released any information about any patient without appropriate patient permission.

B. Occupational exposure

1. Occupational exposure is preventable by following CDC *standard precautions*, and those of your institution or agency.

2. Good handwashing is the single most effective way to prevent transmission of most microorganisms by the nurse, health care worker, patient, and caregiver, and it is an especially helpful adjunct to *standard precautions*.

3. Wash hands before and after providing patient contact.

4. **Wash hands after removing gloves.**

5. Know what type of personal protective equipment (PPE) is appropriate for the task to be performed and consistently use it. **As important as knowing what type of PPE to use is to know where it is located.**

6. The appropriate method to dispose of used needles is to drop them into a hard-wall, puncture-resistant container immediately after use.

C. The nursing process
The nursing process is the same for all patients regardless of their diagnosis or stage of disease.

1. Assessment:

a. The assessment should include an evaluation of:

(1) Signs and symptoms.

(2) Physical status.

(3) Functional level (ability to perform ADLs).

(4) Self-care abilities.

(5) Support systems.

(6) Financial status.

(7) Living environment.

(8) Frequency of infections.

(9) Abnormalities of lymph tissues.

(10) Factors that decrease immune functioning (alcohol and drug use).

b. Review diagnostic tests: CBC, differential, chemistries, CD_4 lymphocyte assays, and other tests specific to disorders suspected.

2. Nursing Diagnoses:

a. Use specific nursing diagnosis for problems identified.

b. Use "High risk for . . . " diagnoses only as supported by assessment findings.

3. Planning

a. Goals:

(1) Protect from infection.

(2) Prevent occupational transmission of HIV.

(3) Instruct patient and significant others in prevention of transmission methods.

(4) Improve health status.

(5) Maintain highest degree of wellness to promote optimal immune functioning.

4. Intervention:

a. Promote adequate and balanced nutrition.

b. Protect from infection.

c. Use and teach good handwashing technique.

d. Psychosocial care to decrease fear, reduce stress, and assist with lifestyle and role changes.

5. Evaluation:

a. Determine if expected outcomes have been achieved.

b. Monitor lab test values for changes in condition.

c. Monitor vital signs and weight.

VIII. Community Care

1. Alert to factors that can facilitate HIV transmission in the community and environment.

2. Teach healthy lifestyle.

3. Identify patients with HIV; plan care to prevent secondary infections and strengthen resistance.

4. Home care and skilled care nurses deal with patients with acute disease processes and also with the chronic disease.

5. Requires careful planning of care.

6. Requires collaboration with other health care team members.

7. Requires ongoing and frequent follow-up with patient and providers.

IX. Elder Care

1. After age 70, there is a definite decline in immune function.

2. Aging does not affect the bone marrow much.

3. There is a decrease in the natural production of CD_4 lymphocytes.

4. The ability to fight infection is diminished.

5. There is an increase of the number of neoplasms in people over 70.

6. People over the age of 55 still have active sex lives.

7. There are now higher numbers of singles over the age of 55. These people need skill building in negotiating safer sex.

8. Older men and women are at higher risk physiologically because of normal changes from aging. Mucous membranes and skin are more fragile in the elderly person, possibly making transmission easier.

9. Referrals to geriatric nurse practitioners for counseling may be appropriate.

CHAPTER 9

Care of Patients with Cancer

OBJECTIVES

Upon completing this chapter the student should be able to:
1. Identify characteristics of neoplastic growth.
2. Identify at least five factors that may contribute to the development of a malignancy.
3. State at least four practices that can contribute to prevention and early detection of cancers.
4. Describe ways to include the recommendations of the American Cancer Society for routine checkups and detection of cancers into patient education.
5. Discuss the pros and cons of the various treatments available for cancer.
6. State the major problems and appropriate nursing interventions for a patient coping with expected side effects of radiation.
7. Devise a general plan of nursing care for the patient receiving chemotherapy.
8. Discuss the teaching necessary for the patient who has bone marrow suppression from cancer treatment.
9. Identify nursing interventions to help the patient cope with the common problems of cancer and its treatment.
10. Describe appropriate nursing interventions to help patients and families deal with the psychosocial effects of cancer and its treatment.

THE IMPACT OF CANCER

Cancer is a group of diseases that characteristically grow in an uncontrolled manner with the spread of abnormal cells. That does not mean that the growth cannot be controlled in many instances by specific treatment. In the early 1900s, there was little hope for survival once cancer was detected. This year four out of ten people who are diagnosed with cancer will be alive 5 years from now.

About 1,382,400 new cases of cancer will be diagnosed in 1997. In addition, about 800,000 people will be told that they have squamous cell skin cancer. Much of the increase in cancer incidence is due to lung cancer. Death rates for many other major cancers have held steady or declined since the 1930s. Although cancer treatment has made progress, cancer still accounts for one in four deaths in the United States and about 560,000 people will die from it in 1997. On the other hand, of the 10 million Americans living who have a history of cancer, 7 million were diagnosed over 5 years ago. Most of these 7 million cancer survivors are

considered "cured," meaning that they have no sign of the disease and now have the same life expectancy as those who have never had cancer.

More people can survive cancer if it is treated in its earliest stages. In fact, the American Cancer Society estimates that early detection and prompt treatment could save the lives of half the people who each year are diagnosed with cancer. Figure 9-1 shows the leading sites of new cancer cases and deaths.

This chapter discusses the prevention and control of cancer, current diagnostic, and screening techniques that help detect cancer in its earliest stages; therapeutic procedures that greatly improve a cancer victim's chances for survival; and the role of the nurse in the control and treatment of malignant diseases.

PHYSIOLOGY OF CANCER

The human body is continuously producing new cells to replace those that are worn out and to repair damage done by illness and injury. An abnormal rep-

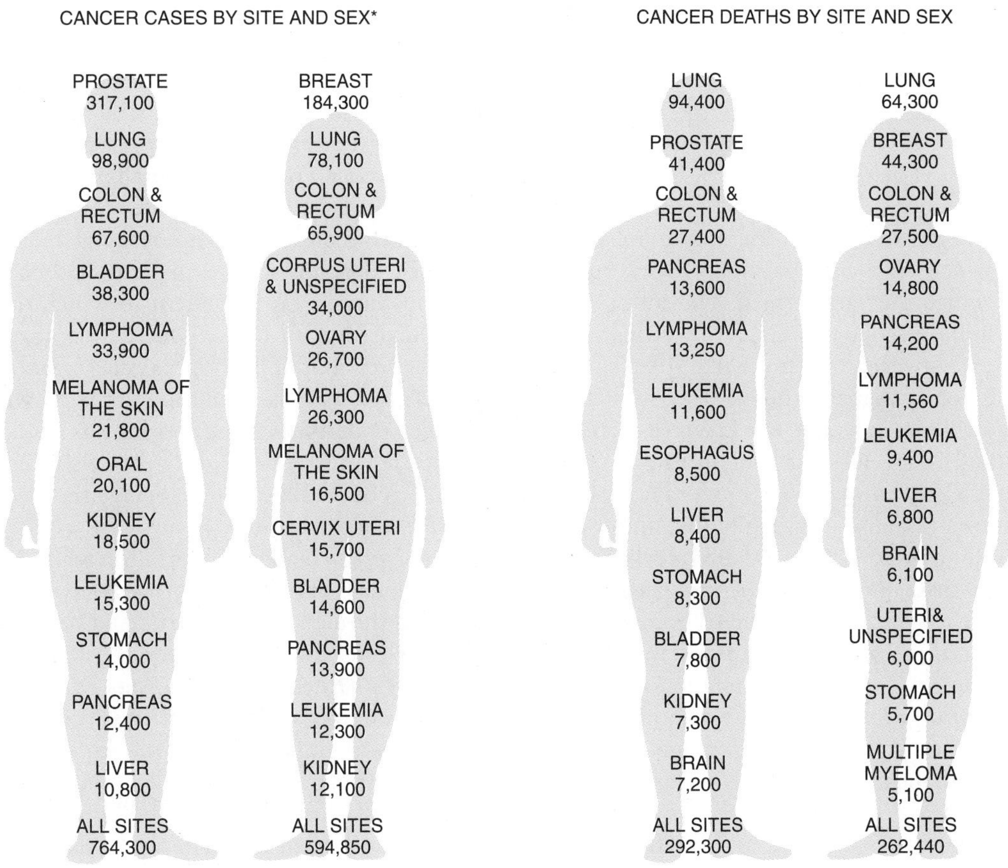

CANCER CASES BY SITE AND SEX*

PROSTATE 317,100	BREAST 184,300
LUNG 98,900	LUNG 78,100
COLON & RECTUM 67,600	COLON & RECTUM 65,900
BLADDER 38,300	CORPUS UTERI & UNSPECIFIED 34,000
LYMPHOMA 33,900	OVARY 26,700
MELANOMA OF THE SKIN 21,800	LYMPHOMA 26,300
ORAL 20,100	MELANOMA OF THE SKIN 16,500
KIDNEY 18,500	CERVIX UTERI 15,700
LEUKEMIA 15,300	BLADDER 14,600
STOMACH 14,000	PANCREAS 13,900
PANCREAS 12,400	LEUKEMIA 12,300
LIVER 10,800	KIDNEY 12,100
ALL SITES 764,300	ALL SITES 594,850

CANCER DEATHS BY SITE AND SEX

LUNG 94,400	LUNG 64,300
PROSTATE 41,400	BREAST 44,300
COLON & RECTUM 27,400	COLON & RECTUM 27,500
PANCREAS 13,600	OVARY 14,800
LYMPHOMA 13,250	PANCREAS 14,200
LEUKEMIA 11,600	LYMPHOMA 11,560
ESOPHAGUS 8,500	LEUKEMIA 9,400
LIVER 8,400	LIVER 6,800
STOMACH 8,300	BRAIN 6,100
BLADDER 7,800	UTERI & UNSPECIFIED 6,000
KIDNEY 7,300	STOMACH 5,700
BRAIN 7,200	MULTIPLE MYELOMA 5,100
ALL SITES 292,300	ALL SITES 262,440

*Excluding basal and squamous cell skin cancer and n situ carcinomas except bladder.

FIGURE 9-1   **Leading sites of new cancer cases and deaths, 1996 estimates.** (*Source:* American Cancer Society. [1996]. *Cancer Facts and Figures—1996.* Atlanta: Author.)

lication of cells results in a *neoplasm,* or new growth of tissue, that is not beneficial and often is harmful to the body.

The word *benign* indicates a neoplasm that is usually harmless. Benign growths are almost always encapsulated, which means they are surrounded by a fibrous capsule that prevents the release of cells and their spread to other parts of the body.

These growths can, however, create problems if they obstruct the passage of fluid and air or if they grow to such a size that they press against and interfere with the normal structure and function of nearby organs.

The cells of **malignant** (uncontrolled growth that can lead to death) growths are quite different from normal cells. Cancer cells are the result of a transformation of normal body cells, probably because of some alteration in the normal cells' deoxyribonucleic acid (DNA). The change in the DNA, which contains the genetic makeup of all future generations of the cell, alters the structure and function of the cancer cell and of its progeny. Hence cancer cells do not look like or behave like normal cells.

The nucleus of a malignant cell is large and irregular. As the cell divides and duplicates itself, it fails to follow the rules that regulate the reproduction of normal cells. Malignant cells do not seem to "know" when to stop multiplying. Their offspring proliferate in great numbers and grow more and more disorganized and uncontrollable. Some take on new characteristics so that they do not in any way resemble the cells of the tissues from which they originated.

Because malignant cell growth is not regulated as it is in normal cells, the malignant cells multiply and form tumorous masses, invade neighboring tissues, and travel to other parts of the body, where they establish another colony of malignant cells. **Their demand for nourishment depletes the supply of nutrients available for normal cells.** This spread of tumor cells is called **metastasis,** a process that is described later in this chapter. **Not all malignant cells metastasize, but the great majority of them do.** This is true because malignant cells are easily broken off from their original mass of tissue and are able to survive on their own until they reach their new home.

Think about . . . Can you compare and contrast the aspects of a benign and malignant tumor for a classmate?

◆ Classification of Tumors

Tumors often are classified according to the organs or tissues from which they first began to grow or the substances of which they are formed. The suffix -*oma* means tumor and is used in the names of various kinds of malignancies. However, remember that -*oma* simply means tumor, not malignant tumor. The suffix can designate any swelling, including one in which there is a collection of fluids, as well as one containing malignant cells. For example, *hematoma* (another word for bruise) is a combination of *hema-*, meaning blood, and -*oma*, meaning a swelling or collection of fluid or cells.

The prefixes used in classifying neoplasms indicate the kind of tissue in which they originate. For example, a tumor arising from fatty (lipid) tissue is called a **lipoma**. A *fibroma* is a tumor composed of fibrous tissue. A *leiomyofibroma* contains both smooth-muscle tissue and fibrous connective tissue. Lipoma, fibroma, and leiomyoma are the most frequently occurring types of benign growths.

Malignant growths are divided into four main types. **Sarcomas** arise from mesenchymal tissues, that is, bone, muscles, and other connective tissues. **Carcinomas** originate in epithelial tissues (skin and mucous membranes). These kinds of cancers make up the majority of glandular cancers of the stomach, uterus, lung, skin, and tongue. Cancers of the blood-forming system comprise the **leukemias** and **lymphomas**. Malignancies of the pigment cells of the skin are called **melanomas**.

These are the main groups of cancers. More precise identification can be made by adding modifying prefixes. For example, *osteosarcomas* arise from bone, and *adenocarcinomas* arise from glandular structures.

◆ Metastasis

The word **metastasis** refers to the movement of cells from one part of the body to another. Bacterial cells metastasize, and so do malignant cells. Malignant growths can invade normal body tissue by penetrating adjacent tissues, thereby destroying normal cells and taking their place. Malignant cells also may separate from the original tissue mass and travel to distant parts of the body. **Metastasis refers to the moving of these cells to another site.** Malignant cells can metastasize by traveling in the blood and lymph, in much the same way as bacterial cells. It also is possible for free malignant cells to be directly transplanted from one organ to another during surgery, when gloves and instruments that have these cells on them serve as vehicles for their transportation. Another way in which malignant cells can "contaminate" normal tissues and organs is by entering a body cavity and coming in contact with a healthy organ. For example, malignant cells may break off from a diseased organ, enter the peritoneal cavity, and attach themselves to an ovary or the mesentery.

The prognosis for a patient with a malignancy depends largely on the extent to which the malignant cells have invaded body tissues. A localized growth is one that remains at the original site *(in situ)* and has not yet released its cells, even though the growth may have invaded underlying tissues. As long as all of the cells are in the area in which the new growth started, the cancer is said to be localized. At this stage the disease is much more easily eradicated.

A *regional* malignancy is one in which cells from the original mass of malignant growth have broken off and traveled through the lymphatic and blood vessels.

The cells' journey has been shortened, however, by the body's protective mechanisms, which trap the foreign cells in the lymph nodes. These cells may continue to grow and multiply, and if the regional cancer is not successfully treated, they will eventually break away and spread throughout the body, producing an *advanced* cancer that is inevitably fatal.

One system in which cancers are classified according to the extent to which the malignancy has spread is the *TNM staging system*. The three basic components of the system are *T* for primary tumor, *N* for regional nodes, and *M* for metastasis. The number written beside each letter indicates the extent to which the malignancy has spread and involves other tissues (Table 9-1). For example, T1, N0, M0 means that the tumor is small and localized (no involvement of regional lymph nodes and no metastasis). A designation of T1, N2, M0 indicates a small (T1) tumor with moderate regional involvement (N2) but no metastasis to distant sites (M0).

CAUSATIVE FACTORS

All cancer results from defects in the DNA of genes. These defects are either inherited or they occur during a person's lifetime from exposure to chemicals or radiation. Several cancer-causing genes, **oncogenes,** are being discovered each year. Oncogenes are like mistakes in the instructions inside a cell. Instead of normal new cells, the defective gene directs the cells to multiply at an abnormal rate. Likewise, *tumor suppressor genes* are being discovered that control the growth of abnormal cells in the body naturally. Each person's body has a different ability to withstand the effects of cancer-causing substances (**carcinogens**), to respond immuno-

TABLE 9-1 ◆ *TNM Staging System for Cancer*

Tumor	
T0	No evidence of primary tumor.
TIS	Carcinoma in situ.
T1 T2 T3 T4	Progressive increase in tumor size and involvement.
TX	Tumor cannot be assessed.
Nodes	
N0	Regional lymph nodes not demonstrably abnormal.
N1 N2 N3	Increasing degrees of demonstrable abnormality of regional lymph nodes. (For many primary sites, the subscript "a," e.g., $N1_a$, may be used to indicate that metastasis to the node is not suspected; and the subscript "b," e.g., $N1_b$, may be used to indicate that metastasis to the node is suspected or proved.)
NX	Regional lymph nodes cannot be assessed clinically.
Metastasis	
M0	No evidence of distant metastasis.
M1 M2 M3	Ascending degrees of distant metastasis, including metastasis to distant lymph nodes.
M4	Multiple organ involvement.

logically, and to repair damaged DNA. It is hoped that some day discoveries in molecular biology will allow individual risk profiles to be drawn that could be used to counsel people to avoid certain occupational and environmental exposures.

Many harmful agents exist in the external environment that are known to be carcinogenic, and others are strongly suspected. **Among these harmful agents are certain chemicals, sources of radiation, and viruses.** In addition to these external causative factors, there are some internal factors that influence an individual's ability to cope with malignant cells. Hormones play an undetermined role in the development and progress of cancer, and although there is no evidence that malignancy follows any pattern of heredity, there is a familial tendency toward the occurrence of cancer in certain organs. This is shown in certain high-risk groups, which are described later in this chapter.

Elder Care Point ... Another factor that enters into the development of a malignancy is age. Although cancer can strike at any age, older people are more susceptible—partially because they have a weakened immune system, perhaps also because their powers of adaptability are weakened and they have been exposed to carcinogens over a longer period than have younger people.

Immunocompetence, or the capability of one's immune system to deal with foreign cells—bacterial, viral, or malignant—is an important factor in the development of cancers.

◆ Chemical Carcinogens

Almost 200 years ago, Sir Percival Pott linked the occurrence of cancer to a substance in the environment when he observed that cancer of the scrotum was common among the chimney sweeps of London. He attributed this high incidence of cancer to repeated accumulations of soot on the skin of these young men, whose occupation required continuous contact with the coal soot in the chimneys they cleaned. Since that time, almost 500 different chemical carcinogens have been identified.

Many of the cancer-producing substances in man's environment are related to occupations that involve repeated exposure to certain substances that are handled or inhaled. **Petroflurocarbons (polychlorinated biphenyls or PCBs) and some pesticides (e.g., DDT) are known carcinogens and other such chemicals decrease immunocompetence.** For example, cancer of the skin often is related to the handling of pitch, asphalt, crude paraffins, and petroleum products. Lung cancer is linked to irritating substances in the air, such as tobacco smoke, asbestos, and chemical wastes from industry and automobiles. Cancer of the bladder is associated with certain substances in aniline dyes, which are present in the environment of workers in that industry. Vinyl chloride, nickel, arsenic, and chromate are linked to cancers in workers in industries that utilize those chemicals. Benzene, an ingredient in older unleaded gasolines, is linked to leukemia. These are but a few of the chemical agents that can contribute to the development of cancer in humans.

Think about ... Can you identify three chemicals used in your home or on your garden that are carcinogenic? How can you reduce your exposure to them and decrease the risk of cancer?

Chewing tobacco has been directly related to cancer of the tongue and structures of the mouth and throat. **Cigarette smoking is a known direct cause of cancer of** the lung and is thought to be linked to esophageal, pancreatic, bladder, and kidney malignancies.

Immunosuppressive drugs used to suppress organ transplant rejection are a cause of non-Hodgkin's lymphoma. Synthetic estrogens are linked to a higher incidence of endometrial cancer. Many of the drugs used to treat cancer affect the immune system and can predispose to other types of cancer. Table 9-2 shows carcinogens that are commonly encountered in the environment.

◆ Promoters

Some agents are not in themselves carcinogenic, but when they are in the person's body along with a known carcinogen, cancer occurs more quickly. Alcohol is such a substance. When in the presence of nicotine, cancers occur at a faster rate in those who are heavy consumers of alcohol than in someone who uses nicotine but does

not drink alcohol. It is thought that about 90% of all head and neck cancers are tobacco plus alcohol related.

◆ Chronic Irritation

In one of the earliest theories about the causes of cancer, a malignancy of the skin and mucous membranes was attributed to long-term chronic irritation of the skin and mucous membranes. Although this condition may be a *contributing cause* of cancer, chronic irritation alone usually does not lead to malignancy. There must be other factors present, particularly a mole and exposure to a chemical carcinogen or ultraviolet rays.

Research is ongoing on a variety of chemicals that may have this same type of influence. The link is most likely that the second substance involved, although not directly carcinogenic, has a depressant or harmful effect on the immune system, making the person more susceptible to growth of malignant cells.

◆ Physical Carcinogens

Radiation   Radiation may originate from x-ray machines and radioactive elements or from the ultraviolet rays of the sun. These rays are capable of penetrating certain body tissues and causing the development of malignant cells in the affected area. The relationship of intense and prolonged exposure to these rays and the production of cancer cells was first discovered when it was noted that there was a high incidence of cancer, particularly leukemia, among people who pioneered studies of x-rays, radium, and uranium. Later it was found that survivors of atomic blasts at Hiroshima and Nagasaki at the end of the Second World War suffered an unusually high incidence of leukemia.

There is continued concern about the dangers that excessive radiation in the environment presents, especially the long-term effects that are not immediately apparent but may eventually prove to be related to malignancy. In addition to leukemia, cancers of the skin, bone marrow, and thyroid are believed to be closely linked to exposure to radiation.

The ultraviolet rays of the sun can produce skin cancer. The deterioration of the earth's ozone layer is causing more ultraviolet rays to reach the earth than in the past, which compounds the problem. The susceptibility of the individual also is a factor. People with fair complexions have less protective pigment and therefore are more likely to develop skin cancer from ultraviolet radiation than are people with darker skin.

Radon gas has been found to be carcinogenic. People who live in areas that have more radon emission from the earth have a higher incidence of malignancy in the population than people in areas that are low in radon.

TABLE 9-2 ◆ *Common Substances That are Carcinogenic*	
Substance	**Type of Cancer**
Asbestos	Lung, peritoneal, pericardial
Benzene	Acute myelocytic leukemia
Tobacco	Lung, mouth, pharynx, larynx, esophagus, pancreas, bladder, kidney
Alcoholic beverages	Mouth, pharynx, larynx, esophagus, liver
Ionizing radiation	Leukemia, tumors of most organs
Sunlight (ultraviolet rays)	Skin
Diethylstilbesterol (prenatally)	Vagina
Estrogens, synthetic	Endometrial
Androgens, synthetic	Liver
Vinyl chloride	Liver
Aromatic amines	Bladder
Arsenic (inorganic)	Lung, skin
Chromium	Lung
Nickel dust	Lung, nasal sinuses
Chronic hepatitis B infection	Liver
Human T-cell lymphotropic virus type I (HTLV-1)	Adult T-cell leukemia and lymphoma
Phenacetin	Renal pelvis, bladder
Alkylating agents (used for chemotherapy)	Acute myelocytic leukemia
Cyclosporine (used to prevent transplant rejection)	Non-Hodgkin's lymphoma

Viruses   In recent years, there has been intensive research directed toward establishing a link between viruses and malignancy. Experiments involving animals have demonstrated that a number of cancers can be produced in animals by injecting them with a filtrate from virus-infected malignant growths. However, few viruses have proved to be directly carcinogenic to humans. **The hepatitis B virus (HBV) is carcinogenic for liver cancer.** The Epstein-Barr virus (EBV) causes Burkitt's lymphoma. Cases of adult T-cell leukemia and lymphoma are caused by human T-cell lymphotropic virus (HTLV). A form of the human papillomavirus (HPV) causes cervical carcinoma. These viruses are known as *oncoviruses* because of their ability to cause cancer.

After the transformation of a normal cell into a precancerous state, the malignant cell probably requires many conditions favorable to its multiplication and growth into a cancerous tumor. **Viruses are capable of introducing new genetic material into a normal cell and transforming it into a malignant one.** Furthermore, cell reproduction can be altered when viruses interact with carcinogens. Viruses can damage the immune system, such as the human immunodeficiency virus (HIV), and decrease immunocompetence, causing the body to become more susceptible to the growth of abnormal cells.

♦ Genetic Predisposition

Research is revealing that there is a genetic predisposition to various types of cancer. It has been known for many years that breast cancer is more likely to occur in women who have a close female relative who developed breast cancer before the age of 65. Genetic markers have been found for a type of colon cancer, one form of breast cancer, and a type of leukemia. In the next decade, genetic markers, or oncogenes, may be found for many other forms of cancer. Such markers could identify high-risk individuals, who then might undergo more vigorous, regular diagnostic testing to detect any malignancy in the very earliest stages. Such early discovery would greatly increase survival rates.

♦ Contributing Factors

Intrinsic Factors   Age, sex, and race are considered "predisposing factors" for certain types of cancers. This simply means that statistically, certain types of cancer strike particular age, sex, or racial groups more frequently than others. For example, prostate cancer is far more common in black males than in white males. The incidence of cervical cancer is higher in black women than in white women. Breast cancer is more prevalent in white women than in Asian women. As for age factors, approximately 50% of cancers occur in people over the age of 65.

Stress   Another factor that seems to play a role in the development of cancer is stress. Considerable stress over long periods has an adverse effect on the immune system, making it less effective in ridding the body of invading organisms and decreasing the body's ability to destroy abnormal cells. Stress is one more factor that can perhaps tip the scales in favor of growth of malignant cells. When one partner of a long-term relationship dies, the stress of the loss and adjustment to life without the person seems to increase the likelihood of cancer in the surviving partner.

Diet and Cancer   **Excessive intake of both saturated and unsaturated fats increases the chance of malignancy of the breast, colon, and prostate.** Studies of various populations throughout the world have shown that colon cancer is more prevalent among groups of people who eat large amounts of fat and very little food fiber. Although there is no universal agreement about the role of fiber in the prevention of malignancy, high-fiber foods, such as fruits, vegetables, and cereals are recommended as a wholesome substitute for fatty foods.

Because the tars in smoke used to prepare smoked and salt-cured meats are carcinogenic, the American Cancer Society recommends limited dietary intake of foods of this kind. There also is evidence that nitrite used in nitrite-cured foods can enhance the formation of nitrosamines, which are potent carcinogens in animals and possibly in humans. Meat processors in the United States have already significantly decreased the amount of nitrite in prepared meats in response to the research findings.

Another dietary recommendation is to reduce the amount of charcoal-broiled meat in the diet. The charred portion of the meat is thought to be carcinogenic. This recommendation is undergoing further study at the present time.

MEASURES TO PREVENT CANCER

The nurse can be very instrumental in educating the public about ways to prevent cancer. Each nurse should teach patients the following measures at every opportunity.

♦ Smoking

Encourage those who smoke to quit. Ninety percent of lung cancers in men and 79% in women are related to smoking. Use of tobacco in conjunction with the intake of alcohol is related to several other types of cancer.

♦ Diet and Nutrition

Encourage maintenance of normal weight. Obesity is considered a risk factor in cancers of the uterus, gallbladder, kidney, stomach, colon, and breast. It also makes early detection of many cancers difficult. One study noted that men and women who were overweight by 40% or more have a 33% and 35% greater risk, respectively, for developing cancer than do persons with normal weight.

Encourage a varied diet. The American Cancer Society has issued nutritional recommendations that are believed to reduce the risk for certain cancers. These recommendations, summarized in Table 9-3, are from a report by a special committee on nutrition and cancer and are based on studies conducted for more than 20 years by the American Cancer Society's Research Program. Although no direct cause-and-effect relationship between diet and cancer has been demonstrated, there is ample evidence that avoidance of obesity and modification of the diet can help prevent some types of cancers.

Total fat intake in the diet should be reduced to 30% or less of the daily total calorie intake. Eating more high-fiber foods, such as whole grain cereals, pasta, breads, vegetables and fruits helps decrease the fat in the diet and may reduce the risk of colon cancer by increasing the bulk in the diet.

The roles of vitamins A and C and betacarotene in the prevention of cancer are not clear. However, human population studies indicate that persons who eat foods high in betacarotene and vitamin A are less likely to develop cancer of the esophagus, larynx, and lung. **However, research has shown that supplemental forms of betacarotene do not have the same effect.** Those who eat foods with a high content of vitamin C also reduce their chances of developing cancer, particularly of the stomach and esophagus. The exact action of the vitamin is not known, and it may be that other constituents of the vitamin C–rich foods exert a protective effect in the upper gastrointestinal tract.

Moderation in the drinking of alcohol is recommended, because drinking often is accompanied by cigarette smoking or the use of smokeless tobacco. It also can lead to liver damage and possibly to liver cancer.

Research has indicated that if foods containing nitrites are eaten in combination with foods containing vitamin C, the formation of nitrosamines is blocked. This means, for example, that if orange juice is consumed along with a meal containing bacon, there is less chance of carcinogenic nitrosamines damaging the body.

Because ground water is so often contaminated with chemicals that have leached into it from fertilizers, pesticides, and industrial wastes, it is wise to know the chemical makeup of the local water supply. If the geographic area is highly contaminated, bottled water might help prevent further damage to immunocompetence and thereby decrease the incidence of cancer.

Think about... Can you identify three specific changes you could make in your personal diet that might decrease your cancer risk? What would you add to the diet or what would you stop eating?

♦ Avoiding and Limiting Exposure to Carcinogens

Knowing which substances used in the household, yard, areas of recreation, and at the place of work are carcinogenic and using protective measures against them can decrease exposure. The use of protective clothing, gloves, and mask as appropriate when spraying pesticides or chemicals or using chemical cleaners or strippers greatly decreases exposure. Being certain the area is well ventilated when using chemical cleaners indoors is protective. Thoroughly washing the hands and any exposed skin after using compounds containing carcinogenic chemicals provides protection. Utilizing an appropriate sunscreen and protective clothing when outdoors, avoiding sunburns, and avoiding tanning salons and sun lamps greatly decreases the incidence of skin cancer.

Avoiding swimming and water sports in contaminated waters and avoiding eating fish from waters that have chemical contamination limit exposure. Washing or rinsing fruits and vegetables before preparing them for eating or cooking decreases exposure to agricultural pesticides.

TABLE 9-3 ♦ *Dietary Recommendations to Minimize Risk for Cancer*

- Eat a varied diet and avoid obesity.
- Reduce total saturated and unsaturated fat intake to 30% of total caloric intake.
- Eat more high-fiber foods: whole-grain cereals, breads, pastas, fresh fruits, and vegetables.
- Include foods rich in vitamins A and C in the daily diet.
- Eat cruciferous vegetables and those containing betacarotene daily: cabbage, broccoli, Brussels sprouts, kohlrabi, cauliflower, carrots, yellow squash.
- Avoid smoked, salt-cured, nitrite-cured, and charred (blackened) foods.
- Keep alcohol consumption moderate; no more than two drinks or two glasses of wine or beer per day.

◆ Identifying High-Risk People

Studies of individuals who have developed cancer, their medical history, lifestyle, and family history, have shown that some people are more likely to develop certain kinds of cancer than others. Table 9-4 shows information on high-risk groups published by the American Cancer Society in order to develop an awareness of the need for frequent and thorough examinations to detect cancer early in those who are susceptible to developing a malignancy.

◆ Detection of Cancer

The purpose of screening large segments of a population is to identify as many susceptible people as possible. Screening clinics often identify individuals who already have developed malignancies but have no symptoms and are not aware that they are suffering from cancer.

Cancer sometimes is called the "great masquerader" because it is capable of causing symptoms similar to those of a variety of diseases. Cancer is, after all, a

---

TABLE 9-4 ◆ *Major Risk Factors for Cancer*

Lung
Heavy smoker over age 50.
Smoked a pack a day for 20 years.
Started smoking at age 15 or before.
Exposure to environmental smoke.
Exposure to asbestos, arsenic, certain chemicals in the workplace.
Radiation or radon exposure.
History of tuberculosis.
Signs: persistent cough, blood in the sputum, chest pain, recurring pneumonia or bronchitis.

Breast
History of breast cancer.
History of some forms of benign breast disease.
Close relatives with history of breast cancer.
Early menarche; late menopause.
Never had children; first child after age 30.
Lengthy exposure to cyclic estrogen.
Higher education and socioeconomic status.
Signs: lump in breast, nipple discharge, thickening, dimpling, nipple retraction, pain or tenderness of the nipple.

Colon-rectum
History of rectal polyps.
Rectal polyps run in family.
History of inflammatory bowel disease.
Signs: blood in stool; alteration in bowel pattern, e.g., constipation alternating with diarrhea.

Uterine-cervical
Frequent sex in early teens or with many partners.
History of HPV or Herpes II virus infection.
Low socioeconomic status.
Poor care during or following pregnancy.
Signs: unusual bleeding or discharge.

Uterine-endometrial
Estrogen therapy.
Late menopause (after age 55).
History of infertility or failure to ovulate.
Diabetes, high blood pressure, gallbladder disease, and obesity.
Pelvic irradiation.
Signs: unusual bleeding or discharge.

Skin
Excessive exposure to sun.
Fair complexion.
Work with coal tar, pitch, or creosote.
Signs: change in the size, color, or appearance of a mole or spot on the skin; scaliness, oozing, bleeding or change in appearance of a bump or nodule; spread of pigmentation beyond the border, or change in sensation of any skin lesion.

Oral
Heavy smoker and drinker.
Use of smokeless tobacco.
Poor oral hygiene.
Signs: white patch in the mouth or on the tongue; nodules.

Ovary
History of ovarian cancer among close relatives.
History of breast cancer.
History of never having children.
Signs: none until well advanced.

Prostate
Over age 65.
Black ancestry.
Signs: difficulty urinating; hesitancy, blood in the urine; need to urinate frequently; pain in lower back, pelvis, or upper thighs.

Stomach
History of stomach cancer among close relatives.
Diet heavy in smoked, pickled, or salted foods.
Some link with blood group A.
Signs: nonspecific; indigestion, feeling of fullnes or pressure; pain and weight loss are late signs.

Pancreas
Smoking.
Signs: None.

Bladder
Smoking.
Signs: painless blood in the urine; need for frquent urination.

Leukemia
Down's syndrome.
Exposure to excessive radiation.
Exposure to benzene (unleaded gas).
HTLV-1 Viral infection.
Philadelphia chromosome.
Signs: frequent infections, easy bruising, fatigue, weight loss, nosebleeds, paleness.

group of diseases. It can strike any organ of the body, affecting different organs with different functions, and therefore can present an untold number of symptoms as it progresses. To be able to identify the symptoms of cancer in its earliest stages, it is important to be aware of its warning signals.

◆ Seven Warning Signals of Cancer

The seven warning signals of cancer are:

- ◆ Change in bowel or bladder habits
- ◆ A sore that does not heal
- ◆ Unusual bleeding or discharge
- ◆ Thickening or lump in breast or elsewhere
- ◆ Indigestion or difficulty in swallowing
- ◆ Obvious change in wart or mole
- ◆ Nagging cough or hoarseness

Elder Care Point . . . Because the incidence of cancer is so much higher in the person over age 65, and because those who have reached old age have been exposed to more carcinogens for a longer period of time, annual screening for cancer is even more important.

In addition to the medical history and thorough physical examination that are essential components of any health status evaluation, the physician also conducts certain tests to determine whether a malignancy is present. Recommendations of the American Cancer Society for routine checkups and early detection of cancer are shown in Table 9-5.

◆ Diagnostic Tests

One widely used and useful technique to detect cancer is to examine cells under a microscope to determine

---

TABLE 9-5 ◆ *Routine Measures Recommended by the American Cancer Society for the Early Detection of Cancer*

Breast
Regular monthly self-examination of breasts for lumps, nodules, or changes in contour; check by physician every three years until age 40, then every year.
Mammogram beginning at age 40 every 1 to 2 years until age 50 when mammogram is recommended yearly.

Colon-rectum
Digital rectal examination as part of annual checkup every year for those over 40.
Proctosigmoidoscopy (after initial negative tests 1 year apart) every 3 to 5 years after age 50.
Stool blood test should be performed every year for those over age 50.

Cervix and uterus
Pelvic exam every year. Pap test for all adult women and high-risk adolescents. After 3 consecutive normal annual examinations, the test may be performed every 2 to 3 years at the discretion of the physician.
Those at high risk for endometrial cancer should have an endometrial tissue biopsy taken at menopause and frequently thereafter.

Testicles and prostate
At age 14, begin performing testicular self-exam (TSE) once a month.
Men age 40 and older should have a digital rectal examination (DRE) annually.
After age 50, prostate-specific antigen (PSA) blood testing should be performed annually.

Skin
Self-examination of skin by all adults once a month to detect new lesions and monitor appearance of moles.
Consultation with a dermatologist if pale, wax-like, pearly nodules, or red, scaly, sharply outlined patches are found.
Melanoma may present as a mole that is asymmetrical one half to the other, have an irregular border, pigmentation that is not uniform throughout the mole, or have a diameter greater than 6 mm. A dermatologist should be consulted if any of these changes are found.

Oral
Regular dental examinations.
Consult physician or dentist if a white patch remains in mouth for more than a week, a nodule is felt on the gums, tongue, or mucous membranes.
Inspect the sides and bottom of the tongue every few months.

High-risk exceptions:
More frequent and thorough examinations recommended for

- ◆ Women with personal family histories of breast cancer.
- ◆ Women who began having sexual intercourse at an early age or those with many partners.
- ◆ Women who have a history of obesity, infertility, failure of ovulation, abnormal uterine bleeding, or estrogen therapy.
- ◆ Men and women who have a personal family history of cancer of the rectum, familial polyposis, Gardener's syndrome, ulcerative colitis, or a history of polyps, and those with a family incidence of melanoma.

Each person is encouraged to confer with a physician and determine whether these recommendations are adequate in light of his or her personal history and risk factors.

whether they are malignant or premalignant. This technique is called **cytology,** and the most widely used cytological test is the Papanicolaou smear.

A *cytological examination* can be done by obtaining a sample of secretions in which there are cells that have been released from adjacent tissue. The technique involves either scraping or brushing a sample of cells from the area or collecting body secretions that contain cells. These secretions may be cervical discharges, sputum, gastric washings, pleural fluid, or urinary washings. The specimen is placed on a slide and sent to a laboratory, where a specially trained technologist or pathologist examines the cells microscopically. If "suspicious" cells are found, the patient is referred to a physician for more extensive diagnostic tests. The "Pap smear," named after Dr. George Papanicolaou, who first developed the procedure, is used in screening for cancer of the uterine cervix.

Another screening technique used for colorectal cancer is the simple test for *occult,* or hidden, blood in the stool. The person simply collects one or more stool specimens, depending on the particular test being used, applies a thin smear on the container provided, and returns the slides to the physician or clinical laboratory. Directions for withholding meat and other foods, vitamins, and drugs from the diet for several days before the test must be clear to the patient. Otherwise, a false-positive or false-negative reading might be obtained. **Occult blood in the stool is not always an indication of cancer of the bowel or rectum.** Other conditions also can produce this symptom.

Biopsy of a tumor and examination of the cells so obtained are the most certain techniques for establishing a diagnosis of malignancy in most neoplasms. Malignancies involving blood cells, as in leukemia, are diagnosed by examining these cells.

Research continues on identifying clonal markers on DNA that might be used to diagnose various types of cancer. Clonal marker tests may soon be available for those at high risk for bladder, cervical, lung, breast, colon, and prostate cancer. If these tests prove reliable, they may well be incorporated into a normal part of routine medical care. Such a test is expected to cost about $50 and the result would be available within one day, but only further research will determine the reliability of the test.

Other procedures used to identify lesions that are possibly malignant include radiological studies, endoscopy, sonography, magnetic resonance imaging, computed tomography, clinical laboratory testing of enzymes and other substances in the blood, and studies specific to the system in which the cancer is suspected.

Biopsy   A **biopsy** is the removal of living cells for the purpose of examining them microscopically. The cells may be removed by surgical excision of a small part of a tumor, by the aspiration of cells through a needle introduced into the growth, or by brush biopsy. If the tumor is small, the entire growth may be removed. The specimen obtained is examined under the microscope.

Ordinarily, the specimen is prepared in the laboratory by placing it in paraffin and waiting 24 hours before examining it. If, however, the sample is taken in the operating room and the surgeon is waiting for the results to determine the extent of surgery needed to remove all the malignant cells, the tissues may be frozen for quick examination. This technique is called *preparing a frozen section.*

New procedures, such as fine-needle aspiration (FNA) and percutaneous large-core breast biopsy, look promising for diagnosing breast cancer without the disfigurement of traditional surgical breast biopsy. Breast biopsy is combined with radiological techniques to verify correct placement of the biopsy needle. Then FNA is combined with computer analysis of the samples obtained.

Radiological Studies   X-ray films are particularly helpful in diagnosing tumors affecting the bones and hollow organs. The respiratory, digestive, and urinary tracts can be visualized by x-ray if a **radiopaque** (not penetrated by the x-rays) substance is used. The substance passes through the hollow organ and, since it is radiopaque, the inner structure of the organ is clearly demonstrated on the x-ray film. A radiopaque substance commonly used is barium, which may be swallowed by the patient or given in an enema. **Mammography** is a radiological examination of the breast that is useful in diagnosing malignant growths.

Another radiologic technique involves the use of a radioactive substance (**radionuclide**) that is given to the patient prior to the x-ray filming. The radionuclide is a "tumor-seeking" chemical that searches for the tumor and may or may not concentrate around it. A special scanning apparatus moves back and forth over the subject's body; as it moves, it records information about the concentration of the radionuclide in the area being examined. If the substance is concentrated in the tumor, the growth shows up as a "hot spot" on the screen of the scanning apparatus. If the tumor does not accept the radionuclide, the normal tissue around the tumor concentrates the radionuclide, and the tumor shows up as a "cold spot." This technique is commonly used in the investigation of thyroid tumors.

A commonly used radiological scanning technique is *computed tomography (CT scanning).* This method is noninvasive and involves relatively small amounts of radiation exposure for the subject. The term *noninvasive* means that no surgical procedures are needed to reveal the size, shape, contour, and density of an organ. The procedure is not uncomfortable for the patient and requires minimal preparation.

In CT scanning, the x-ray source moves past the subject in one direction while the film moves in another. In this way, three-dimensional cross sections, or "slices," of tissue can be obtained. The scanner rotates an entire 180° (half circle) around the area being examined, filming as it rotates 1° at a time. Information received by the scanner is relayed to a computer, which presents an image of the tissues one slice at a time. The "picture" presented by the computer is an interpretation of the varying densities of tissues, fluids, and bones. Tumors, as well as other abnormal structures within the body tissues, can be seen in this way.

Endoscopy   An endoscope is an instrument used for direct visualization of internal body parts. It is designed so that it can be inserted and passed along the interior of hollow organs and cavities. The endoscope has a flexible fiberoptic tube fitted with a lens system so the examiner can view tissues in more than one direction. It has a light to illuminate the area being examined.

Other types of endoscopes include the colonoscope for the colon, the colposcope for the vagina and uterine cervix, the bronchoscope for the trachea and bronchi, the laparoscope for the ovaries or the contents of the abdominal or pelvic cavity, and the cystoscope for the interior of the bladder. During an endoscopy, the physician may take a sample of cells from a suspicious area so they can be examined more precisely under a microscope (biopsy).

Laboratory Tests   Although no one blood test can establish a definite diagnosis of cancer, certain tests are used to ascertain specific information. A complete blood count is helpful in diagnosing leukemia. The presence of a high level of prostate-specific antigen (PSA) may indicate prostate cancer. The PSA test is a recommended part of the routine physical for the male over age 40. The patient must be told not to engage in sexual activity 24 to 48 hours prior to giving the blood sample as ejaculation alters the result. The sample is collected before digital examination of the prostate by the physician. Prostate acid phosphatase (PAA) is a second blood test used to confirm the result of an elevated PSA. Levels of the enzyme *acid phosphatase* in the blood can give information about the extent of cancer of the prostate. The enzyme *alkaline phosphatase* is elevated in many patients with metastatic bone cancer and in some who have liver metastasis.

Specialized tests for tumor markers have been developed in the past few years. These detect biochemical substances synthesized and released into the bloodstream by tumor cells. However, these are not 100% accurate for diagnosing tumors because many of these substances also are produced by normal or embryonic cells and are also found in benign conditions. **Therefore tumor markers are mainly used to** confirm a diagnosis or the response to therapy or to detect a relapse. CA-125 is used to detect the presence of ovarian cancer or its recurrence after therapy. CEA and CA 19-9 are tumor marker tests used to detect the recurrence of gastrointestinal, pancreatic, and liver cancer after initial treatment.

NURSING MANAGEMENT

◆ Assessment

The first step is to find out whether the patient has been informed of his diagnosis and what is known about the illness and treatment. Some patients may suspect they have cancer but do not want to discuss it. Even those who have been informed may choose not to talk about it or ask any questions about their treatment. The fact that a patient cannot discuss his illness and seek help in dealing with the problems it presents should indicate how very frightened he is and how much he needs help and understanding. The nurse must assess how the disease is affecting the patient's body and life to plan comprehensive care.

A thorough assessment of the system in which the cancer is located and a good general physical assessment provide a baseline upon which changes in physical function caused by the cancer can be evaluated. A psychosocial assessment of the patient and family or significant others provides data that point out psychosocial needs, coping abilities and techniques, and resources for support and care.

Finally, the nurse should determine how she can assist the patient to make the most of the personal resources and abilities that he currently possesses. This could mean helping with adjustment to the emotional impact of only recently learning the diagnosis of cancer, or it could require helping the patient to deal with the pain and discomfort of advanced malignancy and to prepare for a peaceful death.

◆ Nursing Diagnosis

Patients with cancer, depending on the stage of the disease, can have a great number of problems, and a large number of nursing diagnoses may be appropriate. Specific diagnoses are chosen for the body systems and functions in which the disease or tumor is causing disruption of homeostasis. Common general nursing diagnoses associated with a diagnosis of cancer are:

- Alteration in nutrition (less than body needs) related to increased metabolic demand and nausea, vomiting, diarrhea, or mucositis.
- Risk for infection related to bone marrow depression from therapy.

- Pain, acute or chronic, related to effects of tumor on body structures or cancer therapy.
- Impaired skin integrity related to surgical or radiation therapy.
- Disturbance in body image related to weight loss or hair loss.
- Risk for injury to patient, staff, and visitors related to exposure to a radioactive implant.
- Impaired physical mobility related to restricted activity secondary to a radioactive implant.
- Diarrhea related to effects of cancer treatment.
- Constipation related to effects of chemotherapy.
- Altered urinary elimination related to radiation therapy or secondary to effects of chemotherapy.
- Activity intolerance related to fatigue.
- Knowledge deficit related to drugs and side effects.
- Self-care deficit related to weakness and fatigue.
- Fear related to the possibility of dying.
- Ineffective individual coping related to denial of significance of cancer.
- Ineffective family coping related to inability to function as a result of anxiety over patient's prognosis.

◆ Planning

Specific expected outcomes are written for each nursing diagnosis chosen as appropriate for the patient. Examples are included in Nursing Care Plan 9-1. Planning is a collaborative process that includes the patient, the family, the physician, the oncologist, the nurse manager, the social worker, and other specialists on the health care team. The home care nurse, the infusion therapy company nurse, and the pharmacist often are involved in care and should be included in the planning process. The nurse manager usually is the one who consults with the others of the team and coordinates the plan of care.

◆ Implementation

Specific interventions are included in Nursing Care Plan 9-1 and in the following sections.

◆ Evaluation

Evaluation is based on determining whether the expected outcomes specified for the patient are being or have been met. Constant assessment for signs of complications, side effects of therapy, nutritional status, and pain status are necessary. The nursing care plan must be changed when the interventions initially chosen are not effective in meeting the desired outcomes. Collaboration with the patient and the other members of the

health care team is important to the success of care plan changes.

COMMON THERAPIES, PROBLEMS, AND NURSING CARE

There are three traditional modes of therapy for malignancies: *surgery, radiation, and chemotherapy. Hormone manipulation, immunotherapy with biological response modifiers, and bone marrow transplant are treatments combined with traditional therapies.* Photodynamic therapy is currently used for bladder cancer and is undergoing trials for lung, esophageal, laryngeal, breast, and other types of cancer.

Each of the modes of treatment may be used singly or in combination with one or more of the other methods available. For example, chemotherapy may be used as an **adjuvant** (assisting treatment) after surgical removal of a tumor. No one method is necessarily better or more effective than another except in regard to the location of the malignancy, its type and extent of spread, and the reaction of the tumor itself and the individual patient. The methods of treatment are chosen after due consideration of many factors and are prescribed with the best interest of the patient in mind.

◆ Surgery

Surgery may be performed to obtain a biopsy specimen; as prophylaxis, such as in the removal of the ovaries of a woman whose mother had ovarian cancer; to determine the effectiveness of therapy by looking to see whether the initial tumor is reduced in size; for palliation as in *debulking* (removing as much as possible) a tumor to prevent pressure on adjacent structures or obstruction of vessels or the gastrointestinal tract; or as an attempt at cure. Reconstructive surgery also is associated with cancer treatment. The woman who has lost a breast to mastectomy may have the breast reconstructed. Other extremely mutilating forms of cancer surgery require reconstructive procedures after the initial procedure. Flap grafts to the patient who underwent radical neck surgery for cancer of the throat is an example.

Surgical removal of a malignant growth is the oldest method of treatment. It works very well for tumors that are easily accessible. Adjacent tissues that may contain malignant cells also are excised. Regional lymph nodes often harbor malignant cells, and these can then travel to distant parts of the body and establish a new cancer site if not removed.

Newer surgical procedures and techniques have significantly reduced the need for extensive surgical removal of adjacent tissues and structures. Radical

Nursing Care Plan 9-1

Selected nursing diagnoses, goals/expected outcomes, nursing interventions, and evaluations for a patient receiving chemotherapy for cancer

Situation: Mr. Pole is receiving chemotherapy for leukemia. This is his third round of weekly intravenous treatments. His platelet count is down to 185,000; he has had difficulty eating as a result of mucositis and anorexia. He states that he is mildly nauseated most of the time. He is 15 pounds underweight.

Nursing Diagnosis	Goals/Expected Outcomes	Nursing Interventions	Evaluation
Risk for infection related to bone marrow suppression. SUPPORTING DATA Receiving chemotherapy drugs that suppress bone marrow.	Patient will remain free of infection.	Monitor WBCs (more susceptible to infection when <3,000 and granulocyte count is <2,000. Assess for signs of infection every shift. Teach good hygiene, mouth care, handwashing before meals and after using bathroom. Restrict visitors; allow no one to visit who has an infection. Use protective isolation techniques if needed. Encourage good nutrition and hydration. Give neupogen as ordered.	WBCs, 3,200; temp. 98.8°F; no signs of infection; visitors monitored; taking sufficient food and fluid; continue plan. Meeting outcome.
Risk for injury related to impaired blood clotting ability. SUPPORTING DATA Chemotherapy treatment lowers platelets and causes extended bleeding time.	Patient will not experience hemorrhage.	Monitor blood count; assess for bleeding of gums or bruising and bleeding into joints q shift. Observe for signs of bleeding: hematuria, melena, etc. Give stool softener as ordered to prevent straining at stool and bleeding. Refrain from needle sticks as much as possible. Do not take temperature rectally. Brush teeth with very soft brush or tooth sponge. Do not floss.	No signs of bleeding; platelet count 180,000; stool softener administered; BM soft; continue plan.
Alteration of nutrition (less than body requirements), related to nausea, vomiting, and mucositis.	Patient will verbalize relief from nausea. Patient will be able to eat with minimal discomfort. Patient will maintain present weight.	Keep room odor free; give mouth care before meals. Give ordered antiemetic before and during chemotherapy. Use distraction, meditation, relaxation techniques. Give small, frequent feedings. Assess mouth and mucous membranes q shift. Give meticulous mouth care every 2 hours. Give antiemetics on a regular schedule before and during chemotherapy treatment times. Encourage added calories in meals and food supplements between meals.	Mouth care: 7, 9, 11, 1, and 3 o'clock; antiemetic 45 min before meals; mucous membranes reddened, but intact; enriched shake between meals taken; has not vomited this shift; continue plan. Meeting outcomes.
Body image disturbance related to alopecia and weight loss. SUPPORTING DATA "I look awful; I don't want any visitors to see me."	Patient will adjust to new body image within 3 weeks as evidenced by verbalization.	Encourage him to maintain sense of humor. Use caps, head bandana, and eyebrow pencil, as needed; assure him that hair will eventually grow back. Encourage verbalization of feelings; focus on strengths. Establish and maintain trusting relationship. Assess spiritual needs; help patient achieve spiritual consolation. Encourage him to obtain clothing that fits.	Has not yet lost hair; checking on purchase of wig; family is bringing head scarfs; talking more about feelings regarding weight loss and appearance; continue plan.
Fear related to diagnosis of cancer. SUPPORTING DATA "Do you really think the treatment will cure my cancer?" "I'm afraid that I'll go through all this and it will just come back in a few months."	Patient will verbalize fears and develop coping mechanisms to decrease fear.	Encourage verbalization and identification of specific fears. Help him to explore ways to cope with fears. Assess spiritual needs; contact minister or other as patient desires. Offer support by active listening, offering hope in some form, and being there for patient. Encourage expression of fears to significant others.	Is verbalizing fears; encouraged to do same with family; used to meditate; encouraged to do so; began teaching imagery techniques; continue plan.

mastectomy, for example, involves removal of the entire breast along with underlying pectoral muscle tissues and lymph nodes under the arm on the affected side. This procedure has been replaced almost completely by a modified radical mastectomy, or lumpectomy, combined with radiation and/or chemotherapy, which is far less traumatic and mutilating. If there is no evidence of metastasis, some patients are good candidates for simple removal of the tumor (**lumpectomy**). The use of radiation during, after, and sometimes before, surgery has decreased the need for extensive removal of adjacent tissues and decreased recurrence.

Laser surgery is an alternative to hysterectomy or conization for the treatment of preinvasive cancer of the cervix. The laser beam vaporizes the water of malignant cells and thus destroys them. The beam provides pinpoint precision for removing diseased tissue, thus saving healthy cells from damage. It is accompanied by minimal bleeding because the laser beam coagulates blood vessels and lymphatics. There also is the advantage of greatly reduced risk for infection, because there is no danger of introducing infectious organisms into the operative site and any bacteria or viruses that might be present are destroyed by the beam. Lasers are used extensively for a variety of types of cancer surgery today.

Surgery of the breast and uterus is discussed in more detail in Chapter 26. Nursing care for patients who have surgical procedures as treatment for malignant growths is discussed throughout this text.

◆ Radiation Therapy

The source for radiation therapy (RT) is either a linear accelerator or a radioactive element or substance. The purpose of radiation is to destroy malignant cells (which are more sensitive to radiation than are normal cells) without permanent damage to adjacent body tissues.

Ionizing radiation can have both an immediate and a delayed effect on malignant cells. It can damage the cell membrane immediately, causing lysis or decomposition of the cell, or it can cause a break in both strands of the DNA in the cell's nucleus. **When a cell is damaged in this way, it will not die until it attempts to divide and replicate itself. The rate at which a particular kind of cell undergoes mitosis determines whether the effects of radiation will occur in a matter of days, months, or years.** This explains the delayed effects and side effects of radiation that might not be evident at the time of treatment but appear later. Normal cells have a greater ability to repair the DNA damage than malignant cells. Some tissues are more sensitive to radiation than others, and this is taken into account when the physicist-physician calculates the dose of radiation needed to eradicate the tumor. The other factors considered are the sensitivity of the tumor to radiation, its location, and its size. The dose once

calculated is fractionalized, meaning it is divided over many days, to deliver the optimum dosage with the least amount of effects to normal tissues. The course of radiation is spread over a period of days to weeks. The *rad*, or *radiation absorbed dose*, is the unit used for measuring dosages of radiation.

Teletherapy and brachytherapy are the two types of radiation delivery for use to treat cancer. Teletherapy is *external*, in which the source of radiation is outside the patient. Bradytherapy is *internal*, in which the source of radiation is a radioactive element or substance that has been implanted or injected into the body.

Because of improvements in tumor localization, beam direction, megavoltage machines, planning and prescribing the field to be irradiated, and determining the precise dosage needed, radiation therapy is far more beneficial and less harmful than it was when it was first pioneered. With the linear accelerator, the damage to normal tissue can be minimized by keeping the dosage or degree of penetration accurate and by aiming the rays from several different angles. The latter technique increases the concentration of the rays in the area of the tumor with a minimum of damage to overlying tissues. Cobalt-60 machines deliver gamma rays and are much more efficient and precise than in the early years of radiation therapy.

External Radiation Therapy   The linear accelerator (Figure 9-2) used for external radiation therapy produces a voltage many times higher than machines used for diagnostic purposes. It produces extremely high energy x-ray and electron beam irradiation that bombards the malignant cells and destroys them. Because malignant cells are dividing at an abnormally high rate, they are more susceptible to destruction than are normal cells.

Modern radiation therapy has improved immensely since the mid-1980s. The use of computers in planning accurate radiation dosage and projectory distributions has decreased the side effects considerably. The use of stereotaxic surgery and the gamma knife (an energy source using gamma rays) is effective for small brain tumors, and research is in progress for other applications. Gamma knife treatment is essentially noninvasive radiosurgery in which the tumor is destroyed by radiation.

Many cancer research institutions have lead-lined surgical suites where radiation therapy is delivered directly to the affected area after tumor removal and before the incision is closed. Depending on the dosage (rads) given, the patient may not need to receive further postsurgical radiation. This method has proven most beneficial for patients with operable pancreatic cancer.

Nursing care of patients undergoing external radiation therapy.   Nursing care goals related to radiation therapy for cancer include (1) helping the

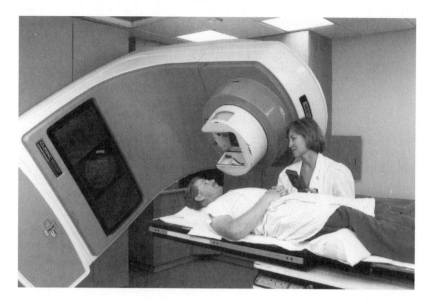

FIGURE 9-2   Linear accelerator used to deliver ionizing radiation to a brain tumor. (Photo by Glen Derbyshire; courtesy of the Cancer Foundation, Santa Barbara, CA.)

patient and family or significant others cope with the diagnosis of cancer and its treatment with radiation therapy; and (2) teaching the patient and significant others how to recognize and manage the expected side effects of radiation.

Helping patients cope with radiation therapy for cancer.   A lack of knowledge about the side effects of radiation and how to cope with them can greatly add to the anxiety and stress that the patient feels. It is not unusual for a layperson to have some misconceptions about how radiation works, whether a patient can present a hazard to others while undergoing treatment, when he will begin to experience its effects, and how long it will be before he begins to recover from them.

Before the first treatment the patient is told what therapeutic effects are anticipated, what it is like to have a treatment, and what is expected of him during the course of therapy. Because the patient will probably be treated on an outpatient basis, he should be encouraged to keep his scheduled appointments and notify the clinic if cancellation is necessary. Assurance that the source of radiation is in the machine only and that it is not possible to "contaminate" others with radioactivity should be provided. Someone should accompany the patient for initial treatments, preferably a family member or a close and trusted friend, who can provide emotional support. It is essential that time be set aside for the nurse to establish a trusting relationship with the patient, to prompt and answer any questions about therapy, and to provide an avenue for communication throughout the course of treatment.

Skin care during radiation treatment.   With the linear accelerator and computerized delivery of radiation, there is a lot less trauma to the skin from radiation therapy than in former years. The patient

should understand that should skin damage occur, it is usually only temporary.

In preparation for radiation therapy the physician will outline the area to be exposed to radiation by marking it with indelible ink. The exposed area will need special care. Most clinics and hospitals have written procedures and precautions to be used to avoid unnecessary trauma to the exposed areas of skin.

In general, the area is not washed with soap any more than absolutely necessary throughout the course of treatments. When the area is cleansed, a mild unscented soap and tepid water are used. Only the hand is used, rather than a wash cloth. The area is gently patted dry with a clean, soft, towel; it is never rubbed. Alcohol, lotions, and salves must not be used, unless prescribed by the physician, as they either dry out the skin or magnify any radiation damage.

The patient should be instructed to avoid lying on the area as much as possible and to avoid wearing tight clothing over it. Only 100% cotton clothing should be worn over the area. He also should avoid exposing it to sunlight and extremes of cold as well as heat, including hot shower water. Men receiving radiation to the head and neck should not shave, or if they must, an electric razor should be used. Should an area of damaged skin begin weeping, it should be cleansed with plain lukewarm water or saline, and a polyethylene film or Vigilon dressing should be applied. Such dressings are removed before the next radiation treatment and then reapplied.

Although skin damage is rare now, the degree of reaction of the skin to radiation is individual and should be assessed daily, either by the patient or some knowledgeable person. In some patients, there may be a reddened area resembling a sunburn about 3 weeks after the first treatment, and the area may be swollen from water in the tissue. Later, the skin may appear dry, scaly, turn plum-colored, and might begin to crack. Most of the time all that is necessary is to protect the skin from further injury and allow it to heal once the course of radiation is completed. If sweat glands are permanently damaged, the skin may remain dry.

Radiation to the chest or upper back may cause pneumonitis. Humidifying the air, maintaining an adequate fluid intake, and carrying out coughing and deep breathing exercises daily can help minimize this problem.

Teaching the patient and significant others how to recognize expected side effects and take an active part in their management is particularly important when the patient is not hospitalized. He will feel less helpless and more in control if he is able to participate in assessing his condition and planning and implementing his care at home. It is unfair to expect either the patient or his significant others to remember everything they are told about his care. Therefore it is essential that they have some written information to refer to once they leave the clinic. They also should be encouraged to write down any questions they might have before the next visit or note any points on which they feel they need more information.

In general, most side effects will not begin before about 3 weeks after the first treatment. This will allow the patient time to assimilate the information given to him and to adjust to whatever changes he might experience. The side effects usually continue throughout the course of therapy and begin to subside about 14 days after treatments end.

Think about . . . Can you list the points to be covered for care of the skin when teaching the patient who is to undergo external radiation therapy?

Internal Radiation Therapy   Radiation from *radioactive elements* has the same ionizing effect as that from linear accelerators; the only difference is the source of radiation. An element that is radioactive is unstable; that is, the nuclei of its atoms decompose naturally and in the process they emit radiant energy. Some elements, such as radium and uranium, are naturally unstable and therefore radioactive. These elements are used as sealed implants. Other elements such as cobalt and iodine can be made unstable by being bombarded with high-energy particles in a nuclear reactor.

Internal radiation therapy involves introducing a radioactive element into the body. The material may be administered in different ways: (1) it can be placed in a *sealed* container and inserted into a body cavity at the site of the tumor or placed directly into the tumor; or (2) it may be administered in an *unsealed* form and taken orally or injected by syringe.

To be effective the radiation source must come into direct contact with the tumor tissue for a specified time. Most implants emit a lower level of radiation than is effective because it is in constant contact with the tumor cells. **Because the radiation source is within the patient, radiation is emitted for a period and can be a hazard to others.**

Not all elements that have been made radioactive by artificial means stay radioactive for very long periods. As soon as an element becomes radioactive, it begins to lose its characteristic of radioactivity. The rate at which it becomes less radioactive is called its *half-life,* which is the amount of time it takes for half of its radioactivity to dissipate. The half-life of radium is about 1,600 years, whereas the half-life of iodine is only about 8 days. It is important that the nurse caring for a patient receiving sealed or unsealed sources of radiation know the element used, its half-life, and the ways in which it might be eliminated from the body. Cesium is a radioactive element frequently used to treat malignancies of the mouth, tongue, vagina, and uterine cervix.

Some isotopes are given orally and others are administered into a body cavity. The isotopes are unsealed sources of radiation. If radioactivity is a hazard, it is only a problem only for the duration of the half-life of the isotope. The substance is eliminated through body secretions such as sweat, sputum, vomitus, urine, or feces. Examples of unsealed sources include iodine 131, which is in a solution and is swallowed by the patient, phosphorus 32, and gold 198, which is administered by injection. Radioactive iodine is useful in the treatment of thyroid malignancies because that gland readily takes up iodine. Thus the radioactive element is delivered to the site of the tumor, where it can be more effective. The major hazard from radioactive iodine is in the patient's urine; therefore special precautions must be taken according to hospital policy. **The nurse must know the half-life of the isotope given to plan appropriate safety precautions. Hospital policies and procedures must be followed when caring for a patient receiving an unsealed source of radiation.**

Nursing care of patients receiving internal radiation. Patients who are treated by internal sources of radiation can be a source of radioactivity. Those who are in close contact with them must therefore take special precautions to protect themselves against unnecessary radiation. Radioactivity is a frightening phenomenon to most people because they do not fully understand it and are misinformed about how it affects the body.

It is important that the nurse know whether the radioactive element is sealed and inserted into the body to remain for a certain time or if it is an unsealed source that may be eliminated through body secretions and excreta. Unsealed sources usually have a very short half-life, which means they are not radioactive for as long as sealed sources are.

Principles of Radiation Protection

In general, the amount of radiation a nurse might receive while caring for a patient being treated with internal radioactive elements depends on three factors: (1) the distance between the nurse and the patient; (2) the amount of time spent in actual proximity to the patient; and (3) the degree of shielding provided.

Distance is an important factor in reducing exposure to radiation. Doubling one's distance from a radioactive element, reduces the exposure to one fourth, and tripling the distance reduces it to one ninth (Figure 9-3).

Time spent near the source of radiation can be controlled by the nurse who plans her nursing care carefully so that she can spend less time with the patient without sacrificing the quality of care given.

Shielding from radiation exposure must take into account the type of rays being emitted. The denser the

shielding material, the less the possibility of penetration by the rays and the better the protection. A lead shield that is 1 cm thick offers the same amount of protection as 5 cm of concrete or 30 cm of wood. Lead aprons give protection from diagnostic x-rays, but do not provide adequate shielding from the *gamma rays* emitted by radium, cesium 137, and cobalt 60. Anyone coming into contact with or in proximity to a source of radiation should wear a radiation dosimeter badge (Figure 9-4). This badge measures the exposure to radiation the individual has received.

Hospitals where sealed sources of radiation are implanted into the body tissues to treat malignancies usually have written policies and procedures to guide personnel who are responsible for patient care. The precautionary measures listed cover general areas of concern:

◆ Place the patient in a private room.
◆ Place a sign on the patient's door indicating that the patient is receiving internal radiation therapy.
◆ Observe principles of time and distance. Limit time spent in the room. Work as quickly and as efficiently

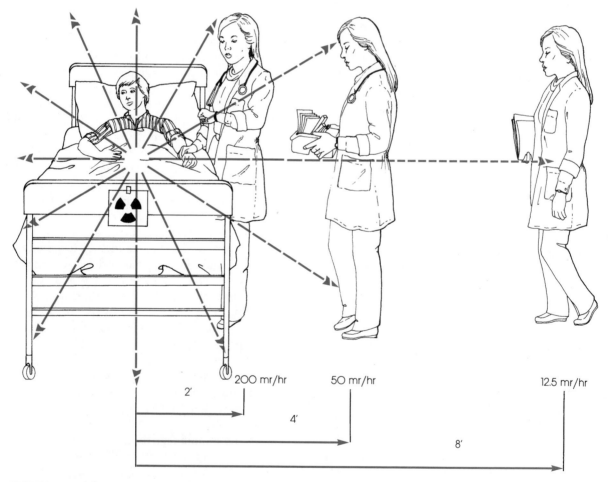

FIGURE 9-3 The nurse nearest the source of radioactivity (the patient) is more exposed; at 2 feet, exposure is more than 15 times that at 8 feet.

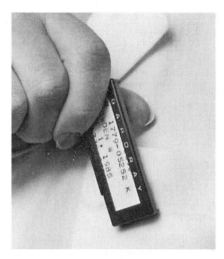

FIGURE 9-4   Badge worn by personnel who might be exposed to radiation. (Photo by Ken Kasper.)

as possible. Avoid standing near the part of the patient's body where the radioactive element is located; stand at the shoulders or the feet depending where the implant is located.

◆ Check all linens, bedpans, and emesis basins routinely to see if the sealed source has been accidentally lost from the tissue.

◆ If a sealed source is dislodged, but has not fallen out of the patient's body, notify the x-ray radiation department at once. If the source has fallen out, *do not pick it up with your bare hands.* Use forceps and place it in a lead container.

◆ Most patients are placed on bed rest and instructed to remain in certain positions so that emanations from the element will reach the correct area.

◆ Visitors will spend limited time in the room.

After the physician removes the source, the patient is no longer in need of special precautionary care. Special observations are necessary, however, in the event a systemic reaction develops.

Some special precautions that should be observed when caring for a patient receiving internal radiation therapy from an unsealed source are:

◆ Observe the principles of time, distance, and shielding for radiation protection.

◆ Wear gloves when handling bedpans, bed linens, and patient's clothes.

◆ Dispose of urine, feces, and vomitus according to policy.

◆ Handle dressings with forceps, and dispose of them according to policy.

◆ Follow hospital procedure for disposal of patient's bed linens and clothing.

Table 9-6 shows the side effects most commonly experienced by patients undergoing radiation therapy. Appropriate nursing care is presented following this section on therapies for cancer treatment.

Think about . . . Can you identify measures you would take to provide psychosocial care for the patient restricted to bedrest with a sealed cervical implant?

◆ Chemotherapy

The oncologist has a wide variety of drugs from which to choose when planning a course of treatment for a patient with cancer. He may choose to give a particular drug alone or in combination with other drugs. Chemotherapy may be used with other forms of therapy, for example, following surgery and before, during, or after radiation treatments, or with immunotherapy.

Among the drugs used to treat malignancies are the *antineoplastic* agents (Table 9-7). **The overall effect of antineoplastic drugs is to decrease the number of malignant cells in a generalized malignancy, such as leukemia, or to reduce the size of a localized tumor and**

TABLE 9-6 ◆ *Common Side Effects of Radiation Therapy*	
Type and Area	**Effect**
External radiation	
Head and neck	Irritaiton of oral mucous membranes with oral pain and risk of infection. Loss of taste. Irritation of the pharynx and esophagus with nausea and indigestion. Increased intracranial pressure.
Chest	Inflammation of lung tissue with increased susceptibility to infection.
Abdomen Pelvis	Nausea, vomiting, diarrhea, anorexia. Diarrhea. Cystitis. Sexual dysfunction. Urethral and rectal stenosis.
General side effects	*Skin:* change in texture and/or color; moist desquamation (rare); alopecia. *Blood:* bone marrow depression with leukopenia, anemia, and thrombocytopenia. Depressed immune function. Fatigue.
Internal radiation	
General effects	Elevated temperature. *Cervical implant:* urinary frequency, diarrhea, nausea, vomiting, anorexia. *Head and neck implant:* mucositis, oral pain and risk of infection, anorexia.

TABLE 9-7 ◆ *Common Antineoplastic Drug Classes, Their Action, and Major Side Effects*

Classification and Examples	Action	Major Side Effects*
Alkylating agents Cyclophasphamide Cisplatin Mechlorethamine Busulfan Chlorambucil Carmustine Melphalan Carmustine Streptozocin Lomustine Triehylene thiophosphoramide	Attach "alkyl groups" or organic side chains to the proteins in the cell, poisoning it; inhibit cell division.	**Bone marrow depression, nephrotoxicity, with some.** Nausea, vomiting, diarrhea, dermatitis; hyperpigmentation. Cisplatin: **Hearing loss.**
Antimetabolites Methotrexate 6 Mercaptopurine 6 Thioguanine 5 Fluorouracil FUDR Cytosine Arabinoside	Interfere with a specific cell phase, thereby preventing replication. Some inhibit enzymes that make essential cellular constituents; others attach to DNA interfering with replication.	**Bone marrow depression, stomatitis,** intestinal ulceration, nausea, vomiting, diarrhea.
Antitumor antibiotics Bleomycin Dactinomycin Doxorubicin Daunorubicin Mithramycin Mitomycin-C Mitoxantrone	Injure cells by direct interaction with DNA, causing distortion. Interfere with DNA or RNA synthesis.	**Bone marrow depression,** some cause cardiotoxicity; stomatitis, alopecia. Bleomycin causes pneumonitis and pulmonary fibrosis.
Mitotic inhibitors Vincristine Vinblastine Vindesine Etoposide	Interfere with mitosis. Act during M phase of cell cycle to prevent cell division.	Vincristine: **peripheral neuropathy, constipation.** Vinblastine: **bone marrow depression**
Miscellaneous agents Altretamine Asparaginase Dacarbazine Etoposide Hydroxyurea Procarbazine Mitotane Teniposide Paclitaxel	These drugs work in a variety of ways; consult information for each drug.	**Bone marrow depression is the major side effect of all except Asparaginase and Mitotane.** Asparaginase: pancreatic dysfunction. Mitotane: central nervous system depression. Paclitaxel: peripheral neuropathy.

*Each drug has specific side effects. Consult information regarding each individual drug before administration.

thereby lessen the severity of symptoms. Antineoplastic drugs are **cytotoxic** (poisonous to cells), and their damaging effects are not limited to malignant cells. However, normal cells do not reproduce in exactly the same way as malignant cells and are able to repair themselves more rapidly and effectively. Steroids often are used in combination with antineoplastic drugs for cancer treatment.

Drugs are combined to treat certain types of cancers because different drugs are effective at different times in the growth and replication cycle of the tumor cell. This method offers the best chance of killing the most malignant cells. Chemotherapy is the preferred treatment for various kinds of leukemias, some lymphomas, multiple myeloma, and many types of tumors resulting from metastasis.

Techniques of administration of antineoplastic agents include intraarterial, intraperitoneal, intraventricular, and intrathecal as well as intravenous infusion. Cancers of the liver, ovary, and brain have sometimes shown better remission with intraventricular or intraperitoneal infusion treatment. An advance in chemotherapy has been the use of lower doses of multiple drugs to treat various types of malignancies. Because side effects are lessened when lower doses of a drug are used, several drugs can be used in combination to hit all phases of the cell cycle, destroying more malignant cells.

Often a central line or implanted injection port is used to administer chemotherapy drugs that are to be given over several weeks or months (Figures 9-5 and 9-6). The nurse cares for the central line and its insertion site according to hospital policy using strict aseptic technique.

Many antineoplastic drugs are **vesicants** (chemicals causing tissue damage upon direct contact) that can cause severe local injury if they escape from the vein into which they are administered. Administration should be only into veins that have good blood flow. If extravasation occurs, the infusion is stopped immediately. The

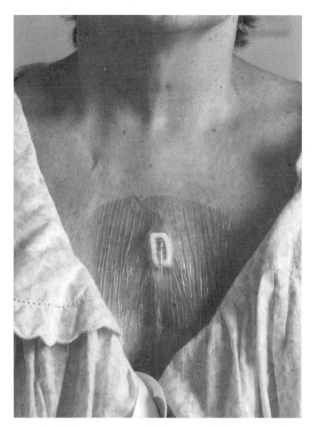

FIGURE 9-6   Implanted infusion port for administration of chemotherapy drugs or continuous morphine drip. (Photo by Glen Derbyshire; courtesy of Leigh Block Hospice and Santa Barbara Visiting Nurse Association.)

type of treatment required depends on the drug that extravasated and the amount that escaped into the tissue. **Consult the pharmacist, the policy and procedure manual, and the physician should extravasation occur.**

Some antineoplastic have toxic effects that must be monitored. Table 9-8 presents the assessments necessary to detect various types of organ toxicity. A new drug, dexrazoxane (Zinecard), appears to be heart protective for patients receiving the cardiotoxic drug doxorubicin (Adriamycin). If a drug is toxic to the reproductive system, the patient should make a decision about banking sperm or eggs before beginning chemotherapy.

Nursing Care of Patients Receiving Chemotherapy

Nursing management of the patient receiving chemotherapy requires special knowledge and skills beyond those of basic nursing. The nurse oncologist is a specialist who is able to give comprehensive nursing care because of years of study and experience. A full discussion of care of the patient receiving chemotherapy is therefore beyond the scope of this text. There are, however, some general principles that can be helpful to

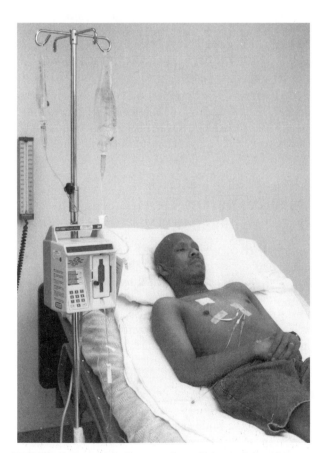

FIGURE 9-5   Patient in outpatient clinic receiving chemotherapy through a central line. (Photo by Glen Derbyshire; courtesy of the Cancer Foundation, Santa Barbara, CA.)

TABLE 9-8 ◆ *Assessment for Toxic Effects of Chemotherapy**	
Side Effect	**Intervention**
Bone marrow suppression	Monitor red and white blood cell count and differential count for numbers of neutrophils and granulocytes; check platelet count.
Cardiotoxicity	Monitor for signs of congestive heart failure, such as pulmonary crackles, shortness of breath, tachycardia, weight gain, and peripheral edema. Monitor EKG.
Neurotoxicity	Monitor for weakness, paresthesias, sensory loss (particularly in feet), and decreased reflexes. Constipation and urinary heistancy are other signs.
Pulmonary toxicity	Evidenced by pulmonary infiltrates and pulmonary fibrosis on x-ray. Monitor respiratory status closely; auscultate for decreased breath sounds and for crackles.
Hepatotoxicity	Monitor liver function tests: AST, ALT, bilirubin.
Nephrotoxicity	Monitor kidney function tests: creatinine and blood urea nitrogen; monitor urine output.
Ototoxicity	Monitor for tinnitus or hearing loss.

*Many antineoplastic drugs are toxic to various organs of the body. Whenever a specific drug has one of the following toxicities, include the specific assessment parameters for that toxicity in your regular assessment.

the nurse who encounters a patient receiving a course of chemotherapy for cancer or experiencing some of the toxic side effects of antineoplastic drugs.

Not all neoplastic drugs produce every toxic side effect, and the oncologist plans therapy so that destruction of malignant cells is maximized and toxicity is kept at a minimum. **The toxicity associated with chemotherapy is most evident in the cells of the body that have a short life span and must continuously reproduce to provide the body with the normal cells it needs. These include the blood cells, hair follicles, and epithelial cells of the mucous membranes lining the digestive tract.**

The more common side effects of chemotherapy and their implications for nursing are summarized in Table 9-7 (p. 224). Some of the side effects of chemotherapy are similar to the expected effects of radiation. Although the causes of the problems are different, assessment of the patient and symptomatic relief mea-

sures are the same. Nursing interventions for selected problems in a patient receiving chemotherapy for cancer are summarized in Nursing Care Plan 9-1 (see p. 218).

◆ Hormone Therapy

Hormone therapy is used as an adjunct to other types of cancer therapy. It can slow tumor growth or prevent recurrence. When a hormone is added to the body, it alters the balance of naturally produced hormones. **Giving large amounts of one hormone prevents the uptake of other hormones. So if the tumor growth is aided by one type of hormone, giving another type prevents the uptake of the growth-promoting hormone and slows the progress of the tumor.** Tamoxifen used against certain types of breast cancer is an example.

Side effects of hormonal therapy depend on the type of hormone used. Androgens and antiestrogen receptor drugs produce masculinizing effects, such as facial and chest hair. Menses may stop and breast tissue will shrink. These drugs cause fluid retention in women. Acne is another side effect of the androgens. Hypercalcemia and liver dysfunction can occur with prolonged therapy. Women taking estrogens and progestins have irregular, heavy menses, fluid retention, and tenderness of the breasts. These drugs increase the risk for thrombus formation in both men and women. In men taking the estrogens or progestins to combat prostate cancer, there is a feminizing effect with decreased facial hair, a redistribution of body fat, breast development (**gynecomastia**), and smoothing of the facial skin. Over time, some testicular and penile atrophy may occur, and it may become more difficult to attain and maintain an erection.

◆ Immunotherapy Using Biological Response Modifiers

Biological response modifiers (BRMs) are agents that manipulate the immune system in hopes of controlling or curing a malignancy with little or no toxic effect on normal cells. These agents either stimulate or suppress immune activity. The BMRs are cytokines, which are small, protein hormones manufactured by the various leukocytes. They essentially make the immune system function better. BMRs stimulate the immune system to recognize cancer cells and to institute action to destroy them. Some BMRs, such as colony-stimulating factor (CSF), work by enhancing a quicker recovery of the bone marrow after radiation or chemotherapy. CSF stimulates bone marrow to function more quickly. Neumega, a drug that stimulates thrombocyte (platelet) production, looks as if it will soon receive FDA approval. Two competing drugs for this purpose may be available soon. These drugs are used to decrease the bleeding tendencies induced by chemotherapy and could help create new chemotherapy protocols that are more effective against cancer cells possible.

There are two types of BMRs used to fight cancer: interleukins and interferons. **Interleukins help the immune system cells recognize and destroy abnormal cells. Interferons slow down cell division in cancer cells, stimulate natural killer cells, inhibit expression of oncogenes, and assist cancerous cells to revert back to more normal cells.** Both interleukins and interferons are manufactured using recombinant DNA technology. Interleukins are undergoing clinical trials on patients with melanoma, renal cell carcinoma, and colorectal cancer. Alpha-2b, an interferon, is used mainly against hairy cell leukemia, but it has been somewhat effective to treat ovarian cancer, renal cell cancer, and cutaneous T-cell lymphoma. Both interleukins and interferons are very expensive to manufacture.

A second group of BMRs includes monoclonal antibodies and tumor necrosis factor (TNF), both of which have direct antitumor effects. Genetic engineering techniques can produce the monoclonal antibodies, and thus this form of therapy holds much promise for the future. A new antibody, HER-2/neu, is undergoing research trials now as a treatment for metastatic breast cancer. One advantage of the therapy is that, other than mild fever, which occurs in 5% to 10% of patients, there are no known side effects. Another BRM, Liposomal MTP-PE, shows promise in treating osteosarcoma. Testing is in combination with multiagent chemotherapeutic drugs to determine if it influences recurrence rates. It can be administered safely in the outpatient setting.

The third group contains miscellaneous agents that have different functions. Some stimulate undifferentiated cells into maturing so that they can be more easily killed; others prevent metastasis.

All the BRMs are undergoing clinical trials to determine effectiveness on various types of malignancies. They are not without side effects, but the most common side effects are fatigue and flu-like symptoms, such as fever, chills, muscle aches, and headache, that are much less life-threatening than some of the side effects of chemotherapy.

◆ Bone Marrow Transplant

Bone marrow transplant (BMT) is mainly used to correct the severe bone marrow damage caused by chemotherapy or radiation. Sometimes whole-body irradiation is used to treat a hematopoietic cancer such as leukemia or Hodgkin's disease. Irradiation of this sort totally incapacitates the body's bone marrow and the patient would die if blood cells could not again be manufactured. BMT is discussed in Chapter 17.

◆ Photodynamic Therapy

Photodynamic therapy (PDT) is currently used for bladder cancer. A photosensitizing agent is given intravenously. This agent concentrates in the tumor tissue, and then a laser beam is used to destroy the cells. The tumor cells are much more sensitive to this light source than normal tissue and therefore can be sought out and destroyed. Clinical trials are in progress to treat lung, esophageal, brain, skin, gynecological cancers and Kaposi's sarcoma common to AIDS patients. The great advantage of PDT is that it selectively destroys malignant cells without toxicity to normal cells or long-term side effects.

◆ Gene Therapy

As research reveals the genes thought to be responsible for various types of cancers, the possibility of gene splicing or replacement becomes a reality. Genetic engineering is still in its infancy, but many scientists are hard at work hoping to make it a reality for cancer patients. The gene $BRCA_1$ is implicated in approximately half of the cases of familial breast and ovarian cancer. Research has shown that when healthy $BRCA_1$ genes are injected into mice who have faulty $BRCA_1$ genes, tumor growth is slowed. This has proven true for other genes implicated in other types of cancer. People with an inherited defect of the MSH_2 gene have a 70% to 90% chance of developing colon or rectal cancer. Women with the defective gene have a 60% to 85% chance of developing uterine or ovarian cancer as well. A defect in gene DPC_4 has been implicated in pancreatic cancer, but it is not yet known whether this is an acquired or inherited defect. Knowing that some people have this increased risk could help save their lives by intensifying cancer screening to detect such malignancies early. Someday gene therapy may be the major treatment for cancer.

◆ Evaluating the Effectiveness of Medical Treatment

The oncologist conducts an ongoing evaluation of each patient's status to determine how effective the prescribed treatment has been and to plan for a future course of therapy should it be needed. It is particularly important to know whether there has been a reduction in the size of the tumor and an abatement of the patient's symptoms. This is the purpose of "second-look surgery."

A test for monitoring the effectiveness of treatment is a measurement of carcinoembryonic antigen (CEA) levels. This particular antigen is a glycoprotein that is produced during fetal life but is not normally present after birth. Its production may resume again, however, and CEA levels can be increased by some kinds of liver disease, heavy cigarette smoking, and benign and malignant tumors. Because of the many and diverse conditions that can elevate CEA levels, the test cannot be used to diagnose cancer. However, it can be used to evaluate the effectiveness of treatment, because CEA levels usually fall to within the normal range about 1 month after successful treatment of cancer. A serum CEA level higher than normal prior to treatment and that remains elevated after treatment suggests that there are malignant cells remaining in the body. The PSA blood test is utilized to track the success of treatment and possible recurrence of prostate cancer.

◆ Common Problems Related to Cancer or Cancer Therapy

The problems that occur in the cancer patient are complex and depend on both the location and type of cancer and the therapy used to treat it. A discussion of the most common problems and the related nursing care is presented here.

Anorexia, Mucositis, and Weight Loss   **Many cancer patients experience an alteration in taste.** Often the first thing noticed is that red meat does not taste good. The taste of sweets also is altered. **Anorexia** (loss of appetite) often is associated with changes in taste and with inflammation of the mouth and tongue, which can cause the patient great difficulty in eating and drinking. The loss of appetite can quickly lead to deficiencies of protein and calories. **The patient with anorexia can experience a significant weight loss (2 or more pounds per week) and suffer from severe malnutrition.** A thorough routine for mouth care to minimize damage and anorexia should be started several days before the beginning of chemotherapy or radiation therapy to the head and neck. Radiation to the head or neck will produce some inflammatory changes in the mouth and often also in the pharynx and esophagus. Measures to combat this expected reaction include frequent oral intake of liquids that are not irritating chemically; the use of artificial saliva; and frequent and consistent mouth care.

Patients are encouraged to drink water as often as they can to help alleviate the discomfort of dryness of the mouth and tongue. The patient should drink water or rinse the mouth every hour while awake. Extra water also helps the body eliminate the debris from destroyed cells. However, drinking water will not completely resolve the problem. Artificial salivas combat mouth dryness in a different way and help keep the mucous membranes soft and moist. They also help buffer the acidity in the mouth and thus reduce irritation of the oral mucosa. They are available in the form of a spray and can be used by the patient as often as desired. If artificial salivas cannot be found at a local pharmacy, they can be obtained from any one of the following pharmaceutical companies: Kingswood Laboratories, Inc., Westport Pharmaceutical, Inc., and First Texas Pharmaceuticals, Inc.

The patient undergoing chemotherapy may experience **mucositis** (irritation and inflammation of the mucosa) in the mouth. A major goal of mouth care, other than protection of the mucosa, is preservation of the teeth and prevention of infections of the gums. To accomplish this, the patient should be encouraged to accept as much responsibility as he can for frequent and consistent oral hygiene. He probably will need to be taught how to brush his teeth using a soft brush or tooth sponges (toothettes) and gentle strokes. He also should be taught how to irrigate his mouth to remove debris and counteract acidity. The solutions most often used for this are normal saline, mild solutions of peroxide (1:5 ratio), or a bicarbonate of soda solution and salt solution (1/4 to 1/2 tsp of baking soda and 1/8 to 1/4 tsp salt in an 8-oz glass of water). A few drops of mouth wash may be added to improve taste. Commercial mouth washes are not necessary and can be chemically irritating and drying. Fluid intake must be increased to 3,000 mL per day. Because of the risk of infection, toothbrushes should be rinsed with a bleach solution or hydrogen peroxide and then rinsed with water before reuse. Running them through the dishwasher is another option.

The mouth is inspected daily for white patches, sores, redness, or a "funny feeling" in the mouth. Mouth washes are used either every 2 hours or four times a day. Lemon-glycerine swabs are to be avoided as they are drying to the mucosa.

Relief of the mouth pain of mucositis or stomatitis is provided by special topical compounds, such as Xylocaine Viscous, that are "swished and spit." Such compounds contain a topical anesthetic and an antiinflammatory agent. **The patient is instructed not to swallow this solution.** The patient should avoid spicy foods, alcohol, and tobacco.

The metabolic demand of malignant growth, anorexia, and mucositis that makes eating difficult all contribute to weight loss. Weight loss also can occur in cancer patients because of disturbances in their metabolism in which the body metabolizes its own proteins for energy instead of using the carbohydrates available in the diet or in body fat. The body has to work hard to repair normal cells after cancer treatment.

Initially, the patient's current weight should be noted and recorded and compared with his ideal weight. His protein intake should be increased to compensate for the fact that cancer patients often metabolize their own tissues for energy, even though glucose may be readily available in the blood. Small, frequent feedings, attention to preferences for foods, and a pleasant and restful environment during meals are often helpful. Supplemental feedings to provide additional protein and calories can help avoid excessive weight loss and protein deficiency. These taste better if they are served in glass or plastic rather than out of a metal container. Table 9-9 shows a sampling of commonly used supplemental feedings. The American Cancer Society has patient pamphlets available on ways to increase nutritional intake.

Nausea, Vomiting, and Diarrhea   Radiation therapy of the abdomen or lower back often produces nausea, vomiting, and diarrhea starting 7 to 10 days after the beginning of treatment. Various antineoplastic drugs also can produce these side effects. Antiemetic agents are started about 12 hours prior to doses of chemotherapy and continued for 24 hours afterward at 4- to 6-hour intervals. Antiemetics are used for nausea and vomiting resulting from radiation therapy as well. A new class of antiemetics, serotonin antagonists, acts on the chemoreceptor trigger zone for vomiting and have proven very beneficial to the chemotherapy patient. Ondansetron (Zofran) is working for previously resistant chemotherapy-induced nausea and vomiting.

Eating before treatment seems to decrease nausea. Eating toast or crackers before arising or engaging in activity during periods of nausea may decrease vomiting. Liquids, liquid supplements, or easily digested foods are given at 3- to 4-hour intervals in small amounts. Foods and liquids should be high protein, high calorie, bland, lukewarm, and to the patient's taste. Meals should be eaten slowly and food chewed thoroughly. Carbonated drinks or tea are tolerated better than other liquids, but should be taken 1 hour before or after meals, not with meals. It is best not to lie down for at least 2 hours after a meal. Caffeine and rich or fatty foods should be avoided for 24 hours before and 72 hours after chemotherapy. The patient's environment should be free of bothersome smells, sights, or sounds. If food odor is nauseating, consider serving cold meals. Chewing gum or sucking on hard or sour candy, or ice, helps reduce nausea in some patients. Nursing care involves providing comfort measures and mouth care. Guided imagery and progressive muscle relaxation helps reduce anxiety and provides some relief from nausea. If nausea strikes, breathing slowly and deeply through the mouth may prevent vomiting. The patient is monitored for dehydration and electrolyte imbalances when excessive vomiting occurs.

Diarrhea may occur from radiation to the abdomen, lower back, or pelvis. Many of the chemotherapy drugs cause diarrhea because they affect the cells of the intestinal mucosa causing inflammation. Treatment involves avoiding high-fiber foods that encourage rapid evacuation from the bowel and adding low-fiber foods such as bananas and cheese to the diet. Cleansing the rectal area and applying petroleum jelly, A&D ointment, or Desitin cream helps decrease discomfort and protects the skin from breakdown. The physician may prescribe a medication to decrease the number and frequency of bowel movements. The nurse must monitor the patient for signs of dehydration and electrolyte imbalance.

Constipation   Certain antineoplastic drugs, such as oncovine, vinblastine, and vindesine, cause constipation. Increasing fluids, as allowed, adding fiber to the diet, administering stool softeners and fiber laxatives, and monitoring vigilantly for the beginning signs of constipation are the usual measures taken. Suppositories or enemas may be necessary. Drug-induced constipation should be treated vigorously at the first signs to avoid fecal impaction.

Cystitis   Cytoxan and infosfamide may cause cystitis. The nurse monitors for hesitancy, urgency, and pain on urination. The urine is checked for cloudiness and signs of **hematuria** (blood in the urine). Fluids are increased to 2 to 3 L a day. The patient is encouraged to empty the bladder frequently. The antineoplastic drug is administered in the morning and/or early afternoon so that most of it can be flushed from the bladder before the patient sleeps through the night.

Immunosuppression, Bone Marrow Suppression, and Infection   Suppression of the bone marrow is the major reason that doses of chemotherapy must be limited.

When the marrow is suppressed, meaning its cell production is slowed, few new erythrocytes,

TABLE 9-9 ◆ *Nutritional Formulas and Preparations for Supplemental Feedings*	
Product	**Company**
Carnation Instant Breakfast	Clintec/Carnation
Delmark Instant Breakfast	Delmark
Forta Shake	Ross
Meritene Powder	Sandoz
Sustacal Powder, Sustacal Liquid	Mead, Johnson
Ensure	Ross
Nutrilan flavors	Elan Pharma
Promote	Ross
Isocal	Mead, Johnson
Prosobee	Mead, Johnson
Resource	Sandoz

NOTE: Other protein products and "energy" booster products are available at health food stores and sporting goods stores. Patients should sample various supplements in liquid and bar form to find the ones that are most pleasing.

leukocytes, or platelets are produced. The reduction of erythrocytes decreases oxygen-carrying power and the patient experiences hypoxia and fatigue. Decreased platelets brings an increased risk of bleeding. A low leukocyte count means lower immune function and ability to fight infection.

All antineoplastic drugs cause some degree of bone marrow suppression, but some can cause severe suppression. The amount of suppression is dose related. This is a life-threatening side effect for the patient. The suppression usually is temporary and improvement in bone marrow function occurs within weeks to months of therapy completion. The white blood cell count (WBC) is monitored for a count of less than 3,000/mm^3, indicating neutropenia. Neupogen is given to raise the neutrophil count and the WBC. Often it is started before the count drops so low.

The resultant anemia places an increased workload on the heart and lungs as they attempt adequately to oxygenate the body. When the platelet count reaches a low of 50,000/mm^3, any small injury can lead to an episode of prolonged bleeding. At 20,000/mm^3, spontaneous bleeding that is difficult to control may occur.

The increased danger of infection is an indication to the nurse to become very attentive to good, frequent, and thorough handwashing and to maintain strict asepsis in all aspects of patient care. If the neutrophil count is below 500 mm^3, follow the policy and procedures for protective isolation to prevent infection. Table 9-10 shows the guidelines for teaching the patient ways to decrease the risk of infection after discharge.

Patients with thrombocytopenia can take measures to help lower the risk of bleeding. Table 9-11 presents the guidelines. An infusion of platelets may be administered if the count falls to 20,000/mm^3. The patient must be handled gently. Using a lift sheet helps in turning and repositioning the patient. Needle sticks for injections, laboratory specimens, and IV starts are kept to a minimum. The smallest-gauge needle possible for the task should be used. Pressure is applied to the site for 5 to 10 minutes or until bleeding stops. All urine and stool should be tested for the presence of blood. Abdominal girth is measured daily to check for internal bleeding. Ice is applied to any area that is bumped or injured.

The diet is modified to avoid irritating foods. Stool softeners are given to keep the stool soft and to prevent the Valsalva maneuver that occurs with constipation. No rectal suppositories or enemas are given and rectal temperatures are contraindicated.

Immunosuppression may be treated with colony-stimulating factors (CSFs), such as GM-CSF, G-CSF, or EPO, to increase leukocytes, granulocytes, and erythrocytes. Granulocyte-stimulating factors are question-

able for patients with a cancer of the blood-forming organs, such as leukemia, unless whole-body irradiation has occurred, as there is a possibility that more abnormal cells will be produced. These agents are used after total body irradiation for Hodgkin's disease, acute

---

TABLE 9-10 ◆ Patient Education: Guidelines for the Patient Prone to Infection Because of Cancer Treatment

◆ Wash your hands well with an antimicrobial soap:
  Before eating.
  After using the toilet.
  After blowing your nose.
  After handling items many people have handled such as railings, money, shopping carts, library books, newspapers, pieces of mail, etc.
  After touching a pet.
  After spending time out in public.

◆ Do not share personal care items (razor, toothbrush, toothpaste, wash cloth, towels, deodorant, hand lotion, lipstick, etc.).

◆ Clean toothbrush by running it through the dishwasher or soaking it in a bleach or hydrogen peroxide solution.

◆ Stay away from people with respiratory or other infections.

◆ Bathe daily if possible; use an antimicrobial soap.

◆ Examine the mouth daily for sores or white patches; perform mouth care frequently.

◆ Examine the skin, especially the feet, for signs of broken areas daily.

◆ Wash dishes, utensils, and items used in cooking in hot sudsy water or run them through a dishwasher.

◆ Drink only fresh, bottled water.

◆ Do not reuse drinking cups or glasses without washing them.

◆ Keep lips moist with lip ice or petroleum jelly to avoid cracking.

◆ Stay out of crowded places.

◆ Eat only canned or cooked foods.

◆ If leukocyte count is extremely low, maintain a low-bacteria diet by avoiding salads, raw fruits and vegetables, undercooked meat, pepper, or paprika.

◆ Do not handle garden flowers, plants, or earth.

◆ Do not clean out cat litter boxes or bird cages.

◆ Have someone change water in flower arrangements if such are allowed.

◆ Monitor temperature daily.

◆ Be careful not to nick or scratch the skin.

◆ Report the following signs of infection to the physician immediately:
  Temperature over 100° F (38° C).
  Persistent cough.
  Colored or foul-smelling drainage from wound or nose.
  Presence of a boil or abscess.
  Cloudy, foul-smelling urine or burning on urination.

TABLE 9-11 ◆ *Patient Education: Guidelines to Prevent Bleeding and Bruising in the Patient with a Low Platelet Count*

- Use a soft toothbrush and brush lightly; do not floss.
- Use only an electric razor or depilatory for shaving.
- Avoid constipation by increasing fluid and roughage in the diet; take a stool softener if needed.
- Caution health care workers not to use a tourniquet to obtain blood specimens.
- Tell health care workers what normal blood pressure is so that cuff is not pumped up excessively.
- Avoid nonprescription drugs that inhibit platelet function: aspirin, ibuprofen (Motrin, Advil), Alka-seltzer. Check for salicylates that inhibit platelet function in all analgesic and cold medicines.
- Move around carefully to avoid bumping into things; avoid contact sports or any sport where falling is a risk.
- If a bump or injury occurs, apply ice to area for 1 hour.
- Avoid tight, constricting clothing or shoes.
- Do not wear jewelry with sharp edges.
- Use ample lubrication for intercourse; avoid anal intercourse.
- Avoid blowing the nose or picking at it; if you must blow, blow gently without occluding either nostril.

lymphocytic lymphoma and non-Hodgkin's lymphoma. They are given after the bone marrow transplant has been completed.

Think about . . . What would you do in this situation? You came to work with a slightly scratchy throat and a drippy nose this morning. The charge nurse has assigned you to a cancer patient who has bone marrow suppression.

Hyperuricemia The antimetabolite drugs cause an increase in uric acid in the blood as cancer cells are destroyed. A high fluid intake helps prevent problems of **hyperuricemia** (high uric acid in the blood) that occurs. Allopurinol may be prescribed to decrease incidence of gout caused by the hyperuricemia; it is started at the beginning of therapy in an effort to prevent the problem.

Fatigue The fatigue occurring from immunosuppression treatment itself requires an adjustment of lifestyle. Frequent rest periods throughout the day should be planned. Maintaining a good nutritional status with high protein intake will help keep up energy levels. Supplemental feedings between meals often are necessary to ensure adequate calorie intake. Fluids should be increased to 3 L per day on day 3 of chemotherapy, unless contraindicated to help flush the waste materials

from killed cancer cells from the body and to decrease the toxicities of the antineoplastic drugs. Explain that fatigue is a normal result of cancer treatment and that it may continue for 2 to 3 months after completion of therapy. Light exercise, such as walking, tends to increase energy level.

Alopecia Hair loss resulting from chemotherapy is temporary. Occasionally radiation therapy to the head causes permanent hair loss. Although some techniques, such as using ice caps or a tourniquet around the scalp during the administration of chemotherapy, have been somewhat effective, they are not recommended by oncologists because the reduction of circulation of the drug to the area may prevent the killing of cancer cells that are harbored in the blood or lymph vessels in the scalp and head.

Hair begins regrowth about a month after the chemotherapy ends. The patient must be told that the new hair may be different in texture and color from the original. Meanwhile the patient should choose a wig or head cover, before hair loss occurs, to wear until the hair is regrown. Some offices of the American Cancer Society have wigs available for loan that have been donated by former patients.

Pain For many cancer patients, pain is a daily reality. Pain reduces appetite, limits activity, and interferes with sleep. Most pain can be relieved or at least controlled by a combination of measures. The Agency for Health Care Policy and Research (AHCPR) has published guidelines for the control of cancer pain. To obtain a copy of *Quick Reference Guide for Clinicians* and a consumer's guide called *Managing Cancer Pain*, call 1-800 4-CANCER. The guidelines direct health professionals to use the assessment techniques and modalities discussed in Chapter 10 to control the patient's pain. Nonpharmacological interventions are combined with oral, topical, and parenteral analgesia to achieve relief or good control of pain. Pain must be assessed and documented regularly. **The main factor in pain treatment is to continue to seek a combination of interventions or different treatments until the pain is under control.** A new drug, strontium-89 (Metastron), is available to treat bone pain for patients with skeletal metastases. Steroids, antidepressants, muscle relaxants, and anticonvulsant-type drugs may be combined with analgesics and opiates to obtain adequate pain control. Constant evaluation of interventions for pain control and their outcomes provides the data needed to adjust the plan of care. **Pain should be reassessed 15 to 30 minutes after parenteral drug administration and 1 hour after oral drugs are given. Medication doses should be scheduled regularly and around the clock to maintain a therapeutic drug level to prevent pain recurrence. The** pain medication employed should be known to be effective for cancer pain. Meperidine, pentazocine, butorphanol, and nalbuphine are not useful for chronic cancer pain. They are sometimes used as a part of combination therapy to control acute pain.

By putting aside worries about addiction to opiates, believing the patient's reports of pain and what relieves it, and concentrating on humane treatment of cancer patients, the nurse can be the instrument for helping the patient achieve a pain-free or pain-controlled existence. Pain control or relief greatly increases the quality of life for the cancer patient.

Think about . . . The pain control regimen for an assigned cancer patient is not working well. Can you write a role-play situation that would show your classmates how you would interact with the physician to obtain better pain control for your patient?

Metastasis   A percentage of cancer patients experience **metastasis** (movement of cancer cells from one organ or body part to a distant location). Table 9-12 shows the most common locations for metastasis for major cancers. Treatment options are the same as for primary cancer. Nursing care becomes more complex as more body systems are affected. All nurses caring for cancer patients should be aware of the possibility of metastasis and be alert for signs that might indicate it has occurred. Periodic assessment of the patient is done by the physician to rule out metastasis. Bone scans are periodically performed to detect metastasis to locations in the skeleton.

Fear and Ineffective Coping   The patient newly diagnosed with cancer faces enormous stress. **Knowledge about the disease, treatment options, and what will be experienced during each type of treatment greatly decreases fear in patients and families.** Knowing what to expect allows people to plan and feel confident that they will have some control over what is happening to them. An assessment of the patient's and family's usual coping techniques is important in formulating the overall plan of care.

When a patient has been diagnosed with cancer, pay attention to the patient's partner. This person's response to the bad news will influence everyone else connected closely to the patient. Give the partner enough knowledge to decrease anxiety and the patient will be calmer. Be honest about the adverse effects of chemotherapy, immunotherapy, radiation therapy, and other treatments, but take a positive approach. Indicating that many patients feel a little nauseated with chemotherapy, but that there is medication that controls that very well is better than telling the patient that there won't be any problems with the chemotherapy.

The nurse must consider psychosocial and spiritual care when working with the cancer patient as the disease will affect every phase of life in some way. The nurse's job is to be supportive, to assist the patient to use strengths in planning and fighting the disease, and to coordinate family strengths in order to support the patient and continue with daily life. Prepare family members for disruption of their normal routines to visit the patient, take care of him, or assume his normal tasks in the household. Praise to family members who are taking on the patient's tasks as well as their own, along with caring for the increased needs of the patient, will be appreciated and help raise spirits. Help the patient realize that family members cannot spend as much time as they would like with him because they are attending to new responsibilities.

Speak with the patient and partner about sexual concerns. Intimacy is to be encouraged. Unless the patient is recovering from surgery, has pathological fractures, or is severely immunosuppressed, sexual intercourse shouldn't be a serious problem. If sexual function has been altered by surgery or treatment, help the patient find other means of sexual expression and gratification.

TABLE 9-12 ♦ *Common Sites of Metastasis for Different Cancer Types*

Cancer Type	Sites of Metastasis
Breast cancer	Bone* Lung* Liver Brain
Lung cancer	Brain* Bone Liver Lymph nodes Pancreas
Colorectal cancer	Liver* Lymph nodes Adjacent structures
Prostate cancer	Bone (especially spine and legs)* Pelvic nodes
Melanoma	Gastrointestinal tract Lymph nodes Lung Brain
Primary brain cancer	Central nervous system

*Most common site of metastasis for the specific malignant neoplasm.
Source: Ignatavicius, D.D., Workman, M.L., Mishler, M.A. (1995). *Medical–Surgical Nursing: A Nursing Process Approach,* 2nd ed. Philadelphia: Saunders, p. 552.

Elder Care Point... The older patient may have developed a fear of cancer from when treatment was so grim and survival so unusual. This person may be reluctant to use the word *cancer*. Respect whatever terminology they choose to use to speak about their condition. Encourage verbalization to decrease fear and increase knowledge of present day treatment and prognosis.

Referral to the social worker may be needed to coordinate resources for treatment and care assistance. Care of the cancer patient is a collaborative process that involves many members of the health care team. Family, friends, individuals, and community groups are among the sources of support and encouragement that the cancer patient might need to care for himself and attain some level of independence and peace of mind.

Local chapters of the American Cancer Society (ACS) and American Lung Association have a wide variety of services available to professionals and laypersons interested in caring for the cancer patient. These include an annotated bibliography of public, patient, and professional information and education materials, pamphlets and booklets, and audiovisual programs. To obtain materials from the American Cancer Society, one can write or call the nearest ACS division. There are more than 3,000 local ACS unit offices in the United States and Puerto Rico. The local telephone directory carries a list of local unit offices in the area. There also may be a regional cancer information service that provides information about local resources for specific problems, such as pain control. Table 9-13 lists some of the organizations that can provide assistance.

TABLE 9-13 ◆ *Resources for the Cancer Patient*

American Cancer Society, 1599 Clifton Road, NE, Atlanta, GA 30329; (404) 320-3333.

Leukemia Society of America, 733 Third Avenue, New York, NY 10017.

National Cancer Institute, Office of Cancer Communications, Building 31, Room 10A24, Bethesda, MD 20892; 1-800-4-CANCER.

National Coalition for Cancer Survivorship, 323 Eighth Street, SW, Albuquerque, NM 87102; (505) 764-9956.

The National Hospice Organization, 1901 N. Fort Myer Drive, Arlington, VA 22209.

National Institutes of Health, Office of Clinical Center Communications, Building 10, Room 1C255, 9000 Rockville Pike, Bethesda, MD 20892.

United Ostomy Association, 2001 West Beverly Boulevard, Los Angeles, CA 90057.

If there is a local hospice program, the services provided might include professional volunteers who visit the terminal patient in his home and provide care the family is not able to give and lay volunteers who help meet the emotional, social, and spiritual needs of the terminally ill patient and his family. Most hospitals and proprietary health care agencies provide coordination with home health care as an extension of hospital care after discharge.

COMMUNITY CARE

More and more cancer patients receive treatment in the outpatient setting. Home care nurses often are employed to perform regular assessment, coordination of care, management of pain and other side effects of the disease or therapy, and to provide patient education on all aspects of the disease and care. Collaboration with the physician, oncologist, dietitian, pharmacist, social worker, physical therapist, and nurse aide is important to the success of the clinical pathway or nursing care plan.

The nurse is the mainstay of the medical support and treatment system for the patient. Cancer is said to be the most treatable of all chronic diseases. Over half of the patients diagnosed in a year will have a normal lifespan. There are some specific ways the patient can make treatment a success. The patient should be encouraged to (1) confront fears; (2) take charge of treatment; (3) know the options; and (4) fight actively.

The way to confront fears is with education, understanding, faith, positive visualization, and relaxation techniques. Connecting with others who have been through the same experience has proven to be of benefit. Support groups that have a positive outlook provide a boost in the active fight against cancer.

Taking charge of treatment means getting at least two opinions on the diagnosis and treatment of the cancer. Referrals to physicians who are experts in oncology should be sought. If in doubt as to whom to contact, the local medical association office can offer a suggestion. Encourage meeting with physicians with a prepared list of questions and having a companion along who will listen and take notes for later review (just forewarn the physician).

Learning as much as possible about the particular kind of cancer advises the patient of available options. Knowledge of the latest and most effective treatments should be gained before making a decision about treatment. Contacting the National Cancer Institute for the latest information is wise.

Throughout treatment the patient should be actively seeking information. The patient must trust the physician and the hospital or treatment facility. Trust is not developed on the basis of someone else's recommendation alone. Encourage the patient to maintain a sense of humor and to look for a little pleasure and enjoyment in life on a daily basis to counteract the hours consumed by treatment.

Nurses working in the radiation oncology center, the oncology floor of the hospital, the oncology outpatient clinic, in the home, or the physician's office can be instrumental in providing support, direction, and hope for the cancer patient.

CRITICAL THINKING EXERCISES

Clinical Case Problems

Read each clinical situation and discuss the questions with your classmates.

1. An acquaintance tells you that she has had a mole on her back for several years and it appears to be getting larger and darker. She states she is worried about the fact that it is getting bigger, but says that she is scared to go to the doctor. She doesn't have health insurance and is worried about paying for the visit.

   a. What is your obligation as a nurse in encouraging this person to see a physician at once?

   b. What suggestions could you make about obtaining a medical opinion without incurring a lot of expense?

2. Ms. Allen went to her physician for a regular physical checkup and was told that she had malignant cells in the cervical secretions obtained from her Pap smear. She had a biopsy of the cervix, and this, too, proved to contain malignant cells. She was admitted to the hospital, cesium was implanted in the cervix, and Ms. Allen was kept in bed in a private room during the treatment.

   a. If you were assigned to give A.M. care to this patient, what special precautions would you take to protect yourself from excessive radiation?

   b. What would be some signs and symptoms that you would watch for to determine whether Ms. Allen is having either a local or a systemic reaction to radiation?

3. Mary is a 19-year-old college student receiving chemotherapy for Hodgkin's disease. Identify psychosocial problems you would expect Mary to have, and state the measures you would suggest to help her deal with them.

4. Mr. Huong, age 66, has metastatic lung cancer. He is to undergo radiation therapy.

   a. What would you tell Mr. Huong the treatments will be like?

   b. What instructions would he need regarding the inked target lines and skin care?

   c. What precautions should Mr. Huong take regarding use of deodorants, type of clothing, and exposure to the sun?

   d. What type of side effects might Mr. Huong experience with radiation therapy to the chest?

   e. What nursing interventions would be appropriate for the expected side effects?

BIBLIOGRAPHY

Almadrones, L., Campana, P., Dantis, E. C. (1995). Arterial, peritoneal, and intraventricular access devices. *Seminars in Oncology Nursing.* 11(3):194–202.

American Cancer Society. (1996). *Cancer Facts and Figures—1996.* Atlanta: author.

Blesch, K. S. (1996). Rehabilitation of the cancer patient at home. *Seminars in Oncology Nursing.* 12(3): 219–222.

Campbell, M. K., Pruitt, J. J. (1996). Radiation therapy: protecting your patient's skin. *RN.* 59(1):46–47.

Charlotte, J. L. (1995). Contemporary approaches of chemotherapy. *Critical Care Nursing Clinics of North America.* 7(1):135–142.

Cotran, R. S., Kumar, V., Robbins, S. L., Schoen, F. J., eds. (1994). *Robbins Pathologic Basis of Disease,* 5th ed. Philadelphia: Saunders.

Davis, J., Sherer, K. (1994). *Applied Nutrition and Diet Therapy for Nurses,* 2nd ed. Philadelphia: W. B. Saunders.

DeVita, V. T., Hellman, S., Rosenberg, S. (1993). *Cancer Principles and Practice of Oncology,* 4th ed. Philadelphia: Lippincott.

Dow, K. H., Hilderley, L. J. (1992). *Nursing Care in Radiation Oncology.* Philadelphia: Saunders.

Dumas, M. A. (1996). What it's like to belong to the cancer club. *American Journal of Nursing.* 96(4):40–42.

Gomez, E. G. (1995). Supporting the families of cancer patients. *Nursing 95.* 25(6):48–51.

Greifzu, S. (1996). Chemo Quick Guide 1: Alkylating Agents. *RN.* 59(2):53–56.

Greifzu, S. (1996). Chemo Quick Guide 2: Antimetabolites. *RN.* 59(3):32–33.

Greifzu, S. (1996). Chemo Quick Guide 3: Antitumor antibiotics. *RN.* 59(4):35–36.

Greifzu, S. (1996). Chemo Quick Guide 4: Hormonal agents. *RN.* 59(5):41–42.

Greifzu, S. (1996). Chemo Quick Guide 5: Plant alkaloids. *RN.* 59(6):36–37.

Held, J. L. (1995). Managing myelosuppression. *Nursing 95.* 25(8):74.

Hoffman, V. (1996). Tumor lysis syndrome: implications for nursing. *Home Healthcare Nurse.* 14(8):595–599.

Houldin, A. D., Wasserbauer, N. (1996). Psychosocial

needs of older cancer patients: a pilot study abstract. *MEDSURG Nursing.* 5(4):253–256.

Ignatavicius, D. D., Workman, M. L., Mishler, M. A. (1995). *Medical-Surgical Nursing: A Nursing Process Approach,* 2nd ed. Philadelphia: Saunders.

Janowski, M. J. (1995). Managing cancer pain. *RN.* 58(9): 30–32.

Kan, M. K. (1995). Palliation of bone pain in patients with metastatic cancer using strontium-89. *Cancer Nursing.* 18(4):286–291.

Koeppel, K. M. (1995). Sperm banking and patients with cancer: issues concerning patients and healthcare professionals. *Cancer Nursing.* 13(4):306–312.

Korinko, A., Yurick, A. (1997). During radiation therapy: maintaining skin integrity. *American Journal of Nursing.* 97(2):41–44.

Lanes, T. I. (1995). Quality of life and symptom distress of cancer patients receiving various anticancer agents. *Oncology Nursing Forum.* 22(2):386.

Lehne, R. A. (1994). *Pharmacology for Nursing Care,* 2nd ed. Philadelphia: Saunders.

Lowdermilk, D. L. (1995). Home care of the patient with gynecologic cancer. *Journal of Obstetric, Gynecologic, and Neonatal Nursing.* 24(2):157–163.

Malarkey, L. M., McMorrow, M. E. (1996). *Nurse's Manual of Laboratory Tests and Diagnostic Procedures.* Philadelphia: Saunders.

McCaffery, M., Ferrell, B. R. (1994). How to use the new AHCPR cancer pain guidelines. *American Journal of Nursing.* 94(7):42–46.

McCarron, E. G. (1995). Supporting the families of cancer patients. *Nursing 95.* 25(6):47–49.

McCorkle, R., Grant, M., Frank-Stromborg, M., Baird, S. B. (1996). *Cancer Nursing: A Comprehensive Textbook.* Philadelphia: Saunders.

McEnroe, L. E. (1996). Role of the oncology nurse in home care: Family-Centered Practice. 12(3):188–191.

McGrath, P. (1995). It's OK to say no! A discussion of ethical issues arising from informed consent to chemotherapy. *Cancer Nursing.* 18(2):97–103.

Meissner, J. E. (1996). Caring for patients with colorectal cancer. *Nursing 96.* 26(11):60–61.

Monahan, F. D., Drake, T., Neighbors, M. (1994). *Nursing Care of Adults.* Philadelphia: Saunders.

National Cancer Institute. (1991). *Eating Hints: Recipes and Tips for Better Nutrition during Cancer Treatment.* Publication no. 87-20079. Bethesda, MD: author.

Page, M. S., Rabbitt, J. E. (1995). Issues in metastatic disease. *Critical Care Nursing Clinics of North America.* 7(1): 135–142.

Pasero, C. L. (1996). Planning for breakthrough cancer pain. *American Journal of Nursing.* 96(6):24.

Rhodes, V. A., Johnson, M. E., McDaniel, R. W. (1995). Nausea, vomiting, and retching: the management of the symptom experience. *Seminars in Oncology Nursing.* 11(4):256–265.

Schreiber, M. J., Hebenstreit, K. M. (1995). Outpatient care in an inpatient setting: innovations in the after hours care of the outpatient bone marrow transplant (BMT) and general oncology patients. *Oncology Nursing Forum.* 22(2):360.

Shaw, K. (1995). Breast cancer and its treatment. *Journal of Practical Nursing.* 45(1):21–29.

Sims, L. B. (1995). Neurologic involvement of systemic cancer. *Critical Care Nursing Clinics of North America.* 7(1): 171–177.

Springhouse Corporation. (1996). *Nursing 96 Drug Handbook.* Springhouse, PA: author.

Stepp, L., Farren, B., and Sosland, J. (1995). The experience of fatigue and the assessment of fatigue in cancer patients. *Oncology Nursing Forum.* 22(2):387.

Symonds, W. C. (1996). A ray of hope for cancer patients: Photodynamic therapy may stop early-stage tumors. *Business Week.* June 10, 1996:104–106.

Tenenbaum, L. (1995). *Cancer Chemotherapy: A Reference Guide,* 2nd ed. Philadelphia: Saunders.

Ulrich, S. P., Canale, S. W., Wendell, S. A. (1994). *Medical–Surgical Nursing Care Planning Guides,* 3rd ed. Philadelphia: Saunders.

Weber, M. S. (1995). Chemotherapy-induced nausea and vomiting. *American Journal of Nursing.* 95(4):34.

Weisman, A. D. (1979). *Coping with Cancer.* New York: McGraw-Hill.

Workman, M, Ellerhorst-Ryan, J., Koenge, V. (1993). *Nursing Care of the Immunocompromised Patient.* Philadelphia: Saunders.

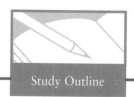

Study Outline

I. The Impact of Cancer

A. Cancer is not a single disease; it is a large group of over 100 diseases that have very little in common.

B. Cancer is the cause of one in four deaths in the United States.

C. Of the 10 million Americans who have a history of cancer, 7 million were diagnosed 5 or more years ago and are considered "cured."

D. More lives could be saved by early detection and prompt treatment.

II. **Physiology of Cancer**

A. Comparison of benign and malignant growths.

1. Benign growths are almost always encapsulated.

2. Benign growths can create problems by pressing against and interfering with functions of adjacent organs, but do not metastasize.

3. Malignant cells are the result of transformation of normal cells, probably because of change in the cells' DNA.

4. Growth of malignant cells is not regulated; they and their offspring are disorganized and uncontrollable by normal mechanisms.

5. Most, but not all, malignant cells metastasize.

B. Classification of tumors.

1. Typed according to the kinds of tissue from which they arise.

2. The suffix -oma simply means tumor. For example, a lipoma is a tumor arising from fatty tissue.

3. Sarcomas arise from mesenchymal tissues; carcinomas from epithelial tissue.

4. Leukemias and lymphomas are cancers of blood-forming organs.

5. Malignancies of pigment cells of skin are melanomas.

6. More precise identification is made by adding modifying prefixes; for example, osteo-(bone) sarcoma.

C. Metastasis: movement of cells to a distant site.

1. Extent to which malignant cells have spread influences prognosis.

a. Localized ("in situ") at original site.

b. Regional, extended to lymph nodes.

c. Advanced, spread throughout the body.

2. Staging system: (T) primary tumor, (N) regional nodes, (M) metastasis.

III. **Causative Factors**

A. All cancer results from genetic defects that are inborn or acquired.

B. Susceptibility influenced by age, familial tendency, exposure to carcinogens, and immunocompetence.

C. There is a relationship between dietary intake and the occurrence of some kinds of cancers.

D. Carcinogens include chemicals, radiation, and physical irritation. Viruses also play a role in cancer development, probably by introducing new genetic material into a normal cell and transforming it into a malignant cell.

E. Some agents, such as alcohol, promote cancer when they are taken in conjunction with a substance such as tobacco.

F. Predisposing factors for the development of cancer:

1. Genetic predisposition is evident in types of leukemia, breast, and colon cancer.

2. Age, sex, and race are predisposing factors for certain types of cancer: black men have more prostate cancer; cervical cancer is higher in black women; breast cancer is more prevalent in white than in Oriental women.

3. Herpes simplex virus 2 (HSV2) and some forms of the human papillomavirus (HVP) that are transmitted sexually are linked to cervical cancer.

4. Stress decreases the efficiency of the immune system and seems to make certain people more susceptible to cancer.

5. Heavy dietary intake of saturated and unsaturated fats increases the chance of malignancy of the breast, colon, and prostate; salt-cured or smoked meats are thought to be carcinogenic, as are foods preserved with nitrites.

IV. **Measures to Prevent Cancer**

A. Education is the key to cancer prevention.

1. Encourage those who smoke to quit.

2. Encourage maintenance of normal weight.

3. Encourage consumption of a varied diet.

B. Avoid and limit exposure to carcinogens.

C. Identify high-risk people.

V. **Detection of Cancer**

A. The purpose of screening is to find cancer in its very early stages.

B. Teach others about the seven warning signals of cancer:

1. Change in bowel or bladder habits.

2. A sore that does not heal.

3. Unusual bleeding or discharge.

4. Thickening or lump in breast or elsewhere.

5. Indigestion or difficulty in swallowing.

6. Obvious change in wart or mole.

7. Nagging cough or hoarseness.

C. Recommendations of American Cancer Society for checkups and diagnostic tests to detect cancer (Table 9-5).

D. Diagnostic tests:

1. Cytological examination of cells is primary method of determining malignancy; cells are obtained by biopsy.

2. Other tests include radiological studies, endoscopy, sonography, magnetic resonance imaging, computed tomography, laboratory testing of blood enzymes, and studies specific to the system in which cancer is suspected.

VI. Nursing Management

A. Assessment:

1. Know whether the patient has been told the diagnosis.

2. General physical assessment and thorough assessment of the body systems the cancer is affecting provides data for determining appropriate care.

3. Psychosocial assessment of the patient and family provides data about coping abilities, needs, and resources for care and support.

B. Many nursing diagnoses may be appropriate, but they must be individualized to the patient (see Nursing Care Plan 9-1).

C. Planning:

1. Specific outcome objectives are written for the chosen nursing diagnoses.

2. Planning is a collaborative process among the patient, the family, the nurse, the physician, and dietitian, the oncologist, the social worker, and other specialists on the health care team.

D. Implementation:

1. Interventions are chosen according to the nursing diagnoses appropriate for the patient's problems that will help achieve the expected outcomes.

2. See Nursing Care Plan 9-1 for specific interventions.

E. Evaluation:

1. Based on determination as to whether outcomes are being met.

2. Requires continuous assessment for response to treatment.

VII. Common Therapies, Problems, and Nursing Care

A. Surgery: removal of malignant growth and adjacent tissue. Newer techniques are less traumatic and mutilating.

1. Biopsy.

2. Removal of tumor.

3. Staging of cancer.

4. Debulking of tumor for palliation of symptoms.

B. External radiation. Sources are linear accelerator, radioactive element such as cobalt 60 housed in a shielded unit; stereotaxic surgery; gamma knife.

1. Nursing care of patients undergoing external radiation therapy:

a. Helping patient cope with side effects of radiation.

(1) Instruct patient and significant others in purpose and goals of radiation therapy.

(2) Assure patient he cannot be a source of radiation for others.

(3) Make sure that patient keeps to scheduled treatments.

(4) Teach patient and significant others how to recognize and take an active part in managing expected side effects.

(5) Most side effects begin a week to 10 days after first treatment and usually continue for several weeks after last treatment.

b. Minimizing trauma to skin.

(1) Avoid friction, sunlight, and application of alcohol, lotions, or salves to exposed areas.

(2) Teach patient to assess degree of reaction daily.

2. Coping with specific side effects of radiation.

a. Radiation to scalp produces alopecia, usually temporary.

(1) Teach patient to avoid harsh treatment of hair and scalp.

(2) Encourage use of wigs, scarfs, hairpieces to maintain self-image until hair grows back.

b. Radiation to chest and upper back causes nausea and indigestion, inflammation of lung tissue.

(1) Humidify inhaled air.

(2) Maintain adequate fluid intake.

(3) Perform coughing and deep-breathing exercises.

(4) Avoid respiratory infections.

c. Radiation to abdomen and lower back cause nausea and vomiting, diarrhea, cystitis.

(1) Increase fluid intake.

(2) Empty bladder promptly.

(3) Avoid irritating foods and beverages.

C. Internal radiation. Source of radioactivity is in the patient's body. Source is either sealed in container or unsealed, as in liquid that is ingested or instilled.

1. Nursing care of patients receiving internal radiation:

a. Nurse should know effects of radiation, source being used, and where it is in the patient.

b. Principles of radiation protection (time, distance, shielding) must be observed.

c. Special precautions and policies and procedures of institution must be followed.

d. If source is unsealed (e.g., radioactive iodine), nurse needs to know how it is excreted and its half-life.

e. Table 9-6 shows common side effects of radiation therapy.

D. Chemotherapy. Use of drugs either alone or in combination with other drugs or other forms of therapy.

1. Overall effect of antineoplastic drugs is to reduce size of tumor and lessen symptoms.

2. Preferred treatment for leukemias, some lymphomas, multiple myeloma, and metastatic cancer.

3. Cell-cycle-specific drugs attack malignant cells at one phase of cell's reproductive cycle.

4. Cell-cycle-nonspecific drugs can destroy cells in all phases.

5. Antineoplastic drugs are used in combinations to destroy malignant cells with the least amount of damage to normal cells and to decrease side effects.

6. Drugs may be administered by intraarterial, intraperitoneal, intraventricular, and intrathecal infusion as well as by intravenous infusion and the oral route.

7. For intravenous infusion a central line or infusion port often is used.

8. Some antineoplastic drugs are vesicants and can cause extensive local tissue damage if they escape the vein or infusion catheter.

9. Consult the pharmacist, policy manual, and the physician should extravasation occur.

10. Assessment of toxic side effects is essential (see Table 9-8).

11. Nursing care of patients receiving chemotherapy:

a. Not all neoplastic drugs are cytotoxic.

b. Toxicity most damaging to cells that have a short life span, such as those in the hair follicles.

c. More common side effects and nursing care are summarized in Table 9-7 and Nursing Care Plan 9-1.

E. Hormone therapy:

1. An adjunct to other types of therapy.

2. May slow tumor growth or aid in prevention of recurrence.

3. Side effects depend on the type of hormone given; androgens have masculinizing effects; estrogens and progestins have feminizing effects.

F. Immunotherapy using biological response modifiers (BRMs).

1. Purpose of BRM therapy is to stimulate, suppress, or assist immune system to combat malignant cells.

2. Three approaches:

a. Active nonspecific immunization: interferons and interleukins, tumor antigens.

b. Second group: monoclonal antibodies and tumor necrosis factor, both of which have direct antitumor effects.

c. Third group: miscellaneous agents that have different functions; some stimulate undifferentiated cells to mature, others prevent metastasis.

G. Bone marrow transplant

1. Utilized to correct severe bone marrow damage caused by chemotherapy or radiation.

2. Follows total body irradiation in treatment of Hodgkin's disease and some types of leukemia.

3. Procedure and nursing care for BMT are in Chapter 17.

H. Photodynamic therapy: photosensitizing agent given intravenously that is taken up by tumor cells; laser light is then used to destroy tumor cells.

I. Gene therapy: once gene defects for specific cancers are identified, gene splicing or replacement may be possible.

VIII. **Evaluating Effectiveness of Medical Treatment**

A. "Second-look" surgery.

B. Reduction in size of tumor, abatement of symptoms.

C. CEA levels, CA-125 levels, PSA levels.

D. Bone scans performed periodically.

IX. **Common Problems Related to Cancer or Cancer Therapy**

A. Anorexia, mucositis, and weight loss.

1. Anorexia: a common side effect. Caused by irritation of mucous membranes of mouth and gastrointestinal tract and changes in taste perception, dryness of mouth, sore tongue.

2. Note current weight, compare with ideal weight.

3. Daily weight to recognize significant (2 or more pounds per week) weight loss.

4. Assess condition of oral mucosa; start oral care program before treatment begins.

5. Give small, frequent feedings; attend to preferences for food; provide restful and pleasant environment.

6. Give supplemental feedings as necessary to maintain adequate protein intake.

7. Radiation to head and neck causes inflammation of oral mucosa, pharyngitis, and esophagitis.
   a. Encourage fluid intake.
   b. Use artificial saliva.
   c. Good oral hygiene, gentle tooth brushing.
   d. Use saline, peroxide, or bicarbonate of soda with salt solution to counteract acidity and cleanse the mouth. Avoid full-strength commercial mouth washes.
B. Nausea, vomiting, and diarrhea.
   1. Produced by chemotherapy or radiation to the abdomen, lower back, or pelvis.
   2. Begin antiemetics 12 hours prior to doses of chemotherapy and continue them for 24 hours afterward at 3- to 4-hour intervals.
   3. Give small, frequent meals; eat before therapy.
   4. Provide odor-free environment.
   5. Provide comfort measures: cold cloth to neck and forehead, mouth care.
   6. Guided imagery and relaxation techniques may help.
C. Constipation:
   1. Increase fluids as allowed, add fiber to the diet, administer stool softeners and fiber laxatives; suppositories and enemas may be necessary.
   2. Treat drug-induced constipation vigorously to avoid impaction or intestinal obstruction.
D. Cystitis: evidenced by frequency and hematuria.
   1. Force fluids.
   2. Empty bladder frequently.
E. Immunosuppression, bone marrow suppression, and infection
   1. Cause of limitation of doses of chemotherapy.
   2. Blood cell production is slowed when bone marrow is suppressed.
   3. Amount of suppression is dose related.
   4. Can be life-threatening.
   5. Improvement in bone marrow function occurs within weeks to months of therapy completion.
   6. A WBC below $3,000/mm^3$ indicates leukopenia and high risk of infection; Neupogen may be given.
   7. Guidelines for decreasing the risk of infection (Table 9-10).
   8. Guidelines for decreasing the risk of bleeding in presence of thrombocytopenia (Table 9-11).
   9. Platelets may be given if the platelet count falls to $20,000/mm^3$.

10. Colony-stimulating factors may be given; anemia may be treated with Epogen.
F. Hyperuricemia: increase in uric acid as cancer cells are destroyed.
   1. Increase fluid intake.
   2. Treat with allopurinol; start along with chemotherapy.
G. Fatigue:
   1. Can alter patient's lifestyle.
   2. Help patient plan realistic goals for periods of rest balanced with activities.
   3. Light exercise may increase energy level.
H. Alopecia:
   1. Hair loss is usually temporary.
   2. Obtain wig before therapy begins if hair loss is expected.
   3. Hair regrowth begins about a month after end of therapy.
I. Pain:
   1. Pain relief or control can be achieved.
   2. Nurse must be an advocate for the patient.
   3. Combinations of analgesics and nonpharmacological measures are very effective.
   4. Combinations of interventions are tried until control or relief is achieved.
   5. The patient is the best source for what the pain is and what relieves it.
J. Metastasis:
   1. Common locations for major cancers (Table 9-12).
   2. Nursing care becomes complex as more body systems are involved.
   3. Treatment modalities are the same as for primary cancer.
K. Fear and ineffective coping:
   1. Diagnosis of cancer is very stressful.
   2. Knowledge of disease, treatment options, and what will be experienced during treatment decreases fear.
   3. Including the patient in the planning of care gives him some control over what is happening to him.
   4. Psychosocial and spiritual care, as well as physical care, is needed for the cancer patient.
   5. Assist the patient and family to identify strengths and coping techniques.
   6. Refer to support groups and services (Table 9-13).
   7. Provide counseling for sexual problems and concerns.
   8. Refer to the social worker for coordination of resources for treatment and care assistance.

X. Community Care
  A. Much of cancer treatment is given in the outpatient setting.
  B. Home care nurses perform assessment, coordination of care, management of pain and side effects of treatment, provide patient teaching, and evaluate effectiveness of care and treatment.
  C. Collaboration with other health team members is important to the success of the nursing care plan.
  D. The patient is encouraged to:
    1. Confront fears.
    2. Take charge of treatment.
    3. Know available options.
    4. Fight actively.

CHAPTER 10

Care of Patients with Pain

OBJECTIVES

Upon completion of this chapter, the student should be able to:
1. Understand the current view of pain as a specific entity requiring appropriate intervention.
2. Review the "gate theory" of pain and its relationship to nursing care.
3. Understand how pain perception is affected by personal situations and cultural backgrounds.
4. Effectively utilize the nursing process in pain management.
5. Effectively use a variety of pain-evaluation tools.
6. Understand the false perceptions that underlie many current ideas about pain and pain management and assist patients to achieve a clearer, more factual understanding.
7. List the different pharmacological approaches to pain management, with examples of each.
8. Recognize common side effects of analgesics and describe techniques for addressing them.
9. List a variety of nonpharmacological approaches to pain management and their appropriate uses.
10. Understand the major differences between acute and chronic pain and their management.

A common link among people who require health care is pain, or the fear of pain. The causes of pain are varied. An illness or injury may cause pain. Surgical intervention and other treatments may cause pain. Anticipation of treatment may foster a fear of pain. People frequently fear that they will not be able to get relief from pain that is occurring or may occur during treatment.

Traditionally, pain was seen as a *symptom* of the illness or injury, something that was temporary and would go away as healing occurred. The physician decided what pain control drug (analgesic) was needed and the nurse administered it according to the physician's order. It was the role of the physician and nurse to determine the presence of pain and to administer appropriate treatment.

Current thinking views pain not as just a symptom, but as a specific problem that needs to be treated. Today we also recognize that the patient must be part of the management team. Although we have equipment that accurately measures such things as blood pressure, heart rhythm, or brain waves, there is no such equipment for measuring pain. Only the patient knows where the pain is and its degree of intensity. Only the patient knows what treatment regimen works and how long it is effective.

THE PATHOPHYSIOLOGY OF PAIN

Pain can be defined as a neurological response to unpleasant stimuli. Pain receptors are abundantly distributed throughout the skin and in many deeper structures of the body. Receptors for pain do not become dulled with repeated stimulation. Indeed, studies indicate that, under some conditions, repeated stimulation results in an increase in the acuteness of the pain sensation.

The actual mechanism of pain is still poorly understood. It is known that pain results from the release of various chemicals from damaged cells. It may be helpful to think of pain being controlled by a "gate" in the central nervous system. When the gate is open, the pain sensation is allowed through, and when it is closed the pain sensation is blocked. The gate control theory also recognizes that stimuli other than pain pass through the same gate. When there is a large volume of nonpainful stimuli competing for the gate, pain impulses may be blocked. A high volume of pain, however, may override other stimuli and pass through the gate, causing the individual to perceive the pain.

Aspects of this theory relate to nursing practice in several ways.

- Two types of nerve fibers carry pain stimuli: small diameter and large diameter.
- Activity in small-diameter nerve fibers seems to open the gate, and activity in the large-diameter nerve fibers seems to close it. Massage and vibration produce activity in the large-diameter nerve fibers.
- High levels of sensory input create brain stem impulses that seem to close the gate. Distraction in the form of activity or social interaction produces these kinds of impulses.
- An increase in anxiety seems to open the gate, and a decrease seems to close it. The fear that pain will not be controlled may actually increase pain intensity, and knowing that pain can or is being controlled may reduce it.

Another way of looking at pain and its management is the idea of "pieces of pain." The more intense the pain, the greater the number of pieces, and therefore a greater number of "pieces" of analgesia will be required to control it. This idea states that inadequate analgesia results in leftover, untreated pain, and relief or control is not achieved.

It is also known that the body produces substances called **endorphins** (endogenous morphine) that can attach to pain receptors and block pain sensation. There are still many questions about endorphins and how they work. Their properties appear to include modification and inhibition of unpleasant stimuli, reduction of anxiety, and relief of pain. They also may produce feelings of euphoria and well-being.

Think about... Can you compare the old view of pain with the new view of pain?

PERCEPTION OF PAIN

The ways in which humans react to pain can vary widely from person to person and in the same individual under different circumstances. People with **chronic pain** (lasting months or years) may have learned adaptive methods that allow them to have some control over it. Coping with pain takes a lot of energy, and patients who are debilitated are less able to withstand pain than are strong, robust people. Fatigue caused by pain can lead to an increase in pain perception.

Pain can cause a variety of physiological responses, including increased respiratory rate, pulse, or blood pressure, muscle tension, sweating, flushing or pallor, frowning or grimacing. Although the presence of any of these factors may indicate pain, their absence does not prove the absence of pain.

A person's cultural background influences feelings about pain. In much of Western culture it is considered valuable to have a high pain tolerance, particularly among men. Some cultures allow for free expression of pain, and moaning, crying, and other actions are considered appropriate. A nurse whose cultural background approves the "stiff upper lip" approach to handling pain may see the patient who outwardly expresses pain as weak or manipulative. Those patients whose cultural upbringing causes them to hide and deny pain may suffer needlessly unless the nurse can intervene by helping them to understand that analgesia will aid the healing process by encouraging movement and decreasing fatigue. Learning to accept without judgment the various ways of coping with and expressing pain is a very necessary process for nurses.

NURSING MANAGEMENT

◆ Assessment

Evaluation of another person's pain is a major nursing challenge. Because there is no technology for accurate measurement, a combination of evaluation methods are used.

Observation

- ***Appearance.*** The face may look tense, drawn, or pale. There may be a grimace or even a look of fear.
- ***Behavior.*** A normally verbal patient may become quiet or withdrawn. One who is normally pleasant may become irritable, demanding, or argumentative. The individual may protect or "cradle" the painful area with the hands or arms. Tears, refusal of food or drink, any behavior which is out of the ordinary for the individual may be an indication of pain.
- ***Activity level.*** A person in pain often reduces activity to a minimum. Staying in bed, creeping slowly from place to place, stooping over during ambulation, and stopping frequently to rest or lean against a support can all indicate pain.
- ***Verbalization.*** Many individuals in pain may verbalize their discomfort. However, it is not always easy to interpret the degree of pain from what is

said. Limited vocabulary, lack of experience in verbalizing abstract concepts, fear of disbelief or disapproval from the caregiver, and fear of becoming addicted to the analgesic can all impair the person's ability to communicate his pain.

♦ *Physiological clues.* These include rapid, shallow or guarded respirations, pallor, diaphoresis, increased pulse, elevated blood pressure, dilated pupils, and tenseness of the skeletal muscles. However, remember that problems other than pain can also cause these to occur. All physiological changes must be fully assessed to determine the cause.

Assessment Tools   A variety of scales and evaluation methods have been developed for use in pain management. Some of the more commonly used are briefly described.

♦ *Number scales.* These use a scale, such as 1 to 5 or 1 to 10, with 1 indicating no pain and the highest number indicating the greatest amount of pain imaginable. The numbers in between show graduated levels of pain. The scale may be simply verbal, or it may actually be drawn on a piece of paper so the person can mark or point to the degree of pain. These can be used very effectively with people who have a good understanding of the numerical concept and who like a strictly logical approach. They are not effective with young children, anyone who has difficulty with numbers, or anyone who is confused or disoriented; and some patients have reported that they cannot relate a numerical scale to something as intensely personal as pain.

♦ *Visual scales.* A variety of these are available. Some use photographs or simple drawings of faces with expressions showing pain-free (happy and smiling) and then progress through a series of faces showing increased discomfort. The final picture shows a face either crying or with an intense grimace.

♦ *Color scale.* A color scale allows the patient to select the colors that represent varying degrees of pain. Colored pieces of paper, crayons or markers, or colored pieces of plastic such as poker chips can be used. The patient selects a color that represents no pain, a color that represents severe pain, and then one, two, or three other colors for pain levels in between. This scale is often used with children, but very young children cannot understand more than three or four possible choices.

♦ *Pieces of pain scale.* This scale uses five poker chips or other identical, plain objects, each one representing a "piece" of pain. The patient can indicate the degree of pain by selecting the number of chips that equals the intensity of pain being experienced.

When using a pain-assessment scale, it is important that the nursing staff use it consistently and that the patient fully understands how to use it. The type of scale being used and any pertinent information about how the patient uses the scale must be included in the patient care plan.

Think about... What is the difference between acute and chronic pain?

Difficulties in Data Gathering   Much of the data gathered when assessing pain comes from conversation with the patient, and this presents a variety of problems. The first is language itself. Concepts of the true meaning of words in the language may vary greatly from person to person. It is important to discuss the words used to describe pain and to agree upon their meaning (Table 10-1). It also is important that documentation include the patient's exact words.

The need to work through an interpreter or deal with language difficulties when the patient speaks a foreign tongue compounds the problem of communication. Whenever possible, use a medical professional with a good knowledge of both languages to interpret. People who do not have a medical background may not give accurate meanings in the translation, and patients may hide personal, embarrassing, or painful information if the interpreter is a family member or personal friend.

Describing the location of pain can be made difficult by the problem of **referred pain** (pain felt in a different part of the body from where it actually originates). Heart pain may be felt in the jaw or radiating down the arm. Gastric pain may center in the area of the heart rather than the stomach. Pain in one area is frequently referred to another area of the body (Figure 10-1).

There also is a tendency not to believe an individual's statement of pain if there is no outward appearance

TABLE 10-1 ♦ *Common Terms to Help Patient to Describe Pain*	
Degree of pain (from least to most severe)	Absent, minimal, mild, moderate, fairly severe, severe, very or extremely severe, exquisite.
Quality of pain	Crushing, tingling, itching, throbbing, pulsating, twisting, pulling, burning, searing, stabbing, tearing, biting, blinding, nauseating, debilitating.
Frequency of the pain	Constant, intermittent, occasional, related to something specific (e.g., only when coughs).

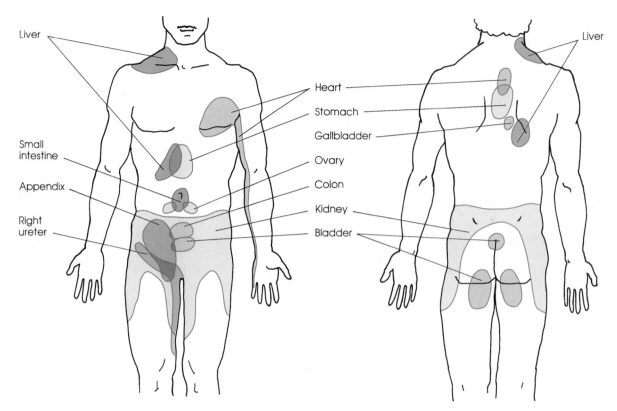

FIGURE 10-1   Referred pain, anterior and posterior regions.

of pain. For example, a patient watching an exciting football game with a friend may enjoy the game even if his surgical incision is quite painful. The lack of a grimace or physiological changes indicative of pain may be viewed as an absence of pain, when in fact the patient is using distraction as a way of coping with the presence of pain. People may fall asleep even though pain is severe, particularly if uncontrolled pain has left them in a state of exhaustion.

◆ Nursing Diagnosis

The nursing diagnosis for pain is frequently "Pain related to" the cause of the pain. An example would be "Pain related to fractured pelvis and fractured left femur."

◆ Planning

Plan the goals of nursing care by indicating actions that will promote the comfort of the patient during treatment and recovery. Planning should be a team effort. Physician input comes as written orders and progress notes and may also be available through direct discussion. In pain management, input from pharmacists, therapists, and other health care professionals should be included. As recovery progresses, the care plan is updated. The type of medication, method of delivery, and comfort measures will change as the patient's needs change.

Planning must address all areas that affect the patient's pain management needs, including family situation, cultural influences, financial constraints, and whether pain is acute or chronic in nature.

◆ Implementation

Actions are always implemented based on the current patient assessment. Therefore, all patients must be reassessed at the beginning of each hospital shift, clinic, or home visit. Appropriate actions would include providing analgesic as ordered, using nonpharmacological measures, such as repositioning or massage (adjunctive measures), and reporting to the physician when measures are not effective or have unwanted side effects. Implementation also includes monitoring effects of treatment and patient and family teaching.

Preventing complications from medications is an important aspect of implementation. Specific actions would include:

◆ Prominent documentation on the chart and medication record of any known drug allergies; and updating of this information should the patient show an adverse reaction to a current medication.

♦ Accurate recording of pertinent information obtained during the initial assessment phase, such as current medications, previous experience with pain, analgesics, and adjuncts to pain relief.

♦ Patient and family teaching regarding dose, frequency, and the need to first consult with the doctor or nurse before taking any other medications to avoid dangerous interactions.

♦ Appropriate monitoring of affects of any medications given and prompt notification of the physician should problems occur.

♦ Accurate and complete documentation of any adverse reactions and communication of that information to other health care providers and to the patient and appropriate family members.

♦ Evaluation

Ask the patient about the effectiveness of the pain-control measures. How quickly did relief occur, how long did it last, to what degree was the pain controlled, were there any unpleasant side effects? Whenever possible, use patient verbalization as the primary evaluation tool. Using a pain-assessment tool and comparing the patient's response to that before the pain relief was given is an effective evaluation technique.

If the patient is unable to verbalize, then evaluate the signs that can be directly observed. For instance, an aphasic stroke patient might thrash, moan, and look fearful when in pain, and evaluation of effective analgesia might include, "Mr. Jones now lying quietly, is free of facial tension, and is watching the activity around him. Did not moan when repositioned one hour after analgesic given."

♦ Documentation

All measures to control pain must be accurately documented:

♦ Initial pain assessment. Document the location, intensity, duration, and method used to assess (e.g., pain scale, patient verbalization).

♦ Measures taken (e.g., analgesic medication, adjunctive measures).

♦ Evaluation of effectiveness.

♦ Physician notification of problems or concerns and physician response, if applicable.

♦ Related patient or family education.

Example. Mrs. Smith states that her pain level following physical therapy is 7 on a 1-to-10 scale. Morphine sulfate 10 mg IM in the right deltoid is given. Forty-five minutes after injection, Mrs. Smith states that her pain level is now 2 to 3. Pulse 72, respirations 16, moving freely in bed. Discussed pain relief needs; suggested that she request pain medication before next therapy session. Mrs. Smith agreed.

Think about . . . What is the value of using a pain scale to evaluate a person's pain?

False Perceptions about Pain   There are many misconceptions regarding pain, and these can affect the ability of the physician and nurse to effectively assess the patient's pain and provide adequate pain relief.

False perception: If pain is really present, there must be a demonstrable cause.

Fact: Pain can be present even though no cause can be found. Although damage to the cells does lead to the release of chemicals that stimulate the pain receptors, in many cases pain may be present although no cellular abnormality can be found. The search for evidence that pain exists is, in the words of Hackett, "fruitless and irrelevant." The patient with a migraine headache may or may not suffer less than one with a brain tumor. We cannot say that, just because the brain tumor can be shown on a brain scan and the headache cannot, the person with the brain tumor has pain and the person with the headache does not.

False perception: The person who has a low tolerance for pain has no self-control and probably is emotionally immature or childish.

Fact: Pain tolerance is a physiological response to pain that is made more complex by psychosocial factors, many of which can be beyond the control of the patient. Tolerance for pain is defined as that duration or intensity of pain the person is *willing* to endure without seeking relief. **Pain tolerance varies greatly from one individual to another and in the same individual from time to time.** Nurses often place a high value on a patient's ability to feel pain without complaining or asking for relief. Those who value a high pain tolerance usually impose their own values on their patients by ignoring or belittling their reports of pain. **The person who should decide how willing he ought to be to tolerate pain is the one who is suffering.**

False perception: The neonate is too neurologically immature to perceive or remember pain, so analgesia is unnecessary in this age group.

Fact: *Neonates do perceive and maintain memory of pain.* They cry and pull away from procedures such as heelstick blood tests. Male infants cry and struggle if they are circumcised. Neonates with medical conditions which require repeated blood tests begin to cry and pull away as soon as someone grasps the foot as if to perform a blood test, indicating a memory of pain from previous heelsticks. **Analgesia is appropriate dur-**

ing procedures or situations which would be known to cause pain in more mature clients.

False perception: Elderly patients have a decreased ability to perceive pain and pain medicines are dangerous for them because of their age.

Fact: *Ability to express pain may be impaired by decreased cognitive function, but acute pain is still perceived.* Age combined with physical impairments such as decreased kidney or liver function may reduce tolerance for various medications, but with appropriate dosage and monitoring, geriatric patients can have good pain management without severe side effects. Untreated pain will interfere with sleep, nutrition, healing, and general well-being.

False perception: Reactions to acute pain and chronic pain are the same.

Fact: In general, acute pain is more often associated with anxiety and chronic pain with depression. The emotional reaction does not cause the pain, but it can intensify it. The management of acute and chronic pain is not the same and is discussed later in the chapter.

False perception: Addiction to pain-relieving drugs is always a hazard, and for the sake of the patient, nurses often must withhold a drug even though the patient asks for it.

Fact: A very small percentage of patients (probably less than 1% and no more than 3%) become addicted to drugs administered for the purpose of relieving acute pain. In spite of an abundance of evidence to the contrary, this mistaken belief about the dangers of addiction persists, causing needless suffering among patients who are denied adequate pain relief.

False perception: Placebos (substances prescribed that contain no medication, such as sterile saline or sugar pills) are very useful in assessing whether a patient actually has pain.

Fact: There is no basis for believing that a patient who finds relief from pain after receiving a placebo is pretending to have pain or that it is "all in his mind." The question of how placebos affect people and why they have a positive response in some and not in others still is poorly understood. However, there has been sufficient study of the subject to show that actual pain is sometimes well relieved by placebos.

Think about . . . What is the most difficult aspect of evaluating someone's pain?

PAIN MANAGEMENT

Effective pain management is not just a matter of giving the right medicine at the right time. It is a combination of pharmacological and nonpharmacological approaches that together give the individual the greatest possible degree of comfort for the longest possible time. This section covers a variety of pain-management tools and adjuncts.

◆ Pharmacological Approaches

- ◆ *Oral Analgesics.* Any substance taken by mouth for the control of pain. These include over-the-counter (OTC) medications, such as acetaminophen, aspirin, and ibuprofen, and prescription medications, such as codeine and morphine.

- ◆ *Intramuscular (IM) analgesics.* Substances which are injected into the muscular tissue to control pain.

- ◆ *Intravenous (IV) analgesics.* Substances injected or infused over a prescribed time directly into the vascular system.

- ◆ *Subcutaneous analgesics.* Medication injected or infused into the **subcutaneous** (fatty tissue just beneath the skin) tissue to control pain.

- ◆ *Patient-controlled analgesia (PCA).* An infusion device controlled by the patient that injects the prescribed dose. The PCA machine is programmed so that the patient can determine when a dose is given, but not exceed the maximum dose or minimum time interval ordered by the physician. PCA analgesia is usually IV, but may also be subcutaneous.

- ◆ *Epidural analgesic.* Medication infused directly into the **epidural** space near the base of the spine using a programmable pump. The infusion catheter is inserted by an anesthesiologist. Patients receiving epidural analgesia need to be monitored for possible delayed respiratory suppression or apnea, bradycardia, hypotension, urinary retention, nausea and vomiting, and allergic reactions, such as itching or hives. Report adverse symptoms to the anesthesiologist immediately.

- ◆ *Antidepressants.* A number of antidepressant medications have been found effective in controlling some specific types of pain, such as nerve root pain. They may be given alone or in combination with other analgesic medications.

- ◆ *Chemotherapeutic agents and other immunosuppressants.* Occasionally drugs such as methotrexate are used for intractable pain in rheumatoid conditions.

Invasive treatments, such as rhizotomies and cordotomies, which sever the nerve conducting the pain, are now uncommon. New advances in pain management, including surgically implanted medication pumps and nerve stimulators, have made these invasive treatments unnecessary in most cases. The medication dosage given directly to the spinal cord (intrathecal) is about 1/100 of the oral dose, so the patient suffers no central nervous system (CNS) side effects. They can work or drive cars while being relieved of severe pain.

Pharmacological analgesics, even OTCs, may be administered to patients in a health care facility only under a doctor's order to prevent unwanted interactions with other prescribed medications. For example, aspirin, commonly taken for occasional headache and arthritis pain, also is a powerful anticoagulant. It can lead to dangerous complications for someone who has a bleeding disorder or who is also on an anticoagulant medication. Acetaminophen in high doses is toxic to the liver, and may therefore be contraindicated in patients with a liver disorder.

Alerting patients that OTC drugs can have serious interactions with their prescribed drugs is an important part of patient education in home care and ambulatory care.

Elderly patients also suffer pain. The idea that pain perception diminishes with age is false. In fact, perception of pain may actually increase with age, as the individual becomes frail and has less resources for tolerating pain.

Elder Care Point . . . The very elderly frequently have reduced tolerance for medications. Smaller doses of analgesics may give effective relief without causing overwhelming sedation or disorientation. Elderly patients on analgesics must be monitored carefully.

Nurses' Responsibilities In addition to following the "five rights" (right patient, right drug, right dose, right route, right time), the nurse has a variety of responsibilities when giving analgesic medications:

1. Document drug, dose, route (including location of injection site on IM or subcutaneous injections), and reason for giving.
2. Monitor the effectiveness of pain relief after 15 to 30 minutes and at 1- to 2-hour intervals. Document the degree and duration of pain relief in the patient record.
3. If the analgesic is ineffective, determine whether a stronger analgesic is available to the patient and administer per physician order. If no other analgesic is available, notify physician that the medication is not effective. Also notify the physician if the medication is initially effective but the duration of effect is too short to maintain patient comfort until the next dose may be given.
4. If the analgesic results in unwanted side effects, (e.g., depressed vital signs, vomiting, or altered level of consciousness), monitor the patient closely and notify the physician before administering another dose.

Table 10-2 lists common analgesics by category and action. Table 10-3 lists common analgesics by route of administration.

◆ Side Effects and Complications of Pain Medication

Probably the most common and one of the most distressing side effects of pain medication is constipation. Analgesics, such as morphine, meperidine, and codeine, slow peristalsis. Fecal material becomes compacted and dry because of the extended time of passage through the intestines. Patients receiving these medica-

TABLE 10-2 ◆ *Analgesic Medications by Type and Primary Action*

Type of Drug and Primary Action	Examples	Nursing Implications
Non-narcotic analgesics, including nonsteroidal antiinflammatory drugs (NSAIDs) **Action:** block pain at the peripheral nervous system level.	Over-the-counter aspirin, acetaminophen, ibuprofen,* ketoprofen,* naproxen.* Prescription naproxen, indomethacin, ibuprofen, ketoprofen.	May be present in combination drugs. Various possible side effects of which to be aware. Educate patients not to use in combination with over-the-counter dosage of same medication.
Narcotics (opioids). **Action:** block pain at the central nervous system level.	Morphine, meperidine, hydromorphone, codeine.	Constipation common, can be severe. Can cause respiratory depression, antidote is naloxone (Narcan).
Medications with nonanalgesic primary actions used as adjuncts to pain control. **Action:** various mechanisms of action.	Antidepressants: amitriptyline, imipramine, trazedone hydrochloride. Anticonvulsants: phenytoin, carbamazepine. Stimulants: caffeine, dextroamphetamine. Muscle relaxants: carisprodol, baclofen.	Varied due to varied mechanisms of action. Always be aware of side effects and possible adverse reactions.

*Nonprescription dose.
Note: Combination drugs are often used. These may combine two forms of analgesic (e.g., acetaminophen and codeine) or an analgesic with another type of medication, such as an antihistamine. It is important to be aware of what is in combination drugs to prevent administration of excessive amounts of one of the components.

TABLE 10-3 ◆ *Common Analgesic Medications by Route*	
Oral	**Injectable**
Acetaminophen	Baclofen
Acetaminophen with codeine	Buprenorphine
Aspirin	Butorphanol
Baclofen	Fentanyl
Carisoprodol	Hydromorphone
Gabapentin	Meperidine
Hydrocodone	Morphine sulfate
Ibuprofen	Nalbuphine
Ketoprofen	
Morphine sulfate	
Morphine sulfate time-released	
Naproxen	
Oxycodone	

*The number of medications available for the control of pain is large and varied. This table gives only some of the more common generic analgesics, including adjunctive medications, currently used.

tions for any length of time should be monitored carefully for regular, normal bowel movements. **Oral fluids must be increased if possible.** Stool softeners and fiber-based laxatives, such as psyllium, can be helpful if approved by the physician.

Some side effects, such as drowsiness and euphoria, generally only last for the first few days and then spontaneously disappear. However, the nurse must always be alert to the possibility of a more serious adverse reaction. Allergic reactions, such as itching and hives, need to be reported immediately. The medication needs to be discontinued and an alternative order obtained. The patient may also need an antihistamine such as diphenhydramine for relief of symptoms.

Narcotic analgesics can depress the respiratory system to the point of apnea (no respiration). Should this occur, resuscitation must begin immediately. In the hospital setting this means providing respiratory support and calling the code team. In settings such as the home, doctor's office, or clinic, it means respiratory support and calling 911. The standard treatment for respiratory suppression from narcotics is Naloxone, an effective narcotic antagonist that can be given IM or IV.

As stated, the most feared side effect, that of addiction to narcotics, in reality almost never occurs. **Patients in pain have a right to expect that effective analgesia will be available to them.**

◆ Nonpharmacological Approaches

A variety of methods exist for relieving pain without medication or as an adjunct to medication. It is probable that the first treatment for pain was the automatic vigorous rubbing of the painful area, as when we rub our head or elbow if we bump it. Using adjuncts can increase the effectiveness of pain medication and may decrease the frequency in which it is needed.

Sleep   Adequate sleep and rest are major factors in healing. Rest increases pain tolerance and improves response to analgesia. Allow adequate time between treatments and other care for naps, and plan night care so interruptions in sleep are kept to a minimum. For instance, take vital signs when the patient is awake to use the bathroom or requests pain medication. It is important to remember that exhaustion will cause a patient to sleep despite severe pain, but such sleep is not as therapeutic. Appropriate analgesia combined with adequate rest promotes healing.

Warmth   Gentle heat is very soothing for many types of pain. Sources include warm compresses, warm blankets, aqua K-pads, hydrocolator pads, whirlpools, tub baths, heat lamps, and chemical self-heating packs. Compresses and packs are usually left in place for 15 to 20 minutes, although gentle heat sources such as aqua K-pads may be used over longer periods. Always check the temperature before applying, and monitor the patient closely for tolerance. The very young and the very old are particularly sensitive to heat. Anyone with an altered level of consciousness or loss of normal sensation may not realize something is too hot, and those with loss of movement may not be able to move away from the heat source when necessary.

Elder Care Point... The skin of the elderly is thin and burns more easily. Stroke patients frequently have areas of lost or diminished sensation. Patients with senile dementia may not recognize that something is too hot. Even the alert and oriented elderly person frequently falls asleep and may be burned without being aware of it. Monitor any heat applications **very** carefully.

Distraction   Any activity that takes a person's attention away from pain is termed a *distraction*. This includes watching TV, talking with friends, or playing a board game. People have an innate ability to distract themselves from their surroundings or situation. Health care workers may mistakenly interpret the patient's ability to do this as proof that there is no pain. Distracting activities can take the patient's mind off the pain momentarily, but they do not stop it. Distraction can be helpful in bridging the time gap between giving an analgesic and the onset of pain relief.

Relaxation   Relaxation also is called "tension release" and involves the conscious relaxation of muscle groups.

It is frequently done as a progression, beginning at the feet and moving up the body, ending with the neck and facial muscles. Initially, the nurse can guide the patient verbally, slowly directing the attention to the next muscle group to be relaxed. After one or two sessions, many patients can effectively provide their own relaxation sequence.

Imagery and Meditation   These methods use mental techniques to induce relaxation. Imagery involves assisting the patient to form mental images of a pleasant environment where they are comfortable and happy. For some, the experience is visual; in their minds they "see" a beautiful place. For others, it is a process of achieving a feeling of comfort and peace. Either is highly effective in giving the patient a brief mental "vacation" from pain. These methods often are used during painful procedures, such as bone marrow extraction.

Meditation involves the use of a focus point, which may be a sound (sometimes called a *mantra*), a repeated phrase, the sound of the breath as it moves in and out of the body, or a visual image. The visual image may be a picture or object that the patient gazes at, or it may be an imagined image.

Hypnosis   Hypnosis, or therapeutic suggestion, should be done by someone trained in the technique. It involves the use of focusing and relaxation to induce a trance-like state during which a patient receives suggestions that may be helpful after returning to a normal level of consciousness. Although people under hypnosis cannot be induced to do things they would ordinarily feel were wrong, this remains a common fear. Reassurance may help the patient to be more accepting, but hypnosis should be used only if the subject is comfortable with the idea and open to its use.

Biofeedback   This specialized technique requires the use of a machine that measures the degree of muscular tension with skin electrodes. The machine has colored lights that change (usually red to yellow to green) and a tone that changes in pitch from higher to lower as the patient relaxes. The patient receives visual and auditory confirmation of self-induced relaxation. This technique is particularly effective with people who are highly competitive because it rewards success and allows them to "win" the game.

Music   Music used alone can be highly effective in bringing about relaxation. It also can be used as a focal point for meditation or to enhance other distracting activities. Nature sounds also can be used to induce relaxation, including audio tapes of the ocean, running streams, breezes, rain, and birds singing. Headphones allow the patient to be immersed in sound without disturbing others.

Cold   Cold is particularly helpful in reducing swelling. It also can be effective in relieving muscle spasms and some types of joint pain. Ice massage of sore muscles can be done by freezing water in a paper cup, then tearing away the edge of the cup to expose the ice, leaving the base of the cup as a handle. Some individuals, however, are very sensitive to cold. If cold applications cause shivering, tensing of the muscles, or an increase in pain or spasm, discontinue their use.

Binders   Binders are helpful for strains, sprains, and surgical incisions. They support the tissues during movement, such as ambulation or coughing, which reduces the pain.

Massage (Cutaneous Stimulation)   Once a mainstay of nursing comfort measures, massage is enjoying a return to popularity. It uses long, firm strokes, short, soft circular strokes, and occasionally gentle pounding with the sides of the hands. It stimulates the circulation, relaxes the muscles, and increases the general sense of well-being. When the painful area has inflammation, a wound or an incision, massaging another area of the body with gentle, but firm pressure, helps the patient direct attention away from the pain. Always be guided by the patient's sense of comfort. Use only the degree of pressure that is pleasant and relaxing.

Simple massage can be done by a family member with just a little instruction, giving them an opportunity to assist in the care in a positive and loving way. Massage should not be used on any area that has been reddened by pressure. This tissue is already compromised and massage can cause further damage through "shearing," the traumatic pulling of tissue layers away from one another.

Acupuncture/Acupressure   Acupuncture originated centuries ago in China and involves the use of tiny needles inserted into the skin at specific points along lines called *meridians*, a concept similar to that of nerve pathways. In recent years it has gained favor in the United States as a pain-control measure. Acupressure involves the use of external finger pressure at the meridian points to achieve similar effects. Both acupuncture and acupressure require extensive training for proper use and should only be done by someone fully trained in these procedures.

Transcutaneous Electrical Nerve Stimulation (TENS)   TENS utilizes a small electrical stimulator attached to the skin with electrodes placed around the area of pain. A low current running between them acts to block pain sensation. The degree of stimulation can be controlled by the patient using dials on the stimulator. The application of TENS requires specific training and must be ordered by a physician. Occasionally a patient will find TENS unpleasant rather than helpful. In such cases, the physician should be notified and an alternative method of pain control selected.

Menthol   When applied to the skin, menthol causes warming and this may have an analgesic effect. Mentholated products are usually massaged into the skin, giving the individual the benefit of both massage and warmth. They are available over the counter, but require a physician's order in a hospital or clinic setting. Do not use with external heating devices, to avoid overheating the skin surface. Caution the patient to wash hands well after applying and to avoid contact of the menthol with the eyes or mucus membranes.

Think about... List nonpharmacological methods for managing pain.

ACUTE VERSUS CHRONIC PAIN

Patients with acute pain are frequently anxious and fearful. This fear and anxiety can take many forms. They may fear something is seriously wrong, that they will not get relief from the pain, or that, if they do, they will become addicted to the pain medication. The anxiety and fear of these patients frequently are alleviated by first providing adequate analgesia to relieve the pain and then by educating them about their pain and the methods that can be used to control pain safely. Being made part of the pain-management team reassures patients that health care professionals believe them and want to make them comfortable so they can focus on getting well and back to normal activity.

Chronic pain, on the other hand, is most commonly associated with depression. People who hurt most or all of the time frequently resign themselves to the idea that they can never again live a normal life. New research

and the work of several outstanding pain centers and nurse and physician specialists now offer much to sufferers of chronic pain. Many people whose lives were previously dictated by their pain now experience good control and have returned to normal, productive lives. Table 10-4 compares both types of pain.

COMMUNITY CARE

Community care can take place in a variety of settings, with varying levels of training among direct caregivers. Nurses working in a hospital setting may be called upon to teach pain-management techniques to those who provide care in the community setting. Nurses working in areas that serve the community directly need a clear understanding of pain care management to assist their clients best.

◆ Extended Care

Extended-care facilities may provide rehabilitative services, long-term care services, or both. Each type of care may include specific pain care management needs.

Patients undergoing rehabilitation often have acute pain related to therapy, particularly in the early phases. It is important that therapy be scheduled to allow for adequate rest and recovery time. It also is important that analgesic medication be given on a schedule that provides the patient with the greatest freedom from pain during therapy sessions. This assists the patient to cooperate with therapy, which in turn encourages a more rapid recovery. Always include the patient in the planning. They know best what medication and what time schedule are giving the best pain relief.

Long-term care facilities, called nursing homes, skilled nursing facilities, and board and care homes, often have patients who live there for the last weeks,

TABLE 10-4 ◆ *Acute versus Chronic Pain*		
	Acute	**Chronic**
Duration	Hours to days.	Months to years.
Prognosis for relief	Good; may resolve spontaneously or in response to analgesic therapy.	Poor unless complicating factors removed; spontaneous relief unusual.
Cause	Relatively easy to identify.	Sometimes cause is known, but diagnosis may be complex or undetermined.
Psychosocial effects	Usually transient or none. May temporarily disrupt normal activites or routine.	Can affect ability to earn a living, enjoy social activities, maintain self-esteem.
Effect of therapy	Medication usually beneficial, surgery often helpful.	Medications may be helpful, but patient may become dependent. Surgery may help, but also may worsen the problem.

months, or even years of their lives. In this setting, the term *resident* is used, rather than patient. They may have pain following a fall, dental work, or during a period of illness; and they may have chronic pain from such conditions as arthritis, degenerative disorders, or cancer.

Residents in these settings may be mentally alert and oriented, alert and confused, or have a decreased level of consciousness. However, each of these individuals can perceive pain and should be given appropriate analgesics when pain exists. The nurse can be of great assistance to the physician in ordering analgesia by providing accurate information about the type of pain, the frequency, the intensity, and precipitating factors. For instance, a resident with degenerative arthritis may have chronic joint pain and benefit from a routine oral analgesic such as acetaminophen or ibuprofen. Those with more severe chronic problems, such as cancer, may benefit from routine time-released medications such as MS Contin (oral morphine sulfate in a time-released tablet). As pain increases, more narcotic may be needed to gain relief, but also remember that the very elderly or debilitated may be more drug sensitive. Monitor all medication carefully and work with the physician to ensure that the resident's pain is being appropriately addressed. Ideally, the patient is comfortable as well as alert and able to participate in activities of choice.

◆ Home Care

The number of individuals receiving skilled and professional nursing care at home is increasing rapidly. Early discharge from the hospital is growing primarily due to (1) the fact that people are generally more comfortable and heal more rapidly in their own environment; and (2) the need to control escalating costs in medical care.

Licensed nurses in the home care setting allow for the use of many of the same pain-management techniques available to the hospitalized patient. People frequently go home from the hospital with peripheral or central IV lines and can therefore receive IV analgesia. PCA is now frequently used in the home care setting. Patient and family education on pain management in the home setting is done by the licensed nurse. Teaching needs to include verbal and written instructions about the medication and any equipment used to dispense it. Telephone numbers that give the patient and family access to 24-hour assistance should be prominently displayed. Many home care agencies now provide a refrigerator door magnet with the telephone number in large, easy-to-read print. Just as in an inpatient setting, home care patients must be evaluated for the continued safe effectiveness of the analgesic medication. The nurse must contact the physician any time the medication orders need to be adjusted. Adjuncts to pain management, such as simple massage, relaxation techniques, the use of pillows, warmth, repositioning, or soft music, are readily taught to patients and families for use in the home care setting.

PCA medications are on occasion given subcutaneously rather than IV, particularly for those patients with poor peripheral venous access who are not candidates for a central line. A tiny needle is placed in the subcutaneous tissue on the abdomen and taped in place. Sites are changed at regular intervals to maintain good absorption of the medication and avoid damage to the tissues. However, the increased use of central IV catheters and ports and the availability of oral timed-release analgesics are making subcutaneous PCA much less common.

Current guidelines for home care by agencies such as Medicare require that case management be done by a licensed professional. This is usually a registered nurse, although the registered physical therapist may fill this role for patients whose only acute need is continued restorative therapy. The role of the LVN or LPN is that of direct patient care under the guidance of the case manager. In many states, LVNs may insert peripheral IVs and infuse standard IV solutions without any additives, but cannot begin an infusion of medications, blood products, or solutions with additives. The LPN may monitor an ongoing infusion and discontinue the infusion as needed, but must report any difficulties immediately to the RN case manager for intervention.

Home care patients may be suffering from pain due to progressive conditions, such as cancer. In such cases, the nurse must always be alert to an increase in pain due to changes in the disease process. The physician needs to be notified of the change so that appropriate measures, including adjusting or changing the medications, can take place.

CRITICAL THINKING EXERCISES

Read each clinical situation and discuss the questions with your classmates.

1. Ann Jefferson, a 43-year-old female, has suffered from shoulder pain from an old healed fracture for several years. Her physician has prescribed an oral narcotic analgesic for her when the pain becomes too severe to be controlled with acetaminophen, but Ann does not want to continue taking drugs that she "might become addicted to":

   a. How would you respond to Ann's statement regarding her fear of addiction to the pain medication?

b. What other measures could you suggest for management of Ann's pain?

2. Fred Hickson had a bowel resection 3 days ago. He is determined to get back to work quickly and is very cooperative about ambulation. He refuses pain medication, stating, "I don't need it". You note that he stops frequently to lean against the wall, walks stooped over, and grimaces when no one is looking.

a. Why might Fred be refusing pain medication?

b. What information might you share regarding pain control and getting well after major surgery?

c. What suggestions might you make to Fred regarding his comfort?

BIBLIOGRAPHY

Benesh, L. et al. (1997). Tools for assessing chronic pain in rural elderly women. *Home Healthcare Nurse.* 15(3): 207–211.

Durham, E., Frost-Haartzer, P. (1991). Relaxation therapy works. *RN.* 54(8):40–42.

Economou, D. (1996). Combining analgesics safely. *Nursing 96.* 26(11):32.

Editors. (1993). *Nurse's guide to O.T.C. analgesics. Nursing 93.* 23(3):66–71.

Ferrell, B. R. (1994). Controlling pain; using placebos ethically. *Nursing 94.* 24(3):28.

Hambelton, N. E. (1994). Dealing with complications of epidural analgesia. *Nursing 94.* 24(10):55–57.

Kemp, C. (1996). Managing chronic pain in patients with advanced disease and substance-related disorders. *Home Healthcare Nurse.* 14(4):255–261.

Lilley, L. L., Guanci, R. (1996). Using high-dose fentanyl patches. *American Journal of Nursing.* 96(7): 18–22.

Magrum, L. C., Bentzen, C., Landmark, S. (1996). Pain management in home care. *Seminars in Oncology Nursing.* 12(3):202–218.

Mattox, L. M. (1996). A working method for pain management outcomes documentation. *MEDSURG Nursing.* 5(4):269–271.

Maxwell, J. (1997). The gentle power of acupressure. *RN.* 60(4):53–56.

McCaffery, M. (1997). Pain management handbook. *Nursing 97.* 27(4):42–45.

McCaffery, M., Beebe, A. (1989). Pain. *Clinical Manual for Nursing Practice.* St. Louis, MO: Mosby.

McConnell, E. H. (1996). About naloxone. *Nursing 96.* 26(8):17. 60(4):53–56.

Melzak, R., Wall, P. D. (1965). Pain mechanisms, a new theory. *Science.* 150:971–979.

Pasero, C. L., Vanderveer, B. L. (1994). Pain control; epidural infusions; not just for labor anymore. *American Journal of Nursing.* 94(12):51–52.

Pasero, C. L. (1996). Alternative use of PCA. *American Journal of Nursing.* 96(10):66–68.

Patterson, J. W. (1994). Banishing phantom pain. *Nursing 94.* 24(9):64.

Peterson, A. M. (1997). Analgesics. *RN.* 60(4):45–50.

Wilkie, D. J. (1995). Relieving cancer pain. *Nursing Clinics of North America.* 30(4).

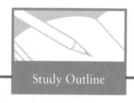

Study Outline

I. Introduction

A. Pain is commonly associated with many of the conditions for which people seek health care.

B. It was traditionally seen as a symptom that would go away when the disease process was cured.

C. Pain is now seen as a specific entity that needs to be addressed directly.

D. Only the patients can perceive the pain, and they must be an active member of the pain-management team.

II. The Pathophysiology of Pain

A. Pain is a neurological response to unpleasant stimuli.

B. Pain receptors are distributed abundantly throughout the skin and many of the deeper structures.

1. These receptors do not become dulled and may even become more acutely sensitive with repeated stimulation.

2. Gate control theory:

   a. Pain is controlled by a neurological gate that allows pain perception when open and blocks pain perception when closed.

   b. Various forms of stimulation compete for access to this gate and may override and block pain perception (e.g., massage and distraction).

    c. Fear can increase pain; knowing that the pain can be controlled may reduce it.

  3. Pieces of pain concept:

    a. More intense pain can be viewed as more "pieces" of pain that will require more "pieces" of analgesic to be controlled.

    b. Inadequate analgesia results in leftover pain.

  4. Endorphins attach to pain receptors and block sensation. They appear to modify and inhibit unpleasant stimuli, reduce anxiety, and produce feelings of well-being.

III. Perception of Pain

A. Pain perception varies widely between individuals and even for the same individual in different circumstances.

  1. Coping with pain requires large amounts of energy.

  2. Robust patients tolerate pain better than debilitated patients.

  3. Fatigue can increase the perception of pain.

  4. A variety of physiological responses may indicate pain. Their absence does not prove the absence of pain.

B. A person's cultural background influences feelings about and reactions to pain.

IV. Nursing Management

A. Assessment.

  1. Observe patients for appearance, behavior, and activity level. Listen to what they say and be alert for physiological changes that may indicate pain.

  2. Assist patients to choose and correctly use an evaluation tool that allows accurate and consistent communication about the degree of pain and pain relief (e.g., number, visual, color, or pieces of pain scales).

  3. Language barriers and the need to find and work through an interpreter can interfere with effective communication.

  4. Referred pain may cause confusion about the actual source of pain.

  5. The lack of outward signs of pain may cause the nurse to doubt the presence of pain.

B. Planning.

  1. The goals of nursing care must include actions to promote comfort.

  2. Planning should be a team effort, including nurse, physician, pharmacist, therapists, and, most important, the patient.

  3. Family situations, cultural influences, financial constraints, and whether pain is acute or chronic must be considered.

C. Implementation.

  1. Actions must always be based on current patient assessment.

  2. Implementation includes monitoring effects of treatment and teaching and the prevention of complications from medications and treatments.

D. Evaluation.

  1. The patient's statement is the best source of information about the effectiveness of pain management.

  2. Use objective observation as the primary source only if the patient is unable to give verbal input.

E. Documentation should include assessment of pain, measures taken, evaluation of effectiveness, any problems or need to contact the physician, and related education.

F. False perceptions about pain can interfere with appropriate pain assessment and management. Review section on false perceptions.

V. Pain Management

A. Effective pain management includes the use of medications.

  1. Medication routes include oral, IM, IV, subcutaneous, PCA, epidural, and intrathecal.

  2. Close observation and proper planning will help prevent serious complications from drug side effects and interactions.

  3. The elderly frequently have reduced tolerance for medication.

  4. Reassessment after pain medication allows for further intervention if the initial treatment was not effective or has undesired side effects.

  5. Constipation is a distressing, common, and preventable side effect of narcotic analgesics.

  6. Narcotic-induced drowsiness and euphoria generally disappear spontaneously after a few days.

  7. Allergic reactions require immediate intervention, including discontinuing the related medication.

  8. Narcotics can cause severe respiratory depression and apnea. Naloxone should always be available when narcotics are being administered.

B. Effective pain management includes the use of adjunctive measures as appropriate.

  1. Adjuncts to pain control that do not require a physician's order include sleep, warmth, distraction, relaxation, massage, music, and imagery and meditation.

2. Adjuncts to pain control that do require a physician's order include hypnosis, biofeedback, binders, acupuncture, acupressure, and TENS.

VI. Acute Versus Chronic Pain

A. Acute pain is frequently accompanied by fear and anxiety.

B. Chronic pain is commonly associated with depression.

VII. Community Care

A. The need for pain management continues in nonacute settings, such as skilled nursing centers, rehabilitation centers, board and care homes, and in the home.

B. Licensed nurses in the community setting allow many of the same techniques available to the hospitalized patient to be used after discharge from the acute care facility.

CHAPTER 11

Care of the Immobile Patient: Preventing Complications

OBJECTIVES

Upon completing this chapter the student should be able to:
1. Identify patients at risk for problems associated with immobility.
2. Describe the effect of immobility on each of the major systems of the body.
3. Assess the status of patients to identify actual problems or risk for problems secondary to immobility.
4. Develop and implement plans for nursing interventions to prevent the adverse effects of immobility.
5. List nursing diagnoses and appropriate interventions to alleviate the problems associated with immobility.
6. Evaluate the effectiveness of nursing interventions to alleviate or prevent the problems associated with immobility for a clinical patient.

Patients are immobilized to varying degrees and for different amounts of time. The multiple trauma patient may be on bedrest for several weeks. The patient with advanced multiple sclerosis may be able to move around only with a wheelchair. The patient who experiences great difficulty breathing from advanced lung disease may have very little energy and does not move around much for that reason. The patient with spinal cord injury or brain damage from a stroke may be immobile for the rest of his life. The patient in traction may be immobilized and on bedrest for several weeks. Patients who have pain or who have arthritic joints that cause pain with movement also tend to be less mobile. Patients who have a disorder requiring bedrest also are at risk. All of these patients are subject to the problems of immobility.

Healthy People 2000 objectives in part aim to decrease the problems that are secondary to disability. The nurse, through action and education of the patient and family, can help prevent the secondary problems and accompanying disability of the immobile patient and thereby help our nation meet the *Healthy People 2000* objectives.

NURSING PROCESS

Nurses must evaluate each patient situation and determine whether the patient is at risk for problems related to immobility. **Even if the patient is going to be immobile for only a few days, measures should be taken to prevent secondary problems.** Table 11-1 presents a list of common disorders that often cause some degree of immobility. Patients with these disorders should be assessed for the degree of risk for the various problems of immobility and interventions to prevent them should be initiated.

> The appropriate nursing diagnosis for patients with limited mobility is "Impaired physical mobility related to . . . " (whatever is the causative factor).

Goals, expected outcomes, and specific interventions are devised to meet individual patient needs. Each problem secondary to immobility is given its own nursing diagnosis and then incorporated into the total plan of care for the patient. Nursing Care Plan 11-1

TABLE 11-1 ◆ *Disorders That May Cause Immobility*

- Multiple sclerosis
- Stroke
- Spinal cord injury
- Lower-extremity amputation
- Head injury
- Multiple trauma
- Fractures of the knee, leg, ankle, hip, pelvis, spine
- Neuromuscular disorders: muscular dystrophy, atrophic lateral sclerosis, poliomyelitis, cerebral palsy, myasthenia gravis, etc.
- Congenital deformities
- Burns
- Advanced metastatic cancer
- Advanced stages of chronic disorders, such as Parkinson's disease, Alzheimer's disease, or Huntington's chorea
- Severe rheumatoid arthritis, osteoarthritis, and other forms of arthritis

presents a sample plan of care for a patient experiencing immobility.

The prevention of problems related to immobility begins the moment a patient first becomes ill or injured.

Preventive actions must continue as long as the patient needs health care, which may be for the rest of her life if she has a chronic illness or a permanent injury.

Some therapeutic purposes of rest and immobility include (1) relief from pain and further injury of a part, as in a fractured bone; (2) reduction of the workload of the heart in a cardiac condition; (3) promotion of healing and repair; and (4) conservation of energy.

The systems of the body work together as a whole. Lack of activity does not affect only one system. The effects vary depending on the general health of the

Nursing Care Plan 11-1

Selected nursing diagnoses, goals/expected outcomes, nursing interventions, and evaluations for an immobilized patient

Situation: Patient is an 83-year-old male with extreme weakness and debilitation and with several chronic diseases. He was transferred to a convalescent center after hospitalization for pneumonia, which has now almost completely resolved.

Nursing Diagnosis	Goals/Expected Outcomes	Nursing Intervention	Evaluation
Impaired physical mobility related to weakness, debility, illness and age. SUPPORTING DATA Unable to turn or reposition self unaided; cannot walk.	Patient will maintain present joint mobility. Patient will do active ROM of arms by discharge.	Perform ROM on all joints tid. Assist to turn and reposition q 2 h round the clock. Place in high Fowler's position for meals; assist to chair for lunch.	ROM: 10, 1, and 5 o'clock; turned: 8, 10, 12, and 2 o'clock; up in chair for lunch; continue plan.
Impaired skin integrity related to immobility and pressure over left trochanter. SUPPORTING DATA Pressure area, stage I, over left trochanter. History of previous pressure ulcers.	No further evidence of pressure damage to skin before discharge.	Position in bed so that one leg is not pressing on the other when patient is on his side; properly support with pillows. Turn more frequently than q 2 h if possible. Keep reddened area clean, clear dressing in place; inspect q shift. Inspect all pressure points q 4 h to identify problems early. Use turning sheet to turn patient.	Turned q 1 h; Tegoderm in place; redness decreasing; other pressure points clear; positioned with pillows.
Alteration in bowel elimination: constipation related to immobility. SUPPORTING DATA Has passed only small amount of hard, dry stool in past 4 days.	Normal bowel pattern by discharge.	Administer oil retention enema as ordered, followed by suppository; monitor results. Give stool softener daily as ordered. Increase fluids to 8 oz every hour while awake. Assist to bedside commode after breakfast each day. Provide privacy. Add bran muffin to breakfast. Offer prune juice nightly.	Taking 4 oz q h; small BM after breakfast; stool softener, prune juice, and bran muffin taken. Continue plan.

Nursing Care Plan 11-1 (Continued)

Nursing Diagnosis	Goals/Expected Outcomes	Nursing Intervention	Evaluation
Risk for injury related to possible falls. SUPPORTING DATA Very weak and debilitated; cannot walk. Tends to be confused after sundown.	Patient will not sustain fall in hospital.	Keep siderails up at all times when not at bedside. Place call light and personal items within reach. Answer call light promptly. Frequently reinforce instructions not to get up without assistance. Assist to bedside commode with two people. Keep low light on in room at night to decrease confusion. Check on patient frequently; anticipate needs.	Siderails up; asking for assistance to get up; night light on during night; less confused.
Risk for impaired gas exchange related to immobility and resolving pneumonia. SUPPORTING DATA Impaired mobility; weakness and debility; lungs just cleared from pneumonia; breathes shallowly naturally.	Patient will perform breathing exercises q 2 h while awake. Lung fields will remain clear.	Auscultate lungs q shift. Assist with sitting position for deep-breathing and coughing exercises q 2 h. Encourage adequate fluid intake. Administer remaining doses of antibiotics as ordered. Encourage him to take deeper breaths during each commercial break when watching television.	Turn, cough, deep-breathe: 8, 10, and 2; lungs clear to auscultation; intake 1,500 mL this shift. Taking antibiotics. Continue plan.
Risk for infection, urinary tract, related to immobility. SUPPORTING DATA Immobility causes stasis of urine; debilitated state makes patient more susceptible to infection; has history of urinary tract infections.	No urinary tract infection, as evidenced by clear urine, no dysuria, no fever. Patient will have fluid intake of at least 2,000 mL per day.	Assess for bladder distention q 4 h; observe characteristics of urine for signs of infection. Measure fluid input and output: encourage fluids every hour while awake.	Urine clear amber; I = 2,650 mL, O = 2,020 mL; taking fluids q h; no bladder distention; continue plan.
Risk for alteration in tissue perfusion related to possible thrombophlebitis from immobility. SUPPORTING DATA Immobile, debilitated, unable to walk. Has moderate peripheral vascular disease.	No evidence of thrombophlebitis or deep vein thrombosis; negative Homans' sign, no swelling of legs.	Encourage active ROM of legs, feet, and ankles q 2 h while awake. Keep TED hose smoothly in place except for 30 min while bathing. Encourage extra fluid intake. Assess for Homans' sign q shift; visually inspect legs for reddening or swelling.	Homans' sign negative; leg exercises: 8, 10, 12, and 2; TEDs in place; taking adequate fluids.

individual, the age, the degree of immobility, and the length of time of inactivity or bedrest. Lack of mobility may begin a vicious circle that can lead only to an ever-increasing loss of independence for the patient. As she becomes less able to move, the patient becomes more dependent, and as she becomes more dependent, she is less able to care for herself—which in turn leads to even more adverse effects from immobility. It is the responsibility of the nurse to avoid the beginning of such a cycle by helping the patient maintain normal functioning of each body system to the highest degree possible.

Elder Care Point... Although a lot of elderly people are physically active daily, many do not engage in much physical activity. When immobilized, these patients quickly lose what strength and flexibility they had as muscle fibers atrophy quickly. It is much more difficult for these patients to regain mobility.

TABLE 11-2 ◆ *Effects and Problems of Immobility*		
Body Part or System	**Effect of Immobility**	**Problem or Complication**
Cardiovascular system	Venous stasis Increased cardiac workload Blood pressure alterations	Thrombus formation Thrombophlebitis Pulmonary embolus Orthostatic hypotension Increased pulse rate
Respiratory system	Stasis of secretions Decreased elastic recoil Decreased vital capacity	Hypostatic pneumonia Bacterial pneumonia Atelectasis Decreased gas exchange
Gastrointestinal tract	Anorexia Metabolic change to catabolism and negative nitrogen balance Decreased peristalsis	Weight loss Protein defficiency Abdominal distention Constipation
Musculoskeletal system	Decreased muscle mass and muscle tension Shortening of muscle Loss of calcium from bone matrix Decrease in bone weight	Fibrosis of connective tissue Atrophy Weakness Joint contracture Osteoporosis Bone pain
Urinary system	Stasis of urine Urinary tract infection Renal stones	Precipitation of calcium salts Frequency Dysuria
Skin	Decreased circulation from pressure Ischemia and necrosis of tissue	Skin breakdown Pressure ulcers
Brain/psychological	Decreased mental activity Decreased sensory input Decreased socialization Decreased independence	Disorientation Confusion Boredom Anxiety Depression Loneliness

Early effects of immobility begin within a few days and include a decrease in muscle strength, generalized weakness, easy fatigue, joint stiffness, decreased coordination, abdominal distention, and various metabolic changes detectable by laboratory test. Table 11-2 presents the more severe problems when lack of activity occurs for more than a few days.

The nurse must thoroughly assess the patient daily, looking closely at each body system in which a problem related to immobility might occur. She must be knowledgeable about the signs and symptoms of each type of problem and understand how to intervene to decrease or prevent it.

CARDIOVASCULAR SYSTEM

◆ Thrombus Formation

Pathophysiology The effects of bedrest on the cardiovascular system include thrombus formation, increased cardiac workload, and orthostatic hypotension.

Blood flow in the veins is decreased when the patient is on bedrest because of external pressure on the veins and lack of the normal muscle contraction and relaxation that occur during activity. The contractions normally squeeze the veins, pushing the blood back toward the heart. When blood flow is sluggish, there is a tendency for it to form a **thrombus** (clot). A thrombus in an extremity impedes blood flow and can irritate the vessel wall, causing a **thrombophlebitis** (clot with inflammation of the vessel wall). Should the thrombus break off and travel in the vascular system, it can become a *pulmonary embolus* (clot lodged in the vessels of the lung).

Assessment Signs and symptoms of a thrombus include swelling of a leg and pain in the calf upon dorsiflexion of the foot while the knee is bent (Homan's sign). Additional signs, such as warmth and redness over the affected area and a temperature elevation, indicate thrombophlebitis. Any of these signs or symptoms should be reported to the physician immediately and the leg should be elevated. **The patient, family, and all health care workers should be warned not to massage the area because of the danger of dislodging the clot.**

Think about . . . Can you describe to a classmate three specific ways in which you would assess a patient for a thrombus in a lower extremity?

Signs of pulmonary embolus include sudden chest pain, difficulty breathing, anxiety, increased pulse rate, bloody sputum, and a feeling of impending doom.

Prevention and Nursing Intervention Interventions to prevent thrombus formation include aspirin therapy, heparin therapy, application of elastic stockings, use of intermittent pneumatic compression devices, changing position frequently, refraining from placing pressure on the posterior knee or deep veins of the lower extremities, and exercising the muscles of the legs with range of motion (ROM) exercises. The patient is taught to flex each leg at the knee and dorsiflex and extend the foot. The ankles are then rotated one direction and then the other. This works the muscles of the thigh and calf, "milking" the veins of the leg and increasing circulation. Fluid intake is increased to 2,500 to 3,000 mL per day, providing fluid to keep the blood as thin as possible and to help prevent clot formation. Ambulation is started as soon as the patient is able to walk as it is the most effective action to prevent thrombus formation. Assessment and nursing intervention for the patient with thrombophlebitis are discussed more thoroughly in Chapter 18.

♦ Increased Cardiac Workload

Pathophysiology The heart works about 30% harder when the patient is in a reclining position. The increased workload has to do with changes in vascular resistance, pressures in the vascular system, gravity changes placing more blood into central circulation, all of which increase stroke volume and cardiac output. This means that the heart has to pump harder. Another factor is that people on bedrest perform the **Valsalva maneuver** 10 to 20 times an hour, tensing their thoracic muscles and holding their breath while exerting themselves and then releasing their breath suddenly. Patients who are confined to bed do this when they use their arms and upper trunk muscles to move themselves about in bed. This maneuver also is done when one strains in an attempt to produce a bowel movement.

When the breath is held and the chest muscles are tensed, exhaled air is pushed against the closed glottis and the flow of blood in the large veins is stopped. This decreases venous return and cardiac output, making the heart work harder to deliver oxygen and nutrients to the tissues. As soon as the muscles are relaxed and the air is exhaled, the blood that has been dammed up in the large veins is suddenly delivered to the heart. **In this way, the workload of the heart is suddenly increased as it must pump out a much larger volume than normal.**

Assessment   A sign of increased cardiac workload is a higher pulse rate. The nurse assesses the patient to see whether the pulse rate is increasing over time and checks to see whether movement in bed occurs without performance of the Valsalva maneuver.

Prevention and Nursing Intervention   Measures to prevent this increase in cardiac workload include placing the patient in a sitting position and teaching exhalation with the mouth open while moving up in bed or attempting to have a bowel movement. Moving the patient with a lift sheet or fitting the bed with a trapeze bar will help the patient refrain from performing the Valsalva maneuver. Providing adequate fiber and fluid in the diet also helps keep the stool soft and prevent straining to defecate. Providing privacy for toileting, helping the patient to the commode, commode chair, or into a squatting or upright position also helps prevent the Valsalva maneuver by preventing constipation.

♦ Orthostatic Hypotension

Pathophysiology   We all probably have experienced weakness and possibly fainting the first time we stood up after having been in bed for several days. The weakness, dizziness, and fainting that may occur is a result of a drop in blood pressure. This condition is called *orthostatic hypotension,* or low blood pressure from standing up straight. It occurs because of decreased muscle tone and because normal compensatory mechanisms have been disrupted by the body being continuously in a lying position on bedrest.

The danger of this situation lies in the possibility that the patient may fall and sustain injuries if there is not sufficient help to support her when she first attempts to get out of bed after prolonged rest.

Elder Care Point . . . The older patient is even more prone to orthostatic hypotension since the vascular system does not respond to position changes as effectively as in younger years. Many elderly patients are taking medications that produce orthostatic hypotension as a side effect. These patients should be supported adequately any time they are repositioned or brought to an upright position.

Assessment   An increase in pulse rate and a drop in blood pressure after a position change from supine to more upright indicates orthostatic hypotension. Dizziness, lightheadedness, seeing spots, or fainting are other symptoms.

Prevention and Nursing Intervention   **Measures to decrease the degree of orthostatic hypotension include getting the patient out of bed as soon as possible, even if only up to a chair.** The patient should change positions gradually. Baseline vital signs are taken with the patient in the supine position. She is slowly raised to a high Fowler's position and her vital signs are taken again to determine increases in pulse rate or decreases in blood pressure. With the nurse present, the patient is left in the high Fowler's position for a couple of minutes to allow the body to adapt to the changes in vital signs. The patient is questioned about dizziness or lightheadedness. When it is determined that her vital signs are stable in this position, she is positioned on the side of the bed with her feet on the floor. Again, she is allowed to stabilize in this position; when there is no dizziness or lightheadedness, she is transferred to the chair. If the patient can stand, she is first raised up on her feet at the bedside, supported, and allowed to stabilize before being assisted to the chair. If she is unable to bear weight, the nurse transfers her to the chair, preferably with the help of an assistant.

If the patient has been on bedrest for a considerable time, the physician may order "tilt" table use before ambulation is attempted. The physical therapist will transport the patient to the physical therapy department and place her on a table that can be tilted by degrees to a more upright position so that the body can adjust slowly to position changes.

Think about . . . Why is a patient who is dehydrated or on diuretic therapy to decrease fluid volume more prone to develop a thrombus when on bedrest?

RESPIRATORY SYSTEM

◆ Pneumonia

Pathophysiology   **When a person's normal mobility is impaired, she does not breathe as deeply or move secretions out of the lungs normally.** If the patient is on bedrest, some portion of the lungs is dependent and full expansion of the chest is blocked by the bed. Secretions collect in the dependent portion of the lung. Stagnant secretions provide a good place for bacteria to grow and the patient may develop hypostatic pneumonia.

Totally immobile patients and those on long-term bedrest become generally weakened; the cough reflex becomes inefficient. When secretions cannot be coughed up, the nurse must maintain a patent airway by suctioning out retained secretions.

Elder Care Point . . . Aging causes a loss of elastic recoil of the lungs, increased airway resistance, and reduced vital capacity, all of which decrease gas exchange. A poor nutritional state is frequently found in the elderly. This predisposes to all types of infections that accompany immobility. Poor nutritional status combined with the effects of bedrest on the respiratory system make the elderly bedrest patient highly susceptible to pneumonia.

Assessment   Signs and symptoms of respiratory problems include gurgling breaths indicating retained secretions, productive cough with colored sputum, fever, pain upon inspiration, dyspnea, decreased breath sounds, and crackles and wheezes heard on auscultation of the lungs.

Additional assessment might include checking bandages and binders to make sure they are not restricting movement of the chest muscles, noting whether abdominal distention is causing pressure against the diaphragm, and determining whether sedatives and other drugs that depress respiration are interfering with normal breathing patterns.

Prevention and Nursing Intervention   **Nursing measures to prevent respiratory problems related to immobility include frequent turning, coughing and deep-breathing exercises, use of an incentive spirometer, adequate fluid intake, and ambulation as soon as and whenever possible.** When it is not possible for the patient to ambulate or sit up in a chair, changing her position to the semi-Fowler's or Fowler's position and from side to side every 2 hours can facilitate the movement of secretions in the air passages.

The patient is asked to deep-breathe and cough at least every 2 hours. She is instructed to take a deep breath in through the nose, hold it for about 10 seconds, and exhale slowly through pursed lips; take another deep breath and exhale slowly again; take a third deep breath and cough as she exhales. This technique prevents excessive fatigue. Incisions should be splinted with a small pillow or the hands when attempting to cough to prevent strain on the incision and decrease pain.

When the patient cannot cough effectively and is accumulating secretions in the nasal-tracheal area, the nurse suctions the secretions from the upper airways using aseptic technique. If the patient has a tracheostomy or endotracheal tube in place, the nurse uses sterile technique to suction the lower airways (see Chapter 16). When the patient has no evidence of retained secretions, deep-breathing without coughing will help prevent atelectasis and improve oxygenation in the immobile patient.

Adequate fluid intake is necessary so that the secretions in the air passages will not become too dry, thick, and difficult to remove by coughing. When the patient has abdominal distention or nausea or is otherwise not inclined to drink fluids, it is better to have him drink small amounts at frequent intervals rather than giving large quantities at a time.

Think about . . . Can you describe why having a patient deep-breathe and cough every 2 hours helps prevent hypostatic pneumonia?

GASTROINTESTINAL SYSTEM

◆ Anorexia

Pathophysiology   Perhaps the most common difficulty experienced by a patient who is immobilized and unable to carry out her usual activities of daily life is that of loss of appetite. Worry, depression, anxiety about dependence on others, and decreased metabolic needs due to inactivity all indirectly contribute to anorexia.

As the food intake decreases, there is a possibility that the patient will develop a protein deficiency. *Hypoproteinemia* is a common disorder in immobilized patients. It can usually be avoided if measures are taken to guarantee a sufficient dietary intake of protein.

Assessment   Patients who are inactive for whatever reason require continual assessment to determine their specific nursing care needs. The care plan should include a schedule for checking the patient's dietary intake and accurately recording the exact amounts and types of food and liquids eaten.

Prevention and Nursing Intervention   Working with the dietitian to provide choices that are agreeable to the patient and offering small frequent meals may increase the appetite. Moving the patient to a chair for meals may also help. Providing a pleasant atmosphere and company for the meal if possible all help to increase appetite.

◆ Constipation

Pathophysiology   **Constipation is the most common gastrointestinal disorder likely to occur in a bedridden, extremely weak, or physically inactive person.** This occurs from slowing of peristalsis and lack of abdominal muscle action and movement. Lower food intake decreases the strength of the gastrocolic reflex that usually initiates defecation. Many patients on bedrest are receiving pain medications for their primary injury

or disorder that are constipating. If constipation is not treated, **fecal impaction** may occur. A sign of this may be diarrhea in the constipated patient. A fecal impaction is the presence of either hardened or puttylike feces in the rectum and sigmoid colon. If the condition is not relieved, intestinal obstruction can occur.

> Symptoms of a fecal impaction include painful defecation, feeling of fullness in the rectum, abdominal distention, and cramps and liquid stools.

Other factors that contribute to constipation include a change in the patient's usual routine and environment. Because of embarrassment, inability to defecate while lying on a bedpan, and weakened muscle tone, the patient may unconsciously ignore the normal urge to have a bowel movement. If the impulse is ignored for a considerable time, the natural urge to defecate is diminished and eventually disappears.

Elder Care Point . . . **Elderly patients must be closely monitored for constipation and fecal impaction when on extended bedrest.** Muscle tone is decreased with aging and combined with the slowing of peristalsis from lack of usual activity, often leads to constipation. Elderly patients often use laxatives or other aids to elimination at home. An assessment of usual bowel patterns and habits is essential to prevent constipation during bedrest.

Assessment   **Bowel status should be assessed daily.** Assess what the patient's usual habits of elimination are. How often during the week does the patient usually have a bowel movement? What time of day? Is she in the habit of taking laxatives or enemas? How frequently? What facilitates her bowel movement? It is not necessary for the patient to have a bowel movement each day, but the absence of stools for more than 3 days should be noted and the rectum examined for possible fecal impaction. The size of the stool also is important, because small amounts of stool may be passing without emptying the rectum and colon, allowing the fecal mass to become increasingly larger.

Prevention and Nursing Intervention   Because embarrassment and inability to use a bedpan with ease are major factors in the development of constipation, **every effort should be made to provide privacy and to help the patient overcome these obstacles to normal elimination.** Whenever possible, a commode chair at the bedside or transfer to a bathroom is preferred to the use of a bedpan in bed. When the patient must remain in bed, he may have less difficulty if he can be helped to a sitting or squatting position on the bedpan.

The prevention of constipation should not depend on such extreme measures as laxatives and enemas (Chapter 20). Increased fluids and added roughage in the diet can help alleviate the problem. If the stools are hard and difficult to pass, stool softeners are indicated.

Once an impaction has developed, the mass of feces must be broken up with a gloved finger. Before digital removal of the mass, it is sometimes helpful to give an oil retention enema to soften the mass. It is best to give an analgesic 1 hour before digital removal of an impaction.

A *bowel training program* should be designed according to each patient's needs (see Chapter 20). The plan of care will depend on the cause of the difficulty in elimination and the patient's physical and mental capacities for cooperation. Adequate fluid intake should be considered, as well as the time and location for elimination. In some cases, exercises to strengthen the abdominal muscles can be employed if the patient's physical condition permits. **Patients need to be informed of the importance of heeding the impulse to defecate so that this normal reflexive action can be preserved and chronic constipation avoided.**

MUSCULOSKELETAL SYSTEM

◆ Range of Motion and Contracture

Pathophysiology   **Even in normal, healthy individuals, confinement to bed for only a few days results in muscle weakness and joint stiffness.** Without exercise, muscle wasting and atrophy will soon occur. The adverse effects of immobility on the bones and joints include demineralization of bone (*osteoporosis* and *hypercalcemia*), decreased range of motion, and joint contractures.

Each of the joints of the body has a range of motion (ROM), that is, the extremes to which the joint may be moved in various directions. Muscular activity maintains that range of motion by allowing the joint to remain flexible and functional.

When there is little or no motion of a joint, its structures change. The muscles lose their elasticity and become shorter. The degree of motion of the joint becomes limited. If range of motion is not maintained, the normal tissue is replaced by fibrous tissue. This adaptive shortening of the muscles and tendons causes a **contracture**—*a joint that is frozen and muscles that have pulled the body part into a contracted position.*

Assessment   As soon as the patient is admitted, the nurse assesses the range of motion of all uninjured joints. Affected extremities are assessed for muscle tone, strength, and dimension; extremity circumference is measured to determine a baseline by which later measurements can be compared during assessment for atrophy.

Prevention and Nursing Intervention   One of the first concerns of the nurse should be to maintain joints in their functional positions so that they are not abnormally flexed or extended. Position maintenance can be accomplished by using a foot board, foot splints, or high-top tennis shoes that keep the feet at right angles to the legs so that foot drop is avoided; by splinting limbs so that they are kept in proper alignment; by using a bed board to prevent curvature of the spine; and by splinting the hands to keep the fingers from drawing up into a tight fist. The nurse refrains from positioning the patient with pillows and pads so that the knees and hips remain in a flexed position.

Each of the joints of the body has a range of motion—that is, the extremes to which the joint may be moved in various directions. Muscle activity maintains that range of motion by allowing the joint to remain flexible and functional.

The purpose of ROM exercises is to put each joint that is at risk for loss of motion through its full range of motion during the exercises. **The major motions are rotation, flexion, extension, abduction, adduction, and hyperextension.**

For the shoulder, internal rotation involves placing the arm at shoulder height, bending the elbow to a 90° angle, and turning the upper arm until the palm of the hand and inner arm face backward; for external rotation of the shoulder, turn the flexed arm until the palm and inner arm face forward. To exercise the hip joint, internal rotation is done by turning the leg inward so that the toes point in the direction of the opposite leg; external rotation involves turning the leg so that the toes point away from the opposite leg. To exercise the elbow, bend the elbow and bring the forearm and hand toward the shoulder; then straighten the arm. Flexion of the hip and knee is performed by flexing the knee and bending the leg toward the hip as far as possible. Abduction of the hip is performed by moving the straightened leg outward from the body as far as possible; for adduction, move the leg toward and slightly past the midline. To hyperextend the hip, place the patient prone and move the straightened leg upward away from the mattress as far as possible. For the hand, extend each finger so that it can lie flat against a surface such as your own finger. Flex by gently curling each finger to the palm.

When there is little or no motion of a joint, its structures change. The muscles lose their elasticity and become shorter. Normal tissue is replaced by fibrous tissue. This adaptive shortening of the muscles and tendons is called a *contracture*. ROM exercises will help the patient maintain optimal function of his joints (Figure 11-1). Active ROM is performed by the patient. Passive ROM is performed for the patient by the nurse, the physical therapist, or another person. If at all possible, the patient should be taught to do these exercises herself or at least to participate in them insofar as she is able. **All joints in the immobilized patient are exercised by active or passive ROM three to four times a day.** If one extremity is paralyzed, the patient is taught how to perform passive ROM on each joint of that extremity herself using her other limb. Many of the motions of ROM are automatically performed when doing activities of daily living.

After certain orthopedic surgeries, frequent passive ROM exercises are necessary to restore the joint's function. Automatic equipment for passive ROM exercise is ordered. The equipment extends an extremity to a prescribed angle for a specified period and then releases the joint. The machine operates continuously while "on." As the patient tolerates the joint movement, the angle may be increased slowly and the time for the use of the machine extended (Figure 11-2).

A progressive exercise program is individualized to each patient's capability. Such an exercise program will gradually reverse the adverse effects of bedrest.

◆ Osteoporosis

Pathophysiology   **Inactivity interferes with the process of building up the bone, causing a depletion of the supply of calcium, phosphorus, and nitrogen in bone.** As a result of this demineralization, the bone becomes porous, hence the name **osteo** (bone) **porosis** (a state of being porous). The soft, spongy bones of osteoporosis are easily deformed or broken.

Assessment   There is no way in which the nurse can assess bone strength or beginning signs of osteoporosis. Only bone density diagnostic studies can detect the signs of osteoporosis.

Prevention and Nursing Intervention   Weight bearing is the best way to prevent osteoporosis. Getting the patient up to a standing position where her legs are supporting her weight is the goal. If this is not possible, exercises in bed, where the feet are pushed against a foot board, and isometric exercises to maintain muscle tone are helpful.

An increase in dietary and supplemental calcium may help prevent osteoporosis, but there is the possibility that in an immobilized patient the increased calcium intake can predispose to the formation of stones

in the urinary system. The calcium content of selected foods is shown in Table 11-3.

The increase in circulating calcium in the blood caused by immobility may lead to hypercalcemia. The elderly seem to be especially prone to the development of this electrolyte imbalance.

Think about . . . Staff nurses have a very busy work schedule. ROM exercises take a lot of time to perform or supervise. How would you incorporate the ordered ROM exercises into your shift work plan for a patient who is paralyzed on the left side from a recent stroke?

URINARY SYSTEM

◆ Renal Calculi and Infection

Pathophysiology   The urinary system is designed so that it functions best when the body is upright. Urine flows from the kidney downward in the direction of the pull of gravity. When the body is in a reclining position, the hilus of the kidney must force urine into the ureters against the pull of gravity. Urine is continually being formed in the kidney, but the peristaltic action of the kidney and ureters is not sufficient to maintain a constant flow of urine. If the body remains in a supine position, even for a few days, the flow becomes sluggish and there is a **stasis** (pooling) in the urinary system.

Sluggish urine flow sets the stage for the formation of stones *(calculi)* and the development of infection. The urinary system must work harder to eliminate the excess amounts of calcium, nitrogen, phosphorus, sodium, and other products of protein breakdown that build up with bedrest. Of these substances, the most troublesome is calcium, the mineral of which most urinary calculi are composed. Stones irritate the tissue and provide a place for bacterial invasion. Stagnant urine also provides a favorable environment for infection to occur.

Assessment   Assess the urine continuously for amount, color, clarity, and odor, checking for signs of infection. Assess the amount of fluid the patient is drinking daily to be certain it is adequate (2,500–3,000 mL for the patient not on fluid restrictions). Question the patient about back or flank pain that may indicate the presence of a renal stone. Observe the urine for a tea color that may indicate the presence of blood related to renal stones.

Prevention and Nursing Intervention   **Adequate fluid intake is an important factor in preventing urinary**

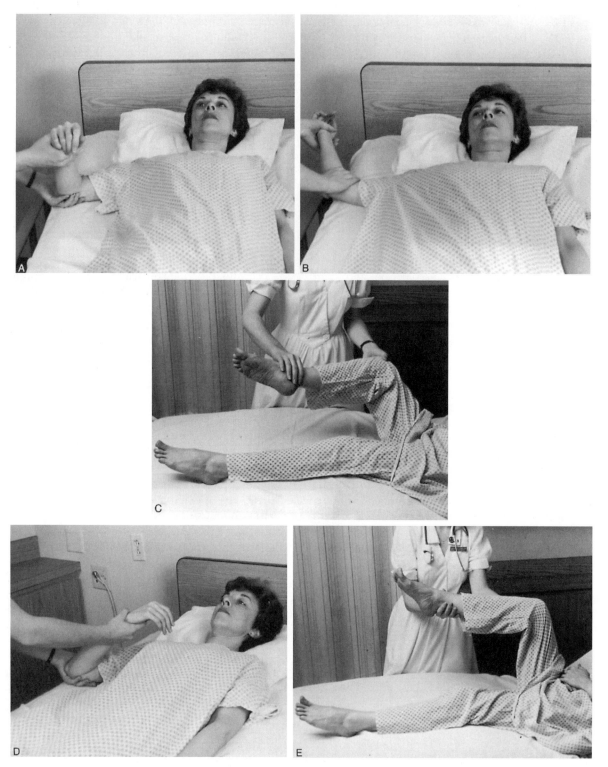

FIGURE 11-1 Range of motion exercises: rotation (A to C), flexion (D and E), extension (F), abduction and adduction (G), and hyperextension (H). (A) Rotation of shoulder. (B) External rotation of the shoulder. (C) Rotation of the hip. Internal rotation. (D) Flexion of elbow. (E) Flexion of hip and knee.

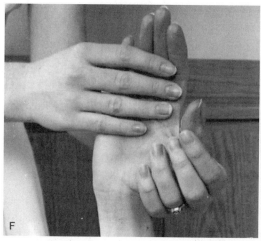

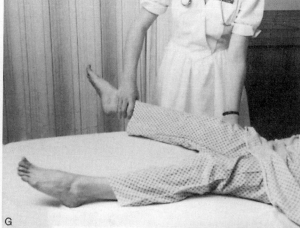

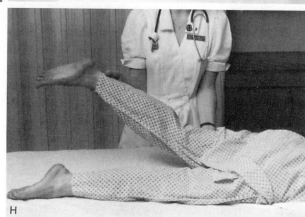

FIGURE 11-1 *Continued*   (F) Extension of fingers. (G) Abduction and adduction of hip. (H) Hyperextension of hip. (Photos by Ken Kasper. From: *Keane's Essentials of Medical Surgical Nursing, 3rd Ed.*)

complications. Ideally, the patient should drink 8 oz of fluid every hour when awake, unless contraindicated. The patient's intake of calcium may be restricted (see Table 11-3 for foods high in calcium). Because most stones are formed in an alkaline environment, the physician may prescribe an acid-ash diet, which is a diet composed of foods and liquids that have an acid residue (Table 11-4). **Contrary to popular belief, citrus fruits,** **such as lemons and oranges, do not make the urine acidic.**

Both infections and calculi can be prevented best by keeping the urine dilute and flowing normally. Bladder catheterization should be used only as a last resort for difficulty with urination because of the ever-present danger of introducing infectious organisms into the urinary tract.

FIGURE 11-2   **Patient using a continuous passive motion (CPM) machine.** (Photo by Glen Derbyshire; courtesy of Goletta Valley Cottage Hospital, Goletta, CA.)

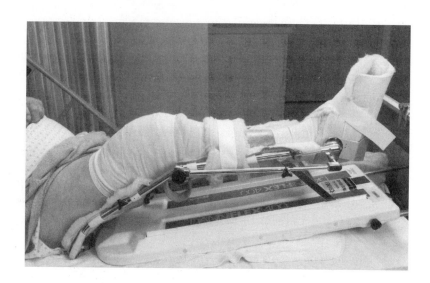

TABLE 11-3 ◆ *Nutrition Point: Foods High in Calcium*

Foods high in calcium may be recommended for the patient who needs extra calcium to help rebuild bone lost from immobility. However, foods high in calcium may be restricted if circulating levels of calcium are too high during periods of immobility or from other causes of electrolyte imbalance. Depending on the situation the patient is counseled either to add or avoid the following foods:

Buttermilk	Oysters
Cheese	Salmon
Cottage cheese	Sardines
Dark green leafy vegetables	Shrimp
Ice cream	Yogurt
Milk	

Note: Most of the listed foods also contain phosphorus, which also is necessary to build bone.

◆ Urinary Incontinence

Pathophysiology   Another effect that lying in bed has on the urinary system is the loss of control of the urinary sphincter muscles and resultant incontinence. **Without the downward pressure of the full bladder against the sphincter muscles, there is less awareness of the need to void. The result is bladder distention and an overflow or dribbling of urine of which the patient is unaware.**

Elder Care Point . . .   The decrease of muscle tone that comes with aging contributes to both urinary retention and urinary incontinence. Vigilant nursing care is necessary because the elderly patient is also at high risk for skin breakdown. Offering a bedpan every two hours during waking hours can help keep these patients dry.

Assessment   The number of times a patient voids and the characteristics of the urine should be accurately recorded. Bladder distention should be monitored, and,

---

TABLE 11-4 ◆ *Nutrition Point: Acid-Ash Foods Used to Acidify the Urine*

Meat
  Meats, eggs, fish, shellfish, fowl, all types of cheese, peanut butter, peanuts
Fat
  Bacon, nuts (Brazil nuts, filberts, walnuts)
Grains
  All types of bread (especially whole-wheat bread), crackers, rice, cereal, pasta, cakes, cookies
Vegetables
  Lentils, corn
Fruit
  Cranberries, prunes, plums

---

if possible, the bladder should be emptied completely at each voiding. Notation should be made of each incidence of incontinence.

Prevention and Nursing Intervention   To assist the patient in completely emptying the bladder, a change in position may be necessary. For a male patient, this may necessitate having him stand and void. If this is not possible, he should be helped to sit upright. Women also should be helped to a sitting position when voiding. Moderate pressure of the hand against the lower pelvic region over the bladder will facilitate emptying.

   The incontinent patient must be kept dry. For the male, a condom catheter often is the best solution. For the female, adult incontinence briefs are helpful. For the patient who only has dribbling, self-adhesive sanitary or incontinence pads placed into underwear work well. Good skin care is essential for the incontinent patient.

INTEGUMENTARY SYSTEM (SKIN)

◆ Pressure Ulcers

Pathophysiology   When a patient is on bedrest, or constantly sitting because of paralysis, pressure against the skin in various areas interferes with circulation, and because cells die very quickly without adequate blood supply, a **pressure ulcer** can begin to develop. **Depending on the patient's general condition, weight, and other factors, skin damage may occur within a few hours to a few days. Areas most prone to pressure ulcer formation are those over bony prominences.** When the patient is placed in a position where the bone is pressing on the skin as it is against the bed, the circulation to that area is compromised (Figure 11-3.)

   Whenever there is pressure against the skin and the underlying blood vessels that supply it, **erythema** (a reddened area) occurs from congestion related to impaired blood flow. If the pressure continues too long, the area of erythema progresses to a skin breakdown and may become a pressure ulcer. A reddened area can occur within an hour or two in a person with healthy skin and adequate circulation. It is even more likely to develop and rapidly progress to an ulcerated stage in persons who are malnourished, obese, aged, or suffering from circulatory disease. **Breakdown of the skin also is more likely to occur if, in addition to continued pressure, the skin is subjected to heat, moisture, and irritating substances, such as those present in decomposing urine, feces, perspiration, and vaginal discharge.**

   Pressure ulcers also are called by the medical term *decubitus ulcer.* The word *decubitus* means "lying down," and an ulcer is a lesion produced by the sloughing of necrotic, inflammatory tissue. A decubitus ulcer is an open wound that is associated with lying in

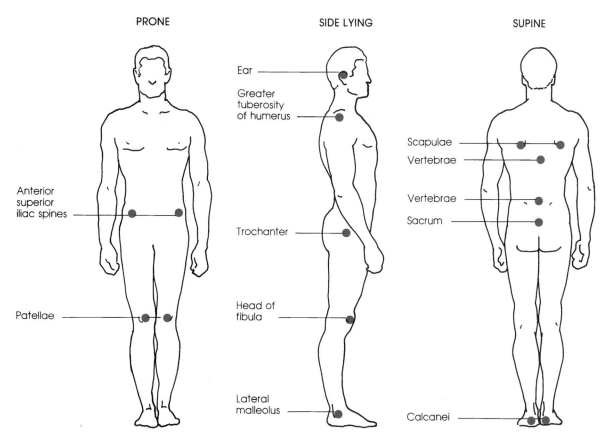

FIGURE 11-3   Bony prominences most susceptible to skin breakdown depending on position.

bed; however, lesions of this kind also can develop in patients who sit in one position for long periods.

Many different factors contribute to the development of pressure ulcers, but the two major causes are prolonged pressure on a specific part of the body, and a *shearing force*, which exerts a downward and forward pressure on tissues underlying the skin. This shearing action takes place when a patient slumps down while sitting in bed or in a chair.

Assessment   The skin should be thoroughly assessed when the patient is admitted. Skin checks are performed every shift on immobile patients, noting the condition of skin over bony prominences. Once every 24 hours, usually during the bath, the skin is totally assessed. When a reddened area is found, it is checked for blanching by pressing gently in the center of the area to see if it turns from red to white or a paler color on darker skin. Blanching usually indicates that the redness is temporary and will resolve when pressure on the area is relieved.

Several kinds of preprinted forms can be used to assess the risk of developing pressure sores. These assessment tools take into account the general condition of the skin, control of urination and defecation, mobility, mental status, and nutritional status and pro-

vide a more systematic approach to evaluating a patient's potential for decubitus ulcer development.

Ascertaining the stage of ulceration can be useful to document that an ulcer was present on admission. Classifying an ulceration also can be helpful to evaluate the effectiveness of treatment and progress toward healing and repair. The Agency for Health Care Policy and Research (AHCPR) of the U.S. Department of Health and Human Services has issued clinical practice guidelines for the prediction and prevention of pressure ulcers and a staging system for classification.

- **Stage I.** An area of reddened, deep pink, or mottled skin. The skin may feel very warm and firm or tightly stretched across the area. The area does not blanch with finger pressure. The redness remains for over half as long as the area was subjected to pressure.
- **Stage II.** Partial thickness skin loss involving epidermis and/or dermis. The skin appears blistered, or abraded, or has a shallow crater. The area surrounding the damaged skin is reddened and probably will feel hot or warmer than normal.
- **Stage III.** The skin is ulcerated. There is a craterlike ulcer, and the underlying subcutaneous tissue is involved in the destructive process. The ulcer may or

may not be infected. Bacterial infection is almost always present at this stage, however, and accounts for continued erosion of the ulcer and the production of drainage.

- **Stage IV.** There is deep ulceration and necrosis involving deeper underlying muscle and possibly bone tissue. At this point the ulcer usually is extensively infected. The ulcer can be dry, black in color, and covered with a tough accumulation of necrotic tissue, or it can be made up of wet and oozing dead cells and purulent **exudate** (drainage). The color photograph collection in the center of the text presents pictures of Stage I through Stage IV pressure ulcers. (See Color Figures 1–4.)

Prevention and Nursing Intervention Preventing pressure ulcers is far more desirable and less time-consuming than treating them. Efforts to preserve the integrity of the skin are the responsibility of the nursing staff, as well as the patient herself if she is able to participate in her own care. Table 11-5 presents interventions for preventing pressure ulcers based on the AHCPR clinical practice guidelines.

> Vigilant nursing care is the main factor in the prevention of pressure ulcers.

Prevention and treatment of pressure sores, pulmonary complications, and other problems of immobility can be greatly facilitated by placing the patient on a special bed such as a continuous-lateral rotation bed, the Roto Rest ® Delta bed, shown in Figure 11-4. Such beds are designed to provide support for patients who must not move, such as the patient with a fractured spine; those who cannot move; and those whose handling, turning, and positioning is

---

TABLE 11-5 ◆ *Guidelines for the Prevention of Pressure Ulcers*

- Assess the skin of all patients at risk at least once a day, paying particular attention to the bony prominences (Figure 11-3).
- Reposition patients every 2 hours; use a written schedule for systematically turning and repositioning each patient.
- Utilize positioning devices, such as pillows, foam wedges, and padding for bedrest patients, to keep body prominences from being in direct contact with one another; include positioning devices in the written plan of care.
- For patients on bedrest who are completely immobile, use devices that totally relieve pressure on the heels, by raising the heels off the bed. Do not use donut-type devices.
- When the side-lying position in bed is used, avoid positioning directly on the trochanter.
- Maintain the head of the bed for bedrest patients at the lowest degree permitted by medical condition. Limit the time the head of the bed is elevated.
- Use lifting devices, such as a trapeze or bed linen, to move rather than drag patients who cannot assist during transfers and position changes.
- For patients with limited mobility, utilize a pressure-reducing device on the bed, such as foam, static air, alternating air, gel, or water matterss. Such devices should be used for any patients at risk for developing pressure ulcers.
- For chair-bound patients, use a pressure-reducing device such as those made of foam, gel, air, or a combination of items. Do not use donut-type devices.
- Positioning of chair-bound patients should include consideration of postural alignment, distribution of weight, balance and stability, and pressure relief.
- Use a written plan for the use of positioning devices and schedules for chair-bound patients.
- Skin cleansing should occur at the time of soiling and at routine intervals based on patient need and preference. Avoid hot water, and use a mild cleansing agent that minimizes irritation and dryness of the skin. Cleanse gently, minimizing the force and friction applied to the skin.
- Any person at risk for developing a pressure ulcer when sitting in a chair or wheelchair should be repositioned, shifting the points under pressure at least every hour; patients who are able should be taught to shift weight every 15 minutes.
- Keep the environment humidity above 40% and avoid exposure to cold. Treat dry skin with moisturizers.
- Do not massage bony prominences.
- Minimize skin exposure to moisture due to incontinence, perspiration, or wound drainage. When sources of moisture cannot be controlled, underpads or briefs that absorb moisture and present a quick-drying surface to the skin should be used. Utilize an incontinence management program for incontinent patients.
- Minimize skin injury due to friction and shear forces by proper positioning and correct transferring and turning techniques. Reduce friction injuries by using lubricants, protective films, protective dressings, and protective padding. Use lift devices to reposition patients rather than sliding them on the bedding.
- Correct inadequate dietary intake of protein and calories with nutritional intervention either by oral supplementation of enteral or parenteral feedings.
- If a potential for improvement of mobility and activity status exists, institute a rehabilitation program. Maintain current activity and mobility status with a range of motion exercise program.

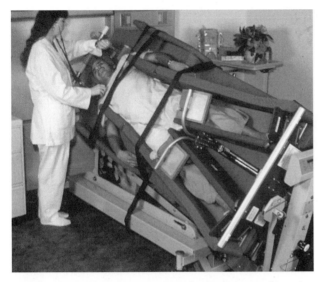

FIGURE 11-4 The Roto Rest® Delta bed is a product of Kinetic Concepts, Inc., San Antonio, Texas. Roto Rest® is a registered trademark of Kinetic Concepts, Inc. for its oscillating support surface. This product is subject to patent and/or pending patent.

painful or difficult, such as a patient with multiple trauma.

Keeping the patient well hydrated promotes good skin turgor that helps decrease the incidence of pressure ulcers. Assess the immobile patient for good hydration by checking skin turgor, the condition of mucous membranes, and amount of liquid intake.

Treatment of pressure ulcers varies from one institution to another and even from one patient care area to another. **Reddened areas are never massaged.** Generally, nursing intervention includes wound culture if the involved area has signs of infection. An infected ulcer is cleansed with an antimicrobial agent such as povidone iodine (Betadine) and then irrigated with normal saline. **Noninfected ulcers are never irrigated with anything other than sterile normal saline.** When further **debridement** (removal of dead tissue) is needed, the patient may have whirlpool baths prescribed along with enzymatic debriding agents and wet-to-dry dressings. Debridement is sufficient when the ulcer bed appears pink, indicating healthy granulation tissue.

The dressing should provide a clean, moist environment to promote healing. Occlusive dressings such as Duoderm or semipermeable films like Opsite are often used. For deep ulcers that are producing a large amount of exudate, karaya powder or absorptive materials are used. Applying a film dressing over a reddened area *before* the skin has broken has proved effective in preventing many pressure ulcers. A more in-depth discussion of pressure ulcers and their treatment is covered in Chapter 29.

Think about . . . Aging causes a loss of elasticity and a thinning of the skin. What other changes that occur with age could contribute to the formation of a pressure ulcer more quickly than in a younger person? How would you change the skin care plan for a patient in his eighties from one of a patient in his forties who is on bedrest?

PSYCHOSOCIAL EFFECTS OF IMMOBILIZATION

Perhaps more than any other consequence of illness and injury, being immobilized and unable to attend to one's own personal needs has a profound and far-reaching effect on mental outlook and social adaptation. In addition to the loss of independence, there is worry over financial matters and concern for family members and friends and how their lives are affected. The immobilized patient may also experience isolation and depression because he is no longer able to go to others to find companionship and social interaction but must wait for them to come to him.

The list of psychological and social problems associated with immobility is almost endless, as are the activities that might be planned to help the patient deal with his problems. These activities are best planned and coordinated by using the entire health care team, including the social worker, psychologist, or occupational therapist.

The inactive person on total bedrest tends to become less mentally active. The elderly person may become disoriented or confused after several days of inactivity. Boredom becomes a problem for the normally mentally active individual. Being confined to bed seriously limits the type of activity in which the patient may participate. Loneliness and isolation should be addressed. Resources such as frequent telephone calls from friends and family, mail, and visits from church or other friends are vital to the patient's psychological well-being.

The primary responsibilities of the nurse in meeting the psychosocial needs of an immobilized patient, no matter what the cause of this immobility, center on (1) preventing the serious physiological consequences that prohibit the patient from regaining some degree of independence; (2) attending to the patient's psychosocial concerns and needs; (3) relating to the patient as a whole person *so that she sees herself as a person of dignity and worth;* and (4) providing diversionary activity to help decrease boredom.

Negative attitudes toward the dependent and disabled are not uncommon, even among health care professionals. Our society as a whole places a high value on youth, productivity, and physical beauty. The nurse who works with immobilized patients, especially those whose outlook for regaining mobility is limited, should be accepting of such patients as worthwhile individuals. Nurses must work with patients to explore strengths so that the patients may regain or maintain their self-esteem and function to their maximum potential.

COMMUNITY CARE

Nurses who work in rehabilitation, home care, or long-term care agencies are challenged daily by immobile patients. **The quality of life of these patients greatly depends on the help of the nurse in preventing or decreasing the problems of immobility.** The nurse must collaborate with family members, nursing assistants, physical and occupational therapists, social workers, dietitians, and others to provide good 24-hour-a-day care for these patients. If care is inconsistent from one shift to another, problems will not be prevented.

In the home care situation where the patient may be alone or attended by family members who are busy with their own lives, it takes great ingenuity to solve the immobile patient's problems at times. Teaching the patient to take charge of her own care and well-being as much as she is physically capable is very important. This is true for patients in rehabilitation facilities also. Written plans that are frequently evaluated for consistency of use and effectiveness are essential in preventing the problems of immobility.

CRITICAL THINKING EXERCISES

Clinical Case Problems

Read each clinical situation and discuss the questions with your classmates.

1. Mr. Herbert, age 26, has had skin grafting done to his abdomen and left leg to treat injuries from a motorcycle accident. He will be on bedrest for at least 10 days. He must be kept flat in bed with the head elevated no more than 20°. Write a nursing care plan that will help prevent disabilities from inactivity.

2. Mr. Cox is admitted to the hospital with a medical diagnosis of cerebral vascular accident (stroke). He has paralysis of his right arm and slight difficulty in moving his right leg. The physician has written an order saying that Mr. Cox may be out of bed twice a day. Taking each system of the body, list nursing activities that should be included in a care plan that is designed to prevent disabilities from inactivity.

BIBLIOGRAPHY

Agency for Health Care Policy and Research. (1992). *Pressure Ulcers in Adults: Prediction and Prevention.* Washington, D.C.: U.S. Department of Health and Human Services.

Braden, B., Bryant, R. (1990). Innovations to prevent and treat pressure ulcers. *Geriatric Nurse.* July/August:182.

Burd, C., et al. (1994). Skin care strategies in a skilled nursing home. *Journal of Gerontological Nursing.* 20(11):28–34.

Carroll, P. (1995). Bed selection: help patients rest easy. *RN.* 58(5):44–51.

Felton, S., Layman, S., McMahon, D. (1996). Reducing pressure ulcers. *American Journal of Nursing* 96(5):22–24.

Hausman, L. L. (1994). Cost containment through reducing pressure ulcers. *Nursing Management.* 25(11):88R–V.

Holm, K., Hedricks, C. (1989). Immobility and bone loss in the aging adult. *Critical Care Nursing Quarterly.* 6:46.

Jacobs, B. W. (1994). Working on the right moves, Part 1. *Nursing 94.* 24(10):58–62.

Jacobs, B. W. (1994). Working on the right moves, Part 2. *Nursing 94.* 24(11):53–54.

Kemp, M. G., Krouskop, T. A. (1994). Pressure ulcers: reducing incidence and severity by managing pressure. *Journal of Gerontological Nursing.* 20(9):11–34.

Mahon, D., et al. (1995). Success stories: reducing specialty bed use. *Nursing Economics.* 13(3):1 114-119.

Makelbust, J., Margolis, D. (1995). Pressure ulcers: definition of assessment parameters. *Advances in Wound Care.* 8(4):6–11.

Murray, M., Blaylock, B. (1994). Maintaining effective pressure ulcer prevention programs. *Medsurg Nursing.* 3(2): 85–93.

Olson, E. V., et al. (1990). The hazards of immobility. *American Journal of Nursing.* 90(3):43.

Potter, P. A., Perry, A. G. (1993). *Fundamentals of Nursing: Concepts, Process and Practice,* 3rd ed. St. Louis, MO: Mosby Year Book.

Regan, M., Byers, P. H., Mayrovitz, H. N. (1995). Efficacy of a comprehensive pressure ulcer prevention program in an extended care facility. *Advances in Wound Care.* 8(3):49, 51–52, 54–55.

Rubin, M. (1988). The physiology of bedrest. *American Journal of Nursing.* 8(1):43–50.

Suarez, C. H., Reynolds, A. (1995). Pressure reduction with a hospitalized population using a mattress overlay. *Ostomy Wound Management.* 41(1):58–63.

U. S. Department of Health and Human Services (USDHHS). (1990). *Healthy people 2000: National health promotion and disease prevention objectives.* Washington, DC: U. S. Government Printing Office.

Wilson, S. F. (1994). Research for practice. Mattresses that spell R-E-L-I-E-F. *American Journal of Nursing.* 94(9):48.

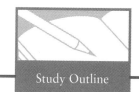

Study Outline

I. Introduction

A. People are immobile to different degrees and for differing lengths of time.

B. Many disabilities arising from immobility can be prevented.

C. *Healthy People 2000* objectives aim in part to decrease the problems that are secondary to immobility.

D. Causes of immobility include paralysis, pain or fear of pain, surgery, physical trauma, weakness, and disease.

E. An appropriate nursing diagnosis for patients with limited mobility is "Impaired physical mobility related to . . ."

F. Each problem secondary to immobility is given a nursing diagnosis and incorporated in the plan of care for the patient.

G. Therapeutic rest is prescribed for cardiac conditions, relief from pain, rest for healing of injury, or reversal of effects of gravity.

H. Body systems are affected singly and in relation to other systems.

II. Cardiovascular System

A. Thrombus formation:

1. Sluggish blood flow from lack of muscle activity makes the patient prone to form clots.

2. When the vessel wall at the site of a thrombus becomes irritated, the patient develops a thrombophlebitis.

3. Signs and symptoms of thrombus formation in a lower extremity include swelling and calf pain.

4. Additional signs indicating thrombophlebitis are redness and warmth over the affected area, plus a temperature elevation.

5. Prevention and nursing intervention:

   a. Aspirin therapy, heparin therapy, application of elastic stockings, intermittent pneumatic compression devices.

   b. Changing position frequently.

   c. Refrain from putting pressure on the posterior knee or deep veins of the lower extremities.

   d. Performing range of motion (ROM) exercises of the legs and feet.

   e. Increase fluid intake to promote good hydration.

B. Increased cardiac workload.

1. Valsalva maneuver produces a sudden increase in blood volume in the heart chambers, thereby increasing its workload.

2. The patient is taught to avoid the Valsalva maneuver.

3. Keep the patient from straining when defecating.

C. Orthostatic hypotension: drop in blood pressure occurring when one stands for the first time after having been in bed for several days or longer.

D. Prevention and nursing intervention.

1. Orthostatic hypotension presents danger of patient's falling and hurting herself. Have sufficient help and support for the patient when she first tries to stand after having been in bed for a long time.

2. Get the patient out of bed as soon as possible.

3. Change the patient's position slowly; allow to sit on side of bed with feet on the floor for a few minutes and allow blood pressure to stabilize before assisting her to stand or transfer.

4. Physician may order "tilt" table therapy.

III. Respiratory System

A. Immobility restricts exchange of oxygen and carbon dioxide.

1. Limits movement of the lungs and muscles of respiration.

2. Decreases normal movement of secretions in tracheobronchial tree.

B. Stagnant secretions provide a place for bacteria to grow, and the patient may develop hypostatic pneumonia.

C. Assess lungs and check bandages and binders to see that they do not interfere with lung expansion.

D. Determine whether abdominal distention is placing pressure on the diaphragm.

E. Determine whether sedatives and other drugs that depress respiration are interfering with normal breathing patterns.

F. Signs of respiratory problems include gurgling breaths, productive cough with colored sputum, fever, pain on inspiration, dyspnea, and crackles and wheezes heard upon auscultation of the lungs.

G. Prevention and nursing intervention.

1. Proper positioning and frequent turning.

2. Teach patient coughing and deep-breathing exercises.

3. Postural drainage.

4. Suction as needed.

5. Ensure adequate fluid intake.

6. Assessment of patient's respiratory status includes rate and depth of respirations; listening for moist, bubbling sounds or wheezing; color of skin.

7. Eventual outcome of unrelieved respiratory depression is hypostatic pneumonia.

IV. **Gastrointestinal System**

A. Anorexia is one of the most common difficulties.

1. Patients often suffer from hypoproteinemia.

B. Elimination of fecal material can be difficult because of embarrassment and inability to use bedpan.

1. Chronic constipation is likely to lead to fecal impaction.

2. Unrelieved fecal impaction can lead to intestinal obstruction.

3. Fecal impaction should be removed digitally; oil retention enema may facilitate removal.

C. Assess food intake, noting patient's preferences in foods and liquids; determine usual bowel pattern and assess on a daily basis.

D. Prevention and nursing intervention.

1. Provide fiber in the diet and adequate fluids.

2. Whenever possible, patient should be allowed to use commode chair at bedside or taken to the bathroom.

3. Prevention of constipation should not depend on laxatives and enemas.

4. Stool softeners may be prescribed.

5. Bowel training programs designed to meet individual patients' needs include adequate fluid intake, time and location best for elimination, and exercises to strengthen abdominal muscles.

V. **Musculoskeletal System**

A. Confinement to bed for even a few days can result in muscle weakness in normal, healthy person.

B. Range of motion lost when there is little or no motion of a joint; consequence of inactivity is *contractures*.

C. Osteoporosis occurs as result of decrease in normal stress on bones that occurs with standing and walking. Bones lose their minerals and become porous, easily deformed, and broken.

D. Assess muscle condition and range of motion at time of admission.

E. Prevention and nursing intervention.

1. Keep joints in their functional position, using foot board, splints, bed board, and other positioning devices.

2. Plan and implement regular ROM exercises.

3. Stand patient up on her feet if at all possible.

4. High calcium diet may lead to formation of urinary calculi.

VI. **Urinary System**

A. System designed so that it functions best when the body is in an upright position.

B. When body remains in supine position, there is a pooling of urine and a sluggish flow.

C. Sluggish urine flow sets the stage for the formation of stones and the development of infection.

D. Distended bladder leads to loss of control of external sphincter muscle.

E. Nursing assessment:

1. Observation for early signs of decreased urinary flow.

a. Check and record number of times patient voids and characteristics of urine.

b. Check for bladder distention.

c. Monitor color, clarity, and odor of urine.

F. Prevention and nursing intervention.

1. Have male patients stand to void whenever possible; if not, have them sit up to void. Females also should void while sitting up rather than while lying on bedpan.

2. Moderate pressure of the hand on the lower pelvic region will assist emptying of bladder.

3. Adequate fluid intake important in prevention of stones and infection (2,500–3,000 mL/day).

4. Calcium intake may be limited.

5. Acid-ash diet may be prescribed.

6. Catheterization used only as a last resort because of the danger of urinary infection.

VII. **Integumentary System**

A. Pressure ulcer are the most common consequence of prolonged pressure from lying or sitting in one position.

1. Pressure against blood vessels deprives tissues of adequate blood supply.

2. Pressure is more intense under bony prominences.

3. "Shearing" action forces a downward and forward pressure on tissues underlying the skin when patient sits in bed or chair and slumps down.

B. Prevention and nursing intervention:

1. Factors placing a patient at risk include:

a. Altered mental status.

b. Incontinence or excessive perspiration.

c. Paralysis.

d. Poor nutritional status.

2. Systematically assess patients for skin changes.

3. Four stages of classification are used to describe pressure ulcers.

4. Institute a plan of care including schedule for changing position, massaging areas likely to break down.

5. Avoid friction against skin, wrinkles in bed clothes.

6. Use bed cradle to support weight of top covers. Use devices to protect heels and keep them off the bed.

7. Flotation pads or special mattresses allow for even distribution of body weight; special beds are available to prevent pressure on any one area for too long.

8. Major factors in success of treatment of pressure ulcers are commitment of nursing staff members and diligence with which they follow program of care.

9. Treatment involves debridement, eliminating infection, and protecting new tissue.

10. An uninfected pressure ulcer is never irrigated with anything but sterile saline.

VIII. Psychosocial Effects

A. Effects on mental state include depression, anxiety, feeling of worthlessness.

B. Social effects include lack of social interaction because of isolation, inability to be physically active.

C. Therapeutic activities may be coordinated by many different members of the health care team.

D. A nurse's responsibilities primarily are:

1. Preventing physiological disabilities that prohibit successful rehabilitation.

2. Helping patient see herself as a person of dignity and worth.

IX. Community Care

A. Quality of life for immobile patients depends on the help of the nurse in preventing the problems of immobility.

B. Proper care depends on collaboration with all health care team members.

C. Care of the immobile home care patient is often a challenge as family members are busy with their own lives.

D. Teaching the patient aspects of self-care is very important in the rehabilitation facility as well as home care.

E. The written plan of care is frequently evaluated for consistency of use and effectiveness.

X. Elder Care Points

A. Other chronic diseases among the elderly augment the effects of immobility.

B. Decreased muscle tone increases likelihood of urinary retention, incontinence, and constipation.

C. Elderly are especially prone to orthostatic hypotension.

D. Elderly often suffer from poor nutrition and are more susceptible to infection.

E. Loss of elastic recoil in the lungs, increased airway resistance, and reduced vital capacity decrease gas exchange.

F. Extended bedrest may cause disorientation and confusion in the elderly person.

CHAPTER 12

Extended Care within the Community: Chronic Illness and Rehabilitation

OBJECTIVES

Upon completing this chapter the student should be able to:
1. State the goals of rehabilitation.
2. Identify the members of the rehabilitation team and the collaborative care-giving process.
3. Describe the types of rehabilitation programs that might be found in a large city.
4. Discuss safety and fall prevention efforts in the long-term care facility.
5. Identify differences in the role of the LPN in a long-term care facility versus the hospital setting.
6. Discuss the general goals for the resident in a long-term care facility and how to meet those goals.
7. List the provisions that must be met for care in the home to be eligible for Medicare reimbursement.
8. Define the roles and functions of the RN and the LPN in home health care.
9. Explain the differences in philosophy and required attitude between the home care setting and the hospital.
10. Differentiate areas of concern for psychosocial care of the home care client and family.

Although some portion of nursing care has always been delivered in the community setting, the focus of today is shifting from the hospital back to home and community agencies. Some clients are transferred to a long-term care facility for recovery after the most acute phase of illness or injury has passed. Many elderly who have several chronic problems and areas of deficit in self-care enter long-term care facilities to obtain the care they need. Other clients are quickly discharged to the home setting after surgery or in-hospital diagnostic tests for major illnesses. These clients need acute, skilled, nursing care for an efficient, uneventful recovery.

Clients with chronic illnesses and disabilities are treated at outclient clinics, rehabilitation agencies, in physician's offices, or in the home setting. Community hospice programs provide care for the terminally ill.

Nurses also work in other areas of the community. Many are employed in physicians' offices, at HMO clinics, as school nurses, as occupational health nurses at various companies, and at state and county health department clinics.

Nurses who work in the community setting need to be skilled in providing care and comfort, promoting coping skills and adaptive living capabilities, promoting self-care for independent living, and fostering quality of life. Nurses entering the community-based health care areas need to be able to work in somewhat less structured settings than acute care settings provide. Nurses in all of these settings are in a position to screen clients for cancer, spot signs of diabetes, screen for hypertension, assess for hearing and vision problems, and teach measures to promote health. The nurse in the community should constantly be alerting clients and family members to the need for recommended cancer screening, teaching about ways to reduce risk factors for heart disease, counseling about quitting use of tobacco, providing information about appropriate nutrition and low-fat diets, and promoting the benefits of regular exercise.

CHRONIC ILLNESS AND REHABILITATION

Chronic illness affects millions of people. Diabetes, hypertension, heart disease, neurological disorders (such as multiple sclerosis and stroke), asthma, arthritis, back disorders, and musculoskeletal deformities and disorders all require continuous care. Although many people with a chronic illness can lead an active and productive life, 34 to 43 million people in the United States have chronic illnesses or disabilities that interfere with normal function. When working with these individuals, the terms *impairment, disability,* and *handicap* are encountered. **Impairment** refers to dysfunction of a specific organ or body system. **Disability** indicates difficulty in performing certain tasks because of impairment, and having a **handicap** means that the person has a social disadvantage that exists because of disability.

Rehabilitation is the process whereby a disabled person is helped to achieve optimal function. A primary goal of rehabilitation is to minimize the deficit from the condition and maximize the abilities that are intact. It involves measures to achieve the highest level of physical, emotional, psychological, and social function and well-being possible. Vocational rehabilitation is job retraining for the disabled to provide a means of contributing to self-support. Rehabilitation, therefore, is concerned with achieving a better quality of life. Funding for rehabilitation is provided by Medicare, Medicaid (state aid), private insurance, and philanthropic groups such as the Shriner's who support children's hospitals and burn centers.

The majority of clients who require rehabilitation services are disabled as a result of a chronic illness. Others have become disabled from trauma incurred during an accident. Several of the objectives for *Healthy People 2000* are rehabilitation oriented. One objective seeks to increase formal education for people with chronic and disabling conditions by including information about community and self-help resources as a part of managing their condition.

Each year about 8,000 spinal cord injuries occur in the United States, and one out of four of the more than 2 million people who suffer head injuries annually have residual deficits. Another objective of *Healthy People 2000* is to reduce the incidence of secondary disabilities associated with injuries of the head and spinal cord. As the population ages, more people suffer heart attacks and strokes, which often leave the person with residual deficits. The need for rehabilitation services will continue to grow rapidly.

THE REHABILITATION NURSE

The nurse who works with rehabilitation clients must be flexible and creative and recognize that the client is the "captain" of the rehabilitation team. The nurse's function is to assist the client to achieve an optimal state of wellness as *defined by the client.* It is very important that the nurse be nonjudgmental and not impose his own values and attitudes on the client.

The rehabilitation nurse must be able to work collaboratively with other health team members. Besides the physician, occupational, physical, speech, and recreational therapists, vocational counselors are part of the team (Figure 12-1). The nurse needs to assist in seeing to it that the client correctly performs exercises and activities as instructed by such therapists and reinforces their teaching. A collaborative care plan or clinical pathway is followed so that each member of the team is aware of what treatment and education the client is receiving. Both short- and long-term goals are

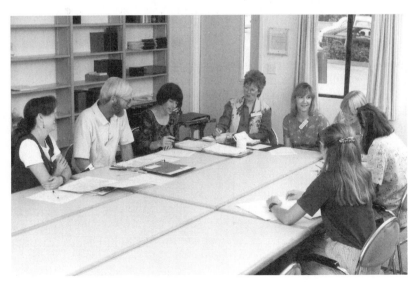

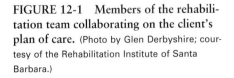

FIGURE 12-1 Members of the rehabilitation team collaborating on the client's plan of care. (Photo by Glen Derbyshire; courtesy of the Rehabilitation Institute of Santa Barbara.)

set. This provides for continuity of interdisciplinary care, recognizing the critical importance of each discipline in promoting positive outcomes for the patient.

The nurse assists the client and family to learn new skills to perform activities of daily living (ADLs). The client and family both undergo considerable stress during the rehabilitation period, and the nurse assists them in developing positive coping techniques and in recognizing their strengths. A good sense of humor, gentle, firm people skills, patience, and the ability to provide solid encouragement are good tools for working with rehabilitation clients.

The philosophy of rehabilitation nursing is based on the recognition of the client's need for independence. The nurse learns to judge when the client should be allowed to struggle to do something on her own and learns to recognize when the client's frustration is reaching a level where the nurse should step in and assist.

The Association of Rehabilitation Nurses (ARN) was founded in 1974. Its journal, *Rehabilitation Nursing*, is a source of current information about techniques, research and devices. Registered nurses (RNs) may become certified in the specialty of rehabilitation nursing.

DETERMINATION OF REHABILITATION NEEDS

A thorough physical and psychosocial assessment is performed for each client to establish a baseline, to determine physical limitations, and to identify present psychosocial difficulties. Physical evaluation includes the relevant data in Table 12-1. The client's home environment also is examined to determine whether physical features of the home, such as stairs or narrow doorways, will present a problem. Questions about the neighborhood, such as the location of shopping centers and types of transportation available, are asked. The nurse inquires about who does the grocery shopping, cooking, errands, and housework for the client.

The client's usual daily schedule and habits of everyday living are explored, including sleeping and waking patterns, eating, elimination patterns, hygiene, grooming, sexual activity, working, and leisure activities. A functional assessment determines how the client's disability has affected his former usual patterns. This focuses on the client's present ability to perform ADLs, such as toileting, bathing, dressing, grooming, ambulating, as well as his ability to use the telephone, shop, prepare food, and perform housekeeping chores. Various assessment tools are used to determine the client's ability to function. A common one, the Katz Index of Activities of Daily Living, assists the nurse to

TABLE 12-1 ♦ *Physical Assessment Points to Consider*

Body System	Relevant Data
Cardiovascular system	Chest pain Fatigue Fear of cardiac failure
Respiratory system	Shortness of breath or dyspnea Activity tolerance Fear of inability to breathe
Gastrointestinal system and nutrition	Oral intake, eating pattern Anorexia, nausea and vomiting Dysphagia Laboratory data (e.g., serum albumin level) Weight loss or gain Bowel elimination pattern or habits Change in stool Ability to get to toilet
Renal/urinary system	Urinary pattern Fluid intake Urinary incontinence or retention Urine culture or urinalysis
Neurological system	Motor function Sensation Cognitive abilities
Musculoskeletal system	Functional ability Range of motion Endurance Muscle strength
Integumentary system	Risk of skin breakdown Presence of skin lesions

Source: Ignatavicius, D. D., Workman, M. L., Mishler, M. A., (1995). *Medical–Surgical Nursing: A Nursing Process Approach,* 2nd ed. Philadelphia: Saunders, p. 220.

evaluate how much assistance the client needs for various activities.

Psychosocial assessment includes evaluating self-esteem and body image. The Baird Body Image Assessment Tool is a good test. Use of defense mechanisms, level of anxiety, and usual coping techniques are explored. To ascertain the client's response to loss, the nurse asks the client to describe feelings related to the loss of a body part or body function. The client's support systems and the family's coping abilities also are determined. As rehabilitation progresses, the nurse performs a vocational assessment so that the vocational counselor can assist the client in finding appropriate training, education, or employment after discharge from the rehabilitation program.

Think about... Can you explain the difference between a physical assessment and a functional assessment?

Some nursing diagnoses that may be appropriate for the client undergoing rehabilitation are:

◆ Impaired physical mobility
◆ Self-care deficit
◆ Risk for impaired skin integrity
◆ Risk for injury
◆ Alteration in urinary elimination
◆ Constipation
◆ Ineffective individual coping
◆ Ineffective family coping
◆ Impaired home maintenance management
◆ Knowledge deficit
◆ Body image disturbance
◆ Altered patterns of sexuality

A collaborative plan of care is devised or a clinical care path is individualized for each rehabilitation client. Often there will be five or more health professionals involved. Periodic care conferences are essential for the members of the health care team to evaluate the progress of the client, share perceptions and ideas, and to revise the plan of care if it is not helping the client to meet established expected outcomes. Depending on the situation, care conferences may occur once every 1 or 2 weeks or once a month.

Sexual concerns should be addressed during the rehabilitation period. The nurse helps the client identify problems and concerns and works to assist in finding means for sexual expression and gratification. If the nurse is not comfortable or knowledgeable in this role, an appropriate referral to a sex therapist is made.

The nurse must be aware that clients with chronic illness, those who have suffered major loss of body function or former roles, and those who have lost most of their independence and social contacts may suffer from depression. Assessing mental outlook is an ongoing nursing function. Should several signs of severe depression become evident, the nurse consults with the physician. The client must be kept safe. Determining suicide potential in the depressed client is important. Chapter 32 discusses depression and suicide.

REHABILITATION PROGRAMS

Most communities that have a hospital have a rehabilitation program for clients with cardiac, respiratory, and musculoskeletal problems. Many communities have rehabilitation programs available for clients who have suffered neurological injury or loss of musculoskeletal function due to amputation, trauma, or disease. Programs often are available for vision or hearing rehabilitation. YMCAs often have rehabilitation programs

TABLE 12-2 ◆ *Resources for Rehabilitation Patients*

Administration on Developmental Disabilities, U.S. Department of Health and Human Services, 370 L'enfant Promenade SW, Washington, DC 20447; (202) 690-6590.

American Diabetes Association, 1600 Duke Street, Alexandria, VA 22314; (800) ADA-DISC.

Clearinghouse on Disability Information, Office of Special Education and Rehabilitation Services, Room 3132, Switzer Building, 330 C Street, SE, Washington, DC 20202; (800) 346-2742.

Information for Individuals with Disabilities, Fort Point Place, 27-43 Wormwood Street, Boston, MA 02210; (617) 727-5540

Mainstream, Inc., 1030 115th Street, NW, Suite 110, Washington, DC 10005; (202) 898-1400.

National Amputation Foundation, 12–45 150th Street, Whitestone, NY 11357; (718) 767-0596.

National Clearinghouse on Postsecondary Education for Individuals with Disabilities, HEATH Resource Center, One Dupont Circle, NW, Washington, DC 20036; (800) 544-3284.

National Council on Disability, 800 Independence Avenue, SW, Washington, DC 20591; (202) 267-3846.

National Rehabilitation Information Center, 8455 Colesville Road, Suite 935, Silver Spring, MD 20910; (800) 34-NARIC.

Office of Vocational and Adult Education, U.S. Department of Education, Policy Analysis Staff, Switzer Building, Room 4525, 330 C Street, SE, Washington, DC 20202-0001; (202) 732-2251.

with water exercise for clients with severe arthritis. Most burn centers have comprehensive rehabilitation programs available for the burn client. Table 12-2 lists resources for the rehabilitation client.

Rehabilitation programs have a philosophy that is based on three beliefs: (1) Each person is unique, whole within herself, and interdependent with her own environment; (2) independence can be achieved within the limits of disability when the person is a full participant in managing her own life; (3) the goal is to enable clients to mobilize their own resources, choose goals, and attain them through their own efforts. Rehabilitation involves the whole person and is a team effort involving a variety of disciplines.

Elder Care Point... The elderly client who has suffered a major loss of body function may not be initially receptive of rehabilitation efforts. It takes a skillful nurse to help motivate the client to want to improve his functional ability. Sometimes introducing the client to someone close to her own age who has been through a similar illness and has managed to regain some functions is the best "medicine." Gentle encouragement with praise for small efforts and accomplishments is better than trying to force the client to perform exercises or practice tasks.

Although rehabilitation begins upon admission to the hospital, clients with chronic problems often are referred to outclient rehabilitation programs. An example of such a program is a respiratory rehabilitation program. Clients referred to such a program are experiencing compromised respiratory function that is affecting their ability to perform ADLs and decreasing their quality of life. Such clients suffer from chronic airflow limitation and are referred to the program by their physician.

A respiratory rehabilitation program teaches self-care techniques to the client that will help her attain a better quality of life. There are generally three components to a respiratory rehabilitation program: (1) breathing exercises; (2) paced walking exercise; and (3) correct use of inhaled medications. Clients are enrolled in the program for a number of weeks and interact with other clients who have the same problems. A nurse or respiratory therapist teaches the various breathing techniques, paced walking, and use of inhalers. The nurse conducts motivational group activities to increase desire to participate in an exercise program and to display the benefits of following the program. Teaching on how to avoid respiratory infections is reinforced. The nurse or respiratory therapist is available to encourage and evaluate progress on using the techniques taught while exercising. Vital signs are monitored periodically to determine the effect of exercise on cardiac and respiratory function. Some rehabilitation centers provide respiratory services by weaning the client from the ventilator and then working with her to improve respiratory function and functional capacity for tasks of daily living.

Paced walking is simply using pursed-lip breathing while walking. The client is taught to inhale through the nose as she takes her first two steps and then exhale slowly through pursed lips as she takes her next four steps. Abdominal or diaphragmatic breathing techniques are used along with the pursed lips. Diaphragmatic breathing techniques are presented in Chapter 16.

One of the main roles of the rehabilitation nurse is to help the client maintain hope that she will regain some autonomy and enjoy an adequate quality of life. The motto is to minimize limitations and maximize capabilities. The nurse must believe in the client and her ability to take charge of her situation and future. The nurse and other health team members are instrumental in guiding the client to the resources needed to improve her quality of life and to gain the skills needed for the greatest degree of independent living possible.

With concerns about health care costs and tightening of Medicare and private insurance expenditures, much rehabilitation care has been transferred to the home setting. Whereas clients with neurological damage from a spinal cord or head injury used to spend several months in a rehabilitation facility, the time has been reduced to about 6 weeks.

LONG-TERM CARE

Nursing home care has come a long way from the turn of the century when the elderly without family and the ill were housed in homes at public expense and were given only custodial care. Today there are several levels of care available. Retirement centers that provide a continuum of care offer apartment complexes combined with central dining facilities, laundry and housekeeping services, and support staff if help is needed. The next level of care is for frail elderly or those recovering from an illness and involves a building complex, usually referred to as a residential care facility for the elderly (RCFE), that provides a room, meals, personal care assistance, and minimal nursing care. Care is provided on a 24-hour basis. When the resident needs assistance with several ADLs or has skilled nursing needs, she moves to a skilled care facility. Skilled care facilities also are called Long-term care facilities, extended-care facilities, or nursing homes.

Clients who need rehabilitation after discharge from a hospital, as well as those who suffer from chronic illnesses and deficits in self-care, often are admitted into a long-term care facility. Some nursing homes provide custodial care for chronically ill elderly who need assistance with several ADLs, such as toileting, bathing, dressing, meals, administration of medications, and movement (unable to ambulate or transfer independently). Many of these elderly have mental health problems, such as dementia, that have become too difficult for the family to handle on a 24-hour basis. Some residents are short term, in that they are there to recover from hip surgery, stroke, or other temporary disability. These residents will return to their home setting within a few weeks or months.

A large percentage of long-term care facilities provide "skilled" care, and professional, licensed, personnel is present around the clock. Skilled facilities are geared to rehabilitative care or to the care of the more helpless resident, such as the ventilator dependent. An RN usually is the director of nurses. Another RN acts as the supervisor for the facility's day-to-day operations. A licensed practical nurse (LPN) often is the charge nurse, and assistants or nurse's aides provide much of the basic direct care to the residents. An occupational therapist, physical therapist, speech pathologist, respiratory therapist, activity therapist, or other professional provides services as needed. A physician supervises each resident's care program. Although the RN ultimately is responsible for the nursing care plan of each resident, the LPN charge nurse often is the person who admits the resident and initiates the plan of care. If the LPN devises a plan of care, collaboration with the RN is necessary to ensure that the plan is appropriate and complete. The LPN performs treatments and wound care, assesses the clients regularly, organizes the shift's workload, administers medications, documents assessment findings and care given, updates the nursing care plans, and delegates care tasks to patient care assistants. The LPN oversees care for a group of residents for a shift. The supervisor manages the care for the entire facility, or if the facility is very large, for a certain number of patient care units on a 24-hour basis. The director of nurses is ultimately responsible for the care given throughout the facility.

The LPN delegates tasks such as assistance with toileting, bathing, feeding, ambulation or range of motion (ROM) exercises, care of the resident unit, and transfer of residents from bed to chair to the patient care assistants. **For any task to be delegated to an unlicensed person, the LPN must be certain that the patient care assistant, or other person, is competent in the task required. The LPN is ultimately responsible for the care delegated to and provided by patient care assistants or other unlicensed assistive personnel under his direction.** Patient care assistants are the "worker bees" of the long-term care facility. The skillful LPN will establish rapport, harmony, and respect among the work team by valuing these workers, appreciating their contributions, and listening to their concerns.

When planning care for clients in a long-term care facility, the nurse keeps in mind that the overall goals of care for the facility are to provide a safe environment, assist the resident to maintain or attain as much function as possible, promote individual independence, and **allow the resident to maintain or achieve as much autonomy as possible.**

◆ Safety

Providing a safe environment for a group of residents, many of whom may not be totally mentally competent, while allowing autonomy and independence is a great challenge. Physical and chemical restraints are used only when a resident is a proven threat to herself or others. (Chemical restraints are tranquilizers or sedatives that calm a resident and alter behavior.) A variety of techniques help provide a restraint-free, yet safe, environment. The techniques depend on the type of population present in a facility. Two of the greatest safety problems often are to keep confused residents within the boundaries of the facility and to prevent falls. Meeting resident safety and independence needs without resorting to chemical or physical restraints requires caring, commitment, and ingenuity on the part of the nurse.

Prevention of Falls   The first step in the prevention of falls is to recognize which residents are at greatest risk.

Risk factors for falls include musculoskeletal disorders that impair normal ambulation or balance, neurological problems such as peripheral neuropathy affecting the feet, balance or gait problems resulting from stroke or inner-ear problems, postural hypotension or dizziness caused by medications, impaired vision, impaired hearing, extreme weakness, and a history of previous falls. Residents who have an oxygen deficit are another group that may suffer from dizziness and loss of balance that can result in a fall.

The second step to prevent a fall is to recognize hazards in the environment that could precipitate a fall. Loose rugs, rugs that do not stay flat, and items to be navigated around in heavily used pathways often are culprits. Pathways should be free of litter and other objects. Shoes or slippers should be placed beneath a piece of furniture rather than left in the pathway. The pathway to and from the bathroom and within the bathroom itself must be adequately lit for nocturnal visits. Lighting must be without glare and of a type that does not produce areas of deep shadow. Any liquid spilled on the floors must be cleaned up immediately. Any piece of equipment with wheels should have the wheels locked when it is not in motion.

Placing the resident's belongings within easy reach of the bed or chair helps prevent falls. **Getting in the habit of always checking to see that the call bell is within the resident's reach and that the resident is aware of where it is located, encourages a call for assistance should there be a need to get up and move around. Promptly answering call lights prevents the resident from arising without needed assistance and reduces the incidence of falls considerably.** Encouraging the use of sturdy, supportive, nonslip footwear helps prevent falls from soles that slide on certain surfaces. All resident areas should have floor covering that is not slippery, not highly patterned, and that is easily navigated in common footwear and with assistive devices. Encouraging ambulatory elderly residents to crouch down to pick up something or to sit to dry their feet, rather than bending from the waist, helps prevent dizziness or loss of balance that can lead to a fall. Grab bars by the toilet, the shower, or tub, along each set of stairs, and in hallways provide stability and can greatly reduce the incidence of falls if clients get into the habit of using them wherever they are available. Chairs that have the proper height and depth help prevent the "calculated fall" into the chair and the bending way forward to catapult oneself out of the chair that sometimes occur when chairs are not of the proper height.

Providing opportunities for exercise and strengthening movements that will increase muscle strength and balance helps decrease debility and the incidence of falls. Clients who are at risk for postural hypotension should rise to a sitting position and dangle for a bit before standing, should hang on to a chair arm or piece of furniture when standing up and stabilize for a few moments before beginning to ambulate once in a standing position. **Assessing all medications a resident is taking to determine the risk of medication-induced postural hypotension or dizziness is a must.** Residents who need glasses for adequate visual acuity must be taught to put them on before arising to ambulate. **Glasses should always be kept clean and close at hand.** Hearing aids should be worn, turned on, and properly adjusted when the resident is up and about to prevent collisions with another simply because the resident did not know the person was in the vicinity. Clothing should be of a sort that will not trip the resident, catching on the heels as she arises or on furniture or door knobs.

Assessing the resident's use of assistive devices for ambulation before allowing unassisted ambulation is vital to safety. It takes considerable practice for a resident to maneuver safely with a cane, walker, or crutches. Besides the coordination and balance required, the resident also must be alert to the path of the device itself to avoid knocking into chair or table legs along the way. If the resident is hooked to an intravenous line, oxygen tubing, or drainage devices, teaching about how to maneuver without tripping on such lines and devices is essential.

The nurse must be alert to the fact that a resident who was previously ambulating safely may be weakened if she has been recently sick with the flu, a bad cold, vomiting, or diarrhea. The resident who is receiving diuretic therapy must be assessed frequently for fluid and electrolyte imbalance that could cause weakness, dizziness, or confusion. **The resident who needs narcotic therapy for pain or sedatives to sleep must be safeguarded.** The resident must be instructed to ring for assistance should the need to arise from the bed or chair occur. The bed should be kept in the low position and the siderails should be raised when the resident is in it. Such residents are at high risk for a fall.

All residents should be taught that, if a fall occurs, they should call for help and not move until assistance comes. After performing an assessment to ascertain that the client has not sustained a serious injury, the nurse can assist with arising from a fall by instructing the client to roll on to the right side, bend the right knee, lever upward to the kneeling position by pressing down on the right forearm. The nurse assists by crouching with one knee on the floor and placing the hands around the back and under the armpits and pulling as the resident pushes. The resident is assisted into a sitting position. The nurse stands, and with the help of a stable base of support and another assistant, assists the resident up and into a chair.

Think about... Can you describe how you would determine just how at risk a new resident is for falls? Can you identify points that should be included in the assessment of a high risk for a fall?

Use of Safety Devices and Techniques   When a resident frequently forgets instructions to call for assistance, repeatedly attempts to get up and falls, or interferes with medical treatment by pulling out ordered tubes or scratching at wounds, the use of restraining or security devices may be necessary. Most states have statutes guaranteeing the resident's right to be free of unreasonable restraints. **The purpose of such statutes is not to outlaw the use of restraints, but to ensure that they are used to protect residents, not just to hinder their movements for the staff's convenience.** All restraints must be ordered by a physician. If a qualified, licensed nurse determines the need for a chemical or physical restraint in an emergency, the need is specifically documented when the restraint is applied. All measures taken to try to correct the situation without the use of restraint prior to its application also is documented. A physician's order for the restraint must be written within 24 to 48 hours. Table 12-3 presents the principles related to the use of security and safety devices.

The resident who is immobilized with a restraining device must be checked visually by the nurse at least every 30 minutes to ensure that her body is in good alignment and that there are no problems. A check of skin color for circulation in the affected body parts is important when rounds are made. Residents must be turned or repositioned every 2 hours. Thorough assessment of skin and circulation is done at that time. Measures to help prevent the need for restraints are listed in Table 12-4.

TABLE 12-3 ◆ *Principles Related to the Use of Security and Safety Devices*

- The use of safety or security devices must help the patient or be needed to continue medical therapy.
- All devices that limit movement or immobilize must be ordered by a physician.
- Restraints must not be used to punish or discipline patients.
- Restraints are applied snugly to a body part, but not so tightly as to interfere with blood circulation or nerve function.
- When used, security or immobilization devices must be removed and the patient's position changed at least every 2 hours. Active or passive exercises are performed for immobilized joints and muscles.
- The physician should be notified as soon as the security device is deemed no longer necessary.

TABLE 12-4 ◆ *Measures Helpful to Prevent the Need for Restraints*

◆ Place the restless or high-risk patient in a room or location close to the nurse's station where the patient can be checked frequently and attempts to get up will be most likely observed.

◆ Use a bed alarm to alert nursing staff that the patient is attempting to get out of bed unassisted.

◆ Remain with the unsteady, agitated, or confused patient when she is up and about.

◆ Leave another person in charge of your patients when leaving the unit for a meal break or other reason; specifically mention which patients need to be visually checked frequently.

◆ If a patient needs to get up at night frequently to urinate and does not call for assistance, restrict fluid intake after 6:00 PM if appropriate.

◆ Provide social and diversional activities to patients confined to a wheelchair or bed so that boredom does not cause the person to try to get up and seek activity.

◆ Move the mattress on to a low platform or the floor so that it is easier for the patient to get in and out of bed more easily without the risk of a fall.

◆ Managing Daytime Confusion and Disorientation

For the resident with mild confusion and disorientation there are various techniques and measures the nurse can use to help her regain a sense of who she is, where she is, and what is happening to and around her. These measures also can help improve an elderly resident's self-esteem. Such measures are part of the resident's plan of care and are used consistently by all personnel. Reality orientation involves both the environment and the persons who interact with the resident and should be followed 24 hours a day. The environment is structured so that the resident has concrete and continual reminders of the year, day, and time of day. Environmental aids include a readable, up-to-date calendar, a clock, and the daily newspaper or local television or radio news. Consistency in mealtimes, scheduled activities, treatments, and daily personal care routine also can be helpful. Limit the number of choices she has to make during these activities. A time schedule for activities and events within the facility is posted in large type where the resident can refer to it frequently. Decorations for the next upcoming holiday give clues as to the current season of the year. Labeling the photographs of the resident's loved ones with their names helps her recall who is who. Place the resident's name in large block letters in her room and on her clothing. Use symbols on signs to help the resident find the bathroom or dining room. Try to assign caregivers who are familiar to the resident and avoid unfamiliar situations, and limit visitors to one or two persons at a time. Older residents usually prefer to be called by title (Mr., Mrs., Miss) and surname. Each resident's preference should be sought and respected. Nicknames such as "Granny," "Pops," "Uncle," or "Dear" are not only demeaning, but also add to a client's confusion and disorientation.

Interaction with staff and family members also can give the resident helpful clues. Sometimes people who do not understand the nature of confusion and disorientation in the elderly think it is a kindness to go along with a confused elderly person. They do not gently correct or remind the client who confuses her daughter with her sister or the nurse with her daughter, nor do they remind the resident where she is when she indicates that she thinks she is at home, rather than at the long-term care facility. A more positive and helpful approach is to respond continuously to the client's confusion with honest and real information. Be certain thoroughly to assess the possibility of a physical cause for the confusion, such as urinary tract infection, constipation, dehydration, or suboptimal pain control.

◆ Dealing with Nocturnal Confusion

Nocturnal confusion (sundowner syndrome) is not uncommon among elderly long-term care residents. Sensory deficits, such as impaired sight and hearing, add to the client's confusion and anxiety at night when the environment becomes stranger because of darkness. Ordinary shapes and sounds can become terrifying, and siderails can be perceived as bars on a jail or a cage. Nursing intervention requires creative adaptations of the environment to decrease the fears of the resident. A night light that gives illumination without shining in the client's eyes or causing frightening shadows, keeping the call bell within reach, frequent visits to calm and reassure, moving the resident closer to the nurses' station, touching, and other signs of caring are all ways in which the nurse can intervene to minimize nocturnal confusion. A bed alarm that alerts the nurse that the resident has gotten out of bed and an alarm system that alerts the staff that the resident has left her room or designated area, may be used in place of physical restraints to keep the confused resident from wandering in unsafe areas. For some residents, keeping the radio on in the room provides company and dispels fears. However this can be done only if it does not disturb other residents.

Keeping the resident active during the day and encouraging physical exercise helps promote sleep at night. If the resident can sleep at night, fewer hours of darkness are spent in confusion and fear. **Listening to the resident to try and determine any possible cause of unrest or fear can help solve the problem.** Sometimes it is just a particular shadow or sound that is disturbing and causing the agitated or confused behavior. Residents who are on diuretics must be continuously monitored for electrolyte disturbances that might cause confusion.

◆ Promoting Independence

The move to a long-term care facility is a major life upheaval for the resident, particularly when it is for life. Research has shown that the more prepared the person is for the relocation, the better the adjustment to nursing home life. Providing choices to the person about which facility, general location of room, room decoration, and personal belongings are ways to maintain both some independence and some autonomy. Bringing favorite photographs, Afghan, pillow, pictures, or special items to the resident's room from home helps with the transition. If permitted, a personal telephone line establishes a link with the outside community and the family and helps the resident feel less isolated. Providing information on other residents who have similar interests and who have had some parallel life experiences in place of residence or occupation is helpful in stimulating interest in making new friends.

Nurses must work with the staff to let the resident choose daily clothing when possible and a say in when they prefer bathing. Options of where to sit in the dining area, if possible, also provides an area for some independence and autonomy. Arranging with family members to set up a schedule with the resident for planned visits helps the resident feel some level of control over his life and provides something to look forward to as the week goes by.

Specific goals should be set with the resident to encourage independence in ADLs and in recreational activity. Perhaps a resident can pursue a former hobby, such as knitting or playing the piano, if one is available. Adaptive devices and a consult with the dietitian may provide all the assistance that is necessary for the resident to feed herself once again (Figure 12-2). **To promote a resident's independence, the staff should refrain from doing tasks that the resident is capable of doing herself.** Table 12-5 lists some common adaptive devices that are very helpful. Often it is quicker for the staff member to bathe the resident or to feed her, but when the goal is to foster independence, refraining from doing the task is the correct intervention.

Elder Care Point... Elderly residents usually prefer to have things in their immediate environment arranged in a particular way. The nurse should not rearrange the resident's belongings for the sake of tidiness without asking the resident's permission as this may cause agitation or anger. The resident's wishes should be respected as long as a safety hazard does not exist.

For the resident who has had a stroke or suffers from debilitating arthritis or other musculoskeletal problem, use of adaptive devices can assist in the promotion of independence, provide some autonomy, and help to maintain function (Figure 12-3).

Encouraging contact with friends outside of the facility is important to the resident's sense of self and her independence. Providing a warm welcome to visitors, assisting the resident to the phone when a friend calls, and providing some privacy for the call if possible, help maintain friendships. Promptly delivering, and reading if necessary, mail to the resident and finding a volunteer

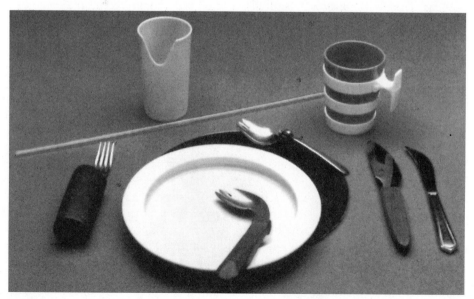

FIGURE 12-2   Adaptive equipment to compensate for limited upper-extremity function.
(Source: Braddom, R. L. [1996]. *Physical Medicine and Rehabilitation.* Philadelphia: Saunders, p. 551.)

TABLE 12-5 ◆ *Uses of Assistive-Adaptive Devices*

Device	Use
Buttonhook	Threaded through the buttonhole to enable clients with weak finger mobility to button shirts. Alternative uses include serving as a pencil holder.
Extended shoe horn	Assists in putting on shoes for clients with decreased mobility. Alternative uses include turning light switches off or on while the client is in a wheelchair.
Plate guard	Applied to a plate to assist clients with weak hand and arm mobility to feed themselves.
Gel pad	Placed under a plate or a glass to prevent dishes from slipping and moving. Alternative uses include placement under bathing and grooming items to prevent their moving.
Foam buildups	Applied to eating utensils to assist clients with weak handgrasps to feed themselves. Alternative uses include the application to pens and pencils to assist with writing or over a buttonhook to assist with grasping the device.
Hook and loop fastener (Velcro) straps	Applied to utensils, a buttonhook, or a pencil to slip over the hand and provide a method of stabilizing the device when the client's handgrasp is weak.
Long-handled reacher	Assists in obtaining items located on high shelves or at ground level for clients who are not able to change positions easily.

Source: Ignatavicius, D. D., Workman, M. L., Mishler, M. A., (1995). *Medical–Surgical Nursing: A Nursing Process Approach,* 2nd ed. Philadelphia: Saunders, p. 228.

to write letters provides a link to friends and the outside world. This also is very beneficial to family members who live far away and cannot visit often. Often residents who have had a stroke are aphasic or have hemiplegia and cannot write. If someone will correspond for the resident and read letters back to her, warm communication can be continued.

If a volunteer group is available, establishing a "buddy" link with a person who is living outside the facility is very special. Such a person can provide many kindnesses for the resident, such as occasional flowers from the garden, homemade cookies, letter writing, holiday decorations, and conversation about community happenings as well as topics of interest to the resident. The volunteer reaps much satisfaction in providing friendship to one who is confined and infirm.

Think about . . . Can you think of three ways to foster independence in your new resident who is still quite weak, has suffered a stroke, and has right-sided hemiparesis. She is right-handed.

◆ Fostering Autonomy

Preserving as much autonomy as possible helps the resident adjust to a long-term care facility better. Working with roommates to provide solutions for such things as wanting to stay up late and watch TV when the other

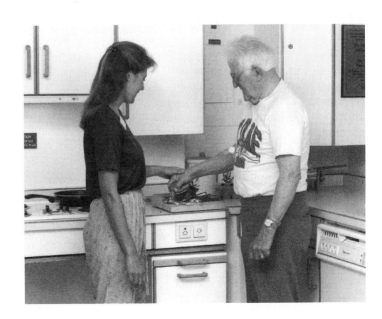

FIGURE 12-3   Occupational therapist working with patient and adaptive equipment to compensate for limited upper-extremity function.
(Photo by Glen Derbyshire; courtesy of the Rehabilitation Institute of Santa Barbara.)

wishes to arise very early in the morning and listen to the radio is necessary to provide autonomy to one without infringing on the privacy rights of the other. Headphones or a pillow speaker device with a headset is one solution to such a problem. Working out an agreement in a shared room about when the shades or curtains will be pulled back to allow more light in the room and a view of the outside can be valuable to both roommates. **The staff must work to encourage honest, but tactful communication, between roommates over such daily living matters and then help them come to satisfactory agreement.**

Allowing the resident a say in goal setting promotes a feeling of power and autonomy. The nurse works to teach the resident about the benefits of various goals that are felt appropriate, discusses any concerns the resident may have about them, and then together, realistic goals are written.

The family also helps maintain the resident's autonomy by continuing to honor her place in the family. Updating the resident on family happenings, seeking thoughts on a family problem, relating family triumphs, and discussing community and family issues all show her that she is still a valued member of the family and society.

It is somewhat difficult not to override a resident's autonomy within an institutional environment. Nurses must step back periodically and evaluate whether the resident is being allowed any autonomy or not. If the hustle and bustle of everyday running of the facility is gravely interfering with autonomy, a care conference is needed to find a solution to the problem that will work within the structure of the institution.

◆ Maintaining Function

Once a functional assessment has been completed, specific goals should be mutually written to maintain the highest level of function possible for the resident. If the resident is ambulatory, exercise should be encouraged daily on a planned basis. If the resident is not ambulatory, ROM exercises should be performed several times a day. Measures to promote continued bowel and bladder continence are essential. Assessing patterns of elimination and providing assistance for toileting as needed is a basic part of promoting continued function and protecting the resident's dignity. If the resident has been temporarily incontinent because of illness or surgery, then a bowel or bladder retraining program is appropriate. Chapters 20 and 23 discusses such programs.

Mental stimulation is essential to maintaining a high level of cognitive functioning. Although resident preference should be considered in group TV viewing areas, the staff should consider planning segments of time to turn on informational programs that are inter-

esting. Scientific shows, travel shows, public television specials, and such can stimulate thinking and encourages the sharing of thoughts on a variety of subjects. Assisting residents to work crossword puzzles is another way to help them keep an active mind. When a resident cannot write or read because of poor vision, group work on a puzzle is an option. Card games promote mental stimulation as well as social interaction.

Computers could be a boon to the mental functioning of long-term care residents. It is hoped that they will soon be inexpensive, small, and easy to use enough that residents will be able to take advantage of the many wonderful things available on CD-ROM disks and possibly even the Internet. This would be an avenue for continued lifelong learning, as well as a place where enjoyment through playing bridge or other games, having a book read to one, or carrying on a conversation with someone miles away is possible for those whose mental faculties are still intact.

CARE TECHNIQUES FOR SAFETY AND REHABILITATION

◆ Transfer Techniques

Clients with impaired mobility will require assistance with transfers from a bed to a chair, to the commode, or into the bath. A thorough assessment is usually performed by the physical therapist to determine the best methods and means of transferring the client. Table 12-6 provides points to remember when transferring a

---

TABLE 12-6 ◆ *Transfers: Points to Remember*

Bed to wheechair
- Position the wheelchair and lock the wheels (patient's strong side should be next to the chair).
- Raise or remove the footrests; remove chair arm closest to bed if possible.
- Lower the bed and siderail; elevate the head of the bed.
- Assist the patient to sit securely on the side of the bed.
- Tell the patient how you will assist or move her.
- Flex your knees and hold on to the patient securely when moving.
- Reposition the patient in the chair so body alignment is correct.
- Position the feet on the footrests and be certain arms are to the inside of the chair before moving.
- Position the wheelchair and lock the wheels.
- Remove the armrest from the wheelchair; raise or remove footrests.

Use of a transfer board
- Powder the transfer board surface.
- Position board under both buttocks.
- Assist the patient to slide.

client. The priority in any transfer is safety for both the client and the nurse.

Clients are moved slowly from a supine to a sitting, and then to a standing position, to decrease the effects of postural hypotension or dizziness and prevent a fall. Maintenance of a normal weight is encouraged to promote greater ease of transfer.

◆ Gait Training

If a client is capable of ambulating, but has suffered a debilitating illness or impairment of mobility from an accident or stroke, gait training can assist her resume safe ambulation. The physical therapist works directly with the client on a gait training program (Figure 12-4). **The nurse reinforces the instructions of the physical therapist and encourages the client to practice.** The goal is independent ambulation with or without an assistive device. Various types of canes, crutches, or a walker may be utilized. A gait belt should be worn by the client until independent ambulation becomes a reality.

If gait training is not a possibility because of neuromuscular impairment, then wheelchair skills are taught to promote mobility. A physical and occupational therapist can teach a wheelchair-bound individual how to get just about anywhere and accomplish most ADLs from the wheelchair.

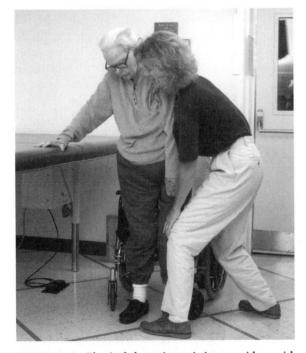

FIGURE 12-4 Physical therapist assisting a resident with weight bearing. (Photo by Glen Derbyshire; courtesy of the Rehabilitation Institute of Santa Barbara.)

◆ Prevention of Hazards of Immobility

The less mobile the long-term care resident or rehabilitation client, the greater the need for interventions to reduce the risk of hazards of immobility. **Preventing skin breakdown is a primary responsibility of all personnel in the agency.** Chapter 11 discusses care of the immobile client. Table 12-7 reviews the potential complications of immobility.

◆ Documentation

Documentation in a long-term care facility is somewhat different from that in the hospital or in home care. An admission assessment and an extensive eight-page Minimum Data Set (MDS) form that is required by the federal government are filled out (Figures 12-5 and 12-6). Bowel and bladder training assessment forms and training program forms, weekly pressure ulcer reports, and 24-hour intake and output records are some of the other documentation forms used in the long-term care facility.

HOME CARE

The majority of care in the community setting is given by home health and hospice agencies. Home health care is the preferred and most cost-effective method of health care delivery. Recent innovations in medical equipment have allowed more complex, high-technology care to be given at home. For the client there are many benefits, both physically and psychologically. **The goal of home care is to keep the client as well as possible and enable her to stay at home.** Home care nursing can prevent an expensive readmission to a hospital or entry into a nursing home. Home health care is family centered, and the family members or significant other are responsible for the ongoing care of the client. The nurse visits to intervene and see that the client is provided comfort, to prevent complications, to improve and promote health, and to assist with rehabilitation. Because home health care is family centered, **the philosophy of the nurse must have a different focus. In the home care setting, the client and family are in charge. The nurse is a guest in the home, acts as a consultant, coordinator of care, provider of skilled care, teacher, and advocate.** This is an instance where the client and family are truly "clients." They are seeking the nurse's services and must be treated as valued customers. The nurse must learn to be nonjudgmental of the client, the family, and the living arrangements. Should the living situation not be ideal, furnishings and equipment lacking, or the home dirty, the nurse must establish trust with the client and family before trying to accomplish major changes. The nurse must be sensitive to the client and family's cultural

TABLE 12-7 ◆ *Prevention of Some Common Hazards of Immobility*		
Body System	**Complication**	**Prevention**
Musculoskeletal	Contractures	Range-of-motion exercises
	Foot drop	Foot support while in bed, range-of-motion acitivities
	Osteoporosis	Range-of-motion exercises
	Susceptibility to fractures	Weight-bearing exercises
	Muscular atrophy	Passive or active range-of-motion exercises
Gastrointestinal	Constipation	Increased activity level
		Increased fluid intake
		Increased fiber intake
Cardiovascular	Decreased cardiac output	Range-of-motion exercises
	Increased venous stasis	Exercise, support hose, or antiembolism stockings
	Thrombus formation	Exercise, support hose, or antiembolism stockings
	Embolism	Avoidance of leg massage
Neurological	Disorientation	Sleep-wake schedule in accord with light–dark pattern
		Reorientation (to person, place, and time)
		Control of sensory stimulation
	Postural hypotension	Avoidance of sudden position changes
Renal/urinary	Calculi	Decreased dietary calcium level
		Increased fluid intake
		Maintenance of acidic urine
Respiratory	Pneumonia	Frequent repositioning
		Respiratory exercises
Integumentary	Pressure sores	Frequent repositioning
		Pressure relief devices
		Skin care

Source: Ignatavicius, D. D., Workman, M. L., Mishler, M. A., (1995). *Medical–Surgical Nursing: A Nursing Process Approach,* 2nd ed. Philadelphia: Saunders, p. 227.

values, financial resources, and specific ways of doing things and not try to impose his own views. **A home care nurse must be very flexible and creative in teaching clients and families ways to accomplish care of the client while abiding by the principles of asepsis and safety** (Figure 12-7).

Safety of the home environment is a priority in home health care. When a client is admitted to the service, the nurse performs a home safety check by looking for fire hazards, level of cleanliness, and potential hazards that could cause a fall. Table 12-8 presents guidelines for the prevention of falls in the home.

The home care nurse must possess good assessment skills. A large percentage of her time with the client is spent evaluating physical and psychosocial status, signs of complications, side effects of medications, and effects of therapy. Both the safety of the home and the quality of nutritional and basic care are evaluated. The nurse is the doctor's eyes and ears, and she spends considerable time consulting with doctors by phone, updating them on client's conditions, seeking new orders, and collaborating about care needs. Each visit to the client includes a physical assessment of the identified problems and of nutritional, home safety, elimination, skin, and psycho-

social status. All findings are documented. The nurse also documents data indicating that home health nursing care is still needed. Between visits the nurse may contact the client or family to check on various aspects of care or to see whether there are any concerns. The client and family may contact the agency or the nurse at any time and phone calls are encouraged.

Other functions of the home health nurse include performing wound care and dressing changes, organizing medications for scheduled administration, monitoring blood sugar, drawing blood samples for laboratory testing, giving injections or teaching injection technique, monitoring pain control, and monitoring enteral feedings. Teaching self-care and rehabilitation techniques and monitoring progress and compliance with treatment are primary nursing functions that help control health care cost and keep the client from needing hospitalization.

The home care nurse provides considerable psychosocial care for the client and family. Sometimes, the nurse is the only visitor the client has. In this instance, the nurse becomes a sort of friend, providing social interaction as well as needed health care. The nurse must become knowledgeable about negotiating the

Text continued on page 291

NURSES' ADMISSION RECORD
(To be completed by the nurse admitting the patient)

Family Name	First Name	Middle Name	Room No.	Bed No.	Admission No.

Attending Physician			Date		Time

Admitting Diagnosis

Take and record temperature, pulse, respiration and weight

Date _____ T____ P____ R____ B.P.____/____ Weight_____ Length _____

Orientation of Patient to Facility

Oriented to functions of call light ☐   Oriented to facility visiting hours ☐
Oriented to procedures of meal times ☐   Oriented to location of room ☐
Oriented to smoking regulations ☐   Facility will do personal laundry ☐
Oriented to activity program ☐   Family will do personal laundry ☐

Patient wears: Dentures ☐   Glasses ☐   Hearing aid ☐   Other_____

SPECIFY

Has prothesis of: Breast ☐   Leg ☐   Arm ☐   Other_____

SPECIFY

General physical appearance_____

General condition of skin_____

Indicate on diagram below all body marks such as, old or recent scars, bruises or discolorations (regardless of how slight), lacerations, decubitus ulcers and other ulcerations or questionable markings considered other than normal:

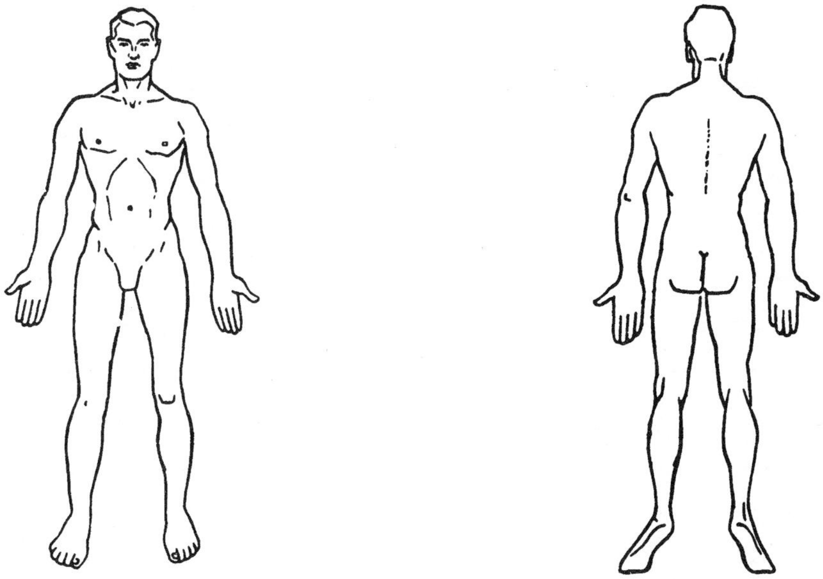

Signed_____

Nursing Assistant

Signed_____

Licensed Nurse

FIGURE 12-5   Nurse's admission record. (Courtesy of Wilshire Nursing and Rehabilitation, Templeton, CA.)

Illustration continued on following page

ALLERGIES: _____

_____

_____

T.B. SCREENING:

Chest X—Ray ☐   Mantoux Test ☐

Date _____   Date _____

Place _____   Neg ☐   Pos ☐

Neg ☐   Pos ☐

Signature _____   Date _____

INCONTINENT ASSESSMENT:

Patient is: Continent ☐   Incontinent ☐
Has Catheter ☐

_____

_____

_____

_____

_____

_____

_____

_____

_____R.N._____
Assessment Completed by   Date

LICENSED NURSES ADMITTING NOTES

_____

_____

_____

_____

_____

_____

_____

_____

_____

_____

_____

_____

_____

_____

_____

_____

Patient Name_____   Room No._____   Attending Physician_____

FIGURE 12-5 *Continued*

MINIMUM DATA SET (MDS) — *VERSION 2.0*
FOR NURSING HOME RESIDENT ASSESSMENT AND CARE SCREENING
BASIC ASSESSMENT TRACKING FORM

SECTION AA. IDENTIFICATION INFORMATION		
1. RESIDENT NAME ⊛	a. (First) b. (Middle Initial) c. (Last) d. (Jr./Sr.)	
2. GENDER ⊛	1. Male 2. Female	
3. BIRTHDATE ⊛	Month — Day — Year	
4. RACE/⊛ ETHNICITY	1. American Indian/Alaskan Native 4. Hispanic 2. Asian/Pacific Islander 5. White, not of 3. Black, not of Hispanic origin Hispanic origin	
5. SOCIAL⊛ SECURITY AND ⊛ MEDICARE NUMBERS [C in 1st box if non Med. no.]	a. Social Security Number b. Medicare number (or comparable railroad insurance number)	
6. FACILITY PROVIDER NO. ⊛	a. State No. b. Federal No.	
7. MEDICAID NO. ["+" if pending, "N" if not a Medicaid ⊛ recipient]		
8. REASONS FOR ASSESS-MENT	[Note—Other codes do not apply to this form] a. Primary reason for assessment 1. Admission assessment (required by day 14) 2. Annual assessment 3. Significant change in status assessment 4. Significant correction of prior assessment 5. Quarterly review assessment 0. *NONE OF ABOVE* b. *Special codes for use with supplemental assessment types in Case Mix demonstration states or other states where required* 1. *5 day assessment* 2. *30 day assessment* 3. *60 day assessment* 4. *Quarterly assessment using full MDS form* 5. *Readmission/return assessment* 6. *Other state required assessment*	
9. SIGNATURES OF PERSONS COMPLETING THESE ITEMS:		
a. Signatures Title Date		
b. Date		

GENERAL INSTRUCTIONS

Complete this information for submission with all full and quarterly assessments (Admission, Annual, Significant Change, State or Medicare required assessments, or Quarterly Reviews, etc.).

⊛ = Key items for computerized resident tracking

▦ = When box blank, must enter number or letter

[a.] = When letter in box, check if condition applies

Code "NA" if information unavailable or unknown.

TRIGGER LEGEND

1 - Delirium	10A - Activities (Revise)
2 - Cognitive Loss/Dementia	10B - Activities (Review)
3 - Visual Function	11 - Falls
4 - Communication	12 - Nutritional Status
5A - ADL-Rehabilitation	13 - Feeding Tubes
5B - ADL-Maintenance	14 - Dehydration/Fluid Maintenance
6 - Urinary Incontinence and Indwelling Catheter	15 - Dental Care
7 - Psychosocial Well-Being	16 - Pressure Ulcers
8 - Mood State	17 - Psychotropic Drug Use
9 - Behavioral Symptoms	17* - For this to trigger, O4a, b, or c must = 1-7
	18 - Physical Restraints

Form 1728HH © 1995 Briggs Corporation, Des Moines, IA 50306 (800) 247-2343 PRINTED IN U.S.A.
Copyright limited to addition of trigger system.

1 of 8

MDS 2.0 10/18/94N

FIGURE 12-6   Minimum Data Set form, pages 1 and 2 of 8. (Courtesy of Wilshire Nursing and Rehabilitation, Templeton, CA. Trigger data used by Permission of Briggs Corporation.)

Illustration continued on following page

MINIMUM DATA SET (MDS) — *VERSION 2.0*
FOR NURSING HOME RESIDENT ASSESSMENT AND CARE SCREENING
BACKGROUND (FACE SHEET) INFORMATION AT ADMISSION

SECTION AB. DEMOGRAPHIC INFORMATION

1.	DATE OF ENTRY	*Date the stay began. Note — Does not include readmission if record was closed at time of temporary discharge to hospital, etc. In such cases, use prior admission date.*

☐☐ — ☐☐ — ☐☐☐☐
Month   Day   Year

2.	ADMITTED FROM (AT ENTRY)	1. Private home/apt. with no home health services 2. Private home/apt. with home health services 3. Board and care/assisted living/group home 4. Nursing home 5. Acute care hospital 6. Psychiatric hospital, MR/DD facility 7. Rehabilitation hospital 8. Other
3.	LIVED ALONE (PRIOR TO ENTRY)	0. No 1. Yes 2. In other facility
4.	ZIP CODE OF PRIOR PRIMARY RESIDENCE	☐☐☐☐☐
5.	RESIDENTIAL HISTORY 5 YEARS PRIOR TO ENTRY	*(Check all settings resident lived in during 5 years prior to date of entry given in item AB1 above.)*

Prior stay at this nursing home	a.
Stay in other nursing home	b.
Other residential facility — board and care home, assisted living, group home	c.
MH/psychiatric setting	d.
MR/DD setting	e.
NONE OF ABOVE	f.

6.	LIFETIME OCCUPA-TION(S) *(Put "/" between two occupations)*	☐☐☐☐☐☐☐☐☐☐☐☐☐☐☐
7.	EDUCATION *(Highest level completed)*	1. No schooling 5. Technical or trade school 2. 8th grade/less 6. Some college 3. 9-11 grades 7. Bachelor's degree 4. High school 8. Graduate degree
8.	LANGUAGE	*(Code for correct response)* a. Primary Language 0. English 1. Spanish 2. French 3. Other b. If other, specify ☐☐☐☐☐☐☐☐☐
9.	MENTAL HEALTH HISTORY	Does resident's RECORD indicate any history of mental retardation, mental illness, or developmental disability problem? 0. No 1. Yes
10.	CONDITIONS RELATED TO MR/DD STATUS	*(Check all conditions that are related to MR/DD status that were manifested before age 22, and are likely to continue indefinitely)*

Not applicable — no MR/DD (Skip to AB11)	a.
MR/DD with organic condition	
Down's syndrome	b.
Autism	c.
Epilepsy	d.
Other organic condition related to MR/DD	e.
MR/DD with no organic condition	f.

11.	DATE BACK-GROUND INFORMATION COMPLETED	☐☐ — ☐☐ — ☐☐☐☐ Month Day Year

▨ = When box blank, must enter number or letter

☐a. = When letter in box, check if condition applies

Code "NA" if information unavailable or unknown.

SECTION AC. CUSTOMARY ROUTINE

1.	CUSTOMARY ROUTINE	*(Check all that apply. If all information UNKNOWN, check last box only)*

(In year prior to DATE OF ENTRY to this nursing home, or year last in community if now being admitted from another nursing home)

CYCLE OF DAILY EVENTS

Stays up late at night (e.g., after 9 pm)	a.
Naps regularly during day (at least 1 hour)	b.
Goes out 1+ days a week	c.
Stays busy with hobbies, reading, or fixed daily routine	d.
Spends most of time alone or watching TV	e.
Moves independently indoors (with appliances, if used)	f.
Use of tobacco products at least daily	g.
NONE OF ABOVE	h.

EATING PATTERNS

Distinct food preferences	i.
Eats between meals all or most days	j.
Use of alcoholic beverage(s) at least weekly	k.
NONE OF ABOVE	l.

ADL PATTERNS

In bedclothes much of day	m.
Wakens to toilet all or most nights	n.
Has irregular bowel movement pattern	o.
Showers for bathing	p.
Bathing in PM	q.
NONE OF ABOVE	r.

INVOLVEMENT PATTERNS

Daily contact with relatives/close friends	s.
Usually attends church, temple, synagogue (etc.)	t.
Finds strength in faith	u.
Daily animal companion/presence	v.
Involved in group activities	w.
NONE OF ABOVE	x.
UNKNOWN — Resident/family unable to provide information	y.

END

SECTION AD. FACE SHEET SIGNATURES
SIGNATURES OF PERSONS COMPLETING FACE SHEET:

a. Signature of RN Assessment Coordinator			Date
b. Signatures	Title	Sections	Date
c.			Date
d.			Date
e.			Date
f.			Date
g.			Date

NOTE: Normally, the MDS Face Sheet is completed once, when an individual first enters the facility. However, the face sheet is also required if the person is reentering this facility after a discharge where return had not previously been expected. It is **not** completed following temporary discharges to hospitals or after therapeutic leaves/home visits.

Form 1728HH   © 1995 Briggs Corporation, Des Moines, IA 50306 (800) 247-2343 PRINTED IN U.S.A.
Copyright limited to addition of trigger system.
2 of 8   MDS 2.0   10/18/94N

FIGURE 12-6 *Continued*

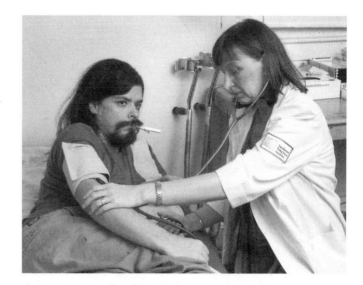

FIGURE 12-7   Home health nurse assessing a client.
(Photo by Glen Derbyshire; courtesy of Santa Barbara Visiting Nurse Association.)

complex medical care system and obtaining supplies, medications, or services when the client does not have money for them. A full knowledge of the community's resources available to the client is essential. Most home health agencies have lists of resources available. The medical social worker who has a liaison with the agency also can be of help. Where the hospital nurse stays out of financial concerns, other than referrals to the social worker, the home care nurse must try to help the client find remedies to financial problems so that stress will be reduced and energies can be directed at healing and learning techniques of self-care.

TABLE 12-8 ◆ *Fall Prevention Guidelines for the Home*

Lights and Lighting

- Eyes tire quickly in improper lighting. Illuminate reading material or the object worked on. Illuminate steps, entranceways, and rooms before entering. Use 70- or 100-watt bulbs, not 60-watt bulbs.
- Avoid glaring light caused by highly polished floors or large expanses of uncovered glass.
- Allow more time to adjust to changes in light levels. When going from a dark to a light room or vice versa, allow a minute or two for the eyes to accommodate to the change in light before proceeding.
- Dirty glasses or outgrown prescription lenses inhibit vision. Keep glasses clean. Have regular eye examinations to identify changes and to get new glasses when needed. If possible, do not use bifocals when walking because you cannot see the ground clearly.
- Ability to see up, down, and sideways decreases with age. Observe the "lay of the land"; learn to look ahead at the ground to spot and avoid hazards such as cracks in the sidewalks. Use canes, walking sticks, and walkers that are prescribed.
- At night, keep a nightlight on in your bedroom and bathroom. When getting out of bed at night, put the light on and wait a minute or two for the eyes to adjust before getting up. Have a telephone in the bedroom so you don't have to get out of bed to answer the phone. Before you go out in the evening or late afternoon, turn a light on for your return.

Activity

- Get up from a chair slowly.
- When getting out of bed, sit up, then wait a minute or two. Move to the side of the bed and wait another minute. Rise after you have sat for a few minutes.
- If you are dizzy, sit down immediately. Sit on a step or a chair, or ease yourself to the sidewalk if you are outdoors.
- Avoid tipping the head backward (extending the neck). Activities to avoid that extend the neck are washing windows, hanging clothes, and getting things from high shelves.
- Use shelves at eye level. Avoid rapid turning of the head.
- If weather is rainy and windy, avoid going out.
- Use alcohol and tranquilizers with caution.
- Exercise programs keep bodies limber. Consult your physician and then engage in an exercise program.
- Shoes and slippers should be flat and rubber-soled. Avoid clothing such as long and loose-fitting garments that may catch on furniture or door knobs.

(Table 12-8 continued)

TABLE 12-8   ◆   *Fall Prevention Guidelines for the Home* (*Continued*)

Around the House

- ◆ Avoid scatter rugs and small bathroom mats that can slide. Repair loose, torn, wrinkled, or worn carpet.
- ◆ Avoid slick, high polish on floors.
- ◆ Put things in easy reach, and avoid reaching to high shelves.
- ◆ Use nonskid treads on stairs and nonskid mats in tub.
- ◆ May wish to install a grab rail in the bath, shower, and also by the toilet.
- ◆ Install handrails on both sides of the stairs. Paint stair edge in bright contrasting color.
- ◆ Remove door thresholds to avoid tripping.
- ◆ Remove low-lying objects, such as low coffee tables and extension cords.
- ◆ Wipe up spills immediately.
- ◆ Watch for pets underfoot and scattered pet food.
- ◆ Check for even, nonglare lighting in every room, with easily accessible light switches.
- ◆ Avoid floor coverings with complex patterns.
- ◆ Avoid clutter in living areas.
- ◆ Select furniture that provides stability and support, such as chairs with arms.
- ◆ Check walking aids routinely, such as rubber tips on canes and screws on walkers.

Source: Chenitz, W. C., Stone, J. T., Salisbury, S. A. (1991). *Clinical Gerontological Nursing: A Guide to Advanced Practice.* Philadelphia: Saunders, p. 310.

Think about . . . Can you explain how you would go about trying to obtain a shower chair for a client who cannot afford to buy or rent one?

A portion of the home care nurse's time is spent interacting with the family. When family members are greatly confined to the home because of the need for constant attendance on the ill person, social contact is reduced. The nurse's visits provide a social contact and are often looked forward to with pleasure. When a family member is totally responsible for extensive 24-hour care for the client, the nurse helps with arrangements for occasional respite care, if available, so that the family member can get out of the house and away for a few days periodically.

The RN acts as case manager and coordinates the care of all of the health care providers involved in the client's care. He is responsible for the plan of care and for seeing that care is delivered in an uninterrupted manner. He must act as a liaison with the other care providers to see to it that all efforts effectively complement one another.

◆ Medicare Requirements for Reimbursement

Funding for care outside of the hospital is mainly determined by Medicare. Outside insurance agencies also parallel Medicare policies of payment for many aspects of care. Home health nursing care must be "skilled." "Skilled" means that only a nurse trained in that care could be expected to safely and adequately deliver the care.

To be eligible for Medicare home care services, the client must meet the following requirements:

- ◆ The nursing care delivered must be necessary and the number of visits per week must be reasonable to deliver the appropriate care and effect a positive outcome for the illness or injury.
- ◆ The client must be *essentially* homebound. There must be difficulty in mobility and the client only leaves the home for medical appointments.
- ◆ The plan of care for Medicare clients must be submitted on HCFA forms 485, 486, and 487. These forms require very specific information on the client's diagnosis, prognosis, medications, functional limitations, and types of services needed and why.
- ◆ Service delivered by the home health agency must be skilled and must be ordered by a physician. A nurse, physical therapist, or speech therapist delivers skilled care. After care has been initiated and skilled services are no longer necessary, an occupational therapist can continue care and qualify the client for the continuation of nonskilled health services, such as bathing and homemaking assistance. Skilled nursing care includes trained observation and assessment, performance of specific skilled procedures, such as wound care, and teaching of new information that the client needs to obtain or maintain health.
- ◆ Skilled care must be on an intermittent or part-time basis. Between visits by the nurse, physical therapist, or speech therapist, the family or significant other provides care for the client. In general, should the client's condition or illness warrant it, Medicare-approved care can be delivered on an intermittent basis for up to 90 days. At the end of that time, documentation must indicate that there is still a need for skilled care to be continued under Medicare

reimbursement. Hospice care by home health agencies also is covered by Medicare.

♦ Case Management

The case manager nurse is the one who obtains and coordinates the services of the other health care providers for the home health client. Contact is made with the physical therapist, the social worker, the home health aide, the intravenous infusion company, the respiratory therapy company, the pharmacist, the physician, and others involved in the comprehensive care of the client.

Generally the LPN working in home care is under the supervision of the RN case manager. The LPN may be providing "private-duty" services for an unconscious client who needs skilled care, performing home visits to change dressings or monitor blood sugar levels, or acting as an in-agency supervisor by coordinating home health aide visits and supervising their work. The role of the LPN in home care is growing monthly. Nurses do not usually provide personal care to clients. The family provides assistance with personal care, and a home health aide may visit a few times a week to bathe the client and shampoo hair. Homemaking is provided by family members, significant others, or a homemaker aide. "Sitters" may be hired to attend to the client's needs at night if the family is not able to provide this service.

Nursing care plans are formulated in collaboration with the client, the family or significant other, and all other health care providers. Teaching and 24-hour needs are considered and often form a large part of the plan. Case conferences are conducted regularly, even if they are done by the case manager on the telephone to the others involved in the client's care. Medicare requires a case conference every 60 days when more than one discipline is involved in the client's care.

♦ Infection-Control Measures

The principles of infection control are the same in the home care environment. Measures are used to prevent the spread of infection and to prevent contamination of the client. *Standard precautions* are followed by all persons involved in the client's care. **Handwashing is the single most important infection-control measure.** Family members and the client are taught the technique and importance of good handwashing. The client should use only her own towel or paper towels for drying the hands. **The nurse should wash her hands before touching the client, before gloving, after removing gloves, and after providing care to the client. Hands should be washed just prior to leaving the residence.** Table 12-9 lists appropriate measures for controlling infection in the home. Table 9-10 presents guidelines for preventing

TABLE 12-9 ♦ *Patient Education: Measures to Prevent the Spread of Microorganisms in the Home*
♦ Washing the hands throroughly and frequently is the best way to prevent transfer of microorganisms.
♦ Wastes, such as secretions from suction catheters, urine, feces, or vomit, can be safely flushed down the toilet. Reusable containers should be cleaned with hot soapy water and rinsed; if blood was in the secretions, a bleach solution of 1:10 bleach to water should be used as well. Gloves are used when handling the containers.
♦ Dishes may be safely washed in hot soapy water or in the family dishwasher. If washed by hand, wash the patient's dishes last, adding hot water as needed.
♦ Clean gloves should be used when changing dressings or handling soiled dressings, linen, incontinence pads, or tissues.
♦ Soiled dressings and disposable items should be placed in sealed plastic bags before being placed in the residence trash container. Items should be moistened with bleach solution in the plastic bag before disposal if they are contaminated with blood or other body fluid requiring special precautions.
♦ Soiled linens should be stored in plastic bags until laundered. Soiled linens and clothing of the patient may be washed in the family washing machine using the hot cycle, detergent, and one cup of bleach. It is preferable to wash the patient's soiled clothes and linens separately from family items. The family dryer may be used without danger.
♦ Blood spills and other body secretions requiring precautions should be cleaned up using gloves and a good household disinfectant, such as alcohol, peroxide, bleach solution, or Lysol.
♦ The bathroom can be safely shared with the patient who has an enteric illness as long as good handwashing is used after toileting and the commode is cleaned with a household disinfectant daily.
♦ Patients with respiratory infections that cause coughing and sneezing should cover the mouth and nose, dispose of used tissues in plastic bags, and wash the hands after each episode of coughing or sneezing.

infection in cancer or other immunocompromised clients.

Working in home health care can be a very satisfying occupation as there is a degree of continuity in client care that is not often found in the hospital. Clients and families appreciate the efforts of the nurse on their behalf. Warmth, humor, and friendliness seem more prevalent in the home care situation. Although the paperwork can seem overwhelming, efforts are being made to decrease the amount of documentation required by Medicare and other government agencies. A paperwork reduction will make this area of nursing even more attractive. Some major home health agencies are using lap-top computers and standardized care plans to maximize the efficiency of the home health nurse.

CRITICAL THINKING EXERCISES
Clinical Case Problems

Read each clinical situation and discuss the questions with your classmates.

1. Mr. Porter has been discharged home and transferred to a home health nursing agency for continued care after suffering a stroke that has left him with left-sided hemiplegia and dysphagia. His wife will be taking care of him, but she has severe arthritis and cannot perform many needed tasks. You are assigned to provide "private duty" care to him as he must have tube feedings.

   a. What assessments would you make each day?

   b. How would you collaborate with the case manager and the physical therapist?

   c. How would you plan care for rehabilitation?

   d. What would you teach Mr. Porter's wife about taking care of the equipment for his tube feeding?

2. Mrs. Robbins is a new resident in the long-term care facility in which you work. She is mentally alert, but needs assistance with bathing, dressing, and toileting because of arthritis and weakness and fatigue from heart failure. She can use a walker to ambulate short distances, but does not like to do so.

   a. How would you promote independence and autonomy for this resident?

   b. How can maintenance of function be promoted for her?

BIBLIOGRAPHY

Antai-Otong, D. (1995). *Psychiatric Nursing: Biological and Behavioral Concepts.* Philadelphia: Saunders.

Ark, P. D., Nies, M. (1996). Knowledge and skills of the home healthcare nurse. *Home Healthcare Nurse.* 14(4): 292–297.

Becker, J. H. (1996). When you need to use restraints. *American Journal of Nursing.* 96(4):59.

Braddom, R. L. (1996). *Physical Medicine and Rehabilitation.* Philadelphia: Saunders.

Carr, P. (1996). Functional limitations. *Home Healthcare Nurse.* 14(4):299, 301.

Chenitz, W. C., Stone, J. T., Salisbury, S. A. (1991). *Clinical Gerontological Nursing: A Guide to Advanced Practice.* Philadelphia: Saunders.

De La Cruz, P. (1996). The role of the interdisciplinary team in subacute care. *Medsurg Nursing.* 5(2):130–131.

deWit, S. C. (1994). *Rambo's Nursing Skills for Clinical Practice,* 4th ed. Philadelphia: Saunders.

Eggland, E. T. (1996). Charting tips: making the transition to home health care charting. *Nursing 96.* 26(3):16.

El-Sherif, C. (1996). How to collaborate with nurse practitioners. *Nursing 96.* 26(1):64.

Foreman, M. D., Zane, D. (1996). Nursing strategies for acute confusion in elders. *American Journal of Nursing.* 96(4): 44–51.

Hoeman, S. P. (1995). *Rehabilitation Nursing: Process and Application,* 2nd ed. St. Louis, MO: Mosby.

Hoffner, R. (1994). *The Rehabilitation Survival Guide.* St. Louis, MO: Mosby.

Hussar, D. A. (1995). Helping your client follow his drug regimen. *Nursing 95.* 25(10):62–64.

Ignatavicius, D. D., Workman, M. L., Mishler, M. A. (1995). *Medical–Surgical Nursing: A Nursing Process Approach,* 2nd ed. Philadelphia: Saunders.

Johnson, S. J., et al. (1996). Evaluating physical functional outcomes: one category of the NOC system. *Medsurg Nursing.* 5(3):157–162.

Keffer, M. J. (1996). Nurse advocate: advocate for whom? *Medsurg Nursing.* 5(2):125–126.

Lange, M. (1996). The challenge of fall prevention in home care: a review of the literature. *Home Healthcare Nurse.* 14(3):198, 200–205.

Loughran, S. (1996). Medication use in the elderly: a population at risk. *Medsurg Nursing.* 5(2):121–124.

Messner, R. L., Lewis, S. (1995). Double trouble: managing chronic illness and depression. 25(8):46–49.

Mignor, D. (1996). Management and evaluation of a care plan. *Home Healthcare Nurse.* 14(3):163–165.

Montgomery, D. (1996). The benefits of wandering. *Nursing 96.* 26(6):24oo–24rr.

Morrison, B. B. (1995). Home health care: staying safe in dangerous times. *Nursing 95.* 25(10):49–51.

Neal, L. J. (1996). Rehabilitation and activities of daily living: the home care client with Alzheimer's disease:Part II, Interventions. *Home Healthcare Nurse.* 14(4):265–267.

Preston, K. (1994). Rehabilitation nursing: a client-centered philosophy. *American Journal of Nursing.* 94(2):66–70.

Senapatiratne, L. (1996). On the road with a home health nurse. *RN.* 59(4):54–57.

Shu, E., Mirmina, Z., Nystrom, K. (1996). A telephone reassurance program for elderly home care clients after discharge. *Home Healthcare Nurse.* 14(3):155–160.

Smith, C. M., Maurer, F. A. (1995). *Community Health Nursing: Theory and Practice.* Philadelphia: Saunders.

Stevens, K. (1993). Portrait of a rehabilitation nurse. *Nursing 93.* 23(11):73, 74, 76, 78.

Ulbrich, S. L. (1995). Cardiac rehabilitation: clearly a lifesaver. *American Journal of Nursing.* 95(9):53.

U. S. Department of Health and Human Services (USDHHS). (1990). *Healthy people 2000: National health promotion and disease prevention objectives.* Washington DC: U. S. Government Printing Office.

Westien, M. J. (1995). Rekindling the flame: what would bring the light back into this injured athlete's eyes? *Nursing 95.* 25(10):94.

Wichowski, H. C. (1995). Improving your client's compliance. *Nursing 95.* 25(1):66–68.

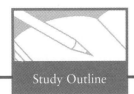

I. Introduction

A. The focus of nursing is shifting to home and community agency settings.

B. Both short- and long-term care clients are treated in rehabilitation programs, long-term care facilities, and in the home.

C. Nurses in the community work in long-term care facilities, rehabilitation centers, physician's offices, outclient clinics, HMO clinics, schools, industrial companies, and state and county health department clinics.

D. Nurses in community settings have many opportunities for health teaching and to screen for health problems.

II. Chronic Illness and Rehabilitation

A. Many people with chronic illnesses have some impairment of body function or disability.

B. Rehabilitation helps a disabled person achieve optimal function.

C. The rehabilitation nurse.

1. Assists the client and family learn new skills to perform activities of daily living (ADLs).

2. Philosophy is based on the client's need for independence.

D. Determination of rehabilitation needs.

1. A physical and psychosocial assessment is performed.

2. An evaluation of the home environment is performed.

3. A functional assessment is completed.

4. The Katz Index of Activities of Daily Living and the Baird Body Image Assessment Tool assist with the assessment process.

5. Vocational assessment is done as rehabilitation progresses.

6. Nursing diagnoses are identified based on the evaluation findings.

7. A collaborative plan of care is devised by all health professionals involved in the care of the client.

8. Care conferences monitor progress and solve problems.

9. Sexual concerns are addressed during the rehabilitation period.

10. Depression is common and assessment of mental outlook is an ongoing process.

E. Rehabilitation programs.

1. Most hospitals have rehabilitation programs for clients with cardiac, respiratory, or musculoskeletal problems.

2. There are rehabilitation programs for people with neurological impairment, burns, cancer, arthritis, visual impairment, hearing impairment, and many other types of disorders.

3. Rehabilitation philosophy.

a. Each person is unique, whole within herself, and interdependent with her own environment.

b. Independence can be achieved within the limits of disability when the person is a full participant in managing her own life.

c. The goal is to enable clients to mobilize their own resources, choose goals, and attain them through their own efforts.

d. Many clients are treated in outclient rehabilitation programs, such as a respiratory rehabilitation program.

(1) Program teaches self-care techniques to attain a better quality of life.

(2) Program consists of breathing exercises, paced walking exercise, and teaching to use inhalers correctly.

e. One role of the nurse is to help the client maintain hope for autonomy and quality of life.

f. The nurse guides the client to resources available to her.

g. Much rehabilitation care is given in the home setting.

F. Long-term care.

1. There are various types of long-term or extended care available.

2. Clients requiring rehabilitation often are admitted to skilled long-term care facilities.

3. Elderly or chronically ill clients who need assistance with more than two ADLs often are residents at long-term care facilities.

4. LPNs often are the charge nurses in long-term care facilities.

5. Care of residents is supervised by a physician.

6. The LPN performs treatments and wound care, assesses residents, organizes the shift's work, administers medications, documents assessment findings and care given, updates the

nursing care plans, and delegates care tasks to the client care assistants.

7. The LPN oversees care for a group of residents for a shift.

8. The LPN must be certain that the person to whom she delegates is competent to perform the task assigned.

9. Goals of care.

a. Provide a safe environment.

b. Assist resident in maintaining or attaining as much function as possible.

c. Promote individual independence.

d. Allow resident to maintain or achieve as much autonomy as possible.

10. Safety.

a. Provide a safe environment for confused or disoriented residents without using physical or chemical restraints is a challenge.

b. Techniques used depend on the type of population in the facility.

11. Prevention of falls.

a. Recognition of residents who are at risk: impaired ambulation or balance, peripheral neuropathy, balance or gait problems, postural hypotension or dizziness, impaired vision, impaired hearing, extreme weakness, history of previous falls.

b. Recognition of hazards in the environment.

c. Making the environment safe; measures to prevent falls.

(1) Safe flooring; nonskid surfaces, nonskid rugs.

(2) Good lighting without shadows.

(3) Belongings within easy reach, including call bell.

(4) Encourage to call for assistance to get up.

(5) Answer call lights quickly.

(6) Clear pathways.

(7) Provision of railings and grab bars.

(8) Supportive, nonslip footwear.

(9) Not bending from the waist to do things; crouch instead.

(10) Proper-height chair seats.

(11) Exercise to strengthen muscles and increase balance.

(12) Reach out to arise slowly and stabilize before ambulating.

(13) Assess all medications for potential to cause postural hypotension or dizziness.

(14) Keep glasses clean and close at hand.

(15) Hearing aid in place and correctly tuned.

(16) Clothing that does not trip or catch on things.

(17) Safe use of assistive devices for ambulation.

(18) Assessment for fluid and electrolyte imbalances.

(19) Appropriate use of siderails.

d. If fall occurs, resident should stay put and call for help.

12. Use of safety devices and techniques.

a. Residents are guaranteed the right to be free of unreasonable restraints.

b. Restraints must be ordered by a physician.

c. All measures tried to keep the resident safe without restraints before a restraint is used must be thoroughly documented.

d. When a restraint is used in an emergency situation, a physician's order for it must be written in 24 to 48 hours.

e. The resident who is immobilized with a restraining device must be checked visually by the nurse at least every 30 minutes.

f. The resident must be turned and repositioned every 2 hours; skin and circulation checks must be documented.

g. Measures to prevent the need for restraints should be followed (Table 12-4).

13. Managing daytime confusion and disorientation.

a. Reorientation techniques help the resident with mild confusion or disorientation.

b. All measures for reality orientation must be used consistently by all staff members.

c. A structured environment and routine helps decrease confusion.

d. Aids to reorientation include a large, easy-to-read calendar, a clock, the daily newspaper or local television or radio news, and holiday decorations indicating the season.

e. Limiting the number of choices the resident must make decreases confusion and agitation.

f. Labeling photos with names of loved ones and labeling signs with symbols for the bathroom, dining room, resident's room, etc., is helpful.

g. Gently correcting the resident about the identity of a person or location of where they actually are is part of the plan.

h. It is not wise to agree with a resident's confused statements.

14. Dealing with nocturnal confusion.

a. Sensory deficits, such as loss of hearing or diminished sight, contribute to confusion and anxiety at night.

b. A night light that gives sufficient illumination without casting deep shadows is necessary.

c. Frequent visits to calm and reassure the resident help.

d. Using touch and caring techniques can be comforting.

e. A bed alarm can alert staff that the resident is trying to get up without assistance.

f. Working with the resident and listening to and exploring fears can sometimes remedy the situation.

g. Keeping the resident active during the day and keeping a nap brief helps with sleep at night.

h. Residents on diuretics that can alter electrolyte and fluid balance must be monitored to prevent imbalance and accompanying confusion.

15. Promoting independence.

a. Allow the resident choice of facility, room location when possible, and items from home to bring for the room.

b. A personal telephone, if possible, maintains independence to some degree.

c. Choices in daily clothing, time of day for bathing, and type of recreational activities help maintain independence.

d. Offer options of where to sit in the dining room.

e. Planned family member visits offer something to look forward to that is not an activity of the facility.

f. Helping the resident set ADL and recreation goals promotes independence.

g. Adaptive devices assist residents in performing ADLs (Table 12-5).

h. The staff should refrain from doing things for the resident that she can do for herself; allow her to do them.

i. Maintaining contact with friends outside the facility promotes independence; assisting the resident to read letters and to write them helps.

j. Linking a resident with a volunteer "buddy" provides a special relationship and increases self-esteem.

16. Fostering autonomy.

a. Working with roommates to come to agreement about personal preferences for TV, radio, light, curtains open, or wake and sleep time helps preserve autonomy.

b. Collaborating with the resident about goal setting provides autonomy.

c. The family contributes to autonomy by continuing to honor the resident's place in the family.

d. Assessment of the resident's autonomy must be periodic.

17. Maintaining function.

a. Exercise is planned and encouraged to maintain muscular strength, ambulation ability, and balance.

b. When the patient is not ambulatory, ROM exercises must be performed several times a day.

c. Assistance for toileting to maintain continence is of prime importance; continence is a major factor in maintaining self-esteem.

d. When continence has been lost, a bowel or bladder retraining program is instituted.

e. Mental stimulation is essential to maintaining cognitive function.

f. Informational TV that stimulates thinking and discussion helps.

g. Crossword puzzles stimulate mental activity.

h. Card or board games can provide mental stimulation.

i. Computer use could be of great benefit to mentally alert residents.

G. Care techniques for safety and rehabilitation.

1. Transfer techniques (Table 12-6).

2. Gait training.

a. Resident works with physical therapist.

b. Nurse reinforces teaching and encourages practice.

3. Prevention of hazards of immobility (Table 12-7 and Chapter 11).

H. Documentation varies according to care setting.

I. Home care.

1. Majority of care in the community is given by home health and hospice agencies.

2. Goal is to keep the client as well as possible and enable her to stay at home.

3. Philosophy is different from hospital: client and family are in charge. Nurse is a guest in the home.

4. Nurse acts as consultant, coordinator of care, provider of skilled care, teacher, and advocate.

5. Clients are to be treated as valued customers.

6. Trust must be established to initiate change.

7. Sensitivity to cultural values and habits is necessary.

8. Home care nurse must be flexible and creative.

9. Safety in the home is a high priority of care.

10. Prevention of falls is important (Table 12-8).

11. Home care nurse must have good assessment skills.

12. The nurse assesses physical and psychosocial status, signs of complications, side effects of medications, and effects of therapy.

13. The nurse consults the physician by phone frequently and collaborates with other members of the health care team by phone.

14. Functions of home care nurses include wound care and dressing changes, organizing medications for scheduled administration, drawing blood samples, monitoring blood sugar, giving injections, teaching self-care, and rehabilitation techniques, and monitoring progress and compliance with treatment.

15. The nurse provides psychosocial care for the client and family.

16. The nurse helps the client and family obtain needed supplies and funding for medications and care by referral to community resources and collaborates with the medical social worker.

17. The RN is the case manager and supervises the LPNs and others.

18. Medicare requirements for reimbursement.

    a. Care delivered must be necessary and reasonable.

    b. Client must be essentially homebound.

    c. Plan of care must be submitted on particular forms.

    d. Service delivered must be skilled and ordered by a physician.

    e. Care in the home must be intermittent.

19. Case management.

    a. Case manager obtains and coordinates services of other health care providers for the client.

    b. The LPN under RN supervision may provide "private-duty" services in the home, perform home visits for procedures, and coordinate care of home health aides.

    c. Nurses do not usually provide personal care for the client in the home.

    d. Nursing care plans are collaboratively formulated with the client, the family or significant other, and all other health care providers.

    e. Case conferences are conducted regularly and must occur at least every 60 days; sometimes they are conducted by phone.

20. Infection control.

    a. Principles of infection control are the same as in the hospital.

    b. Handwashing is single most important measure.

    c. Infection control in the home should be achieved (Table 12-9).

21. Home health nursing can be very satisfying.

CHAPTER 13

Care of the Dying Patient and Hospice Care

All of us know that dying is inevitable. Death is a part of the life cycle. Yet most of us push thoughts of death away, thinking that we'll think about it "later." Most nurses must deal with death and grief on a regular basis. Death causes loss and grief, painful feelings characterized by sadness and emotional distress. Death also can be a blessed relief from a painful, low-quality existence.

Studying death and acknowledging its inevitability can give greater meaning to life. Kubler-Ross called death the final stage of growth. Kubler-Ross, an acclaimed psychiatrist, wrote about the stages of the dying process in her book *On Death and Dying* published in 1969. Other authors who write about dying describe similar phases or stages. Because dying is a unique experience, each individual goes through one or more of these stages in a varying sequence.

The way in which a person experiences death or grief depends on his basic personality, his pre-vious experiences, his cultural attitudes and beliefs, and his spiritual orientation.

Those who are dying experience a series of losses—loss of health, of well-being, of function, of roles, of a pain-free existence, and of independence.

In this chapter we will be talking about the clinical care and support of those patients who are going through the dying process. We will consider the **bereaved**, those who grieve over their loss of a family member, friend, or patient. The moral and ethical issues related to the end of life, such as organ donation, advance directives, and euthanasia also are considered.

The task of the dying patient is to work his way through psychological responses ranging from total disbelief and rejection to whatever resolution he can. **The task of the nurse and other health professionals is to help the dying person live his life as fully as possible, or as much on his own terms as possible, until he dies.**

STAGES OF DYING

In general, the psychological responses to one's impending death begin with denial and progress through anger, bargaining, and depression to an idealized final stage of acceptance.

The stages of dying Kubler-Ross presented may sound familiar because they are the same reactions that people experience when any major change or loss occurs. The way a person reacts to loss depends on his perspective of the loss. The same is true of dying. Each individual perceives dying in his own way. For this reason, a patient may experience one, a few, or all of the stages of dying. There may be progression from one stage to the next, and then a return to a former stage. Not all patients reach the stage of acceptance. Although no two people share the same life experiences or have the same inner resources to deal with life's difficulties, knowing that there are some commonalities shared by people who confront death can be of benefit to those who care for them.

Study of the effect of death on survivors also has shed some light on the stages of grief felt by those whom the dying person leaves behind. In 1964, Dr. George Engel proposed that grief over the loss of a loved one brings about psychological responses not too different from those exhibited by patients who are themselves dying. Moreover, several authors have noted that severely handicapped and disabled persons who must abruptly change their lifestyle might also go through a process in which they move through the four stages of grief from denial, anger, and depression toward acceptance of a new way of life. The manner in which these persons adjust to the "death" of their former selves and the emergence of a new self often bears some resemblance to the adaptive stages of the dying person.

◆ Denial

The initial response to the knowledge that one is dying is shock and disbelief. The person does not seem to be able to believe that death is imminent or inevitable. Most patients initially reject the idea; the typical response to the news that they have a terminal illness is "No, not me. It's not possible." The denial of one's death usually pushes away the shock and reality of the situation so that coping resources can be mobilized.

Denial can be useful if the period is used to find a way to deal with death.

The patient should not be forced to face the reality of his impending death or presented with arguments when he insists he is not dying. **The nurse can encourage him to share his thoughts, feelings, and fears,** and she can be an active listener. This supportive role assists the patient in progressing toward acceptance of his coming death.

Think about . . . Can you think of examples of two behaviors that would indicate the patient is in the stage of denial?

Sometimes asking the right questions will tell you what the patient wants to know. Asking him to tell you about his illness and its effects on him may open the door to a discussion of his feelings. Inquiring about his understanding of the plans for treatment may tell you what he understands and what he is willing to talk about. When trust has been established, asking about adjustments he and his family will need to make as a result of the illness may help him progress through denial.

◆ Anger

A second common and important response to the knowledge that one's life is ending is frustration and anger. The patient no longer denies the fact that he is dying. Instead, he asks, "Why me?" It seems unfair to him, and he retaliates by becoming belligerent, uncooperative, and critical of those around him. Visiting relatives and friends may irritate him; they may visit too often, not enough, or at the wrong time. The physician is not prescribing the right medicines and treatments and might, in fact, be seen by the patient as the one who is responsible for his impending death. Nurses, too, become objects of abuse and criticism. Efforts to comfort the patient, such as a back rub or straightening the bed linen, might be met with an angry outburst or a surly, "Get out of here and leave me alone." **The anger he feels is not directed toward any one person but toward circumstances and events over which the patient has no control and against which he feels helpless.** When a dying patient wants to express his anger and rage, it is best to let him do just that—say whatever he feels, cry, curse, scream, or do whatever he needs to do to release his pent-up feelings. Use active listening and just try to reflect the feelings the patient is expressing such as "you seem to be angry/upset/unhappy this morning" in a nonjudgmental manner.

It should be noted that sometimes the very things nurses do or say to be helpful can be the most annoying to the patient who is terminally ill. For some patients, the efficient, smiling, healthy nurse who bustles cheerfully about the room serves as a source of irritation simply because she *is* healthy and full of life. Through no fault of her own she represents the things he is losing. The patient might see her as a reminder that he is unattractive and no longer free to escape the restrictions his illness has imposed on him.

It is very important that the nurse understand the patient's anger and not take it personally.

Many people *never* get past the anger stage. Anger is certainly the most characteristic and long-lasting response to the certain knowledge of one's own imminent death. Many dying people remain angry while they have the energy and then go into a withdrawal as they become weaker when death approaches.

◆ Bargaining

The bargaining stage, if it occurs, may follow the anger phase closely. The patient says, "Yes, me, but . . ." and then begins to make some kind of arrangement whereby he gives something in order to gain more days of life. Kubler-Ross observes that most bargaining is done with God and that it often is a promise in exchange for prolongation of life. For example, the patient might vow to change his way of life, to become more generous, or to give up something valuable as payment for a few more months or years.

◆ Depression

In another stage, the patient drops the "but" and recognizes that the facts cannot be escaped. "Yes, me . . . ," he says, and by that he means that he knows he is approaching the end of his life. He may become depressed and begin to grieve for all that he knows he will soon lose. When he admits this and can face the reality of his loss, he may be able to grieve and mourn his loss.

Many patients become silent in this stage. They sit quietly, tears rolling down their faces, or sob uncontrollably when they are alone. Many do prefer to be alone in their grief, asking that visitors not come because they do not want to talk with anyone. The patient who is silently grieving may be more difficult to cope with than the one who is venting his anger. There seems to be so little one can say to console him and so little one can do to comfort him. All one can do is listen, to "be there." The nurse can provide companionship and allow him to express his grief in his own way without judgment. She strives to maintain communication with the patient, letting him know by her presence that she is aware of his suffering and that she is concerned for him. She gives him permission to withdraw, accepting his efforts to cope with the problem on his own for a while as a natural process.

◆ Acceptance

In some cases the patient may consciously and openly accept his imminent death and find some degree of peace within himself. He is willing to stop resisting death and to rest quietly. The "acceptance" described by Kubler-Ross is seldom seen in practice.

In the last days or hours of life, the patient may choose to limit contact with others to one person with whom he will share his remaining time. He wants only the comfort of having someone present that he loves or trusts. He may not interact much at all, becoming more and more withdrawn.

THE GRIEVING PROCESS

It is unusual to experience the loss of a loved one without experiencing grief. The grief response has a fairly predictable sequence. **Phases of grief include shock and disbelief; feelings of anger, guilt, and hostility; interruption of life's usual activities, often due to an inability to concentrate and a lack of energy (depression); preoccupation with thoughts of the deceased; and finally a state of acceptance of the loss and a return to psychological and emotional health.** The grief process is individual, and people go through these phases in different orders and at different rates. The nursing diagnosis used for those experiencing normal grief when a loved one is dying is "Anticipatory grief." There are two desirable outcomes of grieving: (1) to come to accept the loss of the loved one and to remember him without severe pain; and (2) to return to participation in life without negating the capacity to love.

The person who is suffering from acute grief is in a state of shock caused by the news of actual or impending death. The physiological signs commonly seen at this time are fainting, a feeling of tightness in the throat, shortness of breath and a need to sigh, waves of nausea or sensations of somatic distress lasting from 20 minutes to more than an hour, a feeling of emptiness in the abdomen, and a strong sensation of tension or pain. **Other signs that a person is suffering from acute grief include inability to sleep, forgetfulness and absentmindedness, and a tendency to repeat the same behavior over and over again. The person may cry uncontrollably or sit withdrawn and unresponsive.**

After the first wave of shock and grief, the bereaved person usually moves into the next phase, in which he experiences powerful emotions that he has difficulty controlling. His attitude is indicative of an attempt to run away or hide from a situation he finds completely repugnant. He may be so angry that he is compelled to withdraw from others, and he will probably try to find someone or something to blame for the catastrophe that has befallen him. He might blame God or some other authority figure such as the physician or nurse. **It is even possible that the bereaved will feel anger against the person who has died or is dying and leaving him, or he might feel terrible guilt, wondering what he might have done to prevent the death.**

Destructive feelings such as anger and guilt need to be admitted to the conscious mind and dealt with by the bereaved. This is necessary so that he can resolve his grief and resume his life without the loved one.

As resolution begins, the person begins to realize that the loved one is indeed dead and will not return, but his loss is not yet fully believed. The person may exhibit searching behavior in which he continues to look for and expects to see and be with the deceased person. He may continue to speak of the person as if he were still alive but simply away for a while. The bereaved will be sad and disconsolate, but he still clings to the hope that by some miracle or clearing up of a misunderstanding he will awaken from a nightmare and find that nothing has really changed. Eventually he *knows* in his mind that the death is a reality, and he is able to speak of the person as dead or "gone." There is overwhelming sadness, but as he progresses through the grief process, there is a gradual emotional detachment and letting go.

The bereaved person begins to reorganize his life and do certain things in order to get on with living. Activities that are typical during this phase of acceptance include cleaning out closets and drawers in the loved one's room and giving away his clothes, books, and tools; changing the listing in the telephone directory; removing wedding rings; redecorating the home; getting a job; and going out to be with others in church, social, and civic gatherings.

♦ Time for Resolution

Persons who are learning to work with the bereaved often ask how long it takes for a person to work through the process to final acceptance and resolution. Sometimes well-meaning friends will tell a grieving person that time heals all things. **However, how much time is needed for resolution and healing depends on the individual, the circumstances of the loss of a loved one, and social and cultural customs.** In many cases acceptance behavior begins 3 to 4 months after bereavement and becomes more evident 6 months to a year later. This is not necessarily a goal or something to be forced on the bereaved. It is simply the average length of time required before resolution can be expected.

The action-oriented person usually begins reorganization behavior earlier than the passive and nonassertive person. It is not so much a matter of how much time it takes to recover from the death of a loved one as what is done with the time the bereaved person has. Arnaldo Pangrazzi, a Roman Catholic priest who serves as a hospital chaplain, has coordinated numerous support groups for the bereaved and has conducted seminars on grief, suggests 10 ways in which a grieving person can use time to recover from the loss of a loved one. The 10 suggestions and a brief explanation of each are presented in Table 13-1.

TABLE 13-1 ♦ *Ten Suggestions for Overcoming Grief*

1. *Take time to accept death.* Facing and accepting death is a necessary condition for continuing with one's own life.

2. *Take time to let go.* Life is a series of letting go—sometimes temporarily, sometimes permanently. Letting go occurs when we are able to endure and accept the feelings that accompany death. It occurs when we are able to tolerate the helplessness and insecurity, when we are willing to face the tears, to wait, trust, and hope again.

3. *Take time to make decisions.* Be patient with yourself and learn to make independent decisions. Start with small decisions; write out a schedule for the day and set up tasks to be done. Planning helps you look forward to visits with friends, eating out, vacations. Making decisions about our life helps us gain control over it and increases self-confidence.

4. *Take time to share.* The greatest need of the bereaved is to have someone to share their pain, their memories, their sadness. Bereaved people need others to give them time and space to grieve.

5. *Take time to believe.* At times our grief can shake up our faith. To survive is to find some meaning in suffering because suffering that has meaning to it is endurable. For many people, religion—with its rituals, promise of an afterlife, and its community support—offers a comforting and strengthening base in the lonely encounter with helplessness and hopelessness.

6. *Take time to forgive.* Forgive yourself for the things you did not do, the words you did not say to the loved one. Forgive others for their hurtful comments or actions, insensitivity or avoidance. Forgive the deceased one who has left you bereaved and angry.

7. *Take time to feel good about yourself.* The death of a loved one does not sentence you to a life of sorrow. It does alter our lifestyle and change our self-image, but grief can help us discover new independence and a new outlook. Explore new interests, develop new hobbies, engage in activities that build self-confidence and provide a feeling of newness, satisfaction, and pleasure.

8. *Take time to meet new friends.* Try to find a new sense of belonging. Take steps to move out of safe boundaries and interact with others. Old friends might be there to offer security and comfort; new friends will be there to offer opportunities.

9. *Take time to laugh.* In life there are as many reasons to laugh as there are to cry. Laughter helps us to survive, to reenter life, to accept our limitations, and develops hope in the present.

10. *Take time to give.* The best way to overcome our loneliness and pain is to be concerned about the loneliness and pain of others. Getting involved with others gives us the feeling that life goes on, and takes us away from self-pity.

Source: Pangrazzi, A. (1983). Overcoming grief: ten suggestions. *St. Anthony Messenger,* June.

People grieve at their own rate. Some coming to resolution quickly, and some continuing to grieve for considerable periods of time. Grief does physically affect the body, and it can depress the immune system, making the person susceptible to infection. If grief is not resolving after 2 years, the person is experiencing a dysfunctional grief process and needs help.

Think about . . . Can you give an example that would indicate dysfunctional grieving?

FEARS EXPERIENCED BY THE DYING PERSON

Dying persons typically experience some specific fears about what is happening to them and how they will be treated by others during their final days and hours. Specific fears expressed by dying patients include:

- Fear of the unknown
- Fear of abandonment and loneliness
- Fear of loss of relationships
- Fear of loss of experiences in the future
- Fear of dependency and loss of independence
- Fear of pain

◆ Fear of the Unknown

Obviously no one can relate to another what actually happens when one dies. The patient's spiritual belief system may provide a belief in continued life in some form. Table 13-2 presents common spiritual beliefs and practices related to death that can give a patient strength and decrease his concerns. **If the patient does not believe in a higher power, the nurse might relieve some fear by relating how those who have had near-death experiences describe a peaceful, joyous, light-**

TABLE 13-2 ◆ *Major Religious Groups in the United States: Concepts and Practices Related to Death*

Religious Group	Afterlife	Rituals	Handling of the Body after Death	"Extraordinary" Life-Prolonging Measures
Eastern Orthodoxy (including Greek and Russian Orthodoxy)	Yes; the soul blends into the spiritual cosmos.	The client's arms are crossed after death, with the fingers set in the shape of a cross. Special prayers are said for those who have been baptized to bless the sick and dying. The last rites must be delivered while the person is still conscious. Holy communion is obligatory.	Autopsy and embalming are discouraged. Organ and body donation are discouraged. Cremation is discouraged.	Encouraged
Judaism	The dead will be resurrected with the coming of the Messiah. A person lives on in the memories of his or her survivors. For Reform Jews, no concept of eternal punishment.	The dying and dead are never left unattended before burial because the soul should depart in the presence of people. The body is ritually washed, sometimes by members of a ritual burial society. Burial is in a wooden casket within 24 hours or as soon as possible after death. Five stages of mourning extend over a year. Funerals are very simple, with no flowers because flowers are a symbol of life.	Orthodox Jews prohibit autopsy and allow no removal of body parts. Conservative and Reform Jews permit autopsy. For Orthodox Jews, no embalming is allowed. Beliefs about organ and body donation vary. Orthodox Jews generally prohibit both but may agree, with rabbinical consent. Cremation is largely prohibited, but beliefs vary. Reform Jews allow cremation but recommend burial of ashes in a Jewish cemetery.	Generally discouraged after irreversible brain damage is determined. Orthodox Jews advocate life support without "heroic measures."

(Table 13-2 continued)

TABLE 13-2 ◆ *Major Religious Groups in the United States: Concepts and Practices Related to Death* (Continued)

Religious Group	Afterlife	Rituals	Handling of the Body after Death	"Extraordinary" Life-Prolonging Measures
Roman Catholicism	The faithful go to heaven, but those who reject God's grace go to hell. The soul goes to Purgatory for a time and is released by prayers and masses. Resurrection occurs at the second coming of Christ.	The family and priest choose prayers. Holy Communion and rites for anointing the sick are mandatory. Confession may be desired but is not mandatory; however, repentance is recommended.	Autopsy is permitted, but all body parts must be buried appropriately. Organ and body donation are unrestricted provided that the donor is not harmed. Cremation is not restricted.	Discouraged
Protestantism	Varies; Episcopalians, Presbyterians, and Lutherans strongly believe in an afterlife, Quakers strongly do not.	Varies; anointing rites, confession, and communion may be available but are not mandatory. Healing services may be available, but there are no official sacraments. The client and family may have a large role in planning services and prayer. Services range from traditional funerals to memorial services. Clergy may minister through prayer, scripture reading, and counseling.	Beliefs about autopsy, organ and body donation, and cremation vary by group from no restriction to individual choice to preferred.	Discouraged
Unaffiliated	Varies.	Spontaneous and individualized, possibly including reading of original or traditional prayers or songs such as Psalm 23. Traditional secular funeral or memorial services are used.	Autopsy, organ and body donation, and cremation are by individual preference.	Individual preference

From Ignataviscius, D. D., Workman, M. L., and Mishler, M. A. (1995). *Medical-Surgical Nursing: A Nursing Process Approach,* 2nd Ed. Philadelphia: Saunders, pp. 204–205.

filled journey. Allowing the patient to talk about his fears and being a sensitive, attentive listener may help to decrease the fear.

◆ Fear of Abandonment and Loneliness

Showing acceptance of the person by just being with him while honoring any desire to be "left alone" helps prevent feelings of abandonment. Sitting quietly in the room or being available in the house or hospital lounge is often best when the patient is withdrawn and very near death. During earlier stages of dying, when the patient is very ill and feels unattractive, but death is not extremely close, it is important that the patient's nurses and loved ones be accepting of his condition and of him as a person. The nurse can be instrumental in helping family members who feel awkward to assist with bits of care and to communicate with the patient. Suggest that family and friends directly ask the patient what he would like done or how he would like to spend time with them.

The dying person needs to know that he has done some things right in his life. Even the most desolate and self-deprecating of patients respond to mention of the positive aspects of their lives. Relatives and friends can be asked to jog their memories and reminisce with the patient about the happy times spent together and the good deeds done by the patient. This can assure him that he will be missed and that others will remember him kindly.

Elder Care Point... Many elderly patients have lost their spouse and most of their lifelong friends. These people have learned to cope with grief and often are ready and accepting of death.

◆ Fear of Loss of Relationships and Experiences in the Future

As the patient accepts the inevitability of his death, he will begin to grieve for the coming loss of his relationships with loved ones and friends. He may grieve over the loss of participation in events that will occur in the future, such as a child's graduation or wedding or the birth of a grandchild. He should be allowed time to grieve but also helped to reminisce about the happy times he has had with the meaningful people in his life.

◆ Fear of Dependency and Loss of Independence

As death approaches and the patient becomes weaker, he becomes more and more dependent on others to meet his basic needs. For people with a high need for control, this is almost intolerable. To help decrease the fear of loss of independence, the patient's opinion regarding treatment and schedules should be sought. He should be reassured that he still is a partner in his own care and that he has the right to refuse specific treatments or care. Reminding him that the nurse will act as his advocate is reassuring.

◆ Fear of Pain

Pain and death are closely linked in the minds of many people. There is no basis for assuming that physiological pain necessarily accompanies death. There is the psychological pain of separation, anxiety, and depression associated with the dying process, but physical agony and mental torment are not inevitable companions of death.

The patient who is terminally ill and does have physical pain must be assured that medication is available to him when he needs it. This assurance is followed up with prompt response to his reports of pain and discomfort. The medication for pain need not cloud the patient's mind and deprive him of meaningful interaction with others. Chapter 10 describes appropriate measures for pain control. Allowing the patient to take part in deciding the frequency and strength of dosage helps diminish the fear that when the pain returns, relief

will not be available. Pain medication regimens are individualized for each patient. The nurse is legally responsible to seek adequate pain relief for the patient.

Noninvasive techniques of pain control can be utilized for pain control in the terminally ill and can be combined with the administration of pain medication. Relaxation techniques, meditation, imagery, therapeutic touch, soft music, massage, and other methods can be very effective in helping to control pain in a majority of patients (see Chapter 10).

Whatever medications and noninvasive techniques are used either to prevent or to control the pain of the terminally ill, they must be administered with compassion and understanding of the experience of pain. **In general, the goal should be to prevent the pain, rather than wait for it to occur and then attempt to relieve it.**

Think about... If you were caring for a patient who is continuing to complain of pain in spite of receiving medication as ordered and the use of relaxation exercises and music, what would you do?

Addiction, which is sometimes a concern of nurses who administer frequent doses of a narcotic, is not a valid concern when there is no hope for recovery from an illness and death is approaching. The nurse should always try to mentally put herself in the patient's shoes when considering pain-control issues.

Relatives and friends of the dying patient often are relieved to know that everything possible is being done so that the patient will not suffer. They also need assurance that the final moments of a person's life are more likely to be tranquil than turbulent, and he is more likely to be unconscious or semiconscious than fully aware of what is happening. Table 13-3 presents the rights of the dying patient.

HOPE AND DESPAIR IN THE DYING PATIENT

The dying patient typically experiences a high level of tension between hope and despair, the will to live and the desire to die. Hope looks to the future and provides comfort in the conviction that whatever is wished for will be attained. Absence of hope can lead to despair and loss of the will to live. The dying patient is particularly vulnerable to feelings of despair, even though hope persists to some degree regardless of what it is that the patient looks forward to.

Clinicians who have studied the emotions and attitudes of the terminally ill tell us that these patients rarely give up all hope of recovery. Even those who have apparently accepted the reality of their impending death

TABLE 13-3 ◆ *Rights of the Dying Patient*

The person who is dying has the right to

- Be treated as a person until death.
- Caring human contact.
- Have pain controlled.
- Cleanliness and comfort.
- Maintain a sense of hope whatever its focus.
- Participate in his care or the planning of it.
- Respectful, caring medical and nursing attention.
- Continuity of care and caregivers.
- Information about his condition and impending death.
- Honest answers to questions.
- Explore and change religious beliefs.
- Maintain individuality and express emotions freely without being judged.
- Make amends with others if desired and settle personal business.
- Terminate with family members and significant others in private.
- Assistance for significant others with the grief process.
- Withdraw from social contact if desired.
- Die at home in familiar surroundings.
- Die with dignity.
- Respectful treatment of the body after death.

seldom deny the possibility of a last-minute reprieve through a newly discovered drug or treatment.

The hopes expressed by these patients lift their spirits during difficult times and can give meaning to the suffering they endure. At first, the patient might want to think that his illness is not really serious or that a wrong diagnosis was made. Later he might hope that a treatment can be found that will cure his illness or at least prolong his life. Finally, he might find assurance in believing that he will continue to exist in life after death. Not every person can accept the concept of an immortal soul that enters into another form of life after this one. For many people the words *everlasting life* have little meaning until they are confronted with the reality of their own death, and even then they might question whether immortality of the soul has any relevance to their own situation. Another patient might believe in reincarnation or a totally different spiritual framework. The nurse must respect the patient's beliefs and not try to impose her own religious beliefs on him.

Whatever the patient chooses to believe and rely on as his source of confidence, he has the right to and a need for the hope of something better than what he is presently experiencing. The nurse can listen to and perhaps share in the patient's experience of optimism, but she must be honest and cannot give him false expectations for recovery or cure when realistically there are none. What she can do is give him hope for a better day tomorrow, hope of a good laugh about something that happens, hope of obtaining a favorite

food or seeing a favorite person, or even hope of seeing an especially beautiful sunrise or sunset. So many pleasurable small things can happen in one day of life. Even hoping for a few small pleasant things can sometimes lift the patient's spirits.

> The creative, thoughtful nurse can find some way to bring a little pleasure and hope to a terminally ill patient's day.

Death itself can be a welcome relief and actively sought by a patient. However, the nurse must be careful not to give the patient the impression that she agrees that his death would be desirable and therefore is willing to "give up" on him. She can empathize with the patient's desire to end the suffering, but she must convey supportiveness.

COMMUNICATION WITH THE DYING PATIENT

Asking the patient if he has questions or thoughts he would like to share allows him to express his feelings and concerns. Being an attentive listener is the nurse's role. Honesty and empathy are the qualities needed for communicating effectively with the dying patient. This is not the place to express reassuring platitudes. Acceptance of the patient's expressed concerns and problem solving about issues for which there are answers can be effective in bringing the patient some comfort. Sometimes the nurse is the only person with whom the patient feels he can express his dismay, fears, and concerns because he doesn't want to upset his family and friends.

Try opening the door to further communication by describing what you see: "You look so lonely and down, I wonder if I can help. Could we talk about it?" Or just acknowledge the struggle: "I'll bet you are tired of being so sick. It's got to be hard. I'm here if you want to talk about it."

Not every patient who is dying wants to talk about himself and what is happening to him, and there are times when even the most outspoken of patients would rather remain silent and aloof. It is important, however, that the patient have opportunities for companionship and conversation and for ventilating his feelings. He should be allowed to choose the time, the topic, and the person with whom he wishes to communicate.

Nonverbal communications can be as meaningful as verbal ones, if not more meaningful. A gentle touch, a willingness to spend time with the patient, and an attitude of patience and acceptance can convey compassion and concern. Terminal illnesses often are accompanied by deterioration of body tissues, unpleasant sights and smells, and messy lesions and discharges. If the patient sees that the nurse is not repulsed by these problems and is willing to make an effort to keep him clean and presentable, he is assured by her actions that she has not chosen to abandon him.

In her dealings with the dying patient it helps both the nurse and the patient if she can maintain a sense of humor in spite of the gravity of the situation. Everyone appreciates occasional comic relief from unrelenting grief and tragedy. Humor and laughter should be natural and healthful parts of everyone's life. The patient who is dying is still living. He still can enjoy whatever contributes to the fullness of his life in his final days, laughing or crying, being creative or appreciating creation, giving love or receiving it.

Nurses who have had extensive experience working with the dying agree that the best way to develop skill in dealing with these issues is through reading actual case histories and through first-hand experience in caring for patients who are approaching death.

THE PATIENT'S RIGHT TO KNOW

A terminally ill patient's right to know his diagnosis and prognosis is directly related to his ability to give informed consent to whatever medical and surgical treatments are being contemplated by health professionals. There seems to be no question that the patient who asks about his condition has a right to know. It is generally agreed that, if the patient is informed about the nature of his illness and the treatments prescribed for it, he will be better able to take care of himself and actively participate in planning his medical and nursing care. Problems arise, however, when members of the health care team do not agree on what or when the patient should be told, do not know what he has been told, or are not aware of or do not care about the patient's wishes in the matter. Some patients do not want to know the seriousness of their condition.

> Every patient has a right to know the expected outcome of his illness, if that is what he wants, but he has a corresponding right not to want to know.

Most patients who are dying already know that they are dying, but not every patient wants to talk about or be completely informed concerning his condition. If it is apparent that the patient does not want openly to admit and talk about his impending death, his wish must be respected. This does not mean, however, that he might not change his mind and ask for information later on. Lines of communication are always kept open so that the patient is always free to ask questions and express his thoughts and feelings.

Some dying patients do want to be fully informed. They want to know approximately how long they have to live and what is likely to happen during the final stages of their illness. Knowing his true status gives the patient an opportunity to maintain some control over his life, plan for his survivors, make peace with his family and his God, if applicable, and settle his business and financial affairs while he is still able to do so.

Everyone in close contact with the patient should be informed as to whether the patient knows his diagnosis and prognosis. If he says he wants to know "the truth" but senses that some people are not being entirely honest with him and are evading his questions, his trust in them will be badly damaged, if not destroyed. Any therapeutic relationship with a patient, dying or otherwise, must be based on mutual trust and respect.

PHYSIOLOGICAL DEATH AND THE DYING PROCESS

Thanatologists (those who specialize in caring for the dying) make a distinction between death and the process of dying. *Dying is a completely subjective and private experience.* For some it is a separation from all hope of companionship; for others it is an opportunity to rejoin those who have gone before them and to be with their God in heaven. Cultural and religious differences can cause us to misunderstand the death-related behavior of others. Those who care for the dying patient must be aware that, to understand what death means to another person, one must listen and observe attentively and nonjudgmentally.

Dying is not, like death, a static event that occurs at a specific moment in time. It is, rather, a physiological and psychosocial process that can take place in a matter of minutes, hours, or months. Dying is actually a stage of life. Thinking philosophically about dying, one might say that we begin the process of dying from the moment we are born. **From the medical point of view, the process of dying begins when a person has a disease that is untreatable and inevitably ends in death or is in the final stages of a disease that is fatal.**

If it is evident that a patient's disease is untreatable and he is considered to be in the terminal stages of disease or from injury, it is the responsibility of the nurse to speak to the physician about the possibility of a "do not resuscitate" (DNR) order. The patient and family should be consulted about **advance directives** (directions for treatments that are to be allowed and those that are not) and about organ donation. **If advance directives are not given and a "do not resuscitate" order is not written in the chart, all medical personnel are legally responsible for making every effort to resuscitate the patient in the event of a cardiac or respiratory arrest.**

The physician should be the one to speak to the patient and family about whether a DNR order should be written. For a terminally ill patient who wishes to be released from his body, going through the process of CPR, which can be both painful and frightening, seems an insult to his dignity and only prolongs his low-quality existence.

Signs that death has actually occurred are the result of the disintegration of cell structures. There is a loss of body heat, stagnation of the blood, and rigidity (**rigor mortis**). Because of the medicolegal and ethical problems associated with continuing life-support systems and obtaining **viable** (able to stay alive) organs for transplantation, it has become necessary to establish some criteria by which to judge whether brain death or irreversible coma is present.

Loss of respiration and heart beat with inability to reestablish them is death. However, because of the use of technology and drugs to sustain critical functions in the very ill, brain death is another criteria for death. **Brain death has occurred when there is loss of response to external stimuli, no pupillary response to light, no corneal reflex, no normal reflexive eye movement, and no gag or cough reflex.** With these criteria, death can be determined even when the patient's respiration and circulation are being maintained artificially.

Repetition of testing is customary, and an electro-encephalogram is recommended to confirm brain death. **If there is a flat encephalogram reading at the time of presumed death and a second flat reading 24 hours later, the person can be declared dead.**

NURSING ASSESSMENT AND INTERVENTION

When a person is terminally ill, all the body systems gradually become less able to maintain their specific functions of protection and adaptation. The patient becomes progressively weaker, more prone to infection and injury, and more likely to suffer some degree of discomfort.

Assessing a dying patient's physiological status and diagnosis of his specific nursing care needs is essentially the same as for any patient with a pathological condition. In the early stages of the process, the patient may be able to do many things for himself and should be encouraged and helped to do so. As he becomes weaker and more dependent, he will need increased support so that he is more comfortable physically and psychologically.

The following nursing interventions are presented according to body systems for convenience. Not every dying patient will have the same needs for nursing intervention.

◆ Integumentary and Musculoskeletal Systems

As the terminally ill patient's physical condition declines, he loses protective fat, his skin becomes more fragile, and he is therefore more subject to pressure ulcers. As his muscles weaken, he is less able to move himself about in bed to relieve pressure and assume a more comfortable position. Nursing interventions to prevent pressure ulcers and how to position the patient for comfort have been covered in Chapter 11. **Whatever is done for the patient should be done with extreme gentleness and care to avoid further damage to the skin.** As death approaches and body systems begin to fail, the skin on the lower extremities may become mottled.

We all move about in bed to get comfortable, even when we are asleep. The terminally ill patient may lack the strength and energy to change his position and must rely on the nurse to do this for him. **Although the process of moving him might cause some discomfort, most patients are more relaxed and better able to rest and sleep when their positions are changed often.** The frequency with which a patient should be turned depends on his general condition and capacity for turning himself without assistance. **All nursing measures to provide comfort, protection, and good personal hygiene should be scheduled as far as possible according to a patient's individual needs, rather than the routine times allotted for bathing, turning, feeding, and other aspects of personal care.** Seek the help of family members or volunteers to help with personal care. Many times family members feel more comfortable around the patient if they can do things for him, rather than just sit and wonder what to say. Both family members and volunteers can be extremely helpful in augmenting the care the staff nurses have time to give to the patient.

Pillows, blanket rolls, towels, and padded footboards are used to support the body and limbs in good alignment. It might be necessary to pad the siderails to prevent bruises and injury to the skin.

Muscular weakness also can lead to urinary and fecal incontinence, and there usually is sweating. All these situations necessitate frequent sponging, partial baths, and changes of linen to keep the patient dry and free of offensive odors. **Good judgment should dictate when the need for rest takes priority over sponging and bathing for the sake of cleanliness and the patient should be allowed to rest undisturbed.**

Dressings should be changed as often as necessary to minimize unpleasant sights and smells. Room deodorizers are helpful, but using one odor to cover up another should never be considered the primary method of dealing with odors. All soiled dressings and linens must be placed in biohazard containers and then removed from the patient's room or bathroom promptly.

It is important to the patient's self-esteem that he not view himself as repulsive to others.

The profuse sweating that often occurs in the final days or hours of life is the result of diminishing blood flow. The perspiration cools the body surface. Body temperature will begin to rise, and the patient is likely to feel hot even though his skin is cold. He may kick away covers and toss or attempt to remove bed clothing that is too hot. Lighter clothes, fresh circulating air, and only a light cover can help make him more comfortable. The top cover should not be tucked tightly over the lower extremities, as this can restrict movement and cause discomfort.

It is difficult for relatives and others less familiar with the dying process to understand that, even though the patient's skin feels cold, he may feel uncomfortably hot. If the patient is able to respond to questions, he can indicate whether he wants more or less warmth. If he is not able to respond, the nurse should look for clues in his bodily movements, such as pulling at covers to remove them or drawing himself up and huddling his body to preserve warmth.

◆ Gastrointestinal System

As muscle tone diminishes, the involuntary muscles of the gastrointestinal tract become more sluggish, causing accumulations of gas and feces and possibly nausea and vomiting. An antiemetic medication might be given to help relieve the nausea. Other measures include taking sips of water or ginger ale, eating ice chips, and frequent mouth care. Care of the patient with nausea and vomiting is discussed in Chapter 5.

Bowel and bladder elimination should be monitored carefully to detect early signs of such problems as abdominal distention, retention of feces in the rectum, or of urine in the bladder, and fecal impaction.

◆ Respiratory System

Because of decreased movement of the muscles involved in respiration, the air passages can become congested with accumulations of mucus, causing or aggravating shortness of breath and producing coughing and general discomfort. Placing the patient in the semi-Fowler's position might help relieve dyspnea. Low doses of oxygen by nasal prongs also could be helpful. Infrequently, secretions that cannot be coughed up by the patient may have to be removed by suctioning and inhalation therapy.

The breathing pattern may alter and become irregular. Those in the room with the patient should be told that this is not unusual. As the patient's condition continues to decline, his breathing may become more difficult and his breath sounds louder. Accumulations of the mucus in the air passages produce a gurgling sound (sometimes called the "death rattle") that can be particularly distressing to family members who are present. An explanation of what causes the sound can be reassuring.

◆ Central Nervous System

The dying patient's senses are often diminished or distorted as death approaches. Although the sensation of touch may be depressed, the dying person can sense pressure. If the patient has exhibited a desire to be touched and derives comfort from being touched by another, simply holding his hand, placing a hand on his arm, or gently stroking him can let him know that he is not alone. However, touch is a very personal thing, and some people who have never been demonstrative do not want or appreciate being touched.

Dying persons are not always comatose or totally unconscious. One who appears comatose or partially conscious should be spoken to in exactly the same way as if he were fully conscious and responsive. He should be told what is going to be done before it is done to him. He deserves an explanation of noises and other unfamiliar sensory stimuli that he could be aware of.

Hearing is thought to be the last sense that is lost when a patient either lapses into deep coma or is close to death. It is imperative that conversations held by others within hearing of the patient be conducted as if he were able to hear and respond. **Whispering is never acceptable; it is rude, and it can increase the patient's anxiety and cause him to distrust those who care for him.**

Nurses who specialize in the care of the dying report that the dying person almost invariably turns his head toward the light. This is probably because as sight and hearing fail the patient strives to see the objects and people near him. Indirect lighting can help avoid unnecessary stimulation. The person sitting with him should be at the head of the bed, near the patient so that the patient can see and hear him more easily. There is a tendency for well-meaning family members to lower the blinds or shades in the room, so that the dying person is in semidarkness. This does the patient a disservice and can increase his discomfort and anxiety. Again, he might feel that he is being hidden or that others are hiding from him because they do not want to confront him and help him deal with his dying. Each person reacts differently during the dying process, and each has needs that are not always shared by every other dying person. Nursing Care Plan 13-1 presents nursing interventions for a terminally ill patient.

◆ Psychosocial Care

Patience, empathy, honesty, and an understanding of the grief process can provide the nurse with the necessary tools to be of help to the terminally ill patient. A variety of interventions have proved helpful to the psychosocial well-being of the patient and the family. Helping the patient to live each day to the fullest and focusing on the best quality of life that can presently be obtained can do much to diminish the fear of death.

The nurse must carefully assess the patient's mood and needs before undertaking the following psychoso-cial interventions. Caution is to be exercised in encouraging the terminal patient to share feelings and deal with issues of death. This should not be done before he is ready. A patient's defenses should never be taken away from him.

Allow the patient to make as many decisions as possible, even if it is over something small, such as

Nursing Care Plan 13-1

Selected nursing diagnoses, goals/expected outcomes, nursing interventions, and evaluations for a terminally ill patient with end-stage renal disease

Situation: Mrs. Cox, age 60, has been ill with renal disease for the past 10 years. In spite of biweekly hemodialysis treatments, her condition has worsened, and she has but a few months to live. She is a widow with three children: two married sons who live nearby and one daughter who lives at home.

When she learned of her prognosis during hospitalization, Mrs. Cox asked to be allowed to go home for her final days. She seems to have resolved her feelings of denial and anger and is moving toward accepting her impending death as inevitable. She is in no great physical distress but does have congestive heart failure, anemia, fatigue, drowsiness, and decreased attention span.

Nursing Diagnosis	Goals/Expected Outcomes	Nursing Intervention	Evaluation
Impaired gas exchange related to fluid in lungs SUPPORTING DATA Bilateral rales, dyspnea, color ashen.	Patient will state that anxiety over difficulty in breathing is lessened.	Maintain in semi-Fowler's or Fowler's position. Administer oxygen via nasal cannula at 3 to 5 L per minute. Auscultate lung fields q shift; suction as needed. Administer morphine as ordered to ease breathing and lessen anxiety.	Oxygen at 3L/min per nasal cannula continuous; suctioned × 3 this shift; morphine at 8, 11, 2; breathing easier; continue plan. Goals partially met.
Anxiety related to feeling of having "unfinished business." SUPPORTING DATA "I'm not ready to die; I have too many things to attend to."	Patient will express sense of having taken care of business and disposal of personal items.	Help patient identify things she wants to take care of and ways in which she can accomplish these tasks. Encourage family members to assist patient and participate in decision making when she requests them to do so.	Made list of tasks to be completed—will, finances, etc.; will meet with attorney tomorrow; daughter included in meeting; continue plan. Goals partially met.
Anticipatory grieving related to impending death. SUPPORTING DATA Crying a lot; states she is very sad and is not ready to say good-bye to family and friends. "It hurts so bad to think of leaving everyone."	Patient will express sense of peace in regard to impending death.	Provide opportunities for verbalization of grief. Support and encourage her to communicate her thoughts and feelings with family members and share love and memories with them. Help patient feel free to cry and express her sense of loss. Establish trusting relationship with patient and family members. Reply honestly to her questions; respect confidentiality of information she divulges. Assess spiritual needs. Help patient identify resources for spiritual solace. Comply with request to call minister, rabbi, or whomever; obtain reading material, and if requested to do so, pray with her. Respect patient's beliefs, values, and philosophic outlook.	Discussed feelings for 15 minutes; is talking with family members and saying goodbye; crying lessened; minister visiting each A.M.; continue plan. Goals partially met.

Nursing Care Plan 13-1 (Continued)

Nursing Diagnosis	Goals/Expected Outcomes	Nursing Intervention	Evaluation
Ineffective family coping, compromised, related to daughter's denial of impending death of mother. SUPPORTING DATA Daughter states: "She's looking much better now." Heard to tell someone on the phone that she feels her mother may be able to go to a relative's wedding 2 months from now.	Daughter participates in physical care and psychological support of mother while dying. Mother expresses deepening bond and sense of unity with daughter and feels more at ease with her.	Help daughter identify personal strengths that make accepting and dealing with her mother's chronic illness less difficult. Allow daughter to express her grief and sense of loss. Encourage her to reminisce with her mother, remember happy times together. Reinforce mother's right to refuse intensive treatment and to choose the place and manner in which she wants to spend her final days.	Daughter assisting with care; talked with her alone for 15 minutes this P.M.; is beginning to realize her mother is terminal; continue plan. Goals partially met.

which arm he would like to have washed first. This is especially important as he loses control over bodily functions, such as defecating and urinating. Seek his input on how and when he wishes to receive visitors and how many he wishes to see. As death approaches, he may prefer to see only one or two close family members or a significant other. At that time a "No Visitors" sign on the door is advisable.

Help the patient maintain his dignity by always providing privacy and showing concern for him during procedures that are embarrassing to him. **When the patient expresses feelings of dependency, loss, anxiety, or despair, help him explore and express those feelings rather than discounting them with a quick reassurance.** Let him live his past or present regrets. Assist the patient in going through a "life review" with a special person or with you. Chronologically reviewing one's life and sharing experiences has proven to be very beneficial to the peace of mind of the dying individual. Be available to listen and encourage family members to share good memories of past events of which the patient was a part.

One of the most difficult parts of dying is to lose relationships. It is appropriate to mourn and grieve over relationships that are to be lost at death. Remembering the positives of those relationships and sharing the memories can be pleasurable. Encourage the patient to give or leave special messages to the people who are most meaningful to him.

Sustaining hope when the end is in sight is important, but the focus shifts to hope for relief from pain, for a time of complete rest, for a visit from a special person, or to complete some task before death.

At an appropriate time, talk with the patient and the family about their wishes regarding organ transplants and artificial means of life support. Discuss their decisions and requests with the physician.

There is as much work to be done with the family as

with the patient as death nears. The family needs to understand that withdrawal emotionally by the patient is a natural occurrence as death approaches. Each family member may be in a different stage of grief.

At the time of death, it is best to ask whether the family wishes you to remain with them. After death has occurred, many times the only honest thing that can be said is, "I'm sorry this has happened," or just "I'm so sorry." It is okay to cry with the family, if the nurse can control her reaction and appropriately stop crying. She must remember that she is there to support the family, not have them support her.

◆ Care of the Body after Death

When the patient has been pronounced dead, the nurse prepares the body for viewing by the family and then for transfer to the mortuary or morgue. The room and bed is straightened and the patient is positioned flat with a pillow under the head. If family members or significant others are present, they may be asked if they wish to help wash the patient. All tubes and lines are removed or cut according to health care policy and the eyes are shut. This is usually done before the family or significant others are brought to the room. The body is washed as needed, the hair combed and pads are placed under the hips and around the perineum to absorb feces and urine that will escape as the sphincters relax. The family or significant others are allowed privacy to perform any religious or cultural customs that they wish. Ask if they wish for you to stay before leaving them alone with the body. If they desire it, notify the hospital chaplain or community religious person of preference. After the family leaves, the body is wrapped in a shroud and identification tags are attached. The final paperwork is completed to ready the body for transfer to the mortuary or morgue.

SUPPORT FOR THE NURSE OF THE TERMINALLY ILL

It is emotionally draining to care for someone who is dying. If the nurse is truly involved in working with the patient as he progresses through the stages of dying, she has needs of her own that must be met. If she is to recover from her personal loss of someone she has grown close to, she needs support and understanding to sustain the inner strength she needs to help other patients.

Someone must be available to listen as she expresses her feelings. Just as the dying patient uses denial to adjust to the news that his life will soon end, the nurse also uses denial as a time to collect herself and gather her strength. She, too, becomes angry and has doubts about her ability and that of her colleagues to provide the kind of care that the patient needs.

The nurse might bargain by asking that she be relieved of some of the duties that bring her into direct contact with the patient. Her feelings of helplessness and inability to cope are understandable. Perhaps she does need relief so that when she returns to the patient, she can be available to him as a caring person.

When the nurse has experienced the loss of a patient, she, too, should have opportunities to grieve without fear of reprisal or ridicule and to have a soft shoulder to cry on, an understanding embrace, words of comfort that say, "Of course you're sad. You too have suffered a loss and by acknowledging it you may develop some insight."

Sometimes it might be necessary for the nurse to have a day off to replenish herself after having given of herself emotionally and physically. Those nurses who are continuously exposed to terminally ill patients might benefit from a temporary transfer to a less stressful assignment. If that is not feasible, they can be assigned to tasks that keep them occupied but do not require prolonged contact with a dying patient.

Nurses need self-esteem, security, love, and respect from their peers no less than any other human beings. Mutual support can help the nurse and her colleagues deal more effectively with death and the natural and expected psychological reactions to it.

HOSPICE CARE FOR THE DYING AND BEREAVED

Hospice originally meant a medieval guest house or way station for pilgrims and travelers. Many of the hospices of twentieth-century England are free-standing facilities unaffiliated with hospitals and autonomous in terms of professional procedures. These hospices were the predecessors of the hospice movement in the United States.

A hospice as currently conceived is not necessarily a specific kind of institution or facility, but a program of care that is specially designed to meet the needs of the terminally ill and their families. The hospice program can be implemented in an institution or in the patient's home. The National Hospice Organization (NHO) was organized in the United States in 1978. The Hospice Nurses' Association was founded in 1986.

Hospice is a concept or philosophy based on universal humanitarianism; it accepts death as a natural part of the life cycle. The purpose of a hospice program is to serve persons with a terminal illness through grief and death and to serve those supporting them through the death process and bereavement. Through an interdisciplinary approach, skilled medical and nursing care is given to meet the medical, social, psychological, and spiritual needs of the patient and significant others.

Generally a terminal prognosis with 6 months or less to live is required for eligibility in a hospice program. The patient must desire supportive care rather than hospital care during these last months of life. A hospice program is concerned with symptom management that maximizes client comfort, enhances feelings of self-worth and well-being, and encourages client participation in decisions affecting his living and dying. Such a program lends support to both the patient and significant others as their activities and relationships undergo change. The support continues into the periods of grief and bereavement.

Most hospices have services that are available on a 7-day-per-week, 24-hour-per-day basis and continue uninterrupted, regardless of the patient's ability to pay for that care. Many home care agencies and the visiting nurse services in large communities have started offering hospice services. Patients and families have been highly satisfied with the care received for both the patient and family.

Think about . . . If your terminally ill patient wishes to be discharged from the hospital and to use a hospice service, how would you help him convince his reluctant family that this is the best thing for him?

The hospice program has been approved and encouraged by the American Medical Association (AMA), the American Nurses' Association (ANA), and other professional organizations.

ETHICAL AND MORAL ISSUES

Nurses have a right and a responsibility to participate in decisions that are made about the effects of certain treatments on a patient's quality of life and the sustaining of life at all costs, even when the patient's prognosis offers no hope for recovery. Nurses are qualified for involvement in the decision-making process because (1) the focus of nursing care is on the patient's responses to health problems; (2) a nurse's education includes social sciences and the humanities, which can contribute to making informed moral decisions; and (3) it is the nurse who has continuous and intimate contact with the patient and is therefore able to provide important insights and speak on his behalf when he is unable to do so.

Participating in deliberations about ethical questions related to death and dying carries with it the responsibility to clarify one's own values and philosophy of life. This can be done by attending seminars and conferences, by informal discussions, and by reading about various points of view. Professional nursing journals frequently carry articles on bioethical and moral dilemmas confronting those who practice in the health care field.

Among the ethical and moral questions surrounding the topics of death and dying and the continued use of life-support systems are:

◆ Who should be the decision makers?

◆ Does hospitalization mean that one is obligated to accept all forms of active treatment?

◆ Is there an appropriate time to let a patient die?

◆ How does one measure rationality or a person's mental competence to decide that he wants life-support measures to be discontinued?

◆ What values should enter into the decision making?

◆ Does the dying patient or his family have the right to allow him to die?

◆ Is there a moral responsibility for a physician or other caregiver not to force the patient and his family into a position where active euthanasia is the only alternative?

◆ Is it always best to act on the side of life?

◆ Should nurses be dedicated to the inherent value of human life?

◆ Is it true that human life that is externally valued (that is, its worth measured in terms of economic, social, and personal considerations) is subject to the whimsy of others?

There are no simple answers to such complex questions. One must know what one believes in and then act accordingly. Modern technology has brought many benefits to humankind, but it also has brought the burden of bioethical dilemmas that were unheard of 30 or 40 years ago.

◆ Advance Directives

In recent years many state legislatures have passed laws that allow an adult to authorize, by means of a written directive, the withholding of life-sustaining measures in the event of his own terminal illness. The living will and durable power of attorney for health care, or similar document, is intended to protect a person's right to die. Such a document spells out exactly what life-saving measures may be used and which he refuses. A sample living will is shown in Figure 13-1.

A durable power of attorney is a most useful document, because, unlike a regular power of attorney, it is not voided when the person becomes incapacitated. It is written so that it can be executed at any time but does not take effect until the person desires or until a specific set of criteria are met (e.g., health decline reaching mental disability or the inability to make decisions on one's own). An example of a durable power of attorney is shown in Figure 13-1.

These legal actions allow patients to control decisions related to life-support procedures. The main features of such laws are (1) a written document that gives directives regarding withholding or withdrawing life-support measures; (2) a definition of "terminal illness"; (3) verification of the patient's prognosis by one or more physicians; and (4) provisions that protect the physician and health care agency against legal action.

Some opponents of the living will argue that it is not necessary, because the patient has an inherent right to die. When a person engages the services of a physician, he retains his right of self-determination. Thus physicians are "servants" rather than "masters" of their patients and must respect their wishes.

Another argument against legislation related to fatal illness is, that although it may give a patient self-determination, lack of such a document signed by the patient may have the opposite effect. In other words, in the absence of a written directive, is the physician obligated to use extraordinary means to prolong life? And if he chooses not to use extraordinary means to sustain life, is he likely to be accused of malpractice or even homicide?

A third objection concerns the length of time between the signing of the will and its application to a specific event at some future time in the patient's life. It is difficult to give informed consent when one does not know what procedures, possible cures, and other conditions might exist years after the will was signed. In answer to this objection, some state legislatures have incorporated a time limit, such as 7 years, during which the document is valid.

Written directives about what should be done in the event of a terminal illness are not the perfect answer to the issue of a person's right to die. They can be a source of conflict among family members and omit some or all of them from the decision-making process. They intrude into the physician–patient relationship and suggest mistrust. However, nurses and other health professionals must ask whether in every instance a person's right

California Medical Association
DURABLE POWER OF ATTORNEY FOR HEALTH CARE DECISIONS
(California Probate Code Sections 4600-4753)

WARNING TO PERSON EXECUTING THIS DOCUMENT

This is an important legal document. Before executing this document, you should know these important facts:

This document gives the person you designate as your agent (the attorney-in-fact) the power to make health care decisions for you. Your agent must act consistently with your desires as stated in this document or otherwise made known.

Except as you otherwise specify in this document, this document gives your agent power to consent to your doctor not giving treatment or stopping treatment necessary to keep you alive.

Notwithstanding this document, you have the right to make medical and other health care decisions for yourself so long as you can give informed consent with respect to the particular decision. In addition, no treatment may be given to you over your objection, and health care necessary to keep you alive may not be stopped or withheld if you object at the time.

This document gives your agent authority to consent, to refuse to consent, or to withdraw consent to any care, treatment, service, or procedure to maintain, diagnose, or treat a physical or mental condition. This power is subject to any statement of your desires and any limitations that you include in this document. You may state in this document any types of treatment that you do not desire. In addition, a court can take away the power of your agent to make health care decisions for you if your agent (1) authorizes anything that is illegal, (2) acts contrary to your known desires or (3) where your desires are not known, does anything that is clearly contrary to your best interests.

This power will exist for an indefinite period of time unless you limit its duration in this document.

You have the right to revoke the authority of your agent by notifying your agent or your treating doctor, hospital, or other health care provider orally or in writing of the revocation.

Your agent has the right to examine your medical records and to consent to their disclosure unless you limit this right in this document.

Unless you otherwise specify in this document, this document gives your agent the power after you die to (1) authorize an autopsy, (2) donate your body or parts thereof for transplant or therapeutic or educational or scientific purposes, and (3) direct the disposition of your remains.

If there is anything in this document that you do not understand, you should ask a lawyer to explain it to you.

1. CREATION OF DURABLE POWER OF ATTORNEY FOR HEALTH CARE

By this document I intend to create a durable power of attorney by appointing the person designated below to make health care decisions for me as allowed by Sections 4600 to 4753, inclusive, of the California Probate Code. This power of attorney shall not be affected by my subsequent incapacity. I hereby revoke any prior durable power of attorney for health care. I am a California resident who is at least 18 years old, of sound mind, and acting of my own free will.

2. APPOINTMENT OF HEALTH CARE AGENT

(Fill in below the name, address and telephone number of the person you wish to make health care decisions for you if you become incapacitated. You should make sure that this person agrees to accept this responsibility. The following may not serve as your agent: (1) your treating health care provider; (2) an operator of a community care facility or residential care facility for the elderly; or (3) an employee of your treating health care provider, a community care facility, or a residential care facility for the elderly, unless that employee is related to you by blood, marriage or adoption. If you are a conservatee under the Lanterman-Petris-Short Act (the law governing involuntary commitment to a mental health facility) and you wish to appoint your conservator as your agent, you must consult a lawyer, who must sign and attach a special declaration for this document to be valid.)

I, ______________________________, hereby appoint:
(insert your name)

Name ______________________________

Address ______________________________

Work Telephone (________) ______________ Home Telephone (________) ______________

as my agent (attorney-in-fact) to make health care decisions for me as authorized in this document. I understand that this power of attorney will be effective for an indefinite period of time unless I revoke it or limit its duration below.

(Optional) This power of attorney shall expire on the following date: ______________________________.

FIGURE 13-1 Living will and durable power of attorney for health care decisions. (*Source:* Reprinted with permission *Western Journal of Medicine.*

to die as he wishes (aside from suicide or active euthanasia) has been honored, and if his rights have been denied, why and how they were denied, and how they could have been protected.

Organ Donation

The Uniform Anatomical Gift Act, which governs organ donation and the determination that life has ceased, requires that health professionals approach the patient or family about the issue of organ donation. Organs for transplantation to other individuals are very badly needed, and nurses are encouraged to seek permission from families of deceased patients for organ harvest. When the patient has made his wishes known via advance directives or by statements on his driver's license, the family may not need to be intruded upon at their time of grief. **If such directives are not in place, the nurse must determine that the patient's illness or condition has left organs suitable for donation before approaching the family.**

Organs must be removed within an hour after death. When a patient has been on life support systems and is declared brain dead, the support systems are usually kept in place until the organs are removed.

Euthanasia

There is great controversy over whether a patient should have the right to decide he is ready to die and to seek assistance in doing so. The patient has reached a point where he does not think that the quality of life he has, or that will soon occur for him, is sufficient to warrant continuing to live. **Euthanasia,** derived from the Greek, means "easy or pleasant death." Euthanasia is illegal in the United States, but is legal in countries such as Sweden and The Netherlands. Those countries allow a

3. AUTHORITY OF AGENT

If I become incapable of giving informed consent to health care decisions, I grant my agent full power and authority to make those decisions for me, subject to any statements of desires or limitations set forth below. Unless I have limited my agent's authority in this document, that authority shall include the right to consent, refuse consent, or withdraw consent to any medical care, treatment, service, or procedure; to receive and to consent to the release of medical information; to authorize an autopsy to determine the cause of my death; to make a gift of all or part of my body; and to direct the disposition of my remains, subject to any instructions I have given in a written contract for funeral services, my will or by some other method. I understand that, by law, my agent may not consent to any of the following: commitment to a mental health treatment facility, convulsive treatment, psychosurgery, sterilization or abortion.

4. MEDICAL TREATMENT DESIRES AND LIMITATIONS (OPTIONAL)

(Your agent must make health care decisions that are consistent with your known desires. You may, but are not required to, state your desires about the kinds of medical care you do or do not want to receive, including your desires concerning life support if you are seriously ill. If you do not want your agent to have the authority to make certain decisions, you must write a statement to that effect in the space provided below; otherwise, your agent will have the broad powers to make health care decisions for you that are outlined in paragraph 3 above. In either case, it is important that you discuss your health care desires with the person you appoint as your agent and with your doctor(s).)

(Following is a general statement about withholding and removal of life-sustaining treatment. If the statement accurately reflects your desires, you may initial it. If you wish to add to it or to write your own statement instead, you may do so in the space provided.)

> I do **not** want efforts made to prolong my life and I do **not** want life-sustaining treatment to be provided or continued: (1) if I am in an irreversible coma or persistent vegetative state; or (2) if I am terminally ill and the use of life-sustaining procedures would serve only to artificially delay the moment of my death; or (3) under any other circumstances where the burdens of the treatment outweigh the expected benefits. In making decisions about life-sustaining treatment under provision (3) above, I want my agent to consider the relief of suffering and the quality of my life, as well as the extent of the possible prolongation of my life.
>
> *If this statement reflects your desires, initial here: _____*

FIGURE 13-1 *Continued*

Other or additional statements of medical treatment desires and limitations: _____

_____

_____

_____

_____

(You may attach additional pages if you need more space to complete your statements. Each additional page must be dated and signed at the same time you date and sign this document.)

5. APPOINTMENT OF ALTERNATE AGENTS (OPTIONAL)

(You may appoint alternate agents to make health care decisions for you in case the person you appointed in Paragraph 2 is unable or unwilling to do so.)

If the person named as my agent in Paragraph 2 is not available or willing to make health care decisions for me as authorized in this document, I appoint the following persons to do so, listed in the order they should be asked:

First Alternate Agent: Name _____

Address _____

Work Telephone (_____) _____   Home Telephone (_____) _____

Second Alternate Agent: Name _____

Address _____

Work Telephone (_____) _____   Home Telephone (_____) _____

6. USE OF COPIES

I hereby authorize that photocopies of this document can be relied upon by my agent and others as though they were originals.

---

physician to administer a lethal dose of medication to a patient who desires to end his life because of pain and suffering. This action is *active euthanasia. Passive euthanasia* occurs when there is omission or withdrawal of treatment that would prolong a person's life. In many states, if a patient has advance directives in place and a durable power of attorney for health care, passive euthanasia is possible.

Many people object to euthanasia or assisted suicide on the basis of religious teachings that state that it is a "sin" to take one's own life. They believe that God is the giver of life and the only one that has the right to end it. However, at the time of biblical writings that created this viewpoint, there were not the medical advances and technology to keep people alive though terminally ill as there are today. Some feel that, because God provided the intelligence to develop these life-sustaining measures, surely he also gave us the intelligence to know when to use them and when to stop using them. Such people feel that, as God has given individuals autonomy over all other aspects of their lives, why would he not desire autonomy for one to choose the end of life at a time when one can no longer be useful to one's self or society?

Think about . . . In a society where we want people to be "humane" to each other and even to animals, does it make sense that we forbid people actively to end their own lives when they have no hope of recovery, no quality of life, and can only continue to suffer each day they exist?

Because active euthanasia is not legal in the United States, some patients are seeking assistance with suicide. Assisted suicide is a topic of great controversy and is not legal in most states. Yet, should a person have the final say over whether he lives or dies or not? Society is working to attempt to find acceptable answers to such questions.

CRITICAL THINKING EXERCISES

Clinical Case Problems

Read each clinical case problem and discuss the questions with your classmates.

1. You are assigned to care for Mr. Ross, age 38, who is terminally ill. He was transferred to your long-term care facility because of the complexity of his needs. He is emaciated, short of breath, and near death. His wife is a nurse who is unable to be with him more than a few hours a day because of her responsibilities at home and at work. Mr. Ross is very difficult to care for because of his belligerent attitude. He refuses to eat and insists that he does not need A.M. care or any other kind of attention. The other health care workers on duty do not go into Mr. Ross's room except when absolutely necessary because "he has asked to be left alone, we are busy, and, anyway, it is depressing to be around him. He is so young to die."

   a. What stage of adjustment do you think Mr. Ross is experiencing?

   b. How can you help him?

   c. What personal attributes and attitudes are lacking in the nurses who choose to leave Mr. Ross alone?

   d. What kinds of physiological needs might Mr. Ross have?

2. The husband of one of your home care patients who has terminal cancer refuses to accept his wife's prognosis and insists that she be kept alive at all costs. The patient has accepted her condition and wishes to discuss her feelings about her approaching death. She asks that you contact a minister but that you not tell her husband about the request. She also asks how you feel about using heroic measures to keep someone alive when he or she is hopelessly ill and willing to accept death.

   a. What would you do about notifying the minister?

   b. How would you answer her second question?

3. Your aunt, age 58, has only recently been widowed. The death of her husband was completely unexpected, and she still has not recovered from the shock. Family members urge you to help her "snap out of it" and get on with her own life. "After all," they say, "he has been dead 6 weeks now."

   a. How would you respond to your relatives who are anxious for your aunt to finish her grieving and look to the future instead of the past?

   b. What behavior might you expect to see in your aunt as she works her way through her grief?

   c. What kinds of support might you give your aunt during her grieving?

BIBLIOGRAPHY

Amenta, M. O., Bohnet, N. L. (1986). *Nursing Care of the Terminally Ill.* Boston: Little, Brown.

American Nurses' Association. (1987). *Standards and Scope of Hospice Nursing Practice.* Kansas City: Author.

Berrio, M. W., Levesque, M. E. (1996). Advance directives: Most patients don't have one. Do yours? *American Journal of Nursing.* 96(8):25–27.

Boles, A. (1995). From hospital to hospice: bridging the gap. *RN.* 58(10):57–59.

Callanan, M. (1994). Back from "beyond." *American Journal of Nursing.* 94 (3):20–23.

Callanan, M. (1994). Farewell messages. *American Journal of Nursing.* 94(5):19–20.

Carter, J. (1996). Can hospice care be provided to people who live alone? *Home Healthcare Nurse.* 14(9):710–716.

Coolican, M. B. (1994). After the loss: offering families something more. *Nursing 94.* 24 (6):60–62.

Diaz, M. R. (1995). When a baby dies. *American Journal of Nursing.* 95(11):54–56.

Dolan, M. B. (1994). Giving closure. *American Journal of Nursing.* 94 (11):66–67.

Ferdinand, R. (1995). "I'd rather die than live this way." *American Journal of Nursing.* 95 (12):42–47.

Fina, D. K. (1994). A chance to say goodbye. *American Journal of Nursing.* 94 (5):42–45.

Goetzke, E. (1995). When your patient is in denial. *American Journal of Nursing.* 95 (9):18–22.

Greve, P. (1994). Has the PSDA made a difference? *RN.* 24 (2):59–64.

Greifzu, S. (1996). Grieving families need your help. *RN.* 59(9):22–27.

Huth, J. (1996). Advance directives and the patient self-determination act: what is a nurse to do? *Journal of Post Anesthesia Nursing.* 10(6):336–339.

Kastenbaum, R. J. (1986). *Death, Society, and Human Experience,* 3rd ed. New York: Macmillan.

Kubler-Ross, E. (1975). *Death: The Final Stage of Growth.* Englewood Cliffs, NJ: Prentice-Hall.

Kubler-Ross, E. (1969). *On Death and Dying.* New York: Macmillan.

Lewis, S., et al. (1989). *Manual of Psychosocial Nursing Interventions: Promoting Mental Health in Medical–Surgical Settings.* Philadelphia: Saunders.

Martocchio, B. C. (1982). *Living While Dying.* Bowie, MD: Robert J. Brady.

McNally, J. C., Bohnet, N. L., Lindquist, M. E. (1996). Hospice Nursing. *Seminars in Oncology Nursing.* 12(3):238–243.

Meyer, C. (1992). Coming to new terms with death. *American Journal of Nursing.* 92(8):19–20.

Murphy, P. A., Price, D. M. (1995). "ACT" taking a positive approach to end-of-life care. *American Journal of Nursing.* 95(3):42–43.

National Hospice Nurses' Association (1989). *Quality Assurance for Hospice Patient Care.* Escondido, CA: Author.

National Hospice Organization. (1982). *Standards of a Hospice Program of Care.* Arlington, VA: Author.

Pangrazzi, A. (1983). Overcoming grief: Ten suggestions. *St. Anthony Messenger,* January.

Parkes, C. M., Weiss, R. S. (1983). *Recovery from Bereavement.* New York: Basic Books.

Reigle, J. (1995). Should the patient decide when to die? *RN.* 58(5):57–61.

Solari-Twadell, P. A., et al. (1995). The pinwheel model of bereavement. *Image: Journal of Nursing Scholarship.* 27(4):323–326.

Taylor, P. B., Ferszt, G. G. (1994). Letting go of a loved one. *Nursing 94.* 24(1):55–56.

Turkoski, B., Lance, B. (1996). The use of guided imagery with anticipatory grief. *Home Healthcare Nurse.* 14(21): 878–888.

Ufema, J. (1994). How to help dying patients feel "safe." *Nursing 94.* 24(10):59.

Vergara, M., Lynn-McHale, D. J. (1995). Withdrawing life support: who decides? *American Journal of Nursing.* 95(11):47–49.

Walsh, S. M. (1995). Resuscitation decisions: showing a family the way. *Nursing 95.* 25(8):51–52.

Zerwekh, J. (1994). The truth-tellers: how hospice nurses help patients confront death. *American Journal of Nursing.* 94(2):31–34.

SUGGESTED READINGS

Carroll, D. (1985). *Living with Dying.* New York: McGraw-Hill.

Craven, M. (1973). I Heard the Owl Call My Name. Garden City, NY: Doubleday.

Gunther, J. (1949). Death Be Not Proud. New York: Harper & Row.

Grollman, E. (1977). *Living When a Loved One Has Died.* Boston: Beacon Press.

Morse, M. (1991). *Closer to the Light.* New York: Ivy Books.

Morse, M. (1992). *Transformed by the Light.* New York: Random House.

Simos, B. (1979). *A Time to Grieve: Loss as a Universal Experience.* New York: Family Service Association of America.

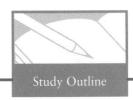

Study Outline

I. Introduction

A. Death is a part of the life cycle; it is inevitable.

B. Death causes loss and grief, painful feelings characterized by sadness and emotional distress.

C. Death is a unique individual experience and people do not experience it in the same way.

D. The task of the dying person is to work his way toward acceptance of his death. The task of the nurse is to help him live his life more fully until he dies.

II. Stages of Dying

A. Theory first proposed by Dr. Elisabeth Kubler-Ross.

B. Each person experiences dying in his own way.

C. A patient may experience one, a few, or all of the stages of dying.

D. The work of Kubler-Ross and other thanatologists has helped caregivers be more sensitive to the needs of the dying person and his family.

E. Death represents change and separation. Stages of dying are similar to responses in other change situations.

   1. Denial and disbelief: "No, not me, it's not possible."

   2. Anger: "Why me?"

   3. Bargaining (usually with God): "Yes, me, but . . ."

   4. Depression: "Yes, me."

   5. Acceptance: person is not happy but appears to have won his struggle with grief and fear.

III. The Grieving Process

A. Phases of grief include: shock and disbelief, feelings of anger, guilt, and hostility; interruption of life's usual activities; preoccupation with thoughts of the deceased; and acceptance of the loss.

B. The grief process is individual, and people progress through phases at their own rate and in their own order.

C. The nursing diagnosis for those experiencing normal grief is "Anticipatory grief."

D. The desirable outcomes of grieving are to come to accept the loss and to remember the person without severe pain; and to return to participation in life with the capacity to love intact.

E. Outward signs of acute grief include inability to sleep, forgetfulness and absentmindedness, and a tendency to repeat the same behavior over and over again.

F. After the initial shock, the grieving person may withdraw and try to place blame for the catastrophe that has occurred to him; he may feel angry toward the deceased for leaving him; he might feel terrible guilt thinking he might have done something to prevent the death.

G. Resolution of grief begins when the finality of the death is accepted; there may be tremendous sadness and apathy for a period, then a gradual emotional detachment occurs; finally the bereaved begins to reorganize his life and get on with living.

H. Grief serves a useful purpose during period of adjustment to new life without loved one.

I. Length of time it takes to work through grief to acceptance is highly individualized.

  1. Action-oriented, assertive person is more likely to begin reorganization behavior earlier than one who is passive and withdrawn.

  2. Ten suggestions for overcoming grief are listed in Table 13-1.

IV. Fears Experienced by the Dying Person

A. Fear of the unknown.

  1. Spiritual belief systems are helpful in presenting answers to the question What happens when you die?

  2. Reading about "life after life" and near-death experiences may comfort those who do not hold strong religious beliefs.

B. Fear of abandonment and loneliness.

  1. Dying persons often express fear that they will be alone when they die and no notice will be taken of their leaving.

  2. Patient should be free to choose whom he wants for companionship and what he needs from others.

  3. Human companionship and contact can give patient a sense of security and calm.

C. Fear of loss of relationships and experiences in the future.

  1. Grieving occurs for the coming loss of relationships with loved ones.

  2. Grief also occurs because of the loss of the chance to participate in future events, such as a child's wedding.

D. Fear of dependency and loss of independence.

  1. As the patient becomes weaker with the approach of death, he becomes more dependent on others to meet his needs.

  2. Consulting the patient about small decisions helps preserve a feeling of some independence.

E. Fear of pain.

  1. Physiological pain does not always accompany dying.

    a. Patient is to be kept comfortable and assured that analgesic medication is readily available.

    b. Combinations of oral and parenteral analgesia or intrathecal analgesia can allow a patient to remain lucid and free of pain.

    c. Use of alternative methods to control pain, such as relaxation exercises, imagery, massage, music, and meditation can augment the degree of relief provided by analgesia.

  2. The goal of pain management is to prevent pain rather than treat it once it has occurred.

  3. Pain control is possible for most patients.

  4. Addiction is not a concern in pain control for the dying.

  5. Pain control is a major nursing function, and the nurse is the patient's advocate in obtaining adequate pain control.

F. Dying person's Bill of Rights (see Table 13-3).

V. Hope and Despair in the Dying Patient

A. There is tension between hope and despair, the will to live and the desire to die.

B. Patients rarely give up all hope. They need a belief in something better to lift their spirits and give them strength to go on. There might be hope for:

  1. A mistaken diagnosis.

  2. Discovery of a cure or some means of postponing death.

  3. Life after death.

  4. Relief from pain.

  5. A better day.

  6. Living for a particular event.

  7. A good laugh.

C. Tension between will to live and desire to die is related to hope and despair.

  1. Death can be a welcome relief and source of hope.

  2. The creative, thoughtful nurse can find some way to bring a little pleasure and hope to a terminally ill patient's day.

VI. Communication With the Dying Patient

A. Patient should be free to express his feelings and needs.

B. The nurse should be honest, empathetic, and an attentive listener when communicating.

C. It is important for caregivers to maintain a sense of humor.

D. There is need for opportunities to relieve tension, release pent-up emotions, and experience grief.

E. Nonverbal communication is very meaningful to the dying.

VII. The Patient's Right to Know

A. The patient should be told about his diagnosis and prognosis if he indicates a need to know.

B. Patient has a corresponding right not to want to know.

C. Most dying patients are aware of the seriousness of their condition, but not every one wants to talk about it.

D. Lines of communication always kept open to give patient an opportunity to ask questions and discuss his condition.

VIII. Physiological Death and the Dying Process

A. Death is an event, a state. It does not have the same meaning for everyone.

1. Dying is a subjective and private experience.

2. It is a dynamic process, a stage of life.

3. Cultural and religious differences can create misunderstanding of death-related behaviors.

B. From a medical point of view, dying begins when the person has an untreatable and fatal disease.

1. When death is inevitable, a "do not resuscitate" (DNR) order is appropriate.

2. Advance directives should be sought regarding life-sustaining measures and organ donation after death.

C. Signs of death are the result of cell destruction: loss of body heat, stagnation of blood, and rigor mortis.

D. Criteria to determine irreversible coma used to make decisions about continuing life-support systems and procuring viable donor organs.

1. Loss of response to external stimuli, no pupillary response to light, no corneal reflex, no normal reflexive eye movement, and no gag or cough reflex and no relationship of these losses to drugs or hypothermia.

2. Cessation of spontaneous movement and breathing.

3. Two electroencephalograms 24 hours apart that are flat decree that the patient has died, even when the respiration and circulation are being maintained by chemicals and equipment.

E. Loss of respiration and heart beat with inability to reestablish them is death.

IX. Nursing Assessment and Intervention

A. Skin and musculoskeletal system:

1. Protective body fat diminishes, skin more fragile. Measures taken to maintain skin integrity, prevent pressure ulcers.

2. Muscle weakness requires repositioning to provide comfort.

3. Nursing intervention to provide comfort, protection, and good personal hygiene is scheduled according to patient's needs.

4. Muscle weakness can lead to urinary and fecal incontinence.

5. Patient and environment kept clean and odor free. Dressing changes, bathing, and mouth care are scheduled to allow patient sufficient rest.

6. Profuse sweating, tossing about, and kicking off covers probably indicate that the patient feels hot, even though his skin may be cold to the touch.

B. Gastrointestinal system:

1. Diminished involuntary muscle function can cause accumulations of feces and flatus.

2. Nausea and vomiting can occur.

3. Nursing intervention should help manage these symptoms.

4. Bowel and bladder elimination are monitored to detect early signs of retention and fecal impaction.

C. Respiratory system: Air passages can become congested. Nursing interventions include positioning to relieve shortness of breath, turning, help with coughing and deep-breathing, and possibly suctioning and inhalation therapy.

D. Central nervous system:

1. Senses become less acute. Touching may or may not be desired by patient.

2. Comatose and semiconscious patient must be talked to and told what is being done to and for him even though he cannot respond.

3. Conversations held within patient's hearing should be held as though patient were fully alert and aware of what is being said.

4. Room should not be darkened or shades drawn.

5. Person sitting with dying patient should sit at head of bed where patient is better able to see and hear the person.

6. Indirect lighting may decrease agitation.

E. Psychosocial care:

1. Help patient to live each day to the fullest.

2. Be cautious; assess mood and needs; defenses should never be taken from patient.

3. Allow patient to make decisions over anything he can, no matter how small.

4. Maintain patient's dignity by providing privacy and showing concern for embarrassing procedures.

5. Help patient express feelings of dependency, loss, anxiety, or despair, and explore them, rather than just offering reassurance.

6. Ask significant others to talk about the worthwhile things the patient has done in his life.

7. Family and friends can reminisce and recall good times spent with the dying patient.

8. Nurse can point out the patient's positive points noted while patient goes through the dying process.

9. Assist patient to go through a "life review."

10. Assist patient to mourn relationships that will be lost.

11. Provide psychosocial support for the family as well.

12. Ask patient and family their preference as to your presence at time of death and respect their wishes.

13. It is okay to grieve and cry with the family as long as the nurse's grief can be controlled; nurse is there to support the family.

F. Care of the body after death:

1. The body is prepared for viewing; remove or cut all tubes according to hospital policy; close the eyes and mouth; straighten the bed and position the patient flat with a pillow under the head; place pads beneath the hips and around the perineum.

2. Ask the family if they you to stay with them in the room or not while they are viewing the body.

3. Inquire whether family members or significant others wish to help prepare the body.

4. Cleanse the body as needed and wrap it in a shroud and tag it per agency policy.

5. Complete the necessary paperwork.

X. Support for Nurses of the Terminally Ill

A. Care for terminally ill can create special needs for support and consolation.

B. Caregiver can experience bereavement and grief over loss of patient.

XI. Hospice Care for the Dying and Bereaved

A. A concept or program of care for the terminally ill and his family.

B. Nurse-coordinated program that can be implemented in an institution or the patient's home.

C. Hospice is designed to meet the medical, social, psychological, and spiritual needs of the patient and significant others.

D. A terminal prognosis with 6 months or less to live is required for eligibility in a hospice program.

XII. Ethical and Moral Issues

A. Nurses have a right and responsibility to participate in moral and ethical decisions about treatments and prolonging life of terminally ill.

B. Some ethical considerations surround reverence for life, the quality of life, and the right to die with dignity and grace.

1. Who should decide?

2. Must one accept all forms of treatment?

3. Is there an appropriate time to let a patient die?

4. Should family and patient be forced into a position where active euthanasia is their only alternative?

C. The optimal time for a family to discuss death is before they must deal with issues of death and dying.

D. Advance directives may include a living will and durable power of attorney.

1. The "living will" is an attempt to document a person's wishes in regard to sustaining his life.

2. A "durable power of attorney" is effective only when the person becomes incapacitated. (Figure 13-1).

E. Nurses are obliged by law to seek permission for organ donation from dying patients and their families.

F. Euthanasia is a topic of controversy.

1. Active euthanasia is prohibited by law.

2. Passive euthanasia is permissible when advance directives are in place.

3. Assisted suicide is not legal in all states, but there is great debate about whether or not a patient should have the final say about the end of his life.

Nursing Care for Specific Medical–Surgical Disorders

In the preceding unit problems common to a variety of disorders were presented. Regardless of the patient's specific medical diagnosis, it is essential that problems of fluid, electrolyte, and acid–base imbalance be corrected, infection be prevented, and healing be promoted and that the hazards of immobility be prevented.

The information presented in earlier chapters is intended to serve as a foundation for safe, competent, holistic, individualized nursing care of adult patients with medical–surgical conditions. The eighteen chapters in this unit present information on caring for patients with specific disorders. The study of disorders is organized primarily by body systems. Each chapter is organized to help you study. The objectives identify major subjects that you will read about. The first part of the chapter is an overview of the anatomy and physiology of the body system in a format that will help you review. Questions are asked about the functioning of the body system, followed by a bulleted list of essential facts you should know. Read the entire section through, then go back and try to answer each question.

After the anatomy and physiology overview, a discussion about health maintenance and prevention of the disorders related to that body system is presented. Health maintenance and disease prevention are important parts of patient education; when you plan patient education sessions, be sure to refer to the health maintenance section for reminders.

In the nursing management section of each chapter, nursing care for the major problems that accompany disorders of the system is presented. Then the specific diseases that affect that organs of each body system are discussed. Although medical science recognizes hundreds of different diseases, only the most prevalent can be discussed in this text. As you continue in your nursing career, you will learn about many other disorders. By learning nursing management of the major problems, you will be able to apply your knowledge for patients with other disorders.

Much emphasis is given to disorders that are particularly common to the elderly, because the older population makes up a large percentage of patients in the hospital. As you read, take also note that nursing care is discussed for patients in their homes, in rehabilitation centers, and in long-term care facilities such as nursing homes.

CHAPTER 14

Care of Patients with Neurological Disorders

O B J E C T I V E S

Upon completing this chapter the student should be able to:

1. Identify four specific ways in which a nurse can contribute to preventing neurological disorders.
2. Demonstrate a "neurological check," and describe the basic neurological nursing assessment.
3. State the appropriate preparation and postprocedure care for patients undergoing lumbar puncture (spinal tap), electroencephalogram, and radiological studies of the brain and cerebral vessels.
4. Develop a nursing care plan for the patient who is experiencing an increase in intracranial pressure.
5. Identify appropriate interactions to meet all basic needs of the patient who has suffered a head injury and is unconscious.
6. Develop and implement a comprehensive nursing care plan for a patient who has suffered a cerebrovascular accident.
7. Describe the appropriate nursing actions and observations to be carried out for a patient experiencing a seizure.
8. Discuss areas of teaching needed by the patient newly diagnosed with epilepsy.
9. List appropriate nursing interventions necessary to provide comprehensive care for a patient who has suffered a C-5 spinal cord injury.
10. Compare the pathophysiology, diagnosis, and treatment of Parkinson's disease, multiple sclerosis, Guillain-Barré syndome, trigeminal neuralgia, and myasthenia gravis.

The nervous system is the communication system of the body. It coordinates all sensory and motor activities by receiving, interpreting, and relaying messages that are vital to the proper performance of all the body's activities. Respiratory, circulatory, digestive, and endocrine functions all depend on an intact and normally functioning autonomic nervous system.

If anything happens to impair the ability of certain nerve cells to receive and conduct impulses, the tissues controlled by the nerve cells cease to function normally. An example of this is trauma to the spinal cord. All parts of the body below the point of injury would be paralyzed and have no sensation of heat, cold, pressure, or pain if the spinal cord had been severed and the flow of impulses interrupted. A basic knowledge of the anatomy of the nervous system and how it works is essential to understand how various disorders affect it. A brief review is provided here as a refresher.

OVERVIEW OF ANATOMY AND PHYSIOLOGY

How Is the Nervous System Organized?

▲ The functional unit of all parts of the nervous system is the neuron, which consists of a cell body, dendrites, and an axon. Neurons react to stimuli, conduct impulses, and influence other neurons.

▲ The nervous system consists of the central nervous system (CNS) and the peripheral nervous system (PNS).

▲ The CNS is made up of the brain and spinal cord (Figure 14-1).

▲ The brain is divided into the cerebrum, diencephalon, cerebellum, and brainstem (Figures 14-1 and 14-2). Table 14-1 lists the functions of the various divisions of the brain.

▲ Different parts of the brain control various functions (Figure 14-2).

▲ The PNS is composed of the sensory organs—eyes, ears, taste buds, olfactory receptors, and touch receptors—12 pairs of cranial nerves, and 31 pairs of spinal nerves and ganglia that link the sensory organs, muscles, and other parts of the body to the brain and spinal cord.

▲ The spinal cord extends from the medulla to the level of the first lumbar vertebra.

▲ The spinal cord is a conduction pathway for impulses going to and from the brain and also serves as a reflex center for nerve impulse transmission. Sensory impulses travel to the brain on ascending conduction pathway tracts; motor impulses travel on descending tracts.

▲ Pyramidal tracts are conduction pathways that begin in the cerebral cortex and end in the spinal cord. These tracts control skeletal muscle movement. All other conduction pathways are extrapyramidal tracts, and they control muscle movements associated with posture and balance.

How Is the Central Nervous System Protected?

▲ The bones of the skull and the vertebral column form the outer layer of protection for the brain and the spinal cord.

▲ The meninges are protective membranes that cover the brain and are continuous with the membranes covering the spinal cord. The meninges consist of the pia mater covering the brain, the arachnoid, which encases the entire CNS, and the dura mater, which is a tough membrane protecting the brain and spinal cord (Figure 14-3).

▲ The subarachnoid space is between the pia mater and the arachnoid membrane and is where the cerebrospinal fluid circulates.

▲ Cerebrospinal fluid (CSF) serves to cushion and protect the brain and spinal cord. It is formed continuously from the blood and is reabsorbed by the arachnoid villi of the arachnoid membrane at the same rate at which it is formed. The volume of CSF normally stays constant.

▲ **Normal CSF pressure is 70 to 125 cm water pressure.** When there is an excess of fluid in the subarachnoid space, the pressure rises above normal.

How Do Nerve Impulses Occur and Travel?

▲ Neurons have a cell body, dendrites that receive impulses, and an axon that transmits impulses. Many axons bundled together and wrapped in connective tissue make up a nerve. Ganglia are collections of nerve cell bodies outside the CNS.

▲ When in a state of polarization neurons have the capacity to become excited (stimulated). They also have the ability to conduct that stimulus along the nerve pathways.

▲ A stimulus is a physical, chemical, or electrical event that changes the cell membrane and initiates conduction of the stimulus as an electrical impulse along the nerve pathway.

▲ The stimulus travels from one neuron to another across a synapse (the space between two neurons).

▲ A neurotransmitter secreted by the neuron is necessary for transmission across the synapse to occur.

▲ Neurotransmitter substances are secreted at the synapse, and these diffuse across to stimulate the postsynaptic membrane on the next neuron. **When normal neurotransmitter is absent or decreased at the synaptic junction, the stimulus cannot travel along the nerve pathways normally.**

▲ Impulses either travel in a reflex arc, going to the spinal cord and traveling back to an effector site, or they travel along nerve pathways to the brain to be interpreted.

⊿ After impulse interpretation, a message may be sent out from the brain via the spinal cord or cranial nerves (PNS) for appropriate action to be taken. In other words, a stimulus produces a response.

⊿ Many axons are surrounded by a myelin sheath that is a white, fatty, covering. The myelin covering is an excellent electrical insulator and it speeds the conduction of nerve impulses. **When myelin is destroyed, impulse transmission is slowed or stopped.**

How Does the Peripheral Nervous System Interact with the Central Nervous System?

⊿ The PNS is subdivided into an afferent division and efferent division. The afferent division carries impulses to the CNS; the efferent subdivision carries impulses away from the CNS.

⊿ The reflex arc is a simple conduction pathway that utilizes a receptor, a sensory neuron centered in the spinal cord, and a motor neuron located in an effector (skeletal muscle). A stimulus travels from the sensory receptor through the spinal cord and back to the effector, causing action (Figure 14-4).

⊿ The cranial and spinal nerves are part of the somatic subsystem and respond to changes in the outside world. Because these nerves initiate voluntary action, the somatic system often is called the *voluntary system.*

⊿ The autonomic system of the PNS is active in maintaining internal body balance (homeostasis) and is automatic (involuntary) in its actions.

⊿ The autonomic system is divided into the sympathetic nerves, which mobilize energy to initiate changes aimed at maintaining or restoring homeostasis, and the parasympathetic nerves, which conserve and restore energy that has been used to maintain homeostasis.

⊿ **Sympathetic and parasympathetic nerves have opposite effects on many organs (Table 14-2).**

What Are the Special Characteristics of the Nervous System?

⊿ Although some cells in the PNS have an outer membrane called the neurilemma that may regenerate after damage, cells of the CNS do not have this capability. **Once destroyed, cells in the brain cannot be replaced.**

⊿ Neurons are very sensitive to oxygen and die quickly when deprived of oxygen. **The brain's neurons cannot survive anoxia for more than 4 to 6 minutes.**

What Changes Occur in the Nervous System with Aging?

⊿ There is a loss of neurons with aging, and brain weight may drop considerably after age 70; there is no loss of intellectual function attributable to this loss of neurons.

⊿ The number of functioning dendrites decreases with aging. The decrease causes slower impulse transmission and resultant slower reaction time in the older person.

⊿ Blood flow to the brain is decreased with advanced age; this makes the elderly more susceptible to permanent damage if blood flow to the brain is further compromised.

⊿ Loss of neurons and slower nerve conduction cause a decrease in efficiency of the autonomic nervous system in old age.

⊿ Body homeostasis is more difficult to maintain or regain in the elderly. Exposure to prolonged, profound cold or to excessive heat may cause death. Adaptation to physiological stress takes much longer, and recovery often is incomplete.

⊿ Recent, short-term memory is affected by the aging process, but long-term, distant, memory is not affected. The ability to learn is not affected by aging, but the learning process is slower. It takes longer to process new information. Abstract reasoning ability slowly diminishes in the very old, and perception may become impaired.

⊿ Decreases in secretion of the neurotransmitters norepinephrine and dopamine occur, and there is an increase in monoamine oxidase (MAO).

⊿ The number of posterior root nerve fibers and sympathetic nerve fibers of the autonomic nervous system declines in the spinal cord. In the PNS the motor nerve fibers and the myelin sheath degenerate with advancing age; reflexes may be diminished or absent in the very old.

⊿ Utilizing the brain and keeping it active promotes continued intellectual function in the healthy elderly.

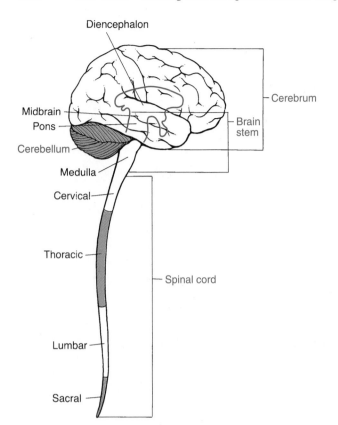

FIGURE 14-1   Main divisions of the central nervous system. (*Source:* Monahan, F. D., Drake, T., Neighbors, M. [1994]. *Nursing Care of Adults.* Philadelphia: Saunders, p. 1451.)

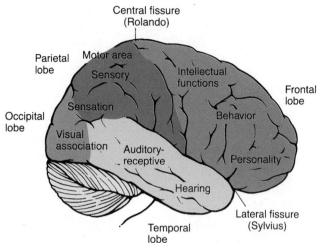

FIGURE 14-2   Specialized functions of the lobes of the cerebrum. (*Source:* Monahan, F. D., Drake, T., Neighbors, M. [1994]. *Nursing Care of Adults.* Philadelphia: Saunders, p. 1451.)

The student is referred to an anatomy and physiology text for a thorough review of this complex system.

CAUSATIVE FACTORS INVOLVED IN NEUROLOGICAL DISORDERS

Many factors can affect neurological function. Genetic and acquired developmental disorders, infections and inflammation, benign and malignant tumors, vascular or neuromuscular degeneration, metabolic and endocrine disorders all can cause damage or interfere with normal function of the nervous system. Chemical or physical trauma often causes permanent damage to the brain or spinal cord. Table 14-3 lists by category the most common neurological disorders in the adult.

PREVENTION OF NEUROLOGICAL DISORDERS

Nurses can help prevent neurological problems in many ways. The goals for *Healthy people 2000: National health promotion and disease prevention objectives*

TABLE 14-1   ◆   *Functions of the Divisions of the Brain*

Division	Function
Cerebrum	Center of intellect and consciousness.
	Receives and interprets sensory information; controls voluntary movements and certain types of involuntary movements; responsible for thinking, learning, language capability, judgment, and personality; stores memories.
Cerebellum	Responsible for coordination of movement, posture, and muscle tone that are the mechanisms of balance.
Diencephalon	Consists of two parts.
Thalamus	Relay center between spinal cord and cerebrum.
Hypothalamus	Controls body temperature, appetite and water balance; links nervous and endocrine systems.
Brainstem	
Midbrain	Mediates visual and auditory reflexes; controls cranial nerves III and IV and certain eye movements.
Pons	Links connecting various parts of the brain; helps regulate respiration.
Medulla oblongata	Contains reticular formation that regulates heart beat, respiration, and blood pressure; controls center for swallowing, coughing, sneezing, and vomiting; relays messages to other parts of the brain.

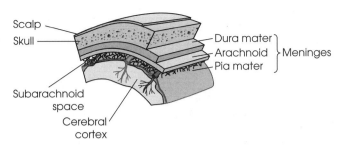

FIGURE 14-3 Meninges of the central nervous system.

encourage health protection through education about safety and responsible self-care. Teaching about head and spine injury prevention involves encouraging people to wear helmets when biking, in-line skating, skate boarding, or riding motorcycles, and when involved in other sports activities that may lead to head injury. Observing safety precautions when diving and swimming, such as never diving into water of unknown depth, helps prevent spinal cord injury. Wearing seat belts in cars and generally consciously trying to avoid accidents, both when driving and walking, decrease the incidence of neurological trauma. Teaching the dangers of recreational drug use, such as the possibility of stroke from the use of "crack" cocaine and the potential for accidents under the influence of some drugs, is another area for public education. Informing the public about the damaging

effect on brain cells of too much alcohol, as well as the increased incidence of accidents, is another area for teaching.

Promoting immunizations against tetanus, poliomyelitis, and infectious diseases that may cause high fever and resultant brain damage is an area where nurses can be effective. **Working to decrease the incidence of hypertension and to provide good control for those afflicted with this disorder can readily reduce the number of strokes and the damage they cause.** Promoting the benefits of a low-fat diet to decrease plaque buildup from atherosclerosis can help reduce the incidence of stroke as well as help to prevent heart disease. Nurses can be effective agents for preventing neurological disorders.

TERMS COMMONLY USED FOR NEUROLOGICAL DISORDERS

As with other medical terms, those used in neurology are combinations of Greek and Latin prefixes and suffixes. The prefixes *a-, dys-, hypo-,* and *hyper-* are probably familiar. Some prefixes and less commonly used suffixes related to disorders of the nervous system may not be so familiar. The following is a list of terms frequently encountered in neurological nursing:

◆ *Aphasia:* loss of the function of speech.
◆ *Dysphasia:* impairment of or difficult speech.
◆ *Dysphagia:* difficulty swallowing.
◆ *Dysarthria:* slurring or indistinct speech articulation.
◆ *Atrophy:* wasting or a decrease in size from lack of use.
◆ *Hypertrophy* of muscle: enlargement of muscle tissue.
◆ *Ataxia:* unsteadiness or lack of coordination.
◆ *Apraxia* or *dyspraxia:* loss or impairment of acquired motor skills.
◆ *Agnosia:* loss of the ability to recognize and interpret sensory information (i.e., unable to recognize use of simple objects).
◆ *Hemianopsia:* blindness for half the field of vision in one or both eyes.
◆ *Hypoesthesia* (sometimes called *hypesthesia*): reduced sensation.
◆ *Hemiparesthesia:* reduced sensation on one side.
◆ *Monoplegia:* weakness of one limb.
◆ *Hemiplegia:* paralysis of arm and leg on one side of the body.
◆ *Paraplegia:* paralysis of the lower limbs.

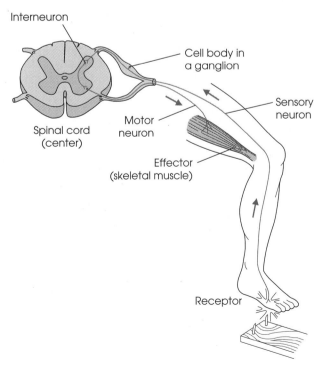

FIGURE 14-4 Components of a generalized reflex arc.

TABLE 14-2 ◆ *Autonomic Effects on Various Organs of the Body*

Organ	Effect on Sympathetic Stimulation	Effect of Parasympathetic Stimulation
Eye		
Pupil	Dilated	Constricted
Ciliary muscle	Slight relaxation (far vision)	Constricted (near vision)
Glands	Vasoconstriction and slight secretion	Stimulation of copious secretion (containing many enzymes for enzyme-secreting glands)
Nasal		
Lacrimal		
Parotid		
Submandibular		
Gastric		
Pancreatic		
Sweat glands	Copious sweating (cholinergic)	Sweating on palms of hands
Apocrine glands	Thick, odoriferous secretion	None
Blood vessels	Most often constricted	Most often little or no effect
Heart		
Muscle	Increased rate	Slowed rate
	Increased force of contraction	Decreased force of contraction (especially of atria)
Coronaries	Dilated (β_2); constricted (α)	Dilated
Lungs		
Bronchi	Dilated	Constricted
Blood vessels	Mildly constricted	? Dilated
Gut		
Lumen	Decreased peristalsis and tone	Increased peristalsis and tone
Sphincter	Increased tone (most times)	Relaxed (most times)
Liver	Glucose released	Slight glycogen synthesis
Gallbladder and bile ducts	Relaxed	Contracted
Kidney	Decreased output and renin secretion	None
Bladder		
Detrusor	Relaxed (slight)	Contracted
Trigone	Contracted	Relaxed
Penis	Ejaculation	Erection
Systemic arterioles		
Abdominal viscera	Constricted	None
Muscle	Constricted (adrenergic α)	None
	Dilated (adrenergic β_2)	
	Dilated (cholinergic)	
Skin	Constricted	None
Blood		
Coagulation	Increased	None
Glucose	Increased	None
Lipids	Increased	None
Basal metabolism	Increased up to 100%	None
Adrenal medullary secretion	Increased	None
Mental activity	Increased	None
Piloerector muscles	Contracted	None
Skeletal muscle	Increased glycogenolysis	None
	Increased strength	
Fat cells	Lipolysis	None

Source: Guyton, A. C., Hall, J. E. (1996). *Textbook of Medical Physiology,* 9th ed, Philadelphia: Saunders, p. 775.

TABLE 14-3 ◆ *Classification of Common Neurological Disorders*

Genetic/developmental disorders
   Cerebral palsy
   Muscular dystrophy
   Huntington's disease
Trauma
   Head injury
   Penetrating brain injury
   Spinal cord injury
   Ruptured intervertebral disc
Cerebrovascular
   Cerebrovascular accident
     Ruptured aneurysm
   Arteriovenous malformation
   Headache
Tumor
   Brain tumor
   Spinal cord tumor
Infection
   Meningitis
   Encephalitis
   Brain abscess
   Poliomyelitis
   Guillain-Barré
Neuromuscular disorders
   Multiple sclerosis
   Myasthenia gravis
   Amyotrophic lateral sclerosis
Degenerative disorders
   Parkinson's disease
   Alzheimer's disease
Cranial nerve disorders
   Bell's palsy
   Trigeminal neuralgia

◆ *Quadriplegia* (sometimes called *tetraplegia*): paralysis of all four limbs.
◆ *Monoparesis:* weakness of one limb.

EVALUATION OF NEUROLOGICAL STATUS

The complete neurological examination performed by the physician, physician's assistant, or advanced practice registered nurse, systematically measures the ability of the body to perform its myriad motor and sensory functions. Mental acuity, memory, and emotional stability also are assessed. The physical examination to identify problems of motor and sensory function is a very long procedure and may be performed in stages over several days. However, gross assessment of the cranial nerves, coordination and balance, muscle strength, and reflexes is standard for every patient with a neurological complaint.

◆Cranial Nerves

The 12 cranial nerves (designated as CN I through CN XII) control both sensory and motor activities within various parts of the body. The patient may be tested for his sense of smell (CN I), sight and pupil constriction (CN II, III), hearing and balance (CN VIII). The ability to change facial expression (CN V, VII, XII), gag reflex and swallowing (CN IX, X), ability to move his eyes (CN IV, VI), and head and shoulder movement (CN XI) also are evaluated. Table 14-4 presents the cranial nerves and their functions.

TABLE 14-4 ◆ *The Cranial Nerves and Their Functions*

Cranial Nerve	Type and Function
Olfactory (CN I)	*Sensory:* smell.
Optic (CN II)	*Sensory:* visual acuity, field of vision, pupillary response (afferent impulse).
Oculomotor (CN III)	*Motor:* eyelid elevation, extraocular eye movement, pupil size, convergence, pupillary constriction (efferent impulse).
Trochlear (CN IV)	*Motor:* extraocular eye movement (inferior and lateral).
Trigeminal (CN V)	*Sensory:* corneal reflex. *Motor:* facial sensation, chewing, biting, lateral jaw movement.
Abducens (CN VI)	*Motor:* extraocular eye movement (lateral).
Facial (CN VII)	*Sensory:* taste. *Motor:* facial muscle movement, including muscles of expression; lacrimal gland and salivary gland control.
Acoustic (CN VIII)	*Sensory:* hearing, sense of balance.
Glossopharyngeal (CN IX)	*Sensory:* sensations of the throat, taste (posterior tongue). *Motor:* gagging and swallowing movements.
Vagus (CN X)	*Sensory:* sensations of posterior tongue, throat, larynx; impulses from heart, lungs, bronchi, and gastrointestinal tract. *Motor:* movement of soft palate, vocal quality of speech, swallowing, gag reflex; parasympathetic activity of the thoracic and abdominal viscera, such as decreased heart rate and increased peristalsis.
Spinal accessory (CN XI)	*Motor:* Shoulder movement and head rotation.
Hypoglossal (CN XII)	*Motor:* Tongue movement, articulation of speech.

◆ Coordination and Balance

This portion of the neurological examination evaluates functions controlled by the higher centers of the brain, the cerebrum and cerebellum. During the examination, the patient is asked to stand with his feet together and close his eyes. If his sense of balance is normal, he will maintain a steady posture and not sway from side to side. He is then asked to walk across the room, and his gait is assessed. Next the examiner stands in front of the patient, holds up a finger, and asks the patient to touch his finger and then his own nose; the examiner moves his own finger to different locations in front of the patient. This tests both the ability to follow directions and coordination.

◆ Neuromuscular Function Testing

Groups of large muscles are tested for strength and coordination. The physician may evaluate the patient's gait while walking, the strength of his hand grip, and the strength of his arms and legs as he pushes against resistance. More sophisticated tests include electromyography (see Table 14-5).

◆ Reflexes

A reflex is an action or movement that is built into the nervous system and does not need the intervention of conscious thought to take place. In other words, it is an automatic response. The knee jerk is an example of the simplest type of reflex. When the knee is tapped, the nerve that receives this stimulus sends an impulse to the spinal cord, where it is relayed to a motor nerve. This causes the quadriceps muscle at the front of the thigh to contract and to jerk the leg upward. This reflex, or simple reflex arc, involves only two nerves and one synapse. The leg begins to jerk up while the brain is just becoming aware of the tap on the knee (Figure 14-4).

The knee jerk, or patellar reflex, tests nerve pathways to and from the spinal cord at the level of the second through fourth lumbar nerves. In addition to testing the patellar reflex, a neurological examination also might include testing the biceps reflex (pathways for the fifth and sixth cervical nerves), triceps reflex (seventh and eighth cervical nerves), brachioradialis reflex (fifth and sixth cervical nerves), and achilles tendon reflex (first and second sacral nerves).

Another reflex action widely used as a diagnostic aid in CNS disorders is the *Babinski reflex,* which is elicited by scraping an object such as a key along the sole of the foot. In a normal response to this stimulus the toes will bend downward. In a *positive* Babinski reflex, the great toe bends backward (upward) and the smaller toes fan outward. A positive Babinski reflex in the person not under the influence of chemical substances indicates an abnormality in the motor control pathways leading from the cerebral cortex (Figure 14-6).

In the unconscious person the physician may perform tests of brainstem function. After ruling out spinal cord injury, the oculocephalic ("doll's eyes") and oculovestibular reflexes are assessed. For the doll's eyes reflex, the examiner places both hands on the sides of the patient's head, using the thumbs to gently hold open his eyelids; while watching the patient's eyes, the head is rotated briskly to one side and eye movement is observed in relation to head movement. If the brainstem pathways are intact, the eyes appear to move in a direction opposite to that of the head movement, that is, if the head is rotated to the right, the eyes appear to move to the left. After ruling out a ruptured tympanic membrane, the oculovestibular reflex is assessed by *caloric* testing. With the patient's head elevated at least 30 degrees, 20 to 200 mL of cold or ice water is instilled into the ear with a catheter-tipped syringe. While the external ear canal is irrigated, the patient's eye movements are observed. Normally the eyes will show nystagmus, darting away from the irrigated ear. Absence of eye movement indicates a brainstem lesion.

◆ Diagnostic Tests

The major diagnostic tests most commonly used to evaluate the neurological system are presented in Table 14-5. Basic physiological testing also is done to rule out disease in some other system that might be affecting the condition of the patient. A chest radiograph, electrocardiogram (EKG), complete blood cell (CBC) count, urinalysis, and basic tests for electrolytes, liver function, kidney function, nutritional parameters, and lipid metabolism (such as are included on a sequential multiple analyzer [SMA] profile) are performed. A nerve or muscle biopsy may be done to determine pathological changes in these tissues. Flexible fiberoptic myeloscopy has been approved by the FDA. This tool can document adhesions, scar tissue, and inflamation around spinal nerves which then can be removed or treated during the procedure. This holds great promise for the treatment of chronic back pain.

NURSING ASSESSMENT OF NEUROLOGICAL STATUS

Neurological nursing requires special training and experience in observation, critical judgment, and specific skills to help patients cope with a myriad of problems. The nurse not only must be aware of subtle changes in the patient's condition but also must recognize the *significance* of these changes and act promptly when medical attention is needed. In a text such as this we can

Text continued on page 334

TABLE 14-5 ◆ *Diagnostic Tests for Neurological Problems*

Test	Purpose	Description	Nursing Implications
Lumbar puncture (spinal tap)	To determine if CSF pressure is elevated; to determine if there is a blockage to the flow of CSF; to inject medication; to obtain fluid for chemical analysis and culture.	Physician performs a sterile puncture into the arachnoid space, using local anesthetic, between L-3 and L-4 or L-4 and L-5; opening pressure is obtained; fluid is aspirated and placed in sterile test tubes labeled 1, 2, 3. Fluid is analyzed for color, pH, cell count, protein, chloride, and glucose; a culture is usually done.	Obtain signature on consent form. Obtain sterile lumbar puncture tray, local anesthetic, sterile gloves, and tape. Assist patient into position with back bowed, head flexed on chest, and knees drawn up to the abdomen. Patient may be lying or sitting. Assist him to maintain position and to hold still during procedure. Reassure patient and provide emotional support. Appropriately label tubes with patient data afterward and transport them to the laboratory immediately. Keep patient flat in bed to reduce headache for 6 to 8 hours after procedure and encourage fluid intake unless contraindicated. Observe the site for signs of drainage and inflammation.
Electroencephalogram (EEG)	To detect abnormal brain wave patterns that are indicative of specific diseases, such as seizure disorder, brain tumor, CVA, head trauma, and infection; to determine cerebral death.	May be performed while asleep, awake, drowsy, or undergoing stimulation such as hyperventilation or rhythmic bright light. Hair should be clean and dry. No sleeping pills or sedatives the night before test; check with physician regarding other drugs to be held; restrict coffee, tea, caffeine, and alcohol for 24 to 48 hours; tracing is taken with patient in reclining chair or lying down. Test takes 45 minutes to 2 hours. Electrodes are applied to the scalp with an electrode paste. If a sleep EEG is ordered, patient may need to be kept up most or all of the night prior to the test; do not keep NPO, as hypoglycemia can affect the test.	Explain purpose of test to the patient; assure him he will not receive an electric shock, the test is not painful, and that the machine does not determine intelligence or read his mind. Test may be done at the bedside or in the EEG lab. Wash hair to remove the electrode paste.
Electromyography (EMG)	To measure electrical activity of skeletal muscle at rest and during voluntary activity to determine abnormalities in muscular contraction. Helpful in diagnosing neuromuscular, peripheral nerve, and muscular disorders.	With the patient sitting in a chair or lying on a table, needle electrodes are inserted in selected muscles. Tracings of electrical activity are taken with the muscles at rest then with various voluntary activities that produce muscle contraction. The test takes 1 to 2 hours depending on how many muscles are tested.	Obtain signed informed consent. Explain the procedure to the patient; tell him that there is discomfort when the electrodes are placed. Check with physician regarding medications to be withheld; muscle relaxants, cholinergics, and anticholinergics can influence test result. There is no food or fluid restriction. If serum enzymes are ordered, they should be drawn before the EMG.

(Table 14-5 continued)

TABLE 14-5 ◆ *Diagnostic Tests for Neurological Problems* (Continued)

Test	Purpose	Description	Nursing Implications
Myelogram	To detect spinal lesions; intervertebral disc problems, tumors, or cysts.	Contrast media is injected into the spinal canal (Fig. 14-5), and fluoroscopic examination and radiographs are made. The study is contraindicated if the patient has increased ICP. The patient is placed prone and strapped to the x-ray table for the spinal puncture; as the contrast medium is injected, the table is tilted. After the test, if oil-base medium was used, it is withdrawn. The patient is kept in bed with head of bed elevated 60 degrees or flat depending on the contrast medium used. Procedure takes 1 hour.	Requires a signed consent. Explain what to expect. Patient may feel a warm flush when contrast medium is injected. Bowel evacuation regimen may be ordered the night before. Keep NPO for 4 to 8 hours prior to procedure. Check for medications to be withheld before and for 48 hours posttest. Assess for allergy to iodine or shellfish. Dress in myelogram pajamas; administer preoperative sedative or analgesic. Posttest: monitor VS q 30 min × 2 h, then 1 h × 4 h. Assess pulses and sensation in extremities; monitor urinary output; catheterize if patient cannot void in 8 h as ordered; encourage increased fluid intake. Observe for signs of meningitis.
Computerized axial tomography (CAT or CT Scan)	To examine the brain from many different angles, obtaining a series of cross-sectional images that provide views from three dimensions. To identify hematomas, tumors, cysts, hydrocephalus, cerebral atrophy, obstruction to CSF flow, and cerebral edema.	May be done with or without contrast dye enhancement. Patient lies on a narrow table with his head cradled and is moved so that his head is inside the circular opening of the machine. A security strap is wrapped snugly around him. CT scanner produces a narrow x-ray beam. Various clicking and whirring noises are heard as the machine rotates the scanner for different views. If contrast dye is used, the patient will feel a warm flush and have a metallic taste in his mouth as it is injected. The test takes 45 minutes to 1½ hours. The patient may need to be sedated if he is prone to claustrophobia; the table can be uncomfortable for those with arthritis or back problems. He will be able to communicate with the machine's operator.	A consent form is required. Explain the procedure and what he will see, hear, and feel. Patient should be NPO for 3 to 4 hours prior to test if contrast dye is to be used to prevent vomiting. Assess for allergy to iodine or shellfish. Remove all hairpins, jewelry, and metal from the head and neck.
Cerebral angiography	To visualize the structure of the cerebral arteries to determine presence of stricture, tumor, aneurysm, thrombus, or hematoma.	Radiopaque liquid is injected through a catheter inserted into the common carotid artery, and a series of radiographs is taken. Fluoroscopy is used during the procedure. Digital subtraction angiography (DSA) is done by utilizing a computer along with the angiography procedure.	Consent form is required. Assess for allergy to iodine and shellfish. Explain procedure; patient will be supine on x-ray table; local anesthetic will be used to introduce the catheter; an IV will be started in case of need for emergency drugs; patient will feel a flush as the dye is injected; test takes 1 to 2

TABLE 14-5 ◆ *Diagnostic Tests for Neurological Problems* (Continued)

Test	Purpose	Description	Nursing Implications
			hours. Should be NPO 8 to 12 hours prior to test; anticoagulants are discontinued beforehand. May be given preprocedure sedative, antihistamine, or steroid to decrease possibility of allergic reaction to dye. Postprocedure: assess for bleeding at site; assess distal pulses; perform neurological checks; monitor vital signs q 15 min × 1 h; q 30 min × 2 h; q 1 h × 4 h or until stable. Assess for dysphagia and respiratory distress that could indicate internal bleeding in the neck. Activities are restricted for 24 hours.
Radionuclide imaging (brain scan)	To detect an intracranial mass: tumor, abscess, hematoma, aneurysm	A radioisotope is administered IV. Abnormal tissue usually absorbs more of the isotope than normal tissue. After a 1- to 3-hour waiting period for absorption, a scintillation scanner is used to image the brain. The test takes ½ to 1 hour.	Explain the procedure; patient will sit or lie on a table; the scanner makes clicking noises; the amount of radioactivity is very low and is not dangerous to the patient or others. Patient will need to lie or sit still during the scanning. A drug may be given the night before to block uptake of the radioactive element by the thyroid and salivary glands. There is no food or fluid restriction; no special aftercare.
Magnetic resonance imaging (MRI)	To visualize soft tissue without the use of contrast media or ionizing radiation; provides excellent images of soft tissue, eliminating bone; can visualize lesions undetected by CT scan. To detect white matter areas in nervous system that represent demyelination, as in multiple sclerosis.	An electromagnet is used to detect radio frequency pulses produced by alignment of hydrogen protons in the magnetic field. Computer produces tomographic images with high contrast of area studied. Cannot be used in the presence of metal. Is quite expensive. A contrast agent often is used for better visualization and definition of specific structures.	Inform patient that the test is painless; no dietary restrictions. Remove all metal objects before test. Screen the patient for hidden sources of metal, such as bullet fragments, iron filings, aneurysm clips. MRI is contraindicated for patients with pacemakers. Patient must be still during test. Explain that body part to be imaged is moved inside large machine; some patients become claustrophobic.
Ultrasound arteriography (Doppler flow studies)	To study flow and determine areas of constriction or obstruction in cerebral arteries. To detect arterial spasm.	Nonivnasive test. Doppler image scanning device is used with computer to visualize anatomy of major cerebral arteries.	Tell patient that the test is painless. A small Doppler wand is positioned over particular "window" areas on the skull (temples), and with the computer, sound waves are directed so as to produce an image of the interior arteries and their blood flow. No special preparation or aftercare.

(Table 14-5 continued)

TABLE 14-5 ◆ *Diagnostic Tests for Neurological Problems* (Continued)			
Test	**Purpose**	**Description**	**Nursing Implications**
Evoked potential studies	To measure response of the CNS to visual, auditory, or sensory stimulus. Helpful in detecting tumor of CN VIII, blindness in infants, or brain stem lesions. Also useful in diagnosing multiple sclerosis.	May be done in conjunction with EEG. Electrodes are used to pick up and transmit impulses to a computer while a stimulus is delivered to the patient. Signals are displayed on an oscilloscope, and data are stored for later interpretation.	Explain the procedure to the patient. Visual evoked responses: stimulus may be a bright flashing light or checkerboard patterns. Somatosensory evoked potentials require stimulation of a peripheral sensory nerve with a mild electric shock. Auditory brainstem evoked potentials utilize various noises or tone bursts through earphones. Discomfort is minimal. Test takes 30 to 60 minutes.
Cerebrospinal fluid analysis and culture	To detect abnormalities that are indicative of specific neurological problems and determine which organism is responsible for infection.	CSF is obtained by lumbar puncture. It is analyzed for color, cell count, protein, chloride, and glucose. The fluid is cultured to detect the presence of organisms; if present, an antibiotic sensitivity test is done to determine which drug will best kill the organism. CSF pressure also is measured. Normal CSF values for the adult are: Color: clear Cell count (WBCs): 0 to 8 cu mm Protein: 15 to 45 mg/dL Chloride: 118 to 132 mEq/L Glucose: 40 to 80 mg/dL Pressure: 75 to 175 mm H_2O	Follow lumbar puncture procedure (above). Label the test tubes #1, 2, 3 and be certain they are filled with at least 3 mL of CSF in this order. Do not refrigerate the tubes; transport to the lab immediately. Maintain *standard precautions*.

cover only the most basic of skills and knowledge required in neurological nursing. It is extremely important that the nurse who is sharing responsibility for the care of a patient with a neurological disorder acknowledge strengths and weaknesses and seek guidance if unsure of his or her ability to observe and evaluate a patient's status.

◆ Patient History

Because neurological disorders can be present in conjunction with or in addition to disorders of other body systems, the nurse should always include questions about neurological status in the initial and ongoing assessments of all patients. For example, a surgical patient could well have had a previous stroke, a history of seizures, or an existing neuromuscular disease such as multiple sclerosis. Although these may not be the primary reason for admission to a hospital, they will certainly influence the course of the illness or injury for which admission occurred.

Questions that the nurse should ask when assessing a patient with an actual or possible neurological problem are presented in Table 14-6.

◆ Physical Assessment

The nurse can perform a basic assessment of neurological function on any patient who is suspected of experiencing a neurological problem. Such an exam is done to alert the patient to the need for a more in-depth examination by the physician. Nurses in long-term care facilities or home care nurses often need to assess the occurrence of cerebrovascular accident (CVA, stroke) or of neurological deficit. Basic neurological assessment includes assessment of the following areas.

Vital Signs   Current vital signs should be compared to those from the previous several days to determine any changes or trends. Look for changes in blood pressure, pulse rate and quality, and in respiratory pattern and for rising temperature.

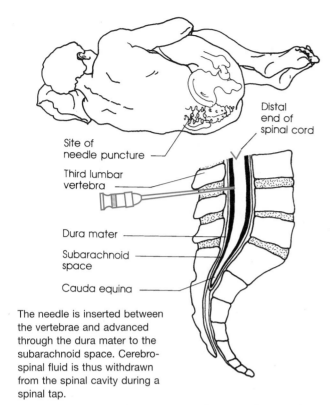

Distal end of spinal cord

Site of needle puncture

Third lumbar vertebra

Dura mater

Subarachnoid space

Cauda equina

The needle is inserted between the vertebrae and advanced through the dura mater to the subarachnoid space. Cerebrospinal fluid is thus withdrawn from the spinal cavity during a spinal tap.

FIGURE 14-5   Lumbar puncture technique. The neurologist may prefer to position the patient sitting on the side of the bed, leaning over the overbed table to expose the lumbar area.

Mental Function   The nurse assesses changes in mental function by asking questions to determine orientation to person, place, and time. What day is today? What month is it? Where are you now? Checking for

TABLE 14-6 ✦ *Nursing Assessment of Neurological Status: Questions to Ask*

When gathering history for the patient who may have a neurological problem, ask the following questions:

- ◆ Do you or any member of your family have any genetic disorder of the nervous system?
- ◆ Have you ever had a seizure or been told you have epilepsy?
- ◆ Have you ever had difficulty in speaking, concentrating, remembering, or expressing thoughts? Have you noticed any changes in these functions?
- ◆ Have you had any changes in muscle strength or coordination?
- ◆ Have you ever injured your head?
- ◆ Have you ever had a really high fever?
- ◆ Have you had any severe sinus, ear, tooth, or facial skin infection?
- ◆ Do you recall any episodes of tremors, muscle spasms, fainting, dizziness, ringing in the ears, or blurred vision?
- ◆ Have you had any "black out" spells?
- ◆ Have you noticed any changes in taste or smell?
- ◆ Do you have any numbness or tingling in the extremities?

memory lapses may be done by asking when the patient was born, what state he is in, what the last major holiday was, and so on. Thinking can be evaluated by asking the patient to add three numbers together; count by 6's; solve a simple puzzle, such as "If a man goes to the store and purchases four oranges at $.40 each, two apples at $.60 each, and two bananas for $.46, how much did he spend? (Allow pencil and paper to be used.) If the patient can read English, hand him a card with a command written on it, such as "walk to the sink" or "turn on your right side" (assuming he is physically capable of performing such a task).

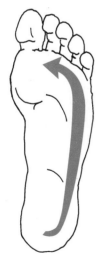

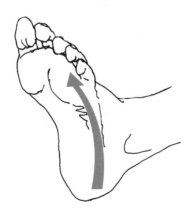

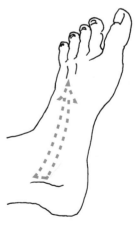

A. Line of stimulation: outer sole, heel to little toe.

B. Plantar (normal) reflex. Toes curl inward.

C. Positive Babinski reflex (always abnormal). Great toe bends upward; smaller toes fan outward.

FIGURE 14-6   Normal and Babinski reflexes.

Judgment can be grossly tested by assessing whether the patient has been making rational choices in his day-to-day life and by asking him what he would do in a particular situation. Asking specifically what he would do if there was a fire in the trash can will provide information about his judgment.

Neurological and Neuromuscular Status   Basic assessment of cranial nerves and motor function can be performed by watching the patient perform morning activities of daily living (ADLs). Does the face move symmetrically when he smiles, is speech clear when he answers questions? Does he move left and right extremities without noticeable problems? Is there anything abnormal about his gait as he moves across the room or down the hall? Does he have difficulty eating or swallowing? Observe the pupils of the eye for size and equality. Can he hear you if you speak to him when his back is turned? Does he seem as alert as usual? Is he having any trouble with balance?

Extraocular muscle movements are also checked. Ask the patient to follow your finger while you move it through the "cardinal points" (Figure 14-7). Note whether both eyes move together (*conjugate*) or one deviates. If there is deviation, it is important to note in which direction the deviation is. It should be noted if there is any quick back-and-forth oscillation (**nystagmus**) of the eye at the end points of each direction. Nystagmus can indicate abnormality or can be a side effect of medication, such as phenytoin (Dilantin).

> An important aspect of neurological assessment is to look for changes in the patient from one day to the next.

◆ Monitoring Neurological Status (the Neuro "Check")

Monitoring the neurological status of a patient with a known neurological disorder includes a "neuro check" on a set schedule. It is performed to determine whether intracranial pressure (ICP) is rising. For example, monitoring is necessary after a traumatic head injury, after ingestion of an overdose of a drug or other chemical, when a stroke has occurred or is suspected, or for any other condition in which the patient has lost or may lose consciousness. A neurological assessment flowsheet is used to chart assessment data so that the trend in function of each area can be quickly identified (Figure 14-8). Four areas are monitored: vital signs, level of consciousness (LOC), pupil reaction, and motor function.

Vital Signs   Assessing and recording temperature, pulse, respirations, and blood pressure are essential. Temperature is important for a number of reasons; an infection may be developing, or there may be damage to the temperature control mechanisms within the brain from increasing ICP.

Changes in blood pressure, particularly a rise in systolic pressure and a widening of pulse pressure, may indicate an ICP increase. The pulse may become slow and bounding, and breathing may become irregular and labored as ICP rises. Changes in breathing pattern often indicate a problem with neurological control of respiration. Any identified change must be reported to the physician promptly.

Level of Consciousness   Changes in the ability of the patient to respond appropriately to whatever is going on around him are not always readily apparent. Patients experience varying levels of awareness and ability to respond. It is necessary to determine where the patient is on a scale of varying degrees of consciousness, the extremes of the scale being alert wakefulness and deep coma (no responsiveness at all).

When observing a patient for LOC, the best assessment is based on established criteria or standards that are understood by the observer as well as by others who will be reading the results of the observations. The Glasgow Coma Scale is a tool that is universally used in one form or another for this purpose (Table 14-7). The nurse gives a rating to the patient in three different categories. The first category is eye opening, the second is best verbal response, and the third is best motor response. A number is assigned for each category

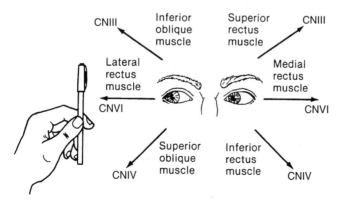

FIGURE 14-7   Cardinal points of eye movement used to check cranial nerves CNIII, CNIV, and CNVI.
(*Source:* deWit, S. C. [1994]. *Rambo's Nursing Skills for Clinical Practice,* 4th Ed. Philadelphia: Saunders, p. 311.)

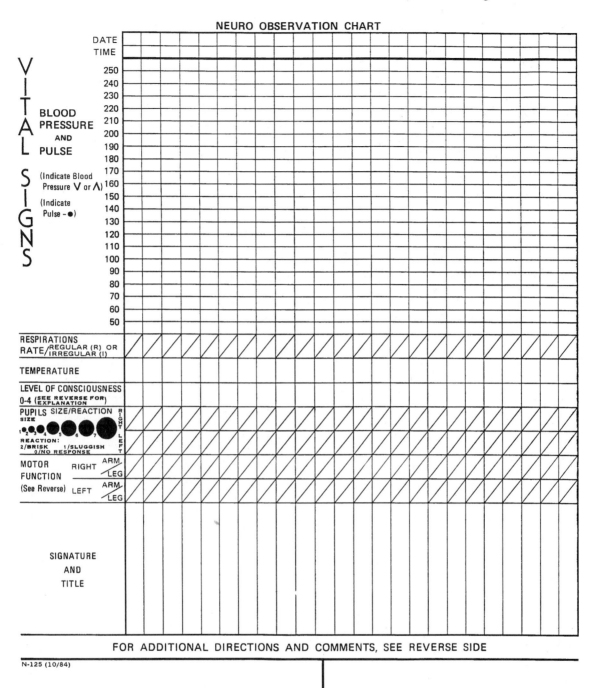

NEURO OBSERVATION CHART

VITAL SIGNS

BLOOD PRESSURE AND PULSE

(Indicate Blood Pressure V or Λ)

(Indicate Pulse - ●)

250 240 230 220 210 200 190 180 170 160 150 140 130 120 110 100 90 80 70 60 50

RESPIRATIONS RATE / REGULAR (R) OR IRREGULAR (I)

TEMPERATURE

LEVEL OF CONSCIOUSNESS 0-4 (SEE REVERSE FOR EXPLANATION)

PUPILS SIZE/REACTION SIZE

REACTION: 2/BRISK   1/SLUGGISH   0/NO RESPONSE

MOTOR FUNCTION (See Reverse) RIGHT ARM/LEG   LEFT ARM/LEG

SIGNATURE AND TITLE

FOR ADDITIONAL DIRECTIONS AND COMMENTS, SEE REVERSE SIDE

N-125 (10/84)

GOLETA VALLEY COMMUNITY HOSPITAL

NEURO OBSERVATION CHART

29A

FIGURE 14-8   Neurological Assessment Flow Sheet. (Courtesy of Goleta Valley Hospital, Goleta, California.)

Illustration continued on following page

depending on what the assessment reveals. Assessment in the first and last category determines whether the patient can respond to voice commands or to pain or doesn't respond at all. Verbal responses are evaluated according to whether the patient is oriented and "mak-ing sense," confused, making inappropriate remarks, incomprehensible, or silent. **The score in each area is added together, and the sum is compared to a score of 15, indicating a fully alert patient, and a score of 3, indicating a totally comatose patient. Coma level is in-**

DIRECTIONS

1). VITAL SIGNS:
   BLOOD PRESSURE – INDICATE ∨ AND ∧
   PULSE – INDICATE ●

2). RESPIRATION:
   RATE – INDICATE NUMBER ◺
   REGULAR OR IRREGULAR ◺R OR ◺I

3). LEVEL OF CONSCIOUSNESS:
   4 = Full orientation for time, place, and person, i.e.; fully conscious.
   3 = Talks and obeys commands, but is confused and disoriented.
   2 = Responds to stimuli with a localized and purposeful movement.
   1 = Responses to stimuli are neither localized nor purposeful.
   0 = Totally unconscious to all forms of stimulation.

4). PUPILS:
   INDICATE SIZE ◺   1● 2● 3● 4●
                     5● 6● 7●
   INDICATE REACTION ◺
   2 / Brisk
   1 / Sluggish
   0 / No response

5). MOTOR FUNCTION
   5 = Full strength
   4 = Mild weakness
   3 = Overcome gravity
   2 = Unable to oppose gravity
   1 = Muscle contractions
   0 = No movement

TIME	DATE	BRIEF COMMENTS (REFER TO NURSING NOTES FOR COMPLETE DOCUMENTATION)

FIGURE 14-8   *Continued*

dicated by a score of 7 or less. Some of the criteria are: Does he awaken easily? Is he oriented to person (himself as well as others), place, and time? Is he able to follow commands? Does he fail to respond to any stimulus, even painful ones? Is he restless? Combative? Does he respond to pain with abnormal posture?

Neuromuscular Responses   This aspect of assessment is concerned with the function of the motor pathways. Each of the upper and lower extremities is tested. Ask the patient to follow verbal commands such as "raise your left leg," "bend your right knee," "touch your left elbow with your right hand," "touch your face with your left hand." Have him push against the palms

TABLE 14-7 ♦ *Glasgow Coma Scale*	
Eye opening	
Spontaneous	4
To sound	3
To pain	2
Never	1
Motor response	
Obeys commands	6
Localizes pain	5
Normal flexion (withdrawal)	4
Abnormal flexion posturing	3
Extension posturing	2
None	1
Verbal response	
Oriented	5
Confused conversion	4
Inappropriate words	3
Incomprehensible sounds	2
None	1

A score of 7 or less indicates coma.
The highest possible score is 15.

of your hands first with one foot then the other to test the strength of the leg muscles. With his arms extended in front of him, press down on each arm one at a time, and ask him to try to raise his arm to test muscle strength.

If the patient has an extremity that is not responding, another stimulus may be necessary to test it. Gentle pressure over the tendons and joints in the extremities is preferred to pinching, deep pressure, and other painful stimuli. **Applying pressure to the nail bed with your own** fingernail or an object such as the cap of a pen is an acceptable alternative.

If the patient does not respond to voice commands at all, the degree of unconsciousness is tested. First use a louder voice to try and arouse the patient; then if he doesn't respond, gently shake him as you would to awaken a child. If that is not successful, painful stimuli are applied for 10 to 20 seconds. First try applying pressure above the eye by placing a thumb under the orbital rim beneath the middle of the eyebrow and pushing upward. If there is no response, pinch the trapezius muscle at the angle of the shoulder and neck; twist the fingers slightly. If there is still no response, the sternum is rubbed with the knuckles of the nurses fist; a twisting motion is used. **This maneuver is only performed on subsequent assessments only if there is good reason to believe that the patient's comatose status is changing, as it causes bruising.**

> The levels of response are (1) purposefully withdrawing from the stimulus or an attempt to push it away; (2) nonpurposeful response, in which the patient may frown or move his arm or leg in a random fashion; and (3) failure to respond at all.

Nonpurposeful responses to pain occur in two ways. Flexor *(decorticate)* posturing, in which one sees extension of the legs and internal rotation and adduction of the arms with the elbows bent upward, occurs with damage to the cortex. In extensor *(decerebrate)* posturing, the arms are stiffly extended and held close to the body, and the wrists are flexed outward. This response means there is damage to the midbrain or brainstem and indicates a very serious injury (Figure 14-9).

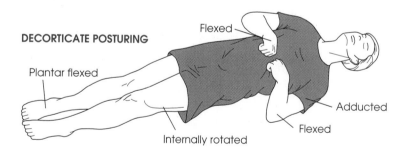

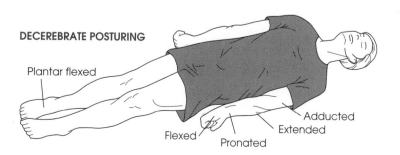

FIGURE 14-9   Decorticate and decerebrate posturing indicating brain stem injury.

The response may be "lateralization," where one side of the body shows typical decorticate or decerebrate posturing.

Pupillary Reactions   Changes in pupil size in response to a bright light are frequently used to determine whether the areas of the brainstem that help control consciousness are functioning normally. Cranial nerves II and III control pupil movement. When ICP rises beyond a certain point, pressure on these nerves cause changes in the pupils. First, if at all possible, one should know the state of the pupils that is normal for the patient. Although pupils of equal size are considered normal, some people have pupils that are unequal in size. The size of the pupils also may vary from person to person. See Figure 14-8 for a chart showing pupil sizes. It is best to measure pupil size rather than estimate it.

The pupils should be checked in a room with low light, in which one would expect the pupils to be dilated. A bright light is then directed into each eye from the side while the other eye is covered. One should observe whether the pupil into which the light is shone constricts and whether it does so briskly or sluggishly *(direct reflex)*. Finally, the light is shone into one eye while watching to see if the pupil constricts in the other eye *(consensual reflex)*. Table 14-8 shows pupil abnormalities and the possible causes. **When pupils have been previously reactive, changes in pupil size or reactivity may signal an emergency, and the physician must be notified immediately.**

If a flowsheet is not being used for charting, normal pupil responses often are charted as "PEARL," meaning "pupils equal and reactive to light."

Pupils that remain dilated and fixed in the presence of a bright light indicate brain damage. One pupil that remains fixed and dilated indicates increased ICP. If both pupils remain constricted, there probably is damage to the pons.

Although changes in the pupils, such as unequal constriction and decreased rate of constriction, indicate increased ICP, sometimes changes in pupils can be caused by medications. For example, atropine and scopolamine can produce dilated pupils, and opiates can cause constriction (Table 14-8).

"Neuro checks" may be ordered as frequently as every 15 minutes or at intervals up to 4 or 8 hours. Often they are ordered to be performed every 2 hours.

TABLE 14-8 ◆ *Pupillary Abnormalities and Possible Causes*		
Assessment Data	**Appearance**	**Possible Causes**
Unilateral, fixed, dilated pupil. Unreactive to light. May be accompanied by ptosis and deviation to side and downward.		Damage to oculomotor nerve related to increased intraocular pressure, compression of oculomotor nerve, head trauma with epidural or subdural hematoma.
Bilateral dilated and fixed pupils that do not react to light.		Hypoxia associated with cardiopulmonary arrest. Pressure on midbrain. Severe CNS disorder. Anticholinergic drug overdose.
Bilateral small, fixed pupils that do not react to light. Accompanied by motor deficits, drowsiness, confusion, headache, vomiting, incontinence when due to damage to diencephalon.		Side effect of opiates such as morphine. Miotic eye drops. Hemorrhage into the pons. Damage to the diencephalon.
Unequal pupil size; both pupils react to light unless there is underlying pathology.		Ocular inflammation. Congenital aberration. Adhesion, as of iris to cornea or lens. Disturbance of neural pathways.

The findings are recorded on the neurological flow-sheet.

Think about... You arrive at the home of an elderly lady who has severe heart disease and is very weak. Her spouse says she is confused and lethargic and that she wouldn't try to eat breakfast. He is worried. As her nurse, what specific assessments would you perform in an attempt to determine whether she has suffered a CVA?

NURSING MANAGEMENT

♦ Assessment

Nursing Diagnosis The most common nursing diagnoses for patients with neurological disorders are listed in Table 14-9. Each nursing diagnosis chosen for the patient should be individualized to fit the situation.

Nursing diagnoses in an active care plan vary according to whether the patient is in the acute stage, recovery stage, or rehabilitative stage of the disorder. Goals and general **expected outcomes** for each nursing diagnosis are presented in Table 14-9 along with appropriate interventions.

♦ Planning

Overall goals for patients with neurological disorders depend on whether there is a physiological possibility that full function may be regained or not. When neurological deficit occurs that will be permanent, such as with many spinal cord injuries, the goal is for the patient to function at the highest level physiologically possible. This requires adjusting to limitations imposed by neurological deficit so that the patient may live his life in as meaningful a way as possible. A goal for all patients with neurological disorders is to prevent injury, whether from complications of immobility, accidents related to

TABLE 14-9 ♦ *Nursing Diagnoses, Goals, Expected Outcomes, and Interventions for Common Problems of Neurological Dysfunction*

Nursing Diagnosis/Goals	Expected Outcomes	Nursing Interventions
Risk for injury related to (1) decreased level of consciousness; (2) paralysis or decreased sensation. **Goal:** no injury will be sustained.	No evidence of injury or trauma.	Siderails up at all times patient is unattended. Bed in low position when patient is unattended. Pad siderails if seizure activity or restlessness indicates need. Provide eye care for unconscious patient and if corneal (blink) reflex is absent; lubrication and eye patch or shield as needed. Position carefully, protecting extremities from contact with siderails. Maintain correct body alignment. Administer anticonvulsants as ordered to prevent seizure activity. Protect from thermal injury. Utilize hand mitts to prevent injury from dislodged tubes.
Ineffective breathing pattern related to neurological disruption of respiration. **Goal:** normal respiration.	Maintain a patent airway. Maintain a pO₂ of 80 to 100 mm Hg. No evidence of pulmonary infection.	Assess respiratory status q 2–8 h depending on patient condition. Position to maximize open airway and to promote chest expansion. Insert oropharyngeal airway as ordered. Suction secretions PRN as ordered. For controlled ventilatory support: auscultate to verify that both lungs are inflating. Check ventilator settings with those ordered. Keep alarm set to "on" at all times. Remove excess water gathering in ventilator tubing as needed. Suction client using sterile technique as ordered PRN. Monitor blood gas values for changes. Provide frequent mouth care, i.e., q 2–4 h. Monitor hydration status.
Impaired physical mobility related to CNS deficit, weakness, paralysis, or fatigue. **Goal:** regain greatest degree of mobility possible.	Maintains mobility of all joints. No evidence of contractures. Regains optimal physical mobility neurologically possible.	Perform passive ROM or supervise active ROM 4 × day. Teach ROM exercises to patient and family. Teach transfer techniques to hemiplegic patient and family. Collaborate with physical therapist to maximize activity.

(Table 14-9 continued)

TABLE 14-9 ◆ Nursing Diagnoses, Goals, Expected Outcomes, and Interventions for Common Problems of Neurological Dysfunction (Continued)

Nursing Diagnosis/Goals	Expected Outcomes	Nursing Interventions
Risk of impaired skin integrity related to impaired mobility, decreased sensory awareness, or decreased sensation. **Goal:** intact, healthy skin.	Intact skin is maintained.	Inspect pressure points for redness, warmth, tenderness, or edema each time patient is turned. Thoroughly inspect skin q shift. Position and pad joints to prevent pressure ulcers. Formulate regular turning/repositioning schedule and stick to it. Use special mattress or special bed to enhance skin protection. Teach patients in wheelchairs to shift the weight every 30 minutes. Teach patient and family to inspect pressure areas and skin for beginning signs of breakdown.
Self-care deficit related to neurological impairment: paresis, paralysis, decreased LOC, or confusion. **Goal:** performs self-care activities without assistance to degree physically and mentally possible.	Self-care needs of hygiene, toileting, feeding, and grooming will be met. Resumes self-care at level physiologically and neurologically possible.	Assist with hygiene, toileting, feeding, and grooming as needed. Assist patient to set small, attainable, goals for self-care. Explain and demonstrate specific ADL in small one-task segments. Obtain and demonstrate adaptive devices to assist with ADLs. Offer patience, support, and encouragement for each attempt at self-care. Maintain chart of self-care improvement to track achievement so that patient can see progress.
Alteration in nutrition related to inability to swallow or danger of aspiration. **Goal:** adequate nutritional intake maintained. Normal weight maintained.	Maintains adequate nutritional status as evidenced by normal weight and adequate levels of serum protein.	Institute tube feeding as needed. Check tube placement before initiating each feeding; aspirate stomach contents; test acidity if there is doubt about origins of aspirated fluid. Check residual before each intermittent feeding or every 4 hours for continuous feedings; if greater than 150 mL or more than ½ of previous feeding, replace and delay next feeding for 1 to 2 hours. Position patient with head of bed up at least 30 degrees when feeding and for 30 to 60 minutes after feeding. Monitor for adverse side effects such as diarrhea. Flush tube with 30 to 60 mL water after each feeding. Instill water between feedings to maintain hydration. Monitor glucose levels after initiation of feedings until blood glucose is stable. Weigh at least 2 × week. Monitor intake and output. **For patient with dysphagia who can take oral feedings:** serve semisoft foods. Provide six small meals per day; provide nonstressful atmosphere with few distractions for meal time; teach to sit upright with head slightly forward and neck flexed; encourage to place food on strongest side of mouth and tongue; remain with patient to decrease fear of choking; keep suction at hand and on during meal; ensure privacy for meal to decrease embarrassment about drooling, dropping food, or choking; encourage to take small bites at a time; provide appropriate tube care (see Chapter 20).
Constipation/diarrhea/bowel incontinence related to decreased level of consciousness, neurogenic impairment, or side effects of medications. **Goal:** maintenance of normal elimination pattern.	Has normal bowel movements as evidenced by soft, formed stool. Attains bowel continence.	Monitor bowel movements and evaluate regularity based on nutritional intake. Administer stool softeners, rectal suppository, or enemas as ordered for constipation. Check for and remove fecal impaction if it occurs, guarding against spinal dysreflexia in the paralyzed patient. Institute bowel training program if needed (Chapter 20). If diarrhea occurs, determine cause and alleviate if possible. Administer antidiarrheal if ordered. Keep rectal area clean and dry; protect rectal mucosa. Monitor hydration status; evaluate intake and output.

TABLE 14-9 ◆ *Nursing Diagnoses, Goals, Expected Outcomes, and Interventions for Common Problems of Neurological Dysfunction (Continued)*

Nursing Diagnosis/Goals	Expected Outcomes	Nursing Interventions
Sensory-perceptual alteration related to decreased level of consciousness. **Goal:** sensory stimulation prompts return to normal level of consciousness.	Responds to family interaction as evidenced by movement, hand squeezing, eye opening, or speech. Returns to alert state as evidenced by proper orientation to person, time and place.	Speak of current events or daily happenings while providing care. Encourage family members and friends to speak to patient of day's occurrences or fun times past. Play music on the radio that is to the patient's taste. Play videotapes on topics of interest to the patient. Turn on the patient's favorite T.V. shows. Ask questions and patiently listen for a response. With a tape recorder, introduce sounds from the patient's home and work environment.
Social isolation related to immobility and intellectual limits imposed by neurological impairment. **Goal:** participation in social relationships.	Has social interaction with visiting friends. Maintains relationships with family members and loved ones. Makes new friends among support group members.	Encourage friends and family to visit. Instruct friends and family on how to interact with the patient. Encourage patient to discuss his feelings regarding social contact. Encourage participation in an appropriate support group. Encourage development of a social network. Encourage participation in church, civic, volunteer, and social groups in community. Provide referrals to community job retraining resources if patient is unable to resume former employment or lifestyle.
Alteration in family processes related to role changes, uncertainty of the future, and financial constraints. **Goal:** each family member regains control over his life. Ongoing, open communication between family members. Shared problem solving.	Each family member demonstrates appropriate coping methods. Each family member regains an optimistic outlook. Each family member accepts the patient in his changed state. Each family member uses referrals to support groups and community resources.	Assess strengths of each family member; look for signs of stress. Provide opportunity for verbalization of fears and concerns; feelings about patient's changed condition. Refer to social worker and community resources for support services. Arrange for psychological counseling or family therapy as needed. Encourage contact with appropriate support group. Initiate interaction and honest communication between patient and family members when patient and each member is ready. Teach problem-solving methods if coping skills are weak.

lack of sensation, aspiration from difficulty in swallowing, or any of the other problems that neurological deficit may cause.

Caring for patients with neurological deficits can be very time-consuming and requires considerable patience and understanding. If the patient has any weakness, paralysis, or decreased sensation in the extremities, is confused, disoriented, aphasic, or otherwise incapacitated, providing care will take more time than usual. Plan accordingly.

When a patient is comatose or paralyzed, try to team up with another person to provide morning care and to turn or reposition the patient. By working together, care is smoother and less taxing for both the patient and the nurse.

◆ Implementation

Interventions for each nursing diagnosis for common problems of neurological disorders are listed in Table 14-9. Interventions are discussed in the following sections on common care problems and with the specific neurological disorders. The nurse provides information, teaches about the disorder and self-care, reinforces positive coping skills, and offers ongoing support.

◆ Evaluation

Evaluation of interventions is performed to see whether goals are being met. Are the interventions chosen helping to meet the specific expected outcomes written? If not, the plan needs to be changed. Progress often is slow in the patient experiencing neurological deficit. It may take a considerable time for improvement to be noted. Long-term goals of a realistic nature are appropriate. The nurse should keep in mind that certain types of neurological deficits, such as those caused by spinal cord severance, may never improve.

COMMON NEUROLOGICAL PATIENT CARE PROBLEMS

Neurological disorders and illnesses cause many of the same problems. Whether the patient has encephalitis, a head injury, is recovering from cranial surgery, has suffered a stroke, has multiple sclerosis or Parkinson's disease, he may need nursing intervention in one or more of the following areas.

◆ Ineffective Breathing

Weakness of the diaphragm, respiratory muscles, or interruption of normal brain function may occur with a variety of neurological disorders. The nurse must monitor the adequacy of respiratory effort and promote patent airway and chest expansion. Elevating the head of the bed 30 degrees lets the diaphragm drop and promotes chest expansion. When consciousness is depressed, the tongue may be flaccid and fall back, blocking the airway. Positioning the patient on the side allows the tongue to fall to the side and opens the airway. An oropharyngeal tube or oral airway also is helpful.

Assisting the patient with deep-breathing and the use of an incentive spirometer can help prevent atelectasis and improve ventilation. Respiratory assessment is performed every shift and includes auscultating the lungs for signs of atelectasis or retained secretions and judging the quality of respiratory effort. If respiratory efforts are considerably impaired, the patient may need intubation and mechanical ventilation. Interventions for the patient undergoing mechanical ventilation are presented in Chapter 16.

◆ Impaired Mobility

The nurse, the physical therapist, and the patient work together to help the patient cope with muscle weakness or paralysis. Activities such as proper positioning and range of motion (ROM) exercises are started immediately to preserve proper alignment of joints and limbs and prevent contractures and muscle atrophy. Assistive devices, such as splints and slings, may be used. The patient who suffers paralysis and loss of sensation in an extremity is taught to become aware of where that arm or leg is when he turns or transfers to a chair to avoid injury to the extremity.

The patient with left hemiplegia from a CVA may neglect his paralyzed side. He must be taught to attend to the affected side of his body by scanning it frequently. To prevent discomfort in the shoulder and arm on the affected side and to prevent dislocation of the shoulder, never pull on the affected arm or shoulder during transfers or ambulation. Support the affected arm with pillows or an armrest to keep it from dangling when the patient is seated. Use a sling for comfort and to promote better balance when ambulating and transferring.

Think about . . . Describe step by step the safest way to transfer a patient with left hemiplegia from the bed to a wheelchair.

The hemiplegic patient is taught how to transfer from the bed to a chair and back and how best to use assistance from others, if needed, for these activities. He is taught how to protect his skin in areas of decreased sensation.

The patient who has **hemiparesis** (one-sided weakness) is taught how to strengthen his muscles and use assistive devices, such as walkers, crutches, or canes, to walk. He is taught the best ways to get out of bed and into and out of a chair.

The **quadriplegic** patient (i.e., with all four limbs paralyzed) is helped to learn to cope with this drastic alteration in his life and how he might direct his energies at different, but attainable, goals.

All patients who have suffered an impairment in mobility need assistance with the grieving process, help in establishing healthy and effective coping patterns, and assistance with depression.

Attention to pain relief and muscle spasm is necessary for the patient to achieve the highest level of rehabilitation of which he is capable. Paralyzed extremities are susceptible to edema and should be elevated when the patient is at rest to decrease this problem. The patient needs to be turned frequently to prevent complications from pressure and sluggish circulation.

Elder Care Point . . . Elderly patients may suffer joint stiffness from arthritis. Assess joints before performing ROM, and be gentle and considerate when turning and repositioning.

Measures to promote skin integrity are instituted. The patient is placed on a special bed or protective mattress cover or pad, pressure points are inspected frequently, and the skin is kept clean and dry. Chapter 11 discusses the effects of immobility on each body system in detail, along with the nursing activities necessary to avoid disabilities resulting from inactivity. The principles and practices presented in that chapter are relevant to the nursing care of a patient with a neurological disorder that produces some type of paresis or paralysis and for the patient who is unconscious.

◆ Self-Care Deficit

Neuromuscular impairment may interfere with the patient's ability to perform hygiene activities or other ADLs. He may need assistance with bathing, grooming, tooth care, dressing, eating, and toileting. The nurse works with the patient as his condition dictates, assisting with techniques to perform self-care in spite of disability when possible, offering encouragement, and praising any effort at accomplishing a self-care task.

Inability to carry out the most basic of self-care activities can erode a person's sense of independence and self-esteem. The ability to feed, clothe, and take care of functions of elimination is an important part of independence. Regaining some level of self-care in these areas is of particular concern to the adult, who, because of neurological dysfunction, may have to relearn ways to perform the simplest of daily activities.

If the patient is unconscious, the mouth must be kept clean to avoid infection of the parotid gland. The lips, tongue, and gums are cleansed and lubricated at frequent intervals as mouth breathing makes them excessively dry. Cleansing may be done by turning the patient to the side, turning on suction to the mouth suction device, and with toothettes or a tongue depressor with gauze taped to it, wiping the oral surfaces. A solution of 50% water, 50% mouthwash, or water with a bit of hydrogen peroxide may be used to moisten the gauze. Too much hydrogen peroxide will cause excessive foaming. Using an irrigation syringe filled with water in one hand and the mouth suction device in the other allows rinsing of the mouth while preventing aspiration of the liquid. It is easiest for two people to work together to rinse the mouth. Each time the mouth is cleansed, the patient should be positioned on the opposite side to ensure thorough cleansing of each side of the mouth. Mouth suction should be available and on any time mouth care is given to a patient who has a weakened gag reflex, cannot swallow normally, or has weakness of the facial muscles.

When the patient cannot shut his eyes, the nurse or patient must provide care to prevent keratitis or corneal ulceration. The eyelids are cleansed with warm sterile water or normal saline every few hours to remove discharge and debris. Artificial tears or a lubricant is instilled as prescribed to prevent dryness. If the corneal reflex is absent, an eye shield or patch is placed over the eye. The eyelid is closed before a patch is applied. The eyes are examined each day for signs of inflammation.

The ability of significant others to learn how to care for the patient and their willingness to do so is an important part of assessing and planning for rehabilitation. Goals for rehabilitation must be realistic and mutually agreed on by the patient, his family, and the nurse.

There are many assistive devices to help patients with neurological deficits feed and dress themselves. Occupational therapists can help the patient relearn how to perform elementary tasks necessary to daily living. Patients are retaught how to feed themselves, how to get in and out of bed or a chair, how to select and put on clothes and fasten them, and how to bathe, brush teeth, and comb their hair.

The nurse provides assistance when the patient cannot do a task completely, and, most of all, she provides encouragement and praise for efforts made. **When pursuing self-help rehabilitation, the nurse needs to remember that the patient tires easily and tasks must be spaced apart so that energy is available to achieve them.** Pushing the patient to try yet another task when he is too tired only sets him up for failure and frustration.

◆ Dysphagia

Every patient who has suffered a neurological insult from head injury, stroke, or intracranial surgery should have his or her swallowing reflex assessed by trying to sip plain water before trying food. Checking periodically that the patient automatically swallows saliva should be done before offering water. Patients who have paresis from a stroke or who suffer from myasthenia gravis or other neurological disorders often have difficulty swallowing (**dysphagia**). Those patients who have difficulty eating are at risk for nutritional disorders. Patients with dysphagia should be sitting upright or in a high Fowler's position to eat. The position should be maintained for at least 30 minutes after the meal. A nonstressful environment without distractions is best as stress makes dysphagia worse (Table 14-10).

When swallowing without choking or aspiration is not possible, tube feeding is necessary. When the patient is receiving nutrients by tube, the caloric intake should be assessed frequently. The patient is weighed twice a week and intake and output are recorded and evaluated. Interventions for the client receiving tube feedings are outlined in Chapter 20.

◆ Incontinence

Many patients with CNS disorders experience temporary or permanent urinary or fecal incontinence. Some patients experience constipation. The patient must be kept clean and dry. A condom catheter for the male or adult diapers or incontinence pads are used for urinary incontinence.

Perhaps the first step in planning and implementing either a bladder or a bowel training program is to convince the nursing staff and the patient and his family that *something can be done* to improve, if not completely relieve, the situation. A negative attitude and lack of persistence can doom a program to failure before it is started. One must be content with small successes at first, setting short-term goals that will eventually lead to a satisfactory resolution of the problem.

TABLE 14-10 ◆ *Nutrition Point: The Patient Who Has Dypshagia*

The patient with dysphagia is in danger of aspiration of food. To help prevent aspiration, teach the patient to:

- Sit up straight to eat and tilt the head slightly forward.
- Place only one teaspoon of food in the mouth at a time.
- If the patient has paresis from a stroke, the food should be placed on the unaffected side of the mouth.
- Place the chin on the chest and swallow; wait a few seconds and swallow again.
- Refrain from taking liquids and solids at the same time.
- Refrain from using a straw.
- Remain in an upright position for 45 to 60 minutes after each meal.

Interventions to assist the patient to eat without aspirating include:

- Plan a 30-minute rest period before each meal.
- Allow plenty of time for a relaxed meal.
- Serve food at room temperature as dysphagic patients often are oversensitive to heat and cold.
- Serve semisolid foods.
- Avoid serving peanut butter, syrup, and bananas because they are sticky and difficult to swallow.
- Avoid serving dry foods, such as rice, popcorn, toast, or crackers.
- Keep the container for liquids no more than two-third full so the patient does not have to tilt the head back too far to drink.

Bladder Training Program   This is a program designed to help a person with some degree of loss of normal bladder function and a resulting disturbance of voiding and bladder control. Loss of control can occur in a variety of neurological disorders, including stroke, spinal cord injury, and tumors and lesions of the spinal cord.

The purposes of a bladder reconditioning program are to prevent urinary complications such as infection and **calculi** (stones) and to allow the patient freedom from fear of embarrassment and loss of self-esteem.

Bladder function is assessed to determine the optimal neural and muscular control that can be realistically expected in view of the physiological cause of loss of control and the patient's mental and emotional ability to cooperate and take an active part in carrying out the program.

The cause of urinary incontinence must be known, and the specific symptoms manifested by the patient must be clearly defined. Significant data would include information about (1) difficulty in initiating voiding; (2) any methods the patient may use to initiate voiding (for example, pressure on the bladder); (3) degree of awareness of the need to void; (4) ability to empty the bladder completely and amount of residual urine; (5) signs of bladder distention and dribbling or over-flow; (6) night incontinence; (7) stress incontinence; and (8) usual times for voiding.

Spinal cord injuries and lesions produce what is known as a *cord bladder* or *neurogenic bladder*. Patients with disorders of this type are not aware of the need to void and must be trained in techniques to initiate voiding and empty the bladder.

The second step in a bladder training program is to keep an accurate record of actual voiding times for a 2- to 3-day period. Some problems of incontinence can be corrected by a simple scheduling of voiding times. Offering a bedpan or getting the patient up to the bathroom one-half hour before times he is usually incontinent may remedy the problem.

A bladder retraining program usually begins with a 2-hour schedule for toileting. The patient should attempt to drink 2,000 to 3,000 mL of fluid between waking up and 6 P.M. Coffee, tea, alcoholic beverages, and soda with caffeine should be avoided near bedtime, because they have a diuretic effect. The patient is toileted before retiring for the night. The maintenance of an accurate retraining record is essential. A trial of 6 weeks is necessary before determining whether the retraining is successful. Various drugs that affect the voiding process, such as oxybutynin chloride (Ditropan) or flavoxate hydrochloride (Urispas), may be helpful for certain types of patients. The nurse must assess whether the medication is beneficial.

Patients who have nerve damage and paralysis are trained in specific techniques to empty the bladder. The Crede technique, in which the open hand is pressed over the bladder and directed toward the suprapubic area, can facilitate emptying a flaccid bladder. Self-catheterization is taught to paralyzed patients so that they are not dependent on an indwelling catheter or on other people for their urinary elimination (see Chapter 23).

Some patients are candidates for the implantation of an artificial sphincter to control bladder release of urine. More and more types of successful devices are developed each year, but these are primarily for the patient who has no neurologic control over the bladder.

Every patient undertaking a bladder retraining program needs a great deal of understanding and encouragement and a positive attitude to be successful. Praise for each small achievement should be given. Accidents should be expected and not looked on as "failures." Achieving total continence takes considerable time and effort, but for many patients it is possible.

Bowel Training Program   Bowel training for the neurological patient is done to correct incontinence or prevent constipation and impaction. The bowel training program begins with an assessment of the specific patterns of elimination. It also helps to know the patient's former bowel pattern before illness or injury. Did he regularly rely on the use of enemas or laxatives? Has he been prone to constipation? Next, the nurse needs to establish whether the patient is aware of the urge to defecate or has any warning that his bowels are about to move.

Bowel training for either constipation or incontinence should incorporate an exercise program that is within the patient's ability, a high-fiber diet, and adequate liquid intake during the day. **An accurate recording of bowel movements correlated with times of oral intake over a 2- to 3-day period will help establish the most opportune times to try to stimulate evacuation and thus establish a habit.** If incontinence has occurred at specific times after eating, toileting 30 minutes sooner and using a rectal suppository or finger to stimulate the urge to defecate may alter the pattern. Gradually the use of the suppository is discontinued.

For the patient who is prone to constipation and then incontinence, increasing liquid intake and administering a stool softener can be effective. Otherwise, a planned regimen of suppository or enema use may be necessary to assist with evacuation at a desired time, thus preventing incontinence.

All patients need to be comfortable when attempting to evacuate the bowel. A raised, padded toilet seat, handrails, and perhaps a footstool can provide enough comfort to allow the patient to relax so that evacuation can occur naturally. Privacy is essential.

Most of all, a positive attitude on the part of staff members that the problem can be overcome is needed. If the nurse and the patient are optimistic and patient, success can be achieved a great deal of the time.

◆ Pain

Many patients with neurological disorders experience pain. The pain often is chronic in nature. **The nurse must work with the patient to identify the characteristics of the pain, its location and spread, its intensity, and how it is affecting the patient's life.** When the patient has suffered a head injury or is experiencing increasing ICP, narcotic analgesics may not be given, as they mask the signs of rising ICP. Other methods of analgesia must be employed.

Pain often causes difficulty sleeping. A trusting relationship between patient and nurse is necessary to assist the patient adequately to deal with pain. Teaching the patient about pain, its relief, the adverse effect of stress, anxiety, and unpleasant stimuli, and the benefits of distraction from the pain become part of the plan. Pharmacological agents and alternative methods for pain control are used (see chapter 10).

Depression often occurs with chronic pain and lack of sleep. The combination of an antidepressant and pain medication often is more effective for chronic pain control than either type of drug used alone.

◆ Confusion

Patients with brain tumors, head injuries, and strokes, as well as degenerative diseases, may experience confusion, deficits in memory, intellectual ability, or judgment. Confusion may be acute and short term, or it may be a permanent state. Confusion also may be mild or severe and may be accompanied by anxiety, agitation, and refusal to cooperate. The person is in a state of disorientation, and until the symptoms subside, he cannot behave rationally. He must be supported and protected, or he may injure himself. In states of severe (acute) confusion (**delirium**) the patient may experience hallucinations, delusions, and severe agitation. This is usually an acute, short-term state caused by fever or metabolic imbalance. Patients who experience confusion after a head injury often become combative as their ICP rises. It is not advisable to restrain these patients, and the nurse must be very careful to stay out of range of flailing arms.

The nurse should be alert to signs of confusion in any patient with a CNS problem. Subjective and objective assessment data include (1) loss of orientation to person, place, or time; (2) inability to cooperate fully with simple tasks and requests, such as eating and bathing; (3) inappropriate statements or inappropriate answers to questions; (4) restlessness and agitation; (5) hostility and anxiety; (6) hallucinations or delusions; and (7) other signs of inability to maintain control over thought processes and behavior.

The patient who is confused needs above all else a stable and calm environment. His thought processes are, in a sense, "fractured" and somewhat beyond his control. Stimuli entering his brain are frightening and threatening to him, and he simply cannot make sense out of most of what is going on around him. A calm, consistent, and orderly approach combined with a set daily routine is most helpful.

Attention to safety of the patient is a priority. Family members must be taught measures to protect the patient who wanders, is disoriented, or who lacks judgment (see Chapter 34).

These patients need a stable, dependable environment and a consistent schedule. If agitation or confusion causes undesirable behavior, the use of distraction can be beneficial. Handing the patient an item, leading him from the area, or decreasing environmental stimuli (turning off the television or radio) can calm the patient.

The patient with memory loss who can read benefits from written instructions and a posting of the day's schedule of activities. Measures to protect the patient and deal with confusion are presented in Chapter 34.

♦ Aphasia

Aphasia is a defect in the ability to express oneself in speech or writing, or an inability to comprehend spoken or written language. It is caused by disease or injury of the brain centers controlling language comprehension and expression.

Aphasia may be *receptive*, *expressive*, or *global*. **The person with receptive aphasia has difficulty interpreting communications to him in either spoken or written form. In expressive aphasia, the person has difficulty expressing himself in speech or writing. Global aphasia is where the person has a combination of receptive and expressive aphasia. Aphasias vary in degree and in type of deficit.** For example, a person may be able to write a message but cannot form the words to say it.

A comprehensive assessment of the patient who has some type of aphasia usually is a team effort carried out under the leadership of a specially trained speech therapist. Nurses and others responsible for the care of the aphasic patient can assist by noting specific abilities or inabilities of the patient to communicate with them. Some important questions the nurse might ask herself while observing and assessing the status of a patient who has difficulty communicating because of a neurological disorder include the following:

- Can he understand yes/no questions? Are his responses of "yes" and "no" reliable (does that seem to be what he means?)?
- Can he point or look toward objects you have named that are in his line of vision?
- Can he name the objects?
- Is he able to follow simple directions (e.g., "Turn your head")?
- Can he repeat simple words? Complex words?
- Can he repeat sentences?
- Can he follow simple written requests?
- Can he write answers to questions?
- Can he write requests?
- Can he read questions or directions?

The patient who suddenly has a problem speaking or understanding words or signs is likely to suffer from isolation and experience extreme frustration unless an effort is made to establish some means of communicating with him as quickly as possible. Once the patient's specific problem is identified (and it could be relatively simple or extremely complex), measures are taken to help the patient communicate as fully as his condition will allow.

Goals for the care of the aphasic patient are focused on stimulating communication without undue frustration and gradually guiding him to appropriate responses and requests. Reaching these goals may take weeks or months, but there are helpful principles and techniques that can be used by all members of the health team and by family members and friends.

Perhaps the most important rule of all is to *avoid talking to the aphasic person as if he were mentally incompetent.* His inability to communicate does not mean a lack of intelligence. He should be spoken *to*, not spoken *about* as if he cannot hear and understand what others are saying in his presence.

Do not shout at the aphasic person. Speak slowly and distinctly as you are facing him. Use body language and sign language to communicate if they seem to be helpful to the patient. Your facial expressions, posture, and gestures can often say more than the words you are saying.

Give the aphasic patient time to respond to questions. Do not ask more than one question at a time. It takes longer for an aphasic person to process what is being said to him. If you need to repeat a statement or question, use exactly the same words. He may have comprehended only half of the sentence the first time. Only one person in the room should speak at a time. Be certain to establish eye contact with the patient before speaking.

It is especially important that the aphasic patient be in an orderly and relaxed environment that is relatively free from distractions that make it difficult to concentrate on communicating.

The speech therapist will plan the patient's therapy program and will share with the nurse the details of how best to work with each individual patient. Some general guidelines include: (1) give praise for attempts at communication and for each correctly expressed word or sentence; (2) do not correct the patient's pronunciation, as he is liable to become too frustrated and give up speaking; and (3) be very patient.

Problems with aphasia sometimes resolve spontaneously in 3 or 4 months after a CVA. Total speech rehabilitation can take many months and may never reach the prestroke level.

Think about . . . Can you identify three specific techniques you might use to assist a patient with expressive aphasia to communicate his needs?

Among the techniques used to stimulate communication and help the patient deal with his problem of aphasia are self-talk, parallel talk, expansion, and modeling. *Self-talk* helps the aphasic person associate activities with specific words and phrases. The nurse or other person talks about what she is doing while performing a task (for example, making the bed). Self-talk is done in the presence of the patient so he can make connection between what is being said and what he sees being done.

Parallel talk describes for the patient what he is doing while he is performing some activity. In *expansion,* the person communicating with the patient completes the patient's sentences when he is able to verbalize but cannot yet speak in complete sentences. No new information is added during expansion. In *modeling,* the patient's sentences are completed, and new information is added.

All of these techniques are helpful in improving communication. They are forms of therapy, however, and are used only in a planned program that has been designed to meet a patient's individual needs. Whatever techniques are chosen, they should not be used in a condescending manner, nor should the patient be treated as a child.

The plan of care for the aphasic patient should not neglect the physical condition of his mouth and tongue. Good oral hygiene is needed to keep the oral mucosa clean and moist and in optimal condition so that it is easier for the patient to form words.

◆ Sexual Dysfunction

Sexual dysfunction from a lesion in neural pathways should be dealt with by allowing expression of the patient's concerns, beliefs, and feelings. Sexual counseling by one skilled in working with patients with neurological deficits should be initiated. Alternate techniques for meeting sexual needs must be explored. Many patients can, with teaching, lead a sexually satisfying life.

◆ Psychosocial Concerns

The multiple stresses, alteration in roles, and changes in body image and self-esteem that results from a chronic neurological disorder can be overwhelming. The patient will need time and assistance in adapting to an altered body image. The nurse must be accepting of the patient's expression of anxiety, anger, denial, regression, and depression. The nurse works to support the patient emotionally, attempting to establish realistic hope for quality of life. Exploring the patient's previous methods of coping with adversity, his support systems, talents, and desires helps to provide clues on how best to help him. Jointly establishing small, accomplishable goals can do much to rebuild self-esteem.

Collaboration with the social worker concerning referral to support groups and interaction with others with similar disabilities who are coping well can prove most beneficial. Contact with community agencies that offer support services and job retraining, if pertinent, is essential. The patient needs a way to be a productive member of society and to contribute to the welfare of his family.

Reentry into the community and a normal social life are other areas for intervention. Often the patient has been out of touch with his normal social circles for many months during his illness and recovery process. Plans should be made before discharge for social contact to be reinstated.

Ineffective Family Coping   A chronic neurological disorder that disrupts normal function for the patient also disrupts normal roles within the family. Family lifestyle is altered, and changes in roles may lead to family conflict. Family members often feel powerless, ambivalent toward the patient, angry, and guilty for having angry feelings. Family members need to be included when educating the patient about his disorder, the possibility of remissions and exacerbations, and the self-care measures necessary. Everyone needs time to adjust to the situation. Referrals to counseling and support groups can be very helpful.

DISORDERS OF THE NEUROLOGICAL SYSTEM

◆ Increased Intracranial Pressure

Diagnosis   Because the skull is a closed bony structure in the adult, it is unable to expand. Any lesion that begins to take up space within the cranial cavity causes an increase in the pressure within the cavity. Therefore any swelling of the brain tissue from injury or surgery, leakage of blood from ruptured cerebral vessels, or tumors, abscesses, or any other lesion within the skull presents an ICP risk. Nerve cells are particularly sensitive to hypoxia and cannot be replaced once they have been destroyed. Pressure against cerebral veins and arteries interferes with the flow of blood, producing a local ischemia and hypoxia. Pressure against the cells themselves can interfere with their vital functions. If it rises very high and remains high for very long, ICP can cause death. Figure 14-10 shows the relationship between the components and the pathological causes of ICP.

When the body can no longer compensate for the increase in volume in the cranial vault, decompensation begins and clinical signs of increasing ICP become apparent.

> The earliest sign of increasing ICP is lethargy and decreasing consciousness, accompanied by a slowing of speech and delay in response to verbal cues.

When ICP rises , it affects the perfusion of the brain and hypoxia occurs. Extended periods of hypoxia cause brain cell death. The body tries to compensate by raising blood pressure to force more oxygenated blood through the brain tissue. If ICP continues to rise, the brain tissue will herniate through the tentorial notch at the midline

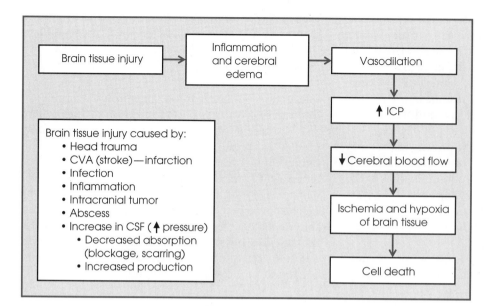

FIGURE 14-10 Pathophysiology of increased intracranial pressure.

of the foramen magnum. This herniation results in pressure on the vital structures of the midbrain, pons, and medulla and causes changes in the vital signs and pupil reactions characteristic of ICP. As brain tissue swells or fluid volume increases in the cranium, pressure is placed on the optic nerve. Pupils begin to react slowly, pupil size becomes unequal, progressing to dilation, and then the pupil size becomes fixed as reflexes disappear.

> The classic signs of ICP are rising systolic blood pressure, widening pulse pressure, bradycardia with a full, bounding pulse, and rapid or irregular respirations.

These tend to be late signs, as are pupil changes, and signal a severe emergency and immediate action to try to prevent the patient's death.

Treatment   The patient with greatly increased ICP is usually placed in an intensive care unit. **Increased ICP is treated with supportive care to keep the pressure from rising further and interventions to decrease the cranial blood or CSF volume.** Osmotic diuretics (mannitol, glycerol), are administered to remove fluid from the body, thereby reducing fluid in the brain. Systemic diuretics, such as furosemide (Lasix), also may be given. Dosage is determined by body weight, and electrolytes are monitored every 6 hours, as mannitol's action can cause electrolyte imbalances. An indwelling urinary catheter is inserted to monitor output. **The patient is kept in a slightly dehydrated state with fluid restriction and a "keep open" IV set at about 50 mL/hour.** Dexamethasone (Decadron) may be given to decrease the inflammatory response and cerebral edema if the ICP is caused by a brain tumor. The patient

is positioned with the head of the bed at 15 to 30 degrees to promote venous drainage from the head. The head and neck must be kept in midline so that venous drainage into the body is not restricted. Hip flexion should be less than 90 degrees.

If ICP is dangerously high, an intraventricular catheter can be inserted into the ventricle, through which CSF can be drained in small amounts to relieve the pressure. A pressure-monitoring device is attached to monitor the ICP changes. Cerebral perfusion pressure (CPP) must be kept above 60 mm Hg to ensure oxygenation of the brain tissue. (CPP = mean arterial pressure − intracranial pressure.) A monitoring device may be used to measure cerebral blood flow.

If the patient is on a ventilator and is extremely agitated, pancuronium bromide (Pavulon) to paralyze skeletal muscle, in combination with sedation, may be used to prevent further increases in ICP. Because carbon dioxide is a vasodilator and can increase blood volume within the cranial cavity, hyperventilation is sometimes used to combat the increased ICP. This is accomplished by increasing the rate of controlled respiration. A CO_2 level between 25 and 30 mm Hg will improve oxygenation to the brain, avoid vasodilation of cerebral vessels, reduce excess blood flow to the brain, and decrease jugular venous pressure. Table 14-11 provides general guidelines for the care of patients with increased ICP.

Barbiturates are sometimes used along with continuous brain wave monitoring when patients do not respond to the more common therapies for reduction of ICP. Their purpose is to induce heavy sedation and slow metabolism thereby decreasing ICP. In general, the short-acting barbiturates are used (for example, pentobarbital [Nembutal] and thiopental [Pentothal]).

TABLE 14-11 ◆ *Do's and Don'ts for Patients with Increased Intracranial Pressure (ICP)*

Do:
- Conduct neurological checks at least once every hour unless more frequent monitoring indicated.
- Report changes immediately.
- Maintain a patent airway and adequate ventilation to ensure proper oxygen and carbon dioxide exchange.
- Elevate the head of the bed 15 to 30 degrees to facilitate return of blood from the cerebral veins.
- Use measures to maintain normal body temperature. Elevations of temperature raise blood presure and cerebral blood flow. Shivering also can increase ICP.
- Monitor intake and output. Restrict or encourage fluids according to physician's order.
- Give passive range-of-motion exercises.
- Space activities apart.

Don't:
- Allow patient to become constipated or perform Valsalva maneuver.
- Hyperextend, flex, or rotate the patient's head.
- Flex the patient's hips (as in female catheterization).
- Place patient in Trendelenburg position for any reason.
- Allow patient to perform isometric exercises.

Temperature control is achieved by placing the patient on a hypothermia blanket for cooling if ICP has affected temperature regulation and the patient is feverish. Fever increases cerebral metabolism and cerebral edema.

Nursing Assessment and Intervention Early recognition of increasing pressure is extremely important to prevent permanent damage to the tissues of the brain, the cranial nerves, and the motor and sensory nerve pathways that are within the cranium. Careful neurological assessment with monitoring of the patient's LOC, pupillary reactions, level of neuromuscular activity, and vital signs is essential accurately to evaluate the patient's progress. "Neuro checks" are performed every 15 minutes to every 2 hours for the acute patient. The following indications that ICP may be rising should be reported immediately:

- Extreme restlessness or excitability following a period of apparent calm.
- Deepening stupor and decreasing LOCs.
- Headache that is unrelenting and increasing in intensity.
- Vomiting, especially persistent, projectile vomiting.
- Unequal size of pupils and other abnormal pupillary reactions.
- Leakage of CSF from the nose and ear.

- Changes in the patient's blood pressure, pulse, or respiration; widening pulse pressure; a slow, bounding pulse.

Table 14-12 summarizes four warning signs that indicate increasing ICP.

The appropriate nursing diagnosis is "**altered cerebral tissue perfusion related to effects of increasing intracranial pressure.**" Goals of care are:

- **Maintain cerebral perfusion.**
- **Reduce ICP.**
- **Maintain adequate respiration.**
- **Protect from injury.**
- **Maintain normal body functions.**
- **Prevent complications.**

Maintaining an open airway and adequate respiration may require suctioning and possibly intubation with mechanical ventilation. (If the patient has sustained a head injury, x-rays to rule out a basilar fracture are necessary before suctioning the patient to prevent the possibility of the suction catheter's entering the cranial vault.) These procedures are necessary if the increasing pressure is affecting the respiratory control centers in the brain. The patient whose consciousness level is decreased and whose gag and swallowing reflexes are impaired is in danger of aspirating blood, vomitus, mucus, and other material into the air passages.

Unless the patient has a tracheostomy or an oral airway in place, he should be positioned on his side or abdomen, not on his back, as the tongue may occlude the airway, and mucus cannot drain naturally. **The unconscious patient requires care for all basic needs.** See

TABLE 14-12 ◆ *Warning Signs of Increasing Intracranial Pressure and Impending Cerebral Disaster*

Sign	Nursing Assessment
Change in level of consciousness	Note change in awareness, whether increasing or decreasing; orientation; decreasing response to stimulation.
Change in limb motion	Extreme restlessness; muscle weakness or paralysis.
Change in pupil size	Bilateral or unilateral dilatation. Unilateral dilatation may be sign of cerebral hemorrhage with rapid deterioration.
Change in vital signs	Slowing pulse rate; widening pulse pressure; labored, irregular breathing; rising body temperature.

Table 14-9 and the section on common care problems for specific interventions.

INFECTIOUS DISEASES

◆ Meningitis

Meningitis is an inflammation of the membranes covering the brain and spinal cord. The membranes can become infected in a number of ways, because infectious agents can be carried (1) through the blood stream or by direct extension from an infected area of the brain, spinal cord, and sinuses; (2) through an opening in the skull in a head injury or from surgery; and (3) by accidental introduction of infectious agents into the spinal canal during spinal puncture.

Many different strains of bacteria and viruses can cause meningitis, but the causative organism is usually *Streptococcus pneumoniae* or *Nisseria meningitidis*. In children the causative organism usually is *Haemophilus influenzae* type B. The disorder frequently follows an upper respiratory infection. Immunization against *H. influenzae* type B is recommended for all infants.

A consequence of bacterial meningitis can be an increase in circulating CSF due to obstruction of normal mechanisms of CSF absorption when bacteria, white blood cells, and debris block the arachnoid villi, resulting in an obstructive **hydrocephalus** (increased CSF in the ventricles of the brain) that increases ICP.

Diagnosis **The most outstanding symptom of meningitis is a severe and persistent headache that is greatly aggravated by shaking the head.** Other signs of meningeal irritation include pain and **stiffness of the neck** (nuchal rigidity), exaggerated deep tendon reflexes, irritability, photophobia, and hypersensitivity of the skin. Meningococcal meningitis often is accompanied by a petechial rash covering the chest and extremities. Seizures frequently are present, as are nausea and vomiting.

When meningitis is suspected, a spinal tap is performed, and the CSF is examined for the number and type of organisms present in it. The CSF pressure usually is elevated. *When meningitis is present, the spinal fluid may appear milky as a result of the increased number of white cells suspended in the fluid.* Other abnormal findings in the CSF include the presence of protein and decreased amounts of glucose. A Gram stain identifies the causative organism.

Treatment Successful treatment of meningitis and prevention of permanent disability depend on early recognition and prompt treatment. Antibiotics are started immediately, and then when the causative organism has been identified, specific antibiotics to which the organism is sensitive are administered. A combination of two drugs is common. The disease usually responds well to IV antibiotic therapy followed by oral doses given for a total of 10 days. Dexamethasone has proven beneficial for many patients if given shortly before antibiotic therapy and continued for 4 days. It decreases the inflammation. Anticonvulsive drugs are administered to control seizures, and aspirin or acetaminophen is given for headache. **Narcotics are rarely used for pain control in patients with increased ICP, as they cause sedation and prevent accurate neurological assessment.** They also can mask signs of increasing ICP. Prophylactic antibiotics are usually given to those in close contact with the patient to prevent the spread of the infection. Mortality occurs in about 20% of cases.

Nursing Assessment and Intervention In addition to noting the specific signs and symptoms of meningitis, the nurse must assess the patient for subjective and objective data relevant to each of the patient care problems that might accompany the disease. Examples include convulsive seizures, elevated body temperature, nausea and vomiting, delirium, pain, increased ICP, and fluid and electrolyte imbalances.

Ongoing, vigilant neurological assessment is a high priority in monitoring for signs of increasing ICP, changes in condition, and response to treatment. Specific nursing interventions in the care of the patient with meningitis are primarily concerned with measures to conserve the strength of the patient, prevent seizures, and promote healing. Preventing the spread of infection includes some precautionary measures. The type of precautions and isolation will depend on the type of meningitis present. Meningococcal meningitis is spread by droplet infection, so the recommended procedure is to use *respiratory precautions*.

The patient's room should be quiet and dimly lit. Sudden noises or bright flashes of light can cause a seizure. It is obvious from outward appearance that the patient with meningitis is acutely ill. Care and treatments are coordinated to allow as much rest as possible. Meningitis often produces mental confusion and delirium, as well as the possibility of seizures. The nursing care for seizures is covered later in this chapter. *Herpes simplex* (fever blisters) frequently accompanies meningitis. The presence of these sores, plus drying of the lips and mouth from high temperature and dehydration, requires special mouth care. Using *standard precautions*, the lips and mouth should be cleansed and lubricated at least every 2 hours during the acute stage of the disease.

Fluid volume deficit often is a problem; thus the patient's intake and output should be measured and dehydration prevented. Excessive vomiting or outward signs of early dehydration should be reported promptly so that fluids may be given IV when necessary.

A decrease in the peristaltic action of the intestines often occurs in meningitis and can lead to an accumulation of flatus and fecal material with severe abdominal distention. The patient's abdomen should be checked for distention and his bowel sounds noted and recorded. Rectal tubes, suppositories, or *small, low* enemas may be ordered for relief. Large amounts of fluid should not be given rectally, because they may increase ICP by being absorbed into the body's fluid compartment and causing fluid excess or by initiating the Valsalva maneuver for defecation.

The patient will need support and reassurance from the nurse, because the severity of this illness is frightening. If he is confused, he will need frequent orientation. The family also will need information and reassurance.

Once the acute stage of the disease is over, the patient is allowed to resume his former activities gradually. Residual effects of the disease, such as paralysis, deafness, and visual defects sometimes occur, but these sequelae of meningitis do not usually occur if the disease is diagnosed and treated in the early stages before permanent damage is done.

◆ Encephalitis

Encephalitis is an inflammation of the tissues of the brain that causes cerebral edema and diffuse nerve cell destruction. The disease is most often caused by a virus or the toxins produced by the organisms that cause chickenpox, measles, and mumps. Some chemicals, such as lead and arsenic, also can produce encephalitis or encephalopathy.

The severity of the illness may be mild or fatal. The two most common types of viral encephalitis in the United States are the Western equine encephalitis and herpes simplex encephalitis. Neurological impairment is caused by direct infection of neural cells. Western equine encephalitis is spread by the mosquito and occurs most frequently between May and September. Herpes simplex encephalitis spreads from neural tissue to the CNS. It can be a primary or secondary infection and can occur from reactivation of latent virus. If **treatment for the herpes simplex type I is not started before coma occurs, death is almost certain.**

Diagnosis   The onset of encephalitis may be either **sudden or insidious and is characterized by headache, high fever, stiff neck or back, muscular weakness, and extreme restlessness or lethargy.** Then CNS signs appear usually 1 to 4 hours after the other symptoms. Mental confusion, visual disturbances, and disorientation may be present. The lethargy may progress to coma. The patient with herpes simplex encephalitis may start with flu-like symptoms that rapidly progress to lethargy, confusion, and coma. Diagnosis is confirmed by the presence of the virus in the CSF or blood stream. The CSF in herpes simplex encephalitis will show an elevated WBC count, a small increase in protein, and normal glucose levels.

Treatment   The treatment of encephalitis is primarily symptomatic, with general supportive measures to maintain cardiac and respiratory function, keep the strength of the patient up, promote healing, and prevent complications. Herpes simplex type is treated with antiviral acyclovir.

Nursing Assessment and Intervention   Specific nursing measures are essentially the same as for any patient who is subject to seizures, high fever, delirium, or altered LOC.

◆ Guillain-Barré Syndrome

Guillain-Barré syndrome is a relatively rare disease that affects the peripheral nervous system, especially the spinal nerves outside the spinal cord. It also can affect the cranial nerves. Pathological changes include **demyelination** (loss of the fatty sheath around the nerves), inflammation, edema, and nerve root compression. These changes bring about the paresthesia, pain, and progressive, ascending paralysis typical of the syndrome.

The cause of Guillain-Barré syndrome is not known, but it usually follows a viral respiratory infection or gastroenteritis within 10 to 21 days. Because one-half to two-thirds of patients with the syndrome report a febrile condition before its clinical onset, some authorities believe that the disease is related to an autoimmune response.

Diagnosis   Objective and subjective symptoms of **Guillain-Barré syndrome include mild sensations of numbness and tingling in the feet and hands, followed by muscle pain, tenderness, and aching, especially in the shoulder, pelvis, and thighs. There is progressive muscle weakness, usually starting in the lower extremities and moving upward over 24 to 72 hours.** However, it also can affect the facial muscles first and move downward. Sensory loss can also occur, but is not as common as motor loss.

Diagnosing Guillain-Barré syndrome is difficult because its characteristic signs and symptoms are similar to those of several other diseases. Analysis of the CSF is helpful. Typically there is an elevated protein content that tends to rise as the disease progresses, peaking in 4 to 6 weeks. The number of leukocytes remains within normal limits, as does CSF pressure. For the most part, the physician must depend on the clinical picture presented by the patient to diagnose Guillain-Barré syndrome.

Treatment   Medical treatment is mainly supportive. Plasmapheresis, in which the patient's plasma is removed and "washed" to remove antibodies, hastens recovery in some patients and decreases the time ventilatory support is needed (see Chapter 16). The use of IV immune globulin to hasten recovery is under investigation.

Nursing Assessment and Intervention   There are three stages in Guillain-Barré syndrome, each demanding different kinds of monitoring and intervention. **During the *acute phase,* the goals are to sustain life, prevent complications related to immobility, and promote rest and comfort.** Respiratory problems are particularly troublesome and may require suctioning, tracheostomy care, artificial ventilation, and other life-support measures.

Vital signs must be checked frequently. Alterations in the autonomic nervous system can cause drastic changes in blood pressure, particularly hypotension. Cardiac arrhythmias also frequently occur.

The paralysis and loss of control that take place with Guillain-Barré syndrome come on so suddenly and are so overwhelming that the patient becomes very frightened. Because the course of the disease usually extends for months with a very slow recovery, the patient begins to have feelings of hopelessness, despair, and isolation. If the respiratory muscles are affected, the patient will be placed on a ventilator.

The *static* phase is a kind of plateau the patient reaches 1 to 3 weeks after the onset of his illness. During this time the motor loss and paresthesias no longer progress, and the patient's condition becomes somewhat stabilized; he gets no better or no worse. This phase can last from a few days to months.

Think about... What problems requiring specific nursing interventions would you expect to encounter for the patient with Guillain-Barré syndrome who is now stable but has paralysis of the lower extremities and paresis of the upper extremities?

During the *static phase,* nursing care is concerned with preventing complications of immobility and helping the patient deal with his feelings of anger, depression, and anxiety. Exercises are usually begun, but are limited to passive and gentle ROM and stretching exercises. There must be a balance of rest and exercise and no sudden changes in posture or position, lest blood pressure suddenly drop.

Meticulous skin care is essential. Monitoring for thrombophlebitis is important, as this is a frequent complication. Elastic stockings or sequential intermittent compression devices applied to the legs are used, along with anticoagulant therapy, to try to prevent thrombophlebitis.

The final phase, *rehabilitation,* is one of gradual recovery. The patient may become elated over the change in his condition and must be prevented from overexertion, which can lead to a relapse. As muscle function returns, the level of exercise and activity is slowly increased. It may take up to 2 years for maximal improvement. Approximately 80% to 90% of patients have little residual deficit.

◆ Poliomyelitis and Post-Polio Syndrome

Poliomyelitis destroys the motor cells of the anterior horn of the spinal cord, the brainstem, and the motor strip located in the frontal lobe. It is caused by a virus and can be prevented by immunization with the Salk or Sabin vaccine. It is rare in the United States, but outbreaks still occur in other parts of the world. It is mentioned here because some people who had poliomyelitis have developed post-polio sequelae (PPS) or post-polio syndrome. A new onset of weakness, pain, and fatigue occurs in people who had the disease over 30 years ago. Disability may be temporary or permanent. Treatment is geared toward making lifestyle modifications to preserve energy and physiological function. Swimming in warm water has been found to promote comfort and help maintain flexibility.

◆ Brain Abscess

A brain abscess is a purulent infection in an area of the brain where pus forms. A bacterial infection that has traveled from the sinus, ear, or mastoid region usually is the cause. An abscess can form from bacteria introduced at the time of skull injury or during surgery. **Signs and symptoms are generally headache, fever, and progression to lethargy and confusion.** If the abscess is not treated, ICP will rise as the size of the abscess increases. **The nurse must teach patients who experience sinus infections with purulent drainage to seek treatment if symptoms last for more than a few days to prevent brain abscess.**

HEAD INJURIES

Head injuries are the most frequent cause of death in people between the ages of 1 and 35 years. Those who survive initial head injury require meticulous observation and care so that damage to the brain cells can be kept at a minimum.

◆ Types of Injuries

A blow to the head may cause *open* injuries, with lacerations of the skin and scalp and fracture of the skull, or *closed* injuries, in which the scalp and skull remain intact, but the underlying brain tissue is damaged.

> The term concussion is used to describe a closed head injury in which the brain is compressed by a portion of the skull at the time of the blow and temporary ischemia of the brain tissue results. In a contusion, the brain tissue is bruised and blood from broken vessels accumulates, causing increased ICP.

A coup-contrecoup injury, also called an acceleration-deceleration injury, occurs when the head is moving rapidly and hits a stationary object, such as a windshield. The contents within the cranium hit the inside of the skull (coup) and then bounce back and hit the bony area opposite the site of impact, causing a second injury (contrecoup).

Subdural hematoma is a common result of head injury. A **hematoma** is a blood-filled swelling. When a blow is delivered to the head, it may rupture the blood vessels that lie between the delicate arachnoid membrane covering the brain and the tough, fibrous dura mater. As the blood leaks under the dura mater (subdural), the hematoma grows in size, pressing against the softer arachnoid and the brain tissue it is covering (Figure 14-11).

An *epidural hematoma* rarely occurs, but when it does, it is caused by rapid leakage of blood from a relatively large artery, which quickly elevates ICP. This constitutes a medical emergency. A craniotomy is needed to repair the damaged vessel and relieve pressure.

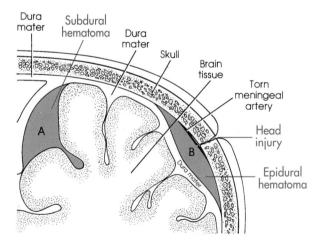

FIGURE 14-11 Subdural and epidural hematoma. *A,* Subdural hematoma. As a result of trauma to the head, small ruptured blood vessels leak blood into the space under the dura mater. The hematoma forms between the dura mater and the arachnoid membrane. *B,* Epidural hematoma, the result of a head injury that tears a large meningeal artery, causing the collection of a large amount of blood above the dura mater. The large epidural hematoma compresses brain tissue. If not relieved, subdural and epidural hematomas can be fatal.

Diagnosis   The severity of brain damage from a head injury is best judged by the symptoms presented by the patient, neurological assessment, the history of the type of blow received, and whether the victim lost consciousness and for how long. No head injury should be considered completely harmless. All are potentially dangerous because there may be a delayed reaction in which there is hemorrhage into the brain tissues or the formation of a blood pool or clot, a subdural hematoma. This condition builds up over time and results from weakening and rupture of the small blood vessels in the brain. Sometimes the bleeding is so slow that it takes weeks or even months for the symptoms of pressure within the skull to appear.

The outward symptoms of head injury are fairly obvious; these include bruising, swelling, lacerations, and bleeding. However, the symptoms indicating a buildup of pressure within the skull are more subtle and less easily detected. The patient is observed for signs of increased *ICP,* as well as other pathological changes.

The diagnostic tests and examinations commonly used to determine the extent of head injury include a radiograph of the skull, a computed tomographic (CT) scan, cerebral angiography, electroencephalography, and brain scanning.

Treatment   The patient with a head injury usually is treated conservatively at first, unless a serious emergency that greatly increases ICP arises or a compound fracture of the skull demands surgical debridement of the wound and removal of splintered bone from the brain tissues.

Subdural hematoma is removed surgically either via burr holes or by craniotomy incision. Epidural hematoma, which can occur with skull fracture, necessitates immediate craniotomy to stop the bleeding and evacuate the hematoma to prevent death from increased ICP.

Nursing Assessment and Intervention   *Leakage of spinal fluid* should be watched for in all patients with head trauma, as well as in those who have had brain surgery. To be sure that drainage is spinal fluid, it may be tested for sugar with a glucose monitor such as Accuchek. *Spinal fluid will show a reading for sugar; mucus or nasal secretions will not.* If blood is mixed in the fluid, the test is not reliable, as blood contains glucose.

Cerebrospinal fluid may leak from the nose, the ear, or both. It appears as a clear fluid that might be slightly blood-tinged. If the fluid leaks onto the pillowcase or sheet, there often is a "halo" effect; that is, it has a pinkish center surrounded by a ring of a lighter shade. When this is noticed, the piece of linen should be set aside for the physician to see.

If it has been determined that there is indeed leakage

of spinal fluid through the nose, ear, or an open head wound, special precautions must be taken to prevent infection. These include the following:

◆ Keep the patient on absolute bedrest with the head of the bed elevated 30 degrees.

◆ Cover a draining ear with a sterile gauze square, changing it periodically to look for drainage.

◆ Instruct the patient *not* to blow his nose or pick at it.

◆ Remind the patient that he is not to change his position in any way unless he has been told it is all right to do so. Specific nursing diagnoses are listed in Nursing Care Plan 14-1.

Observation of a patient treated in an emergency department for head injury and released to go home requires specific techniques. Table 14-13 includes instructions for the patient's family.

Think about . . . If a family member is knocked unconscious for a few minutes by a baseball and suffers a concussion, what specific assessments would you continue to perform after discharge from the emergency room?

◆ Brain Tumors

Neoplasms within the confines of the skull are space-occupying lesions and thus create problems of increasing ICP by compressing adjacent tissues. If the tumor arises from cells of the brain, the cranial nerves, or the pituitary gland, the neoplastic cells can infiltrate and destroy these structures. Many brain tumors are benign. However, because of the increased ICP it causes and the way it can invade brain tissue, a benign tumor presents a serious condition.

Intracranial tumors may begin in the substance of the brain itself, or they may begin in the meninges, cranial nerves, or pituitary gland. Primary malignant brain tumors rarely metastasize outside the brain, but an intracranial tumor may be secondary to malignant lesions outside the skull, such as a malignancy of the breast, lung, or melanoma of the skin.

Diagnosis   There can be as many symptoms of intracranial tumors as there are functions of the structures within the skull. The symptoms depend on location and may appear gradually, or, if the tumor is a highly malignant, fast-growing type, they may appear suddenly. In a slow-growing type of tumor, the patient may first show personality changes, disturbances in judgment and memory, loss of muscular strength and coordination, or difficulty in speaking clearly. Headache, vomiting, visual problems, and other signs of increased ICP also may occur. Approximately 20% to 50% of adults with brain tumors develop seizure activity.

Diagnostic procedures to identify the site and extent of intracranial tumors include MRI, arteriography, and CT scan.

Treatment   The four modes of therapy for intracranial tumors are the same as those for neoplastic diseases elsewhere in the body: surgery, radiation therapy, chemotherapy, and immunotherapy. These are discussed more thoroughly in Chapter 9.

Whenever possible, intracranial tumors are removed surgically, and the other modes of treatment are used to destroy remaining cells. Sometimes, however, the tumor has infiltrated vital parts of the brain that must not be traumatized by surgical procedures. If the tumor is located in the cerebrum, an operation called a *craniotomy* is done. A flap of scalp and bone is cut and pulled down, the dura is opened, and the tumor is removed. Tumors in or near the *cerebellum* are removed through an incision under the occipital bone. This is called a *suboccipital craniectomy,* in which part of the skull is permanently removed, leaving a defect in the skull. In this case, IV mannitol, an osmotic diuretic, and dexamethasone (Decadron), a corticosteroid, are given to reduce inflammation and fluid volume, thereby lowering ICP.

If the tumor is found while it is still very small, a stereotactic or gamma knife procedure can destroy it. This procedure uses a domed steel head covering with ports through which gamma radiation is directed. Measurements are calculated by a computer to precisely locate the tumor, and the radiation is delivered only to the tumor. This procedure also can be used for small recurrent tumor growth (Figure 14-12).

If all of the tumor cannot be removed, a portion of the tumor may be removed to relieve compression of the brain against the skull. This procedure is only a temporary measure to relieve the patient's symptoms. Obstruction of CSF flow may require a shunting procedure to reduce CSF pressure. A shunt is a tube attached to a small manual pump that moves excess CSF fluid from the ventricles to the peritoneal cavity or into the atrium of the heart.

An Ommaya reservoir may be implanted between the scalp and the skull. It consists of a port attached to a catheter that is placed in the lateral ventricle of the brain. Chemotherapy drugs can be injected into the port and instilled into the CSF in the ventricle. In this way the chemotherapy drug is carried to the tumor cells in greater quantity than can be achieved by infusion of the drugs into the bloodstream. In patients for whom chemotherapy and radiation have previously failed, implantation of carmustine (BiCNU) wafers into a glial cell tumor is under trial. Gliadel is inserted into brain tissue after removal of glioma to fight the malignancy and slow or prevent regrowth. Experiments for a vaccine that will allow the patient's im-

Nursing Care Plan 14-1

Selected nursing diagnoses, goals/expected outcomes, nursing interventions, and evaluations for a patient with a head injury

Situation: A 16-year-old male who suffered a head injury in an automobile accident is assigned to you. He is groggy but arousable.

Nursing Diagnosis	Goals/Expected Outcomes	Nursing Intervention	Evaluation
Alteration in cerebral tissue perfusion related to increased intracranial pressure from head injury. SUPPORTING DATA Alteration in LOC; confused as to where he is, what day it is; somewhat combative; hit head on dashboard on right side.	No further increase in ICP.	Monitor neurological status q 2 h using Glasgow Coma Scale; notify physician of any pupil changes or signs of increasing ICP, such as widening pulse pressure, change in respiratory pattern, slowing of pulse, increase in temperature, or decrease in LOC. Monitor for seizure activity; institute seizure precautions. Keep head of bed at 30 degrees and body in correct alignment; turn side to side q 2 h. Maintain IV at 50 mL/h; keep room calm and softly lit; do not disturb more than necessary; talk to patient while giving care; allow rest periods between any invasive procedures; monitor intake and output; reorient frequently.	PEARL; still groggy; no change in blood pressure and pulse; no sign of seizure activity; states name, age; still confused as to place; continue plan.
Self-care deficit related to confusion, grogginess, and increased ICP. SUPPORTING DATA Falls asleep during attempts at bath, etc. Is confused about how to use ordinary objects such as toothbrush.	Adequate hygiene, nutrition, activity will be maintained. Patient will resume own self-care by discharge.	Provide assistance with all ADLs while groggy and confused. Inspect when turning; place foam pad on bed. As level of consciousness improves, encourage self-care activities.	Assistance for all ADL provided; skin intact; turned 8, 10, 12, and 2; voiding quantity sufficient; able to drink liquids; continue plan.
Ineffective family coping related to anxiety about patient's condition. SUPPORTING DATA Mother states she is afraid he will die. She keeps trying to arouse him when she is in the room.	Mother's anxiety will decrease as she gains information about her son's condition and prognosis. Patient will resume own self-care by discharge.	Explain to family that confusion and grogginess are usual after head injury. Explain that the danger is if the ICP keeps increasing; tell what measures are being done to minimize increasing ICP; explain all procedures; explain that calm, rest, and positive talk in the room will help. Encourage family members to share their fears and concerns with each other. Call hospital chaplain or own minister if family desires. Keep family informed of changes in patient's condition.	Discussed condition with mother; states she understands the need for quiet and vigilance; appears less anxious.

TABLE 14-13 ◆ *Patient Education: Instructions for Home Care after Head Injury*

- Avoid strenuous physical activities for at least 24 hours after injury.
- Apply icebag to areas of swelling—continue for at least 24 hours after injury.
- Light diet for 24 hours after injury.
- Arouse patient every 2 hours, day and night, for at least 24 hours.

Call doctor immediately or return to emergency department if:

- Patient becomes confused, irrational, disoriented, "talks out of head," doesn't know where he is.
- Unable to arouse patient.
- Patient continues to be nauseated and/or vomits more than once, especially if projectile.
- Patient has trouble with his balance.
- Patient complains of double or blurred vision.
- Headache persists or becomes more intense 12 hours after the injury.

Source: Courtesy Emergency Department, St. Mary's Hospital, Athens, GA.

mune system to recognize and destroy the cells of glioblastoma are about to begin trials in humans. The vaccine blocks the ability of brain tumor cells to secrete a substance that hides glioblastoma cells from the patient's immune system, allowing them to be recognized and destroyed.

Nursing Care of Patients Undergoing Brain Surgery

Preoperative care.   Unless an emergency exists, the patient who is scheduled for intracranial surgery receives essentially the same care as other surgical patients. The exceptions are physical preparation, neurological assessment, and intervention to manage such problems as altered LOCs, seizures, and increased ICP. Psychological preparation also is important.

The operative site usually is not shaved until the patient is under anesthesia in the operating room. A shampoo may be ordered the evening before surgery. Any scalp lesions or other unusual conditions that are noted at this time should be reported. Usually the entire head is not shaved only the operative area, and, if the patient has long hair, any hair that is cut off may be saved to be used as a hairpiece until the patient's hair grows back.

Postoperative period.   During the immediate postoperative period, the patient will be in the intensive care unit for continuous monitoring and attention. Essentially, his care will be the same as that for a patient who has had a head injury. Additional specific points in the postoperative care of the patient who has undergone intracranial surgery are as follows:

- Position the patient according to written orders from the attending surgeon. *Make no exceptions.*
- Keep the neck in midline and prevent excessive hip flexion.
- Use nasal suctioning *only* if there is a written order allowing this.
- Watch carefully for signs of leakage of CSF from the nose, ear, and operative site, and report evidence of leakage immediately. Use aseptic technique in applying dressings to collect the drainage.
- Provide a quiet, nonstimulating environment.
- Do not restrain the patient unless absolutely necessary and only if there is a written order.

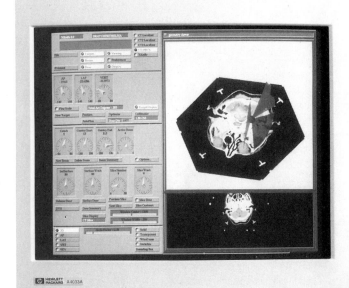

FIGURE 14-12   Stereotactic surgery plotted by computer for correct radiation dosage to tumor site. (Photo by Glen Derbyshire; Courtesy of the Cancer Foundation, Santa Barbara, California.)

◆ Administer only those treatments, comfort measures, and medications for which there are specific written orders.

◆ Report promptly any changes in the neurological status of the patient.

HEADACHE

Headaches are the most common cause of pain in people. Headaches are commonly caused by allergy and related sinus problems, tension, or are vascular in origin. Arthritis, cervical spondylitis, and temporomandibular joint syndrome may also cause headaches. The pain of a headache may be minor or severe. Persistent headache requires testing to rule out organic problems such as anemia, brain tumor, or cerebral aneurysm.

Treatment for severe, recurrent headaches begins with determining the cause, if possible, and identifying factors that seem to precipitate the headache. Mild headaches usually are relieved by rest and a mild analgesic.

◆ Migraine Headaches

It is thought that constriction and subsequent dilatation of cerebral arteries cause migraine headaches. Attacks occur irregularly and may begin with visual disturbances such as "spots before the eyes" (**scotoma**). The visual "aura" may take other forms and often occurs up to an hour before the onset of pain. Pain usually begins on one side of the head and is throbbing in character. Migraine headache often is accompanied by nausea and vomiting. Symptoms may last for several hours or a day or more. Light increases the pain and for some sufferers, certain types of light set off the headache.

Lying in a darkened, quiet room that is odor free with the eyes closed decreases the symptoms. Sometimes doing this at the very beginning of symptoms can prevent a full-blown migraine headache.

Treatment consists of ergotamine derivatives by suppository, often in combination with caffeine, analgesic for pain, medication for vomiting if it is severe, and sumatriptan (Imitrex) by self-injection. Cold compress to the temple, eye, and occiput on the side of the headache is helpful. For some people, compression of the temporal artery on the side of the pain is beneficial. Identifying any food or other substance that seems to trigger an attack is very important. If migraine headache tends to occur around the time of menses, taking a diuretic for 3 days prior to onset of menstruation may be effective in preventing the headache. Divalproex (Depakote) has been released for use in preventing migraines. It doesn't stop the headache once it has begun though.

CEREBROVASCULAR ACCIDENT (CVA, STROKE)

◆ Incidence and Causes

Stroke is a common disease, more common than many of us realize. There are over 3 million stroke survivors living in the United States today, and stroke is the leading cause of disability. An average of one person per minute suffers a stroke in the United States. The incidence is about 19% higher in males than in females. For people over age 55, the incidence of stroke more than doubles with each successive decade. Although the incidence of stroke has been decreasing despite the lengthening life span for the general population, stroke is the third leading cause of death in the United States. The decrease in the incidence of stroke can be attributed to successful preventive measures such as those presented here. An increase in public education could result in lessened disability and death from stroke. Table 14-14 lists the risk factors for stroke.

> Control of high blood pressure, quitting cigarette smoking, decreasing intake of cholesterol and controlling blood lipids, maintaining a normal blood sugar level, avoiding excessive alcohol intake, getting sufficient exercise, avoiding obesity, and living a lifestyle that helps prevent heart disease all can help reduce the risk of stroke as well.

A CVA usually is the result of an interruption of blood flow to a specific area of the brain (that is, *cerebral ischemia*). Ischemia of cells directly causes cellular ne-

---

TABLE 14-14 ◆ *Patient Education: Risk Factors for Stroke*

Nurses should educate all patients about the risk factors for stroke and encourage measures to alter those factors that can be changed.

Risk factors that can be treated
◆ Cigarette smoking
◆ Heart disease (especially atrial fibrillation)
◆ High blood pressure
◆ High red blood cell count (polycythemia)
◆ Transient ischemic attacks (TIAs)

Risk factors that cannot be changed
◆ Age over 65
◆ Asymptomatic carotid bruit (indicates atherosclerosis, which increases stroke risk)
◆ Diabetes mellitus
◆ Heredity (family history of stroke increases individual risk)
◆ Prior stroke
◆ Race (African Americans have a 60% higher risk rate)
◆ Sex (incidence is 30% higher in men)

crosis (death) and **infarct** (area of tissue that has become necrotic from lack of blood supply). The ischemia can be caused by (1) cerebral thrombosis (formation of a blood clot in a cerebral artery); (2) intercerebral bleed (the blood vessel ruptures and leaks blood into brain tissue); (3) an **embolus** (occlusion of a cerebral vessel by a traveling clot, tumor, fat, bacteria, or debris); or (4) pressure on a blood vessel causing ischemia. Figure 14-13 shows the events causing stroke (CVA).

The carotid arteries supply a major portion of the blood that goes to the brain (Figure 14-14). **If plaque forms in these arteries as a result of atherosclerosis, the person is at risk for a stroke as blood supply to the brain is diminished or stopped.** Less common causes of stroke are arterial spasms and compression of cerebral vessels by a tumor, local edema, rupture of a cerebral aneurysm, and other disorders.

Think about . . . How many risk factors for stroke are present for each member of your family?

◆ Stroke Prevention

Many strokes can be prevented by either surgical procedures or medical management of diseases that predispose a person to a CVA.

Surgical procedure for the prevention of a major stroke is reserved for carotid arteries that are 70% to 99% occluded and involves the removal of plaque laid down on the inner wall of the carotid artery (**carotid endarterectomy**). There is controversy about whether the surgery is more effective than medical treatment. As angioplasty has been effective for coronary arteries, studies are under way to determine whether this is an option for opening carotid arteries. Laser surgery and clot dissolution with enzyme solutions, such as t-PA used for coronary thrombosis, has just been approved for clot dissolution. About one-third of all strokes can be traced to obstruction of any one of the four arteries in the neck that supply blood to the brain. These arteries are readily accessible, so the surgeon can open the artery and remove the obstruction. He then sutures the vessel wall or sews a Dacron patch over the incision, leaving the vessel larger than before. Care for patients undergoing vascular surgery is presented in Chapter 18.

Medical preventive measures are aimed at eliminating or managing some of the conditions that predispose a person to stroke. Control of hypertension and the effective treatment of rheumatic heart disease, cardiac dysrhythmias, and atherosclerosis have significantly reduced the incidence of stroke. Instructing the public about the danger of stroke from cocaine use must continue. Teaching people to seek assistance immediately when signs of stroke occur may allow medical

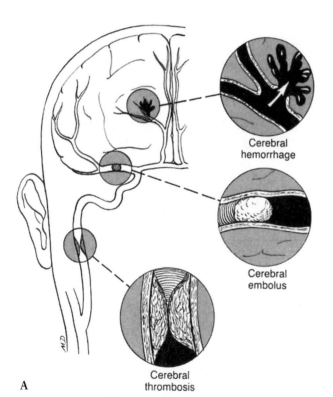

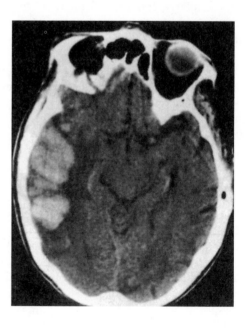

A   B

FIGURE 14-13   (A) Events causing stroke. (B) An MRI showing hemorrhagic stroke in the left cerebrum.
(*Source:* Black, J. M., Matassarin-Jacobs, E. [1993]. *Luckmann and Sorensen's Medical-Surgical Nursing: A Psychophysiologic Approach,* 4th ed. Philadelphia: Saunders, p. 706.)

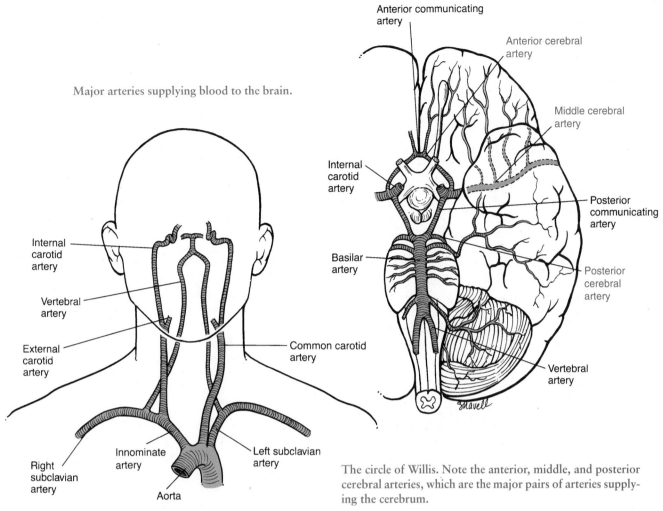

Major arteries supplying blood to the brain.

The circle of Willis. Note the anterior, middle, and posterior cerebral arteries, which are the major pairs of arteries supplying the cerebrum.

FIGURE 14-14   Major arteries supplying blood to the brain. Blockage of any major artery precipitates a CVA. (*Source:* Monahan, F. D., Drake, T., Neighbors, M. [1994]. *Nursing Care of Adults.* Philadelphia: Saunders, p. 1449.)

intervention that will decrease permanent neurological deficit (Table 14-15).

Medications that reduce platelet aggregation and decrease the chance of thrombosis often are used. Low-dose enteric-coated aspirin or ticlopidine is pre-

scribed for patients who have transient ischemic attacks or to prevent the recurrence of stroke from thrombosis.

Another factor to prevent the devastating neurological effects of a stroke is early detection and prompt treatment of the early warning signals. Many patients with a narrowing of the lumen of the arteries supplying the brain experience what are called *transient ischemic attacks* (TIAs). Although they usually are not recognized as such, TIAs often are warnings that a more serious neurological event is likely to occur. During the attack, the person may feel a weakness or numbness on one side of the body, slurring of speech or inability to talk, visual disturbances, such as blindness or double vision, and staggering or uncoordinated walking. These symptoms last from a few minutes to 24 hours. Unless the person has been told about them and their importance, he usually will not seek medical treatment and will not further investigate. About 5% to 20% of those persons who experience TIAs will eventually have a complete stroke within a year.

TABLE 14-15 ◆ *Patient Education: Warning Signs of Stroke*

Teach people to seek immediate medical attention from their physician or the emergency room if any of the following warning signs of stroke appear:

◆ Sudden weakness or numbness of the face, arm, or leg on one side of the body.
◆ Sudden dimness or loss of vision, especially in one eye only.
◆ Loss of speech, difficulty talking, loss of understanding when someone else is speaking.
◆ A sudden, severe headache for no known reason.
◆ Dizziness, loss of balance, a sudden fall that is not related to the side effects of medication, fever, or other known reason—particularly if it occurs with any of the other signs.

Cerebral ischemia caused by thrombosis causes signs that progress slowly. Thrombosis develops in an area of the vessel where there is atherosclerotic plaque. Lodging of an embolus in a major cerebral vessel causes sudden neurological deficit. Emboli most often are the result of heart disease and resultant *atrial fibrillation*, a cardiac dysrhythmia. Intracerebral bleeding from a disrupted vessel may occur from aneurysm rupture, rupture of an arteriovenous malformation, or because the vessel has been weakened by long-term hypertension.

◆Cerebral Aneurysm and Arteriovenous Malformation

An **aneurysm** is an abnormal ballooning or blister on an artery. It may be congenital or caused by a weakening of the artery wall from chronic hypertension. Rupture of the aneurysm causes bleeding into the subarachnoid space or into the ventricles. An arteriovenous (A-V) malformation is a congenital abnormality and is a tangled mass of malformed, thin-walled, dilated vessels that form an abnormal communication between the arterial and venous systems. An A-V malformation can leak, causing an intracerebral bleed. Vasospasm often occurs after intercerebral bleeding, leading to further ischemia of the brain tissue and more neurological impairment. **Subarachnoid hemorrhages (SAHs), which refers to bleeding in the brain below the arachnoid, often causes rapid onset of neurological deficit and loss of consciousness.** A leaking cerebral aneurysm may cause a severe headache. However, some bleeding is slower, producing a more gradual progression of headache, neck stiffness, and other neurological signs, such as blurred vision.

Diagnosis   In addition to a complete physical and neurological examination, the physician may order a CT scan, cerebral angiogram, or magnetic resonance imaging (MRI) scan to determine the specific cause of the stroke. An electroencephalogram is then performed, and brain scans or Doppler flow studies of the carotid arteries may be ordered. Positron emission tomography (PET) or single photon emission computed tomography (SPECT) has not yet proven to be more revealing than a CT or MRI scan.

Once the specific cause of the CVA has been determined, the physician is able to plan a more effective regimen of care. For example, anticoagulant therapy is indicated when cerebral thrombosis is present but is initially contraindicated if the patient is suffering from cerebral hemorrhage. Nimodipine (Nifidipine) is given to decrease arterial spasm if the stroke is from subarachnoid hemorrhage. Testing of new drugs continues in an effort to find a way to decrease the resultant damage from a CVA. Pro-urokinase, a modified form of a naturally occurring enzyme that dissolves clots is undergoing trials. t-PA, tissue plasminogen activator, has just been approved by the FDA for use in dissolving clots and emboli in nonhemorrhagic stroke. It must be given within 3 hours of the onset of symptoms. Tirilazad (Freedox) has recently been released and is helpful in limiting neuronal degeneration after a stroke. It is an antioxidant. Another neuroprotective drug being tested, citicoline, which appears to limit the size of the stroke, speed recovery, and improve the victim's mental functioning is promising.

Testing for blood levels of glutamate may alert physicians to patients whose condition is likely to rapidly deteriorate. Glutamate lowering drugs may possibly limit further brain damage in some stroke victims.

Treatment   Immediately after a person is suspected of having suffered a stroke, it is especially important to maintain an open airway. All constricting clothing around his neck should be removed, and the patient should be turned to one side to prevent aspiration of saliva and obstruction of the air passages. No attempt should be made to move the person until an ambulance has arrived. Reassure the patient regardless of whether he is able to respond. If he is conscious, elevate the head slightly to reduce ICP.

Nursing Assessment and Intervention   The neurological effects of stroke can range from mild motor disturbances to profound coma. Figure 14-15 shows some control zones of the brain and some motor and sensory functions likely to be affected by a stroke. When the stroke patient is first admitted to the hospital, the general state of health is assessed as well as effects of the stroke. The Agency for Health Care Policy and Research has issued Clinical Practice Guidelines for Post-stroke Rehabilitation. Standardized, validated assessment tools are used to determine deficits and to measure progress toward recovery.

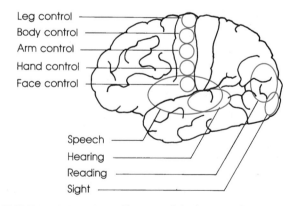

FIGURE 14-15   Control zones of the brain. When a cerebrovascular accident deprives brain cells of their blood supply, the area of the body controlled by the affected cells becomes **unable to function.** (Redrawn from Strokes: A guide for the Family. © American Heart Association.)

Care of the stroke patient can be divided into three phases: *phase one,* or initial care; *phase two,* which is concerned with rehabilitation efforts; and *phase three,* during which plans are made for continuity of care once the patient returns home. These are not phases in the sense that one begins only after another is finished. There is much overlapping of activities in each phase. Because about 80% of all stroke victims survive the first or initial phase of their illness, rehabilitation and plans for self-care are of the utmost importance. Chapter 12 discusses concepts of rehabilitation.

Phase 1.   Initial care of the stroke patient requires careful assessment to determine the extent to which neurological functions have been affected. Complete hemiplegia is a common effect of stroke. **Paralysis on the left side indicates focal damage to the right side of the brain because the motor pathways cross to the opposite side before extending down to the spinal cord. Aphasia often indicates ischemia of the brain cells on the left side and is usually accompanied by right-sided hemiplegia.** Figure 14-16 illustrates deficits often experienced by damage to the left or right side of the brain.

Nursing diagnoses for the patient who has experienced a CVA commonly include:

- Risk of injury related to weakness, paralysis, confusion, decreased consciousness, or dysphagia.
- Impaired physical mobility related to weakness or paralysis.
- Altered nutrition that is less than body requirements, related to impaired swallowing and hemiparesis or hemiplegia.
- Self-care deficit related to inability to perform ADLs (feeding, bathing, grooming) without assistance.
- Urinary incontinence, related to neurological deficits.
- Bowel incontinence, related to impaired mobility and neurological impairment.
- Risk for impaired skin integrity, related to decreased mobility, paresis, or paralysis.
- Impaired verbal communication, related to inability to clearly verbalize or inability to comprehend communication.

LEFT-SIDED BRAIN DAMAGE
Slow and cautious in behavior
Speech problems, aphasia
Difficulty in following verbal commands
Apraxia
Difficulty in performing simple tasks

RIGHT-SIDED BRAIN DAMAGE
Quick and impulsive in behavior
Short attention span
Neglects left side
Easily distracted

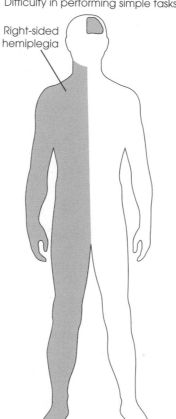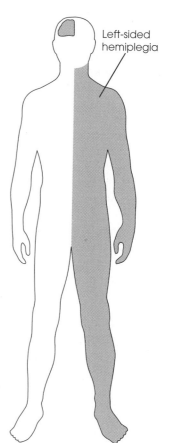

Right-sided hemiplegia

Left-sided hemiplegia

FIGURE 14-16   Comparison of deficits and behaviors related to damage to the left and right side of the brain.

- Unilateral neglect related to neurological damage and hemiplegia.
- Sensory/perceptual alteration: visual, related to loss of vision in parts of visual field; kinesthetic, related to decreased sense of touch on one side of the body.
- Self-esteem disturbance related to alteration in body image and dependence on others.
- Depression related to loss of usual lifestyle, neurological deficits, and dependence on others.

The amount of activity permitted a stroke patient during the initial acute stage of his illness depends on the cause of his CVA. If there is danger of continued hemorrhage from a ruptured artery and resultant increase in ICP, physical activity will necessarily be limited, and the patient care problems will not be the same as for a patient with stroke from another cause. When there is no danger of further damage to his brain, the patient usually is encouraged to become active as soon as his condition has stabilized. Bedrest for the first 24 hours is usual for all stroke patients.

Once the patient is stabilized, assessment is conducted in a systematic way, considering the possibility that any of the above problems could be present. Assessment of and nursing intervention for the patient with problems of immobility, incontinence of urine and feces, aphasia, delirium or confusion, and altered LOC are discussed in the section Common Neurological Patient Care Problems. Measures to prevent complications, such as subcutaneous heparin injections and elastic stockings to prevent deep vein thrombosis, skin care to minimize the risk of skin breakdown, physical therapy and splinting to prevent contractures and spasticity, and measures to prevent falls are included in the plan of care. To reduce the possibility of recurrence of a stroke, risk factors are identified, and teaching is begun to modify them.

When a CT scan has ruled out an intracerebral bleed and the stroke is found to be from a thrombus, continuous heparin infusion may be ordered to prevent an increase in the size of the thrombus and to prevent further thrombus formation. If t-PA is used first, heparin is not started for 24 hours after the administration of the t-PA. After a few days an oral anticoagulant is started and the heparin infusion is tapered and then stopped. Antihypertensive drugs are ordered as appropriate. Care for the patient receiving heparin is presented in Chapter 18. Clopidogrel, a new anticlotting drug has been found to be more effective than aspirin in preventing stroke recurrence.

Planning for specific goals must take into account the individual patient's previous lifestyle, age, general health or illness status, and specific problems of care. The 80-year-old retired person will not have the same goals for rehabilitation and recovery as the 47-year-old mother of three who had been working full time as a schoolteacher before her attack.

Major goals during the first phase are (1) to establish baseline data regarding vital signs, LOC, neuromuscular function, and neurological status; (2) to preserve joint and muscle function; and (3) to prevent complications that may interfere with rehabilitation.

Phase 2: Rehabilitation. Plans for rehabilitation should begin the moment the patient is admitted. This means maintenance of an adequate airway and aeration of the lungs, proper positioning, ROM exercises for affected limbs, adequate nutrition and fluid intake and output, prevention of pressure ulcers, and all other nursing measures directed toward maintaining normal body functions until the patient is able to maintain them on his own (Clinical Pathway 14-1).

If the patient suffers from *homonymous hemianopia,* he has a visual defect affecting the same half of the visual field in each eye. He will not be able to see past the midline toward the side opposite the lesion and must turn the head to scan that side. The problem may cause accidents when ambulating. The patient must be taught ways to deal with this visual problem.

If dependent disabilities from inactivity are avoided, rehabilitation has a much better chance of success. During phase 2, various members of the health care team collaborate with the patient and his family to help resolve both psychosocial and physical problems. Among the team members helping the stroke victim may be the physical therapist, speech pathologist, social worker, psychologist, and occupational therapist. The patient usually is transferred from the hospital to a rehabilitation facility.

During phase 2, the patient is encouraged to strengthen his muscles as well as his resolve to help himself. He will need to exercise his muscles actively and retrain them. *The stroke has not directly affected his muscles, but it has damaged the centers that control muscular activity.*

There are many ways to encourage the patient. Instead of feeding him every item on his tray, let him hold bread and other "finger foods," suggesting that he feed himself these things. Chewing may be slow at first; the patient should not be hurried, nor should he be allowed to chew to the point of exhaustion. Eating often is difficult and messy, and privacy must be provided. If hemiplegia is causing the patient to "pocket" food in the folds of the mouth, the mouth should be checked after meals.

Combing and brushing the hair is good exercise for the arm and shoulder, as are brushing the teeth and washing the face and hands. The patient may not be able to carry all these procedures through to completion at first, but with encouragement he can gradually improve until he is able to perform much of his own personal care.

Text continued on page 368

CLINICAL PATHWAY 14-1 ◆ *Cerebral Vascular Accident (CVA)*

ICD-9 Code 014

ELOS 4 days

Nursing Diagnosis/ Collaborative Problem	Expected Outcome (The Patient Is Expected to . . .)	Met/Not Met	Reason	Date Initials
Altered cerebral tissue perfusion	Maintain baseline vital and neuro signs			
Sensory perceptual alteration	Have minimal complications and remain free of injury			
	Be oriented to environment			
Impaired physical mobility	Ambulate with or without assistive/ adaptive devices			
Self-care deficit	Perform own self-care with or without assistive/adaptive devices			
	Family member has received instruction on how to assist the patient			
Impaired verbal communication	Utilize communication strategies via speaking, communication board, or voice synthesizer			
Impaired swallowing	Eat meals without aspiration			
	Have an adequate nutritional status			

Aspect of Care	Date _____ Day 1	Date _____ Day 2	Date _____ Day 3	Date _____ Day 4
Assessment	Systems assessment with attention to neuro and cardiovascular system ◆ Change in LOC ◆ Visual field deficit ◆ Cognitive and language deficit ◆ Cranial nerve deficit ◆ Heart sounds and rhythm Evaluate need for Foley cath VS and NS q 4 h Monitor for complications ◆ Aspiration ◆ Paralytic ileus ◆ DVT, PE, SIADH, DI ◆ Atrial fibrilation, dysrhythmias ◆ Increased ICP, hydrocephalus Monitor for bleeding if on anticoagulant	Same as Day 1 Systems assessment q 8 h Assess pulmonary status before and after meals for aspiration pneumonia Assess for risk of falling	Same as Day 2 Assess for depression and emotional lability	Same as Day 3 VS q 8 h

Continued on following page

CLINICAL PATHWAY 14-1 • *Cerebral Vascular Accident (CVA) (Continued)*

Aspect of Care (Continued)	Date Day 1	Date Day 2	Date Day 3	Date Day 4
Teaching	Orient to unit and hospital	Prepare for diagnostic tests	Same as Day 2	Same as Day 3
	Prepare for diagnostic tests	Continue education regarding diagnosis	Begin bowel and bladder program, if incontinent	Instruct regarding meds to be administered at home
	Provide information about diagnosis	Begin ADL training	Teach lifestyle modification	◆ Route, time, action, side effects
	Involve family in care of patient as appropriate	◆ Communication	◆ Diet	
	Review care plan/critical pathway with patient and family	◆ Visual field deficits	◆ Exercise	
		◆ Muscle strengthening	◆ Quit smoking	
		◆ Swallowing		
		Continued family involvement		
		Right hemisphere stroke:		
		Teach to scan to left side		
		Have visitors sit on patient's left side, provide tactile stimulation to left side		
		Eliminate distraction of TV/radio		
		Left hemisphere stroke:		
		Communication skills		
Consults	Dietician	Rehab services: PT/OT/SLP	N/A	N/A
	Neurologist	Swallowing evaluation		
	Social worker			
Lab Tests	CBC with diff	APTT, if on heparin	APTT, if on heparin	INR(PT)
	U/A	Serum albumin, total protein	INR(PT), if on oral anticoagulants	
	Coag studies			
	Serum electrolytes			
	ESR			
Other Tests	CT/MRI	Ultrasonic or Doppler study	N/A	N/A
	Chest x-ray	*Embolic stroke:*		
	ECG	◆ Echocardiogram		
	Cerebral angiogram if hemorrhagic stroke	◆ Holter monitor		
		EEG		
Meds	*If cause other than hemorrhagic stroke:*	Same as Day 1	Change heparin to oral anticoagulant	Same as Day 3
	◆ Heparin continuous infusion			
	◆ ASA one tab or dipyridamole			
	Anticonvulsant			
	Calcium channel blocker, if stroke due to subarachnoid hemorrhage			
	Antihypertensive			
	Diuretic			
	Opioid or nonopioid analgesic			

Treatments/Interventions	Strict I & O Elevate HOB 30 to 45° Thigh-high antiembolism stockings Seizure precautions Daily wts Place call light in easy reach Suction as needed Mouth care q shift Develop communication system Prevent from injury Speak slowly, using short, simple sentences	Same as Day 1	Same as Day 2	I & O Thigh-high antiembolism stockings Elevate HOB 15–30° Continue with communication system Prevent from injury and falls
Nutrition	NPO	DAT ◆ Check for swallowing deficit ◆ Semisolid or pureed Assist with meals ◆ HOB elevated 90° ◆ Tilt head slightly forward ◆ Use spoon	Same as Day 2	Same as Day 3
Lines/Tubes Monitors	Continuous IV fluids Monitor for dehydration or overhydration	Same as Day 1	Convert IV to saline loc	D/C saline loc
Mobility/Self-Care	Bed rest TCDB q 2 h Active or passive ROM to all extremities q 4 h Maintain body alignment and support extremities with pillows, minimize stress on joints Skin assessment and care Use footboard, boots to prevent foot drop	*Same as Day 1 except:* OOB to chair TID ◆ Monitor for hypotension Arm sling to affected arm Muscle strengthening program Use assistive/adaptive devices for ambulation/transfers	*Same as Day 2 except:* Begin ambulation as tolerated with assistive devices as needed	Same as Day 3
Discharge Planning	Social worker to assess need for social services, financial status, health insurance and coverage, home environment, need for placement, and family support	Identify placement for discharge ◆ Rehab facility ◆ ECF ◆ Home	Begin discharge instruction and notes for ECF or rehab facility *or* Ensure that home has been equipped with assistive/adaptive devices and that family and patient know how to use them	Continue as Day 3 Arrange for follow-up visit with MD

The patient who has suffered brain injury becomes fatigued very quickly, and this must be kept in mind when encouraging self-care activities. Encouragement and praise for the smallest accomplishment can help the patient's tattered self-esteem.

The stroke patient is prone to rapid mood swings and spontaneous weeping. All health care workers must be patient and accepting, and an explanation to the patient and family that this is very common after a stroke can ease his embarrassment. Further information on rehabilitation programs is located in Chapter 12.

Phase 3. Plans are made for discharge and referral to individuals and agencies outside the hospital who will help the patient and his family adjust to his new way of life. A visiting nurse often is assigned for some time to coordinate rehabilitation efforts, assist with teaching, and assess the patient's status. The patient continues rehabilitation as an outpatient under the physician's supervision.

◆ Seizure Disorders and Epilepsy

A seizure or convulsion is an attack of uncontrollable muscular contractions that may affect all (*generalized seizure*) or part (*partial* or *focal seizure*) of the body. With *tonic* convulsions, there is continued contraction of all muscles and the body becomes rigid. *Tonic-clonic* convulsions are characterized by alternate contraction and relaxation of the muscles, which give the affected part a rhythmic, jerking motion. A *tonic-clonic* convulsion is typical of the grand mal organized seizure.

Epilepsy is a condition wherein recurrent seizures occur with altered consciousness, motor activity (convulsions), or sensory disturbances. Over 1 million people in the United States have some form of epilepsy. A brain tumor, scar tissue from head trauma or brain surgery, infection or irritation of the brain, or a progressive neurological disease may cause seizures.

There are several ways to classify epilepsy. The International Classification of Epileptic Seizures defines four groups: partial seizures, generalized seizures, unclassified seizures (because of insufficient data), and status epilepticus. The first group, partial seizures, is further divided into three subgroups: simple partial seizures, in which consciousness is not impaired but there are other motor, sensory, autonomic, or psychological symptoms; complex partial seizures, in which there is some impairment of consciousness with or without *automatisms* (repetitive, automatic actions such as lip smacking); and partial seizures that become generalized as the seizure continues.

Generalized seizures have symptoms or activity that is bilaterally symmetric and include absence, myoclonic, clonic, tonic, tonic-clonic, atonic, and infantile spasms (usually caused by fever). **Absence seizures are** called *petit mal* and tonic-clonic seizures are called *grand mal.*

The third major group, unclassified seizures, simply means that not enough data have been obtained to determine which type of seizure the patient is experiencing.

The fourth designation, status epilepticus, indicates prolonged partial or generalized seizure without recovery between attacks.

Seizures can be symptomatic of a large number of disorders. Brain injury, infectious diseases with high fever, end-stage renal disease with uremia, toxicity (such as that occurring in eclampsia during pregnancy or in drug poisoning), epilepsy, and tetanus are but a few examples of seizure-producing disorders. **Seizures also can occur any time the brain is deprived of oxygen.**

Epilepsy is a chronic disturbance of the nervous system characterized by recurrent seizures that are the result of abnormal electrical activity of the brain. In epilepsy there is an excessive firing of brain cells, but this abnormal discharge occurs only occasionally; at other times the firing is normal.

Partial seizures also are called *simple* or *focal* seizures and result from an abnormal localized cortical discharge. Partial seizures with complex symptomatology, also called *psychomotor* or *temporal lobe seizures,* usually, but not always, originate in the temporal lobe of the brain. Partial seizures can be unilateral, with involvement on only one side of the brain and activity only on one side of the body.

Generalized seizures are bilaterally symmetrical (affecting both sides of the body equally) and *do not* have a local onset; that is, they do not typically begin in one part of the body.

In classifying epileptic seizures on the basis of origin, seizures are grouped as either idiopathic or symptomatic. *Idiopathic* epilepsy has no known cause. *Symptomatic* epilepsy has a known physical cause (e.g., brain tumor, injury to the head at birth, a wound or blow to the head, or an endocrine disorder).

Diagnosis   The manifestations of epilepsy depend on the area of the brain where the abnormal firing occurs. *Absence* or *petit mal* seizures last only a few seconds. **The onset is sudden, with no aura or warning and no postictal (after-seizure activity) symptoms.** Seizures of this type usually affect children between 5 and 12 years of age and disappear during puberty. There usually is a twitching about the eyes and mouth. The person remains standing or sitting and appears to have had no more than a lapse of attention or a moment of absent-mindedness.

Grand mal or *tonic-clonic* seizures usually begin with bilateral jerks of the extremities or focal seizure activity. There is loss of consciousness and both tonic and clonic convulsions. The patient may be incontinent during the attack, and there is danger of biting the tongue. In the postictal phase the person is confused and drowsy.

Atonic or *akinetic* seizures are characterized by loss of body tone that results in nodding of the head, weakness of the knees, or total collapse and falling— "drop attacks." The person usually remains conscious during the attack.

Status epilepticus **is a grave condition in which there is a rapid, unrelenting series of convulsive seizures without intervening periods of consciousness and absence of respiration. Irreversible brain damage can occur if the seizures are not controlled.** Treatment of status epilepticus depends on its cause. Many times patients who are known to have epilepsy arrive in the emergency department with status epilepticus because, for one reason or the other, they stopped taking the medication that controls their seizures. Treatment in this instance would involve administering diazepam, phenytoin, or phenobarbital in a dose sufficiently high to stop the seizures.

Uncontrolled seizures secondary to hypoglycemia (as in improperly controlled diabetes mellitus) can be relieved by IV administration of 50% dextrose. If the unrelenting seizures are caused by chronic alcoholism or withdrawal, treatment consists of IV administration of thiamin. Although these kinds of seizures are known as status epilepticus, they should not be confused with chronic epileptic seizures.

A diagnosis of epilepsy is confirmed by electroencephalogram and MRI. These tests help locate the site, or *locus,* and possibly the cause of the seizures. Skull radiographs also are part of the diagnostic workup when epilepsy is suspected.

Treatment   When the cause of seizures is known, as in cases of high fever or drug toxicity, medical treatment is aimed at controlling or eliminating whatever is responsible for the seizures. However, when there are recurrent seizures, as in epilepsy, the condition usually is managed with anticonvulsant drug therapy.

The major antiepileptic drugs are phenytoin (Dilantin), phenobarbital, primidone (Mysoline), carbamazepine (Tegretol), Vigabatrin (Sabril), and lamotrigine (Lamictal) for complex partial tonic-clonic seizures and valproic acid (Depakene), ethosuximide (Zarontin), and clonazepam (Klonopin) for absence epileptic seizures. Lamictal is used with Depakene as an adjunct for partial seizures. Felbamate (Felbatol) is a new drug that provides better seizure control for patients who have had poor control with older drugs. Gabapentin (Neurontin) is a new drug for adult epilepsy that can be added to the patient's drug regimen to achieve better seizure control. Fosphenytoin (Cerebyx) was approved early in 1997 for injection, replacing injectable Dilantin. It can be injected IM as well as IV and produces fewer local reactions. It is compatible with most IV solutions, can be infused faster than Dilantin and does not cause tissue sloughing and necrosis if the IV solution infiltrates. Anticonvulsants are capable of interacting with other drugs and decreasing or enhancing their specific action. Among the drugs that interact with anticonvulsants are warfarin, digoxin, aspirin, certain antibiotics, antacids, folic acid, and narcotics.

All of the anticonvulsant drugs can produce some unpleasant side effects, such as fever and leukopenia and, in the case of phenytoin, gingival hyperplasia and rash. Physical dependence can become a problem for patients taking either phenobarbital or primidone, which is largely converted to phenobarbital in the bloodstream. Toxic side effects such as ataxia, drowsiness, nausea, sedation, and dizziness are not uncommon. Because of these and other toxicities associated with anticonvulsant therapy, patients taking these drugs regularly must have periodic laboratory tests performed and must remain under close supervision.

Patient education is extremely important, because the patient will need to report any untoward effects to the physician or nurse clinician so the dosage can be adjusted or the drug changed.

Through the efforts of the Epilepsy Association of America, the general public has become increasingly aware of the true nature of epilepsy. Research continues in an effort to find the cause and cure for this disease. In the meantime, we all have a responsibility to help those afflicted with epilepsy gain steady employment and lead useful, active lives. Most individuals who suffer from epileptic seizures are perfectly normal between seizures; they are not mentally retarded and are quite capable of becoming contributing members of our society if only they are given the chance to prove their worth.

Surgical treatment of epilepsy is an alternative for about 5% of all persons who have the disorder. The procedure involves removing the portion of brain tissue that is the source of the seizures. Surgery of this kind is not without danger and is reserved for those patients whose seizures cannot be managed by medical treatment and in whom the focus of the seizures is accessible. It is most successful for temporal lobe seizures.

A NeuroCybernetic Prosthesis has been approved as an implant in the chest with a wire tunneled to stimulate the vagus nerve. It acts similar to a pacemaker and provides a tiny stimulus every 5 minutes which stimulates the brain to interrupt seizures. It provides great hope for the 200,000 Americans, and others, whose seizures cannot be adequately controlled by medicine.

Nursing Assessment and Intervention   Patients with a known seizure problem usually are treated on an outpatient basis. However, these patients also are seen in hospitals or long-term care facilities and must be assessed carefully to provide optimal safety and care. Significant information includes the kind of seizures they experience, whether they have any sensation (**aura**) just before the appearance of clinically observable signs, what medications they are taking, and what measures are known to be helpful either to prevent a seizure or to assist while they are having a seizure and afterward.

When caring for a patient who is likely to experience a seizure during an acute illness, the nurse should periodically observe the patient for tremors, unexplained sensory or motor changes, mental changes that indicate confusion or disorientation, and restless or agitated behavior. **In many cases, a change in the neurological status of a patient can signal the possibility that a seizure might occur.** Nursing care of patients with epileptic seizures is concerned with immediate care during and after a seizure and long-term management and control of seizures and their psychosocial implications. Assessment should include any factors that could have triggered the seizure (e.g., hyperventilation, bright lights [photosensitivity], alcohol and other drugs, fluid and electrolyte imbalances, lack of sleep, and emotional stress).

A major concern of those caring for a patient subject to seizures is to protect him from injury. Although witnessing a seizure for the first time can be a frightening experience, the movements the person is making are just exaggerations of normal body movements.

> The nurse's first responsibility is to stay calm, remain with the patient, and send for assistance.

The environment of a patient at risk for seizure should be made as safe as possible. If the patient is very likely to have seizures, the siderails and headboard of the bed are padded. The nurse should never try to pry open the mouth or insert something into it as teeth may be broken and the airway may be obstructed.

If a seizure comes on without warning, the patient should be left wherever he is lying. If he is on a hard surface, his head should be protected from injury by placing a pillow or a rolled blanket or coat under it. The head should be turned to the side, if possible, to prevent aspiration. Do not attempt to restrain the patient's movements or to move him to a bed or chair during the seizure. If supplemental oxygen is near, it should be administered. When the seizure is over, turn the patient to the side.

Observations during a patient's seizure should include as much of the following as possible:

- The time the seizure began, whether the patient experienced an aura, and the length of time the seizure lasted.
- What the patient was doing just before the seizure.

- Where in the body the seizure began and what parts of the body were involved; which side the eyes move toward or other eye movement.
- The character of the movements (tonic or clonic) and whether they changed during the seizure.
- Whether the head or eyes turned to one side and, if so, which side.
- Whether there was incontinence of urine or stool; vomiting, bleeding; or foaming or frothing at the mouth.
- If the eyes are open, in which direction they were positioned.
- The effects of the seizure on the patient's vital signs.
- Changes in skin color or profuse perspiration. *Postictal (after seizure) assessment after establishing an open airway* should include information about the presence of lethargy, confusion, headache, speech impairment, and muscle soreness. The patient should be allowed to sleep or rest after the seizure.

The long-term management of epileptic seizures is primarily focused on providing the patient with the information and support he needs to care for himself and avoid recurring and debilitating seizures.

Patient education. Self-care for the epileptic requires that he understand the nature of his disorder, the purpose of his prescribed medications, their side effects, and the signs of toxicity that should be reported to the physician. He must understand the necessity for compliance with the prescribed regimen to avoid recurrent seizures. He will need assistance in developing coping mechanisms to deal with the psychosocial impact of having epilepsy.

The teaching plan also should include information about possible seizure-triggering mechanisms and the importance of avoiding them whenever possible. Alcohol is especially contraindicated for the patient with seizures, as it interferes with the effectiveness of the medications, causes excessive sedation, and may trigger seizures. Fatigue also can make the patient more prone to seizure activity. He must be helped to plan for adequate rest each day.

The patient is taught not to swim or participate alone in activities that could have dangerous effects if he had a seizure and was alone. Women need to know that menstruation puts additional stress on the body, and they are more prone to seizures during this period each month. Persons with epilepsy should wear a Medic-Alert bracelet or necklace and carry a list of the medications they are taking and names and phone numbers of their physician and others to be notified in an emergency.

Psychosocial support is necessary to encourage the patient to talk about his fears and concerns. Lifestyle changes will have to be made if he is not permitted to drive. Most states allow resumption of driving when a patient has been seizure free for 1 year. A referral to the local epilepsy society for connection with a support group can be very helpful for both the patient and his family.

Think about . . . What would you teach a 22-year-old male who has just been diagnosed with grand mal epilepsy regarding safety?

◆ Cerebral Palsy

Cerebral palsy includes a group of paralytic disorders in which muscle coordination is lost as a result of cerebral damage that is generally thought to occur at or near the time of birth. The exact cause is not known, but the condition is believed to be associated with oxygen lack. Current research also has indicated that low thyroid levels at birth may be a factor.

Diagnosis   Although cerebral palsy can cause a wide variety of muscular disorders and some disturbances of sensory perception, it can be categorized into three general types: (1) *spastic paralysis*, in which there are exaggerated reflexes, increased deep tendon reflexes, and muscle spasms; (2) *athetoid type*, in which there are random and purposeless movements and a high degree of muscle tension; and (3) *ataxic type*, in which there is a disturbance of coordination with poor balance and a staggering gait. The patient also may suffer from defects of hearing, vision, or speech. The impairment may be severe or minimal.

Treatment   There is no cure for cerebral palsy, but early muscle training and special exercises can be of benefit if they are started before a child develops faulty habits of movement and incorrect muscle patterns. In some cases, orthopedic surgery and devices such as braces and casts can be used to correct orthopedic deformities and disabilities. Treatment is lifelong and individualized, attempting to prevent complications and to help individuals lead the fullest life possible, limited only by the imposed muscular and sensory disturbances.

◆ Attitudes toward Cerebral Palsy Victims

Most victims of cerebral palsy, be they men, women, or children, long to be treated as normal, sane individuals. For some reason, many people assume that the speech difficulties and uncoordinated movements characteristic of cerebral palsy indicate mental retardation or total disability. Although the cerebral palsy victim may be somewhat slow and clumsy in accomplishing relatively simple tasks or difficult to understand when he is talking, he can be fairly independent if one is patient with him and willing to make the effort to communicate. Patients who have entered hospitals for an unrelated illness and are sufferers of cerebral palsy often are treated in a humiliating and degrading manner by personnel who assume that, because the patient is uncoordinated in his movements and cannot speak clearly, he too is mentally retarded, unable to comprehend what is happening to him, and unaware of the fact that he is not thought of or treated as a rational, thinking human person. A young patient wrote the following after being admitted to a hospital for an appendectomy: "There were many depressing moments during my hospital stay. Some could not have been avoided; others might have been if personnel had known that what I needed most was to be treated as any patient would be—as the 19-year-old adult I am."

MUSCULAR DYSTROPHY

Muscular dystrophy is a disorder that affects both the nerves and the muscles. It is an inherited, progressive disease that takes several forms. It is not certain whether the disorder is due to a disturbance in nerve–muscle interaction or to muscle cell degeneration. Symptoms usually begin in infancy, and many of the patients do not survive past early adulthood. There is no cure. Treatment is corrective surgery and the use of braces along with exercise programs to prevent deterioration of muscle capability and to correct contractures.

HUNTINGTON'S DISEASE

Huntington's disease is a genetically transmitted degenerative neurological disorder characterized by abnormal movements (chorea). It is accompanied by decline in intellectual capacity and emotional disturbances. Signs usually become evident during the fourth or fifth decade of life, but may occur earlier. Women and men are equally affected. The disorder is progressive and causes disability and then death within 15 to 20 years after signs appear. Genetic transmission is by an abnormal gene on the short arm of chromosome 4. It is an autosomal dominant disorder, meaning that 50% of the children of a person who has the disease will inherit it. If a child does not inherit the disease, the gene is not passed on to the next generation.

The person progresses from being fidgety and restless to a state of constant movement. There is no specific test for the disease, and there is no known treatment to alter its course. Voluntary movement deteriorates until the patient is totally helpless. Intellectual decline causes depression, suspiciousness, and eventual dementia.

CRANIAL NERVE DISORDERS

◆Trigeminal Neuralgia (TIC Douloureux)

This disorder involves one or more branches of the fifth cranial (trigeminal) nerve. The three branches of this nerve are the ophthalmic, the mandibular, and the maxillary (Figure 14-17). The disorder most commonly affects people over age 50. In most cases of trigeminal neuralgia the ophthalmic nerve is not involved. The motor and sensory functions affected by trigeminal neuralgia include chewing and facial movements and sensations of the face, scalp, teeth, nasal cavities, and ear drum.

The cause of trigeminal neuralgia is not known, although it can be related to pressure on the nerve root by a tumor or to a lesion of the blood vessels.

Diagnosis   The most notable symptom of trigeminal neuralgia is severe pain, which is described as sharp and intense, lasting for 1 to 2 minutes, and located along the pathway of one of the branches of the trigeminal nerve. The pain is localized on one side of the face, rarely affecting both sides. It can extend from the midline of the face across the cheek and jaw to the ear.

Attacks are usually triggered by exposure to cold drafts or drinking cold or very hot liquids, chewing, brushing the hair, shaving, or washing the face. Between acute flareups the patient may experience no pain, or he may report a dull ache. The pain during the acute phase is so severe that many patients live in constant fear they will do something to provoke an attack.

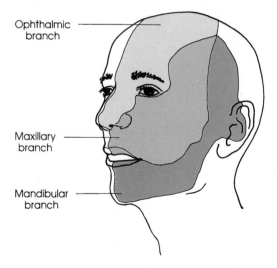

FIGURE 14-17   Areas of innervation by each of the three branches of the trigeminal nerve.

Diagnosis is based on the patient's history and chief complaint and tests to rule out cerebellopontine angle tumor. There is no test to confirm the diagnosis, and there are no observable pathological changes.

Treatment   Medical management usually is preferred to surgical intervention, because the latter involves dissection of nerve rootlets with resultant loss of motor and sensory function. Microsurgical techniques to decompress the fifth cranial nerve at its entrance to (or exit from) the brainstem provide relief in about 73% of cases. Percutaneous radiofrequency rhizotomy may be used to coagulate specific divisions of the nerve that is causing pain. Laser surgery is another option. The procedure decreases facial sensation as well as relieves pain.

The drugs most frequently prescribed to prevent or relieve spasmodic pain are the anticonvulsants carbamazepine (Tegretol), or phenytoin (Dilantin) and the muscle relaxant baclofen (Lioresal). Relief of severe pain usually can be obtained by injecting either alcohol or glycerol into the terminal branch of the trigeminal nerve.

Nursing Assessment and Intervention   Observing the patient between acute attacks can help identify clues to affirm the presence of trigeminal neuralgia. The patient may not wash his face or shave, and he will guard his face or hold it immobile to avoid an attack. He is very sensitive to any contact with his face and will indicate the area of pain by pointing to, but never touching, it.

The universal nursing diagnosis for patients with trigeminal neuralgia is, of course, pain. Because chewing can provoke an attack of pain, the patient may be susceptible to nutritional deficit. Small, frequent feedings consisting of food that is moderately warm can help provide adequate nutrition and at the same time avoid precipitating an acute attack.

Nursing intervention for the patient who is being treated medically includes instruction about the expected actions and adverse side effects of the drug he is taking. Phenytoin can produce ataxia, skin eruptions, overgrowth of the gums, and nystagmus. Carbamazepine can damage the bone marrow and produce such hematological reactions as leukopenia, aplastic anemia, and decreased platelet count. Skin eruptions also can occur as a reaction to carbamazepine or baclofen. The patient's blood count and liver function must be closely monitored to detect early signs of drug toxicity. Baclofen may cause transient drowsiness, nausea, weakness, or fatigue.

Surgical treatment of trigeminal neuralgia brings about problems related to potential for damage to the cornea when the ophthalmic branch is dissected. The patient must be taught to avoid rubbing his eyes or exposing them to foreign objects because the normal protective corneal reflex is no longer functional. He should get into the habit of wearing protective goggles when there is the possibility of getting dust and debris in his eyes and to try to blink his eyes often to cleanse their surface.

Dissection of the second or third branches of the trigeminal nerve produces problems of potential damage to the oral mucosa and teeth. The patient cannot feel hot liquids and foods and could be burned, he could bite the inside of his mouth without realizing it, or he may have dental caries that will not cause pain. Good oral hygiene and periodic dental examinations are particularly important when the body's natural warning system is not operative.

BELL'S PALSY

Bell's palsy is weakness or paralysis of the muscles supplied by the facial nerve. It usually affects only one side of the face. The cause is unknown, and it occurs in people over age 30. It is most likely viral in origin. Exposure to cold is a risk factor. Sometimes it occurs during pregnancy. **Signs and symptoms are numbness and partial or total paralysis of the facial muscles suddenly or over a few days.** Treatment consists of closing and patching the eye if it loses the blink reflex. Artificial tear eye drops also are used to prevent dryness of the cornea. Corticosteroids are given if they can be started right after the beginning of symptoms. They are ineffective if delayed more than 4 days. Recovery is individual; those with total paralysis may not achieve full recovery but will improve as inflammation declines.

DISORDERS OF THE SPINE AND SPINAL CORD

◆ Spinal Cord Injury

Diagnosis   A person may suffer from injury to the spinal cord in a number of ways. Automobile accidents, gunshot wounds, and other forms of violence often inflict severe damage to the spinal cord, but tumors, degenerative disease, and infections also can impair the functions of the spinal cord and its branches. When sufficient force is applied to the spinal cord, damage occurs. Fracture, dislocation, or subluxation of the vertebral column often results in cord damage. Penetrating trauma from gunshot or knife wounds or other type of accident may cause severance of the cord, or compression, or contusion. Extreme flexion or hyperextension of the neck, or falling on the buttocks, which causes flexion of the lower thoracic and lumbar spine, all may cause spinal cord damage. Tumor growth may compress or destroy spinal cord tissue.

Generally speaking, spinal cord injuries are classified according to their anatomic location; that is, cervical, thoracic, or lumbosacral. Whatever the cause of spinal cord injury, the clinical manifestations of the injury are the same.

> A complete severance of the cord results in a total loss of sensation and control in the parts of the body below the point of injury. If the cord is severed in the cervical region, the paralysis and loss of sensory perception will include both arms and both legs. Severe injury to the cord above the level of the fifth cervical vertebra often is fatal if emergency care is not immediate because the phrenic nerves originate in the third, fourth, and fifth cervical segments. Branches of these nerves play a major role in the control of respiration, and when they are severed, respiration must be maintained by artificial means.

Interruption of the thoracic spine through L-1 and L-2 causes **paraplegia** (paralysis of both legs). Table 14-16 presents activities possible at varying levels of cord injury.

Injury to the spinal cord that does not involve complete severance of the cord may result in a temporary paralysis, which may subside as the spinal cord recovers from the swelling and initial shock of the injury.

Treatment

> There are four main objectives in the treatment and nursing care of the patient with an injury of the spinal cord: (1) to save the victim's life; (2) to prevent further injury to the cord by careful handling of the patient; (3) to repair as much of the damage to the cord as possible; and (4) to establish a routine of care that will improve and maintain the patient's state of health and prevent complications, so that eventual physical, mental, and social rehabilitation is possible.

Immediate care.   As soon as a person suffers a sudden injury to the spinal cord, he must be handled with extreme care. Because a nurse or doctor may not be at the scene of the accident to supervise the moving of the victim, laypersons should learn the proper emergency care of such injuries. Any time an accident suggests that the victim may have suffered a neck or back injury, the victim complains of neck or back pain, cannot move his legs or has no feeling in them, he must be treated as if he has a spinal cord injury. **Anyone with a head injury is treated as if he has also suffered a spine injury until proven otherwise.**

The neck is immobilized before moving the person. This can be done when no cervical collar is available by using a shirt, towel, coat, or other material rolled and

TABLE 14-16 ◆ *Level of Spinal Cord Damage, Function Present, and Activities Possible*

Level of Injury	Function Present/Neurological Deficit	Activity Possible
C-1–C-3	No respiratory function; usually fatal unless immediate emergecy help is available to establish respiration.	Respirations stimulated with phrenic pacemaker. Can manipulate electric wheelchair with breath, chin, or voice control.
C-4	Loss of diaphragm movement; breathe with assistance. Quadriplegia.	May live if assisted respiration is begun immediately. Can use a mouthstick to turn pages, type, or write.
C-5	Partial shoulder movement; partial elbow movement.	Can turn head. Able to feed self with special adaptive devices. Able to move wheelchair for short distances; moves well with electric wheelchair. Can assist a bit with self-care.
C-6	Retains gross motor function of arms; partial shoulder, elbow, and wrist movement possible. Paraplegia.	Needs adaptive devices; may be able to propel wheelchair. Independent in feeding and with some grooming with adaptive devices. Can roll over in bed. Can drive a car with hand controls. Can assist in transfer. Can self-catheterize the bladder.
C-7	Shoulder, elbow, wrist, hand partial movements possible; paraplegia.	Manipulate wheelchair with arms; transfer to and from chair; may drive specially fitted car. Excellent bed mobility. Independent in most ADLs.
C-8	Normal arm movement; hand weakness. Paraplegia.	Bed and wheelchair independent. Can perform most activities of daily living and may achieve vocational and recreational goals. Performs self-catheterization.
T-1–T-10	Normal arm movement and strength; loss of bowel, bladder, and sexual function.	T-6–T-10 may achieve walking with braces. Able to perform ADLs and achieve vocational and recreational goals.
T-11 and below	Loss of bowel, bladder, and sexual function.	Wheelchair not essential. Able to perform ADLs, work, and recreation.

Note: Each level can also perform the activities of the levels above it.

placed around the neck as a collar to keep the neck as straight as possible, preventing it from flexing or hyperextending. If the victim must be moved to safety, he should be rolled like a log, as one straight piece, onto a flat surface, such as a piece of plywood or a door removed from its hinges. He is rolled as one piece onto his side, the flat surface placed beside him, and then he is carefully rolled back onto the board. This is done slowly and carefully to avoid twisting or bending the spinal column.

Transfer of the patient to the hospital should be done only by trained emergency medical technicians or others qualified to administer first aid. **A cervical collar is applied if there is any question of neck injury.** The victim is log-rolled onto a stretcher or board and taken directly to the hospital. His back must be kept straight and be well supported. **To avoid flexion of the neck, *no pillow or other kind of support is placed under the head.***

In the emergency department of the hospital, the patient's condition is stabilized and a thorough examination is conducted to establish the extent of his injuries. A large dose of methylprednisolone may be given as soon as the examination and diagnosis of cord injury is made. If given within 8 hours of injury it minimizes further injury and improves the return of both motor function and sensation. Tirilazad (Freedox) may be infused to prevent or limit neural damage after cord injury. **Cervical spinal cord injury usually is treated with traction to immobilize the affected vertebrae and maintain them in alignment.** Traction can be accomplished by a head halter; skeletal traction using Crutchfield or Gardener-Wells tongs with ropes, pulleys, and weights (Figure 14-18); or a halo ring and fixation pins (Figure 14-19).

Care of the pin sites is performed every shift initially and then twice a day. Sterile technique is used and is performed according to agency policy. Solutions, such as saline or hydrogen peroxide, or ointments, such as povidone-iodine or bacitracin, may be used. Weights for traction with cervical tongs must be kept hanging free to be effective. If the patient is wearing a halo fixation device, skin care must be given frequently and the skin checked to see that the jacket or cast is not causing pressure areas. One finger should be able to slip easily beneath the cast or jacket. The patient is never moved or turned by holding or pulling on the halo device. **The halo jacket is never unfastened unless the patient is supine or head movement will immediately occur.**

Selecting the type of bed to be used for a patient with spinal cord injury depends on many factors. Some

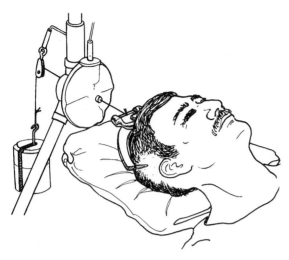

FIGURE 14-18 Crutchfield tongs for cervical traction.

physicians and nurses prefer placing the patient in a special bed designed to prevent the problems of immobility while maintaining traction. If halo traction is used and the patient has no severance of the spinal cord, a standard orthopedic bed may be used. Figure 14-19 shows a patient in cervical traction with halo fixation that can maintain stability of the cervical vertebrae while the patient is in or out of bed. "Log-rolling" the

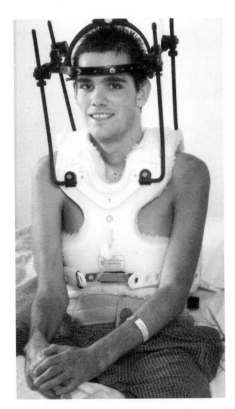

FIGURE 14-19   Halo ring and apparatus for stabilization of the cervical spine. (Photo by Glen Derbyshire; Courtesy of Rehabilitation Institute of Santa Barbara, California.)

patient must be done with extreme care to avoid twisting the vertebral column and further damaging the spinal cord (Figure 14-20).

Once the patient is in bed, the true test of nursing care begins. All the nursing measures designed to prevent the disabilities that may result from immobility, to promote healing, and to avoid complications are used to help the patient achieve the goals of rehabilitation. Bladder and bowel training programs, as well as instruction in moving from bed to chair and other aspects of self-care, may be necessary. Realistic goals should be set for the patient and every effort made to achieve them.

Spinal shock (neurogenic shock).   The disruption in the nerve communication pathways between upper motor neurons and lower motor neurons immediately causes spinal shock. It is characterized by flaccid paralysis, loss of reflex activity below the level of the damage, bradycardia, hypotension, and occasionally paralytic ileus. Spinal shock may last for a few days to several months. Treatment is aimed at maintaining adequate blood pressure and heart rate.

Muscle spasms.   Immediately after a cord injury, the patient will usually have a flaccid type of paralysis. Later, as the cord adjusts to the injury, the paralysis will become *spastic,* and there will be strong, involuntary contractions of the skeletal muscles.

These muscle spasms, which may be violent enough to throw the patient from his bed or wheelchair, must be anticipated and the patient secured so that accidents can be avoided. If the upper extremities are involved, he is likely to tip over glasses, water pitchers, or anything within reach of his arms when he is seized with uncontrollable muscle spasms.

The patient and his family may interpret these spasms as a return of voluntary function of the limbs and will thus have false hopes of complete recovery. It is best if the nurse in charge or the physician explains to them that such is not the case.

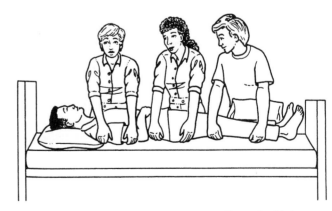

FIGURE 14-20   Log-rolling a patient with a spinal injury. (*Source:* deWit, S. C. [1994]. *Rambo's Nursing Skills for Clinical Practice,* 4th ed. Philadelphia: Saunders, p. 127.)

To avoid stimulating the muscles when moving the patient and thereby precipitating a spasm of the muscles, the nurse should avoid grasping the muscle itself. The palms of the hands are used to support the joints above and below the affected muscles. The administration of antispasmodic medications such as baclofen (Lioresal) may decrease the severity of the spasms.

Autonomic dysreflexia (hyperreflexia). Autonomic dysreflexia (AD) is an uninhibited and exaggerated reflex response of the autonomic nervous system to some form of stimulation. It is a response that occurs in 85% of all patients who have spinal cord injury at or above the level of the sixth thoracic vertebra (T-6). The response is potentially dangerous to the patient, because it can produce vasoconstriction of the arterioles with an immediate elevation of blood pressure. The sudden hypertension can, in turn, cause a seizure, hemorrhage into the retina of the eye, or a stroke. Less serious effects include severe headache, changes in pulse rate, sweating and flushing above the level of the spinal cord lesion, and pallor and "goose bumps" below the level of injury.

It is important for nurses and others participating in the care of a patient with quadriplegia and other kinds of spinal cord disorders at or above the T-6 level to be aware of the circumstances that can trigger AD, its manifestations, and the correct measures to take if it happens. The problem can occur any time after a spinal cord injury; in some cases it has first appeared as late as 6 years after the injury.

There are many kinds of stimulation that can precipitate AD. Most are related to the bladder, bowel, and skin of the patient. For example, catheter changes, a distended bladder, the insertion of rectal suppositories, enemas, and sudden changing of position can provide the stimulation that results in AD.

Once the patient exhibits symptoms of AD, an emergency exists. Efforts should be made to lower blood pressure by placing him in a sitting position or elevating his head to a 45-degree angle. If the cause of the stimulation is known—for example, an impacted bowel, overdistended bladder, or pressure against the skin—the stimulus should be removed as gently and quickly as possible. The physician should be notified immediately so that the appropriate medications can be prescribed and administered. Patients who experience repeated attacks of AD may require surgery to sever the nerves responsible for the exaggerated response to stimulation.

Pyschological impact. The short-term and long-term psychological changes brought about by spinal cord injury and paralysis are difficult, if not impossible, to measure. Adjustment to such a drastic change in one's lifestyle is a continuous process that may well last a lifetime.

It is fortunate that today many health care professionals other than the physician and the nurse are prepared to counsel and guide the patient in his efforts at adjustment. Nurses who feel uncomfortable and unknowledgeable about the best way to help a patient deal with emotional and psychosocial problems should discuss feelings with other professionals and seek their assistance.

Legislation in the last decade to protect the rights of Americans with disabilities has done much to make the life of a person with a neurological deficit better. Most buildings, theaters, and restrooms, are now wheelchair accessible, allowing handicapped individuals to enjoy eating out and social activities, as well as promoting their independence in taking care of their own business matters. Most cities have public transportation available that can accommodate a wheelchair. Individuals cannot be terminated from or refused a job on the basis of their neurological deficit as long as they are capable of performing the tasks required. Vocational training is available to anyone who is unable to return to a former occupation because of neurological deficit.

One area of concern to the patient and his family members that has formerly been ignored for the most part is that of sexual function and sexuality following spinal cord injury. Discussions of sexual conduct and the larger concept of human sexuality are not easily approached and participated in by many individuals. The nurse who wishes to help a patient deal with problems of sexuality must first come to terms with her own feelings and attitudes and clarify her own values. She should also try to be uncritical and nonjudgmental in her dealings with her patients. The patient and his partner must be encouraged to verbalize their concerns and questions and should be given guidance in alternative ways to express sexuality and meet sexual needs.

There often is a tendency to treat a physically disabled patient as if he were something less than a "whole" person with the same desires, hopes, and anxieties that all humans share. The nurse can best serve her patients by reacting to and interacting with them in an open and honest manner. When the nurse feels unprepared to handle a certain problem, there is no reason not to admit embarrassment, confusion, or lack of information readily and seek assistance from other members of the health care team. Rehabilitation of the patient with spinal cord injury is also discussed in Chapter 12.

BACK PAIN AND RUPTURED INTERVERTEBRAL DISC ("SLIPPED DISC")

Back pain occurrence is only surpassed by headache pain. Low-back pain causes 40% to 50% of all "sick" days taken from work. It is estimated that the cost of low-back pain for the 8 to 10 million people who experience it is at least $16 billion a year in the United States. Needless to say, it is a major health care problem. Carelessness and incorrect methods of lifting contribute to a large percentage of back problems. On-the-job accidents and resultant trauma to the spine are another cause. Obesity contributes to the stress placed on the back muscles and to the occurrence of injury or the severity and duration of pain.

Preventing back pain and disorders begins with proper posture and the use of correct lifting techniques. The use of a lumbar corset brace when lifting is known to decrease the incidence of injury. Maintaining one's weight within normal limits also helps prevent back strain. Sufficient physical exercise that maintains the condition of the back muscles and specific exercises to strengthen the abdominal and back muscles can greatly decrease the repeated incidence of back pain. Back pain can occur from a sprain or strain of the muscles or can be due to herniation of the *nucleus pulposus*.

The bodies of the vertebrae lie flat on one another like a stack of coins. Between the vertebral bodies there is a disc of fibrous cartilage that acts as a cushion to absorb shocks to the spinal column. This disc may be ruptured by an injury, such as strain caused by lifting a heavy object or wrenching or falling on the back. When the disc ruptures, part of it squeezes out from between the vertebrae and pinches the adjacent nerve root by pressing it against the bone (Figure 14-21). Thus the person suffers from what is sometimes called a "slipped disc." Another name for this condition is *herniated nucleus pulposus* (HNP).

Diagnosis About 95% of all ruptured or slipped discs in the lower back occur at the fourth and fifth invertebral spaces in the lumbar spine. The patient experiences pain in the lower back radiating down the back of the leg to the foot. Walking is extremely painful, and the discomfort is aggravated by coughing, sneezing, or straining. Many times young patients give a history of "feeling something give way" in their backs.

When the ruptured disc is located in the cervical region, the patient complains of pain in the neck, shoulder pain radiating down the arm into the hand, and tingling and numbness of the hand and fingers. Diagnosis usually is confirmed by radiographs, CT scan, MRI scan, or myelography.

Treatment In most instances, the physician will treat back pain initially with conservative measures in the hope that surgical correction will not be necessary. The Agency for Health Care Policy and Research has issued Clinical Practice Guidelines that suggest the following measures.

The patient is placed on a firm mattress with bed boards under it. The bed is kept flat, and the patient is placed on bedrest for 2 to 3 days. During this period, the patient is encouraged to get up and walk around every 2 to 3 hours while awake even if this causes pain. When he is turned off his back, he is taught to turn without bending his back. To accomplish this, the arms are brought up to the chest, the knee opposite the side on which he is to turn is flexed, and the patient eases himself over.

Ice packs are applied for 5 to 10 minutes at a time each hour for the first 48 hours to reduce muscle spasm

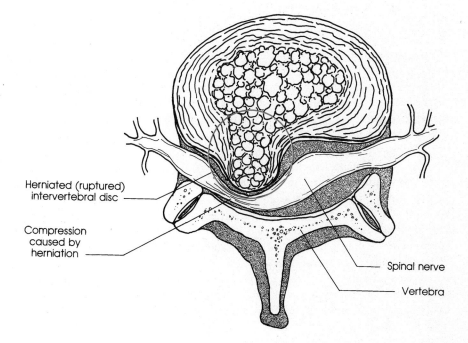

FIGURE 14-21 Cross section of intervertebral disc with herniation pressing against spinal nerve.

Herniated (ruptured) intervertebral disc

Compression caused by herniation

Spinal nerve

Vertebra

in the back. After 48 hours heat may be more helpful. Heating pads, hot packs, and hot showers work well. Heat is applied for 20 minutes every 1 to 2 hours. Pelvic traction may be ordered by some physicians, and mild exercises are usually ordered. These treatments are performed under the guidance of a physical therapist. Specially designed corsets or back braces are sometimes used to maintain proper alignment of the spine when the patient is allowed out of bed. The patient is cautioned not to lift anything heavier than 2 to 5 lb and not to twist when reaching for things. The patient should be up moving about frequently rather than sitting for long periods. Walking for short distances frequently is very beneficial. An adjustment by a chiropractor may also help relieve pain. If pain continues beyond 3 to 4 weeks, there is evidence of neurological deficit, or pain is worsening, surgery may be indicated.

Surgical procedures. For those patients who cannot find relief through conservative measures, surgical removal of the damaged disc may be the only alternative. A diskectomy often is performed. This is a microsurgical technique that utilizes a very small incision through which the herniated intervertebral disc material is dissected and extracted. If the area cannot be handled with microsurgery, an open incision diskectomy or laminectomy, which involves removal of the posterior arch of the vertebra along with the disc, is done. A spinal fusion is necessary in some patients to stabilize the spine. In a spinal fusion, a piece or pieces of bone from the iliac crest are grafted onto the vertebrae to strengthen them. This procedure may be done for conditions other than a ruptured disc, for example, for such degenerative diseases of the spine as Pott's disease (tuberculosis of the spine), for fractures of the spine, and for spinal dislocation. Once a laminectomy has healed, the fused vertebrae are immobile.

Nursing Assessment and Intervention Preoperatively, a baseline neurological assessment is performed and documented. Other preoperative care is the same as for other types of general surgery. The major concern after spinal fusion, laminectomy, or diskectomy is to keep the spinal column in alignment so that healing can take place and no further injury is done to the spinal cord. If the surgeon allows the patient to be turned on to his side, he must be log-rolled to avoid twisting the spine. Sometimes the surgeon will allow the patient to be positioned only on his back or abdomen. Whenever the patient's position is changed, there should be ample help to move him. The patient who has had cervical spine surgery is placed in a cervical collar and continues to wear a collar for several weeks.

After spinal surgery a small bedpan is used, and the patient's back is firmly supported while he is resting on the pan. His back and legs should be supported so that all of his body is on the same plane. To promote healing, circulation to the back, head, and neck can be stimulated by gentle massage.

When the patient is allowed out of bed, the physician may order a back brace or corset to support the spinal column until complete healing has occurred. The patient is not allowed to sit for any length of time for several weeks. He must stand or lie down. The microdiskectomy patient is usually up and about the day after surgery. However, weeks to many months of exercises and physical therapy are necessary before recovery is complete.

DEGENERATIVE AND AUTOIMMUNE NEUROLOGICAL DISORDERS

◆ Parkinson's Disease

Parkinson's disease (PD) is named after James Parkinson, who first described the syndrome in 1871. It is a degenerative disorder with symptoms that are neurological in nature and become progressively more incapacitating. It has sometimes been called "shaking palsy," because the outstanding manifestation is a tremor or involuntary motion of the muscles.

Parkinson's disease is considered a major health problem because of its crippling effects; it is considered by some to be the third most crippling disorder in the United States, where about 50,000 people per year are affected. It is a progressive disorder, beginning rapidly at first and then advancing more slowly. It affects more men than women and occurs most frequently around age 60.

Classification of the syndrome may be based on the causative factor. It is a disorder of the part of the brain that controls balance and coordination. The most common type of Parkinson's is *idiopathic*, that is, the primary or specific cause is not known. The syndrome can be drug-induced, especially by some tranquilizers, and may be related to toxic substances such as mercury or pesticides. Some feel that there is probably an infectious cause. Degeneration of the cells in the brain that produce dopamine leads to degenerative changes in the neurons in the basal ganglia. The basal ganglia are grey matter that is scattered throughout the white matter of the cerebrum beneath the cerebral cortex. These degenerative changes produce the symptoms of the disorder.

Diagnosis Two groups of symptoms are characteristic of Parkinson's. The first, *tremor*, occurs when the body is at rest, decreases when there is voluntary movement, and is absent when the patient is asleep. The tremor is most often of a "pill rolling" motion of the thumb against the fingers. If the patient suffers stress and emotional tension, the tremor becomes more pronounced. The second symptom *bradykinesia* (slow movement) is required for diagnosis. Bradykinesia produces poor body balance, a characteristic gait, and difficulty initiating movement. The gait is shuffling with short steps that become quicker. Normal swinging of the arms when walking is absent. A foot may drag or may be stiff. In advanced stages there is a stiff bent-forward posture when walking. Earlier the patient may lean slightly to one side. The third symptom is *rigidity* affecting the skeletal muscles and contributing to postural changes and difficulty in movement. The facial expression becomes blank or mask-like in appearance with little or no expression. Speech becomes low in tone, monotonous sounding, and slow; enunciation becomes difficult. Drooling may occur. The patient may experience decreased tearing, constipation, incontinence, excessive perspiration, heat intolerance, and decreased sexual ability. Parkinson's disease does not usually affect intellect; however, a small percentage of patients do develop a dementia similar to that of Alzheimer's disease. Mood disturbance does occur, and depression is a problem. Stress tends to make symptoms worse.

The specific cause of PD is uncertain, but leads to a dopamine deficiency in the brain. The characteristic symptoms of the disease are used to diagnose the disorder. Laboratory tests usually reveal findings within normal ranges. Morever, CT scans of the brain may be performed to rule out other neurological disorders.

Treatment

Treatment of PD usually includes drug therapy, physical therapy, and considerable emotional support. Drug therapy aims to provide dopamine to the basal ganglia. Levodopa, anticholinergics, dopamine agonists, and a monoamine oxidase (MAO) inhibitor drugs are used to control symptoms. For patients in the early stages of the disease who have no disability, Selegiline (Deprenyl) has just been approved and is given in an attempt to prevent worsening of the patient's condition. When disability is present, L-dioxyphenylalanine (L-dopa, or levodopa) or a combination of levodopa and carbidopa (Sinemet) is given. Sinemet is given in increasing doses until control of the symptoms is achieved. It is not without side effects, however. Other drugs used either along with L-dopa or sometimes alone to treat early stages of PD or to minimize the side effects of L-dopa, include antispasmodic and anticholinergic drugs. Bromocriptine mesylate (Parlodel) or pergolide (Permax) also are prescribed for PD patients as they activate postsynaptic dopamine receptors. Common anticholinergics prescribed include trihexphenidyl (Artane), benztropine (Cogentin), procyclidine (Kemadrin), and ethopropazine (Parsidol). These help control tremor, rigidity, and drooling. The antihistamine diphenhydramine (Benadryl) may be added if the patient suffers from insomnia. Table 14-17 presents the major nursing implications specific to these drugs.

Stereotactic neurosurgery may be done if the drug therapy fails. In this procedure the area in the thalamus that is causing the involuntary movements is destroyed. The surgery only relieves the symptoms; it is not a cure. Depression is frequent in Parkinson's patients, but most respond well to a tricyclic antidepressant.

Recent research has shown some success in relieving symptoms by transplanting tissue from the adrenal medulla into the brain or by implanting embryonic cells that produce dopamine from tissue cultures of a fetus. There is much controversy about this procedure because of the issues related to abortions from which fetuses are obtained. A growth factor called GDNF injected into the brain of monkeys has significantly relieved Parkinson's disease symptoms and shows hope for the possibility of treatment of PD in humans.

The FDA has approved the Activa brain implant which controls tremors on one side of the body by constant electrical shocks that block them. It is hoped that the device will lessen symptoms that interfere with daily functions.

Nursing Assessment and Intervention

Nursing care focuses on preventing complications of PD and drug therapy, enhancing voluntary movement, and safety. Constipation is a problem and requires the addition of fiber to the diet and an increase in fluids to at least 2,000 mL/24 hours. Grasping coins or another object may decrease tremors. Walking is improved by thinking about an imaginary line down the pathway. An exercise program is instituted to maintain muscle function and promote joint mobility. The patient is taught to assume correct posture consciously. Not using a pillow when resting helps prevent flexion of the spine. Learning to sleep prone also is beneficial.

The nurse needs to remember that the PD patient needs extra time to finish tasks. A warming tray can be used to keep food hot during meals so that the patient can take rest periods while eating. Considerable patience and understanding are necessary to help the patient deal with the frustration of his deteriorating body and inability to do things easily that he formerly could.

Falls are common, and safety is a major factor. Using a cane or walker will decrease the incidence of falls. Leg braces or foot braces often are helpful. Loose carpets should be removed from the home and grab bars and a raised toilet seat should be installed. Patients with tremor must be cautioned against carrying hot liquids. Information in the section on Common Care Problems in this chapter discusses measures to help with dysphagia, confusion, and other problems experienced by the PD patient.

TABLE 14-17 ♦ *Major Nursing Implications for Pharmacological Management of Parkinson's Disease*

When giving a drug for Parkinson's disease, the nurse should:

- Follow the "five rights" of medication administration to prevent errors and injury to the patient; pay special attention to dosage amount as therapy is individualized for each patient.
- Check other medications the patient is receiving for interactions with anti-Parkinson drugs.
- Administer the drugs as closely to the time ordered as possible to maintain a consistent blood level of each drug.
- Carbidopa/levadopa can cause many neurological disturbances, including psychiatric problems; discuss any onset of new symptoms that occur after initiation of the medications with the physician.
- Administer anticholinergic medications with meals to decrease gastrointestinal irritation.
- Selegiline may increase the side effects of carbidopa/levodopa; if this occurs, seek an order to decrease the dosage.
- Monitor for effectiveness of each drug by observing for a decrease in Parkinson's symptoms, such as tremor, rigidity, or drooling; assess for decrease in side effects of carbidopa/levodopa when anticholinergic drugs are given for that purpose.
- Continually assess the patient for worsening of symptoms that may be due to disease progression, side effects of medication, or failure of medication.

Regarding possible side/adverse effects of the drug, the nurse should:

- Monitor patients taking carbidopa/levodopa, amantadine, bromocriptine, or pergolide for orthostatic hypotension.
- Monitor patients taking carbidopa/levodopa, amantadine, or an anticholinergic drug for urinary retention; this is especially a problem in men with an enlarged prostate gland.
- Assess patients for excessive or inappropriate sexual behavior who are taking carbidopa/levodopa.
- Bromocriptine may cause changes in mental status; report observed changes to physician.
- Amantadine and pergolide may cause insomnia and should not be administered at bedtime.
- Anticholinergics are contraindicated in patients with acute angle glaucoma; consult with physician if patient has this disorder.
- Anticholinergics cause dry mouth and constipation; increase fluids to 3,000 mL per day; treat constipation as needed per orders; add fiber to diet.
- Monitor blood pressure and pulse during initiation and adjustment of anticholinergic medication; report tachycardia to physician.
- Consult pharmacology book or drug insert for specific side effects of each particular drug.

The nurse should teach the patient taking anti-Parkinson drugs that:

- Selegiline may cause dizziness; warn patient to move cautiously during the initiation of therapy.
- Orthostatic hypotension causes dizziness and can precipitate falls; it is important to allow the blood pressure to stabilize in a sitting position before standing; stabilize while holding on to something when standing before walking.
- Carbidopa/levodopa will turn the urine dark.
- Constipation is a problem with the anticholinergic drugs; increases in dietary fiber, plenty of fluid, and exercise can help control constipation; bowel movement frequency should be monitored to prevent impaction.
- Adjustment of dosages and combination of medications that will control symptoms with the least amount of side effects takes weeks or months to accomplish sometimes.

♦ Multiple Sclerosis

Multiple sclerosis (MS) is a neuromuscular disorder that affects primarily the CNS. It usually, but not always, tends to be progressive. Its cause is not known, although many believe it is an autoimmune disorder. Others feel that it is triggered by a virus. There is no cure. Symptoms most often appear in young adults in their teens and twenties. Usually MS is diagnosed when these individuals are between 20 and 40 years old. It affects females more often than males. The neuromuscular dysfunctions characteristic of MS are unique to each person and can vary greatly from time to time in the same person.

Clinical signs and symptoms reflect the pathological changes that occur as a result of inflammation and subsequent scarring of myelin covering the nerves. Myelin, the protective sheath around the axons that transmit electrical impulses from one neuron to the next, acts as a thick, protective insulator. **When myelin is eroded by inflammation and replaced by scar tissue (demyelinization), nerve impulses cannot travel along** the damaged neurons. Thus the muscles served by the affected nerves do not receive the impulses they need to perform in a well-coordinated and useful manner.

Diagnosis   No laboratory test will definitively establish a diagnosis of MS, although most patients have elevated gamma immunoglobulin (IgG) levels in their spinal fluid with the presence of oligoclonal bands. An MRI scan usually shows characteristic white matter lesions scattered through the spinal cord and brain, which confirms the diagnosis of MS. However, the clinical signs and symptoms presented by a patient usually are sufficiently characteristic of the disorder to allow the neurologist to make a diagnosis that the patient possibly or probably has MS. The clinical manifestations of the disease reflect the extent to which inflammation and scarring of the myelin have occurred.

The disorder typically follows a course of unpredictable flareups that unaccountably are followed by periods of partial or complete remission. The very nature of the disease affects a patient's life in terms of ability to make a living, maintain satisfying interpersonal relationships with family and friends, and maintain a positive self-image.

The more common manifestations of MS are as follows:

- *Motor dysfunction* can include weakness or paralysis of limbs, trunk, and head; diplopia caused by oculomotor weakness; and spasticity of the muscles.
- *Sensory dysfunction* might include numbness, tingling, burning, and painful sensations; patchy or total blindness or blurring of vision in one or both eyes; dizziness; ringing in the ears and hearing loss; and Lhermitte's sign (a sensation like an electric shock down the spine when the neck is flexed).
- *Problems of coordination* include ataxia, intention tremor of limbs and eyes, slurring speech, and dysphagia.
- *Mental changes* usually are limited to depression and possibly inappropriate euphoria. Intellectual function is *not* adversely affected.
- *Fatigue* is a characteristic of MS and is worsened by heat; for example, a hot bath or hot weather.
- Other problems that occur late in the disease are related to urinary and bowel incontinence and disordered sexuality: loss of male and female self-esteem, physical impotence in the male, and diminished sensation.

Treatment   Interferon Beta-1B is a drug that is effective for many ambulatory patients with relapsing-remitting MS. It reduces MS attacks by one-third and decreases the number of severe attacks. It is not a cure, and not all patients respond to it. Interferon beta-1a (Avonex, Biogen) is a new drug and causes fewer injection site reactions. It also is very expensive. Injections of adrenocorticotropic hormone (ACTH) may curtail an episode of increased symptoms.

Because there is no specific preventive treatment or cure for MS, most therapeutic efforts are centered on supportive measures to maintain resistance to infection, reduce muscle spasticity, and manage specific symptoms, such as diplopia, speech disorders, muscle weakness, and others listed.

In addition, the patient should be provided the support and physical and psychological means necessary to develop a positive and hopeful outlook. A positive and affirming mental attitude can have beneficial physiological and biological effects on the MS patient. There is an understandable tendency to become depressed and pessimistic about one's future when confronted with the realities of muscle weakness, incontinence, sexual impotence, and any combination of disabilities likely to be experienced during the course of MS.

Nursing Assessment and Intervention   Appropriate care for the patient with MS depends on the severity of the disease and the symptoms. Care is individualized for each patient. During the diagnostic phase the patient and family need a great deal of emotional support, as most patients know that there is no cure.

Ongoing care focuses on safety, prevention of complications, assistance with physical therapy, and emotional support. The patient should not be exposed to excessive heat or hot baths, as this causes his weakness to become much worse. Care of the particular common problems of the neurological patient was covered earlier in this chapter. The importance of proper nutrition with adequate fluids and roughage in the diet should be stressed to maintain proper bowel function and decrease the likelihood of urinary tract infections.

The nurse helps the patient and family establish a consistent daily routine that will promote optimum levels of functioning for the patient. The routine should include daily physical exercise balanced by rest periods to prevent fatigue.

Patient teaching involves (1) education about the unpredictability of the disease and the need to avoid stress, infections, and fatigue to maintain independence as long as possible; and (2) referral to the National Multiple Sclerosis Society and local support groups. (Additional information and local sources of help for the patient with MS and his family can be obtained by writing to the National Multiple Sclerosis Society, 205 East 42nd Street, New York, NY 10010.)

◆ Alzheimer's Disease

Alzheimer's disease is a form of dementia due to pathological changes in the brain tissue of the patient. Unfortunately the changes can be detected only at autopsy. The cause of Alzheimer's disease is unknown, and considerable research is in progress better to define this disease. It can occur during middle age or during the later decades of life and causes devastation to the patient and family. The disease has a slow onset, progresses at varying rates of speed through several stages, and is eventually fatal.

Early signs and symptoms are those of beginning mental deterioration: forgetfulness, recent memory loss, difficulty learning and remembering, inability to concentrate, and a decline in personal hygiene, appearance, and inhibitions. Later the patient becomes quite confused and unable to make judgments, has difficulty communicating, suffers losses in motor function, and becomes dependent on others. PET scanning can detect brain damage caused by Alzheimer's. A new test, AD7C, checks levels of neural thread protein in cerebrospinal fluid. This substance is up to 10 times higher in people with Alzheimer's. However, the test costs about $1000.

Testing for pupil dilation in response to a mydriatic such as Tacrine, is another screening test.

There is no cure or specific treatment for Alzheimer's disease. Aricept (donepezil) has just been approved to help alleviate mild to moderate symptoms. It is a cholinesterase inhibitor that increases levels of acetylcholine. Acetylcholine is necessary for normal thinking. Tacrine has been shown to improve symptoms in some patients. Selegiline is effective in controlling both behavioral symptoms and in improving cognition in many patients. Care is supportive and is directed at assisting the patient to maintain as much ability to perform ADLs for himself for as long as possible. Preserving dignity is another goal for these patients. More information on the care of the Alzheimer's patient is found in Chapter 34.

◆ Amyotrophic Lateral Sclerosis

Amyotrophic lateral sclerosis (ALS), also called *Lou Gehrig's disease,* is a progressive neuromuscular disease characterized by degeneration of the gray matter in the anterior horns of the spinal cord and the lower cranial nerves. It has an estimated incidence about 5 per 100,000 people. It most often occurs in persons between the ages of 40 and 70 years and equally affects males and females. Although some persons with ALS can survive for many years, the disease usually progresses rapidly, producing a prognosis of death within about 3 years of the onset of symptoms.

Diagnosis   One of the first clinical manifestations of ALS is weakness of the voluntary muscles, especially of the distal muscles of the extremities. Some patients may notice difficulty swallowing and speaking clearly because of oropharyngeal weakness. As the disease progresses there is atrophy of the muscles. Until atrophy is complete, however, there may be spontaneous contractions or spasticity of the muscles and abnormal sensations (**paresthesias**), such as tingling or prickling. The patient also may report pain, which is probably caused by undue strain on weakened muscles.

Only the motor neurons are affected in ALS; therefore the patient remains mentally alert and has no sensory impairment. Mental depression is relatively common as a result of the unrelenting progression of muscle weakness and atrophy.

There is no laboratory test to confirm a diagnosis of ALS, electromyelography in combination with muscle biopsy provides data for positive diagnosis. Other neuromuscular disorders such as multiple sclerosis, myasthenia gravis, and progressive muscular dystrophy must be ruled out.

Treatment   There is no known cause of sporadic ALS, although there is a genetic familial variety. There is no satisfactory treatment for control or cure. Eventually the muscle paralysis renders the patient totally dependent because of inability to move, swallow, speak, and, ultimately, breathe. Rilutek (riluzole) just approved by the FDA has been shown to extend survival.

Nursing Assessment and Intervention   During her first contact with the ALS patient, the nurse conducts a thorough assessment of his neurological status. As the disease progresses, periodic assessments can identify specific needs. Nursing diagnoses likely to be associated with ALS are those related to difficulty with respiration, all problems of immobility, dysphagia, impaired ability to communicate, pain, ineffective coping, and depression.

In the latter stages of ALS the patient and his family will probably need more assistance and guidance to maintain some level of independence and comfort for the patient. Rehabilitation efforts include obtaining equipment and devices such as a walker, wheelchair, hospital bed, suction machine, and nasogastric or gastrostomy tube-feeding supplies.

Because of the nature of the disease, problems related to terminal illness, death, and the grieving process are likely to be present (see Chapter 13). The services of a visiting nurse or a hospice program can provide appropriate instruction and physical and emotional support.

◆ Myasthenia Gravis

The words *myasthenia gravis* literally mean "grave muscle weakness." The disease is a chronic disorder manifested by fatigue and exhaustion that are aggravated by activity and relieved by rest. The muscular weakness can be so mild that it causes a minor inconvenience or so severe that it is life-threatening because of its effect on breathing and swallowing.

Myasthenia gravis is believed to be an autoimmune disease in which circulating autoantibody is directed against the postsynaptic acetylcholine receptors at the neuromuscular junction (the point at which nerve impulses are transmitted to muscle tissue). The antibody reduces the number of functional receptor sites and thereby interferes with total neural stimulation of the muscle, which in turn produces muscle weakness.

Diagnosis   Symptoms of myasthenia gravis include **ptosis** (drooping eyelid), **diplopia** (double vision), and difficulty chewing and swallowing. The voice tends to be hoarse, and volume decreases toward the end of a sentence. Severe muscle weakness is the outstanding symptom of the disorder. Any of the skeletal muscles might be involved; intestine, bladder, and heart muscles are not affected.

The onset is gradual, and muscle weakness often is first noted when the patient tries to walk upstairs, get up from a sitting position, raise his arms over his head, or lift a heavy object. The fatigue is relieved by rest but soon returns and is more severe than expected from the amount of exertion put forth.

Diagnosis is established by administering an injection of edrophonium (Tensilon); a marked increase in muscular strength is noted within 1 minute of injection if the patient has myasthenia gravis.

Treatment   There are two main modes of therapy, the choice depending on the severity of the symptoms. In milder cases the physician may manage the disease by dealing with the specific symptoms, rather than trying to induce a remission of the disease. In more severe cases efforts are made to manage the underlying cause of the symptoms by inducing remission.

Because 80% to 90% of myasthenia gravis patients have autoantibodies against acetylcholine receptors, plasmapheresis can be an effective treatment for short-term control. It is particularly helpful for severe illness where the patient is dependent on a ventilator. The purpose of the plasma exchange is to remove the circulating autoantibodies from the patient's blood (see Chapter 17). This mode of therapy may bring clinical improvement in some patients, but it is not a cure for myasthenia gravis.

Anticholinesterase therapy is the earliest form of treatment for myasthenia gravis. Anticholinesterase agents inactivate acetylcholinesterase, a substance that prevents accumulations of acetylcholine at the neuromuscular junction. Acetylcholine must be present at the neuromuscular junction. Acetylcholine must be present at the point where nerve impulses are transmitted to muscle for sustained repetitive muscle contraction to occur. Anticholinesterase agents temporarily increase muscle strength by inhibiting the enzyme acetylcholinesterase and allowing the acetylcholine to work, but they do not cure the problem. Two drugs commonly used as anticholinesterase agents are neostigmine (Prostigmin) and pyridostigmine (Mestinon). Pyridostigmine is more commonly used, because it can be taken orally.

The dosage of anticholinesterase drugs is precisely calculated for each patient, the aim being to achieve a delicate balance between too much and too little acetylcholine at the neuromuscular junction. Stress can quickly alter a patient's need for acetylcholine; hence overmedication or undermedication can occur rather suddenly. Unfortunately, the symptoms of too much medication are quite similar to those of too little medication, so it is often difficult to adjust the dosage correctly.

Another method of treatment is to remove the thymus gland, which decreases the antibody production. Immunosuppression also is a form of therapy for myasthenia gravis, inasmuch as it is believed to be an autoimmune disorder. The patient may, therefore, be given corticotropin (also known as adrenocorticotropic hormone [ACTH]), prednisone, azathioprine, or cyclophosphamide (Cytoxan). Treatment with IV immunoglobulin (IVIG) for 5 days may produce a favorable response for 30 to 60 days.

Nursing Assessment and Intervention   As with other neurological disorders, nursing care of patients with myasthenia gravis will be based on the specific nursing problems. When a person with this disorder is admitted to the hospital, special care and precautions must be taken, whether or not he was admitted for a condition related to his myasthenia gravis.

Infection, surgery, and other physical and emotional stresses can precipitate a myasthenic crisis. During the crisis frequent monitoring is essential. The patient's ability to swallow and breathe on his own can be seriously compromised. Suctioning, tracheostomy, and artificial ventilation may be necessary to maintain life until the crisis is over.

Education of the patient and his family must include instruction about the nature of the illness and the adverse effects of emotional upsets, respiratory infections, and similar stresses. Rehabilitation goals include education and support for the patient and family so that the patient remains as independent as possible.

Because he can become critically ill and need immediate medical attention at any time, the patient with myasthenia gravis should at all times wear a Medic-Alert emblem that identifies him as having the disease. The patient, as well as members of his family and the nurses who care for him in the hospital or at home, should know the symptoms of improper dosage of anticholinesterase agents. These include dyspnea; poor tongue control, which produces difficulty in chewing, swallowing, and speaking; generalized muscle weakness; and neurological symptoms, such as restlessness, anxiety, and irritability. If any of these symptoms occur, the physician should be notified immediately.

In addition to being affected by problems arising from the anticholinesterase drugs, the myasthenic patient also can suffer from exaggerated and bizarre effects from a variety of drugs. These include the steroids and thyroid compounds; sedatives and respiratory depressants, such as morphine; tranquilizers, such as the phenothiazines; the mycin antibiotics; and some cardiac drugs, such as quinine and quinidine. Because so many drugs are potentially dangerous to a patient with myasthenia gravis, it is imperative that the nurse check with the physician ordering a medication to be sure he is aware that the patient has myasthenia gravis and that she give the prescribed drugs with great caution.

The Myasthenia Gravis Foundation, whose headquarters is in Chicago, promotes research to discover the cause and cure for the disease and distributes information through its local chapters.

COMMUNITY CARE

After leaving the hospital, patients with neurological problems often are cared for in long-term care centers, rehabilitation programs, outpatient clinics, and in the home. Nurses who work in long-term care facilities must be confident in caring for post-stroke patients and patients with Parkinson's disease, as a large percentage of residents in these facilities have these disorders. Because elderly patients often have more than one chronic illness, it is essential that the nurse be knowledgeable about medication interactions and side effects. Each patient's medications must be continually assessed for possible adverse effects as well as for data indicating that each medication is producing a sufficient therapeutic effect to warrant continued administration. A close working relationship with the pharmacist can assist the nurse in judging these matters. Collaborative care between the pharmacist, nurse, nurse aides, physical therapist, social worker, and others who interact with the patient is needed to provide the best plan of care for these complex patients.

The nurse who works with patients who have neurological deficits that cause some degree of immobility is constantly trying both to prevent the complications of immobility and to achieve as high a level of function for the patient as possible.

The home care nurse interacts with the entire family and needs to continually offer support as the difficulties of learning to live with someone who has a neurological deficit are met. Family roles often are altered, and the period of adjustment for the patient and family is lengthy. It often is difficult for the family to cope with the personality changes that occur in the patient who has suffered brain injury or who has a degenerative neurological disorder. Referral to community support groups is often helpful for both the patient and the family members. The following agencies can provide materials, information, and support for patients with neurological disorders. The local library can provide current addresses and phone numbers of both national and local offices:

- American Cancer Society
- American Heart Association
- American Parkinson Disease Association
- Epilepsy Foundation of America
- Guillain-Barré International Foundation
- Myasthenia Gravis Foundation
- National Head Injury Foundation

- National Institute of Neurological and Communicative Disorders and Stroke
- National Multiple Sclerosis Society
- National Parkinson Foundation
- National Spinal Cord Injury Association
- Parkinson's Disease Foundation
- The Stroke Foundation

Cultural Point

A Japanese patient who had suffered a head injury in an automobile accident was ready for discharge from the hospital to the outpatient rehabilitation program. The gentleman had residual paralysis on the left side of the body. The physical therapist felt that the patient needed help with his exercises at home. A grandson had been living in the household for 2 years while attending college. He was chosen to help because of his availability and his basic understanding of the scientific principles involved.

Each day the student came in to assist his grandfather with the exercises. However, the grandfather expressed doubts at his grandson's ability to help him. The grandfather balked when his grandson gave him instructions, and anytime the grandson corrected the position of his extremity during an exercise, the grandfather became offended.

After exploring the situation, it was revealed that the grandfather is a traditional Japanese. He has great respect for the wisdom of elders. Therefore, it was difficult for him to take direction from a person so much younger than himself. The solution was to find an old family friend who could be properly trained to help with the gentleman's exercises.

CRITICAL THINKING EXERCISES

Clinical Case Problems

Read each of the following clinical situations and discuss the questions with your classmates.

1. Mr. Lawson is to have several diagnostic tests done to determine the cause of his neurological symptoms, which include headache, visual disturbance, muscular weakness, and personality change.

   a. How would you explain an EEG to Mr. Lawson? A lumbar puncture? CT scan? MRI?

2. Mary is a 22-year-old college student who has suffered a head injury in an automobile accident. She had no illnesses prior to her accident. She was stabilized in the emergency department and admitted to the neurological intensive care unit. She is confused and groggy and has leakage of spinal fluid (CSF) from one ear and irregular respirations.

a. What assessments would you do on Mary.?

b. What specific nursing measures would you include in your care plan concerning the leaking CSF?

c. What measures would you take to provide appropriate respiratory care?

3. Mr. Foster is a 77-year-old retired teacher who complained of a severe headache during dinner and then slumped over the table, unconscious. He was rushed to the hospital, and a tentative diagnosis of cardiovascular accident (CVA) was made.

a. What diagnostic tests might be appropriate for Mr. Foster.?

b. What emergency care could you have given Mr. Foster if you had been present at dinner?

Mr. Foster's diagnostic tests indicate a subarachnoid hemorrhage (SAH) from a ruptured aneurysm. He is comatose; his pupils are equal and reactive to light; and he responds to pain with decorticate posturing, opens his eyes at random, and seems to be paralyzed on the right side.

c. Write a nursing care plan for Mr. Foster, including appropriate nursing actions for each nursing diagnosis.

4. Gus Berrini is a 40-year-old truck driver who received a severe spinal injury when he was shot in the back by a hitchhiker. The bullet severed the spinal cord at the sixth thoracic vertebra.

a. What kinds of activities should Mr. Berrini eventually be able to perform?

b. How would you plan his care during the acute stage of his illness so that efforts at rehabilitation might be successful?

c. What other members of the health care team might participate in his care and rehabilitation?

BIBLIOGRAPHY

American Heart Association. (1997). *Heart and Stroke Statistical Update*. Dallas: Author.

Allen, T. G. (1994). Parkinson's disease: helping your patients. *Nurseweek*. (6):10–11.

Applegate, E. J. (1995). *The Anatomy and Physiology Learning System: Textbook*. Philadelphia: Saunders.

Arbour, R. (1996). What you can do to reduce increased I.C.P. *C. E. Test Handbook*, Volume 7:17–22.

Black, J. M., Matassarin-Jacobs, E. (1997). *Medical-Surgical Nursing: Clinical Management for Continuity of Care*, 5th ed. Philadelphia: Saunders.

Callahan, S. W. (1996). Arteriovenous malformations. *American Journal of Nursing*, 96(12):30–31.

Chiocca, E. M. (1995). Meningococcal meningitis. *American Journal of Nursing*. 95(12):25.

Cole-Arvin, C., Notich, L., Underhill, A. (1994). Identifying and managing dysphagia. *Nursing 94*. 24(1):48–49.

Copstead, L. C. (1995). *Perspectives on Pathophysiology*. Philadelphia: Saunders.

Cramer, J. A. (1994). Quality of life for people with epilepsy. *Neurologic Clinics*. 12(1):1–12.

Crawley, W. K. (1996). Case management: improving outcomes of care for ischemic stroke patients. *MEDSURG Nursing*. 5(4):239–244.

Crigger, N., Forbes, W. (1996). Assessing neurologic function in older patients. *American Journal of Nursing*. 97(3):37–40.

Dambro, M. R. (1996). *Griffith's 5 Minute Clinical Consult*. Baltimore: Williams & Wilkins.

Darovic, G. (1996). Assessing pupillary responses. *Nursing 97*. 27(2):49.

Fowler, S., Durkee, C. M., Webb, D. J. (1996). Rehabilitating stroke patients in the acute care setting. *MEDSURG Nursing*. 5(5):327–332.

Grant, J. S. (1996). Home care problems experienced by stroke survivors and their family caregivers. *Home Healthcare Nurse*. 14(11):892–902.

Garrett, C. G., Bechtel, G. A. (1996). The efficacy of Bobath neurodevelopmental interventions at home for patients after postcerebrovascular accidents. *Home Healthcare Nurse*. 14(6):435–440.

Guyton, A. C., Hall, J. E. (1996). *Textbook of Medical Physiology*, 9th ed. Philadelphia: Saunders.

Habel, M., Strong, P. (1996). The late effects of poliomyelitis: nursing interventions for a unique patient population. *MEDSURG Nursing*. 5(2):77–85.

Held, J. L. (1994). Identifying spinal cord compression. *Nursing 94*. 24(5):28.

Hickey, J. V. (1992). *The Clinical Practice of Neurological and Neurosurgical Nursing*, 3rd ed. Philadelphia: Lippincott.

Huston, C. J. (1995). Autonomic dysreflexia. *American Journal of Nursing*. 94(6):55.

Ignatavicius, D. D., Hausman, K. A. (1995). *Clinical Pathways for Collaborative Practice*. Philadelphia: Saunders.

Ignatavicius, D. D., Workman, M. L., Mishler, M. A. (1995). *Medical–Surgical Nursing: A Nursing Process Approach*, 2nd ed. Philadelphia: Saunders.

Janowski, M. J. (1996). A road map of stroke recovery. *RN*. 59(3):25–30.

Johnson, C. C. (1995). After a brain injury: clearing up the confusion. *Nursing 95*. 25(11):39–45.

Kane-Carlson, P. A. (1995). Managing patients with T.I.As. *C. E. Test Handbook*, Volume 6:62–67.

Kelly, C. L., Smeltzer, S. C. (1994). Betaseron: the new MS treatment. *Journal of Neuroscience Nursing*. 26(1):52–56.

Kelly, M. (1995). Status epilepticus. *American Journal of Nursing*. 95(8):50.

Kelly, M. (1995). Transient ischemic attack. *American Journal of Nursing*. 95(9):42–43.

Kernich, C. A., Kaminski, H. J. (1995). Myasthenia gravis: pathophysiology, diagnosis and collaborative care. *Journal of Neuroscience Nursing*. 27(4):207–215.

Kirton, C. A. (1996). Assessing for a carotid bruit. *Nursing 96.* 26(10):55.

Latham, L. (1994). When spinal cord injury complicates med/surg care. *RN.* 57(8):26–29.

Lehne, R. A. (1994). *Pharmacology for Nursing Care,* 2nd ed. Philadelphia: Saunders.

Long, L., McAuley, J. W. (1996). Epilepsy: A review of seizure types, etiologies, diagnosis, treatment, and nursing implications. *Critical Care Nurse.* 16(4):83–92.

Monahan, F. D., Drake, T., Neighbors, M. (1994). *Nursing Care of Adults.* Philadelphia: Saunders.

Matteson, M. A., McConnell, E. S. (1997). *Gerontological Nursing: Concepts and Practice,* 2nd ed. Philadelphia: Saunders.

Meissner, J. E. (1995). Caring for patients with meningitis. *Nursing 95.* 25(7):50–51.

Meissner, J. E. (1994). Caring for patients with multiple sclerosis. *Nursing 94.* 24(8):60–61.

Moore, K., Trifiletti, E. (1994). Stroke: the first critical days. *RN.* 57(2):22–27.

Mower, D. (1997). Brain attack: Treating acute ischemic CVA. *Nursing 97.* 27(3):34–46.

Nayduch, D., Lee,. A., Butler, D. (1994). High-dose methylprednisolone after acute spinal cord injury. *Critical Care Nurse.* 14(8):69–78.

Neal L. (1996). Is anybody home? Basic neurologic assessment of the home client. *Home Healthcare Nurse.* 15(3):156–167.

Nussbaum, E. (1996). Migraines: The latest on symptom relief and prevention. *American Journal of Nursing.* 96(10):36–37.

O'Hanlon-Nichols, T. (1996). Intracranial tumors. *American Journal of Nursing.* 96(4):38–39.

Parker, C. D. (1995). Fast action for subarachnoid hemorrhage. *American Journal of Nursing.* 95(1):47.

Polaski, A. L., Tatro, S. E. (1996). *Luckmann's Core Principles and Practice of Medical-Surgical Nursing.* Philadelphia: Saunders.

Prociuk, J. L. (1995). Management of cerebral oxygen supply–demand balance in blunt head injury. *Critical Care Nurse.* 15(8):38–44.

Rakel, R. E., ed. (1994). *Conn's Current Therapy 1994.* Philadelphia: Saunders.

Robinson, K. S. (1994). Early signs of epidural hematoma. *American Journal of Nursing.* 94(4):37.

Scheinberg, L., Holland, N. (1987). *Multiple Sclerosis: A Guide for Patients and Families,* 2nd ed. New York: Raven Press.

Shantz, D., Spitz, M. C. (1996). What you need to know about seizures. *C. E. Test Handbook,* Volume 7:11–16.

Shellenbarger, T., Stover, J. (1995). ALS demands diligent nursing care. *RN.* 58(3):30–32.

Specht, D. M. (1995). Cerebral edema: bringing the brain back down to size. *Nursing 95.* 25(11):34–38.

Stolley, J. (1994). When your patient has Alzheimer's disease. *American Journal of Nursing.* 94(8):34–41.

U.S. Department of Health and Human Services, Agency for Health Care Policy and Research. (1994). *Acute Low Back Problems in Adults: Assessment and Treatment.* Rockville, MD: Author.

U.S. Department of Health and Human Services, Agency for Health Care Policy and Research. (1995). *Post-Stroke Rehabilitation.* Rockville, MD: Author.

Wirtz, K., La Favor, K. M., Ang, R. (1996). Managing chronic spinal cord injury: issues in critical care. *Critical Care Nurse.* 16(4):24–37.

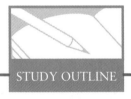

STUDY OUTLINE

I. Introduction

    A. The nervous system coordinates all sensory and motor activities by receiving, interpreting, and relaying messages.

    B. When something happens to impair the ability of the nerves to send or receive impulses, the tissues controlled by those nerves cannot function normally.

II. Causative Factors Involved in Neurological Disorders

    A. Genetic and developmental disorders affect neurological function.

    B. Infection and inflammation may damage the nervous system.

    C. Benign and malignant tumors cause neurological damage and dysfunction.

    D. Metabolic and endocrine disorders may cause neurological dysfunction; vascular or neuromuscular degeneration may cause neurological deficit.

    E. Trauma from chemical or physical causes may disrupt neurological function or cause permanent neurological deficit.

III. Prevention of Neurological Disorders

    A. Education about safety and responsible self-care care help prevent neurological dysfunction:

1. Prevent head and spine injury by wearing helmets when biking, skating, or riding motorcycles.
2. Observe safety precautions when diving and swimming.
3. Wear seat belts.
4. Avoid recreational drug use and excessive alcohol.
5. Promote immunization against tetanus, poliomyelitis, and infectious diseases.
6. Promote prevention and control of hypertension to prevent heart disease and stroke.
7. Promote a healthy, low-fat diet to prevent atherosclerosis and stroke.

IV. **Neurological Terminology Combines Prefixes and Suffixes Often Used in Medical Terminology.**

V. **Evaluation of Neurological Status**
   A. The neurological examination includes motor and sensory functions, mental acuity, memory, and emotional stability.
   B. The 12 cranial nerves are tested for normal function (see Table 14-4).
   C. Specific tests for coordination and balance are done to determine whether problems exist in the cerebellum.
   D. Neuromuscular function tests assess muscle strength and coordination.
      1. Strength of muscles, grip, pushing against resistance.
      2. Reflexes
         a. Knee jerk reflex tests innervation of spinal cord at the second, third, and fourth lumbar levels.
         b. Biceps reflex and brachioradialis reflex test innervation at the fifth and sixth cervical levels.
         c. Triceps reflex tests innervation at the seventh and eighth cervical levels.
         d. Achilles tendon reflex tests innervation at the first and second sacral levels.
         e. The Babinski reflex indicates abnormality of motor control pathways.
         f. Oculocephalic ("doll's eyes") and oculovestibular reflex assess brainstem function.
   E. Diagnostic tests are listed in Table 14-5.

VI. **Nursing Assessment of Neurological Status**
   A. Objectivity important in observing and recording findings; vague terms should be avoided.
   B. Patient history; see Table 14-6.
      1. Past and current neurological disorders.
      2. Symptoms noticed by patient.
      3. Observations of nurse.
   C. Physical assessment.
      1. Vital signs.
      2. Mental function: questions to determine orientation to person, place, and time.
      3. Assessment of cognition; ability to follow commands.
      4. Assessment of judgment.
      5. Neurological and neuromuscular status.
         a. Cranial nerve testing.
      6. Observing for changes on a day-to-day basis.
   D. Assessment of patient with diagnosed neurological disorder: monitoring neurological status.
      1. Four major components of "neuro check."
         a. Level of consciousness (LOC).
         b. Neuromuscular responses: ability to move limbs in response to stimulus.
         c. Pupillary reactions to light, equality in size.
         d. Vital signs.
      2. Glasgow Coma Scale (Table 14-7) used to determine LOC.

VII. **Nursing Diagnosis (see Table 14-9)**
   A. Expected outcomes are individualized for each patient.

VIII. **Planning**
   A. Goals depend on whether there is a physiological possibility of full recovery or not from a neurological deficit.
   B. Goals include adjustment to changes in lifestyle and physical limitations when necessary.
   C. A primary goal is to prevent further injury.
   D. Caring for patients with neurological deficits is very time-consuming and requires patience and understanding.

IX. **Implementation**
   A. Table 14-9 presents interventions for common nursing diagnoses associated with neurological disorders.
   B. Interventions focus on maintaining safety, providing information, teaching about the disorder and self-care, reinforcing positive coping skills, and providing support.

X. **Evaluation**
   A. Evaluation of the effectiveness of interventions is performed to determine whether expected outcomes and goals are being met.

XI. **Common Neurological Patient Care Problems**
   A. Ineffective breathing.
      1. Promote lung expansion; raise head of bed up 30 degrees.

2. Position unconscious patient who is not on a ventilator on side to prevent tongue from blocking airway.

3. Assist with deep-breathing exercises and incentive spirometer use.

B. Impaired mobility: help patient cope with muscle weakness or paralysis.

1. Prevent contractures and muscle atrophy with positioning, splints, and ROM exercises.

2. Teach use of assistive devices and techniques to promote mobility.

3. Teach to attend to paralyzed extremities to prevent injury.

4. Assist with grieving process; treat for depression.

5. Review problems of mobility and nursing care from Chapter 11.

C. Self-care deficit.

1. Provide assistance with bathing, grooming, dressing, eating, and toileting.

2. Teach adaptations for self-care.

3. Provide scrupulous mouth and eye care for the unconscious patient.

4. Teach family or caregiver techniques for necessary care.

5. Work with occupational and physical therapist to achieve highest level of self-care possible.

6. Work with the energy level of the patient; neurological disorders cause easy fatigue.

D. Dysphagia.

1. Assess the swallowing reflex before offering food or liquid by mouth.

2. Seat in upright position for feeding.

3. Maintain upright position for 30 minutes after a meal.

4. Maintain a nonstressful environment for feeding.

5. Teach techniques to assist swallowing; see Table 14-10.

E. Incontinence.

1. Bladder training program.
   a. Assess bladder function and patterns of incontinence; determine optimal neural and muscular function that can be expected.
   b. Design program according to patient's needs; try different techniques until successful.

2. Bowel training program.
   a. Assess former and present bowel patterns.
   b. Determine expected neural and muscular capability for bowel elimination.
   c. Set objectives with patient.
   d. Increase fiber and fluids in diet; employ rectal suppositories for retraining if needed.
   e. Keep accurate record of bowel movements.

F. Pain.

1. Identify characteristics of the pain, its location and spread, its intensity, and how it is affecting the patient's life.

2. Pain may cause difficulty sleeping; use all measures to promote sleep.

3. Depression may result from chronic pain; antidepressant combined with pain medication may be most effective.

G. Confusion.

1. Cause may be organic or temporary, secondary to illness, or toxicity.

2. Assess degree of problem; may fluctuate from day to day.

3. Use principles of reality orientation.

4. Provide calm, stable environment; help patient focus on what he is able to do; give instructions one step at a time.

H. Aphasia.

1. Assessment: note specific abilities and disabilities of patient in area of communication.

2. Nursing intervention.
   a. Goals focused on stimulating communication without undue frustration for patient.
   b. Helpful principles and techniques to be used by nurses, family, and all others who deal with patient.
   c. Good oral hygiene helps patient form words more easily.

I. Sexual dysfunction.

1. Recognize problems and need for sexual counseling.

2. Assure that a sexually satisfying life may well be possible.

J. Psychosocial concerns.

1. Assist with mental adjustment; treat depression.

2. Build self-esteem and help integrate new body image.

3. Provide emotional support and encouragement.

4. Refer for vocational rehabilitation if appropriate.

5. Plan with patient for renewed social life.

K. Ineffective family coping.

1. Goal is for patient to assume as much responsibility for his care as he can.

2. The nurse should assess the patient's capabilities and the family's ability and willingness to assist him.

3. Goals must be realistic and agreed on by patient and family.

4. Referrals to counseling and support groups are helpful.

XII. Disorders of the Neurological System

A. Increased intracranial pressure (ICP).

1. Any lesion taking up space in the cranial vault causes increased ICP (Figure 14-11).

2. Earliest signs of increasing ICP are subtle and include restlessness and change in LOC.

3. Classic signs of increasing ICP are decreasing LOC, widening pulse pressure, and slow, bounding pulse, but these occur very late (see Table 14-12).

4. Pupils that are unequal in size, sluggish to react, or dilated and will not constrict signal an emergency, and the physician should be notified immediately.

5. Goals of care.

   a. Maintain cerebral perfusion.

   b. Reduce ICP.

   c. Maintain adequate respiration.

   d. Protect from injury.

   e. Maintain normal body functions.

   f. Prevent complications.

XIII. Infectious Diseases

A. Meningitis: inflammation of coverings of the brain.

1. Causative organisms: bacteria and viruses.

2. Symptoms and medical diagnosis.

   a. Headache, stiffness of neck, irritability, photophobia.

   b. Spinal tap and analysis of spinal fluid for definitive diagnosis.

3. Medical treatment: symptomatic; antibiotics and anticonvulsants.

4. Nursing assessment directed toward accompanying problems, such as increased ICP, seizures, fever, nausea and vomiting, delirium, pain, electrolyte imbalance.

5. Nursing interventions directed at decreasing ICP and supportive measures to prevent complications and promote healing.

B. Encephalitis: inflammation of brain tissue.

1. Causative organism usually viral; lead, arsenic, and other heavy metals also can cause encephalitis.

2. Symptoms: headache, fever, extreme restlessness, lethargy, confusion, visual disturbances, delirium.

3. Treatment is symptomatic.

C. Guillain-Barré syndrome: inflammatory disease affecting myelin, with edema and compression of the nerve root.

1. Symptoms: paresthesia, pain, and progressive paralysis.

2. Diagnosis difficult because it mimics many other disorders.

3. Spinal fluid shows elevated protein levels, but leukocyte count is normal.

4. Nursing assessment and intervention.

   a. During acute phase, goals are to sustain life, prevent complications of immobility, and promote rest and comfort.

   b. Vital signs monitored frequently.

   c. Avoid stimulation and the Valsalva maneuver; otherwise extreme changes in blood pressure can be triggered.

   d. Static phase: patient gets no worse and no better; provide a balance of rest and activity (passive exercise and ROM).

   e. Rehabilitation phase: gradual recovery.

D. Poliomyelitis and post-polio syndrome.

1. Polio is caused by a virus that destroys motor cells in the spinal cord, brainstem, and frontal lobe.

2. It is preventable by immunization and is rare in the United States.

3. Post-polio syndrome causes a new onset of weakness, pain, and fatigue in people who had polio years ago.

4. Treatment is based on conserving energy by lifestyle modifications.

E. Brain abscess.

1. Pocket of infection in the brain; causes headache, fever, and change in LOC.

2. If untreated, ICP will rise and may cause brain damage.

3. Treated with antibiotics.

XIV. Head Injuries

A. Brain is encased in rigid skull, with very little room for expansion.

B. Types: open fracture and closed injuries.

1. Closed types include concussion, contusion, and hematoma.

2. Symptoms and medical diagnosis.

   a. Outward signs: evidence of fracture, bleeding, scalp laceration, etc.

   b. Increased ICP.

   c. Skull radiograph, angiogram, electroencephalogram (EEG), and brain scan.

3. Medical and surgical treatment: treated conservatively at first. Surgery may be necessary to relieve intracranial pressure or debride wound.

4. Nursing assessment and intervention (see Nursing Care Plan 14-1).
   a. Maintain open airway and adequate ventilation.
   b. Raise head of bed at 30 degrees, and position patient properly.
   c. Frequent assessment per Glasgow Coma Scale, neuro check, and vital signs.
   d. Observe for leakage of cerebrospinal fluid (CSF).
   e. Instruction of patient and family when head injury has been treated and patient released from emergency department.

C. Treatment for increased ICP.
   1. Administration of IV mannitol and furosemide to promote fluid excretion.
   2. Fluid restriction.
   3. Mechanical ventilation with hyperventilation to decrease levels of CO_2 and promote vasoconstriction.
   4. Insertion of cerebral perfusion monitor.
   5. Intraventricular catheter to drain small amounts of CSF.
   6. Surgical removal of hematoma by burr holes or craniotomy.

XV. Brain Tumors

A. Symptoms: headache, vomiting without nausea, visual problems, personality changes, and disturbances in judgment, memory, coordination, and speech.
B. Medical treatment: surgical removal, chemotherapy, radiation, stereotactic surgery.
C. Nursing care: preoperative psychological preparation and thorough baseline neurological assessment.
D. Postoperative care: position only per orders, watch for CSF leak, monitor for increasing ICP.

XVI. Headache

A. Most common cause of pain.
B. Migraine headaches thought to be due to constriction and subsequent dilatation of cerebral arteries.
   1. May be accompanied by an aura, such as spots before the eyes.
   2. Pain often causes nausea and vomiting.
   3. Treatment consists of medication, cold compresses, rest, and decreasing stress.
   4. The patient should try to identify any triggers that bring on the headaches.

XVII. Cerebral Vascular Accident (CVA, Stroke)

A. Cerebral ischemia caused by thrombosis, hemorrhage, or occlusion of cerebral blood vessel by embolus.
B. Persons most at risk: those with hypertension, atherosclerosis, heart disease, obesity.

C. Stroke prevention.
   1. Incidence of stroke has decreased as a result of better control of hypertension, better management of heart disease, early recognition of impending stroke. A small dose of aspirin per day may be protective.
   2. Surgical procedures include removal of plaque, rerouting of blood around obstructed carotid artery; and repair of aneurysm.
D. TIA causes temporary symptoms; provides warning that stroke may occur.
E. Medical diagnosis: CT scan, angiogram, EEG, MRI scan, and occasionally lumbar puncture.
F. Emergency treatment: loosen constricting clothing, turn head to side, elevate head slightly, monitor pulse and respirations.
G. Stabilize vital signs, promote adequate respiration, decrease ICP.
H. t-PA or heparin is given for thrombosis.
I. Aneurysm repair if needed.
J. IV mannitol is administered to decrease ICP.
K. Nursing assessment and intervention.
   1. Closely monitor neurological status.
   2. Prevent complications; decrease ICP.
   3. Assist with rehabilitation.
   4. See Clinical Pathway 14-1 for care of the stroke patient.

XVIII. Epilepsy: Chronic Disturbance of Electrical Activity of the Brain

A. Idiopathic: no known cause.
B. Symptomatic: related to brain tumor, injury, endocrine disorder, etc., which cause the seizures.
C. Seizures classified under four major groups: (1) partial; (2) generalized; (3) unclassified; and (4) status epilepticus. Each has various subgroups.
D. Symptoms and medical diagnosis.
   1. Absence or petit mal: usually only slight twitching around mouth or eyes, no loss of consciousness.
   2. Grand mal or tonic-clonic: bilateral jerks of the limbs; loss of consciousness, incontinence.
      a. Tonic convulsions: continued muscle contraction.
      b. Clonic convulsions: alternate contraction and relaxation of muscles.
      c. Atonic or akinetic seizures: loss of body tone, weakness of knees, or total collapse and falling; usually no loss of consciousness.
   3. Status epilepticus: unrelenting series of convulsions. An emergency is treated with anticonvulsants and diazepam. If seizures are caused by hypoglycemia or alcohol with-

drawal, treatment may consist of IV 50% dextrose or IV thiamin.

    4. Diagnosis confirmed by EEG or CT scan.

E. Medical and surgical treatment.

    1. Antiepileptic drugs.

    2. Surgical removal of abnormal brain tissue.

F. Nursing assessment and intervention.

    1. Two major areas: assessment and care of patient during seizure and long-term support for management of seizures and coping with psychosocial effects of epilepsy.

        a. Education of patient about nature of illness, importance of compliance, side effects, and symptoms of toxicity of medications.

        b. Avoidance of factors that trigger seizures.

        c. Information about community resources for social interaction and information.

XIX. Cerebral Palsy: A Type of Paralysis Accompanied by Poor Muscle Coordination

A. Caused by cerebral damage possibly stemming from lack of oxygen at birth, traumatic birth, premature delivery, or infection.

    1. Symptoms: exaggerated reflexes, poor coordination of voluntary muscles, high muscle tension, and sometimes defect of speech, hearing, or sight.

    2. Treatment: early muscle training and special exercises; orthopedic surgery, braces, or casts can correct some deformities and disabilities.

    3. Patient instructed in self-care.

XX. Muscular Dystrophy

A. Affects both the nerves and the muscles; an inherited, progressive disease.

B. Symptoms begin in infancy; there is no cure; death frequently occurs in early adulthood.

C. Treatment focuses on preventing deterioration of muscle capability and contractures.

XXI. Huntington's Disease

A. Genetically transmitted degenerative neurological disorder characterized by chorea.

B. Progressive disorder with signs appearing in the fourth or fifth decade of life.

C. No known treatment; patient becomes totally helpless.

XXII. Cranial Nerve Disorders

A. Trigeminal neuralgia (tic douloureux).

    1. Pain along pathways of one or more branches of the trigeminal nerve.

    2. Sometimes caused by tumor or vascular disease, but most often cause is not known.

    3. Symptoms: acute attacks of severe, sharp pain localized on one side of the face and extending from the midline of the face across the cheek and jaw to the ear.

        a. Acute attacks often are triggered by exposure to heat or cold, chewing, brushing the teeth, or washing or shaving the face.

    4. Medical treatment: administration of anticonvulsant, such as phenytoin (Dilantin), carbamazepine (Tegretol), or baclofen (Lioresal).

    5. Surgical treatment: dissection of trigeminal nerve branch rootlets.

    6. Nursing intervention.

        a. Help patient avoid triggering attack. Instruct about side effects of prescribed medication.

        b. Following surgery, patient may need instruction to avoid damage to cornea, inside of mouth, and teeth, depending on branch of nerve removed.

B. Bell's palsy.

    1. Weakness or paralysis of the muscles supplied by the facial nerve.

    2. Signs: numbness and partial or total paralysis of the facial muscles.

    3. Treatment: protect eye if blink reflex is lost; corticosteroids if these can be started at onset of symptoms.

    4. Recovery is individual; some may not achieve total recovery.

XXIII. Disorders of the Spine and Spinal Cord

A. Spinal cord injury.

    1. Degree of motor function depends on level of injury.

    2. Immediate care: move victim only after neck and back have been splinted.

    3. Traction may be applied to stabilize spinal column; Gardner-Wells tongs, Crutchfield tongs, halo may be used.

    4. Patient may be placed on special bed (Rotorest; Stryker frame) to facilitate care.

    5. Muscle spasms and autonomic dysreflexia require skilled nursing assessment and intervention.

    6. Goals of medical and surgical treatment.

        a. Stabilize vital signs.

        b. Prevent further cord damage by splinting and traction, and give large doses of corticosteroid to decrease inflammatory response and swelling.

        c. Repair damage to spine and cord as much as possible.

        d. Prevent complications and maintain as much function as possible.

        e. Promote rehabilitation.

7. Efforts of health care team members necessary to help patient and family deal with psychosocial impact of paralysis.

8. Spinal shock: flaccid paralysis, loss of reflex activity below level of damage, bradycardia, hypotension, and occasionally paralytic ileus.

   a. Treatment aimed at maintaining adequate blood pressure and heart rate.

   b. May last a few days to several months.

B. Ruptured intervertebral disc ("slipped disc").

1. Fibrous cushion between vertebrae slips out of place (herniates) and pinches adjacent nerve.

2. Symptoms and medical diagnosis.

   a. Pain in lower back radiating down leg; history of feeling something "give way."

   b. Cervical ruptured disc: pain in neck and shoulder, radiating down arm.

3. Diagnosis confirmed by myelography, MRI.

4. Medical and surgical treatment.

   a. Bedrest on firm mattress with bed board; heat, cold, pelvic or head traction, mild exercises, back brace.

   b. Muscle relaxants, antiinflammatory agents, and analgesics for muscle spasm and pain.

   c. Surgical procedures: microdiskectomy or laminectomy; may do spinal fusion.

   d. Must be "log-rolled" for turning; back must be kept straight; physical therapy exercises.

XXIV. **Degenerative and Autoimmune Neurological Disorders**

A. Parkinson's disease.

1. Characterized by a group of symptoms, including tremor, poor coordination, rigidity of muscles; most often idiopathic.

2. Treatment with dopamine, anticholinergics, dopamine agonists, and monoamine oxidase inhibitors to control symptoms; physical therapy to promote mobility and self-care.

3. Stereotaxic neurosurgery on area of thalamus may control symptoms if drugs are ineffective.

4. Research with embryonic tissue transplants into the brain have been promising; ethical issues are the problem.

5. Nursing intervention.

   a. Prevent complications.

   b. Monitor drug therapy; control side effects.

   c. Promote safety.

   d. Enhance mobility.

   e. Prevent constipation or diarrhea.

B. Multiple sclerosis: a neuromuscular disorder affecting primarily the CNS. Most often affects those between 20 and 40 years of age.

1. Symptoms and diagnosis.

   a. Clinical manifestations reflect inflammatory changes and demyelinization of the spinal cord nerves and neurons in the brain.

   b. Clinical manifestations indicate diagnosis.

   c. Symptoms include motor dysfunction, sensory changes, problem of coordination, mental changes (depression and inappropriate euphoria), and fatigue worsened by heat.

C. Medical treatment: no cure. Supportive measures taken to prevent infection, reduce muscle spasticity, and manage specific symptoms.

   a. Beta-1B is effective for many ambulatory patients with relapsing-remitting MS.

   b. ACTH injections may curtail an episode of increased symptoms.

2. Nursing assessment and intervention.

   a. Identification of specific problems related to immobility, incontinence, diplopia, and other visual problems, speech disorders, sexual impotence, muscle spasticity, and other manifestations of disorder.

   b. Intervention requires well-coordinated planning with patient, family, and appropriate members of health care team.

D. Alzheimer's disease: pathological changes that cause a dementia.

1. Slow onset; progresses through stages at varying speeds; eventually fatal.

2. Symptoms progress from forgetfulness and memory loss to decline in personal hygiene and inhibitions; later, severe confusion, helplessness, and difficulty communicating, until totally dependent.

3. Goals: promote ability to perform ADLs as long as possible; protect from injury; preserve dignity.

E. Amyotrophic lateral sclerosis (Lou Gehrig's disease).

1. Progressive degeneration of gray matter in the anterior horn cells and lower cranial nerves.

2. No known cause and no satisfactory treatment for control or cure.

3. Symptoms: voluntary muscle weakness, usually beginning in hands. Difficulty speak-

ing and swallowing. Eventually patient is unable to move, speak, swallow, and finally breathe. There is some pain; patient remains mentally alert and continues to have sensation.

4. Nursing assessment to determine patient's level of optimal physical activity and specific problems related to muscle paralysis.

5. Nursing intervention aimed at providing physical comfort, emotional support to patient and family, and full utilization of resources for maximum independence of patient within the limitation of his disability.

F. Myasthenia gravis: chronic disorder manifested by fatigue and exhaustion that are aggravated by activity and relieved by rest. Believed to be an autoimmune disease with circulating antibodies acting against neuromuscular receptor sites.

1. Symptoms and medical diagnosis.

a. Severe muscle weakness is the principal symptom; also ptosis, diplopia, and difficulty in chewing and swallowing.

b. Diagnosis established by injection of edrophonium (Tensilon) followed by marked increase in muscle strength.

2. Medical treatment.

a. Anticholinesterase therapy.

b. Plasmapheresis to remove autoantibodies mechanically.

3. Nursing intervention.

a. Monitor hospitalized patient frequently for signs of myasthenic crisis.

b. Educate patient and family about the disease.

XXV. **Community Care**

A. Neurological patients often continue care in rehabilitation centers, long-term care facilities, outpatient clinics, or in the home.

B. Because elderly patients often have other chronic disorders, careful assessment of medication interactions and observation for side effects is very important.

C. Prevention of the complications of immobility is a major nursing concern when caring for patients who have paralysis, paresis, or who are unconscious.

D. Collaborative care involving the whole health care team, the patient, and the family is essential in formulating an effective plan of action.

E. Referral to community support groups and agencies that can provide materials, information and support for the patient and family is most helpful.

XXVI. **Elder Care Points**

A. The elderly often suffer from arthritis; assess joints, and be gentle when performing ROM exercises.

B. The elderly cannot adapt to physiological stress as well as younger people and are subject to hypothermia and hyperthermia.

C. Older patients often have other diseases and conditions that affect the neurological system: arthritis, hearing loss, visual loss, diabetic neuropathy, etc.

CHAPTER 15

Care of Patients with Upper Respiratory Tract Disorders

The throat has been described as the "crossroads of the human body." It has openings leading from the nose and ears and also serves as a passageway for food and air (Figure 15-1). It is little wonder that inflammation of the throat *(pharyngitis)* is such a common condition considering the exposure of the throat to the hordes of bacteria present in our environment.

The other common disorder of the oral cavity and larynx is tumor growth. Laryngitis usually accompanies infections of the lower respiratory tract (for example, laryngotracheobronchitis involving the larynx, trachea, and bronchi). Tumors of the larynx are less common than neoplasms in other parts of the body and, like other tumors, can be either benign or malignant. There will be an estimated 30,750 cases of cancer of the oral cavity and pharynx in 1997.

The study of disorders of the upper respiratory system requires a basic understanding of the anatomy and physiology of the system. A brief overview is presented to refresh the student's memory.

OVERVIEW OF ANATOMY AND PHYSIOLOGY

What Are the Functions of Each of the Structures of the Upper Respiratory System?

- On its way to the lungs, air passes through the nose, mouth, pharynx, larynx, and the trachea (Figure 15-1).
- The nasal cavity is lined with mucous membrane that warms and moistens the air as it passes through; moisture protects the cilia.
- The mucous membrane secretes mucus, which traps dust particles and bacteria.
- The cilia, small hair-like projections, propel the mucus toward the larynx where it can be swallowed or expectorated.
- Olfactory cells are located in the roof of the nose.

- The paranasal sinuses (maxillary, frontal, sphenoid, and ethmoid) are air-filled cavities lined with mucous membrane and situated among the facial bones around the nasal cavity.
- The sinuses reduce the weight of the skull, produce mucus, and influence voice quality.
- **When allergy or infection affects the membranes or the sinuses, inflammation and swelling occur. If drainage is obstructed by swelling, pressure builds, resulting in a sinus headache.**
- The pharynx is about 5 inches long and extends from the back of the mouth to the esophagus.
- The pharynx serves as a passageway for the respiratory tract and the gastrointestinal system, moving air to the lungs and food to the esophagus.

- The larynx is important to the formation of the sounds of speech.
- The tonsils, which are part of the lymphatic system, are located in the larynx; if they become inflamed and enlarged, they may interfere with breathing.
- The larynx sits between the pharynx and the trachea. The vocal cords are located in the larynx.
- The trachea extends from the larynx to the bronchi; it is the "windpipe" and carries air to the lungs.
- The trachea is made up of cartilage, smooth muscle, and connective tissue and is lined with mucous membrane.

How Does the Epiglottis Protect the Airway?

- The epiglottis forms a hinged "door" at the entrance to the larynx.
- When swallowing is initiated, the epiglottis closes over the larynx, preventing food from entering it. The food is then directed into the esophagus.
- The epiglottis prevents aspiration of food and secretions into the lungs.
- When the swallowing reflex is weak or missing, aspiration is a risk.

How Is Speech Produced in the Larynx?

- The vocal cords are made up of mucous membrane attached to the front and back of the larynx.
- The glottis is the space between the folds.
- When air from the lungs passes through the larynx, it causes rapid opening and closing of the glottis.
- Movements of the mouth, lips, jaws, and tongue convert the sounds made by the rush of air into speech sounds.
- Swelling or growths on the vocal cords cause hoarseness and alteration of normal speech.

What Age-Related Changes Affect the Upper Respiratory System?

- The decrease in the immune system's efficiency makes the elderly more susceptible to upper respiratory infections.
- The cough reflex is weaker because of weakened respiratory muscles, thoracic wall rigidity, and decreased ciliary movement, making the potential for aspiration greater.

PREVENTION OF UPPER RESPIRATORY DISORDERS

The best way to prevent infection and inflammation of the upper respiratory system is to wash the hands frequently, stay out of crowds especially during cold and flu season, refrain from smoking; and avoid known allergens as much as possible. Maintaining adequate nutrition and obtaining sufficient rest help keep the immune system healthy and thereby decrease the frequency of upper respiratory infections (URI). Tobacco smoke is not only irritating to the mucous membranes, but also is a co-factor in the occurrence of throat

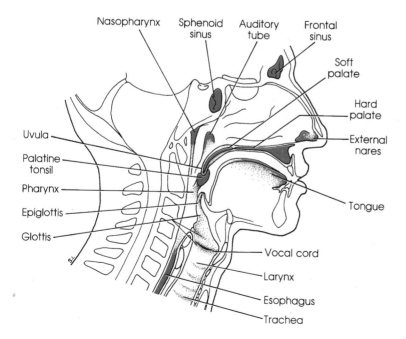

FIGURE 15-1   Upper respiratory tract.

cancer. **About 90% of throat cancer occurs in people who both smoke and immoderately drink alcohol. Refraining from excessive alcohol intake is very important in preventing throat cancer.** Teaching the public to seek medical assessment when hoarseness or a sore throat lasts longer than 2 weeks assists in the early detection of throat malignancy.

Allergy to substances that are airborne causes the mucous membranes of the nose and sinuses to become irritated and inflamed. When these membranes are inflamed, bacteria and viruses can more easily invade the cells and cause infection. Control of allergies decreases the incidence of URI.

Elder Care Point... People over 80 years old or those elderly who suffer from chronic disease of the respiratory system should take care not to be exposed to people with upper respiratory ailments. The elderly should not be exposed to children with colds and coughs. The elderly person who is mostly confined to the house or long-term care facility and does not mingle with the public much does not have the immunity to common viruses and bacteria that younger, more socially active people do.

DIAGNOSTIC TESTS AND EXAMINATIONS

◆ Visual Examination of the Nose, Mouth, and Throat

The interior of the nose, mouth, pharynx, and the tonsils can be inspected by an examiner using a tongue blade and a good source of light. The nose is inspected for redness, swelling, discharge, and lumps. With the head tilted upward, the inside of the nares are inspected for pallor, redness, swelling, and polyps and for mucus color, consistency, odor, and amount. The examiner obtains a better view if a nasal speculum is used. The hard and soft palates are inspected, and the mobility of the soft palate is evaluated by asking the patient to say "ah." The pharynx can be brought into view by asking the patient to say "ee." The examiner is looking for signs of inflammation, lesions, plaques or exudates. The paranasal sinuses are assessed by observing for purulent discharge in the nares and by palpating over the sinus areas for tenderness. Sometimes sinus radiographs are ordered.

◆ Laryngoscopy

Inspection of the larynx is done in one of two ways: by *indirect laryngoscopy* or *direct laryngoscopy*. Indirect laryngoscopy is a relatively simple office procedure that does not require local anesthesia unless the patient has a very sensitive gag reflex. The patient is placed in a sitting position directly in front of the examiner. A warm laryngeal mirror is placed at the back of the throat, and the soft palate is gently lifted up. The examiner wears a head mirror, which reflects light from a source near the patient's head. While the throat is at rest the examiner can see only the upper part of the epiglottis, the base of the tongue, and the back of the pharynx. The larynx is brought into view by asking the patient to make an "ee" sound. During indirect laryngoscopy the examiner is looking for inflammation, ulceration, mucosal irregularity, tumors, and polyps on the vocal cords. Polyps can be removed easily at the time of direct laryngoscopy.

The procedure requires the use of a fiberoptic endoscope (laryngoscope) introduced through the mouth and past the pharynx to the larynx. It may be performed on an outpatient basis. Direct laryngoscopy permits visualization of areas that cannot be seen by indirect laryngoscopy. During the procedure, specimens of exudate or tissue can be obtained or foreign bodies removed.

Direct laryngoscopy may be done to obtain a biopsy or to locate benign lesions, malignant tumors, or strictures that interfere with breathing.

Direct laryngoscopy requires local or general anesthesia. The patient is prepared by withholding food and drink for 6 to 8 hours before the test. The procedure and its purpose should be explained to the patient. A mild sedative usually is administered, along with atropine to reduce secretions. The patient should know that the room will be darkened. The laryngoscope is passed through the mouth, but it will not obstruct breathing.

After the procedure, nursing intervention is similar to that for a patient undergoing a bronchoscopy. The patient's vital signs are monitored, and he is watched carefully for signs of adverse reaction to the anesthetic and medications administered before and during the test. Laryngeal edema and discomfort are reduced by applying an ice collar. Any signs of airway obstruction from edema, epiglottitis, or laryngospasms must be reported immediately.

Foods and fluids are restricted for 4 to 8 hours or until the gag reflex has returned. The patient should be given an emesis basin and instructed to expectorate saliva rather than swallow it. Saliva and other secretions from the mouth are observed for blood, which should not be present in more than very small amounts. The patient also is instructed not to cough or clear his throat, especially when a biopsy has been done. To do so may initiate fresh bleeding from the biopsy site.

Loss of the voice (*aphonia*), hoarseness, and a mild sore throat are expected after laryngoscopy, but these discomforts should not last more than a day. Warm saline gargles and throat *lozenges* (medication that dissolves when sucked on) can be soothing but are not allowed until the gag reflex has returned.

CT and MRI scans may be ordered to locate tumors and pathological abnormalities of the esophagus and larynx.

◆ Throat Culture

The most common reason for culturing pharyngeal secretions is to establish a definitive diagnosis of infection with *Streptococcus pyogenes*. A culture permits prompt and appropriate treatment of a potentially dangerous infection that can have such **sequelae** (following result) as rheumatic heart disease and glomerulonephritis. The incidence of rheumatic fever has increased considerably since 1985. A throat culture also is sometimes done to identify carriers of various organisms or to establish a diagnosis of diphtheria, meningitis, or whooping cough. These diseases can be particularly harmful to elderly, debilitated, or very young patients and therefore require prompt diagnosis and treatment.

NURSING ASSESSMENT

◆ History Taking

Infections and inflammations of the throat and larynx frequently are treated on an outpatient basis. The patient often will have a history of exposure to a specific person who had a respiratory infection or to a large group of people at school or work where there are likely to be frequent occasions for contact with infected persons.

The patient's personal history also might include recurrent respiratory infections and sore throats, known allergies, or chronic sinusitis.

Subjective and Objective Data   The patient is questioned about frequency of URI, known inhalant allergies, and sinus problems. **Patients with sinus problems complain of headache, malaise, a bad taste in the mouth, nasal congestion or obstruction, and purulent drainage from the nose.** There may be facial puffiness over the affected sinus. Those with pharyngitis usually report a sore or "scratchy" throat, malaise, headache, and sometimes a cough. Dysphagia also might be a problem for patients with pharyngitis, because swallowing involves pushing the food back against the inflamed oropharynx. **Hoarseness and loss of the voice are common symptoms of laryngitis.**

However, if either dysphagia or hoarseness persist for more than 4 to 6 weeks and there are no other signs of infection or inflammation, a tumor should be suspected.

Objective data include fever and other signs of infection, productive or nonproductive cough, and hoarseness. Palpation of the neck may reveal enlarged lymph nodes.

NURSING MANAGEMENT

Appropriate *nursing diagnoses* for patients with upper respiratory disorders depend on the type of problem and the stage of the disorder. The most commonly used nursing diagnoses include:

- Impaired verbal communication
- Pain
- Risk for aspiration related to impaired swallowing
- Ineffective airway clearance related to physical alteration in airway (tracheostomy)
- Risk for infection related to surgical procedure
- Body image disturbance related to loss of voice or disfiguring surgical procedure
- Ineffective individual coping related to changes in body image and roles

Expected outcomes are written based on individual condition and needs.

Planning for the patient with an upper respiratory disorder should consider comfort measures, time needed for eating or feeding, use of strict asepsis for wound and tracheostomy care, provision of measures to provide a means of communication, time for patient education, and consideration of psychosocial needs.

Interventions are included in Nursing Care Plan 15-1 and within the discussion of the various disorders. *Evaluation* is based on gathering data regarding the result of the interventions carried out and achievement of expected outcomes. If the plan is not succeeding in meeting goals and expected outcomes, the plan should be changed.

Nursing Care Plan 15-1

Selected nursing diagnosis, goals/expected outcomes, nursing interventions, and evaluations for a patient with a laryngectomy

Situation: Mr. Cato had a supraglottic laryngectomy 5 days ago. He is withdrawn and having difficulty adjusting to his tracheostomy and states, with pencil and paper, that he doesn't feel he can learn to speak again.

Nursing Diagnosis	Goals/Expected Outcomes	Nursing Intervention	Evaluation
Ineffective airway clearance related to discomfort and secretions resulting from surgery and tracheostomy. SUPPORTING DATA Unable to cough secretions out of tracheostomy tube; becomes anxious when secretions build up, decreasing air flow.	Tracheostomy will be cleared by suctioning as needed. Patient will learn to suction own tracheostomy effectively by discharge. Patient will learn to clear tracheostomy by coughing effectively.	Suction as needed, at least q 4 h. Encourage patient to assist with procedure: hold water for moistening catheter, turn on suction. Teach to attach catheter to suction tubing; teach to suction self using mirror. Praise for all attempts. Point out advantages of not being dependent on others for care of airway. Medicate for discomfort and encourage patient to cough to remove secretions without suctioning.	Suctioned approximately q 2 h; assisting with equipment; first teaching session on suctioning complete; will cough on command. Continue plan.
Impaired skin integrity related to surgical incisions. SUPPORTING DATA Supraglottic laryngectomy and tracheostomy.	No infection at incision sites as evidenced by no redness, swelling, or purulent discharge. Skin integrity is intact within 6 weeks.	Clean incision lines with H_2O_2; apply antibiotic ointment as ordered q shift. Clean around tracheostomy with acetic acid or normal saline and change gauze pad as needed. Change tracheostomy ties q 24 h, being very careful not to dislodge tracheostomy tube. Observe for signs of infection.	Incision cleaned with H_2O_2; antibiotic ointment applied; trach cleaned and dressed; stoma reddened, without signs of pus or excessive swelling; continue plan.
Impaired verbal communication related to loss of larynx. SUPPORTING DATA Laryngectomy and tracheostomy.	Patient will show interest in learning new style of speech within 6 weeks.	Assist him to use Magic Slate or paper and pencil for communication; show patience. Obtain order for visit from rehabilitated laryngectomy patient who has mastered some form of speech. Encourage affiliation with community support group for laryngectomy patients.	Using Magic Slate for communication; becomes frustrated with time it takes to communicate; spoke to physician about referral to Lost Cord group.
Anxiety regarding aspiration when tries to swallow; doesn't feel he'll be able to eat by mouth again. SUPPORTING DATA Chokes when tries to swallow saliva; tends to aspirate.	Lungs will remain clear. Patient will learn to swallow without aspirating within 6 weeks.	Teach patient to hold his breath and perform the Valsalva maneuver while swallowing; teach him to keep his neck relaxed forward when swallowing and forcibly exhale after swallowing.	Still very anxious when tries to swallow; still coughing a lot with each attempt; get consult with speech therapist for swallowing exercises; continue plan.

DISORDERS OF THE UPPER RESPIRATORY SYSTEM

◆ Upper Respiratory Infection (the Common Cold) and Rhinitis

The common cold is an inflammation of the upper respiratory tract caused by a virus. It is the most prevalent infectious disease among people of all ages. So many different strains of viruses can produce the symptoms of a common cold that total immunity is difficult to achieve. Avoiding exposure to those who have a cold and maintaining a state of good health are the only ways one can avoid catching a cold.

◆ Symptoms

The common cold usually starts with a mild sore throat or a hot, dry, prickly sensation in the nose and back of the throat. Within hours after the onset of a cold, the nose becomes congested with increased secretions *(rhinitis)*, the eyes begin to water, and sneezing and an irritating, nonproductive cough appear. There usually is no elevation of temperature; if a fever does develop, it is low grade.

Allergic rhinitis may be seasonal. The treatment also is symptomatic. Antihistamines, steroids, and sprays that stabilize the mucous cell membranes often are prescribed. The patient is taught to avoid the offending allergens as much as possible. If the disorder is severe, an allergy evaluation is indicated so that a desensitization program can be started.

Medical Treatment and Nursing Intervention
There is no cure for the common cold. However, zinc lozenges have proven effective in limiting a cold's duration for many people if started at the first signs of symptoms. A major goal in the care of a common cold is prevention of a secondary bacterial infection. For their own sake as well as that of people around them, persons with a cold should avoid contact with others so as to avoid picking up a bacterial infection or giving their viral infection to someone else. A person with a cold is contagious for about 3 days after his symptoms first appear.

Colds are spread by droplet infection, and most people realize that coughing and sneezing can send literally millions of viruses into the air. Some are also aware of the danger of spreading a cold by sharing drinking glasses and cups with others. They might not know, however, that a cold can be transmitted by hand. Coughing and sneezing into tissues does limit the viruses' travel by air, **but they are also very likely to be on the person's hands, where they can be transferred to anything he touches. Handwashing, then, is an impor-**tant part of teaching patients about preventing the spread of their cold to others.

The patient should stay indoors, preferably in bed or resting during the first few days of the illness. Fluid intake should be increased. Fruit juices are recommended, especially citrus juices, because of their vitamin C content.

Aspirin or some other mild nonprescription analgesic can help relieve the muscle aches and headache of a cold. Nose drops or sprays for the relief of nasal congestion can have a rebound effect, leaving the nose "stuffier" than before if used for more than 3 days. Antibiotics do not cure a common cold, which is a viral infection.

If a "cold" persists for more than a week to 10 days, or if the patient begins to feel worse, has a temperature of 102°F (38.9°C), and develops chest pains or coughs up purulent sputum, a bacterial infection that should be treated medically is present.

◆ Sinusitis

Sinusitis is an inflammation of the mucosal lining of the sinuses. Causes include infection that has spread from the nasal passages to the sinuses and blockage of normal sinus drainage routes. Sinusitis often occurs after colds or other respiratory infections. People with a deviated nasal septum or allergy problems tend to have recurrent sinusitis. Symptoms include headache, fever, tenderness over sinuses, malaise, and purulent drainage from the nose.

Treatment of sinusitis is directed at relieving pain, promoting sinus drainage, controlling infection, and preventing recurrence. Hot, moist packs over the sinus area can be helpful. Inhaling moist steam and increasing fluid intake to thin secretions helps promote drainage. Medications are prescribed to promote vasoconstriction, reduce swelling, and promote drainage. Decongestants also may be used. Infection is treated with an antibiotic or antiinfective agent. Rest, reduced stress, a balanced diet, and control of allergies can help prevent recurrence. Analgesics are given for pain.

Think about . . . How would you know if you, or a patient, has a sinus infection rather than just an ordinary cold?

Acute or chronic sinus infection should not be ignored, as the infection can cause a variety of complications, including septicemia, meningitis, or brain abscess.

◆ Epistaxis

Epistaxis (nosebleed) is a common occurrence and usually involves minimal blood loss. Nosebleeds may occur for many reasons. Decreased humidity, excessive nose blowing, allergy with inflammation, and nose picking are some causes. They usually result from crusting, cracking, or irritation of the mucous membrane covering the front of the nasal septum and can easily be stopped by the application of pressure. Nosebleeds also can result from trauma, hypertension, and blood disorders such as leukemia.

When epistaxis occurs, the patient should sit forward and apply direct pressure by pinching the nose for 10 to 15 minutes (Figure 15-2). This is done to avoid having blood run down the back of the throat, where it is either swallowed or aspirated into the lungs. Cold compresses or ice, which will constrict the blood vessels, may be applied to the nose or face. The patient is asked to rest quietly for a few hours and warned not to blow the nose, pick at it, or rub it for 4 to 8 hours after the nosebleed has stopped. If needed, the nose may be loosely packed with gauze along with the application of pressure. The gauze should be left in place for several hours and then very gently removed and pressure applied again for several minutes. If a nosebleed cannot be stopped in this manner, the patient should go to the emergency department, where a physician will cauterize the bleeding vessels or solidly pack the nose to stop the bleeding. Otherwise the patient will continue to hemorrhage slowly.

◆ Pharyngitis

Inflammation of the pharynx, usually called a *sore throat*, is such a common occurrence that almost everyone has experienced it at one time or another. The symptoms familiar to us all include a dry, "scratchy" feeling in the back of the throat, mild fever, headache, and malaise. Dysphagia is also present, with greater discomfort when swallowing one's own saliva than when swallowing food. Unfortunately, pharyngitis is

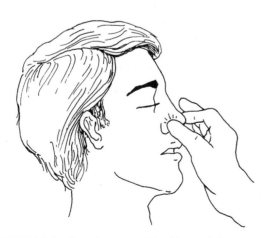

FIGURE 15-2   Stopping a nosebleed by applying pressure to the nose.

TABLE 15-1 ◆ *Patient Education: Warning Signs of Cancer of the Larynx or Throat*

Teach patients to seek medical attention if the following signs of cancer of the larynx or throat occur:

◆ Hoarseness lasting more than 2 weeks.
◆ Sore throat that lasts more than 2 weeks.
◆ Pain on swallowing that persists for more than 2 weeks.
◆ Difficulty swallowing or pain when swallowing.
◆ Coughing up of bloody sputum.
◆ Lumps or knots on the neck indicating enlarged cervical lymph nodes.

accompanied by a constant urge to swallow. The usual course for uncomplicated pharyngitis is 3 to 10 days. All patients should be assessed for the warning signs of cancer of the larynx and throat; the signs are listed in Table 15-1.

The diagnosis of pharyngitis is confirmed by clinical signs and symptoms, such as those previously mentioned and a red and inflamed throat. A throat culture is sometimes done to confirm or rule out streptococcal and other bacterial infections.

Medical Treatment and Nursing Intervention   Uncomplicated viral pharyngitis usually responds to such conservative measures as rest, warm saline gargles (one-half to one teaspoon of table salt to a glass of warm water), throat lozenges, plenty of fluids, and a mild analgesic for aches and pains. Antiseptic sprays and lozenges help provide relief from discomfort.

Bacterial pharyngitis requires antibiotic therapy, particularly if the infecting organism is *Streptococcus*. Chronic pharyngitis may require diagnostic procedures to determine the underlying cause (for example, an infection elsewhere in the respiratory tract) and therapeutic measures, such as humidification and filtering of environmental air.

◆ Tonsillitis

An inflammation of the tonsils usually is caused by streptococci or staphylococci and is completely different from pharyngitis, even though the symptoms may be somewhat alike. Acute tonsillitis may occur repeatedly, especially in those who have a low resistance to infection. Chronic tonsillitis usually produces an enlargement of tonsillar tissue and adjacent adenoidal tissue as well.

Symptoms   *Acute tonsillitis* occurs most often in young children. There is an elevation of temperature, sore throat, general malaise, and chills. Inspection of the throat reveals redness and swelling of the tonsils and surrounding tissues.

Chronic infection of the tonsils produces symptoms that may not be as dramatic as those of acute tonsillitis but most certainly are capable of making the person uncomfortable. The child with chronic tonsillitis and enlarged adenoids has frequent colds and appears to be in poor health. He may give the impression of being dull or mentally retarded, because he constantly holds his mouth open to breathe and often has difficulty in hearing.

Treatment and Nursing Intervention

A throat culture is done before treatment is begun to check for the presence of *Streptococcus*, which can cause rheumatic fever or glomerulonephritis if not treated promptly. Acute tonsillitis is treated with hot saline throat gargles and the administration of specific antibiotics to destroy the causative organism. Bedrest, nursing measures to reduce the fever, and a liquid diet to minimize trauma to the tonsils are also included.

Surgery is used to treat tonsillitis when it is recurrent or when enlargement of the tonsils and adenoids obstructs airways. **The physician's rule of thumb is usually to consider surgery if the patient has more than five episodes of tonsillitis per year.** Surgery is performed after the acute infection has cleared.

Nursing Care of the Patient Undergoing a Tonsillectomy and Adenoidectomy

Preoperative care. These procedures are generally done on an outpatient, same-day surgery basis. Preliminary laboratory testing and patient education begin before the patient is admitted. Physical preparation of the patient involves administration of preoperative medications as ordered and restriction of the patient's diet for 6 to 8 hours prior to surgery. It is especially important that the patient be observed for signs of fever. An elevation of temperature or any signs of an upper respiratory infection should be reported. Surgery is usually postponed if these signs are present. When tonsillectomy is performed with a laser, there is very little swelling and little bleeding. The patient also has an easier time swallowing postoperatively.

Postoperative care.

Following tonsillectomy or adenoidectomy, the nurse's chief concern is observation for hemorrhage.

Although tonsillectomy and adenoidectomy patients usually recover from surgery rapidly and rarely suffer any complications, nurses should be vigilant because hemorrhage is a real danger. **Vital signs are checked frequently, and the patient is observed for frequent swallowing, which may indicate bleeding in the throat. Restlessness can be another clue to excessive bleeding.** An ice collar may be placed around the neck to reduce swelling and prevent the oozing of blood from the operative site.

Although it is difficult to keep a child in one position for very long, he should be kept on his side or abdomen as long as there is drainage from the surgical wound. If the child is thrashing about in the bed when recovering from the anesthesia, it is best to collect secretions from the mouth in a large towel rather than use a metal emesis basin, which may injure him. Older children may sit up in a semi-Fowler's position after they have recovered from the anesthesia and are often more comfortable this way. A younger child usually can be kept calm and quiet if someone holds him and rocks him. He needs to keep as quiet as possible to prevent hemorrhage from the operative site, and he also needs love and affection to reassure him at a time when he is frightened and uncomfortable.

The postoperative diet usually consists of ice-cold liquids, popsicles, and gelatin, progressing to ice cream, custards, and other semisolid foods for the first 24 hours. Citrus fruits, hot fluids, and rough foods should be avoided until the throat has completely healed. Written instructions are sent home when the child is discharged from the same-day surgery unit. The parents are given a phone number to call in case of emergency or if they have questions.

Think about . . . What sign would alert you to the probability that the tonsillectomy patient was experiencing bleeding and that the blood was running down the throat where you cannot see it?

◆ Cancer of the Larynx

Cancer of the larynx occurs most often in men in their sixties to eighties, but it can strike anyone, especially those over the age of 18. It is one of the most easily cured of all malignancies because of its location and adjacent tissues, and about 90% of all patients treated by early radiation and/or surgery are cured. The cause of cancer of the larynx is not known, but there is some evidence that predisposing factors are cigarette smoking, alcohol abuse, chronic laryngitis, abuse of the vocal cords, and a familial tendency to cancer. Exposure over long periods to environmental pollutants, such as asbestos, diethyl sulfate, mustard gas, or wood dust, also is considered a risk factor.

Medical Symptoms and Diagnosis

Because the larynx, sometimes called the voice box, is directly involved with the production of vocal sounds, a tumor of the larynx will quickly produce persistent hoarseness that does not respond to usual methods of treatment. After the cancer has spread beyond the vocal cords (and is much more difficult to treat), the symptoms may include difficulty in swallowing or breathing, a sensation of having a lump in the throat, cough, enlarged lymph nodes in the neck, and pain in the region of the Adam's apple.

Diagnosis is established by visualizing the larynx via a laryngoscope, CT scan of the larynx and throat, MRI scan, and microscopic examination of a sample of tissues taken from the tumor.

Medical and Surgical Treatment   Often radiation alone may be utilized to treat early cancer of the larynx. Radiation may be combined with laser surgery for certain types of lesions. Several types of surgical procedures may be performed to treat laryngeal malignant disease. Most often this disorder can be treated on an outpatient basis. If the tumor is large or not restricted to the vocal cords, the surgeon may perform a *partial laryngectomy* in which the thyroid cartilage is split, and only the tumor and involved portion of the vocal cords are removed. A partial laryngectomy does not permanently eliminate voice sounds. A tracheostomy may be done to facilitate breathing temporarily, but the opening made for the stoma eventually is closed, and the patient may resume talking after the affected area is healed completely.

Microlaryngoscopy combined with laser is now the method of choice for removing vocal cord polyps and carcinoma in situ. Cure rates for malignancy of the true vocal cords treated by laser are about 90%. Other advantages include the absence of mechanical trauma and swelling when laser is used, which means that the patient returns to normal activities within about 3 days. There is, however, no need for extended voice rest; 2 days is usually sufficient.

A total laryngectomy is done if the tumor has progressed to the point of paralyzing the vocal cords. The surgeon excises the entire larynx, epiglottis, thyroid cartilage, hyoid bone, cricoid cartilage, and two or more rings of the trachea.

If the tumor has extended to the lymph nodes, a radical neck dissection also is performed on the side of the lesion. All the muscle, lymph nodes, and soft tissue from the lower edge of the mandible to the clavicle and from the top of the trapezius muscle to the midline are removed. A tracheostomy is performed at the same time. The trachea is diverted to a surgically constructed opening (**stoma**) in the neck. The patient then has a permanent tracheostomy with no connection between the nose and mouth and the lower respiratory system; he must depend on the stoma for breathing (Figure 15-3). A laryngectomy tube, which is shorter and wider than a tracheostomy tube, is put into place before discharge. After the stoma is completely healed and matured, about 6 weeks after surgery, the tube can be left out as long as there is no compromise of the airway. Care of the

patient with a tracheostomy is presented in the next chapter.

A thin feeding tube is placed during surgery for postoperative use for about 10 to 14 days. The patient has only IV fluids initially but then progresses to regular tube feedings. When healing is far enough along that the danger of contamination of the operative site is not a concern, training in eating and swallowing is begun. When the patient is discharged from the hospital, a visiting nurse or clinic nurse will work with the patient on eating skills. Some patients have to rely on a feeding tube, as they cannot master the swallowing procedure without aspiration. The indwelling tube may then be replaced with a tube that the patient can insert and then remove after feedings.

Nursing Intervention   The patient who has had a laryngectomy will require adequate instruction in the care of his stoma and laryngectomy tube. He will need help and guidance in facing a future in which he will not be able to speak until he learns esophageal speech or uses an artificial "voice box" (Figure 15-4). He also may have difficulty eating and swallowing until he gets accustomed to the sensations of choking and gagging that frequently occur after a laryngectomy. Table 15-2 presents guidelines for assisting the partial laryngectomy patient to eat.

Immediate postoperative care focuses on maintaining a patent airway and observing for hemorrhage. **If the patient has a tracheostomy, it will need to be suctioned very frequently during the first 24 to 48 hours. His air exchange is dependent on the nurse's maintaining a patent airway for him.** *Totally aseptic technique* **must be used when suctioning to prevent lung infection.** Special care must be taken when the ties that hold the tracheostomy tube in place are changed; otherwise the tube may be dislodged by coughing, which movement of the tube tends to cause (see Chapter 16 for tracheostomy care). Good aseptic technique is a must when caring for the tracheostomy and the neck incisions to prevent infection of the incision areas.

The patient will go through a grief process over losing his natural voice if a total laryngectomy has been done. A radical neck dissection creates further problems with alteration of body image, as the procedure is somewhat disfiguring. Depression is a common problem initially, but contact with others who have had the surgery and are leading full productive lives may help the patient focus on the benefits of the surgery in saving his own life.

Protection of the tracheal opening from dust and lint can be accomplished through the use of a simple gauze covering or high-necked clothing. The patient also should be told to avoid swimming and to use care when taking a shower or tub bath so that water is not

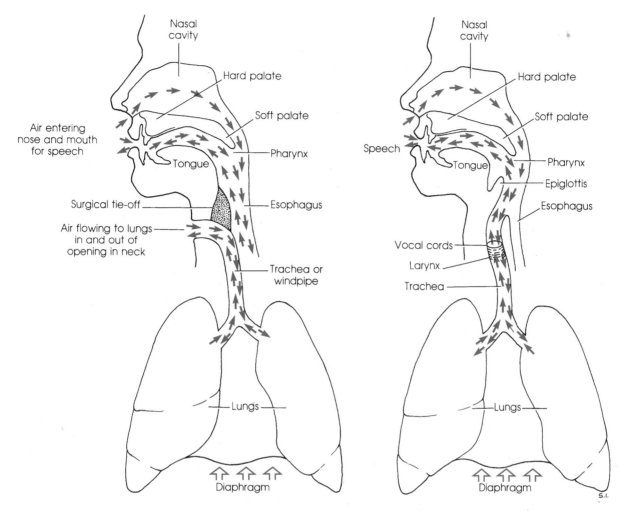

FIGURE 15-3 Airflow after laryngectomy *(left)* and in a normal respiratory tract *(right)*.

aspirated through the opening. To protect the patient from inhalation of extremely cold air (he no longer breathes through his nose and mouth, which normally warm the inspired air) the patient may wear a small scarf over the opening during the winter.

Proper rehabilitation of the patient plays a very important part in his acceptance of surgery and its consequences. Nursing Care Plan 15-1 (p. 398) lists some problems and nursing interventions for the laryngectomy patient. The speech therapist works closely with the patient to help him master a new form of speech. Many people are able to learn esophageal speech in which they first master the art of swallowing air and then moving it forcibly back up through the esophagus. They then learn to coordinate lip and tongue movements with the sound produced by the air passing over vibrating folds of the esophagus. The sounds may be somewhat hoarse, but they can be understood as speech and are more natural than the sounds produced by an artificial larynx. For patients who cannot master esophageal speech in this manner, a tracheoesophageal prosthesis can be implanted. A fistula is created by

connecting the esophagus and the trachea. A silicone prosthesis is inserted after healing has taken place. The patient can cover the opening of the prosthesis with a finger or close it with a special valve that diverts air from the lungs up through the trachea into the esophagus and out of the mouth. Speech is formed by the lip and tongue movement as the air is expelled.

A mechanical vibrator device known as an electronic artificial larynx can be used externally when applied to the skin of the esophagus to simulate speech. These are battery powered; they do not produce voice-like speech, but they do provide understandable sounds and make it possible for the patient to communicate (Figure 15-4). An electronic speech aid with a small tube device inserted into the mouth attached to a pocket-sized power pack can also be used. A button device that can be occluded with a finger can be implanted in the throat, allowing the patient to use diaphragmatic speech. New devices are under development.

In various parts of the United States, several groups have organized for laryngectomy patients who wish to get together for social and rehabilitation purposes.

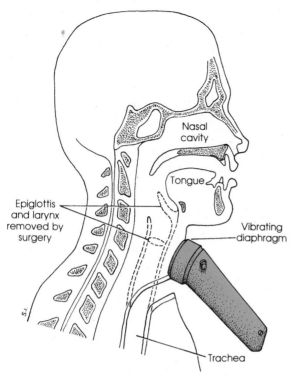

The vibrating cap of the electronic larynx is held against the throat with sufficient pressure to maintain firm contact. Sound vibrations are transmitted into the lower portion of the pharynx and transformed into speech by the normal movements of the tongue, lips, and teeth.

FIGURE 15-4   External larynx.

These clubs have names such as Lost Cord, New Speech, New Voice, and Esophageal Speech. Information regarding these clubs and other aspects of postlaryngectomy rehabilitation can be obtained by writing to

---

TABLE 15-2 ◆ *Nutrition Point: Assisting the Partial Laryngectomy Patient with Eating*

To assist the patient to eat, practice in swallowing is necessary. The following guidelines are helpful in teaching the patient to swallow, thereby maintaining an adequate nutritional status.

- Explain that swallowing food without choking is possible.
- Obtain a visit from a partial laryngectomy patient who has mastered the procedure.
- Begin practice with soft or semisolid foods.
- Supervise initial practice and expalin that someone needs to be with the patient when he eats until swallowing without choking is mastered.
- Teach to swallow by asking the patient to:
  - Take a deep breath and bear down to close the vocal cords.
  - Place a small bite of food in the mouth.
  - Tip the chin toward the chest and swallow.
  - Emit a cough to rid the throat of any food particles.
  - Swallow again.
  - Cough again.
  - Begin breathing normally again.
- Offer encouragement for each effort.

---

the American Speech-Language-Hearing Association, 10801 Rockville Pike, Rockville, MD 20852. Local chapters of the American Cancer Society also are good sources of information and assistance for the laryngectomy patient and his family. Further information regarding care of the laryngectomy patient who has cancer can be found in the chapter on care of the cancer patient.

Think about . . . Can you identify all of the health care professionals who would be involved in the collaborative care of the patient undergoing a total laryngectomy and radical neck dissection?

COMMUNITY CARE

One of the primary aspects of community care for nurses is to promote immunization for influenza. It also is important to remind the public, now that everyone is so used to having antibiotics to clear up infections, that the best way to prevent infections is through hygiene measures such as frequent handwashing and covering the mouth when coughing or sneezing.

Home care nurses supervise the follow-up care for the patient recovering from a severe respiratory infection. Reviewing the correct methods of deep-breathing and coughing is an important nursing function. **Reminding patients to take all of their prescription antibiotic to adequately kill all causative microorganisms is very important in preventing the development of disease-resistant strains of bacteria.** The home care nurse will also be very instrumental in helping the patient with throat cancer recover. Attention to nutritional concerns, wound care, supervision of self-care techniques for care of a tracheostomy, and psychosocial support are the keys to prompt recovery for the laryngectomy patient.

Tracheostomy care in the home setting is a little different from in the hospital. Suction catheters may be used longer and can be disinfected at home for reuse. Once the stoma is healed, the patient learns to adapt supplies to his needs. The patient's economic status may dictate what type of supplies and which type of tracheostomy tube will be best for him.

Long-term care facility nurses must be vigilant for signs of URI in residents to prevent the spread of infection to others. Refraining from coming to work with a contagious URI or diligently wearing a mask and washing hands, can help prevent introducing URI organisms into the environment. Working to assist residents to maintain adequate nutrition helps promote immunity .

Referring cancer patients who have had a laryngectomy to the support services of the American Cancer Society can help provide hope of a more normal life to these patients. Contact with other individuals who have experienced this disease, adjusted, and gone on to continue with a productive, happy life is the best medicine the patient can receive.

CRITICAL THINKING EXERCISES

Clinical Case Problem

Read the following clinical situation and discuss the questions with your classmates.

1. Mr. Kim has undergone diagnostic procedures to confirm suspected cancer of the larynx. He has been admitted to the hospital for a hemilaryngectomy.

   a. Describe the teaching plan that would be used for a patient undergoing a direct laryngoscopy.

   b. What diagnostic tests would have been done on Mr. Kim?

   c. Devise a postoperative nursing care plan for Mr. Kim, including interventions for psychosocial problems.

   d. What resources in the community could be suggested to help Mr. Kim adjust to his laryngectomy?

BIBLIOGRAPHY

American Cancer Society. (1996). *Cancer Facts and Figures.* Atlanta: Author.

Applegate, E. J. (1995). *The Anatomy and Physiology Learning System: Textbook.* Philadelphia: Saunders.

Baker, C. A. (1992). Factors associated with rehabilitation in head and neck cancer. *Cancer Nursing.* 15(6):395–400.

Bennett, J. C., Plum, F. (eds.). (1996). *Cecil Textbook of Medicine,* 20th ed. Philadelphia: Saunders.

Boucher, M. A. (1996). When laryngectomy complicates care. *RN.* 59(8):40–44.

Chiocca, E. M. (1996). Actionstat: Epiglottis. *Nursing 96.* 26(9):25.

Dambro, M. R. (1996). *Griffith's 5 Minute Clinical Consult.* Baltimore: Williams & Wilkins.

Green, J. (1992). Recognizing epiglottitis. *Nursing 92.* 22 (8):33.

Haynes, V. L. (1996). Caring for the laryngectomy patient. *American Journal of Nursing.* 96(5):16B–16K.

Ignatavicius, D. D., Workman, M. L., Mishler, M. A. (1995). *Medical–Surgical Nursing: A Nursing Process Approach,* 2nd ed. Philadelphia: Saunders.

Kersten, L. D. (1989). *Comprehensive Respiratory Nursing: A Decision Making Approach.* Philadelphia: Saunders, 1989.

Lockhart, J., Troff, J., Artim, L. (1992). Total laryngectomy and radical neck dissection. *AORN Journal.* 55(2): 458–479.

Monahan, F. D., Drake, T., Neighbors, M. (1994). *Nursing Care of Adults.* Philadelphia: Saunders.

Polaski, A. L., Tatro, S. E. (1996). *Luckmann's Core Principles and Practice of Medical-Surgical Nursing.* Philadelphia: Saunders.

Smalley, P. J. (1990). Lasers in otolaryngology. *Nursing Clinics of North America.* 25(3):645–656.

Ulrich, S. P., Canale, S. W., Wendell, S. A. (1994). *Medical–Surgical Nursing Care Planning Guides,* 3rd ed. Philadelphia: Saunders.

Weber, M., Reiner, M. (1993). Laryngectomy: grieving, disfigurement and dysfunction. *The Canadian Nurse.* 89(3): 31–34.

Weimert, T. A. (1992). Common ENT emergencies: the acute nose and throat, part 2. *Emergency Medicine.* 24(6): 26–28, 31–32, 34–36.

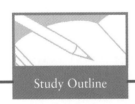

Study Outline

I. Prevention of Upper Respiratory Disorders

A. The best way to prevent URIs is to wash hands frequently, stay out of crowds, refrain from smoking, and avoid known allergens.

B. Refraining from excessive alcohol intake, especially if one smokes, helps prevent throat cancer.

C. Immunization against influenza helps prevent URI.

II. Diagnostic Tests and Examinations

A. Inspection of nasal passages with nasal speculum and light.

B. Visual examination of mouth and throat.

   1. Requires only a tongue blade and good light.

C. Laryngoscopy: visualization of larynx.

   1. Indirect laryngoscopy: relatively simple office procedure.

      a. Examiner uses a warm laryngeal mirror, head mirror, and light source.

      b. No anesthetic required unless patient has strong gag reflex.

   2. Direct laryngoscopy: endoscopic examination of larynx.

      a. Local or general anesthetic required.

      b. Patient fasts 6 to 8 hours prior to examination.

      c. Postexamination care similar to that for bronchoscopy.

d. Resuscitative equipment must be close at hand in case of laryngeal edema, epiglottitis, or laryngeal spasm.

e. Hoarseness, aphonia, and mild sore throat expected.

D. CT and MRI scans are performed to locate tumors and other pathological abnormalities of the larynx and esophagus.

E. Throat culture: usually to establish or rule out streptococcal infection.

III. Nursing Assessment

A. History taking: recent exposure to infectious agents, known allergies, chronic sinusitis. (Many cases of pharyngitis and other throat infections treated on outpatient basis.)

1. Complaints of headache, malaise, bad taste in the mouth, nasal congestion, purulent drainage from nose indicate possible sinus infection.

2. A thorough history of smoking and of alcohol intake is very important in determining the risk of throat cancer.

B. Subjective and objective data: sore throat, malaise, fever, dysphagia, hoarseness, aphonia, cough, enlarged lymph glands.

1. Persistent hoarseness and dysphagia should be further investigated for possible malignancy (Table 15-1).

IV. Nursing Management

A. Nursing diagnoses appropriate depend on the type of problem and the stage of the disorder.

B. Expected outcomes are individualized to the patient.

C. Interventions are instituted to prevent complications, promote safety, promote nutrition, relieve pain, promote oxygenation, and provide psychosocial support (see Nursing Care Plan 15-1).

D. Evaluation is performed to determine the effectiveness of the actions and progress toward meeting expected outcomes.

V. Disorders of the Upper Respiratory System

A. Common cold and rhinitis.

1. Caused by many different viruses.

2. Rest, fluids, mild analgesics for aches and pains.

3. If cold persists or high fever develops, patient should obtain medical attention.

4. Rhinitis may be allergic in origin. If it interferes with lifestyle or productivity, desensitization is an option.

B. Sinusitis: inflammation and infection of the sinuses.

1. Symptoms: headache, fever, tenderness over sinuses, purulent drainage from nose, malaise.

2. Uncontrolled sinus infection can lead to meningitis or brain abscess.

3. Treated with 10 to 14 days of antibiotics; control of allergies.

4. Surgery is sometimes necessary to open drainage tract and clear purulent material.

C. Epistaxis: nosebleed; caused by many factors: irritation from nose blowing, hypertension, trauma, blood dyscrasias, decreased humidity, and nose picking.

1. Apply direct pressure to nose for 10 to 15 minutes to stop bleeding.

2. Cold compresses or ice are helpful.

3. If bleeding does not stop, a physician's attention is necessary to prevent slow hemorrhage.

D. Pharyngitis: inflammation of the pharynx or sore throat

1. Sore throat accompanied by headache, malaise, and mild fever with difficulty swallowing.

2. Rest, warm saline gargles, throat lozenges, and a mild analgesic are the usual treatment for viral pharyngitis.

3. Bacterial pharyngitis may require a throat culture and administration of an antibiotic.

E. Tonsillitis: inflammation of the tonsils; usually streptococcal or staphylococcal infection

1. Symptoms: fever, sore throat, chills, malaise.

2. Chronic infection can lead to enlargement of tonsils and adenoids.

3. Treatment and nursing intervention: warm saline gargles, throat lozenges, rest, antibiotics. Surgery indicated in some cases.

4. Nursing care of patient undergoing tonsillectomy and adenoidectomy:

a. Preoperative care routine. Monitor for elevated temperature.

b. Postoperative care: vital signs checked frequently, patient kept on side or abdomen as long as there is drainage from the throat; diet limited to soft, nonirritating foods until throat is no longer sensitive.

c. Observe for frequent swallowing, which may indicate blood running down the throat.

F. Cancer of the larynx

1. Most easily treated of all malignant diseases.

2. Predisposing factors: smoking, alcohol use, chronic laryngitis, abuse of vocal cords.

3. Symptoms: persistent hoarseness at first; later, pain in throat, dysphagia, lump in throat, pain in region of Adam's apple.

4. Surgical treatment: laser tumor treatment, partial or total laryngectomy, radical neck dissection.

a. Patient who has had partial laryngectomy retains function of speech.

b. Total laryngectomy patient has permanent opening in trachea and must learn new speech pattern.

5. Nursing intervention: special care problems (see Nursing Care Plan 15-1).

VI. Community Care

A. Primary aspect: promote immunization for influenza.

B. Teach prevention of infection by hygiene measures: proper handwashing; covering the mouth when coughing or sneezing.

C. Supervise home patients in coughing and deep breathing techniques.

D. Remind to take all of prescription antibiotics prescribed.

E. Teach home techniques for tracheostomy technique.

F. Prevent introducing URI into long-term care environment.

G. Referral of laryngectomy patients to support groups in the community.

VII. Elder Care Points

A. The cough reflex is weakened in the elderly, creating a potential for aspiration. Weakened muscles predispose to aspiration.

B. The immune system is less efficient in the elderly, making them more prone to contracting URI.

C. Elderly men with a long history of smoking and heavy alcohol use are most likely to develop throat cancer.

D. People over 80 years of age should take care not to be exposed to others with URIs, as immunity is decreased.

CHAPTER 16

Care of Patients with Lower Respiratory Tract Disorders

OBJECTIVES

Upon completing this chapter the student should be able to:

1. Identify three measures people can take to prevent respiratory disorders.
2. Describe the pre- and posttest care for the patient undergoing the following: chest radiograph, bronchoscopy, pulmonary function testing.
3. Describe the procedure for nursing assessment of the respiratory system.
4. Compare and contrast commonalities and differences in nursing care for patients with bronchitis, influenza, pneumonia, pleurisy, and empyema.
5. List at least three nursing interventions appropriate for care of patients experiencing the following: persistent cough, increased secretions in the respiratory tract, dyspnea, alteration in nutrition and hydration related to respiratory disorder, and fatigue related to hypoxia.
6. Complete a nursing care plan, including home care, for the patient with chronic airflow limitation (CAL).
7. List four ways a nurse can contribute to prevention and prompt treatment of tuberculosis.
8. Describe the specifics of nursing care for the patient who has had thoracic surgery and has chest tubes in place.
9. Devise a nursing care plan for the tracheostomy patient on oxygen therapy and on a mechanical ventilator.

Breathing is essential to life. When a problem interferes with the ability to breathe or with the diffusion of gas across the lung membranes, homeostasis of the whole body is affected. For *ventilation* to take place there must be sufficient oxygen in the air, muscle ability to lower the diaphragm and draw in a breath, a stable bone structure of the chest wall, nonobstructed airway passages, and functioning alveolar membranes. **Perfusion** (blood flow) also is an essential part of respiration because it is the bloodstream that carries the oxygen to the cells of the body. Blood must be pumped past the alveolar

membrane for oxygen and carbon dioxide diffusion to take place. Blood must circulate to the many parts of the body for the oxygen taken in through the lungs to reach the cells. Many problems can interfere with the structural units of the body needed for a healthy respiratory system. Trauma or disease can affect the structures of the respiratory system or the nerves controlling respiration. To understand these problems, a basic knowledge of the anatomy and physiology of the respiratory system is essential. A brief overview is provided to refresh the student's memory.

OVERVIEW OF ANATOMY AND PHYSIOLOGY

How is Oxygen Delivered to the Alveolar Membrane Where It Can Diffuse into the Blood?

⅄ After passing through the nose, pharynx, larynx, and trachea of the upper respiratory system, the air enters the left and right bronchi branching off of the trachea.

⅄ The bronchi bring air into the lungs; the right lung has three lobes, and the left lung has two lobes.

⅄ The main bronchi divide into smaller, and smaller bronchi and then divide into bronchioles that deliver the air to the alveoli (Figure 16-1).

⅄ The alveoli are lined with membrane that allows passage of oxygen into the blood and the passage of carbon dioxide from the blood into the alveoli.

How Is the Lung Protected?

⅄ The pleural sac, which encloses each lung and protects it, is an airtight compartment. Pressure within the pleural cavity is less than that of the outside atmosphere. **If the pleural sac is punctured, air will rush into the pleural cavity and collapse the lung.**

⅄ The *pleura* is a serous membrane of two layers. One layer covers each lung, and the other lines the inner wall of the chest cavity.

⅄ A fluid between the two layers of pleura lubricates the pleural cavity and prevents friction between the pleural layers from occurring when the lungs expand and deflate.

⅄ The pleural cavity is a potential space between the pleural layers.

⅄ The mucous membrane lining the bronchial tree contains tiny hairlike projections, *cilia*, that trap and help remove small foreign particles that are inhaled.

⅄ The mucous membrane secretes mucus, which assists the cilia in cleansing foreign substances from the respiratory tract.

⅄ The alveoli contain macrophages that quickly phagocytize inhaled bacteria and other foreign particles.

⅄ The mucus and cilia propel the foreign substances toward the entrance of the respiratory tract; the cough reflex works to expel the secretions.

⅄ Disorders that interfere with the cough reflex lead to retained secretions and the potential for pneumonia.

How Is Respiration Controlled?

⅄ The regulatory mechanisms that control breathing patterns do so in response to metabolic demands and increasing cardiac output and are very complex.

⅄ The central nervous system controls both involuntary and voluntary respiration. The vagus nerve supplies the pharynx, larynx, respiratory airways, and lungs.

⅄ The brainstem chemoreceptors are sensitive to changes in carbon dioxide and hydrogen ions in the cerebrospinal fluid; the chemoreceptors in the aorta and the carotid arteries are sensitive to low oxygen levels in the blood.

⅄ The signals of changing levels of hydrogen ions (indicated by pH), carbon dioxide, and oxygen trigger the respiratory center to send signals through the spinal cord to the phrenic and intercostal nerves that control the diaphragm and respiratory muscle contractions.

⅄ When CO_2 and hydrogen ion levels in the cerebrospinal fluid become higher than normal, the central receptors in the brainstem signal the nerves to initiate faster respiration to blow off the excess CO_2. Carbon dioxide levels give the primary signals for respiration.

⅄ When arterial blood O_2 levels fall below normal, the respiratory centers in the arteries signal the nerves to cause the lungs to inflate more fully, making the person breathe more deeply and at a faster rate. Chemoreceptors respond to changes in arterial blood gases (see Table 16-1 for normal values).

⅄ When CO_2 levels are constantly high, as occurs with chronic lung disease, the respiratory drive comes from the receptors for low arterial oxygen. If these patients are given too much oxygen, their respiratory drive is suppressed and they will stop breathing.

How Do the Bones of the Thorax and the Respiratory Muscles Affect the Respiratory Process?

⅄ Inspiration (inhalation), and expiration (exhalation) occur by movement of the diaphragm and the muscles in the chest wall.

⅄ Contraction of the diaphragm and the chest muscles draw the diaphragm downward, expanding the lungs and creating a greater area of negative pressure. Air from the atmosphere, which has a higher pressure, flows into the lungs.

⅄ When the muscles relax, the lungs are allowed to return to a resting position that has a smaller internal volume and air is pushed out in exhalation.

⅄ **During normal breathing, about 500 mL of air moves in and out of the lungs with each breath.**

⅄ The respiratory muscles depend on nerve impulses from the spinal cord. **If damage to the spinal cord occurs above the level where the respiratory nerves are located, voluntary respiration ceases.**

⅄ If the muscles of the diaphragm and chest are paralyzed, **apnea** (absence of breathing) occurs.

⅄ The thoracic cage, composed of the thoracic vertebrae, the sternum, and the ribs, forms a stable unit that allows the respiratory muscles to function correctly.

⅄ If the ribs, the sternum, or any bones of the thorax or chest wall, are injured or fractured, breathing becomes difficult and **dyspnea** occurs.

⅄ **Compliance** describes the elasticity of the lungs; it refers to how easily the lungs inflate; when compliance is decreased, the lungs are more difficult to inflate.

⅄ **Arthritis of the rib cage may cause decreased compliance.**

⅄ **Weakness of the respiratory muscles, such as occurs with neuromuscular diseases, also causes decreased compliance.**

⅄ **Kyphosis** (inward curvature and collapse) of the spine constricts the thoracic cavity and restricts the capacity of the lungs to expand fully.

How Does Oxygen and Carbon Dioxide Exchange across the Alveolar Membrane?

⅄ Oxygen mixed in air enters the alveoli through the alveolar ducts that extend from the bronchioles.

⅄ The alveoli are lined with a permeable membrane.

⅄ Surfactant is secreted by cells in the alveoli; surfactant decreases surface tension on the alveolar wall, allowing it to expand more easily with inspiration and preventing alveolar collapse upon expiration. This provides an adequate surface across which diffusion of oxygen and carbon dioxide can take place.

⅄ **When surfactant levels are low, alveoli cannot properly expand and oxygen and carbon dioxide cannot cross the membrane adequately.**

⅄ When interstitial edema occurs in the lung tissue, the alveolar membrane is thickened and gases cannot diffuse across the membrane as easily. If fluid fills the alveoli, such as occurs with an inflammatory process in the lung, the gases cannot diffuse across the membrane.

⅄ Edema in the lungs occurs with infectious processes such as pneumonia and in disorders such as congestive heart failure.

How Does Oxygen Get to the Tissues and How Does Carbon Dioxide Travel from the Cells to Be Exhaled by the Lungs?

⅄ The blood transports both oxygen and carbon dioxide. Erythrocytes (red blood cells) play the major role in transporting these gases. The plasma also transports a portion of each gas; about 3% of oxygen is dissolved in the plasma. About 7% of carbon dioxide is transported dissolved in the plasma.

⅄ The major portion of the oxygen, about 97%, attaches to the heme portion of the hemoglobin molecule carried by the erythrocytes and forms *oxyhemoglobin.*

⅄ Oxyhemoglobin carries the majority of the oxygen to the cells of the body.

⅄ Carbon dioxide (CO_2), a cellular waste product, combines with water in the red blood cell, forming carbonic acid; dissociation (uncombining) occurs forming hydrogen ions and bicarbonate ions.

⅄ About 77% of carbon dioxide is transported in the blood plasma in the form of bicarbonate ions.

⅄ The remaining 23% of CO_2 combines with hemoglobin and is carried to the lungs in that manner.

⅄ In the lung the process reverses and the bicarbonate ions reenter the red blood cells and combine with hydrogen ions to form carbonic acid, which then dissociates into water and carbon dioxide. The carbon dioxide diffuses across the alveolar membrane and is exhaled.

What Changes in the Respiratory System of the Elderly Predispose Them to Problems?

⅄ Adults age 70 and older have some degree of alteration of connective tissue that causes decreased elasticity and affects lung function and ventilation.

⅄ Total body water decreases to 50% after age 70, which means that the mucous and respiratory membranes are not as moist as in younger individuals. Mucus becomes much thicker.

⚠ There is some degree of impairment of the ciliary action in the airways, which makes it more difficult to remove mucus, and retained mucus provides a breeding ground for bacterial infection.

⚠ There is a loss of normal elastic recoil of the lung during expiration, and the patient must use muscle action to complete expiration.

⚠ Connective tissue changes and loss of elastic tissue in the alveoli cause the alveolar membranes to become thickened, decreasing the ease with which gases can diffuse across the membranes. Oxygen saturation decreases, with pO_2 dropping to 75 to 80 mm Hg from the usual 80 to 100 mm Hg.

⚠ Essentially these changes mean that the elderly patient has less respiratory reserve. The body cannot meet demands made for increased oxygenation.

CAUSES OF RESPIRATORY DISORDERS

The respiratory system is particularly susceptible to harmful substances in the environment. Inhalation of bacteria and other organisms can quickly produce an infection in either the upper or lower respiratory tract. Tobacco smoke, allergens, poisonous gases, and other toxic substances cause irritation and inflammation of the air passages and can eventually lead to chronic inflammation, obstructive diseases, and tumors.

Because adequate exchange of oxygen and carbon dioxide depends on sufficient blood supply to lung tissues, cardiac disease, emboli, and other disorders of the heart and pulmonary blood vessels eventually cause problems in the respiratory system. Aside from infection of the respiratory tract, there are two major types of ventilatory diseases: *restrictive* and *obstructive*. Each group has different causative factors and pathophysiological effects.

Restrictive diseases **are a group of disorders characterized by decreased lung capacity.** They are not necessarily primarily lung disorders, but their eventual effect is to limit expansion of the lung and chest wall, and they can include a large variety of illnesses. Examples include scoliosis and kyphosis, both of which decrease the size of the chest cavity; arthritis, which increases stiffness of the chest wall; pneumothorax (collapsed lung), which diminishes lung space; neuromuscular disorders that weaken the strength of the muscles of respiration (e.g., myasthenia gravis); and disorders of the lung that increase stiffness and decrease lung volume (e.g., pneumonia, atelectasis, and fibrosis).

Obstructive pulmonary diseases **are characterized by problems moving air into and out of the lungs.** Narrowing of the openings in the tracheobronchial tree

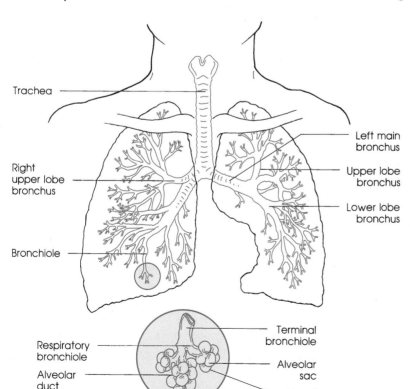

Trachea

Right upper lobe bronchus

Bronchiole

Left main bronchus

Upper lobe bronchus

Lower lobe bronchus

Respiratory bronchiole

Alveolar duct

Terminal bronchiole

Alveolar sac

Alveoli

FIGURE 16-1   Lower respiratory tract and alveoli.

TABLE 16-1 ◆ *Normal Range for Arterial Blood Gases*	
pH	7.35–7.35
pO_2	80–100 mm Hg
pCO_2	35–45 mm Hg
HCO_3	22–26 mEq/L

increases resistance to the flow of air, making it difficult for oxygen to enter and contributing to air trapping, as exhalation also is difficult. Asthma, emphysema, and chronic bronchitis are examples of obstructive lung diseases.

PREVENTION OF RESPIRATORY DISEASES

Elimination of such widespread respiratory diseases as the common cold and influenza is hardly possible, considering the many daily contacts a person has with viruses and other infectious organisms. There are, however, certain common sense measures that can reduce one's chances of catching a respiratory infection. These include adequate rest and good nutrition, especially during the time of year when respiratory infections are most prevalent. In addition, it is important to practice good personal hygiene, such as frequent handwashing and avoiding as much as possible direct contact with people who have a respiratory infection. Following airborne and droplet precautions while caring for patients whose condition indicates possible exposure can help protect the nurse from unnecessary infection.

For some persons, particularly the elderly and the chronically ill, immunization against influenza is an effective means of reducing the incidence of respiratory disease. The U.S. Public Health Service Advisory Committee on Immunization recommends annual immunization for high-risk persons. Immunization against pneumococcal infection that occurs secondary to viral infection also is recommended on a one-time basis to high-risk persons. Those considered at high risk are people over 65 years of age, those confined to extended-care facilities, and persons with (1) chronic respiratory disorders; (2) congenital or chronic cardiovascular disorders; (3) chronic renal disease; (4) diabetes mellitus and other chronic metabolic disorders; and (5) conditions compromising the immune response. Physicians, nurses, and others involved in providing health care, and therefore often exposed to influenza viruses, also should be immunized.

Although there is some danger in taking the vaccine, the benefits far outweigh the risks. Among the more serious reactions to influenza vaccine are allergic reactions, fever, malaise, muscle soreness, and possibly the development of Guillain-Barré syndrome. This latter reaction occurs in only about 1 in 100,000.

Immunization against influenza is not recommended for children under the age of 8 years. **Persons who are allergic to eggs, chicken protein, or feathers should not be given the vaccine either because it is prepared from chicken embryos.**

Other actions that can be taken to avoid serious respiratory disease include prompt treatment of upper respiratory infections, especially in children. **An acute respiratory infection that is not completely eliminated can develop into a chronic disorder and cause problems throughout the person's life.**

Perhaps one of the most important preventive measures is to avoid prolonged and repeated inhalation of irritating substances. Such substances include tobacco smoke, industrial gases, coal dust, soot and other carbons, and air polluted by automobile exhaust. Stopping smoking does decrease the incidence of respiratory ailments.

Think about . . . Can you think of three changes in lifestyle that might prevent a family member from developing a chronic or serious respiratory disorder?

TERMS COMMONLY USED IN RESPIRATORY CARE

As with other specialties in health care, some terms are used almost exclusively in respiratory care. A selection of these terms and their definitions follow:

◆ *Apnea:* absence of respiration.
◆ *Diffusion:* the movement of oxygen and carbon dioxide across the alveolar-capillary membrane. It takes place between the gas in the alveolar spaces and the blood in the pulmonary capillaries.
◆ *Elastance:* the extent to which the lungs are able to return to their original position after being stretched or distended.
◆ *Lung compliance:* the ability of the lungs to distend in response to changes in volume and pressure of inhaled air. Lung compliance first increases and then decreases with age as the lungs become stiffer and the chest wall more rigid.
◆ *Hypoxia:* a broad term meaning diminished availability of oxygen to the body tissues.
◆ *Hypoxemia:* deficient oxygenation of the blood.

- *Resistance:* the force working against the passage of air. The major determinant is the radius of the airway.
- *Respiratory failure:* an abnormality of gas exchange with either an excess of carbon dioxide or a deficit of oxygen, or both.
- *Perfusion:* the passage of a fluid through the vessels of a specific organ. **Perfusion of blood through the pulmonary vessels is an essential function of respiration. The other two essential functions are ventilation and diffusion of gases.**
- *Shunting:* turning aside or diverting. **Intrapulmonary shunting is the diverting of blood so that it does not take part in the gas exchange at the alveolar sites.** When intrapulmonary shunting occurs, blood enters the left side of the heart without being oxygenated. It is, therefore, a possible cause of hypoxemia.
- *Surfactant:* a complex lipoprotein produced by cells lining the alveoli and essential to ventilatory func-tion. Its primary purpose is to lower surface tension within the alveoli. It prevents collapse of the lung by stabilizing the alveoli and decreasing capillary pressures.
- *Ventilation:* the movement of air from the external environment to the gas exchange units of the lung. It can be spontaneous or done by a mechanical ventilator.

DIAGNOSTIC TESTS AND PROCEDURES AND NURSING IMPLICATIONS

A complete blood cell (CBC) count with hemoglo-bin and hematocrit determinations is done to detect any deficiency in oxygen-carrying capacity of the blood. Pulmonary function tests (PFTs) are useful in screening gross abnormalities in the respiratory sys-tem. Table 16-2 lists the specific tests for respiratory problems.

TABLE 16-2 ◆ *Diagnostic Tests for Respiratory Problems*

Test	Purpose	Description	Nursing Implications
Chest radiograph (x-ray)	To determine pathological condi-tions in the lungs, such as pneumonia, lung abscess, tu-berculosis, atelectasis, pneumo-thorax, and tumor. Also gives indication of heart size.	Front, back, and lateral views are taken; fluoroscopy may be used to visualize lung and diaphragm movement. Tomo-grams, which give enhanced pictures of "slices" of lung tissue, may be done; tomo-grams better define location and size of known lesions in the lung. More sophisticated tomograms can be obtained by CT.	Tell patient he will need to re-move his clothes down to the waist and put on an x-ray gown so that it ties in back. Will be asked to take a deep breath and hold it while the radiograph is taken. Radio-graphs take 15 to 45 minutes.
Bronchogram (rarely used)	Visual anatomy of the bronchial tree; evaluate presence and severity of bronchiectasis.	Chest radiographs are taken after bronchial instillation of a radio-paque dye. A topical anesthetic is used. The patient is placed in various positions to coat the bronchial tree with the dye.	Requires a consent form. NPO for 6 to 8 h before test. Assess for iodine allergy. Pro-vide good oral hygiene before test to decrease bacteria. A sedative and atropine are ad-ministered 1 h beforehand. Pharynx and trachea will be sprayed with topial anesthetic. Catheter is introduced via the nose into the trachea, and contrast dye is administered. Postprocedure nebulization treatment may be given, fol-lowed by postural drainage to drain the dye. Check gag reflex before giving anything by mouth.

(Table 16-2 continued)

TABLE 16-2 ◆ *Diagnostic Tests for Respiratory Problems* (*Continued*)

Test	Purpose	Description	Nursing Implications
Lung ventilation and perfusion scan (V-Q scan)	To assess lung ventilation and lung perfusion; to locate pulmonary embolism and diagnose tumor, emphysema, bronchiectasis, or fibrosis.	*Perfusion scan:* An IV injection of radioactive dye is given. Decreased blood flow to any part of the lung is shown by decreased radioactivity in that area. *Ventilation scan:* Radioactive gas is inhaled and, when scanned, presents a pattern of ventilation in the lungs.	Assess for allergy to iodine. Ask patient to remove all metal jewelry from around the neck. Assure him that amount of radioactivity used is very small and is not harmful. Either iodine- or technetium-based dye is used. An IV access will be inserted. Patient will be asked to hold breath for a short period for the ventilation scan. Images are viewed by use of a scintillation scanner.
Pulmonary angiography	To visualize pulmonary vasculature; to locate pulmonary embolus or other abnormality.	Radiopaque dye is injected via a catheter into the right side of the heart or the pulmonary artery. Radiographs are taken; fluoroscopy is used.	Check consent form. Assess for allergy to dye. Explain that patient may feel warm flush as dye is injected. Posttest: monitor vital signs and check pressure dressing for signs of hemorrhage.
Bronchoscopy	To inspect bronchi; to remove foreign objects or mucus plugs; to biopsy lesions.	Preoperative sedation (benzodiazepene) is usually given. Throat is sprayed with local anesthetic. With neck hyperextended, a flexible fiberoptic bronchoscope is guided into bronchi; biopsies are taken if needed. Oxygen is administered; a patent IV line is necessary in case emergency drugs are needed.	NPO for 6 h prior to test. Check consent form; administer preoperative sedative. Give mouth care just before test. Posttest: monitor vital signs and for bleeding, dyspnea, and swelling of face and neck; sputum will be slightly blood-tinged at first. Position patient on side until gag reflex has returned. Check for return of gag reflex by having patient take small sips of water. When gag reflex has returned, throat lozenges may be used for sore throat.
Pulmonary function tests (PFTs)	To determine integrity of mechanical function and gas exchange function of the lungs: volume of air lung can hold, rate of flow of air in and out of the lung, and the elasticity, or compliance, of the lung.	Patient breathes in as much air as possible and then breathes out as much air as possible into a spirometer indicating the forced vital capacity (FVC); Forced expiratory volume in 1 second (FEV_1) is measured. Other measurements include total lung capacity (TLC), vital capacity (VC), tidal volume (TV), functional residual capacity (FRC), and residual volume (RV).	Should not be done within 1 to 2 h of eating; explain procedure to patient. Posttest: monitor vital signs and allow patient to rest, as test can be fatiguing.
Arterial blood gas analysis (ABGs)	To determine if there is adequate exchange of carbon dioxide and oxygen across the alveolar membrane; to determine acid–base balance within the body; to determine hypoxemia.	Useful for patients with respiratory disorders, problems of circulation and of blood distribution, body fluid imbalances, and acid-base imbalances. Arterial blood sample is drawn and tested for pH, Pao_2, $Paco_2$, and HCO_3.	Explain procedure to patient; arterial puncture is briefly painful. Apply firm pressure for 5 to 10 minutes after specimen is drawn. Compare lab results to normals: pH: 7.35–7.45 Pao_2: 80–100 mm Hg $Paco_2$: 35-45 mm Hg HCO_3: 22–26 mm Hg

TABLE 16-2 ◆ *Diagnostic Tests for Respiratory Problems (Continued)*

Test	Purpose	Description	Nursing Implications
Sputum analysis	To examine sputum from lower respiratory tract for bacteria, bacilli, or malignant cells; to determine color, consistency, and sensitivity of bacteria to specific antibiotics.	Sputum specimen is examined and cultured for bacteria; acid–fast stain and Gram stains are done for tuberculosis bacillus; cytological studies may be done to search for malignant cells. If bacteria are present, sensitivity studies to antibiotics are performed.	Explain that specimen is desired from lower areas of lungs; may require respiratory therapy to obtain proper specimen or coaching in proper coughing technique. Best specimen is obtained in A.M. before eating or mouth care. Provide mouth care after obtaining specimen. Specimen is expectorated into sterile container.
Oximetry (O_2 sat)	To noninvasively monitor arterial oxygen saturation (Sao_2). To allow comparison of oxygenated hemoglobin to total hemoglobin.	Device attaches to earlobe, pinna of ear, or fingertip. Sensor warms skin, increasing capillary blood flow. Light beam is used to obtain reading, which is displayed by number on oximeter monitor.	Explain equipment to the patient. Keep sensor intact on patient. Monitor Sao_2 readings and record. Report readings persistently below 95% to physician.
Thoracentesis	To remove pleural fluid, instill medication or obtain fluid for diagnostic studies.	With local anesthetic, a large-bore needle is inserted through the chest wall into the pleural space, and fluid is withdrawn with a large-bore syringe. Aseptic technique must be used. Specimens are obtained for culture, microscopic examination, and stains. Medication may be instilled. Usually done at the bedside (Figure 16-2).	Explain procedure to patient. Take baseline vital signs. Position patient sitting, facing side of bed, and leaning over the overbed table with arms crossed on it; pillows or the back of a chair can also be used. Monitor respirations and skin color during procedure. Assist patient to remain still. Chest radiograph may be ordered after procedure. Monitor vital signs q 15 min for 1 h or until stable, then routinely. Auscultate breath sounds frequently. Rapid breathing, cyanosis, changes in breath sounds, and tachycardia should be reported immediately. Chart amount and appearance of fluid and condition of patient.

Figure 16-3 compares a normal spirogram with one of a patient with an airway obstruction. The *forced vital capacity* (FVC) is affected by diseases that restrict lung motion. *Forced expiratory volume in 1 second (FEV$_1$)* gives some estimate of the amount of *obstruction* to the patient's airflow. The FEV$_1$ is lower in obstructive pulmonary diseases such as emphysema and chronic bronchitis.

The results of spirometry tests often are recorded in the following terms:

- *Total lung capacity (TLC):* the volume of gas the lung can hold at the end of a maximal inspiration.

- *Vital capacity (VC):* the volume (amount of gas) that a person can exhale after inhaling as much air as he can (maximal inspiration).

- *Tidal volume (TV):* the volume of gas either inspired or exhaled during each breath.

- *Functional residual capacity (FRC):* the volume of gas remaining in the lungs when the lungs and chest

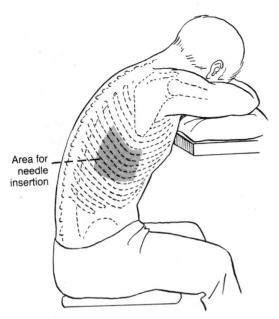

Area for needle insertion

Arms are raised and crossed. Head rests on folded arms.

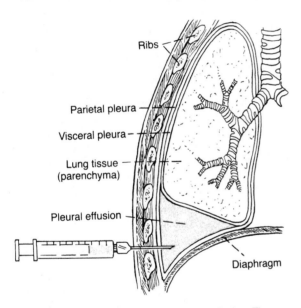

Ribs

Parietal pleura

Visceral pleura

Lung tissue (parenchyma)

Pleural effusion

Diaphragm

Site for needle insertion for a right-sided effusion. The site may vary.

FIGURE 16-2   Thoracentesis position. (*Source:* Black, J. M., Matassarin-Jacobs, E. [1993]. *Luckmann and Sorensen's Medical-Surgical Nursing: A Psychophysiologic Approach,* 4th ed. Philadelphia: Saunders, p. 938.)

wall are at resting end-expiratory position (that is, at rest at the end of a normal expiration).

◆ *Residual volume (RV):* the volume of gas remaining in the lungs after a person has exhaled as much air as he can (maximal expiration).

Figure 16-4 shows the various subdivisions of total lung capacity. Magnetic resonance imaging (MRI) is sometimes used to better define the extent of a lesion found by other diagnostic tests.

NURSING MANAGEMENT

◆ Assessment of Respiratory Status

History Taking   Information is gathered about the patient's past and current respiratory status and is used to plan systematic and goal-oriented nursing care. If the patient is in obvious respiratory distress, only a few questions about his present illness and chief complaint are asked. Later, during a formal admission interview and informal discussions with the patient and his family, more information can be obtained to plan individualized nursing care. Some of the more pertinent areas to be covered in a thorough respiratory disease history are listed in Table 16-3.

Physical Assessment   Assessment of respiratory status demands careful and frequent observation of the patient. Begin by having the patient sit up, if possible, so that the bed or back of the chair is not interfering with chest expansion. What is the rate and character of respirations? Is the patient breathing deeply or shallowly? Fast (**tachypnea**)? or slow (**bradypnea**)? Are there any signs of respiratory distress? Note whether both sides of the chest expand equally when a breath is taken. Is the patient using any accessory respiratory muscles to breath? Are there intercostal retractions? Does the patient seem restless or confused? **If so, this may indicate an oxygen deficit.**

Is the shape of the chest normal, or is it "barrel" shaped? Obstructive disorders can cause enlargement of

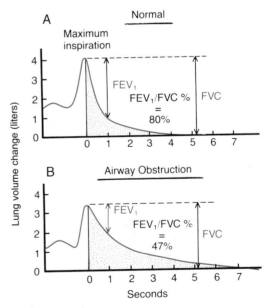

FIGURE 16-3   Normal spirogram compared to spirogram of a person with an airway obstruction. (*Source:* Guyton, A. C., Hall, J. E. [1996]. *Textbook of Medical Physiology,* 9th ed. Philadelphia: Saunders, p. 539.)

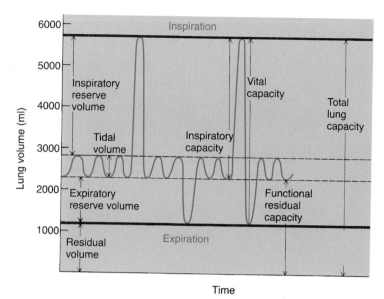

FIGURE 16-4 This diagram shows the subdivisions of total lung capacity. During normal breathing a person inhales and exhales approximately the volume of air represented by *tidal volume*. In a healthy person, a maximum inspiration and maximum expiration involve a much greater volume of air. (*Source:* Guyton, A. C., Hall, J. E. [1996]. *Textbook of Medical Physiology,* 9th ed. Philadelphia: Saunders, p. 483.)

the front-to-back (A-P) measurement of the chest wall, giving a barrel-like appearance to the chest because of the presence of trapped air in the lungs and inadequate recoil. These forces prevent the chest from returning to its original position at the end of each expiration. Over time there is a gradual elevation of the resting level of the diaphragm, which produces an increase in the size of the chest wall. Is there kyphosis or scoliosis, which may cause restriction of the thoracic cavity?

Note the posture of the patient, the amount of effort exerted to breathe, the way abdominal muscles and other accessory muscles of respiration are used, the number of words that can be said between breaths, and, of course, the rate and depth of breaths.

A patient with chronic obstructive pulmonary disease (COPD) may lean forward in a sitting position and use the abdominal muscles to force air out of the lungs. Other movements during ventilation indicating difficulty are elevating the shoulders and ribs, tensing the neck and shoulder muscles, and flaring of nostrils. Exhaling through pursed lips is another clue to obstructive disorders. A retraction of the spaces below and around the sternum also might be observed in a patient in respiratory distress. Note the number of pillows the patient uses to prop up in bed or if the head of the bed needs to be raised to facilitate breathing. Other indications of respiratory difficulty are extreme restlessness and agitation.

Note skin color as it can be significant in a respiratory assessment, but cyanosis of the skin is not a reliable indicator of hypoxemia. Cyanosis occurs late in the process of oxygen depletion and, as explained, could indicate problems of circulation or hemoglobin deficiency. **The skin of a person with emphysema can have a pinkish color in spite of the fact that there is inadequate oxygenation in the blood.** Pallor may indicate anemia, which can affect the respiratory system because inadequate oxygen may be reaching the cells of the body.

Look at the hands to see whether there is clubbing of the fingers (Figure 16-5), which is frequently seen in patients with chronic respiratory or heart disease. The fingers are wider than normal at the distal end, similar in shape to a club. There also is marked rounded curvature of the fingernails. These physical changes

TABLE 16-3 ◆ *Respiratory Assessment*	
Area	**Specifics**
Present illness: chief complaint	When started; exposure to infection; history of respiratory infections? Description of symptoms. Dyspnea? Orthopnea?
Precipitating factors	Any allergies? Sinusitis? Asthma? Emphysema? Chronic bronchitis? Exposure to dust or other irritants?
Risk factors	Smoke? Number of packs per day for how many years? Exposure to occupational air pollutants? Exposure to tuberculosis?
Cough	Type of cough? When occurs? Productive? Quantity and color of sputum? Odor and taste?
Dyspnea	Any shortness of breath? On exertion? Any wheezing? Use of accessory muscles?
Measures for symptom relief	Humidifier? Over-the-counter medicines? Antihistamines? Decongestants? Cough medicines? Bronchodilators? Other medications?

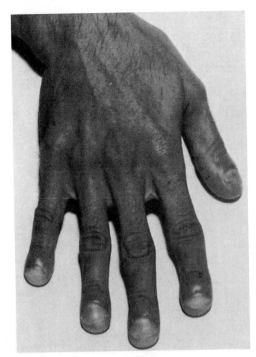
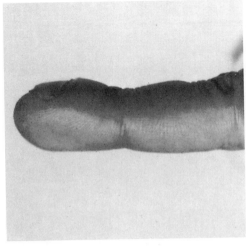

FIGURE 16-5   Clubbed fingers of patient with diffuse interstitial lung disease. (*Source:* Hinshaw, H. C., Murray, J. F. [1980]. *Disease of the Chest.* Philadelphia: Saunders.

result from inflammatory changes in the bones of the fingers.

Does the patient have a cough? Is it deep and moist sounding? or dry and hacking? What seems to set it off? How long has it been present? Is there sputum production? What is the amount, character, and color of the sputum? Is there any blood in the sputum? Is there pain, breathlessness, or dyspnea, a change in vital signs, or fatigue with coughing?

A *productive* cough is moist and deep, often accom-

panied by bronchial crackles or wheezing, and ends in producing quantities of sputum. A *nonproductive* cough is dry and harsh and no sputum is produced. **Sputum** refers to material brought up from the bronchial tree. It is not mucus from the sinuses, nasal secretions, or saliva. Table 16-4 shows various characteristics of sputum and the implications of each.

Next, auscultate the lungs. Ask the patient to remain quiet and to breathe slowly and deeply through the mouth. Turn off the radio or TV. Listen to one full breath in each location (Figure 16-6). Place the stethoscope diaphragm with moderate pressure against the skin. Move from one side of the midline of the chest to the equivalent location on the other side of the midline, comparing one side's sounds with the other. Begin above the clavicles and progress downward in the intercostal spaces to above the sixth rib. On the back, start above the scapula and progress along the sides of the spine, inside the scapular area, on down and then toward the lateral areas above the tenth thoracic vertebra. Laterally, listen in the mid-axillary line in three descending locations to just above the diaphragm. If the patient is short of breath, begin posteriorly at the bases and work upward as the patient may not be able to cooperate for the full sequence. Table 16-5 presents sounds normally heard in various locations.

Listen for abnormal sounds. Are there any wheezes? Wheezes are a whistling, musical, high-pitched sound produced by air being forced through a narrowed airway. It is common in patients with asthma. Rhonchi are coarse, low-pitched, sonorous, rattling

TABLE 16-4 ◆ *Characteristics of Sputum and Possible Causes**	
Characteristic	**Possible Cause**
Thick, tenacious, and "ropey"; difficult to cough up	Chronic bronchitis, emphysema
Scant, sticky, rust-colored	Pneumococcal pneumonia
Frothy, pinkish or blood-tinged	Pulmonary edema
Yellow, yellow-green, or grayish-yellow, with foul odor or taste	Pulmonary infection
Blood-tinged, bloody, or blood-streaked	Tuberculosis, or ulcerated pulmonary vessel, or bronchogenic carcinoma
Large amounts	Pneumonia or bronchitis
Scanty	Asthma
Very thick and viscous	Inadequate hydration

*Normal sputum is white and slighty viscous and has no odor or taste.

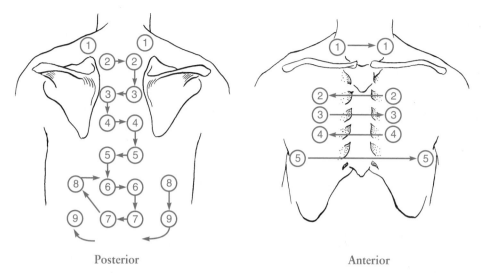

Posterior   Anterior

FIGURE 16-6   Sites for auscultation of the lungs.

sounds caused by secretions in the larger air passages. Crackles are produced by air passing through moisture in the smaller airways. Crackles are either fine or coarse. Fine crackles are high in pitch and can be heard in patients who have atelectasis, fibrosis, pneumonia, or early congestive heart failure. **Crackles sound similar to the sound produced by rubbing hairs between the fingers close to the ear.** Coarse crackles are louder and low in pitch and are heard in patients with bronchitis, pulmonary edema, and resolving pneumonia.

Stridor ("croaking" sounds) can be heard when there is partial obstruction of the upper air passages. They are typically heard in children with croup, but can also occur in adults with some kind of obstruction. The inflammation that is producing the obstruction often also affects the larynx, producing hoarseness.

Another abnormal, or **adventitious,** sound is that of a *pleural friction rub,* which is a grating or scratchy sound similar to creaking shoe leather or an opening, squeaky door, that occurs when irritated visceral and parietal pleura rub against each other.

Learning to detect abnormal breath sounds takes practice, and the only way to get that is by listening to lungs. Practice on friends and relatives and listen to each patient available. Table 16-6 presents a guide for performing physical assessment.

◆ Nursing Diagnosis

Nursing diagnoses associated with respiratory symptoms or disorders are:

- ◆ Ineffective airway clearance
- ◆ Ineffective breathing pattern
- ◆ Impaired gas exchange
- ◆ Risk for infection
- ◆ Activity intolerance related to hypoxemia
- ◆ Anxiety related to dyspnea
- ◆ Fatigue related to hypoxemia
- ◆ Altered health maintenance related to inability to stop smoking

Other diagnoses may be included in the care plan as they relate to secondary problems.

TABLE 16-5 ◆ *Normal Lung Sounds*		
Type of Sound	**Location Where Normally Heard**	**Description of Sound**
Vesicular breath sounds	Over lung tissue to level of sixth intercostal space.	Low to medium pitch with a soft whooshing quality; inspiration is two to three times the length of expiration.
Bronchovesicular breath sounds	Over the mainstem bronchi below the level of the clavicles beside the sternum; posteriorly: between the scapulae.	Moderate to high pitch with a hollow, muffled quality; equal time of inspiration and expiration.
Bronchial breath sounds	Over the trachea above the sternal notch (these sounds are abnormal elsewhere and often indicate atelectasis).	High pitch with a loud, harsh, tubular quality; inspiration half as long as expiration.

TABLE 16-6 ◆ *Guide to Physical Assessment of the Lower Respiratory System*

Observe for
- Skin color
- Posture: need to be upright or to lean forward
- Shape of chest
- Use of accessory muscles for respirations: intercostal retractions
- Shape of fingers
- Rate of respiration, depth, rhythm
- Character of respiration: how deep are the breaths?
- Restlessness or agitation
- Symmetrical chest expansion
- Cough: frequency, characteristics
- Sputum: amount, character, color, presence of blood

Auscultate
- Systematic pattern of auscultation
- Listen for abnormal breath sounds or absence of breath sounds
- Any wheezes?
- Any crackles?
- Any rhonchi?
- Any "rubs"?
- Do abnormal sounds clear when patient coughs?

◆ Planning

The goals for the patient with a respiratory disorder are to:

- Promote oxygenation
- Prevent infection
- Prevent further lung damage
- Promote rehabilitation

Specific *expected outcomes* are individualized for each patient.

◆ Implementation

Examples of interventions and teaching necessary for the patient with respiratory disorders are presented in Table 16-7. Interventions also are listed in the Clinical Pathway and Nursing Care Plan presented in this chapter. Interventions are discussed in the sections on Common Care Problems, with the specific disorders, and in the section Therapeutic Measures. Working with patients who have dyspnea requires that the nurse plan extra time to accomplish treatments and care. A patient who is hypoxic moves more slowly, takes more time to answer questions, and has less energy. Rest periods between treatments or activities of daily living (ADLs) are often necessary. Teaching is a major part of nursing care for the respiratory patient.

◆ Evaluation

Effectiveness of interventions and treatment of the patient with a respiratory disorder is based on improving breathing pattern, arterial blood gases values, and lung sounds. Decreases in coughing, sputum production, wheezing, and signs of infection are other parameters that indicate improvements. Lessened dyspnea, more energy and ability to perform more of own self-care, and other activities indicate that interventions are effective.

COMMON RESPIRATORY PATIENT CARE PROBLEMS

◆ Ineffective Airway Clearance

A cough usually is a reflex triggered by a foreign substance or some other irritant in the respiratory tract. Coughing can be beneficial if it is effective in clearing the air passages and removing accumulations of stagnant mucus. It can be harmful if done excessively, because it can exhaust the patient and traumatize the respiratory tissues and thoracic structures. A chronic cough can greatly limit one's activities, even eating, because the person hesitates to do anything that might trigger a bout of severe coughing.

Effective coughing techniques usually must be taught to the patient. The nurse should explain that deep-breathing and coughing maneuvers are the most effective ways to remove sputum. Table 16-8 presents teaching guidelines for effective deep-breathing and coughing.

Cough medicines are administered either to assist with thinning the sputum so that it can be coughed up and expectorated or to suppress the cough. **Antitussive** agents inhibit the cough reflex in the cough center in the brain. Many sedative cough mixtures contain codeine or other drugs that decrease the desire to cough. The liquefying agents and diluents discussed later in this chapter are examples of expectorants.

Cough syrups are given to soothe the nerve endings in the upper respiratory mucosa. These medications are given in small doses to coat and protect the throat. **Water should not be taken immediately after a cough syrup.**

In bacterial infections and chronic respiratory diseases, the sputum often is foul smelling, leaving a bad taste in the mouth and offensive breath odor. Frequent oral hygiene is important for patients with this problem. Mouth care is especially needed before meals, when the taste or odor of the sputum may adversely affect appetite. **Frequent mouth care also helps remove pathogenic microorganisms from the oral cavity and thereby**

TABLE 16-7 ◆ *Common Nursing Diagnoses, Expected Outcomes, and Nursing Interventions for Patients with Lower Respiratory Disorders*

Nursing Diagnosis	Goals/Expected Outcomes	Nursing Interventions
Impaired gas exchange related to decreased airflow and respiratory muscle fatigue.	Patient will utilize modified breathing techniques to facilitate ventilation. Patient will display increased ability to tolerate nonstrenuous activity by walking short distances without breathlessness.	Instruct in techniques of pursed-lip, diaphragmatic breathing, deep breathing, and effective coughing; teach relaxation techniques. Review medication dosages and schedule with patient and proper technique for use of measured dose inhaler; assess effectiveness and compliance. Encourage use of incentive spirometer. Begin stepped exercise program to improve muscle function and promote efficient oxygen use by muscles. Help formulate plan for pacing activities of daily living. Assess sputum and obtain culture for infective organism if need indicated.
Ineffective airway clearance related to viscous sputum.	Thinner mucus that is easier to cough up. Fluid intake will increase to 2,000 mL/day. Patient will demonstrate proper use of nebulizer.	Explain effect of inadequate fluid intake on liquidity of mucus; assess what fluids patient likes, advise to drink 8 oz. of fluid every hour while awake, suggest use of room humidifier at home; review technique for using nebulizer and mucolytic agents. Obtain peak flow readings before and after nebulizer treatment.
Risk for respiratory infection related to compromised respiratory system and decreased resistance.	Patient will have no more than one respiratory infection per year.	Review ways to decrease contact with respiratory infectious organisms: avoiding those with colds, flu, and other infections; frequent hand washing. Teach to avoid respiratory irritants; stay in house when air pollution index is high; avoid smoke, dust, and cold air. Observe sputum for changes in color, consistency, odor, and amount; call clinic promptly if signs of infection occur. Give influenza and Pneumovax vaccines. Encourage to maintain adequate nutrition.
Disturbance in self-concept related to inability to do much of anything	Patient will express improvement in self-concept within 3 months. Patient will be able to resume favorite hobby within 3 months.	Allow to verbalize concerns; assist to focus on activities possible; explore ways of continuing favorite activities using modifications. Give encouragement and praise for efforts in stepped exercise program.
Activity intolerance related to dyspnea.	Patient will be able to perform bathing and dressing without dyspnea within 3 months. Patient will participate and comply with stepped exercise program.	Encourage use of pursed-lip and diaphragmatic breathing Begin stepped exercise program as soon as acute respiratory infection has resolved. Alternate activity with rest periods, beginning with small increments of activity. Utilize oxygen as prescribed at 2–3 L/min during acute episodes of dyspnea.
Anxiety related to hypoxia and dyspnea.	Patient will verbalize that anxiety has lessened within a week.	Allow to verbalize concerns within ability to speak without becoming dyspneic. Encourage use of pursed-lip and diaphragmatic breathing to decrease dyspnea. Teach best positions to decrease dyspnea. Teach relaxation techniques; encourage practice. Interact with calm, reassuring manner.
Altered health maintenance related to continued smoking.	Patient will look at alternative ways to quit smoking within a week. Patient will begin a stop smoking program within three weeks.	Explain the harmful effects of continued smoking. Motivate patient to quit smoking by emphasizing benefits of increased stamina and decreased dyspnea if smoking is halted. Introduce to various methods and programs for quitting smoking. Introduce to people with equivalent lung disease who have quit smoking. Praise any effort at decreasing or quitting smoking.

TABLE 16-8 ◆ *Patient Education: Guidelines for Effective Deep-Breathing and Coughing*

Instruct to deep-breathe
- Clear the nasal passages.
- Sit with the feet spread about shoulder-width apart.
- Lean forward with the hands or elbows on the knees and the arms and hands completely relaxed.
- Take a deep breath, allowing the diaphragm to drop as you inhale; feel the abdomen expand. Exhale slowly.
- Continue to take several slow, deep breaths.

Instruct to cough effectively
- Position tissues or a basin for expectoration.
- While in a sitting position with the feet supported, deep-breathe several times.
- Bend the head forward, and slightly hunch the shoulder forward.
- Take in a deep breath, and slowly exhale coughing three times in succession with exhalation. (The first cough mobilizes secretions and the next two bring secretions up to be expectorated.)
- Repeat process if secretions are still audible in lungs.
- Rest in between attempts at coughing.

For the patient who will not effectively cough
- After deep-breathing, encourage to take a deep breath through the nose and then forcibly exhale through the mouth. Repeat the process producing "huffs" that move secretions upward until they can be expectorated.

diminishes the possibility that they will be aspirated deep into the air passages.

Mechanical suctioning of excessive amounts of secretions in the respiratory passages is indicated when the patient cannot clear her airway. Removing secretions from the nose, mouth, and throat (nasopharyngeal suctioning) is a relatively safe and simple procedure. Deep tracheal suctioning, whether through the nose, mouth, or endotracheal tube, however, should only be performed using strict aseptic technique by someone experienced in the correct procedure.

The need for suctioning should be determined on an individual basis when suctioning is ordered PRN. Some patients may require suctioning only once or twice daily to remove deeply situated pools and plugs of mucus that cannot be brought up by coughing. Others require suctioning every 10 to 15 minutes to clear their air passages. It should be remembered that the purpose of suctioning is to facilitate breathing and to allow for an adequate exchange of carbon dioxide and oxygen in the lungs. Even though the procedure may be necessary, the suctioning process removes oxygen, which is the very substance the patient needs to relieve his distress.

Some basic guidelines should be helpful to the nurse in avoiding the serious consequences of removing oxygen by suctioning:

- Select the proper-size suction catheter; preoxygenate the patient before suctioning by (1) using a ball-valve bag attached to 100% oxygen for 2 minutes or the setting on the ventilator that will briefly hyperoxygenate the patient. Repeat this procedure after suctioning and between repeated sessions of suctioning.
- Suction no longer than 10 to 15 seconds; counting silently while suction is applied is one way to avoid suctioning too long.
- The suction gauge pressure should be between 80 and 100 mm Hg when the tubing is unoccluded; no higher pressure should be used.
- If tachycardia or bradycardia develops during suctioning, stop and hyperoxygenate unless the airway is badly occluded by secretions.

See Nursing Procedure 16-1 on how to suction a tracheostomy.

◆ Ineffective Breathing Patterns

Dyspnea or Breathlessness   The patient who must struggle for breath or feels that she is smothering suffers from mental anxiety as well as physical stress. Unfortunately, the mental anxiety can only aggravate the situation and increase the distress.

> Nursing actions that can help relieve dyspnea and its consequences include proper positioning so that the respiratory passages are able to function as best they can, administering oxygen as prescribed by the physician, and assuring the patient that everything possible is being done to bring relief.

The position that best facilitates breathing is the high Fowler's position. Proper positioning and support allow the respiratory muscles to function at maximum efficiency.

For severe dyspnea, the orthopneic position is most effective. The term *orthopnea* means the ability to breathe only in the upright position (Figure 16-7). The patient should sit upright, lean over the overbed table, which is padded with pillows, and elevate and round the shoulders to allow maximum expansion of the lungs.

Another factor to be considered in caring for the dyspneic patient is that of pressure from organs below or near the lungs and diaphragm. A full stomach can contribute to dyspnea by limiting the amount of space available for expansion of the lungs. For this reason, **small, frequent feedings are preferred to three large meals a day.** Abdominal distention due to a collection of flatus and fecal material also can make breathing more difficult. Pursed-lip and diaphragmatic breathing may lessen dyspnea.

Nursing Procedure 16-1

Tracheostomy and Endotracheal Suctioning: It is difficult for a patient with an endotracheal tube to cough out secretions. For this reason, suctioning is needed periodically to clear the airway. Many patients with tracheostomy tubes can learn to cough out secretions, but others cannot. The tracheostomy tube must be kept free of secretions for the patient to receive oxygen. **Endotracheal or tracheostomy suctioning are sterile procedures.**

To perform endotracheal or tracheostomy suctioning, the nurse first identifies the patient, washes the hands, explains what is to be done to the patient, provides privacy, arranges needed supplies, and dons goggles to protect the eyes from secretions before beginning the following steps.

Supplies needed
- ◆ Sterile disposable suction catheter
- ◆ Sterile solution container
- ◆ Sterile normal saline
- ◆ Suction source
- ◆ Sterile gloves
- ◆ Connecting tubing
- ◆ Manual resuscitation bag

Steps	Rationale
1. Connect tubing to suction source, turn on suction, and check the pressure setting.	Verify that suction is functioning by occluding end of suction tubing and watching pressure on gauge rise. Set pressure according to agency protocol. Wall suction unit pressure is generally set at 80–120 mm Hg.
2. Open supplies and don sterile gloves. With gloved dominant hand, attach the catheter to the connecting tubing. The hand holding the connecting tubing is no longer sterile.	Supplies catheter with suction.
3. Have an asistant oxygenate using the manual resuscitation bag attached to the oxygen source with 2 to 3 large volume inspirations. Or use the setting on the ventilator that delivers short-term 100% oxygen. Check agency protocol for desired way to preoxygenate the patient.	Preoxygenation prevents hypoxia during suctioning.
4. Moisten the catheter tip in the sterile saline solution, disconnect the ventilator tubing if ventilator is in use. Immediately introduce the catheter into the endotracheal tube or tracheostomy tube using only sterile gloved hand: **do not use suction while placing the catheter** (Figure P16-1).	Moisture lubricates the catheter and makes it easier to introduce. Suction would only draw out oxygen. Holding the catheter at a 90-degree angle to the tube to enter it helps prevent contaminating the catheter by touching the patient's face or neck. Standing slightly to the side of the patient will prevent getting splattered by any coughed-out secretions during the suctioning process.

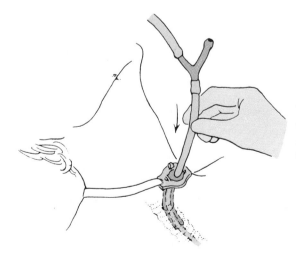

FIGURE P16-1   Inserting the suction catheter into the tracheostomy tube. (*Source:* deWit, S. C. [1994]. *Rambo's Nursing Skills for Clinical Practice,* 4th ed. Philadelphia: Saunders, p. 1052.)

Continued on following page

Nursing Procedure 16-1 *(Continued)*

Steps	Rationale
5. Push the catheter quickly into the tube until resistance is reached (6–10 inches); pull back slightly at this point. Apply suction as you withdraw the catheter for 5 to 10 sec. Rotating the catheter between your fingers helps catch secretions around the circumference of the trachea and tube (Figure P16-2). The patient may cough; offer reassurance.	Counting silently to 10 slowly while applying suction ensures that you do not suction too long. Rotating the catheter turns the eye openings to another part of the trachea or tube. Placing the thumb over the suction valve opening provides suction. The distance the catheter should be introduced depends on whether you are suctioning an endotracheal tube or a tracheostomy tube. The distance will be less for a tracheostomy tube.

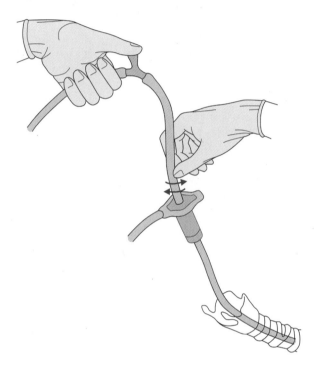

FIGURE P16-2   Twisting the suction catheter while applying suction. (*Source:* deWit, S. C. [1994]. *Rambo's Nursing Skills for Clinical Practice,* 4th ed. Philadelphia: Saunders, p. 1052.)

Steps	Rationale
6. Reattach the patient's tube to the oxygen source and allow a rest period before suctioning again. Keep the catheter sterile while waiting; use the nonsterile hand to reattach the oxygen source. Auscultate the lungs when finished to be certain that secretions have been adequately cleared.	Suctioning draws out oxygen as well as secretions and may cause hypoxia. Hyperoxygenation should be done again before each suctioning as in Step 3.
7. Suction the nasopharynx if needed.	Secretions may collect above the cuffed tracheostomy tube and need to be removed.
8. Discard the catheter by holding it in your gloved hand and pulling the glove off over it. Discard it according to *standard precautions.*	A sterile catheter must be used each time tracheobronchial suctioning is performed. Sterile catheters must be kept at the bedside for immediate use.
9. Rinse the connecting suction tubing.	Prevents occlusion by secretions.

Suctioning with a sleeved catheter

Steps	Rationale
1. Open catheter package without disturbing protective sleeve covering the catheter.	Sleeve maintains sterility of catheter so that it can be reused several times.
2. Attach catheter to suction tubing. Slide sleeve back and lubricate catheter with sterile normal saline.	Lubrication with sterile saline makes inserting the catheter into the trachea easier.
3. As catheter is inserted via endotracheal tube or tracheostomy, slide the sleeve back, and advance the catheter as far as possible.	Positions the catheter into the trachea and bronchus for suctioning.

Nursing Procedure 16-1 *(Continued)*

Steps	Rationale
4. Apply suction while rotating and withdrawing the catheter; allow the sleeve to recover the catheter as it is withdrawn.	The sleeve will prevent the catheter from becoming contaminated from outside the trachea.
5. Rinse the connecting tubing with sterile normal saline when finished. Auscultate lungs when finished to be certain that secretions have been cleared sufficiently.	Clears the connecting tubing.
6. Empty or replace the suction container at the end of each shift using *standard precautions.*	Disposes of contaminated secretions.

7. Chart the procedure.	**Documentation example:**
	    2:30 P.M.: coughing, gurgling sounds auscultated. Suctioned twice with sterile technique and preoxygenation. Moderate white secretions obtained; lungs clear; reattached to ventilator; no signs of dysrhythmia._____
	                                 Nurse's Signature

Respiratory Failure Hyperventilation and hypoventilation were discussed in Chapter 5, as was the effect of either of these abnormal breathing patterns on the acid–base balance of body fluids. **Hypercapnia** (also called *hypercarbia*) is the retention of excessive amounts of carbon dioxide. It is the result of hypoventilation, during which the usual amount of carbon dioxide is not eliminated by exhalation.

Carbon dioxide is a respiratory stimulant; hence the body responds to excessive levels of carbon dioxide by increasing the rate of respirations in an effort to "blow off" larger quantities of the gas. If, however, the respiratory centers in the brain are exposed to higher-than-normal levels of carbon dioxide over a long time, they cease to react and a drop in the respiratory rate occurs. The patient then becomes mentally confused, her senses become less acute, and eventually she may fall into a coma. **The heart rate increases to meet the tissues' need for more oxygen. Mental confusion and an increase in pulse and heart rate are indicators of inadequate oxygenation of the blood and tissues.** If the slowing down of respiration is not corrected, the accumulation of carbon dioxide continues, and a vicious cycle begins. The final outcome can be cardiac arrest from respiratory acidosis—a result of respiratory failure.

Respiratory failure is defined by arterial blood gases. It has occurred when the paO_2 is below 50 mm Hg and *the pCO_2 is over 50 mm Hg.*

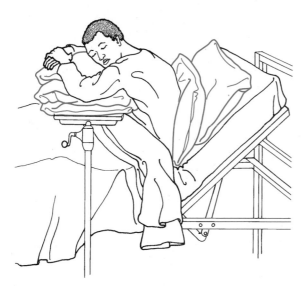

Pillows are used to support the back.

Other pillows are placed on an overbed table to support the weight of the arms, shoulders, and head.

FIGURE 16-7   Orthopneic position.

Blood gas analysis is the best way to determine whether respiratory acidosis is either threatening or already present. Results of the analysis will show a high level of $PaCO_2$, high bicarbonate (HCO_3) level, and a low pH (acidosis) if the condition has been present for several days.

Respiratory Acidosis and Respiratory Alkalosis

Hypocapnia, which is a deficit of carbon dioxide, occurs as a result of hyperventilation and eventually produces respiratory alkalosis. Conditions associated with hypocapnia include (1) those in which there is an increased metabolic rate, such as thyrotoxicosis, persistent fever, and hysteria; (2) salicylate overdosage; and (3) improper use of mechanical ventilation.

Clinical signs of respiratory alkalosis include hyperactive neuromuscular reflexes, tetany, vertigo, blurred vision, and diaphoresis. Blood gas analysis will show a low $PaCO_2$ and a high pH (alkalinity).

Other abnormal respiratory patterns are as follows:

* *Biot's respiration:* respiration that is characterized by irregular periods of apnea alternating with periods in which four or five breaths of identical depth are taken. A respiratory pattern of this kind is seen in patients with increased intracranial pressure.
* *Cheyne-Stokes respiration:* breathing characterized by rhythmic waxing and waning of the depth of respiration, with regularly recurring periods of apnea. This kind of respiration is often seen in patients in coma resulting from a disorder affecting the central nervous system.
* *Kussmaul's respirations* (also called *air hunger*): respiration characterized by a distressing difficulty in breathing that occurs spasmodically at irregular intervals. This abnormal breathing pattern is often seen in patients with diabetic acidosis and coma.
* *Apneustic respiration:* prolonged gasping inhalation, followed by short, ineffective exhalation. The pattern is indicative of damage to the respiratory centers in the brain.

Think about... Can you name four nursing interventions that can ease breathing for your patient suffering from dyspnea?

♦ Risk of Infection

Many acute upper respiratory infections are transmitted by droplet infection; that is, the causative organisms are expelled along with the liquid secretions released during coughing and sneezing. Cores of the droplets expelled from the nose or mouth continue to float in the air after the liquid evaporates. These cores are called *droplet nuclei,* and they are teeming with bacteria or viruses when an infection is present.

The patient with a chronic respiratory disorder and the nurse should carefully avoid contamination. Staying out of crowded places where people are coughing and sneezing is advised. Washing the hands frequently, particularly after being out in public places and touching items that are likely to be contaminated, decreases the likelihood of infection. Keeping the hands away from the face and mouth also decreases risk. Patients and family members should be instructed in the proper ways of handling and disposing of secretions. Standing to the side of a person who is coughing and sneezing reduces contamination. **After each contact with a person with a respiratory disorder that produces airborne or droplet secretions or with articles contaminated by secretions the hands should be washed thoroughly.**

Most people are not offended by tactfully being told to place a folded tissue over the nose and mouth while sneezing and to turn the head away whenever they are in close contact with another. Tissues should be disposed of following *standard precautions,* that is, placed in a plastic or waxed paper bag that is sealed before disposal. Gloves should be used when handling used tissues.

♦ Alterations in Nutrition and Hydration

Anorexia and inadequate nutrition are not uncommon in patients with respiratory disorders, particularly when the disorder is chronic in nature.

Reasons for this are that (1) the senses of taste and smell may be impaired by nasal congestion; (2) the patient might be afraid that chewing and swallowing will bring on an attack of coughing; (3) purulent sputum leaves a bad taste in the mouth and can cause nausea; and (4) fatigue can deprive the patient of the will to expend the energy needed to feed himself.

Nursing intervention to help overcome the problem of loss of appetite and poor nutrition should start with the environment in which the patient eats meals. The room should be kept clean, uncluttered, and orderly. Used tissues are disposed of promptly, and sputum cups are kept covered and out of sight.

Frequent oral hygiene and mouth care before meals can help diminish mouth odor and nausea and improve taste. Smaller, more frequent feedings of nutritious liquids and foods are preferable to three large, heavy meals.

Because there is an increased energy expenditure when breathing is difficult, many patients have difficulty maintaining weight even when they do take in normal amounts of calories. Supplements are now available that have an increased fat content and provide more calories in smaller quantities than can be accomplished with carbohydrate substances. Pulmocare is one such supplement. **When a patient is receiving mechanical ventilation her caloric needs rise considerably.** Sometimes total parenteral nutrition (TPN) or lipid infusions are necessary to prevent malnutrition in a patient with severe chronic airflow limitation (CAL).

A fluid deficit is likely in patients with respiratory disorders because there is an increased loss of fluid in respiratory secretions. The patient usually breathes through the mouth and exhales large amounts of moisture from the body. Without adequate replacement of these fluids, the patient becomes dehydrated very quickly. Unless contraindicated, an intake of at least 3,000 mL of liquid should occur each day. This may include low-sodium bouillon, fruit juices, and other liquids in addition to water.

Humidifying the air breathed by the patient is an effective way to minimize dehydration and liquefy secretions in the air passages. It is especially important to the patient whose secretions are thick and tenacious and difficult to cough up. Humidification of inhaled air is covered under Common Therapeutic Measures later in this chapter.

◆ Fatigue

Hypoxia, which is an oxygen deficit in the tissues, produces a loss of energy because it causes a disturbance in cellular metabolism. Patients with respiratory disorders often have hypoxia and, to make matters worse, must use the little energy they have to struggle for breath and cough up secretions.

Patients with respiratory disorders, whether acute or chronic, have some degree of intolerance to physical activity and therefore need periods of rest throughout the day. Treatments and medications should be scheduled so that the patient can rest without interruption. As with any inflammation, repair of damaged tissue is facilitated resting the affected part. To rest the lungs, the patient should lie down for short periods. Long naps during the day are not recommended, because they interfere with a restful sleep at night. Although rest is needed, the dangers of physical inactivity and the disabilities that can result cannot be ignored. The goal of nursing care, therefore, should be to achieve a satisfactory balance of rest and activity.

Deep-breathing exercises and coughing techniques should be planned whenever the patient is able to do them with or without some assistance. These activities should be followed by good mouth care and a short period of uninterrupted rest. The problem of fatigue in the patient with chronic lung disease is covered later in this chapter.

DISORDERS OF THE LOWER RESPIRATORY SYSTEM

◆ Acute Respiratory Disease

Acute Bronchitis   Acute bronchitis frequently is an extension of an upper respiratory infection involving the trachea (tracheobronchitis) and usually is viral in origin. Causes other than infectious agents are physical and chemical agents inhaled in air polluted by dust, automobile exhaust, industrial fumes, and tobacco smoke.

Acute bronchitis is most often encountered in small children and the elderly and debilitated. It is particularly dangerous in the very young, because their bronchi are smaller and more easily obstructed.

Symptoms and Medical Diagnosis. Early symptoms of acute bronchitis are similar to those of the common cold. In acute bronchitis the symptoms progress to chest pain, fever, and a dry, hacking, and irritating cough. Later the cough becomes more productive of mucopurulent to purulent sputum. The fever may be moderate and accompanied by chills, muscle soreness, and headache. The physician relies on history and signs and symptoms for diagnosis.

Treatment. Acute bronchitis is treated conservatively; antibiotics are used only as indicated by sputum that contains specific organisms. Symptomatic treatment includes the use of humidification using either warm or cool moist air, cough mixtures and aerosols to reduce coughing and soothe the irritated tracheal and bronchial mucosa, and bedrest to promote healing. Nutrition and fluid balance should be maintained. A period of rest is recommended to avoid progression of an acute condition to a chronic one.

Influenza   Influenza is an acute, highly infectious disease of the respiratory tract and is caused by any of three major types (A, B, and C) and numerous subtypes of viruses. It occurs as isolated cases or in epidemics. The most virulent form is type A, which usually affects young adults first and then spreads to the very young and very old in the community.

Influenza is spread by direct and indirect contact with infected persons by coughing and sneezing and by sharing items such as drinking and eating utensils or towels.

Diagnosis. The first symptoms of influenza appear 2 to 3 days after exposure. They come on rather suddenly and include dry, hacking cough, headache, fever, chills, muscle aches, sore throat, fever blisters, and red and watery eyes.

Chest radiograph and auscultation usually show no abnormality. The white cell count is normal or slightly below normal. Diagnosis is based on clinical findings, as there is no specific laboratory test for influenza.

Treatment. Uncomplicated influenza usually is managed more effectively by nursing intervention than by drugs or other forms of medical treatment. Antibiotics are given only if there is evidence of bacterial infection secondary to the viral infection.

If a person is known to be at high risk for influenza and has been exposed to type A influenza, the physician may choose to provide prophylaxis with an antiviral agent such as amantadine hydrochloride (Symmetrel) or rimantadine (Flumadine). Prevention of influenza was discussed under Prevention of Respiratory Diseases.

Nursing interventions for patients with these kinds of problems might include the following:

- Administer suppressant cough medicine at bedtime and during the night as prescribed.
- Mouth care at least every 4 hours, before each meal, and more frequently if patient reports bad taste in mouth or has halitosis from sputum.
- Cater to patient's food and drink preferences within limits of dietary restrictions.
- Schedule procedures and medications to allow periods of uninterrupted rest.
- Give antipyretics and perform sponge bath and other measures to reduce fever.
- Increase oral intake to at least 3,000 mL per 24 hours.
- Humidify inhaled air.
- Splint chest and abdomen with pillow during coughing attacks.
- Administer cough medicine and analgesics promptly.
- Encourage patient to take analgesics when discomfort first appears.
- Apply emollient to lips and nares as needed.
- Clear nostrils as much as possible to prevent mouth-breathing.

Pneumonia   Pneumonia is an extensive inflammation of the lung with either consolidation of the lung tissue as it fills with exudate or interstitial inflammation and edema. It can affect one or both lungs or only one lobe of a lung (lobar pneumonia). There are two general types of *infectious* pneumonia: typical, or bacterial, pneumonia, and *atypical* pneumonia, which can be viral or due to *Mycoplasma pneumoniae*. Bacterial pneumonia usually produces exudate leading to consolidation. It most commonly affects only one lung. Viral pneumonia does not produce exudate; it causes interstitial inflammation. The most common causative organism of bacterial pneumonia is *Streptococcus pneumoniae*, which also is called *pneumococcus*. However, some

pathogenic microorganisms are always present in the upper respiratory tract. They usually cause no harm unless resistance is lowered by some other factor, such as chronic disease, alcoholism, physical inactivity, or extremes in age (very young or very old). Patients who are weak are particularly susceptible to pneumonia. Figure 16-8 presents a diagram of the pathophysiology of pneumonia.

Pneumonia also can result from inhalation of poisonous gases *(chemical pneumonia),* accidental aspiration of foods or liquids that causes a pneumonitis progressing to pneumonia *(aspiration pneumonia),* or a blow or injury to the chest that interferes with normal respiration *(traumatic pneumonia)*. *Hypostatic pneumonia,* which results from lying in bed for extended periods, always is a threat to those with impaired mobility. Lack of physical exercise and inadequate aeration of the lungs are major factors in the development of hypostatic pneumonia, where retained secretions cause inflammation.

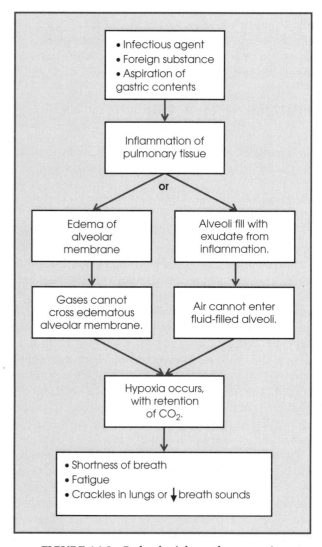

FIGURE 16-8   Pathophysiology of pneumonia.

Prevention

Elderly, weak, debilitated, and immobilized persons are all prime candidates for pneumonia, as are those who have some kind of chronic pulmonary disease. Weakened elderly patients are at high risk for aspiration as well.

A variety of nursing interventions can help prevent pneumonia. These include (1) using nursing intervention to strengthen the patient's natural defenses and avoid infection; (2) frequent turning, coughing, and deep- breathing for postoperative patients or those who are otherwise unable to ventilate their lungs adequately; (3) carefully watching and properly positioning those vomiting patients who are in decreased states of consciousness, such as patient's recovering from anesthesia; (4) elevating the head of the bed when administering tube feedings and when assisting a patient to eat and leaving the head elevated for 30 to 60 minutes after the feeding; (5) avoiding giving liquids to patients who are prone to aspiration; (6) faithfully following principles of cleanliness and asepsis when caring for debilitated patients and those most susceptible to infection; and (7) administering pneumonia vaccine when prescribed for those most at risk for developing the disease.

Nosocomial pneumonia is a major problem that considerably lengthens hospital stays, increasing the cost of health care. Vigilant nurses who provide aggressive respiratory care can greatly decrease the incidence of hospital-acquired pneumonia.

Diagnosis. Symptoms of pneumonia vary according to type. In typical, infectious pneumonia there usually is a high fever accompanied by chills, a cough that produces rusty or blood-flecked sputum, chest pain that is made worse by respiratory movements, and a general feeling of malaise and aching muscles. **Diagnosis is confirmed by chest radiograph, which reveals densities in the affected lung.**

The diagnosis of atypical pneumonia might be missed because of a lack of symptoms usually indicative of pneumonia. Body temperature can be normal or subnormal, breath sounds can be good with perhaps only occasional crackles and wheezes, there may be no pleural involvement and therefore no pain, dry cough, or feeling of extreme fatigue. Chest radiograph reveals diffuse, patchy areas of density. Cytomegalovirus has become a cause of pneumonia in immunocompromised patients, particularly those with AIDS or transplant patients on immunosuppressive drugs.

Treatment. Typical pneumonia is treated with IV or oral antibiotic agents such as penicillin, erythromycin, cephalosporins, aminoglycosides, ciprofloxicin (Cipro), or clarithromycin (Biaxin) depending on the type of bacteria responsible and the degree of sensitivity to various antibiotics. Atypical pneumonia caused by *Mycoplasma* usually is treated with either erythromycin or tetracycline. Viral, atypical pneumonia requires no antiinfective therapy. *Pneumocystis carinii* pneumonia (PCP) associated with AIDS is treated with aerosolized and intravenous pentamidine, trimethoprim/sulfamethoxazole (Bactrim), trimetrexate glucuronate (NeuTrexin), Dapsone, Clindamycin, or Atovaquone. Some patients require mechanical ventilation.

Think about . . . Can you identify five signs or symptoms found on assessment that might correlate with a diagnosis of pneumonia?

Nursing Assessment and Intervention The nursing care plan for a patient with pneumonia should include interventions to promote oxygenation, control elevated temperature, maintain nutritional and fluid intake, provide adequate rest, monitor vital signs and respiratory status, relieve pain and discomfort, provide good oral hygiene and care for "fever blisters" (herpes), prevent irritation of the lungs by smoke and other irritants, and avoid secondary bacterial infections. The patient should deep-breath and cough five to ten times each hour while awake. It is important that the nurse assess for signs of increasing impairment of gas exchange. Because abdominal distention, nausea, and vomiting also may accompany pneumonia, nursing intervention to deal with these problems may be indicated. Other problems that could be presented by the patient include altered states of consciousness (delirium and confusion) and the development of such complications as empyema (see later) and congestive heart failure. Convalescence with rest should extend for at least a week after acute symptoms subside for the young adult. The older adult needs several weeks, and the elderly may require 6 to 12 weeks to feel able to do usual activities without undue fatigue.

Elder Care Point . . . Confusion often is the most obvious sign of atypical pneumonia in the elderly. The elderly patient may never quite regain the former level of wellness after a serious episode of pneumonia. This is why it is even more important to teach the elderly to seek medical attention quickly if symptoms of pneumonia occur.

Atelectasis Atelectasis is an incomplete expansion, or collapse, of alveoli. It may occur from compression of the lungs from outside, a decrease in surfactant, or bronchial obstruction that prevents air from reaching the alveoli. Postoperatively it occurs from retained secretions that accumulated during anesthesia, positioning on the operating room table for an extended period without movement, and hypoventilation related to surgical pain. It usually is a reversible condition. Treatment consists of ridding the bronchial tree of excess secretions by coughing and providing air to the depths of the lung by deep-breathing. Aerosolized surfactant may be used in those instances where there is a surfactant deficiency, such as in adult respiratory distress syndrome (ARDS).

Pleurisy   Pleurisy is an inflammation of the pleural membranes surrounding the lungs. In *pleurisy with effusion,* there also is an increase in the amount of serous fluid within the pleural cavity. The most outstanding symptom of pleurisy is a sharp, stabbing pain in the chest. The pain is aggravated by taking a deep breath. Pleurisy may occur alone or in conjunction with another disease of the respiratory system.

The patient with pleurisy is placed on bedrest and observed carefully for signs of development of a respiratory tract infection. Nonsteroidal antiinflammatory drugs (NSAIDs) are used to decrease inflammation and control pain and offer some relief.

When pleurisy is accompanied by effusion of serous fluid, the physician may perform a thoracentesis (removal of fluid from the pleural cavity) for diagnostic tests or symptom relief. It is not uncommon for as much as 500 mL to be removed at one time during a thoracentesis (see Table 16-2 for further information on this procedure).

Empyema   When the fluid within the pleural cavity becomes infected, the exudate becomes thick and purulent, and the patient is said to have *empyema.* The organisms causing the infection may be staphylococci or streptococci.

Empyema is treated by eliminating the infection through specific antibiotics and by removing excess fluid from the pleural cavity by inserting an empyema tube. A specimen of the fluid is sent to the laboratory for a culture and sensitivity study. This test determines which exact antibiotic will most effectively destroy the organism causing the infection.

Fungal Infections   *Pneumocystis carinii* pneumonia (PCP) has a high incidence in AIDS patients. *P. carinii* is a protozoon. It is found only in immunocompromised patients and is highly lethal. (see Chapter 8).

Histoplasmosis and coccidioidomycosis are fungal lung infections caused by the inhalation of spores. Both can cause pneumonia. They are diagnosed by history, signs and symptoms, and skin test reaction to the fungus. Treatment is IV amphotericin B.

Sarcoidosis   Sarcoidosis is a group of interstitial lung diseases characterized by granulomas. These diseases cause fibrotic changes in the lung tissue over time. They affect other tissues in the body as well. A cellular immune response seems to be responsible for the tissue changes. Sarcoidosis is ten times more common in blacks than in whites, and most cases occur between ages 20 and 40. The fibrotic changes cause a reduction in function in lung tissue.

♦ Chronic Airflow Limitation (CAL, Chronic Obstructive Pulmonary Disease, COPD)

Chronic airflow limitation (CAL) was formerly called chronic obstructive pulmonary disease (COPD). The terms may be used interchangeably. The term is used to describe a condition that is common to three diseases: *pulmonary emphysema, chronic bronchitis,* and *bronchial asthma.* Although the clinical history, manifestations of the specific illness present, treatment, and course of each of the diseases may vary, the term *CAL* describes one condition that is common to all three. This condition is *obstruction of the small airways.* The condition also is sometimes called *chronic obstructive lung disease* (COLD) or *chronic airway obstruction* (CAO).

> CAL ranks fourth among the major causes of death in the United States, and the number of its victims is increasing.

About 20% to 30% of the adults in the United States are affected by CAL. This represents billions of dollars in economic loss as a result of inability to work and the expense of repeated visits to the physician and hospitalizations. The American Lung Association estimates that about 20 million Americans suffer from CAL.

The dramatic increase in the rate of morbidity and mortality due to CAL is attributed to increases in habitual cigarette smoking and rising levels of air pollution. A third factor is genetic susceptibility to the destruction of lung tissue. A serum protein, *alpha$_1$-antitrypsin* (AAT) is deficient in certain people, and the deficiency runs in families. This protein inhibits the activity of the enzyme *elastase,* which tends to break down lung tissue. In the absence of AAT, lung tissue is more easily destroyed by the enzyme. Patients with a deficiency of AAT may develop severe lung disease at an early age.

Pulmonary Emphysema   Emphysema is characterized by a permanent distention of the bronchioles and destruction of the walls of the alveoli (Figure 16-9). It is essentially a disease of the *terminal* respiratory units. Air that is inhaled becomes trapped, causing the victim to work harder to *exhale* air than to inhale it.

As pulmonary emphysema progresses, the patient suffers further loss of lung elasticity. The diaphragm becomes permanently flattened by overdistention of the lungs, the muscles of the rib cage become rigid, and the ribs flare outward. This produces the "barrel chest" that is typical of many patients with CAL.

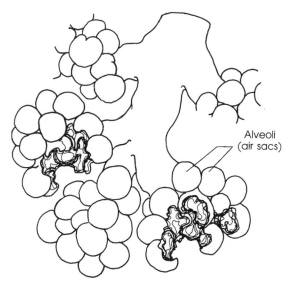

Alveoli (air sacs)

Irreversible breakdown of the walls of individual air sacs creates large air spaces.

Small air tubes collapse, trapping air and making exhalation difficult.

FIGURE 16-9   Emphysematous alveoli.

To compensate for the loss of muscular action that normally aids respiration, the patient begins to use other muscles, mainly those of the neck and shoulders. She holds her shoulders high in an attempt to enlarge the space in which her lungs can expand. Her facial expression conveys the anxiety and tension that result from her struggle to get enough air into her lungs.

The patient with almost pure emphysema, that is, no asthma and very little bronchitis, has only a small amount of mucus. The skin is a pinkish color, even though hypoxia may be present. Carbon dioxide is usually not retained, and therefore an acid–base imbalance is unlikely.

Chronic Bronchitis   Inflammation of the bronchi is considered chronic when the recurrent cough is present for at least 3 months of each year for at least 2 years. Chronic bronchitis can range from a mildly irritating "cigarette" cough in the morning with production of small amounts of sputum to a severe disabling condition. The latter extreme is characterized by increased resistance to airflow, hypoxia, and frequently hypercapnia and *cor pulmonale*. Cor pulmonale is a heart condition characterized by pulmonary hypertension and an enlarged right ventricle, both of which are secondary to chronic lung disease. Cor pulmonale places the patient at risk for right-sided heart failure.

The primary clinical characteristics of chronic bronchitis include a productive cough due to hyperplasia of the bronchial glands and increased secretion of mucus, and the breathing difficulties typical of obstructive lung disease. Pulmonary function testing reveals an increased residual volume due to the premature closure of the narrowed airways during exhalation. The patient has a marked increase in his $PaCO_2$ levels and a marked decrease in PaO_2 levels. **The retention of carbon dioxide and deficiency of oxygen give the skin a reddish-blue color.** The reddish color also is due to an increase in the red blood cell count (**polycythemia**). Laboratory tests will show elevated hemoglobin and hematocrit levels. The increase in production of red blood cells is an attempt by the body to compensate for the chronic hypoxia. Table 16-9 presents a comparison of emphysema and chronic bronchitis.

Asthma

Diagnosis.   Asthma is a chronic lung disease characterized by reversible airway obstruction, airway inflammation from edema or swelling, and increased airway sensitivity to a variety of stimuli. The person with asthma has a hypersensitivity of the trachea and bronchi to various kinds of stimuli (Figure 16-10). Most likely no single cause is responsible for the group of symptoms known as asthma. Among the factors implicated in the development of asthma are allergens, viruses and other infectious agents, occupational and environmental toxins, exercise, and psychological disturbances. Table 16-10 presents the various types of asthma.

The symptoms of asthma are due to constriction of the bronchi, inflammatory changes in the mucosa, accumulations of secretions in the lumen of the bronchi, and changes in the elastic recoil of the lungs (Figure 16-11).

Symptoms of asthma can be simulated by breathing only through a straw for one minute. Some asthmatics are without symptoms between attacks, but pulmonary

TABLE 16-9 ◆ *Comparison of Pulmonary Emphysema and Chronic Brochitis*		
Clinical Feature	**Pulmonary Emphysema**	**Chronic Bronchitis**
Onset of signs and symptoms	Age 50–75	Age 40–50
Body build/appearance	"Pink Puffer," Thin, barrel chested, weight loss; obvious difficulty breathing; may use accessory muscles; pursed lip breathing. Often has marked weight loss and appears emaciated.	"Blue Bloater." Stocky build; may have slight increase in chest A-P diameter; uses accessory muscles in late stages.
Chief complaint	Shortness of breath	Sputum production
Sputum	Scanty, mucoid	Copious mucopurulent
Carbon dioxide retention	Uncommon	Common
Cor pulmonale	Occasional	Common
Health history	Generally healthy, smoking	Frequent respiratory infections, smoking

function tests may occasionally reveal some abnormalities, even though there is no wheezing, coughing, or other outward signs. Cough is a common symptom of asthma in adults and usually indicates obstruction of the larger airways. Dyspnea, another common symptom, is indicative of edema or mucus in the smaller airways.

Because asthma is a chronic disease, the patient should know the intended effect of medications. Ideally, the patient will eventually be able to adjust dosage and therapy as symptoms change, using guidelines provided by the physician or nurse. As with any chronic disease, the patient with asthma periodically consults the physician for continued management of the illness. Both

patients and nurses need to know that a severe, acute, asthma attack can cause death from hypoxia.

Treatment. Because emphysema, chronic bronchitis, and asthma often are seen in combination in patients with CAL, the first step in designing therapy is to determine which aspects of these diseases the patient displays. Treatment is aimed at managing the underlying symptoms.

The goals of medical treatment are to (1) minimize irritation of the air passages and relieve obstruction by secretions, edema, or bronchospasm; (2) prevent or control infection and allergy; (3) increase the patient's tolerance for activity; and (4) determine the best drug

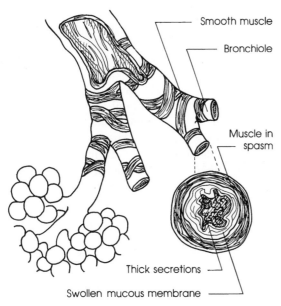

The bronchiole is obstructed during expiration by muscle spasms, swollen mucous membranes, and secretion of thick mucus within air tubes and sacs.

FIGURE 16-10   Bronchial asthma.

TABLE 16-10 ◆ *Types of Asthma*		
Types of Asthma	**Precipitating Factors***	**Mechanism or Immunologic Reaction**
Extrinsic		
Atropic (allergic)	Specific allergens	Type I (IgE) immune reaction
Occupational	Chemical challenge	Type I immune reactions
Allergic bronchopulmonary aspergillosis	Antigen (spores) challenge	Type I and III immune reactions
Intrinsic		
Nonreaginic	Respiratory tract infection	Unknown; hyperreactive airways
Pharmacological (e.g., aspirin-sensitive)	Aspirin	Decreased prostaglandins, increased leukotrienes

*All types may be precipitated by cold, stress, exercise. All have hyperreactive airways.
Source: Robbins, S. L., Schoen, F. J., eds. (1994). *Robbins Pathologic Basis of Disease,* 5th ed. Philadelphia: Saunders, p. 690.

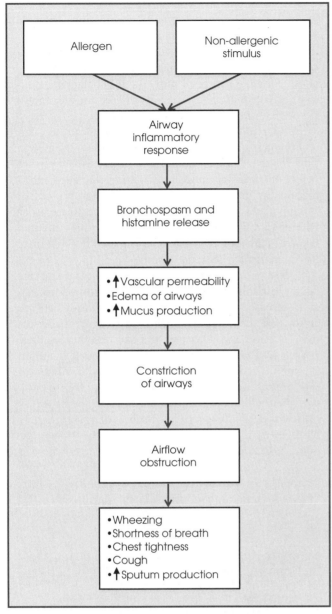

FIGURE 16-11 Pathophysiology of asthma.

combination in the least amounts that will control symptoms.

Bronchodilators in the form of beta-adrenergic agonists, theophyllines, or anticholinergic agents such as ipratropium bromide (Atrovent) are used as the main form of therapy. Corticosteroids, mucolytics, and antibiotics also may be prescribed (see Common Therapeutic Therapies section).

Oxygen is prescribed for moderate and severe hypoxemia. For acute episodes of CAL with hypoxemia, oxygen is given to raise the PaO_2 above 60 mm Hg. Oxygen is used in patients with chronic CAL who have consistent PaO_2 levels less than 55 to 59 mm Hg. Oxygen always is used cautiously in patients with CAL, as they have adjusted to high levels of CO_2, which

normally provides the drive to breathe, and are dependent on low oxygen levels to stimulate breathing. **If too much oxygen is given, the patient may cease to breathe and require mechanical ventilation.** Oxygen also is prescribed for moderate and severe cases of dyspnea. Patients who continue to experience exertional dyspnea after discharge may be taught to administer their own oxygen at home. A portable oxygen tank can be used to allow the patient to increase her level of activity without triggering severe and frightening episodes of dyspnea.

Nursing Assessment and Intervention **Rehabilitation and education of the patient and family are the chief long-term goals of nursing intervention.** With proper home care the patient with CAL can live longer and have a higher quality of life, reduce the number of hospitalizations and visits to her physician, and have fewer psychosocial problems related to inactivity and a feeling of hopelessness.

It is very important that the family, as well as the patient, be educated so that there will be an understanding of the need for appropriate exercise and activity and of the desire for independence. Families often tend to become very overprotective of the patient because of their fear of episodes of dyspnea. Rehabilitation needs to be a joint effort by the patient and family to help the patient attain as high a quality of life as possible while avoiding the complications of CAL.

The major problem of chronic, diffuse, and irreversible obstruction of the airways must be dealt with in a systematic way. This means working with the patient, identifying specific difficulties she is experiencing, assessing current ability to cope with them, and devising plans to accomplish specific goals for improvement. In general, no matter what the primary cause of the disorder, patients with CAL will require some nursing interventions to help them (1) maintain optimal health status; (2) achieve a balance of maximal exercise and adequate rest; (3) use techniques to facilitate breathing (for example, breathing through pursed lips and diaphragmatic breathing); and (4) cough effectively to remove secretions. To prevent frequent hospitalizations for acute flareups of her disease, the patient will need to be taught how to avoid bronchial irritation and infection and prevent such complications as right-sided heart failure (cor pulmonale). Tables 16-8, 16-11, and 16-12 show some helpful techniques and pointers for the patient with CAL.

Encouragement to quit smoking is of major importance for those with CAL who still smoke. Continued smoking will seriously compromise the extent and quality of life for this patient. The American Lung Association has both literature and community programs directed to assist CAL patients with this problem.

The asthma patient is taught to use a peak flow meter to determine the drug dosage needed to control

TABLE 16-11 ◆ *Patient Education: Pursed-Lip Breathing and Diaphragmatic Breathing*

Instruct the patient with obstructive lung disease to breathe with pursed lips, to promote better exhalation and decrease air trapping.

Pursed-lip breathing
- Sit up tall and move the back away from the chair; place the feet about shoulder-width apart. Lean forward slightly with hands or elbows on the knees.
- Close the mouth, and breath in through the nose.
- Purse the lips as though to whistle or blow out a candle.
- Breathe out slowly without puffing out the cheeks; control the flow of exhaled air as if you wanted to cause a candle to flicker, but not extinguish.
- Take twice as much time to let the breath out as it did to take it in.
- Tense the abdominal muscles to force as much air from the lungs as possible.
- Use pursed-lip breathing during any physical activity.
- Refrain from holding your breath when lifting objects or performing other physical activities.

Abdominal ("belly") or diaphragmatic breathing
- Initially practice lying down.
- Lie on the back with the knees bent. Take a deep breath through the nose with the abdomen relaxed and with the palm of one hand feel it rise. Exhale slowly to a count of four.
- Exhale slowly through pursed lips, tightening the abdominal muscles that push the diaphragm up, forcing more air out of the lungs.
- Once comfortable with the abdominal breathing technique, use it when standing or sitting. This type of controlled breathing will provide more endurance during physical activity.

the asthma, to predict the effectiveness of therapy, and to detect airflow obstruction buildup before it becomes serious and requires hospitalization. Peak flow monitoring is based on the greatest airflow velocity that can be produced during a forced expiration that starts from fully inflated lungs. It assesses airflow obstruction. Readings are recorded, and, once a baseline for the patient's personal best peak flow is set, readings are compared to it. If a reading is 80% below the patient's best, treatment should be adjusted.

Psychosocial concerns are another area for nursing intervention. The patient often needs help with adjustment to alterations in roles and lifestyle. He may have problems with self-esteem, body image, and sexuality that stem from his chronic disease. A trusting relationship between nurse and patient opens the way for discussing the most personal concerns and provides a means to explore possible solutions or adaptations for problems in these areas. Referral to community support groups also can be beneficial, as the patient then has an opportunity to see and hear how others in his situation have learned to cope and adapt.

The teaching plan for the CAL patient is extensive and includes (1) management of medications and side effects; (2) use of respiratory therapy measures and care of equipment; (3) management of dyspnea; (4) control of the immediate environment and avoidance of allergens; (5) maintenance of nutrition; (6) balancing exercise and adequate rest; (7) signs of complications; and (8) need for close medical supervision.

Education of the patient and family can be overwhelming if it is not planned carefully, allowing enough time for them to gain confidence in one aspect of care before introducing more information. Detailed information on nursing intervention and the specifics of teaching are found in the section Common Respiratory Patient Care Problems presented earlier in the chapter. Clinical Pathway 16-1 presents the collaborative care for the patient with acute asthma.

Most patients with CAL have difficulty getting sufficient rest and sleep because of their dyspnea, anxiety, and decreased mobility. Sedatives and tranquilizers are contraindicated, because they tend to depress respiration. Tension and anxiety often can be relieved if the patient is taught some relaxation techniques. It should be emphasized that these techniques must be *taught to the patient.* Simply telling her to relax or to stop worrying will not be helpful; she is using almost every muscle in her body to struggle for breath or is extremely tense in anticipation of an attack of breathlessness. Some patients become very agitated and talkative if dyspnea is not too severe. It is best to display a calm attitude, stay with the patient, hold a hand, and state, "Shh—we'll talk in a minute. Catch your breath first."

TABLE 16-12 ◆ *Patient Education: Instructions for the Patient with CAL*

- To make mucus more liquid and easier to cough up, drink at least 2 and preferably 3 quarts of liquid every day.
- When you exert yourself, as in lifting something or getting up from your chair, exhale slowly through pursed lips rather than holding your breath. You should do the same thing when you are walking for exercise. It is natural for all of us to hold our breath when we exert ourselves, so you may need practice to get into the habit of exhaling on exertion.
- Eat three or four small, balanced meals rather than one or two large ones each day.
- Practice your breathing exercises every day without fail.
- Try to avoid crowds during the flu and cold seasons.
- Do not take over-the-counter drugs. They can interact with your prescribed drugs, and some may be harmful because of their effects on your breathing. Antihistamines can dry out the mucus even more and make it more difficult for you to clear your air passages.
- Don't smoke or inhale the tobacco smoke of others.

Note: Normal sputum is white and slightly viscous and has no odor or taste.

CLINICAL PATHWAY FOR ACUTE ASTHMA ♦ *ICD-9 Code 097 ELOS 3 days*

Nursing Diagnosis/ Collaborative Problem	Expected Outcome (The Patient Is Expected to . . .)	Met/Not Met	Reason	Date/Initials
Ineffective breathing pattern	Resume baseline breathing pattern and respiratory rate with a peak flow >70% of baseline.			
Ineffective airway clearance	Clear airway without difficulty.			
Activity intolerance.	Resume ADLs living with good exercise tolerance.			
Ineffective individual and family coping	Identify successful coping strategies and participate in plan of care.			

Aspect of Care	Date _____ Day 1	Date _____ Day 2	Date _____ Day 3
Assessment	Systems assessment q shift with focus on respiratory. Adventitious breath sounds and accessory muscle utilization. Vital signs q 4 h Sputum for color, tenacity, and amount. Skin assessment for color, temperature, and diaphoresis. Anxiety, fear, and fatigue levels; family support and resources. Assess response to therapy. Assess need for mechanical ventilation. Monitor for complications: hypoxemia; pneumonia; respiratory acidosis.	Same as Day 1.	Same as Day 2. Vital signs q 8 h.
Teaching	Orient to hospital and unit. Prepare for diagnostic tests. Instruct on use of peak expiratory flow meter, nebulizer, and metered dose inhaler. Provide information on diagnosis and medications. Involve family in care of patient as appropriate. Review plan of care/clinical pathway with patient and family.	Stress reduction techniques, need for adequate rest and sleep. How to recognize and prevent respiratory infection, irritants. Adaptive breathing techniques (pursed lips, pushing/pulling during exhalation) and energy-conserving measures.	What to do during acute asthma attack when to seek emergency care. Medication administration and use of metered dose inhaler. Importance of diet and fluids. Assess knowledge about factors that trigger asthma and how to pretreat before exposure to trigger. Provide information concerning medications that may trigger asthma.
Consults	Respiratory therapy. Pulmonologist. Social worker.	N/A.	N/A.
Lab tests	Complete blood count with differential, electrolytes. Arterial blood gases. Theophylline level. Total immunoglobin E. Sputum culture.	Theophylline level (while on IV or if dosage changes).	Same as Day 2.
Other tests	Chest x-ray. ECG (if >40 years of age). Pulmonary function tests.	N/A.	N/A.

Continued on following page

CLINICAL PATHWAY FOR ACUTE ASTHMA ◆ *ICD-9 Code 097 ELOS 3 days* (Continued)

Aspect of Care	Date _____ Day 1	Date _____ Day 2	Date _____ Day 3
Meds	Bronchodilator or beta₂ agonist metaproterenol, albuterol via nebulizer q 4 h. *or* IV bronchodilator (aminophylline) via continuous drip. Corticosteroids IV q 6 h.*or*	Nebulizer q 4 h. Consider changing to PO if patient is stable. Taper dosage and change to PO.	Discontinue nebulizer and place on metered dose inhaler. Theo-Dur PO. Prednisone PO bid.
Treatments/ interventions	O_2 per NC or Ventimask at 2 L to maintain SaO_2 >90%. Pulse oximetry. Peak flow before and after nebulizer treatment Bronchodilator via nebulizer or metered dose inhaler q 4 h. Position to facilitate breathing. Elevate head of bed to 45°–90°. Allergen-free pillow. Frequent oral care. Provide periods of uninterrupted sleep and rest. Daily weight.	Same as Day 1.	Discontinue O_2. Pulse oximetry. Peak expiratory flow q 8 h. Incentive spirometer tid. Aerosol inhalation qid. Position to facilitate breathing. Oral care as needed.
Nutrition	DAT (low Na^+ if steroid dependent) Encourage fluid intake to 2,000 mL/day (restrict if on steroids).	Same as Day 1.	Same as Day 2.
Lines/tubes/ monitors	IV fluids for hydration and medications.	Discontinue IV fluids; change to saline loc	Same as Day 2. Discontinue saline loc
Mobility/self-care	Bedrest with bathroom privileges. Sit on side of bed or up in bed leaning on overbed table.	Out of bed and ambulate as tolerated.	Same as Day 2.
Discharge planning	Assess need for home respiratory equipment.	Refer to support group. Continue as Day 1 with attention to home needs, modification of environment to reduce allergens.	Arrange for follow-up visit with physician.

Source: Clinical Pathway for acute asthma. From: Ignatavicius, D. D., Hausman, K. A. (1995). *Clinical Pathways for Collaborative Practice.* Philadelphia: Saunders, pp. 78–81.

Relaxation exercises can be learned, but it takes a bit of practice to call them into practice whenever relaxation is needed. Table 16-13 presents the script from which the patient can make a "relaxation" tape.

Think about... Can you list five nursing interventions that might help your CAL patient avoid episodes of dyspnea?

Bronchiectasis Bronchiectasis is a chronic respiratory disorder in which one or more bronchi are permanently dilated. It is thought to occur as a result of frequent respiratory infections in childhood. It often is classified with CAL, and its management is similar.

Cystic fibrosis (CF) is a major cause of bronchiectasis. It is a genetic disease in which there is excessive mucus production because of exocrine gland dysfunction. The lungs, intestines, sinuses, reproductive tract, sweat glands, and pancreas are all affected. It is diagnosed by history, physical examination, and a positive sweat test.

Lung damage occurs in cystic fibrosis patients as a result of excessive secretion of abnormally thick mucus, impairment of ciliary action in the lungs, airway obstruction, and repeated infections, which cause scarring. Cystic fibrosis eventually results in CAL. It was once solely a pediatric disease, because children with cystic fibrosis died before reaching adulthood. Today 20% of cystic fibrosis patients are adults. A few cystic

TABLE 16-13 ♦ *Relaxation Exercise*

This exercise is performed by recording the script onto audiotape and following the instructions as the tape is played. Using the exercise regularly over a period of weeks makes it easier to call on these techniques to induce relaxation during an exam or at other times you feel particularly tense.

Slowly read the script in a soft, firm, voice. Allow sufficient pauses between segments for the instructions to be followed. Sit in a chair, or lie down to do the exercise. Decrease outside noise and distractions as much as possible.

Script

♦ Close your eyes and find something to focus on mentally. It might be a spot of light, your pulse, a visual image, or whatever you choose. Try to hold it constant.

♦ Breathe in slowly and deeply; hold it a moment, and slowly breathe out. Now breathe normally, slowly, in and out.

♦ Tighten your face and neck muscles as firmly as you can, while clenching your teeth. Feel the tension. Hold it; slowly relax the muscles. Feel the relaxation in your face, jaw, and neck.

♦ With less tension, tighten the muscles in the face, jaw, and neck again. Feel this level of tension. Let go and relax. Notice the feeling of relaxation.

♦ Tighten your chest muscles firmly. Hold it; feel the tension. Let the chest muscles relax. Notice the difference between the tension and relaxation.

♦ Tighten the chest muscles again with less tension. Now let the muscles relax. Feel the relaxation.

♦ Tighten the fists and arm muscles as hard as possible. Hold the tension a moment. Slowly relax the muscles. Notice the difference in feeling between tension and relaxation.

♦ Tighten the fists and arm muscles again with less tension. Hold it. Let the muscles relax. Feel the relaxation.

♦ Tighten the abdominal muscles firmly. Hold the tension, noting the feeling. Relax the muscles, noting the difference between tension and relaxation.

♦ Tighten the abdominal muscles again with less tension. Hold it. Allow the muscles to relax completely. Notice the feeling of relaxation.

♦ Tighten the muscles in your right leg and foot. Hold the tension. Note the feeling. Allow the muscles to relax. Notice the difference between tension and relaxation.

♦ Tighten the muscles in your right leg and foot again with less tension. Hold it. Completely let go of the tension in the muscles and relax. Feel the relaxation.

♦ Tighten the muscles in your left leg and foot firmly. Hold it. Note the tension. Allow the muscles to relax. Focus on the difference between tension and relaxation.

♦ Tighten the muscles in your left leg and foot again with less tension. Hold it. Completely let go of the tension in the muscles and relax. Notice the feeling of relaxation.

♦ Breathe in and out deeply and slowly five times, focusing on your breathing.

♦ When you are ready, open your eyes.

Source: deWit, S. C. (1994). *Rambo's Nursing Skills for Clinical Practice,* 4th ed. Philadelphia, Saunders, p. 209.

fibrosis patients live into their thirties and forties because of aggressive respiratory treatment and antibiotics. The new drug, dornase alfa (Pulmozyme), reduces the frequency of respiratory infections and improves pulmonary function in patients with CF. This may extend the present average lifespan of the CF patient considerably.

Research has finally identified the gene responsible for cystic fibrosis. Work is continuing on ways to isolate and replace the missing gene to prevent or cure the disease.

♦ Tuberculosis

Pulmonary Tuberculosis **Pulmonary tuberculosis (TB) is an infectious disease of the lung characterized by lesions within the lung tissue.** The lesions may continue to degenerate and become necrotic, or they may heal by fibrosis and calcification. The causative organism is the true tubercle bacillus *Mycobacterium tuberculosis.*

Contrary to popular beliefs, tuberculosis is *not* highly contagious. Infection most often occurs after prolonged exposure to the tubercle bacillus, but not everyone contracts the disease, even after close and extensive contact with infected persons.

Tuberculosis still is a major health problem in many countries throughout the world, and unfortunately its incidence is rising again in the United States. The increase in the immune incompetence of AIDS and the influx of immigrants who are infected are the two major causes of the increase. Poor living conditions, especially in urban areas, and malnutrition all increase susceptibility to the tubercle bacillus. The increase in this population is another reason why the disease is spreading.

Diagnosis. Early detection of tuberculosis is of great importance because (1) the anti-TB drugs are more effective in the early stages of the disease; (2) the period of disability is much shorter; and (3) the complications are fewer.

Skin testing (intradermal tests). Skin testing for tuberculosis may be done by the *Mantoux* test. The multi-puncture test is no longer approved. In this test, 0.1 mL of purified protein derivative (PPD) tuberculin containing 5 tuberculin units is injected intradermally. The test is *positive* when the swelling at the site of injection is more than 10 mm in diameter 48 to 72 hours after injection.

A positive tuberculin test indicates that the person has been infected with the tubercle bacillus. It does not indicate whether the disease is active or inactive at that time, only that the body tissues are sensitive to tuberculin. A positive reaction indicates a need for further evaluation.

Radiographs.   An x-ray examination of the chest may or may not reveal tubercular lesions in the lung, but calcified and healed lesions, as well as active lesions, usually can be seen on radiographs. **A diagnosis of active tuberculosis is established when the tubercle bacillus has been found in the sputum.** Because people are quite likely to swallow sputum rather than expectorate it, a sample of stomach contents may be examined if the patient cannot produce an adequate sputum specimen (gastric analysis). A new laboratory test is able to identify tubercle bacillus in the sputum within 4 hours whereas the older tests took about 6 weeks for definitive results.

The onset of tuberculosis is gradual; a patient may have an active and progressing lesion before symptoms appear. Typical symptoms are cough, low-grade fever in the afternoon, anorexia, loss of weight, fatigue, night sweats, and sometimes hemoptysis.

Treatment.   Before the advent of anti-TB drugs, patients with pulmonary tuberculosis were treated in sanatoria, where they were isolated to avoid spreading the disease. In the 1960s, the trend was to treat patients with active tuberculosis in general hospitals for a short time and then send them home on medication. Now uncomplicated pulmonary tuberculosis is managed in the outpatient setting. People in close contact with the patient have usually been exposed before the disease was diagnosed. After 2 weeks on medication, the sputum of the patient usually is not infectious. Close contacts are monitored with skin testing. Effective cure can be obtained within 6 to 9 months for most patients with pulmonary tuberculosis. Medication is continued for at least 2 months after recovery is complete to make certain that residual organisms are killed. There is an increase in the incidence of multiple-drug-resistant TB, and these patients do not fare so well. If recovery is achieved, medications are continued for several years to prevent relapse.

Tuberculosis was once greatly feared, because it was considered to be highly contagious, and the treatment and confinement to an institution could last for years. Now, however, it is considered far less threatening. This change in attitude has come about because of the chemotherapeutic agents that quickly render the patient with drug-susceptible TB noninfectious. A second factor is the knowledge that tuberculosis is essentially an airborne infectious disease that requires respiratory precautions rather than strict isolation of the patient. Information about drugs commonly used in the treatment of tuberculosis is summarized in Table 16-14. The drugs are prescribed in combinations of two or three anti-TB agents (for example, the primary drug INH and a secondary drug, such as RMP).

Chemotherapy is the preferred method of treatment for most patients with tuberculosis, but some may require surgery if the disease has progressed to an advanced stage, or if drug-resistant infection has developed. Surgical treatment involves the removal of the affected lung tissue.

Nursing Assessment and Intervention   Because tuberculosis is an infectious disease, nursing goals are similar to those for other diseases of this type. Nursing objectives concerned with prevention and control of infectious diseases are (1) to control the spread of the infectious agent; (2) to promote immunity to infectious diseases; and (3) to support and strengthen the capacity for recovery in a patient who has an infectious disease.

Control of infection.   Pulmonary tuberculosis is transmitted principally by way of the respiratory tract. Airborne precautions in addition to *standard precautions* are recommended for the patient who has an active case of tuberculosis and is just beginning drug therapy. The patient is placed in a well-ventilated room, and a HEPA respirator mask is required for all personnel when caring for the patient. A gown is worn if the patient is coughing and splattering of clothing is likely. The patient is encouraged to rest as fatigue is common during the active phase of infection and the beginning of medication treatment. The home care patient does not need these precautions because family members have already been exposed by the time of diagnosis. The patient is taught to cover the mouth when coughing or sneezing, dispose of tissues in plastic bags, and to wear a mask when in contact with crowds until medication effectively suppresses the infection. Sputum examinations are required every 2 to 4 weeks; when two consecutive sputum cultures are negative, the patient is considered no longer infectious and may resume work and other usual social activities. Another aspect of infection control is the identification and prompt treatment of potential and active cases of tuberculosis.

Promotion of immunity.   A vaccine is available that is made from live, attenuated bacilli. It is called BCG (bacille Calmette-Guérin) and offers some protection from tuberculosis but cannot be depended on to provide complete immunity. The BCG vaccine has the disadvantage of causing a positive reaction to the tuberculin test (this interferes somewhat with the usefulness of tuberculin testing programs). Public health officials in this country advise the administration of BCG vaccine only to those who live in an environment that has a very high rate of tuberculosis. In countries where there are high rates of tuberculosis, the World Health Organization strongly recommends the widespread use of BCG, which is credited with having a favorable impact in reducing the morbidity of tuberculosis.

Fortunately, tuberculosis is one of the most easily avoided of all serious respiratory illnesses. The body's innate immune system cannot work well, however, when a person is malnourished, physically debilitated,

TABLE 16-14 ◆ *Drugs Commonly Used in the Treatment of Tuberculosis*

	Dosage		Most Common Side Effects	Test for Side Effects	Remarks
	Daily	**Twice Weekly**			
Primary drugs Isoniazid (INH)	5–10 mg/kg up to 300 mg PO or IM	15 mg/kg PO or IM	Peripheral neuritis, hepatitis, hypersensitivity, jaundice	AST/ALT (not as a routine)	Bactericidal. Pyridoxine 10 mg as prophylaxis for neuritis; 50-100 mg as treatment
Ethambutol	15–25 mg/kg PO	50 mg/kg PO	Optic neuritis (reversible with discontinuation of drug; very rare at 15 mg/kg), skin rash	Red-green color discrimination and visual acuity	Use with caution with renal disease or when eye testing is not feasible
Rifampin (RMP)	10–20 mg/kg up to 600 mg PO	Not recommended	Hepatitis, febrile reaction, purpura (rare)	AST/ALT (not as a routine)	Bactericidal. Orange secretion color. Affects action of other drugs
Streptomycin	15–20 mg/kg up to 1 g IM	25-30 mg/kg IM	VIIIth cranial nerve damage, nephrotoxicity; hypersensitivity	Vestibular function, audiograms; BUN and creatinine	Use with caution in older patients or those with renal disease
Pyrazinamide	15–30 mg/kg up to 2 g PO	Not recommended	Hyperuricemia, hepatotoxicity	Uric acid, AST/ALT	Under study as first-line drug in short-course regimens
Secondary drugs Kanamycin	15–30 mg/kg up to 1 g IM	Secondary drugs are not recommended for twice-weekly dosage.	Similar to streptomycin	BUN, creatinine	Increase hydration; evaluate hearing before therapy starts
Capreomycin	15–30 mg/kg up to 1 g IM		Similar to streptomycin	BUN, creatinine	Periodic hearing evaluation needed
Cycloserine	10–20 mg/kg up to 1 g PO		Depression, psychosis, hypersensitivity	Neurologic exam	Warn to avoid alcohol; monitor serum blood levels of drug
Ethionamide	15–30 mg/kg up to 1 g PO		Peripheral neuritis, GI distress, dermatitis	AST/ALT	Pyridoxine used for neuropathy Give with meals; avoid alcohol
Para-amino salicylic acid	150 μg/kg up to 12 g PO		GI distress, hepatotoxicity, hypersensitivity	AST/ALT	Give with meals; monitor for hepatotoxicity

ALT, Alanine aminotranferase; AST, aspartate aminotransferase; BUN, blood urea nitrogen.
*May use as thrice-weekly schedule.
Source: Adapted from American Thoracic Society. (1994). *Treatment of Tuberculosis and Tuberculosis Infection in Adults and Children 1994.* American Lung Association.

and subject to extreme physical and emotional stress. Improvement of living conditions and carrying out sound health practices are essential to maintaining a natural resistance to tuberculosis.

Preventive therapy with isoniazid (INH) has been particularly successful in reducing the transmission of tuberculosis. It is estimated that the drug is 85% effective in reducing the chances of contracting tuberculosis by persons who are most exposed. The drug is given prophylactically once daily for a full year. Those for whom a course of INH therapy is recommended include (1) those living in the house with or closely associated with a person who is newly diagnosed as having tuberculosis; (2) people who have positive skin reactions but normal chest radiographs; (3) positive skin reactors who suffer from a chronic disease (for example, diabetes mellitus), are taking steroids, or have had a gastrectomy; and (4) those who have recently shown a positive skin reaction in spite of a history of negative reactions.

Support. Even though studies of the effectiveness of INH and RMP consistently show a very high success rate (98%) in the control of drug susceptible tuberculosis, many people still dread the disease. When a person first learns that she has tuberculosis, she will need reassurance and continued support in sorting out her feelings and overcoming any fears and misinformation she might have.

In addition, it is important that the patient name all close contacts so that they can be reached and started on preventive therapy. Giving the names of contacts may be very difficult for the patient because of the social stigma that is still attached to tuberculosis in certain cultural groups.

The vast majority of newly diagnosed tuberculosis patients are treated on an outpatient basis. Only those who are very debilitated or suffering from another chronic illness are hospitalized. Because much of the responsibility for care probably rests on the patient and possibly on family members, health education is a major intervention in the management of tuberculosis.

Education of the patient, the family, and close contacts should include information about how the disease is transmitted, how it affects the lungs, the importance of taking prescribed medications continuously and without fail, and the risks involved in failing to take both therapeutic doses and preventive doses of medication.

Instruction in personal hygiene and nutrition is included in the program of health care teaching if the patient needs this information. Specifically, the patient and family are taught measures to cope with a cough, handle secretions properly, and observe sputum and report any change in its characteristics. A balance of rest and physical activity also should be stressed if it appears

that the patient is overexerting himself either by working or by indulging in a debilitating social life.

Extrapulmonary Tuberculosis   It is possible for the tubercle bacillus to attack and damage parts of the body other than the lungs. This is called *extrapulmonary tuberculosis.* The areas most frequently affected are the bones, meninges, urinary tract, and reproductive system. Tuberculosis of the spine, called *Pott's disease,* is now quite rare in the United States. The deformity most commonly seen in Pott's disease is *kyphosis,* or "hunchback."

◆ Lung Cancer

In 1930, the death rate from lung cancer for males was 3.6 per 100,000 population; in 1996 the rate had increased to approximately 70 per 100,000. Today, whereas death rates from other forms of cancer are decreasing or remaining stable, lung cancer has become the leading cause of cancer deaths worldwide. Cigarette smoking in women has caused lung cancer to surpass the incidence of breast cancer. Contributing factors are increasing air pollution, more cigarette smoking by young people, and the growing numbers of older people in the population. Approximately 85% of lung cancer is thought to be directly linked to cigarette smoking. Lung cancer is found most often in people 40 years of age or older. About 13% of patients diagnosed with lung cancer survive more than 5 years.

Diagnosis.   Most lung tumors begin in the epithelial lining of the bronchi. There are few symptoms at first, usually only a cough and some wheezing. As the tumor grows larger, the patient may have some pain or discomfort in the chest, exertional dyspnea, and expectoration of blood-streaked sputum. More specific symptoms depend on the location and size of the malignant tumor and the areas to which it has metastasized. If, for example, the malignancy has involved the esophagus, there will be ulceration, bleeding, and dysphagia. Tumors pressing against the trachea can produce hoarseness and paralysis of the vocal cords.

The oncologist may choose from a variety of diagnostic tests and procedures to establish a definite diagnosis of lung cancer. These include chest radiograph and cytology, which is an examination of cells obtained by mediastinoscopy, bronchoscopy, thoracentesis, and needle biopsy of the tumor. Lung scans also are used to diagnose lung cancer.

Treatment.   It may be possible to remove the affected area of the lung by surgery if the malignancy is in its earliest stages and is localized. Radiation may be used after surgery; however, some types of lung cancers are radioresistant. Small cell tumors respond dramatically to chemotherapy, but the malignancy tends to recur as metastasis has almost always occurred by the time it is diagnosed. Large cell lung cancer is very aggressive and difficult to treat. Unless it is caught in the very early stages, the prognosis is not good. There is a new drug available, vinorelbine (Navelbine), which is a new vinca alkaloid with lower neurotoxic effects and it has extended lifespan during clinical trials.

A new experimental treatment for lung cancer is photodynamic therapy (PDT). The patient is given a drug that is taken up by the tumor cells, making them very sensitive to light and/or heat. The tumor is then exposed to a laser beam that destroys the malignant cells. The laser is introduced into the bronchi via a bronchoscope. Tumors in the main bronchi are particular targets for this type of therapy. Immunotherapy also is undergoing evaluation as a treatment option to be combined with chemotherapy or radiation. As with other forms of cancer, the oncologist chooses specific therapies on the basis of the type of malignancy affecting the lung and its stage of development.

Nursing Assessment and Intervention   Care of the patient undergoing thoracotomy for cancer of the lung follows later in the chapter. See Chapter 9 for nursing care of the patient with cancer.

◆ Sleep Apnea

Sleep apnea affects 4% to 8% of the adult population in the United States. It is characterized by repetitive episodes of upper airway occlusion during sleep associated with decreased arterial oxygen saturation. Signs and symptoms are excessive daytime sleepiness, loud snoring, complaints of disrupted sleep, tiredness upon awakening, awakening during the night short of breath, and morning headaches. Apneic episodes must last at least 10 seconds and occur 10 to 15 times an hour to be clinically significant. Diagnosis is by polysomnogram, sleep studies, with O_2 saturation testing. If the problem occurs only while the patient is lying on the back, wearing a fanny-pack with tennis balls in it may cure the problem by preventing that position. Otherwise surgery to correct upper airway deformities and obstructions may be necessary or continuous positive airway pressure (CPAP) or biphasic positive airway pressure therapy at night may be employed. This involves using a face mask or nasal cannula during sleep that is attached to a portable ventilator.

◆ Chest Injuries

Injury to the chest wall and underlying structures can range from minor bruises to major trauma to the pulmonary and cardiovascular systems. Thoracic trauma is a major cause of accidental death, exceeding head and facial injuries. Whenever there is evidence of chest injury, a very real state of emergency exists, because the condition of the victim can rapidly deteriorate to death.

The major complications of chest trauma involve either the lungs and air passages or the heart and major blood vessels, or both. Pneumothorax and hemothorax frequently occur as a result of a blunt (nonpenetrating) or penetrating injury to the chest wall. These conditions can cause partial or total collapse of one or both lungs. There also can be contusion of the myocardium, rupture of the aorta, and tracheobronchial or tracheo-abdominal injuries. The procedure to correct pneumothorax or hemothorax is to insert a thoracostomy tube (chest tube) (Figure 16-12).

> Major concerns in the care of patients with chest injuries are (1) maintenance of an airway; (2) assurance of adequate ventilation; and (3) treatment of circulatory problems to ensure circulation of oxygenated blood.

Flail Chest   When a patient experiences severe chest trauma in an automobile accident or fall, often several ribs are broken. When three or more ribs are broken in two or more places, the chest wall becomes unstable. This condition is called *flail chest*. It produces "paradoxical respirations." When the patient breathes in, the fractured portion of the chest is drawn inward instead of expanding outward as the rest of the chest does; when he exhales, the flail portion expands outward as the rest of the chest collapses normally. This process interferes with oxygenation, as the lungs cannot expand normally. Emergency treatment consists of turning the patient onto the affected side so that the ground or bed will act as a splint and reduce the pain of breathing. The patient is observed for signs of external and internal bleeding, pneumothorax, and shock. The fractured ribs may cause tissue damage to the lung.

Once the patient is in an emergency facility, flail chest is treated by intubation and mechanical ventilation while the ribs heal. This causes considerable pain, and the patient usually has to be given a neuromuscular blocking agent such as pancuronium bromide (Pavulon) to prevent fighting the action of the ventilator. In addition, IV morphine or meperidine is given for pain control and sedation to decrease anxiety over being totally paralyzed. The patient should never be left totally alone without a nurse or personnel in sight as the fear of being paralyzed and having something go wrong with the ventilator or tubing connections when totally alone is terrifying.

Penetrating Wounds   Victims of stabbing can have an open chest wound that creates serious respiratory difficulties. An open, or "sucking" chest wound is one in which pneumothorax results from penetration of the

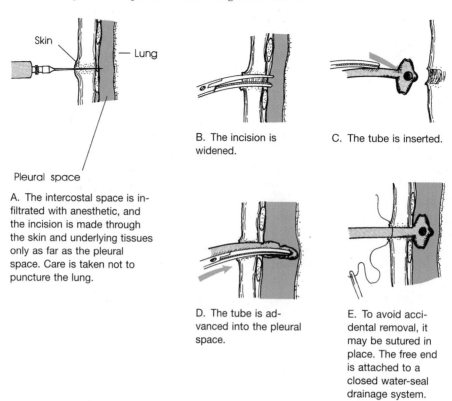

A. The intercostal space is infiltrated with anesthetic, and the incision is made through the skin and underlying tissues only as far as the pleural space. Care is taken not to puncture the lung.

B. The incision is widened.

C. The tube is inserted.

D. The tube is advanced into the pleural space.

E. To avoid accidental removal, it may be sutured in place. The free end is attached to a closed water-seal drainage system.

FIGURE 16-12   Insertion of a thoracostomy tube (chest tube).

pleural cavity, which allows air and gas to accumulate there. Symptoms of pneumothorax include labored, shallow respirations and lack of movement on one side of the chest when the person inhales and exhales. A sucking chest wound should be covered at the end of a forceful expiration with an occlusive dressing—that is one made of plastic wrap, aluminum foil, Vaseline covered gauze, or any other material that seals the wound and prohibits the flow of air into the pleural cavity. **One corner of the dressing is left unsealed to allow accumulated air to escape.** Place the patient in a semi-Fowler's position if possible.

If a knife or other item is stuck into the chest cavity, do not remove it; stabilize it so that it does not move around and cause more damage as the patient is transported to an emergency facility. The object may be wedged against severed vessels preventing them from bleeding; removing it may cause hemorrhage.

Pneumothorax and Hemothorax   The space within the pleural membranes is an airtight compartment. Pressure within this compartment is less than that of the atmosphere and therefore is called a *negative pressure*. This negative pressure is necessary to allow sufficient space for normal breathing in which the tidal movement of air in and out of the lungs inflates and deflates them. If, however, there is a break in the airtight compartment, either along the surface of the lung or from outside the pleural sac, air rushes in and collapses the lung. The

presence of air or gas within the pleural cavity is called **pneumothorax** (Figure 16-13).

Pneumothorax always is a threat in chest injury, as well as in the period following chest surgery. However, the condition also can occur spontaneously when there is a pathological opening on the surface of the lung that allows a leakage of air from the bronchi into the pleural cavity. This condition is called a *spontaneous pneumothorax*. Treatment for spontaneous pneumothorax may

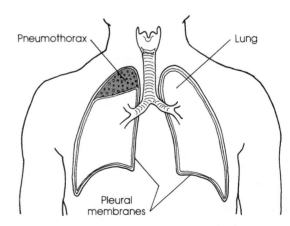

Air within the pleural cavity has entered some of the space normally occupied by the lung, thus preventing its expansion and causing partial collapse. A chest tube for the drainage of the air would be located in the upper chest.

FIGURE 16-13   Pneumothorax.

require nothing more than rest and the administration of oxygen to relieve discomfort. A chest tube is inserted to remove the air and allow reexpansion of the lung.

Tension pneumothorax develops when air enters the pleural space on inspiration but remains trapped there rather than being expelled on expiration. It can occur from trauma, mechanical ventilation, or rib fracture during CPR. The air in the pleural space increases with each breath, and the pressure within the chest builds, which gradually collapses the lung. If unrelieved, this increasing pressure will cause a *mediastinal shift*, resulting in a decrease in cardiac output and blood pressure. Mediastinal shift means that the structures in the mediastinum—the heart, great vessels, trachea, and esophagus—are all shifted to the unaffected side of the chest. In this case, a flutter valve needle is inserted until a chest tube can be placed to remove the air from the pleural cavity.

Hemothorax is the presence of blood within the pleural cavity. It can occur as a result of laceration of the lung, heart, and blood vessels within the thorax. The accumulation of blood in the pleural cavity can have the same effect as accumulations of gas or air, that is, it fills up space and causes partial or total collapse of the lung. There also is the possibility of mediastinal shift in hemothorax and the likelihood of impaired venous return in the pulmonary blood vessels. The blood is removed by chest drainage.

Assessment of a patient for pneumothorax, hemothorax, or a combination of the two (hemopneumothorax, Figure 16-14), includes awareness of the patient's history in regard to acute or chronic respiratory disease, accidental injury to the chest, or chest surgery. The condition is suspected when the patient complains of sudden chest pain or a feeling of tightness in the chest. There will be an increase in both pulse rate and rate of respirations, a drop in blood pressure, and the absence of normal chest movements on the affected side when the patient breathes.

Think about... You come upon an automobile accident and stop to assist. You are on your way to work and have your stethoscope with you. Name three assessment criteria that would lead you to believe that the driver of the vehicle has suffered a pneumothorax.

◆ Pulmonary Edema

Acute pulmonary edema is a medical emergency. Congestive heart failure, particularly of left ventricular failure, is a major cause of pulmonary edema. Signs and symptoms include severe dyspnea, orthopnea, noisy respirations, frothy sputum, crackles heard on auscultation in the bases of the lungs extending upward, abnormal blood gases, anxiety, restlessness, and possibly confusion. Diagnosis is based on ruling out other disorders, such as pneumonia, asthma, pulmonary embolism, and on determining the cause. Treatment depends to some degree on whether the edema is a result of heart problems or from another cause (see ARDS).

Both IV morphine sulfate and furosemide are given for fluid diuresis. The morphine reduces anxiety and the workload on the heart. Oxygen is started immediately. Aminophylline may be ordered to relax the bronchial smooth muscle. Drugs for the underlying heart disorder also are ordered.

Nursing care involves providing reassurance to the patient to decrease anxiety, closely monitoring fluid intake and output, administering drugs, and performing continuous respiratory and cardiac assessment to evaluate the effectiveness of treatment.

◆ Adult Respiratory Distress Syndrome (ARDS)

Adult respiratory distress syndrome (ARDS) is a form of pulmonary edema that is not heart related. It results from pulmonary changes that occur in connection with many disorders, including sepsis, trauma, cardiac or other major surgery, and any critical illness. It is a particular danger when a patient has multisystem disorders. Mortality is 30% to 60%. **The hallmark for diagnosis is a paO$_2$ below 70 mm Hg even with 100% oxygen delivery.** Pulmonary edema and lung stiffness occur, resulting in severe hypoxemia. Treatment is ventilatory support and treatment of the underlying disorder, careful fluid and electrolyte management, and total care for basic needs. Liquid ventilation may become the favored treatment for ARDS. It is presently

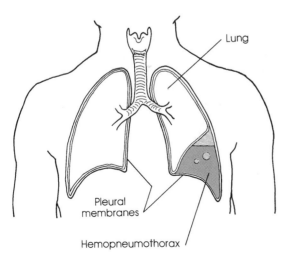

A collection of air and blood in the pleural space causes inadequate lung expansion. A chest tube would be placed in the lower chest to drain the blood and air.

FIGURE 16-14   Hemopneumothorax.

under investigation at six centers in the United States. See the section on Modes of Ventilation.

◆ Pulmonary Embolism

Pulmonary embolism (PE) occurs when a pulmonary vessel is plugged with a mass or clot. Emboli can occur in solid, liquid, or gas forms and can occur from fracture of a long bone (fat embolus), from amniotic fluid during childbirth, from air introduced through a central line, and from clots formed elsewhere in the body, such as from a deep vein thrombosis or thrombi that form in the heart when the patient has dysrhythmias. Regardless of the origin of the embolus, the result is the same: interference with blood flow in the lung distal to the point where the embolus lodges. The obstruction causes shunting to occur at the alveoli that are no longer filling with air. Blood flows past without receiving oxygen or giving up carbon dioxide and hypoxia results.

Elder Care Point . . . The elderly are especially prone to developing deep venous thrombosis when they are immobilized from surgery or for a major illness. Preventing dehydration in these patients helps prevent thrombus formation. Many elderly patients with heart disease suffer cardiac dysrhythmias that predispose to the formation of thrombi in the heart. The dysrhythmia atrial fibrillation when uncontrolled is a direct cause of pulmonary emboli. The discovery of a new irregularity of heart beat upon assessment of the elderly patient should be reported to the physician promptly.

Symptoms depend on the size and location of the clot and whether there is one clot or multiple small clots. **The general symptoms are respiratory distress with dyspnea, chest pain, cough, hemoptysis, and anxiety.** Hypotension and tachycardia may occur. **A sudden onset of dyspnea in a patient at risk of thrombus formation is very suggestive of PE.** The consequences of pulmonary embolism can be minor or life-threatening.

The nurse should stay with the patient, raise the head of the bed to a high Fowler's position, begin low-flow oxygen therapy if there is oxygen in the room, assess vital signs, notify the physician of the patient's symptoms, and administer heparin when it is ordered.

Diagnosis is made by ruling out other problems, such as heart failure, and by tests to support a diagnosis of pulmonary embolus. Arterial blood gases are drawn, a 12-lead EKG and chest radiograph are ordered, and an echocardiogram will most likely be done. If the data seem to indicate that the cause of symptoms is PE, a ventilation/perfusion scan is performed. A pulmonary angiogram is the "gold standard" for detecting a PE, but it is an expensive procedure that is invasive and not without risk as it involves a right-sided heart catheterization.

Treatment depends on the size and location of the embolus. Intravenous heparin is usually begun and continued for 7 to 10 days. Warfarin (Coumadin) is initiated several days before discharge and is continued at home for up to 1 year. Some physicians are performing trials with thrombolytic therapy using streptokinase, urokinase, or t-PA. There is concern about whether the benefits of lysing the clot outweigh the risk of bleeding complications. Pulmonary embolectomy is a last resort because the surgery carries a high mortality rate.

COMMON THERAPEUTIC MEASURES

◆ Intrathoracic Surgery

Many kinds of surgical procedures require opening the chest wall and entering the pleural cavity. For example, in addition to resection of lung tissue and other pulmonary structures, intrathoracic surgery also is necessary to repair the heart and great vessels and to correct defects of the esophagus.

Today *endoscopic thoracotomy*, also called video thoroscopy, is replacing the traditional standard thoracotomy for many surgical procedures in the chest cavity. About 70% of thoracic procedures can be performed endoscopically, including pulmonary resections, biopsy or resection of mediastinal tumors or masses, and drainage of pleural effusions. An endoscope equipped with a multichip minicamera, along with intense lighting, magnifies the image of the cavity and structures and transmits it to a video monitor. Instruments can be guided through the endoscope to biopsy or remove tissue and to place surgical staples. One to four 1-inch incisions are used to accommodate the endoscope, instruments, and suction.

Preoperative Care   Assessment of the patient's respiratory status prior to chest surgery depends on whether the surgery is elective or in response to accidental trauma. If there is time, history taking and obtaining subjective and objective assessment data will be essentially the same as described earlier.

Preoperatively efforts are made to improve the respiratory status of the patient as much as possible. Special exercises may be prescribed to strengthen chest and shoulder muscles and accessory muscles of respiration and to remove accumulated secretions from the air passages.

When standard thoracotomy is to be performed, arm and leg exercises are also taught preoperatively to avoid thrombophlebitis in the lower extremities and problems with movement of the arm on the operative side. Movement of the arm may be very painful, because of either the position in which the patient was placed during surgery or the surgical involvement of muscles that control the arm. If the arm is not moved in spite of discomfort, the patient may develop a "frozen" (immobile) shoulder. Patients undergoing endoscopic thoracotomy do not have this complication.

Preoperative patient education focuses on teaching the patient techniques to use after surgery to improve lung ventilation. Information about chest tubes, suctioning, mechanical ventilation, use of an incentive spirometer, and any other procedures that are anticipated as part of postoperative care is given.

Postoperative Care   During the immediate postoperative period, nursing assessment and intervention focus on special observations (in addition to routine postoperative ones), positioning, routine turning, coughing and deep-breathing, and attention to chest tubes and the closed drainage system. In spite of the tubes and machines used postoperatively, the patient with chest surgery usually must ambulate early. An advantage of endoscopic thoracotomy is that the patient is out of bed and into a chair within 4 to 6 hours of surgery. Because pain is less, the patient is better able to move around and can more quickly resume normal activities. Where the standard thoracotomy patient has a 4- to 6-week recovery, the endoscopic thoracotomy patient resumes ADLS in 3 to 4 days and can even return to work within 1 week.

Interpleural analgesia may be used for the postoperative standard thoracotomy patient. An analgesic agent is administered through a catheter that has been placed percutaneously in the interpleural space or is introduced via an injection lumen of the chest tube. Suction is turned off for 15 minutes when medication is instilled. Injections are given every 4 to 6 hours rather than on a PRN basis.

Assessment   Special observations include watching for signs of pneumothorax, hemothorax, or both; symptoms of respiratory distress; and auscultation and palpation of the upper chest and neck for swelling caused by *subcutaneous emphysema*, which is an accumulation of air or gas under the skin. It usually occurs after thoracic surgery when air leaks into the tissues around chest tubes. It could be a sign of malfunctioning of the drainage system and should be reported. Inspecting the drainage system for signs of air leak is essential. Assessing signs of infection, both respiratory and incisional, is very important.

Gastric distention and paralytic ileus also are possible complications of standard thoracic surgery. **Distention of the stomach and intestines is particularly hazardous for the postthoracotomy patient, as it can cause these organs to push up on the diaphragm and impair ventilation, which is already severely compromised by the surgery.**

Positioning. Positioning for comfort, optimal ventilation, and adequate drainage of the operative site is an important aspect of postthoracotomy care. In most cases the patient is allowed to lie on his back and operative side. Many surgeons do not permit lying on the unaffected side, because this position diminishes the expansion of the good lung. There is also danger of infection of the good lung by drainage from the side of the affected lung if the patient lies with the operative side uppermost. When the patient has a tube inserted for drainage from the operative site, lying on the operative side facilitates the flow of drainage. **Care must be taken when positioning the patient to prevent kinking the chest tubes.**

A pneumonectomy patient is never turned on to his unoperated side, because first, tension pneumothorax and mediastinal shift could occur, and second, the bronchial stump where the lung was removed could leak and the patient could drown in accumulated fluid.

When in doubt about positioning a patient who has had chest surgery, it is always best to check the physician's orders before turning the patient or raising the head of the bed.

Chest Tubes and Closed Drainage.   Of all the special procedures and techniques used to care for a patient who has had chest surgery, the use of tubes and a drainage system to allow reexpansion of the lung is probably the most anxiety-producing for many nurses (Figure 16-15).

Care of patients with chest tubes and closed drainage.   Chest tubes inserted during surgery may be attached to any of a variety of drainage systems. Among these are *disposable plastic water-sealed drainage systems* and bottle systems with one, two, or three bottles. **Whatever system is used, its purposes are (1) to provide for drainage of air and blood from within the pleural cavity; and (2) to allow for gradual reexpansion of the**

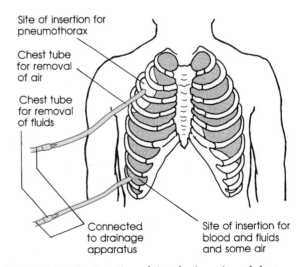

Site of insertion for pneumothorax

Chest tube for removal of air

Chest tube for removal of fluids

Connected to drainage apparatus

Site of insertion for blood and fluids and some air

FIGURE 16-15   Location of sites for insertion of chest tubes for drainage of air and fluids.

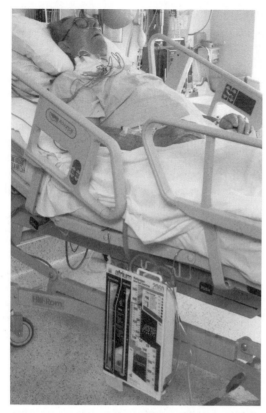

FIGURE 16-16 Disposable water seal drainage system hooked up to chest tube of postsurgery patient. (Photo by Glen Derbyshire; courtesy of Goleta Valley Cottage Hospital, Goleta, CA.)

lung. Figure 16-16 shows a disposable system. Note that the water in the left-hand chamber serves as a seal to avoid the return of air to the chest cavity. **The water level will fluctuate as the patient breathes.** There should not be bubbles in this chamber. The collection chamber, located on the far right of the device, is calibrated for more accurate measurement of drainage from the chest. It also contains float valves, which prevent the entry of air or fluid back up into the chest. Suction can be attached to the device to better facilitate removal of air and secretions from the lung. Specialized chest drainage systems are used to collect the patient's blood from the chest after surgery so that it can be reinfused in an autologous transfusion.

A flutter valve may be substituted in closed chest drainage systems. This valve permits the flow of air and fluid from the pleural space into a collection area, but prevents the return flow of air or fluid and is inserted between the chest tube and the drainage collection apparatus.

Caring for a Closed Drainage System

The following should be kept in mind:

- Remember that the pleural cavity is an airtight compartment. The apparatus and all connections must remain airtight at all times; all connections should be taped.
- Do not allow the tubing to become kinked or obstructed by the weight of the patient.
- Never pin the tubing to the bed clothes.
- Do not empty thoracotomy drainage containers. Replace the container when the drainage chamber is full.
- Dressings may be reinforced but are not changed except by order of the surgeon.

Special aspects of patient care. Monitor the patient who has a chest tube regularly and frequently. There are three major areas of assessment: (1) the respiratory status of the patient; (2) the site at which the tube is inserted into the chest and the length of the tube for kinks; and (3) the amount and character of the drainage in the collection chamber.

The patient is assessed for ease of breathing, pain or discomfort, level of consciousness and orientation, and anxiety and restlessness. The rate and character of respirations are noted, as are breath sounds. The entry site is assessed for unusual drainage, integrity of sutures, and the presence of subcutaneous emphysema.

The drainage tubing must be patent at all times, unless clamped off by the surgeon or momentarily in an emergency when there is leakage of air. It cannot be occluded by kinks, compression, or dependent loops; otherwise gas, air, and fluid have no way of escaping from the pleural cavity. It must be airtight; otherwise air will enter the pleural cavity and collapse the lung.

In addition to respiratory distress in the patient, conditions that require immediate attention are:

- Persistent bubbling in the underwater seal that indicates a leak in the system. Fluid in the chamber *should* fluctuate as the patient breathes air in and out.
- Fluid drainage through the chest tube accumulating at a rate of more than 100 mL per hour.
- A "puffed-up" appearance caused by leakage of air (subcutaneous emphysema) into the subcutaneous tissues in the upper chest and neck. (This feels like bubble wrap when palpated.)
- Leakage of air around the junctions in the chest tube and drainage tube and disposable drainage device.

The patient should be medicated 30 to 60 minutes before removing a chest tube. When the surgeon removes the chest tubes, he will cover the incision with a dressing containing sterile petroleum jelly to close off the opening so that air does not enter the pleural space. Eventually the incision will seal itself. A sample plan for care of a patient having thoracic surgery is shown in Nursing Care Plan 16-1.

Nursing Care Plan 16-1

Selected nursing diagnoses, goals/expected outcomes, nursing interventions, and evaluations for a patient having thoracic surgery

Situation: A 58-year-old male smoker with a diagnosis of early lung cancer is scheduled for a right thoracotomy and lobectomy. He has no other medical problems except mild arthritis, for which he occasionally takes aspirin.

Nursing Diagnosis	Goals/Expected Outcomes	Nursing Intervention	Evaluation
Knowledge deficit related to postoperative care for thoracotomy SUPPORTING DATA "I've never had surgery before."	Patient will demonstrate leg and arm exercises. Patient will verbalize understanding of postoperative routine of frequent monitoring of vital signs, chest tube care, and respiratory treatments.	Teach deep-breathing, coughing, arm and leg exercises; obtain return demonstration. Explain kind and purpose of tubes, drainage appratus, and oxygen equipment. Explain need for early ambulation. Describe methods of pain control.	Returned demonstration of turning, coughing, exercises, and deep-breathing; states tubes he will have postoperatively; verbalizes understanding of pain control method with patient-controlled analgesia (PCA) pump.
Postoperative period: Risk of impaired gas exchange related to surgical removal of portion of lung and possible complications. SUPPORTING DATA Thoracotomy and lobectomy.	Patient will display normal respiratory rate and normal blood gas exchange within 36 hours.	Position patient on back or operative side; turn, cough, and deep-breathe using incentive spirometer q 2 h; splint incision with small pillow to minimize pain. Administer humidified oxygen as ordered. Monitor vital signs q 4 h and respirations frequently; auscultate lung fields q shift; monitor blood gas levels. Pulse oximetry readings q 1 h × 4, then q 2 h. Report SaO$_2$ <90%. Medicate adequately for pain control to promote better cooperation with respiratory therapy, coughing, and deep-breathing, but avoid oversedation and respiratory depression. Maintain intact, functioning closed chest drainage system. Observe for signs of subcutaneous emphysema; assess for signs of pulmonary embolism. Monitor abdomen for signs of distention or ileus, which could cause pressure on diaphragm.	Turn, cough, and deep-breathe 8, 10, 12, and 2; splinting with pillow; oxygen per nasal cannula on continuously; lung fields clear to auscultation; using PCA appropriately; chest tube system intact, fluid fluctuating properly; SaO$_2$ 92%; blood gases: P$_{O_2}$, 76; P$_{CO_2}$, 46; HCO$_3$, 26. resp., 26 min; continue plan.
Risk for infection related to surgical incisions and chest tubes. SUPPORTING DATA Thoracotomy and lobectomy; chest tube in place.	No signs of infection as evidenced by clean incision, temperature in normal range, normal white blood cell (WBC) count, and clear breath sounds.	Use aseptic technique for dressing changes and care of chest tube. Assess temperature trends q 24 h; monitor WBCs. Auscultate lungs q shift. Observe wound for signs of infection. Protect from people with infections; maintain adequate nutrition and fluid intake.	Incision clean and dry; temperature, 100° F; WBC, 10,000; breath sounds clear bilaterally; continue plan.
Anxiety related to diagnosis of cancer of the lung, treatment, and prognosis. SUPPORTING DATA "I'm scared. I don't want to die of cancer. Will I have to have chemotherapy? Will there be a lot of pain?"	Patient will cope positively with diagnosis of cancer by determined attitude to do whatever he can to fight the cancer by discharge.	Establish trusting relationship; use active listening. Encourage verbalization of fears and concerns; answer questions honestly. Establish hope; discuss what patient can do to optimize chances of survival: quit smoking, exercise program, diet, relaxation techniques, stress reduction. Advise that oncologist will discuss modes of treatment after full pathology report is back. Focus on positives of his life now and for each day in the future; assure him that pain control is possible.	Asking questions about radiation therapy; has quit smoking; wants to learn relaxation techniques; continue plan.

Think about... What would you do if you went to assess your first-day postop standard thoracotomy patient and the water in the closed drainage system was not fluctuating with the patient's breathing?

◆ Medications

A wide variety of drugs are used to treat respiratory disorders. Patients often take several drugs simultaneously, and **it is vitally important that the nurse monitor side effects and drug interactions.** Current treatment is mainly by inhalation, but some drugs are taken orally.

Bronchodilators are drugs that act directly on the smooth muscle of the bronchi to relax them and thereby relieve bronchospasms. Among the bronchodilators are *aminophylline, epinephrine hydrochloride* (adrenalin and Vaponefrin), *isoproterenol hydrochloride* (Isuprel), *ephedrine sulfate,* and adrenergic drugs such as *metaproterenol* (Alupent), *terbutaline* (Brethine), and *salmeterol xinafoate* (Serevent). See Table 16-15 for general nursing implications for these drugs. Theophylline preparations are tolerated better if they are taken after meals so that there is less stomach upset. **The pulse should be assessed before and after the patient takes this medication. If the pulse increases more than 20 to 30 beats, the physician should be notified.** Patients taking theophylline derivatives should have serum drug levels assessed periodically; therapeutic range is 8 to 20 g/mL. Patients receiving IV aminophylline must be monitored for hypotension.

Liquefying agents and *diluents* help to thin the bronchial secretions, making them more liquid and less tenacious. Preparations of this type include *acetylcysteine* (Mucomyst), distilled water, and *tyloxapol* (Alevaire).

Antiinfectives are helpful in controlling infectious agents in the respiratory tract. These include the tetracyclines, penicillin, cephalosporin antibiotics (cephalothin, Keflin), clarithromycin (Biaxin), ciprofloxacin (Cipro), streptomycin, and the sulfa drugs.

Corticosteroids are a major part of inhalation therapy for patients with CAL. However, acute respiratory problems are sometimes treated with oral corticosteroids.

When corticosteroids are part of drug therapy, the patient must be closely watched for infection, as steroids may mask signs and symptoms. She must be cautioned never abruptly to stop taking a steroid drug; it is to be slowly tapered over several days to prevent the serious problems of abrupt steroid withdrawal. Potassium loss must be replaced and monitoring for elevated blood glucose performed.

Antihistamines are used to treat respiratory symptoms of an allergic disorder. They reduce the secretions

of the nasal and bronchial mucosa. *Decongestants* are prescribed for symptoms of the common cold and sinusitis.

In 1996 a new class of asthma drug was approved. Accolate (Zafirlakast) helps control symptoms by blocking the activity of substances that mediate inflammation called *leukotrienes.*

TABLE 16-15 ◆ *General Nursing Implications for the Administration of Bronchodilators*

When giving a bronchodilator drug, the nurse should

◆ Check the ID band of the patient before administering each dose to ensure that the right patient receives the drug.
◆ Follow the "five rights" of medication administration to prevent errors and injury to the patient.
◆ Verify allergies and inquire about previous adverse reaction to the drug.
◆ Auscultate the lungs to ascertain types of lung sounds present.
◆ Take pulse and count respirations to establish ranges prior to drug administration.
◆ Use these drugs cautiously in patients with cardiac disease as they affect heart action.
◆ Consult physician before administering a bronchodilator to a patient who has a current cardiac dysrhythmia.
◆ Give the drug with a full glass of water or with meals to decrease the possibility of gastrointestinal upset.
◆ Give each dose of the drug as close to the ordered time as possible to maintain a steady blood level of the drug.
◆ When patient is taking theophylline, check therapeutic drug serum levels; therapeutic range is 10 to 20 µg/mL. Withhold drug if level is above 20 µg/mL and notify the physician.
◆ Warn elderly patients that the drug may cause dizziness and to take precautions when changing positions.
◆ Monitor the patient for effectiveness of the drug by performing a respiratory assessment.

Regarding possible side effect or adverse effects of the drug, the nurse should

◆ Warn the patient about the possibility of paradoxical bronchospasm and advise to consult the physician if this happens before administering another dose.
◆ Tell the patient to chew sugarless gum or suck on hard candy to relieve dry mouth.
◆ Monitor the patient for specific side effects of each drug; general side effects of bronchodilators are: dry mouth, insomnia, nervousness, dizziness, palpitations, gastrointestinal upset, changes in blood pressure.

The nurse should teach the patient taking a bronchodilator drug to

◆ Take the drug with a full glass of water; if it causes gastrointestinal upset, take the drug with a meal.
◆ Take the drug 15 to 60 minutes before exercising (check specific time for individual drug as time depends on form of the drug (i.e., inhalant or oral tablet).
◆ Follow correct procedure for inhaling the drug: shake the inhaler gently before using; clear the nose and throat; take a deep breath, relax, and completely exhale before inhaling drug.

Metered dose inhalers (MDIs) are used to deliver a variety of drugs to the respiratory patient. The patient should be taught to exhale completely, insert the mouthpiece of the inhaler into his mouth, and depress the cylinder while inhaling deeply. The breath is then held for a few seconds before exhaling. **It is important to have the patient demonstrate how she uses an inhaler to determine whether her technique is correct.**

Bronchodilators, liquefying agents, and some anti-infectives may be administered directly onto the mucous membranes of the respiratory tract by means of nebulizers and mechanical ventilators.

◆ Humidification

Aerosols are fine suspensions of very small particles of a liquid or solid that constitute a gas. Water is the most important of all aerosols in respiratory therapy. Without adequate humidity, mucous secretions become extremely thick and tenacious, and the mucous membranes become dry, crusted, and irritated. They are then more susceptible to invasion by pathogenic microorganisms. Aerosols other than water include a variety of bronchodilating or mucolytic drugs.

The four general purposes of aerosol and humidity therapy are (1) relief of edema and spasms of the bronchi; (2) liquefaction of bronchial secretions; (3) delivery of medication; and (4) humidification of the respiratory mucosa.

Aerosol Jet Nebulization therapy is used to deliver medication or large amounts of liquid to help liquefy respiratory secretions so that they can be mobilized. *Aerosol* means liquid or solid particles suspended in a gas. Aerosols are delivered by a *nebulizer*. There are several types of nebulizers: (1) a metered-dose device (inhaler); (2) a handheld nebulizer; and (3) an intermittent positive pressure breathing (IPPB) device. Aerosol is delivered by face mask, face tent, or tracheostomy collar. Most aerosols are produced in a jet nebulizer in which a high-velocity gas shatters the liquid into small aerosol particles. Many CAL patients have been switched from IPPB nebulization treatments to handheld nebulizers to deliver their aerosol medications. In the hospital the nebulizer is attached to oxygen so that hypoxemia can be treated as medication is being administered. There are a variety of home nebulizer units in use, such as the Puritan nebulizer or the Ohio Deluxe nebulizer. Nebulizer treatments are usually 20 to 30 minutes long and are given two, three, or four times a day.

The patient is taught to breathe through the mouth during the treatment. She should sit in a comfortable chair. Halfway through the treatment and after the treatment, deep-breathing and coughing are performed to raise loose mucus. Equipment is cleaned and dried before storing.

When a handheld nebulizer is used, the patient should sit upright with the chin pointed slightly upward. The nebulizer cartridge should be shaken before beginning the treatment. The patient fully exhales, begins inhaling, and depresses the cartridge fully, continuing to inhale slowly and as deeply as possible. She should hold her breath for a few seconds and then slowly exhale. Equipment should be cleaned after each treatment to minimize the risk of infection.

◆ Pulmonary Hygiene

Patients with chronic pulmonary disease can benefit from a program of pulmonary hygiene that is designed (1) to remove secretions for more efficient exchange of oxygen and carbon dioxide; and (2) to help them control their breathing so that it is more effective in moving air in and out of the lungs. Pulmonary hygiene programs are achieved by administering prescribed drugs, humidification of the air inhaled, nebulizer and MDI therapy, chest physiotherapy, and breathing exercises.

Chest physiotherapy includes postural drainage when possible and percussion and vibration. *Postural drainage* involves positioning the patient so that the forces of gravity can help remove secretions deep in the bronchi and lungs (Figure 16-17). The nurse who assists a patient with postural drainage should obtain specific directions from the physician or physical therapist so that the patient can be positioned properly. Tapping, clapping, and vibrating techniques sometimes are used during postural drainage. These measures are carried out for the purpose of dislodging mucus plugs so that they can be coughed up more easily. They must be done with precision and only by someone who has received adequate instruction in the proper technique. Family members can be taught the procedures if they are to be continued after the patient goes home.

Because there is likely to be some gagging during coughing episodes that take place during postural drainage, it is best to carry out the procedure before meals, when the stomach is relatively empty and vomiting is less likely.

Elder Care Point... The elderly patient usually tolerates vibrating techniques during postural drainage better than clapping. Elderly patients with osteoporosis are at risk for fractures of the vertebrae and ribs and clapping should not be used on these patients.

If the patient is to have postural drainage only once a day, it should be done in the morning when he

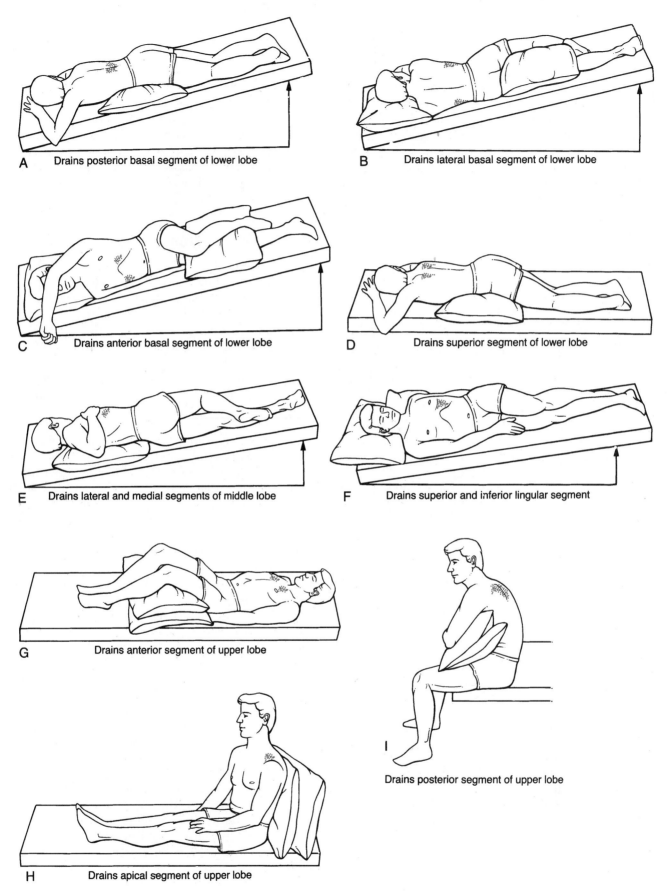

A Drains posterior basal segment of lower lobe

B Drains lateral basal segment of lower lobe

C Drains anterior basal segment of lower lobe

D Drains superior segment of lower lobe

E Drains lateral and medial segments of middle lobe

F Drains superior and inferior lingular segment

G Drains anterior segment of upper lobe

I Drains posterior segment of upper lobe

H Drains apical segment of upper lobe

FIGURE 16-17 Positions for postural drainage. The patient assumes various positions to facilitate the flow of secretions from various portions of the lung and the bronchi, trachea, and throat so that the secretions can be expectorated. The drawing shows the various positions used to drain each segment of the lung. (*Source:* Monahan, F. D., Drake, T., Neighbors, M. [1994]. *Nursing Care of Adults.* Philadelphia: Saunders, p. 444.)

awakens. At this time, secretions that have accumulated during the night can be removed. After postural drainage is completed, good mouth care, including tooth brushing and a refreshing mouth wash, should be given.

The most important aspects of breathing exercises include blowing through pursed lips, exhaling slowly, and *not* forcing the air out of the lungs (this can bring about the collapse of the airway structures). Breathing through pursed lips is described in Table 16-11.

The mechanics of respiration can become less efficient as chronic respiratory disease progresses. The patient suffers a loss of lung elasticity, a flattened diaphragm, and fixation of the rib cage as she becomes more and more dependent on the muscles of her upper chest and neck for breathing. Difficulty in breathing causes respiratory muscle fatigue.

> The purpose of breathing exercises is to help correct this situation by strengthening the abdominal muscles so that they can push upward against the diaphragm and assist in the expiration of air from the lungs.

These exercises also help overcome rigidity of the thorax so that the lungs can inflate and deflate more easily.

Patients who follow the exercises prescribed for them often find that they can lead more active and useful lives than formerly possible because their exertional dyspnea is less severe. This means that they can make better use of all the muscles of their body and are less likely to develop complications that accompany immobility. (Chapter 11). They are also better able to cough up secretions that would otherwise remain in the lower bronchi and serve as a growth medium for bacteria or as a cause of atelectasis. The psychological value of being able to indulge in ordinary activities that once left the patient breathless cannot be overestimated. Abdominal and diaphragmatic breathing are described in Table 16-8.

◆ Oxygen Therapy

Because oxygen acts as a drug, it must be prescribed and administered in specific doses to avoid oxygen toxicity. The dosage of oxygen is stated in terms of *concentration* and rate of *flow*.

High concentrations (above 50%) may be prescribed to treat acute conditions in which the patient can benefit from prompt treatment of hypoxia, as in cardiovascular failure and pulmonary edema. The rate of flow may be as high as 12 L per minute.

Moderate concentrations of oxygen usually are prescribed when increased metabolic rate raises the consumption of oxygen or when there is poor distribution of oxygen because of either congestive heart failure or pulmonary embolism. **The concentrations of oxygen** given in a moderate dosage are about 23% at a rate of flow of 4 to 7 L per minute.

Low concentrations of oxygen of about 23% delivered at a rate of 1 to 3 L per minute are indicated when the patient needs oxygen over an extended period. Patients with chronic respiratory insufficiency who can utilize only a minimum amount of oxygen in a given period usually are given low doses of oxygen.

The above percentages and rates of flow are approximate amounts. The exact dosage depends on the method of administration and the patient's individual need for additional oxygen supply.

> Short-term oxygen therapy, which is the administration of oxygen to treat hypoxemia, is indicated when (1) there is an inadequate intake of oxygen because of obstruction or restriction of airflow through the air passages; (2) oxygen is not distributed throughout the body because of circulatory failure; (3) there is an inadequate supply of hemoglobin to transport the oxygen; and (4) carbon dioxide or other gases displace the oxygen in the blood. Objective criteria for oxygen needs include PaO_2 less than 60 mm Hg or SaO_2 less than 90%.

Outward signs of hypoxia vary in patients and therefore cannot be completely relied on as indications that additional oxygen is needed. Dyspnea and confusion are the most common signs seen. More reliable indicators are the results obtained from blood gas analysis and determination of the blood pH. Not all patients with hypoxia can benefit from oxygen therapy.

Long-term oxygen therapy for patients with CAL is used (1) to relieve hypoxemia; (2) to reverse tissue hypoxia and its signs and symptoms; and (3) to allow the patient to function better mentally and physically, thereby allowing greater self-reliance. Home oxygen units and portable units are available for patients who require long-term therapy.

The patient with CAL obtains signals to breath from oxygen levels in the blood. **If this patient is given too much oxygen, it will depress respiration.**

Even though oxygen is essential to life, excessive amounts are toxic and can have serious adverse effects on the tissues of the body. High concentrations of inhaled oxygen can bring about collapse of the alveoli, because the oxygen displaces some of the nitrogen there. Another effect of high oxygen concentration is an interruption in the production of *pulmonary surfactant,* a substance that stabilizes the alveoli and prevents atelectasis.

Modes of Administration   The manner in which additional oxygen is supplied to a patient depends on his particular need for oxygen and his physical condition.

Methods of administration are divided into high-flow and low-flow systems.

Low-flow systems. Low-flow systems use a flow rate of less than 5 L per minute and are often not humidified.

Oxygen by nasal cannula. This is the simplest, most convenient, and most commonly used means of administering oxygen (Figure 16-18). The two-pronged nasal cannula is inserted one-fourth to one-half inch into each nostril, **with the curved prongs pointing downward.** *This method does not provide sufficient oxygen concentration for a patient with severe hypoxemia.*

Oxygen by mask. Care must be taken to ensure that the mask fits snugly and follows the contour of the face. The mask should be removed briefly periodically so that the patient's face can be washed to prevent skin irritation.

The patient inhales from the mask, which is connected to 30% to 60% oxygen at a flow rate of 5 to 10 L per minute. The mask is used for short-term therapy.

Oxygen by partial rebreathing mask. The partial rebreathing mask (Figure 16-19) is similar to the face mask, but has a reservoir bag attached to it. Oxygen-rich air plus some room air from the exhalation ports in the mask is inhaled from the reservoir bag. The mask provides 40% to 60% oxygen at 6 to 10 L per minute and is used for acutely ill patients. The bag should not deflate completely.

Oxygen by nonrebreathing mask. This device has a one-way valve between the mask and the reservoir bag that prevents exhaled air from entering the bag. There also are flaps or valves on the sides of the mask to allow air to be exhaled out into the room, but no air from the room can be inhaled through these openings.

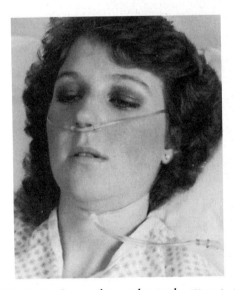

FIGURE 16-18   Oxygen by nasal cannula. (Photo by Ken Kasper.)

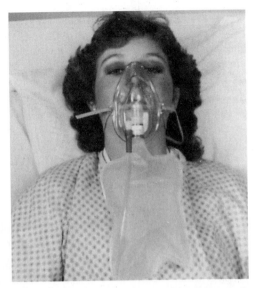

FIGURE 16-19   Oxygen by partial rebreathing mask. (Photo by Ken Kasper.)

The patient breathes pure oxygen from the reservoir bag. This mask provides 90% to 100% oxygen. **The patient should be kept on this mask for as brief a time as possible to restore adequate PaO$_2$, as oxygen in this concentration can cause toxicity.**

High-Flow Systems

Oxygen by Venturi mask. This mask can deliver the most precise dose of oxygen. It has a circle of holes on the sides and a flexible tube attached to the bottom of it. A concentration of 24% to 50% oxygen is mixed with room air in the flexible tubing. The amount of room air is controlled by an orifice whose opening can be adjusted. The exhaled air exits through the side exhalation ports. This mask can be used for both short- and long-term therapy.

Other high-flow systems. The face tent, aerosol mask, tracheostomy collar, and T-piece for the tracheostomy are high-flow systems. They are used to deliver high humidity. A face tent fits over the patient's chin with the top extending to a halfway point across the face.

Transtracheal Oxygen Therapy This is a method for delivering oxygen directly into the lungs for long-term therapy when nasal prongs are irritating or the patient does not like the cosmetic appearance of the prongs. A small, flexible catheter is inserted into the trachea via a small incision under local anesthesia. The catheter is then attached to an oxygen source.

Nursing Considerations The nurse checks the **oxygen-delivery system at the beginning of the shift and then periodically to verify that the flow is set according to the physician's order.** Tubing is checked to see that it is not kinked, blocking the flow of oxygen. This is particularly important whenever the patient is repositioned. Oxygen should be humidified before delivery to the patient, especially if the flow rate is more than 3 L per minute. Oxygen is *not* explosive. However, it does support combustion, which means that a spark or flame can cause a major fire in a short time. **Smoking is not allowed when oxygen is used.**

The tubing should be kept off the floor and the connections should be handled aseptically to prevent contamination of the system. Microorganisms grow easily in a warm, moist, environment.

When oxygen therapy is discontinued, it is usually done gradually. The patient is "weaned" from dependence on oxygen by reducing the dosage and then alternating periods of breathing room air with periods of breathing low concentrations of oxygen.

Think about . . . Can you describe the respiratory assessment points you would cover at the beginning of the shift for a patient who is receiving oxygen therapy?

◆ Mechanical Ventilation

Mechanical ventilation is needed when the patient cannot maintain adequate ventilation because of respiratory, neurological, or neuromuscular problems or trauma. There are two major types of basic ventilators used to give support to patients with ventilatory problems: negative-pressure and positive-pressure ventilators. Negative-pressure ventilators are mainly used for patients with normal vital capacities who have neuromuscular disease, central nervous system disorders (e.g., spinal cord damage), and CAL. Negative-pressure ventilators include the iron lung, cuirass, poncho, and body wrap ventilators.

Positive-pressure ventilators are seen far more frequently. There are several types of positive-pressure ventilators: (1) pressure-cycled; (2) time-cycled; (3) volume-cycled; and (4) high-frequency ventilation machines. These work by delivering a positive driving pressure to the patient's airway. The pressure delivered is greater than that within the airway and alveoli; therefore gas flows into the lungs either assisting or controlling inhalation. When the pressure is released, exhalation takes place without effort on the part of the machine or the patient.

Types of Ventilators *Pressure-cycled* ventilators are those in which cycling primarily depends on a buildup of pressure within the patient's lungs and are rarely used.

Time-cycled ventilators deliver air into the lungs for a preset length of time. The volume of gas delivered may vary. The Babybird and the Siemens Servo are examples of this type. These are mainly used for infants and children.

Volume-cycled ventilators deliver a preset volume of gas to the bronchi and lungs. Pressure limits also are set. If the ventilator meets with too much pressure to deliver the selected volume of gas, an alarm sounds to tell the nurse that the patient is not receiving the correct tidal volume. Most commonly this occurs because there is a buildup of secretions in the lungs and the patient needs to be suctioned. Ventilators of this type are most often used in a critical care setting, in which severe chest disease or surgery has severely compromised normal respiratory function. This type of ventilator will deliver adequate tidal volume even when airway resistance is great (for example, in patients suffering from severe obstructive lung disease). Examples of volume-cycled ventilators include the MA-1 and the Bear-2.

Microprocessor-controlled ventilators are becoming more common as high-tech features are integrated into the various types of ventilators. They are mainly used for patients with ARDS, major burns, or multisystem failure.

High-frequency jet ventilation is used to supplement volume ventilation. It provides good ventilation of the patient with the use of relatively small tidal volumes at very high respiratory rates. The oxygenation and ventilation are accomplished by gas diffusion and convection rather than a high flow of gas. Because the intrathoracic pressures needed for this type of ventilation are much lower, there are fewer complications (e.g., barotrauma, hypotension, and pneumothorax) than with other types of ventilation.

Modes of Ventilation   There are several modes used for positive-pressure ventilation. In *controlled-mode* ventilation, the machine is set to deliver a fixed number of breaths per minute, no matter how the patient tries to breathe. This is used during periods of central nervous system depression, such as during anesthesia and drug overdose.

In *assist mode,* the frequency of ventilation is determined by the patient. When she takes a breath, the machine is triggered to deliver a set tidal volume. This mode is not used alone in the clinical setting, but is combined with the control function to provide an *assist-control mode.* If the patient's respiratory rate falls, the machine will deliver a set number of breaths per minute; if the patient is breathing within the set rate, the machine assists only by delivering the set tidal volume. This mode is mostly used in the clinical setting. It considerably decreases the work of breathing for the patient.

Intermittent mandatory ventilation (IMV) and *synchronized intermittent mandatory ventilation* (SIMV) are the most common modes of ventilation found in critical care settings. These allow the patient to breathe spontaneously and yet provide a preset number of ventilator breaths at a preset tidal volume to ensure adequate ventilation without respiratory muscle fatigue.

For example, IMV can "stack" breaths when the machine delivers a breath at the end of normal inspiration on the part of the patient, and SIMV is activated by the patient's own breath and is therefore synchronized with her breathing pattern. One of the main advantages of these modes is that the respiratory muscles do not become as weak during mechanical ventilation from lack of use, and it is then easier to wean the patient from the ventilator by steadily decreasing the number of mandatory breaths per minute.

Positive end-expiratory pressure (PEEP) also can be delivered by most ventilators. When using PEEP, the pressure in the airways never falls below a certain level (usually between 5 and 15 cm H_2O). This has the effect of holding the smaller air passages open, thus limiting atelectasis. It also holds alveoli in expansion so that there is more time for gas to diffuse across the alveolar membrane and, correct hypoxemia. It is used for adult respiratory distress syndrome and respiratory failure where there is a PaO_2 less than 50 and a PCO_2 greater than 50.

Inverse-ratio ventilation. This new mode of ventilatory support supplies controlled breaths with an inspiratory to expiratory duration ratio of 1:2, 1:3, or 1:4. The rationale is that a prolonged inspiratory time will open stiff alveolar units and a shorter exhalation time will not allow them time to recollapse. It is an alternative to PEEP. A disadvantage of this mode is that it is often uncomfortable for the patient, it requires sedation or the use of a neuromuscular blocking agent. Monitoring the patient requires observing for signs of compromised cardiac action related to the prolonged inspiratory pressures.

Pressure support ventilation. This mode provides pressure support only during inspiration. The patient controls both the duration and volume of inspiration. It is designed to eliminate the pressure or work required by the patient to draw airflow through the ventilator tubing during spontaneous efforts, preventing tiring. It has proven very beneficial during weaning from IMV because it minimizes the workload. The other form of pressure support ventilation is support ventilation max or PSV_{max}. It also is used during weaning and provides higher pressures to produce tidal breaths equivalent to those on conventional positive pressure ventilation.

Liquid ventilation. This mode is under investigation for treatment of respiratory distress syndrome, RDS, and ARDS. The ventilator mixes air with perflubron liquid which is capable of dissolving and carrying large quantities of oxygen. The method gently expands the alveoli and transfers the oxygen into the blood and removes carbon dioxide. Perflubron is a cousin to Teflon

and does not trigger any side effects because it does not chemically react with anything in the human body. The method is proving to be life saving for both premature infants with RDS and adults with ARDS.

Continuous positive airway pressure. Continuous positive airway pressure (CPAP) can be used for patients who are breathing spontaneously but are showing signs of hypoxemia. It is used for infants with mild respiratory distress syndrome and for adults in the early stages of respiratory failure. The patient does not have to be intubated for CPAP to be used. It can be given with nasal prongs.

Nursing Intervention   Nursing responsibilities for patients on mechanical ventilation include checking the physician's order each shift and then the ventilator for the proper settings: mode, FIO_2 (oxygen concentration delivered), respiratory rate, tidal volume, peak inspiratory pressure, and PEEP. Alarms are checked to see that they are turned on. **Alarms should not be turned off when disconnecting the patient in order to suction as they may not be reactivated.** Tubing should be kept clear of pooled water.

The patient is observed for signs of complications, such as gastric distention, pneumothorax, and impaired cardiac output from decreased venous return, and the need for increasingly higher pressures to deliver the set tidal volume, which can indicate stiffening of the lungs (decreased compliance). **The nurse auscultates the lung fields to be certain that both lungs are being ventilated.** Arterial blood gas levels are monitored to determine the effectiveness of ventilation treatment.

For ventilation to be effective, the lungs must be kept clear of secretions. Many patients can cough up secretions and do not need to be suctioned; others may need suctioning as frequently as every 15 minutes. **Endotracheal and tracheal suctioning must be done with strict aseptic technique.** Mechanical ventilation places the patient at considerably greater risk of respiratory infection because of its invasive nature.

The intubated patient on the ventilator cannot talk and must be given an alternative means of communication such as a Magic Slate or paper and pencil. Being hooked up to a ventilator is very frightening for most patients, and it is important that the nurse assure the alert patient that he will not be left alone.

Any time a patient is turned or repositioned, the endotracheal or tracheal tube must be checked to be certain that the ventilator tubes are not pulling on it too much.

Attention must be paid to adequate nutrition, as the patient cannot eat by mouth when she is connected to a ventilator. Additional calorie intake is needed just to maintain weight when a ventilator is used. Continuous enteral feeding is the method most often used to prevent malnutrition in these patients; but whatever method is

TABLE 16-16 ♦ *Dangers of Mechanical Ventilation*	
Danger	**Manifestations**
Barotrauma	Sudden increase in peak inspiratory pressure; absent breath sounds over one area of lung; pneumomediastinum; pneumothorax; subcutaneous emphysema; high-pressure alarm goes off frequently.
Oxygen toxicity	Parenchymal damage and absorption atelectasis; alveolar membrane damage; nonproductive cough; decreasing vital capacity; decreased compliance; increased peak inspiratory pressure.
Impaired cardiac output	Decreased BP, poor peripheral perfusion; decreased level of consciousness.
Infection	Change in sputum color, quantity, and consistency; crackles and rhonchi; increased white blood cell count; fever; infiltrate on chest radiograph.
Fluid retention	Increasing body weight; fluid intake more than output; peripheral edema; crackles in lungs or diminished breath sounds.
Gastric distention	Increasing abdominal girth; complaint of distention; tender to palpation.
Gastrointestinal bleeding	Positive stool guaiac; "coffee grounds" aspirate from gastric suction; dropping hemoglobin; black or bloody stool.

used, the nurse should keep an eye on nutritional parameters to assess whether nutrition is adequate.

If a ventilator alarm sounds and the problem cannot be located quickly, the patient should be disconnected from the machine and ventilated with a manual resuscitator bag and oxygen until the problem is solved. Table 16-16 summarizes the dangers of mechanical ventilation.

Care for a patient who is being ventilated artificially by a ventilating machine is extremely complex. No one should care for such a patient without extensive training and supervised practice. The patient will require protection from infection, continuous monitoring of the vital signs, observations for hypoventilation and hyperventilation, measurement of intake and output, and prevention of the disabilities of inactivity (Chapter 11).

Think about . . . You have just assisted another nurse in turning a patient who is attached to a mechanical ventilator. The patient has been positioned on the left side and the ventilator is on the right side of the bed. What would you check before you leave the bedside?

Endotracheal Intubation and Tracheostomy   Endotracheal intubation means that an endotracheal tube is inserted into the trachea via the nose or the mouth. An endotracheal tube is placed for airway protection against aspiration when there is upper airway obstruction and when mechanical ventilation is necessary. Endotracheal tubes are used for short-term respiratory support, such as during anesthesia or for a few days postoperatively.

A *tracheostomy* is a surgical incision into the trachea for the purpose of inserting a tube through which the patient can breathe.

Tracheostomy is done for the following reasons: (1) to assist or control ventilation by mechanical means over a prolonged period of time; (2) to facilitate suctioning of secretions in the air passages of patients unable to cough; (3) to prevent aspiration of oral and gastric secretions (as in unconscious or paralyzed patients); and (4) to bypass a constricted or obstructed upper airway (as results, for example, from edema of the larynx, presence of a foreign body or tumor, surgical procedures involving the neck, severe burns, facial trauma, or chest trauma).

Tracheostomy may be an emergency procedure or an elective operation. When passing an endotracheal tube through the nose or mouth is impossible or extremely difficult, a tracheostomy may be done to provide an airway. Because of changes in the structure of the throat, some patients will need a tracheostomy tube for the rest of their lives. In general, an endotracheal tube is used when the patient is expected to be able to breathe normally within a few days or a week, such as after surgery. A tracheostomy tube is inserted when the patient is expected to need an artificial airway for an extended period (Figure 16-20).

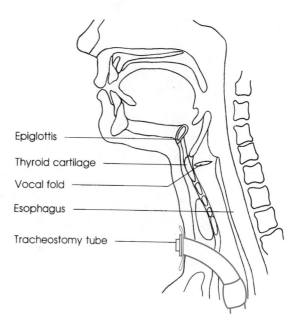

Epiglottis
Thyroid cartilage
Vocal fold
Esophagus
Tracheostomy tube

FIGURE 16-20 Tracheostomy with tube in place.

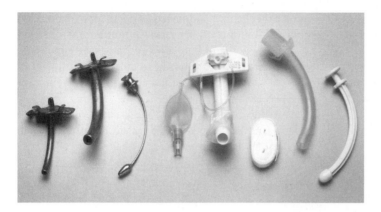

FIGURE 16-21   Metal and plastic tracheostomy tubes of varying sizes; some have an obturator and an inner cannula. (Photo by Glen Derbyshire; courtesy of Goleta Valley Cottage Hospital, Goleta, CA.)

Types of tracheostomy tubes.   Tracheostomy tubes are available in a variety of materials and styles. Most of the newer models are made of plastic or rubber. Tubes made of metal alloys are used chiefly for patients who need a tracheostomy for an extended time. The three styles of tracheostomy tubes are single-cannula, double-cannula, and fenestrated tubes. *Single-cannula* tubes are made of pliable materials that conform to the shape of the trachea more easily than do double-cannula tubes. In a *double-cannula* tracheostomy tube, the outer cannula acts as a sleeve for the inner cannula, which can be removed for cleaning (Figure 16-21). Newer tracheostomy tubes have no need for an inner cannula (the

tube) or have a disposable inner cannula that can be replaced rather than cleaned. The obturator is used during insertion as a guide (the olive tip extends beyond the end of the tube) and to protect against scraping the sides of the trachea with the sharp edge of the tube.

Fenestrated tubes have a small opening in the outer cannula that allows some air to escape through the larynx. This helps prepare the patient for the time when the tracheostomy tube will be removed and he breathes normally again (Figure 16-22).

A one-way tracheostomy valve box can be fitted into the tube opening. It allows air to be inhaled through the tracheostomy opening, but the valve closes when the

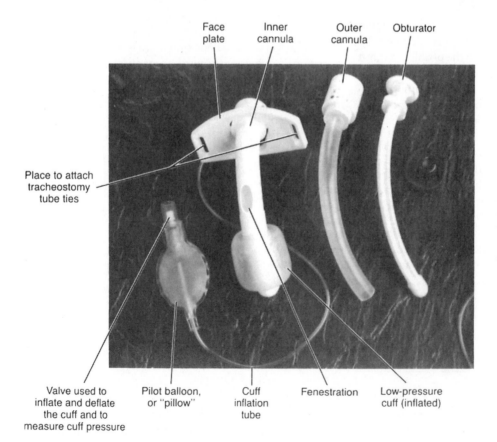

FIGURE 16-22   The Shiley fenestrated low-pressure cuffed tracheostomy tube. (Courtesy of Malinokrodt Medical. Shiley Tracheostomy Products, Irvine, CA.)

patient exhales. This diverts the exhaled air through the larynx and enables the patient to speak. Other types of speaking tracheostomy tubes are now available for the patient who must have the tracheostomy for the rest of her life.

The *cuffed tracheostomy tube* has a small balloon encircling its tracheal end (Figure 16-22). It is sometimes called a *balloon tracheostomy tube*. When the balloon is inflated, it fills the space between the outside of the tracheostomy tube and the trachea, thereby providing a seal and preventing the escape of air around the tube. When positive-pressure artificial ventilation is administered, the air passes through the tracheostomy tube *only*, thus providing sufficient pressure to inflate the lungs. **The cuffed tracheostomy tube also reduces the chance of aspiration of mucus and fluids by those patients whose protective reflexes in the larynx and trachea are impaired.**

Foam-cuffed tracheostomy tubes have the cuff bonded to the tube and, of course, do not need to be inflated and deflated. They are disposable and cause minimal tissue necrosis.

Because the lumen of the tube is the only source of air for the patient, she must be watched closely for signs of obstruction of the tube. If the lumen is not suctioned frequently and kept open, the patient will suffocate. To avoid depression of the surface blood vessels in the tracheal wall and resultant necrosis, the cuff must be inflated just enough to seal the trachea without causing extreme pressure against the tracheal wall. Cuff pressure is checked each shift and each time the cuff is reinflated.

Nursing Intervention   A patient with a new tracheostomy requires very specialized nursing care, especially if she is receiving artificial ventilation through the tube.

> During the first 24 hours, the patient is monitored continuously for signs of respiratory distress. If the patient is unable to cough to remove mucus and drainage, tracheal suctioning is necessary. However, adequate humidification of the inhaled air helps reduce the need for such frequent suctioning.

The lungs should be auscultated (1) before suctioning to assess the need; and (2) afterward to verify that the procedure successfully cleared the airways. Suctioning is done with a sterile suction catheter, sterile normal saline, or water to lubricate the catheter, sterile gloves, and a hookup to suction with a drainage container. Sterile technique is important, as the patient with a tracheostomy is very susceptible to respiratory infection. Suctioning technique is presented in Nursing Procedure 16-1 and is discussed in the section under Ineffective Airway Clearance.

Preventing infection is another nursing responsibility. The incision is an open wound with minimal dressings, is frequently exposed to sputum that is coughed up, and is an ideal entryway for infectious organisms. Tracheostomy care is a sterile procedure until the stoma (opening) is well healed.

If the patient is to go home with a tracheostomy, techniques for suctioning and providing the necessary tracheostomy care are taught to both the patient and a family member or caregiver.

The stoma wound usually is cleaned with normal saline, hydrogen peroxide, or acetic acid solution, removing all secretions. The slit gauze pad is replaced as frequently as needed, and the twill tape ties that hold the tube in place are replaced whenever they become soiled. **It is best to have two people help change the ties, as movement of the tube can easily cause the patient to cough and expel the tube from the stoma.** The tube must be securely held in place while the ties are loose. The nurse will quickly learn that it is best to stand to the side of the patient, as coughing frequently takes place and mucus is expelled during the cleaning procedures.

No nurse should suction a patient without supervised practice in this technique to the point of competence. Considerable skill is necessary to maintain sterile technique while suctioning, yet perform the maneuver quickly and efficiently.

Psychological support of the tracheostomy patient and the family is an essential component of nursing care. The patient has to learn to breathe in a totally different way and cannot speak or call out for help. Continued reassurance is needed both verbally and by actions that show that the nurse is aware of the patient's apprehension and readily available should help be needed. Some means of communication must be devised until the patient is able to speak again. Explanations about what is being done, and why, are given each time tracheostomy care is provided. Teaching begins as soon as the patient is alert after the tracheostomy tube is placed.

COMMUNITY CARE

Many patients in long-term care facilities have chronic respiratory disorders. Home care nurses see a large number of respiratory patients, and outpatient clinic nurses frequently see patients with respiratory infections as well as those with chronic respiratory disorders. Home care nurses often monitor patients for signs of pulmonary edema and must become adept at detecting the signs of fluid in the lungs. All nurses must have a solid knowledge of the care required by respiratory patients. Careful assessment techniques can often catch a respiratory problem before it becomes serious.

Teaching the techniques to promote better breathing and more effective coughing is a simple measure that can greatly improve the life of the patient with CAL. Working with patients to promote compliance with their exercise and medication regimen is a primary function of the nurse in the community. Teaching use of the peak airflow meter and the metered dose inhaler (MDI) can save considerable health care dollars by decreasing serious episodes of acute respiratory dysfunction.

Rehabilitation of the chronic respiratory patient is directed at (1) improving breathing; (2) improving activity tolerance; (3) decreasing infection; (4) preventing acute episodes. Rehabilitation issues are covered in Chapter 12.

CRITICAL THINKING EXERCISES

Clinical Case Problems

Read each clinical situation and discuss the questions with your classmates.

1. You are assigned to take care of Linda Grey, a 16-year-old who has pneumococcal pneumonia. She is receiving oxygen by nasal cannula at 5 L/minute. She is on bedrest with bathroom privileges. She is receiving nebulization, chest physiotherapy, and postural drainage treatments from respiratory therapy. She is very weak and runs a temperature of 104.6° F in the afternoons and evenings, which sometimes seems to cause delirium.
   - What would be an appropriate plan of care for Linda?
   - How would you evaluate the effectiveness of the nursing interventions listed on the plan of care?
   - What psychosocial problems might Linda have? How would you help her with these?

2. Mrs. Wester is 62 years of age. She has suffered from emphysema for several years but has not sought help in coping with the problems it presents. While in the hospital with an acute respiratory infection, she becomes very depressed and says she will never be able to take care of herself again because of her breathlessness. She is not willing to give up smoking and has not been taught any techniques for pulmonary hygiene.
   - What do you think might be the attitude of some health care professionals in regard to Mrs. Wester's problems?
   - Devise a teaching plan to help her with her problem of fatigue and breathlessness.
   - List interventions that would be appropriate in helping with her nutritional and hydration needs.

3. Mr. Cohen is admitted to the hospital for pneumonectomy. His diagnosis is early lung cancer. He is 56 years old and has worked in a cotton mill since he was 16. He is slightly underweight but is physically strong and has an optimistic outlook about his surgery and chances for recovery.
   - What special preoperative instruction would you expect Mr. Cohen to need?
   - What nursing interventions would you expect to be on his postoperative nursing care plan?
   - How would you help Mr. Cohen deal with the diagnosis of cancer, treatment, and prognosis?

BIBLIOGRAPHY

American Cancer Society. (1996). *Cancer Facts and Figures—1996.* Atlanta: Author.

American Lung Association. (1996). *Facts in Brief about Lung Disease.* New York: Author

Anastasi, J. K., Thomas, F. (1994). Dealing with H.I.V.–related pulmonary infections. *Nursing 94.* 24(11):60–64.

Applegate, E. J. (1995). *The Anatomy and Physiology Learning System: Textbook.* Philadelphia: Saunders.

Bennett, J. C., Plum, F., eds. (1996). *Cecil Textbook of Medicine,* 20th ed. Philadelphia: Saunders.

Black, J. M., Matassarin-Jacobs, E. (1997). *Medical-Surgical Nursing: Clinical Management for Continuity of Care,* 5th ed. Philadelphia: Saunders.

Bolton, P. J., Kline, K. A. (1994). Understanding modes of mechanical ventilation. *American Journal of Nursing.* 94(6):36–42.

Borkgren, M. W., Gronkiewicz, C. A. (1995). Update your asthma care from hospital to home. *American Journal of Nursing.* 95(1):26–34.

Brenner, Z. R., Addona, C. (1995). Caring for the pneumonectomy patient: challenges and changes. *Critical Care Nurse.* 15(10):65–72.

Calianno, C. (1996). Actionstat: Aspiration pneumonia. *Nursing 96.* 26(10):47.

Calianno, C. (1995). Guarding against aspiration complications. *Nursing 95.* 25(6):52–53.

Calianno, C. 1996). Nosocomial pneumonia. *Nursing 96.* 26(5):34–39.

Calianno, C., Clifford, D. W., Titano, K. (1995). Oxygen therapy: Giving your patient breathing room. *Nursing 95.* 25(12):33–38.

Carroll, P. (1995). Chest tubes made easy. *RN.* 58(12):46–48, 50, 52–55.

Carroll, P., Milikowski, K. (1996). Getting your patient off a ventilator. *RN.* 59(6):42–47.

Carroll, P. (1994). Safe suctioning. *RN.* 57(5):32–36.

Carroll, P. Tradition or science? Spotting the difference in respiratory care. *RN.* 59(5):26–29.

Carroll, P. (1997). Using pulse oximetry in the home. *Home Healthcare Nurse.* 15(2):88–95.

Collins, P. M., Benedict, J. L. (1996). Pleural effusion. *American Journal of Nursing.* 96(7):38.

Copstead, L. C. (1995). *Perspectives on Pathophysiology.* Philadelphia: Saunders.

Dabbs, A. D., Olslund, L. (1994). The new alternatives to intubation. *American Journal of Nursing.* 94(8):42–45.

Dambro, M. R. (1996). *Griffith's 5 Minute Clinical Consult.* Baltimore: Williams & Wilkins.

deWit, S. C. (1994). *Rambo's Nursing Skills for Clinical Practice,* 4th ed. Philadelphia: Saunders.

Dirkes, S. (1996). Liquid ventilation: New frontiers in the treatment of ARDS. *Critical Care Nurse.* 16(3):53–58.

Eisenbeis, C. (1996). Full partner in care: Teaching your patient how to manage her asthma. *Nursing 96.* 26(1):48–51.

Finkelstein, L. E. (1996). TB or not TB? How to interpret a skin test. *American Journal of Nursing.* 96(12): 12–13.

Gaedeke, M. K., Cross, J. (1996). Actionstat: Blunt chest trauma. *Nursing 96.* 26(2):33.

Glass, C. A., Grap, M. J. (1995). Ten tips for safer suctioning. *American Journal of Nursing.* 95(5):51–53.

Grimes, D. E., Grimes, R. M. (1995). Tuberculosis: what nurse's need to know to control the epidemic. *Nursing Outlook.* 43(4):164–173.

Guyton, A. C., Hall, J. E. (1996). *Textbook of Medical Physiology,* 9th ed. Philadelphia: Saunders.

Hamner, J. (1995). Challenging diagnosis: adult respiratory distress syndrome. *Critical Care Nurse.* 15(10):46–51.

Harwood, K. V. (1996). Non-small cell lung cancer: an overview of diagnosis, staging, and treatment. *Seminars in Oncology Nursing.* 12(4):285–294.

Held, J. L. (1995). Caring for a patient with lung cancer. *Nursing 95.* 25(10):34–43.

Hilderly L. J. (1996). Radiation therapy for lung cancer. *Seminars in Oncology Nursing.* 12(4):304–311.

Howland, W. A. (1995). Defending your patient against nosocomial pneumonia. *Nursing 95.* 25(8):62–63.

Ignatavicius, D. D., Hausman, K. A. (1995). *Clinical Pathways for Collaborative Practice.* Philadelphia: Saunders.

Ignatavicius, D. D., Workman, M. L., Mishler, M. A. (1995). *Medical-Surgical Nursing: A Nursing Process Approach,* 2nd ed. Philadelphia: Saunders.

Iyer, P. W., Taptich, B. J., Bernocchi-Losey, D. (1995). *Nursing Process and Nursing Diagnosis,* 3rd ed. Philadelphia: Saunders.

Jarvis, C. (1996). *Physical Examination and Health Assessment,* 2nd ed. Philadelphia: Saunders.

Johannsen, J. M. (1994). Chronic obstructive pulmonary disease: current comprehensive care for emphysema and bronchitis. *Nurse Practitioner.* 19(1):59–67.

Keep, N. B. (1995). Identifying pulmonary embolism. *American Journal of Nursing.* 95(4):52.

Kelly, M. (1996). Acute respiratory failure. *American Journal of Nursing.* 96(12):46.

Knebel, A., Strider, V. C., Wood, C. (1994). The art and science of caring for ventilator assisted patients: learning from our clinical practice. *Critical Care Nursing Clinics of North America.* 6(4):819–829.

Laskowski-Jones, L. (1995). Meeting the challenge of chest trauma. *American Journal of Nursing.* 95(9):23–29.

Lavell, D. R., Higgins, V. R. (1995). Lung surgery: when less is more. *RN.* 58(7):40–45.

Lazzara, D. (1996). Why is the Heimlich chest drain valve making a comeback? *Nursing 96.* 26(12).

Lehne, R. A. (1994). *Pharmacology for Nursing Care,* 2nd ed. Philadelphia: Saunders.

Majoros, K. A., Moccia, J. M. (1996). Pulmonary embolism: targeting an elusive enemy. *Nursing 96.* 26(4):26–31.

Malarkey, L. M., McMorrow, M. E. (1996). *Nurse's Manual of Laboratory Tests and Diagnostic Procedures.* Philadelphia: Saunders.

Martin, V. R., Comis, R. L. (1996). Small cell carcinoma of the lung: An "updated" overview. *Seminars in Oncology Nursing.* 12(4):295–303.

Mathews, P. J. (1997). Ventilator associated infections: Reducing the risks Part 1. *Nursing 97.* 27(2):59–61.

Matteson, M. A., McConnell, E. S., Linton, A. (1996). *Gerontological Nursing: Concepts and Practice,* 2nd ed. Philadelphia: Saunders.

Mays, D. A. (1995). Turn ABGs into child's play. *RN.* 58(1):36–39.

Mee, C. L. (1995). Ventilator alarms: how to respond with confidence. *Nursing 95.* 25(7):61–64.

Misasi, R. S., Keys, J. L. (1994). The pathophysiology of hypoxia. *Critical Care Nurse.* 14(8):55–64.

Monahan, F. D., Drake, T., Neighbors, M. (1994). *Nursing Care of Adults.* Philadelphia: Saunders.

McConnell, E. A. (1995). Assisting with chest tube removal. *Nursing 95.* 25(8):18.

McConnell, E. A. (1996). Administering oxygen by nasal cannula. *Nursing 96.* 26(3):14.

McConnell, E. A. (1995). Using a handheld resuscitation bag. *Nursing 95.* 25(9):18.

McConnell, E. A. (1997). Your role in thoracentesis. *Nursing 97.* 27(3):76.

McGaffigan, P. A. (1996). Hazards of hypoxemia: How to protect your patient from low oxygen levels. *Nursing 96.* 26(5):41–47.

McGregor, R. J., Schakenbach, L. H. (1996). Lung volume reduction surgery: A new breath of life for emphysema patients. *MEDSURG Nursing.* 5(4):245–252.

McKinney, B. (1994). COPD and depression: treat them both. *RN.* 57(4):48–50.

O'Hanlan-Nichols, T. (1995). Adult respiratory distress syndrome. *American Journal of Nursing.* 95(8):42.

O'Hanlon-Nichols, T. (1996). Commonly asked questions about chest tubes. *American Journal of Nursing.* 96(5): 60–63.

Pfister, S. M. (1995). Home oxygen therapy: indications, administration, recertification, and patient education. *Nurse Practitioner.* 20(7):44, 47–52, 54–56.

Polaski, A. L., Tatro, S. E. (1996). *Luckmann's Core Principles and Practice of Medical-Surgical Nursing.* Philadelphia: Saunders.

Powell, S. G. (1994). Medication compliance of patients with COPD. *Home Healthcare Nurse.* 12(3):44–50.

Repasky, T. M. (1994). Tension pneumothorax. *American Journal of Nursing.* 94(9):47.

Risser, N. L. (1996). Prevention of lung cancer: The key is to stop smoking. *Seminars in Oncology Nursing.* 12(4):260–269.

Rokosky, J. M. (1997). Misuse of metered-dose inhalers: Helping patients get it right. *Home Healthcare Nurse.* 15(1):13–21.

Ruben, R. L. (1994). Tuberculosis is making a comeback. *Journal of Practical Nursing.* 44(4):47–56.

Rutter, K. M. (1995). Tension pneumothorax: how to restore normal breathing. *Nursing 95.* 25(4):33.

Ryan, L. S. (1996). Psychosocial issues and lung cancer: A behavioral approach. *Seminars in Oncology Nursing.* 12(4):318–323.

Samuel, J. R. (1997). Management of recurrent spontaneous pneumothorax and recurrent symptomatic pleural effusion with chest tube pleurodesis. *Critical Care Nurse.* 17(1):28–32.

Shawgo, T. (1996). Thoracoscopic surgery: A new approach to pulmonary disease. *Crit Care Nurse.* 16(2):76–82.

Sinski, A., Corbo, J. (1994). Surfactant replacement in adults and children with ARDS—An effective therapy? *Critical Care Nurse.* 14(12):54–58.

Somerson, S. J. et. al. (1996). Mastering emergency airway management. *American Journal of Nursing.* 96(5):24–30.

Springhouse Corporation. (1996). *Nursing 96 Drug Handbook.* Springhouse; PA: author.

Tasota, F. J., Wesmiller, S. W. (1994). Assessing A.B.G.s: maintaining the delicate balance. *Nursing 94.* 24(5):34–44.

Turner, P., Glass, C., Grap, M. J. (1997). Care of the patient requiring mechanical ventilation. *MEDSURG Nursing.* 6(2):68–77.

Ulrich, S. P., Canale, S. W., Wendell, S. A. (1994). *Medical-Surgical Nursing Care Planning Guides,* 3rd ed. Philadelphia: Saunders.

Walsh, K. (1994). Guidelines for the prevention and control of tuberculosis in the elderly. *Nurse Practitioner.* 19(11):79–84.

Weilitz, P. B., Dettenmeier, P. A. (1994). Back to basics: test your knowledge of tracheostomy tubes. *American Journal of Nursing.* 94(2):46–50.

White, V. M. (1996). t-PA for pulmonary embolism. *American Journal of Nursing.* 96(9):34.

Whitney, L. (1995). Chronic bronchitis and emphysema: airing the differences. *C. E. Test Handbook.* Vol. 6:89–95.

Wolf, Z. R. (1996). Positioning your patient for better breathing. *Nursing 96.* 26(5):10.

Zimmerman, H. E. (1996). Ventilation therapy flashback. *RN.* 59(12):26–31.

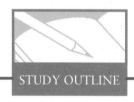

STUDY OUTLINE

I. Causes of Respiratory Disorders

   A. Inhalation of infectious organisms and chemical irritants.

   B. Cardiac disease and other conditions that interfere with blood supply to the lungs and distribution of gases.

   C. Two major types of ventilatory diseases: restrictive (decreased lung volume) and obstructive (narrowed air passages).

     1. Restrictive disorders decrease lung capacity. **Scoliosis and kyphosis are restrictive disorders.**

     2. Obstructive disorders cause problems moving air in and out of the lungs (chronic airflow limitation [CAL]). **Asthma, emphysema, and chronic bronchitis are obstructive disorders.**

   D. Tumors may cause obstruction of airways and destruction of lung tissue.

II. Prevention of Respiratory Diseases

   A. Good health practices: rest, nutrition, personal hygiene.

   B. Vaccination against influenza and pneumococcal pneumonia.

   C. Prompt treatment of respiratory infections.

   D. Avoidance of irritants such as tobacco smoke, industrial pollutants. **Stopping smoking decreases the incidence of respiratory ailments.**

III. Terms Commonly Used in Respiratory Disease Nursing.

IV. Diagnostic Tests and Procedures and Nursing Implications (Table 16-2)

V. Nursing Management

   A. Nursing assessment of respiratory status.

     1. History taking (see Table 16-3).

     2. Physical assessment.

       a. Posture, amount of effort to breathe, use of abdominal muscles and other accessory muscles of respiration, rate, depth, and character of respirations.

       b. Skin color: cyanosis appears late in oxygen depletion.

c. Shape of chest: barrel-shaped? Kyphosis? Scoliosis?

d. Clubbing of fingers.

e. Any cough? Characteristics? Sputum production?

f. Auscultate for breath sounds; any abnormalities?

  (1) Auscultate lungs in systematic manner.

  (2) Abnormal sounds: wheezing, "croaking" or stridor, hoarseness.

  (3) Rhonchi: coarse, rattling sounds due to secretions in the air passages.

  (4) Crackles: produced by air passing through moisture. Dry crackles are produced by thick secretions.

B. Nursing diagnosis: nursing diagnoses commonly associated with respiratory disorders: Ineffective airway clearance, ineffective breathing pattern, impaired gas exchange, risk for infection, activity intolerance, anxiety, fatigue, altered health maintenance.

C. Planning.

  1. Goals for the patient with a respiratory disorder include: Promote oxygenation, prevent infection, prevent further lung damage, promote rehabilitation.

  2. Expected outcomes are individualized for each patient and each nursing diagnosis.

D. Implementation.

  1. See Table 16-3, Clinical Pathway 16-7, and Nursing Care Plan 16-1.

  2. Interventions are discussed in the sections Common Care Problems, on specific disorders, and Therapeutic Measures.

E. Evaluation.

  1. Effectiveness of interventions and treatment is based on improvements in breathing pattern, arterial blood gas values, and lung sounds.

  2. Decreased cough, sputum production, wheezing, and dyspnea are other parameters.

  3. Greater activity tolerance is an evaluative criteria.

VI. **Common Respiratory Patient Care Problems**

A. Ineffective airway clearance.

  1. Productive or nonproductive of sputum.

  2. Events that trigger cough; time of day; measures that help relieve; other symptoms occurring simultaneously, such as fatigue, dyspnea, change in vital signs.

  a. Cough medicines either thin sputum or suppress the cough.

  b. **Water should not be taken immediately after a cough syrup.**

3. Sputum (see Table 16-4).

  a. *Standard precautions* plus airborne and droplet precautions to prevent spread of infection.

  b. Teach patient proper handling and disposal of secretions.

  c. Frequent oral hygiene.

  d. Observe amount and characteristics of sputum.

  e. Suctioning may be necessary to remove secretions.

  f. See Guidelines for suctioning and Nursing Procedure 16-1.

B. Ineffective breathing pattern.

  1. Dyspnea or breathlessness.

  a. Positioning in high Fowler's or sitting with shoulders hunched and arms resting on knees with legs apart eases breathing.

  b. The orthopneic position is used for severe dyspnea.

  c. Pursed-lip and diaphragmatic breathing help relieve dyspnea.

  d. Relieve abdominal distention.

  e. Avoid overfilling stomach.

  2. Respiratory failure.

  a. Hyperventilation.

  b. Hypoventilation.

  c. Excessive levels of CO_2 cause an increase in respiratory rate to blow off the excess.

  d. When oxygenation is low, heart rate increases; mental confusion may occur.

  e. Respiratory failure: pO_2 less than 50 mm Hg and pCO_2 over 50 mm Hg.

  3. Respiratory acidosis and respiratory alkalosis.

  a. Signs of respiratory acidosis: excessive pCO_2, rapid respirations.

  b. Signs of respiratory alkalosis: tetany, vertigo, blurred vision, diaphoresis; low pCO_2 and high pH.

  4. Other abnormal patterns: Biot's respirations; Cheyne-Stokes respirations; Kussmaul's respirations; apneustic respirations.

C. Risk of infection.

  1. Respiratory infections are transmitted by airborne or in droplet manner.

  a. Cover mouth and nose when coughing or sneezing.

  b. Wash hands frequently.

  2. Maintain adequate nutrition and rest to increase immunity.

  3. Immunize against influenza and pneumonia.

D. Alterations in nutrition and hydration.

  1. Anorexia is common in patients with chronic respiratory disease.

2. Nursing intervention: clean, odor-free environment; good oral hygiene; small, frequent feedings; supplements (Pulmocare).

3. Fluid deficit not uncommon because of increased secretions and abnormal breathing patterns.

4. Patient should drink at least 3,000 mL per day.

5. Humidification of air can help prevent fluid deficit.

E. Fatigue.

1. Hypoxia produces a loss of energy.

2. Dyspnea causes an increase in the work of breathing.

3. Alternate activity with rest periods.

4. Breathing exercises can decrease fatigue.

VII. Disorders of the Lower Respiratory System

A. Acute respiratory disease.

1. Acute bronchitis: symptoms: chest pain, fever, dry, hacking cough progressing to productive cough.

   a. Treated with humidification and rest; antibiotics only if sputum contains specific infectious organisms.

2. Influenza.

   a. Highly infectious: symptoms: dry cough, headache, fever, chills, muscle aches, sore throat, red, watery eyes.

   b. Treated with rest and fluids. Antiviral medication may be given if started immediately at onset of symptoms. Comfort measures.

3. Pneumonia: extensive inflammation of lung tissue with consolidation. Various causes, ranging from infectious agents and chemicals to atelectasis.

   a. Prevention: nursing intervention to avoid hypostatic and aspiration pneumonia.

   b. Diagnosis by radiograph.

   c. Typical pneumonia responds to antibiotic therapy.

   d. Atypical pneumonia caused by *Mycoplasma* treated with erythromycin or tetracycline. Viral atypical pneumonia requires no antiinfective therapy.

   e. *Pneumocystis carinii* pneumonia (PCP) associated with AIDS; treated with pentamidine and combinations of other medications (See Chapter 8).

   f. Nursing care plan should include measures to control fever, maintain fluid and electrolyte balance, meet needs for nutrition, rest, and comfort; avoid irritating substances and secondary infections. Abdominal distention, nausea and vomiting, and altered states of consciousness are frequent problems.

4. Pleurisy: inflammation of pleural membranes.

   a. Pleurisy with effusion: an increase in serous fluid in pleural cavity.

   b. Symptoms: sharp, stabbing pain in chest.

   c. Treatment includes bedrest and prevention of infection. Thoracentesis may be needed to remove excess fluid.

5. Atelectasis: common after surgery or during bedrest. Treated with deep-breathing and coughing to remove secretions and open alveoli.

6. Empyema: thick and purulent fluid within pleural cavity.

   a. Treated by antibiotics and thoracentesis: empyema tube.

7. Fungal infections: *Pneumocystis carinii*: high incidence in AIDS patients; histoplasmosis and coccidioidomycosis caused by fungus.

   a. Sarcoidosis: interstitial lung disease characterized by granulomas.

VIII. Chronic Airflow Limitation (CAL, Chronic Obstructive Pulmonary Disease, COPD)

A. Ranks fifth among major causes of death in the United States.

B. Increased incidence from tobacco smoke and air pollution.

1. Pulmonary emphysema is essentially a disease of the terminal respiratory units. Walls of the alveoli are damaged, bronchioles permanently distended.

   a. Patient has more difficulty exhaling because of loss of lung elasticity.

2. Chronic bronchitis: increased residual volume due to premature closure of the airways during exhalation.

3. Asthma: hypersensitivity of trachea and bronchi to various stimuli. Bronchospasm usually reversible with drug therapy.

4. Bronchiectasis: bronchi become dilated; caused by frequent respiratory infections and cystic fibrosis.

   a. Adult cystic fibrosis patients have form of CAL.

C. Medical treatment goals.

1. Minimize irritation of air passages and their obstruction by secretions, edema, etc.

2. Prevent or control infection.

3. Increase tolerance for physical activity.

D. Nursing intervention.

1. Rehabilitation and education of patient for self-care are major goals.

2. Techniques and pointers for patient with CAL listed in Tables 16-8, 16-11, and 16-12.

IX. Tuberculosis

A. Pulmonary tuberculosis.

1. Infectious disease caused by tubercle bacillus. *Not* highly contagious; opportunistic and therefore has increased incidence in AIDS patients.

2. Categories can help identify those needing treatment or preventive therapy.

3. Symptoms: cough, low-grade fever in the afternoon, weight loss, night sweats, hemoptysis.

4. Diagnostic tests: tuberculin skin tests, chest radiographs, examination of sputum and gastric contents for causative organism.

5. Treatment, rest, good nutrition, proper handling of secretions, control of coughing.

6. Specific anti-TB drugs: isoniazid (INH), rifampin (RMP), pyrazinamide, ethambutol, and streptomycin. Drugs selected according to sensitivity of organisms in sputum.

7. Preventive therapy for selected groups. INH and RMP are 85% effective in preventing the development of tuberculosis in high-risk persons.

8. Nursing intervention is primarily concerned with education of patient and family to ensure control and prevent transmission.

B. Extrapulmonary tuberculosis: bacillus affects organs other than the lungs.

X. Lung Cancer

A. A leading cause of cancer deaths in males and females; major factor is smoking.

B. Tumors usually begin in epithelial lining of bronchi.

C. Symptoms appear late in disease.

D. Treatment includes surgery, chemotherapy, and radiotherapy.

XI. Sleep Apnea

A. Episodes of upper airway occlusion during sleep that interfere with sufficient rest.

B. Causes hypoxia.

C. Treated by surgery, CPAP, or BPAP.

XII. Chest Injuries

A. Can be life-threatening because of possible damage to respiratory and cardiovascular systems.

B. Major concerns are:

1. Maintaining airway.

2. Ensuring adequate ventilation.

3. Controlling circulatory problems.

C. Pneumothorax and hemothorax are two major complications. Unrelieved tension pneumothorax can lead to mediastinal shift and can be fatal. Treatment: insertion of chest tubes and closed chest drainage.

D. Penetrating wounds: Do not remove penetrating object; stabilize it.

E. Flail chest requires intubation and mechanical ventilation.

XIII. Pulmonary Edema

A. Medical emergency: lungs fill with fluid.

B. Signs and symptoms: severe dyspnea, orthopnea, noisy respirations, frothy sputum, crackles heard on auscultation, anxiety, restlessness, and confusion; abnormal blood gases.

C. Treated with IV morphine to reduce workload of heart and ease anxiety; treat underlying cause. Diuretics given.

D. Provide reassurance; continuous respiratory assessment; close monitoring of intake and output.

XIV. Adult respiratory distress syndrome (ARDS)

A. Noncardiac pulmonary edema; accompanies other serious illness or injury.

B. Mortality is high. Treat with ventilatory support and correction of underlying problem.

XV. Pulmonary Embolism (PE)

A. Mass or clot occludes pulmonary vessel; can be a mild problem or fatal.

1. Many types of emboli: blood, fat, amniotic fluid, air.

2. Symptoms depend on site and location of embolus; dyspnea, chest pain, cough, hemoptysis, and anxiety.

3. Stay with patient, position in high Fowler's, start oxygen, assess vital signs, notify physician.

4. Treatment: oxygen, anticoagulation, lysis of clot.

XVI. Common Therapeutic Measures

A. Intrathoracic surgery: Standard thoracotomy or endoscopic thoracotomy.

1. Preoperative care: assessment of patient's respiratory status; arm and leg exercises; explanation of chest tubes, closed drainage system, suctioning, any other procedure anticipated.

2. Postoperative care: special observations, positioning, and chest tubes.

3. Care of patients with chest tubes and closed drainage.

   a. Apparatus can be one-, two-, or three-chamber system for closed drainage or disposable self-contained unit.

b. Purpose is to allow for gradual reexpansion of lung and to prevent hemothorax and pneumothorax.

c. System must be airtight at all times; tape connections.

d. Note conditions that require immediate attention:

(1) Persistent bubbling in underwater seal.

(2) More than a 100-mL drainage per hour.

(3) "Puffed-up" appearance in chest and neck; feels like bubble wrap.

(4) Leakage of air around connection.

e. See Nursing Care Plan 16-1.

B. Medications: antihistamines, bronchodilators, liquefying agents and diluents, antiinfectives; cromolyn sodium, corticosteroids.

C. Humidification: aerosol and humidity therapy; nebulizers.

1. Relief of bronchial edema and spasms.

2. Liquefaction of secretions.

3. Delivery of drugs.

4. Moisten mucous membranes.

D. Pulmonary hygiene: purposes are (1) removal of secretions in the air passages; and (2) breathing control.

1. Chest physiotherapy includes postural drainage, percussion, and vibration.

2. Breathing exercises and effective coughing.

E. Oxygen therapy:

1. Indicated when there is either inadequate intake or poor distribution of oxygen.

2. Oxygen toxicity: damage to cells from excess O_2 in their environment.

a. Concentration and rate of flow must be specific.

3. Administration by low-flow and high-flow systems: nasal cannula, mask, and tent.

4. Special considerations to avoid fire hazards; measures to control infection.

5. Patient is "weaned" from oxygen dependence.

F. Mechanical ventilation:

1. Two types of ventilators: positive-pressure and negative-pressure.

2. Positive-pressure ventilators: pressure-cycled, time-cycled, volume-cycled, high-frequency.

3. Modes of delivery:

a. Controlled artificial ventilation for patient who cannot breathe on his own.

b. Assisted ventilation helps patient breathe more deeply.

c. IMV allows patient to breathe spontaneously between controlled breaths.

d. PEEP delivers pressure at the end of expiration; for patients who have been intubated and require assisted ventilation.

e. Inverse-ratio ventilation: longer inspiration period than expiration; helps keep alveoli from collapsing.

f. Pressure support ventilation: decreases work of inspiration by providing positive pressure; helpful for weaning from ventilator.

g. CPAP delivered continuously to patients who are breathing spontaneously.

h. All ventilators humidify inspired air and measure expired volumes.

4. Nursing intervention.

a. Check physician's orders and compare with settings on ventilator.

b. Ventilator settings: mode, FIO_2, respiratory rate, tidal volume, peak inspiratory pressure, PEEP.

c. Keep alarms turned on.

d. Keep tubing clear of water.

e. Assess patient for signs of complications: pneumothorax, gastric distention, impaired cardiac output, decreased compliance.

f. Auscultate lung fields frequently.

g. Monitor arterial blood gas levels.

h. Suction with aseptic technique.

i. Provide means of communication.

j. Assess nutritional adequacy.

G. Aerosol therapy by jet nebulization for humidification and medication.

H. Endotracheal intubation and tracheostomy: an artificial airway.

1. Types of tubes: single-cannula, double-cannula, fenestrated.

2. Cuffed tracheostomy tube allows air to pass through the tube only.

3. Patient care requires specific instruction and supervised practice. Major concerns are:

a. Maintaining open airway.

b. Preventing infection.

c. Maintaining integrity of skin around stoma and mucous membranes of respiratory tract.

d. Providing psychological support of patient and family.

XVII. Community Care

A. Many long-term care residents have respiratory disorders.

B. Home care nurses treat a large number of respiratory patients.

C. Nurses in outpatient clinics frequently see patients with respiratory disorders.

D. Respiratory assessment is an important skill to hone for all nurses.

E. Teaching techniques for better breathing and more effective coughing improves the life of the patient with chronic airflow limitation.

F. Teaching the use of a peak air flow meter and proper use of MDIs saves health care dollars by decreasing serious episodes of acute respiratory dysfunction and wasted medication.

G. Rehabilitation of patients with chronic respiratory disorders focuses on improving breathing and activity tolerance, decreasing episodes of infection, and preventing acute flareups.

XVIII. Elder Care Points

A. Confusion may be a sign of atypical pneumonia in an elderly patient with a respiratory infection.

B. Pulmonary emboli in the elderly may result from venous thrombosis developing during periods of immobilization or from emboli related to atrial fibrillation.

C. Elderly patients with osteoporosis are at risk for fractures from clapping during chest physiotherapy; use vibration instead.

D. The elderly patient may be taking medications for other disorders and all medications should be checked for interactions.

CHAPTER 17

Care of Patients with Hematological and Lymphatic Systems Disorders

OBJECTIVES

Upon completing this chapter the student should be able to:

1. Compare the functions of the lymphatic system with those of the blood.
2. Identify ways in which the nurse might help prevent blood and lymphatic disorders.
3. Describe the steps to be taken to obtain a sample of blood for a diagnostic test.
4. List at least five different kinds of information that can be obtained from a complete blood count (CBC).
5. Outline the factors considered when performing nursing assessment of hematological and lymphatic status.
6. From the NANDA list of nursing diagnoses, identify at least four nursing diagnoses that are commonly used for a patient with a blood or lymphatic disorder and choose appropriate nursing interventions for each.
7. Considering the goals of care, write expected outcomes for each of the appropriate nursing diagnoses for a patient with a blood or lymphatic disorder.
8. Describe the pathology and clinical signs and symptoms of anemias, sickle cell disease, leukemia, hemophilia, and Hodgkin's disease.
9. Describe how hypovolemic shock occurs, ways to prevent it, and the measures to take when it occurs.
10. Describe the nursing interventions used to prevent infections in patients with leukopenia.

Blood sustains life for every cell of the body. The cardiovascular system is composed of blood, the heart pump that propels the blood throughout the body, and the veins, arteries, and capillaries that form an interconnecting network for carrying blood to the cells. The lymphatic system brings fluid from out in the tissues (**interstitial fluid**) back to the cardiovascular system. Any disorder that affects blood, blood-forming organs, or the lymphatic system interferes with the vital functions the blood and lymph perform.

This chapter discusses disorders that affect the blood and its formed elements, the organs that produce the various blood cells, and the lymphatic system, which drains the fluid from the spaces around each cell and channels it into the circulatory system.

OVERVIEW OF ANATOMY AND PHYSIOLOGY

What Are the Functions of Blood?

⅄ Blood transports water, oxygen, nutrients, hormones, enzymes, and medications to the cells.

⅄ Blood transports carbon dioxide and other waste products away from the cells.

⅄ The 6 to 7 L of blood in the body help regulate fluid volume and electrolyte distribution.

⅄ Blood assists in regulating body temperature.

What Are the Components of Blood?

⅄ Blood is a connective tissue composed of formed elements (cellular components) and plasma (Figure 17-1).

⅄ About 45% of the blood is made up of various types of cells and the remainder of the blood is plasma.

⅄ Plasma contains proteins, water, salts, dissolved gases (such as CO_2), bicarbonate (HCO_3), hormones, glucose, and wastes.

⅄ The plasma proteins are albumin, globulins, and fibrinogen.

What Are the Functions of the Plasma Proteins?

⅄ Albumin raises osmotic pressure at the capillary membrane, preventing fluid from leaking out into the tissue spaces.

⅄ The alpha and beta globulins work as carriers for drugs and lipids combining with them and transporting them throughout the body; gamma globulins act as antibodies.

⅄ Fibrinogen is essential to the formation of blood clots.

How Does the Body Produce Blood Cells?

⅄ Blood cells develop from stem cells located in the bone marrow through **erythropoiesis** (Figure 17-2).

⅄ The kidney produces the majority of erythropoietin-stimulating factor, which prompts erythropoietin to be released from the liver for erythrocyte production.

⅄ Erythropoiesis requires iron, vitamins B_{12}, C, and E, folic acid, and amino acids from proteins.

What Are the Functions of the Red Blood Cells?

⅄ Red blood cells (RBCs, erythrocytes), the most numerous of the blood cells, contain hemoglobin, which carries oxygen to the cells and a portion of carbon dioxide away from the cells.

⅄ The normal range for adults for RBCs is 4.2 to 6.2 million/mm³.

⅄ The normal range for hemoglobin in adults is 12.0 to 18.0 g/dL.

Decreased numbers of RBCs or decreased hemoglobin results in a reduction in the amount of oxygen that can be carried to the cells of the body.

⅄ Red blood cells live for approximately 120 days.

⅄ Old, damaged, red cells are removed by the spleen.

What Are the Functions of the White Blood Cells?

⅄ White blood cells, also called WBCs or leukocytes, provide the first line of defense against microbial agents.

⅄ The normal adult range for total leukocytes (WBCs) is 4,500 to 11,000/mm³.

⅄ Leukocytes are divided into granulocytes and agranulocytes, meaning with and without granules in the cell nucleus (Figure 17-2).

⅄ Leukocytes function out in the tissues and are carried where they are needed by the bloodstream (Table 17-1).

⅄ Granulocytes are divided into neutrophils, eosinophils, and basophils.

⅄ Neutrophils make up 50% to 70% of the white blood cell count (WBC) and work by engulfing and destroying bacteria by the process of *phagocytosis*.

An infection in the body stimulates increased production of neutrophils, resulting in a higher-than-normal white blood cell count, or leukocytosis.

⅄ Eosinophils, which make up 1% to 5% of the total WBCs, help detoxify foreign proteins; they increase in number during allergic reactions and in response to parasitic infections.

⅄ Basophils, which comprise up to 1% of the total WBC, release histamine in response to allergens and help prevent clotting in the small blood vessels.

- Agranulocytes consist of lymphocytes and monocytes.
- Lymphocytes comprise 25% of the WBCs and occur as B-cells and T-cells. B-cells synthesize antibodies. T-cells are called killer cells and help B-cells destroy foreign proteins (See Chapter 7).
- Monocytes become macrophages when out in the tissues and are active as phagocytes, fighting infection and ridding the body of foreign substances.
- A differential blood cell count gives information about the numbers of different types of leukocytes present in the blood and about the type of inflammatory process that is occurring.

What Are Platelets and What Is Their Function?

- Platelets, also called thrombocytes, are fragments of megakaryocytes that are produced by the bone marrow.
- Platelets provide the first line of protection to prevent bleeding by promoting clotting when the wall of a blood vessel has been damaged.
- Fibrin strands derived from the plasma protein fibrinogen attach to aggregated platelets to help form a clot.
- **The normal adult platelet count range is 150,000 to 350,000/mm³; the lifespan of a platelet is about 10 days.**

Although the body can withstand a substantial drop in the number of platelets, when the platelet count is low, there is risk of spontaneous bleeding into the skin, kidney, brain, and other internal organs.

How Does the Lymphatic System Interact with the Vascular System?

- The lymphatic system provides a route for fluid to flow from the tissue spaces into the circulatory system.
- The lymphatic system consists of lymph nodes, lymph channels, the spleen, and the thymus gland (Figure 17-3).
- The spleen, located in the upper left abdominal cavity below the diaphragm and behind the stomach, filters the blood, removing pathogens, old blood cells, and debris, and produces lymphocytes.

- The spleen is a reservoir for extra blood; in response to hemorrhage it contracts, adding blood to the cardiovascular system.
- If the spleen is removed its functions are taken over by other lymph tissue and the liver.
- Lymph nodes, located along the lymphatic vessels, produce lymphocytes and filter out leukocytes and cell debris from inflammations and infections.
- Lymphocytes are divided into B-lymphocytes and T-lymphocytes and are active in the immune responses of the body (see Chapter 7).
- T-lymphocytes produce antigen-reactive cells, thereby reacting against invading antigens.
- B-lymphocytes can change into plasma cells that produce the immunoglobulins responsible for the humoral immune response.
- **Malignant cells can move via the lymphatic system when they metastasize and often involve the lymph nodes along the way.**

Think about . . . *The CBC of your patient shows the following values:*

RBC	4.8 mil/mm³
WBC	6.7 mil/mm³
Hbg	10.2 g/dL
Platelets	250,000/mm³

What abnormalities, if any, do these results show?

What Changes Occur with Aging?

- Plasma volume decreases after age 60; the older person has less blood volume.
- Bone marrow activity decreases by about 50% as years advance; the marrow becomes infiltrated with fat and fibrotic tissue.
- New cells are produced at a slower rate and correction of anemia is a longer process.
- When blood loss occurs, the elderly patient is at greater risk for hypovolemia and shock.
- Blood is more prone to coagulate because platelets tend to aggregate more with advancing age and there are alterations in clotting activity. **The increased incidence of thrombosis in coronary and cerebral arteries may be related to changes in clotting activity.** Daily low-dose aspirin sometimes is prescribed to counteract this phenomenon.

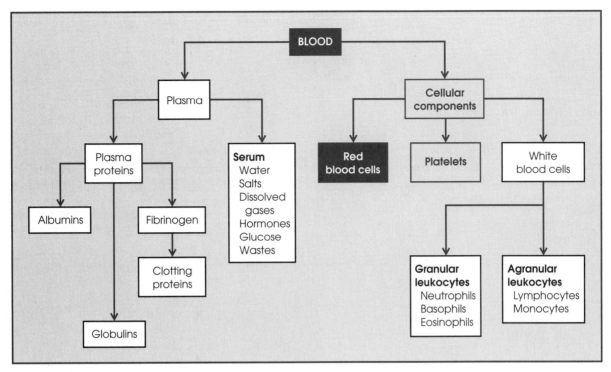

FIGURE 17-1   Components of blood. (*Source:* Redrawn from Solomon, E. P. [1992]. *Introduction to Human Anatomy and Physiology.* Philadelphia: Saunders.)

CAUSES OF HEMATOLOGICAL AND LYMPHATIC DISORDERS

Several disorders that interfere with normal function of the blood are inherited. Hemophilia, sickle cell disease, and certain types of anemias are examples. Accidental tearing or cutting of the vessels of the cardiovascular system and surgery cause bleeding and loss of blood. Blunt trauma to the spleen, such as might occur in an automobile accident, may cause tearing and massive internal hemorrhage. Chemicals and transfusions of the wrong blood type can cause **hemolysis** (destruction) of blood cells.

Some blood disorders are **iatrogenic;** that is, they are brought on by medical treatment. For example, blood **dyscrasias** (imbalance in numbers of types of cells) or other pathological conditions of the blood can be induced by drugs through at least three kinds of actions: (1) bone marrow suppression, which interferes with the production of blood cells; (2) interference with normal cell function; and (3) destruction of the blood cells by cytotoxic drugs.

Some antineoplastic drugs, for instance, act to depress the bone marrow, which inevitably causes a reduced supply of blood cells. Other drugs, such as phenytoin (Dilantin), primidone (Mysoline), barbital derivatives, and oral contraceptives, can produce ane-mia by interfering with the absorption and utilization of folic acid, a substance needed to produce red blood cells (Table 17-2).

Diuretics such as furosemide (Lasix) and hydro-chlorothiazide (Hydrodiuril) sometimes cause de-creased numbers of white cells (**leukopenia**), **aplastic anemia** (deficient red cell production due to a bone marrow disorder), and abnormally low counts of plate-lets and granulocytes. Procainamide hydrochloride (Pronestyl) and quinidine, which are used to correct dysrhythmias of the heart, also can cause **thrombo-cytopenia** (too few platelets), agranulocytosis, and aplastic anemia. Keep in mind that most drugs are powerful chemicals that are capable of producing un-desirable side effects, even though they can be of great value.

Nutritional deficiencies can interfere with erythro-poiesis and normally functioning blood cells. Abnormal red cells are more prone to rapid destruction, which can result in anemia. Bone marrow damage from toxic substances may also interfere with the production of blood cells.

Malignant conditions such as leukemia, lym-phoma, Hodgkin's disease, and multiple myeloma cause growth of abnormal blood, plasma, or lymph cells and interfere with the production of normal cells. Table 17-3 presents factors that alter hematological or lymphatic system function.

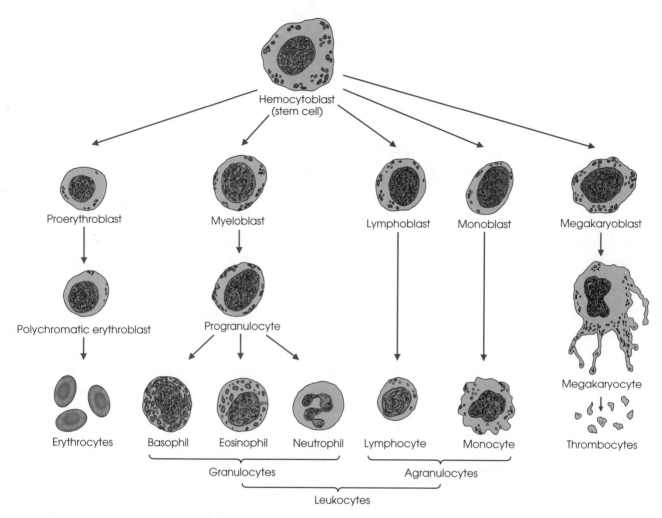

FIGURE 17-2   Development of the formed elements of blood, originating from stem cells in the bone marrow. Erythrocytes (RBCs), leukocytes (WBCs), and thrombocytes (platelets) are the end products.

TABLE 17-1 ◆ *Leukocytes and Their Functions*	
Cell Type and % of Leukocytes	**Function**
Granululocytes	
Eosinophils (1%–5%)	Detoxify foreign proteins; increase in allergic reactions and in parasitic infections.
Basophils (0%–1%)	Prevent clotting in small vessels; release histamine in response to allergens.
Neutrophils (40%–70%)	Engulf and destroy bacteria via phagocytosis.
Agranulocytes	
Monocytes (2%–10%)	Change into macrophages, move out into tissue, and perform phagocytosis.
Lymphocytes (20%–40%)	Divided into B-lymphocytes and T-lymphocytes; B-lymphocytes change into plasma cells that produce immunoglobulins responsible for the humoral immune response. T-lymphocytes fight antigens and are responsible for the cell-mediated immune response.

PREVENTION OF BLOOD DISORDERS

When considerable blood is lost through hemorrhage, the patient becomes anemic. Hemorrhage can occur from an accidental cut or tear to an artery, from a surgical incision, from trauma to internal organs, or during childbirth or spontaneous abortion. Sometimes excessive blood loss can occur during menstruation. **The nurse can often prevent hemorrhage after surgery or childbirth by vigilantly assessing the amount of blood loss and by instituting measures to stop the loss if it is excessive.**

The nurse can help prevent anemia by promoting proper nutrition and educating the public about the possibility of nutritional anemia. Nutritional anemia is a particular concern for individuals who subsist mostly on "fast food."

Cautioning the public about the dangers of exposure to ionizing radiation and harmful chemicals can decrease the incidence of blood disorders related to harmful substances. Genetic counseling regarding the

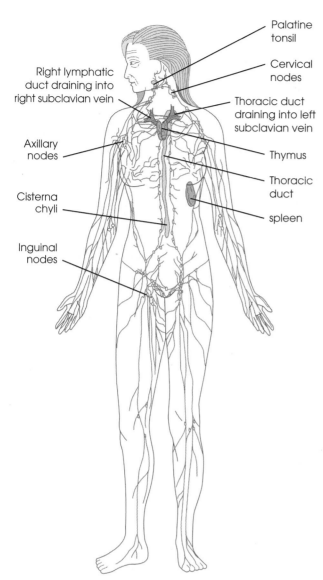

Palatine tonsil

Cervical nodes

Right lymphatic duct draining into right subclavian vein

Thoracic duct draining into left subclavian vein

Axillary nodes

Thymus

Thoracic duct

Cisterna chyli

spleen

Inguinal nodes

FIGURE 17-3   The lymphatic system.

TABLE 17-2 ◆ *Commonly Prescribed Drugs That May Cause a Blood Disorder*
Antineoplastic drugs that suppress the bone marrow
Barbital derivatives
Chloromycetin
Furosemide (Lasix)
Hydrochlorothiazide (Hydrodiuril)
Oral contraceptives that interfere with folic acid absorption or use.
Phenytoin (Dilantin)
Primidione (Mysoline)
Procainamide hydrochloride (Pronestyl)
Quinidine

of studies include those done on the plasma to measure the rate at which RBCs settle out from plasma (called the *sedimentation rate*) and to separate and classify various kinds of proteins, including antibodies, in the plasma.

The nurse's responsibility with blood tests is to explain the venipuncture procedure and the purpose of the test to the patient. Many patients have a great fear of needles. Others are concerned about having what seems like a lot of blood withdrawn. A few words of

TABLE 17-3 ◆ *Factors That May Alter Function of the Hematological or Lymphatic System*
Genetic Disorders
Hemophilia
Sickle cell disease
Agranulocytosis
Hemorrhage (anemia)
Surgical blood loss
Blood loss from childbirth or spontaneous abortion
Traumatic blood loss
Anemia
Iron deficiency
Folic acid deficiency
Pernicious anemia
Chronic slow blood loss
Hemolysis
Blood transfusion reaction
Genetic types of anemia
Bone marrow suppression
Antineoplastic agents used in treatment of cancer
Radiation treatment used for cancer
Excessive exposure to ionizing radiation
Exposure to toxic chemicals that damage the bone marrow
Drugs that suppress the bone marrow
Bone marrow proliferation or abnormality
Leukemia
Lymphoma
Hodgkin's disease

possibility of transmitting a genetic blood disorder to offspring is another nursing action that helps prevent blood disorders.

Monitoring patients for drug side effects and alerting the physician should blood-related side effects occur, can prevent a serious blood disorder from developing. Carefully monitoring blood transfusions and promptly reporting any untoward reaction may decrease the incidence of hemolysis from a transfusion reaction.

DIAGNOSTIC TESTS AND PROCEDURES

A surprising amount of information can be obtained from a stained blood film using only a 5-mL sample of uncoagulated blood. Each of the formed elements can be studied for shape, maturity, and number. Other kinds assurance and explanation can do much to relieve anxiety about a needle stick and promote cooperation. If the nurse is to perform the venipuncture, *Standard Precautions* and aseptic technique must be followed, and the correct tubes for each sample must be used. Rubber gloves must be worn by the nurse any time a venipuncture is performed, and equipment must be disposed of according to *Standard Precautions* (see Nursing Procedure 17-1).

Leukocyte counts provide information about infection and possible immune disorders. Data about the number of platelets are valuable in diagnosing a variety of diseases affecting or affected by the clotting of blood.

There are at least 12 different types of hemoglobin in human blood. The types are designated by letters—for example, hemoglobin A is normal adult hemoglobin, hemoglobin F is normal fetal hemoglobin, and

Nursing Procedures 17-1

Venipuncture and drawing a blood sample using a Vacutainer system: Performing blood tests is one of the most common diagnostic procedures. Nurses must be proficient at drawing blood efficiently with as little trauma to the patient as possible. The Vacutainer system is the most common method used to obtain blood samples and for that reason is presented here. Blood can also be drawn using a syringe and needle with this venipuncture technique.

Steps	Rationale
1. Check the physician's order for the tests to be done.	Verifies that the patient needs a blood sample drawn.
2. Gather the equipment: Vacutainer holder, Vacutainer needle, tourniquet, alcohol swabs, sterile 2 × 2 gauze squares, tape, appropriate test tubes for the desired tests, labels for the tubes, laboratory requisition slip, appropriate latex gloves (impermeable to blood), biohazard sharps container and a biohazard bag.	Gathering equipment prior to beginning procedure promotes efficiency and saves time.
3. Identify the patient by checking the armband or verifying name verbally. Explain the procedure.	Ensures samples are taken from the correct patient. Explaining the procedure decreases anxiety.
4. Fill out a label for each test tube.	Properly identifies sample and prevents need for repeating the venipuncture procedure.
5. Attach the Vacutainer needle to the Vacutainer tube holder by inserting it into the narrow end and screwing it securely in place.	Prepares the system for use.
6. Wash your hands.	Helps prevent infection at the puncture site.
7. Select an appropriate venipuncture site, avoiding scars, lesions, or a vessel in which an IV infusion is running (Figure 17-4). The best distal site on the vein should be used first.	Scar tissue is difficult to puncture; a puncture over a lesion may introduce microorganisms into the blood; IV fluids may alter the test results.

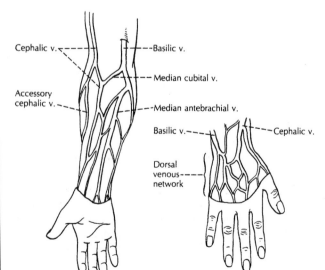

Cephalic v.
Basilic v.
Median cubital v.
Accessory cephalic v.
Median antebrachial v.
Basilic v.
Cephalic v.
Dorsal venous network

FIGURE 17-4   Venipuncture sites. (*Source:* Lammon, C. B., et al. [1995]. *Clinical Nursing Skills.* Philadelphia: Saunders, p. 139.)

Nursing Procedures 17-1 *(Continued)*

Steps	Rationale
8. Place the Vacutainer tube inside the holder, but do not push it onto the needle; position the Vacutainer holder and tubes within easy reach.	Preparing the system for use allows you to pick up the equipment after you have stabilized the vessel with one hand.
9. Put on the latex gloves.	Latex gloves are impermeable to blood and are required for *Standard Precautions.*
10. Lower the extremity so the site is below the heart.	A dependent position enhances blood flow to the site.
11. Apply a tourniquet to the extremity 2 to 4 inches above the venipuncture site. It should be moderately tight. Ask the patient to make a fist.	The tourniquet obstructs blood flow out of the vessel and causes the vein to fill with blood. A distended vein is easier to palpate and puncture. Making a fist aids in vein distention.
12. Cleanse the site with 70% alcohol in a circular motion outward, and allow the area to dry.	Alcohol decreases the number of microorganisms on the skin, preventing their transfer to the blood.
13. Pick up the Vacutainer holder and tube in your dominant hand and remove the needle cover.	Prepares the unit for venipuncture.
14. Anchor the vein with the thumb of your nondominant hand far enough below the site so that the needle will not touch the thumb as it enters the vessel.	Stabilizes the vein so that it doesn't roll when venipuncture is performed.
15. Hold the Vacutainer unit with the needle bevel facing up and position it at a 45-degree angle over the desired venipuncture site.	Allows a parallel insertion of the needle in the vein and decreases the risk of running the needle through the back side of the vessel.
16. Puncture the site, and, while stabilizing the Vacutainer unit, press the tube stopper onto the needle; blood running into the tube indicates successful venipuncture.	Stabilizing the unit prevents pushing the needle through the vein when pressing the tube stopper onto the Vacutainer needle.
17. Allow the tube to fill completely.	Ensures a sufficient quantity of blood to perform the test.
18. Loosen the tourniquet, and withdraw the needle from the vein.	Loosening the tourniquet before withdrawing the needle will decrease the amount of bleeding that occurs.
19. Immediately apply a dry gauze pad with pressure to the vein to stop the bleeding.	A dry pad aids coagulation of the blood, and pressure constricts the vessel, decreasing bleeding.
20. Apply a small adhesive bandage over the puncture site.	Decreases entrance of microorganisms at the site and helps prevent further bleeding.
21. Carefully remove and dispose of the Vacutainer needle in a biohazard sharps container.	Prevents accidental needle sticks.
22. Remove and label the tube of blood, and place it in a biohazard bag.	Correctly identifies the patient's blood. A biohazard bag prevents blood contamination should the tube become broken.
23. Fill out the laboratory requisition slip, and attach it to the blood sample; send it to the laboratory.	Identifies the correct test to be done for the right patient.
24. Remove the gloves and wash your hands.	Decreases microorganisms on the hands.
25. Chart the procedure, noting the time, site of venipuncture, type of specimen obtained, and that it was sent to the laboratory.	Verifies that the ordered blood sample was drawn and sent to the laboratory.

hemoglobin S is found in sickle cell disease. A **hematocrit** is a test that measures the volume of blood cells in relation to the volume of plasma. When there has been a loss of body fluids but no loss of cells, as in dehydration, the cell volume is high in proportion to the amount of liquid (plasma) in the bloodstream (i.e., the hematocrit rises). On the other hand, when either hemorrhage or anemia has depleted the supply of cells, the blood is "thinned" and the cell volume is low. Table 17-4 presents the most common diagnostic tests and related nursing care for the hematological and lymphatic systems.

TABLE 17-4 ◆ *Diagnostic Tests for Disorders of the Hematological and Lymphatic Systems*

Test and Normal Range	Purpose	Description	Nursing Implication
Complete blood count (CBC)	Determine whether abnormalities are present in the numbers of blood cells or types of blood cells; assess the amount of hemoglobin present. Useful to diagnose anemia.	Fill a lavender-top tube containing EDTA with a venous sample of blood. Use a site where there is little chance of dilution from IV solution. Mix the blood and the EDTA by gently rotating the tube.	Warn the patient that a "stick" is about to occur, but that the pain will be short-lived. Apply pressure directly to the puncture site after withdrawing the needle; at the antecubital space do **not** have patient flex the arm as this tends to cause a hematoma.

Erythrocytes
    Hemoglobin: females: 12.0–15.5 g/dL; males: 13.00–16.5 g/dL
    Red blood cell count: females: 4.0–5.9 mil/mm^3; males: 4.8–5.5 mil/mm^3
    Hematocrit: female: 37%–48%; male: 40%–45%
Leukocytes
    White blood cell (WBC): 4,000–9,000/mm^3
Differential count
    Granulocytes
        Neutrophils: 60%–70% of WBCs
        Eosinophils: 0%–5% of WBCs
        Basophils: 0%–3% of WBCs
    Agranulocytes
        Lymphocytes: 30%–40% of WBCs
        Monocytes: 0%–5% of WBCs
    Thrombocytes (platelets): 150,000–450,000/mm^3 of blood
    Mean corpuscular volume (MCH): 26–34 pg/cell
    Mean corpuscular Hb concentration (MCHC): 32–36 gm/dL
    Mean corpuscular volume (MCV): 80–96 μm^3

Test and Normal Range	Purpose	Description	Nursing Implication

Sedimentation rate
  <age 50 15–20 mm/hour
  50–85 20–30 mm/hour
  >age 85 30–42 mm/hour
	To detect inflammation and infection.	Fill a blue-top tube with venous blood. The laboratory determines the rate at which the RBCs settle.	Explain that this test helps diagnose an inflammatory process but is nonspecific.

Hemoglobin electrophoresis
  Hemoglobin A1C: 3%–5%
  Hemoglobin A2: 1.5%–3%
  Hemoglobin F: <1%
	Useful in diagnosing various types of anemia.	Performed on venous sample using lavender-top tube with EDTA.	Same as for CBC.

Tests for anemia
  Iron: 75–175 μg/dL total
    iron binding capacity:
    240–410 μg/dL
  Saturation 20%–55%
	Detect reason for anemia.	Performed on a venous blood sample.	Same as for CBC

Coagulation tests
  Prothrombin time (PT):
    12–28 sec
  Partial thromboplastin time
    (PTT): 20–35 sec
  Activated partial thromboplastin time (APTT):
    16–25 sec
  Bleeding time, ivy: 2.75–8.0 min.
	Determine abnormalities of clotting time.	Performed on a venous blood sample; use a blue-top tube	Same as for a CBC; pressure may need to be applied longer than usual if the patient has an abnormal clotting time or is on heparin or coumadin therapy.

TABLE 17-4 ◆ *Diagnostic Tests for Disorders of the Hematological and Lymphatic Systems* (Continued)

Test	Purpose	Description	Nursing Implication
Sickledex: 0	Test for the presence of hemoglobin S.	Performed on a venous blood sample; use a lavender-top tube.	Client may be anxious about the result; be sensitive to feelings. Positive result indicates need for genetic counseling.
Bence-Jones protein test	Assist in the diagnosis of multiple myeloma.	Obtain a 10-mL fresh morning specimen of urine in a clean container. Must be refrigerated or tested immediately. Presence of Bence-Jones Proteins in the urine is abnormal.	Explain the procedure to the patient.
Schilling test ≥7% excreted within 24 hrs.	Determine ability to absorb vitamin B_{12}; used to diagnose pernicious anemia.	Radioactive B_{12} is given orally, followed in 2 hours by an IM injection of B_{12}. A 24-hour urine specimen is collected.	Assess kidney function. Requires an 8- to 12-hour fast. No B vitamins for 3 days prior; no laxatives for 24 hours. Subnormal levels of B_{12} in the urine indicate the lack of intrinsic factor, which facilitates absorption of vitamin B_{12}.
Lymphangiogram Normal size vessels and nodes without filling defects.	Detect abnormalities in the lymphatic system, especially cancer.	Dye is injected intradermally between the first three toes of each foot while the patient is supine. Local anesthesia is injected and an incision is made in the dorsum of the foot to inject iodine contrast material directly into a lymphatic vessel over a 1½-hour period. X-rays are taken of the abdomen, pelvis, and upper body.	Repeat films are taken in 24 hours. Obtain written consent. Assess for allergy to iodine or shellfish. Explain procedure. Postprocedure elevate legs to decrease swelling for 24 hours. Assess for signs of infection and oil embolism q 4 h × 24 h.
Spleen sonogram Proper size, shape and position.	Detect structural abnormalities of the spleen.	An ultrasound wand is moved over the abdomen in the area of the spleen with the patient supine on the examining table.	Explain that the test takes about 30 minutes.
Spleen scan Even distribution of labeled erythrocytes throughout the spleen.	Detect anatomic changes in the spleen; determine invasion of Hodgkin's or metastatic disease. Usually done in conjunction with a liver scan.	A radioactive nuclide colloid is injected intravenously. After about 20 minutes a minimum of three views are obtained. Radiation exposure is about 0.5 rads (equal to about 1 year of natural radiation exposure to the body). Schedule scan before tests using barium.	Explain that a substance will be injected and after about 20 minutes scanning begins. Radiation exposure is minimal. The test takes about 60 minutes.

(Table 17-4 continued)

TABLE 17-4 ◆ *Diagnostic Tests for Disorders of the Hematological and Lymphatic Systems* (Continued)			
Test	**Purpose**	**Description**	**Nursing Implication**
Bone marrow aspiration and biopsy Normal cell counts	To help diagnose blood disorders.	Cells are withdrawn by needle from the sternum or iliac crest. Leukocytes, platelets, and erythrocytes are examined in the various stages of development to determine abnormalities. Assists in identifying certain anemias, leukemia, and thrombocytopenia.	Explain that the aspiration is done at the bedside. Seek an order for prebiopsy medication to decrease the discomfort. Explain that there is a feeling of pressure when the needle is inserted and sharp, brief, pain when the marrow is aspirated. The area of aspiration is surgically prepped. The patient must hold perfectly still. Pressure is applied to the site afterward to prevent hematoma formation. Posttest observe for swelling and tenderness indicating continued bleeding or infection.

Note: Normal values differ between laboratories.

Think about . . . When caring for a patient who has been in an automobile accident and has sustained trauma to the central body, what laboratory values should the nurse check daily?

NURSING ASSESSMENT

◆ History

The nurse assesses patients for signs and symptoms that indicate abnormalities in the blood and in the lymphatic system. **Abnormal symptoms result from too little circulating blood or too little hemoglobin, too few platelets, deficiency of normal neutrophils or lymphocytes, and from too many abnormal blood cells. When there is insufficient hemoglobin to carry oxygen to the cells, signs of oxygen deficit occur.** Asking the following questions will provide an appropriate history concerning factors pertinent to the blood and lymphatic system.

- Do you or anyone in your family have a genetic blood disorder, such as hemophilia, thalassemia, sickle cell trait or disease, aplastic anemia, agranulocytosis, or thrombocytopenia purpura?
- Have you ever been told you had anemia?
- Do you have frequent sore throats or other infections?

- Do you frequently feel like you have a fever?
- Do you ever have night sweats?
- Are your joints painful? Do they swell?
- Do you bruise easily or develop pinpoint blood spots?
- Do you suffer from itching?
- Have you noticed any swollen lymph nodes or lumps in the neck, armpits, or groin?
- Do you ever have tingling or numbness in the extremities?
- Do you have frequent headaches? Palpitations?
- Have you become more irritable than usual?
- Do you get dizzy frequently? Do you suffer fainting spells?
- Do you get short of breath when you walk a ways or when you climb stairs?
- Do your gums bleed when you brush your teeth? Does your tongue get sore? Do you have frequent mouth sores?
- Do you have any difficulty eating?
- Do colds or other infections seem to last a very long time for you?
- Do you frequently feel fatigued even when you haven't been doing much?
- Have you been exposed to chemicals, such as pesticides, cleaning agents, or industrial chemicals of any kind?
- Have you ever noticed that you have black, tarry-looking stool or smokey or brown urine?

- Do you have stomach pain or indigestion? Have you ever had an ulcer?
- Are your menstrual periods unduly heavy (if appropriate)?
- What do you usually eat for each meal?
- Are you often cold when others are not?

♦ Physical Assessment

In addition to the usual initial and ongoing assessment conducted by the nurse caring for a patient, some special observations are relevant for patients with blood or lymphatic disorders. Table 17-5 provides a guide for physical assessment.

Skin   Although pallor may be a sign of anemia, it is not the most reliable sign. Many other factors can affect a person's complexion and skin color, including thickness of the skin, amount of skin pigment, and number and distribution of blood vessels near the surface of the skin. Pale conjunctiva of the eye or pale mucous membranes is a better indicator. A very ruddy complexion with a red, florid appearance is typical of an excessive number of red blood cells (**polycythemia**).

Jaundice, or a yellowing discoloration of the skin and sclera of the eyes, can occur as a result of excessive destruction of red blood cells (**hemolysis**). When red blood cells are ruptured, bilirubin is released. The pigment eventually finds its way into the bloodstream, where it causes jaundice. If hemolysis is occurring, the urine will often contain bilirubin, giving it a brown tea color.

TABLE 17-5 ♦ *Guide to Focused Physical Assessment of the Hematological and Lymphatic Systems*

Head and neck
Color of conjunctiva and sclera or eye
Condition of gums and oral mucous membranes; condition of tongue
Presence of enlarged cervical lymph nodes

Skin
Color (pallor, jaundice, ruddy, flushed face)
Check conjunctiva, palms of hands, and roof of the mouth in people with dark skin.
Condition of fingernails (brittle)
Presence of ecchymoses or petechiae
Presence of red streaks around lymph nodes

Chest and abdomen
Presence of swollen lymph nodes in armpits or groin
Rapid respirations; shortness of breath upon exertion
Rapid pulse rate at rest
Epigastric tenderness

Extremities
Presence of swollen or painful joints

Bruises and small red patches (**petechiae**) are typical of thrombocytopenic purpura, a hemorrhagic disease sometimes associated with a decrease in the number of circulating platelets. In dark-skinned people, check the palms of the hands and soles of the feet for petechiae. Bleeding under the skin and formation of bruises in response to the slightest trauma frequently occur in anemias, leukemias, and diseases affecting the bone marrow and spleen. These appear as darker areas on brown-skinned people.

Elder Care Point... The elderly bruise more easily because of thinner skin and greater fragility of blood vessel walls. Aspirin or other drug therapy also may make them more prone to bruising. Therefore bruising is not necessarily an unusual sign in this age group.

Cyanosis, or a bluish tint to the skin, can indicate hypoxia resulting from inadequate numbers of circulating erythrocytes. The roof of the mouth is the best place to check for a bluish color in dark-skinned people.

Mucous Membranes   Nutritional deficiencies contributing to anemia and resultant hypoxia may cause sore and painful gums and tongue. The patient may have difficulty chewing and eating. Bleeding of the gums (**gingivitis**) may occur with tooth brushing when the platelet count is low.

Abdomen   Stomach pain or nausea can be caused by bleeding ulcers, a frequent cause of chronic blood loss. Black, tarry, or coffee-ground stools indicate gastrointestinal (GI) bleeding. Hiatal hernia also can cause a chronic blood loss.

Swollen and Painful Joints   Bleeding into the joints (**hemarthrosis**) is not uncommon in certain kinds of anemia, such as sickle cell disease or in hemophilia. This might be evidenced by swelling and slight redness in the area of the joints, or the patient may move more slowly and with obvious discomfort.

Lymph Tissue Involvement   Enlarged lymph nodes occur in a number of different blood disorders as well as in infections and immune disorders. The nodes most often inspected and palpated are those under the arm, in the neck, and in the inguinal (groin) region. Lymph node enlargement is often found while bathing a patient or helping him with activities of daily living (ADLs). Note any red streaks on the skin that may indicate lymphadenitis.

Enlargement of the spleen, which also accompanies polycythemia and several other blood disorders, might be described by the patient as a feeling of fullness on the left side of the upper abdomen.

Mental State   Irritability and mental depression are often found in patients with blood disorders. **Irritability, dizziness, difficulty in concentrating, and headache may be caused by a decreased supply of oxygen to the brain.** Depression often accompanies the chronic lack of energy, difficulty in eating and enjoying food, and the many other problems from which patients with blood disorders often suffer.

Activity Intolerance   Physical activity increases the demand for oxygen, but if there are not enough circulating RBCs to carry the necessary oxygen, the patient becomes physically weak and unable to engage in physical activity without severe fatigue. Note whether the patient is able to do things for herself or needs help to complete specific ADLs.

Think about...

- Can you name four signs or symptoms that you might encounter when taking a patient's history that could indicate your patient may be anemic?
- How can the conjunctiva and the sclera of the eye provide information about anemia or jaundice?
- What signs and symptoms might indicate that the patient is suffering a chronic blood loss?

◆Nursing Diagnosis

Nursing diagnoses for hematological and lymphatic disorders are based on the problems caused for the patient. Nursing diagnoses commonly associated with hematological and lymphatic disorders are listed in Table 17-6.

TABLE 17-6 ◆ *Common Nursing Diagnoses and Intervention for Patients with Blood Disorders*

Nursing Diagnosis	Goals/Expected Outcomes	Intervention
Alteration in nutrition, less than body requirements, related to:		Teach the patient about foods that meet required needs. Obtain dietary consult as needed Administer iron preparation; if liquid, give through straw.
Iron deficiency from inadequate intake or blood loss	Hemoglobin levels will be within normal range within 3 months.	Give with vitamin C–containing juice or food. Warn that stool may be greenish-black.
Vitamin B$_{12}$ deficiency	The patient will administer his own B$_{12}$ injections on a regular schedule.	Administer vitamin B$_{12}$ as ordered; advise that lifetime therapy is needed.
Inflammation of mucous membranes	The patient performs mouth care diligently on schedule. Patient displays normal-appearing mucous membranes. CBC shows increasing RBCs and Hbg within 3 weeks.	Give gentle mouth care before meals and q 2 h. Provide bland, easily chewed foods. Monitor CBC count for evidence of increase in RBCs and Hgb.
Activity intolerance related to decreased RBCs or Hgb A	Patient is using oxygen as ordered. Patient alternates activities with rest. Patient seeks assistance with ambulation when dizzy.	Administer oxygen by nasal cannula at 3 to 6 L/minute as ordered for patient with sickle cell crisis. Space activities, allowing rest periods for patient with fatigue. Assist with ADLs to prevent fatigue. Maintain skin integrity. Turn frequently. If dizzy, caution to change position slowly; call for assistance with ambulation.
Pain related to ischemia and swollen joints.	Patient verbalizes that pain is controlled by analgesics. Patient verbalizes that pain has decreased within 48 hours.	Elevate swollen joints, and apply hot or cold packs. Encourage high fluid intake. Monitor IV fluid therapy. Teach to avoid strenuous exercise. Use bed cradle to support bed covers. Administer analgesics as ordered PRN.

TABLE 17-6 ◆ *Common Nursing Diagnoses and Intervention for Patients with Blood Disorders* (Continued)		
Nursing Diagnosis	**Goals/Expected Outcomes**	**Intervention**
Risk of injury, related to low platelet count	Platelet count within safe limits after platelet administration. Patient will have no new hematoma formation or other evidence of bleeding.	Assess for signs of internal bleeding; bruises, urine, stool; measure abdominal girth q day. Minimize trauma; handle gently. Apply ice packs and gentle pressure if hematoma seems to be forming. Monitor administration of platelets PRN. Use small-guage needle for injections; rotate sites. Apply pressure to puncture site for 10 minutes.
Risk of infection, related to decreased leukocytes	Patient will have no evidence of infection.	Observe for early signs of infection and report. Use strict aseptic technique for wound care and invasive procedures. Use protective isolation as needed. Teach patient good personal hygiene. Maintain integrity of skin and mucosa. Administer antiinfectives precisely as ordered.
Knowledge deficit, related to substances that damage bone marrow	Patient verbalizes knowledge of drugs and chemicals that are harmful to the bone marrow within one week.	Assess for exposure to substances that could have damaged the bone marrow. Teach about drugs and chemicals that are harmful to bone marrow and how to prevent damage. Seek feedback to validate understanding of content taught.
Anxiety related to unknown outcome of diagnostic tests and knowledge of disease, treatment, and prognosis	Patient verbalizes purpose and expected experience for each diagnostic test ordered. Patient verbalizes fears regarding disease, treatment, and prognosis.	Provide teaching regarding each diagnostic test. Encourage verbalization of fears. Offer emotional support to patient and family.
Self-esteem disturbance, related to inability to perform usual activities	Patient defines ways to cope with physical limitations. Patient verbalizes strengths. Patient discusses possibility of seeking counseling.	Assist to cope with limitations of the illness. Help plan ways to maintain appropriate activity. Help to focus on the things he can still do. Obtain counseling referral if psychological disturbance indicates need.
Risk of ineffective family coping, related to expense of treatment and possible death of patient	Patient and family seek assistance from community resources as needed. Patient and family verbalize understanding of disease, treatment modalities, and their implications.	Refer leukemia patient and family to community resources, such as the American Cancer Society, for assistance. Assist family and patient to understand the disease, treatment modalities, and their implications. Encourage attendance for all family members in a support group. Obtain referral to social worker for further assistance. Encourage open communication within family.

◆ Planning

Planning care for a patient with a blood or lymphatic disorder focuses on preventing infection, conserving energy, control of pain, and correction of the underlying disorder if possible.

Nursing care should be planned to provide rest periods for the patient. Planning dietary teaching or consult with the dietitian is important for patients with nutritional anemias. **The patient with a blood or lymph abnormality is at higher risk for infection and using aseptic techniques is extremely important.** Such patients should not be exposed to people who are ill with contagious diseases, such as colds or influenza, whether they are the health care workers or visitors.

Nursing goals include:

- ◆ Prevent infection.
- ◆ Conserve patient's energy and prevent undue fatigue.
- ◆ Correct nutritional deficiencies.
- ◆ Provide treatment to halt or slow disease process.
- ◆ Control pain or discomfort.

Specific expected outcomes are written for individualized nursing diagnoses. Examples are included in Nursing Care Plan 17-1.

◆ Implementation

Nurses should handle patients with blood dyscrasias gently to prevent bruising and hematomas. Care is taken to apply sufficiently long pressure after injections. Good skin care is essential, as the skin acts as a protective barrier against infection. Teaching about nutrition and medication administration, prevention of infection, and measures to prevent bleeding is a major part of the nursing care for these patients. Pain control is important for the patient with sickle cell anemia in crisis, the hemophiliac with hemarthrosis, and for the advanced leukemia and lymphoma patient.

Specific interventions for patients experiencing blood and lymphatic disorders are listed in Table 17-6. Other interventions are included in the discussion of the various disorders.

◆ Evaluation

The evaluation process provides data to determine whether the specific outcome criteria are being met for each patient. Monitoring laboratory values for blood counts and determining whether counts are improving is vital to determine if treatment and nursing actions are meeting the patient's needs. Assessing for side effects and evaluating how the patient is tolerating the medication or other treatment for the underlying disorder is important. **When a patient with leukemia or lymphoma** is undergoing chemotherapy, evaluate the blood count results to determine that safe levels of leukocytes and platelets are present before administering another dose of a drug that inhibits their production.

It is important that each home care nurse evaluate how closely the patient is following the prescribed treatment plan. The nurse also determines whether the treatment is effective, and, if it isn't, should initiate collaboration with the physician to change the plan.

DISORDERS OF THE HEMATOLOGICAL SYSTEM

◆ Anemia

In a healthy person, a balance is maintained between the production of new cells and the disposal of old, "worn-out" cells. When something happens to upset this balance or interfere with maturation of cells, anemia results. **There aren't enough healthy blood cells to carry sufficient oxygen throughout the body.**

Pathophysiology   **Oxygen transport depends on the number and condition of the red cells and the amount of hemoglobin they contain.** Anemia is a state in which there are insufficient numbers of functioning red blood cells or a lack of hemoglobin to meet the demands of the tissues for oxygen (Figure 17-5).

> There are three major classifications of anemia according to cause: (1) anemia resulting from blood loss; (2) anemia resulting from a failure in blood cell production; and (3) anemia associated with an excessive destruction of red cells.

A blood loss that leads to anemia may result from severe trauma to the blood vessels and massive hemorrhage or may be more gradual, as from a small, bleeding peptic ulcer that causes a chronic blood loss.

Anemia caused by a failure in cell production is the result of either a deficiency of certain substances necessary for the formation of red blood cells or abnormal function of bone marrow. Examples of this type of anemia are (1) nutritional anemia, in which there is an inadequate intake of foods containing proteins, folic acid, and iron; (2) anemia caused by bone marrow suppression by toxic substances; and (3) pernicious anemia, in which there is faulty absorption of specific nutrients, such as vitamin B_{12}.

In *pernicious anemia,* the intrinsic factor is missing from the gastric juices, so the iron and protein taken into the stomach cannot be properly absorbed. The result is that the red cell production is decreased, and those red cells that are produced are abnormal in structure and function. To correct this condition, the physician will order the administration of vitamin B_{12}.

Nursing Care Plan 17-1

Selected nursing diagnoses, goals/expected outcomes, nursing interventions, and evaluations for a home care patient who has leukemia.

Situation: Jason Shubert, a 38-year-old male, has acute myelogenous leukemia (AML). He is undergoing outpatient chemotherapy and is being followed at home by a home care agency nurse.

Nursing Diagnosis	Goals/Expected Outcome	Nursing Interventions	Evaluation
Risk of infection related to low WBC. SUPPORTING DATA WBCs 2,000/mm³.	Patient will remain free from infection.	Monitor temperature daily. Report temperature elevation >100.4°F (>38°C) that lasts for more than 24 hours. Teach patient and family to wash hands frequently. Use meticulous handwashing when caring for patient. Have patient deep-breathe q 2 h while awake. Administer transfusion of granulocytes as needed.	Temperature remains at 99.2°F (37.3°C). Demonstrated handwashing technique; patient and wife using correct technique. Maintaining strict asepsis for care. Using incentive spirometer 4 × a day only. Granulocytes not yet needed.
Fatigue related to decreased RBCs SUPPORTING DATA States has no energy. Frequently falls asleep. RBCs 3.2 mil/mm³. Hct 33 mL/dL.	Fatigue will lessen as evidenced by ability to perform more self-care activities.	Administer packed RBCs to restore normal erythrocyte level as needed. Administer Epogen as ordered. Provide assistance for ADLs. Provide spaced rest periods.	1 unit of RBCs transfused; RBCs rising. Epogen × 2 given this week. Mother assisting with ADLs when wife is not home. Napping after morning care and after lunch.
Self-care deficit related to fatigue. SUPPORTING DATA Unable to bathe self with extreme fatigue. Becomes short of breath when performing ADLs.	Patient will be able to bathe and dress self without assistance.	Provide bathing assistance 3 × a week. Encourage resting between care activities. Encourage to perform ADLs in small segments.	Bath aid given × 3 this week. Patient allowed to rest for 10 minutes between bath and dressing. Able to comb own hair and brush own teeth with rest period in between.
Ineffective family coping related to alteration in roles. SUPPORTING DATA Patient unable to work; wife is searching for full-time position to support family.	Patient's wife will cope effectively as primary wage earner.	Assist wife with defining alternatives for employment. Arrange consult with social worker to coordinate patient's care at home when wife returns to work. Suggest community resources that might help wife find employment.	Discussed job skills today. Called social worker to advise of consult. Gave wife list of community resources for women returning to work.
Risk of injury related to decreased platelet count. SUPPORTING DATA Platelets 120,000/mm³	Patient will not experience episodes of bleeding.	Monitor CBC and platelet counts. Instruct to report oozing of blood from the gums. Instruct to observe stool and urine for signs of bleeding. Use small-gauge needle for injections. Administer stool softener to prevent constipation. Instruct to use soft toothbrush or toothettes to clean teeth. Instruct to use an electric razor to shave.	CBC remaining stable; platelet count down to 119,000. States has no oozing from gums and no signs of bleeding elsewhere. Epogen administered IV through port. Taking stool softener daily; no constipation. Using soft toothbrush and electric razor. Progressing toward goals; continue plan.

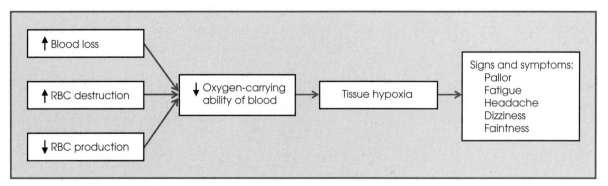

FIGURE 17-5   Pathophysiology of anemia.

Anemias associated with excessive destruction of red blood cells are exceedingly rare. They are known as *hemolytic anemias* (**hemolysis** means the destruction of red blood cells). Some of the hemolytic anemias, such as *thalassemia*, are inherited, whereas others are caused by exposure of the erythrocytes to poisonous agents, such as chemicals or certain bacterial toxins.

Anemia occurs in end-stage renal disease patients when there is a deficiency of production of *erythropoietic renal factor,* a substance necessary to stimulate the production of red blood cells in the bone marrow.

The microscopic appearance of the red cells on a film of blood that has been spread over a slide gives information about abnormalities in size, shape, and color of erythrocytes circulating in the patient's bloodstream.

The prefix *normo-* refers to normal, the suffix-*cyte* refers to cell, and the suffix-*chrom* refers to color. Thus a normocytic, normochromic anemia is characterized by cells that are normal in size and color but have a deficiency in the number of RBCs and in the hematocrit. **This type of anemia usually occurs as a result of sudden blood loss.**

A hypochromic, microcytic anemia is characterized by decreased levels of hemoglobin (not enough color) and small (micro) cells. **This type of anemia is typical of an iron deficiency anemia.**

Elder Care Point... Anemia is not a normal part of aging. In the older age group, anemia is more commonly the result of poor nutrition. If the patient has an intestinal disorder, the anemia may be due to decreased absorption of nutrients or from pernicious anemia.

Hemorrhagic or Hypovolemic Shock **Rapid, severe bleeding leads to anemia from blood loss,** *hypovolemia* **(decreased volume of circulating blood), and shock.** The bleeding may be external, or it may be internal and therefore more difficult to detect. The amount of blood loss that leads to hypovolemic shock varies depending on the ability of the patient's body to compensate for the lost fluid volume. A blood loss of 500 to 2,800 mL in an adult who had normal circulating volume causes hypovolemic shock.

The elderly may develop shock with smaller blood loss because of decreased vascular tone and impaired cardiac function.

Shock from hemorrhage results from trauma, surgery, bleeding esophageal varices, or a ruptured aortic aneurysm, excessive bleeding during childbirth, or from a coagulation disorder.

When discovered and treated early, hypovolemic shock is reversible. Unrecognized or untreated shock often progresses to death. Table 17-7 presents techniques to control bleeding from accidental trauma.

TABLE 17-7 ◆ *Techniques to Control Bleeding*

Severe bleeding can lead to irreversible hypovolemic shock from loss of intravascular fluid and to circulatory collapse. Blood loss from an artery is bright red and will gush forth in spurts at regular intervals as the heart contracts. Blood loss from an artery is more rapid than that from a vein. Blood from a severed or punctured vein leaks slowly and steadily and is dark red.

Procedure

Position the body part that is bleeding over a firm surface and immobilize the part.

Place a sterile dressing or clean cloth over the wound.

With the flat palm of the hand or several fingers, apply direct pressure on the wound continuously for 5 minutes.

Check for stoppage of bleeding after 5 minutes; if bleeding is occurring, apply pressure continuously for another 10 minutes.

When bleeding has stopped, gently remove hand pressure and apply a pressure dressing over the cloth or dressing by folding another dressing or piece of cloth several times and tying it firmly over the wound.

Check circulation distal to the wound to be certain that the pressure dressing is not so tight that circulation below the wound is cut off.

Reinforce the dressing as needed by applying yet another layer of dressing as blood soaks through; do not remove previously applied dressings.

If direct pressure will not stop the bleeding, and bleeding is considerable, apply pressure over the artery leading to the wound. **(Cut off arterial flow only as a last resort).**

Check for adequate pressure over the artery by determining a lack of pulse distal to the wound and a sensation of tingling and numbness in the wound area.

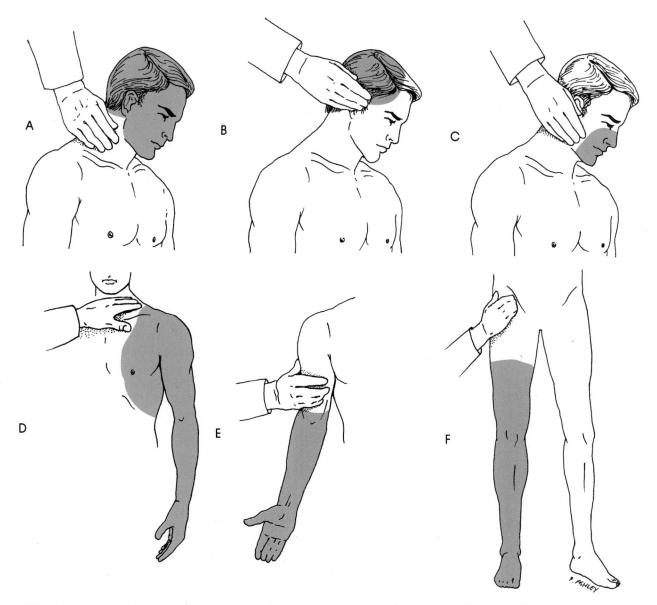

FIGURE 17-6   Locations of commonly used digital pressure points to stop hemorrhage. The screened areas are those within which hemorrhage may be controlled by pressure on a specific artery. (A) Carotid artery. (B) Temporal artery. (C) External maxillary artery. (D) Subclavian artery. (E) Brachial artery. (F) Femoral artery.

The classical signs and symptoms of hypovolemic shock are falling blood pressure; rapid, weak pulse; cool, damp skin; thirst; decreased urine output; and restlessness progressing to decreased consciousness.

Treatment. Finding the cause of the bleeding and stopping it is essential. The best treatment is to restore blood volume with fluids and blood by transfusion, thereby restoring tissue perfusion. Of primary importance is an open and functioning airway. A large-bore IV line and fluids are started immediately. Fluids administered include normal saline, dextrose in water, Ringer's solution, packed blood cells, plasma, or plasma substitutes (dextran, perfluorocarbons, or hetastarch). During fluid administration, the patient is assessed for signs of fluid overload, such as crackles in the lungs heard upon auscultation. Supplemental oxygen is administered to counteract oxygen deficit. The patient is positioned with the legs elevated 45 degrees or less with the knees straight, the trunk flat or raised very slightly, and the head level with the chest or slightly higher. Leg elevation promotes venous return from the lower extremities, improving cardiac output. Vasoconstrictor or vasodilator drugs may be used to assist the treatment of shock depending on the individual situation. If vasoconstrictors are used, the goal is to keep the systolic blood pressure at 70 to 80 mm Hg. Vasodilators may be used when fluids have been infused and there is still persistent vasoconstriction. Table 17-8 outlines nursing actions for the patient in hypovolemic shock.

TABLE 17-8 ◆ *Nursing Actions for the Patient in Hypovolemic Shock*

- Locate the cause of bleeding and stop it.
- Increase the rate of IV fluid flow if an IV is hanging.
- Reassure the patient that the situation is being remedied; do not leave the patient alone.
- Monitor vital signs closely.
- Notify the physician of your assessment findings and of the patient's status.
- Start a large-bore IV line if one does not exist already, and initiate fluid therapy to expand volume.
- Place the patient flat with the legs raised 45 degrees or less and the knees straight; the head may be raised slightly.
- Keep the patient warm.
- Administer supplemental oxygen by face mask at 4 to 5 L a minute; use a flow rate of 2 to 3 L a minute for patients with known lung disease.

Signs and Symptoms

Signs and symptoms of anemias from causes other than rapid bleeding include pallor, fatigue, headache, and dizziness or faintness.

These all relate directly to the decreased ability of the blood to transport sufficient oxygen to the tissues.

Treatment   Anemia from chronic, slow blood loss is treated by correcting the underlying problem and then building replacement blood cells with good nutrition and iron intake. Anemia caused by inadequate iron, folic acid, or protein intake is managed with oral iron supplements, vitamins, and diet adjustment. If the anemia is serious, iron supplementation may be administered IV with iron dextran, Imferon.

Pernicious anemia is treated by regular injections of vitamin B_{12}, as the deficiency of intrinsic factor prevents adequate absorption of this vitamin from food. Table 17-9 presents the medications most com-

TABLE 17-9 ◆ *Medications Commonly Prescribed for Disorders of the Hematological And Lymphatic Systems*

Classification	Action	Nursing Implication	Patient Teaching
Mineral Ferrous sulfate (Feosol, Fer-in-Sol) Ferrous glugonate (Fergon) Ferrous fumarate (Feostat, Ircon) Iron dextran (Imferon)	Increases elemental iron as a component in the formation of hemoglobin. Used to treat iron deficiency anemia.	May cause GI upset: nausea, diarrhea or constipation; monitor for constipation. Tell patient that oral form will turn stool black. Do not give with milk as it reduces absorption. Dilute elixir in juice and give through a straw to prevent staining of the teeth. Do not crush enteric-coated or sustained-release tablets or capsules. For IM form give with at least a 3″, 19- to 20-gauge needle and use "Z" track technique to prevent staining of the skin. Change needles after drawing up the solution. When given IV, monitor closely for anaphylactic reaction. Flush line with 10 mL saline post-infusion.	Tak oral form with orange juice or other vitamin C–rich food. Avoid taking iron with milk products. Keep out of reach of children as it is toxic. Have Hgb checked according to physician's schedule to check response to medication. Eat foods high in iron. Increase fluids and roughage if constipation occurs.
Vitamins Folic acid (Folvite)	Promotes normal erythropoiesis; used in certain types of anemia.	May interfere with anticonvulsant blood levels. Chloramphenocol interferes with absorption. Increase foods high in folic acid.	Have blood count monitored according to physician's schedule to determine effectiveness of therapy.

TABLE 17-9 ◆ *Medications Commonly Prescribed for Disorders of the Hematological And Lymphatic Systems* (Continued)

Classification	Action	Nursing Implication	Patient Teaching
Vitamin B$_{12}$ Cyanocobalamin (Rubramin, Anacobin)	Acts as coenzyme for cell replication and hematopoiesis. Used in pernicious anemia, other GI disorders that decrease vitamin B$_{12}$ absorption and in cases of dietary deficiency.	Give SC or IM daily for 5 to 10 days and then once monthly for maintenance. Can cause anaphylactic reaction when given IV. Deficiency more common in strict vegetarians.	Teach importance of maintaining monthly injections for life for prevention of further episodes of pernicious anemia. Encourage increased intake of vitamin B$_{12}$ in diet if deficiency is diet related.
Antimetabolite Hydroxyurea (Hydrea)	Inhibits DNA synthesis. Used to reduce episodes of sickling in sickle cell anemia. Used to irradicate abnormal cells in leukemia, myeloma, and some solid tumors.	Discontinue if WBC is <2,500/mm^3 or platelet count is >100,000/mm^3. Capsule granules may be mixed with water if taken immediately. May cause GI stomach upset, stomatitis, vomiting, diarrhea.	Use cautiously in presence of renal dysfunction. Radiation therapy increases toxicity. Monitor intake and output. Monitor for infection. Monitor blood counts for neutropenia and thrombocytopenia; bone marrow suppression. Caution to avoid exposure to infection and to report signs or symptoms of infection promptly. Increase fluid intake to maintain adequate hydration. Give mouth care every 4 hours to prevent stomatitis. Report bleeding to the physician.
Biological response modifiers Epoetin alfa; erythropoietin (Epogen, Procrit)	Controls rate of red cell production; a natural hormone produced by recombinant DNA techniques. Stimulates the bone marrow, functioning as a growth factor. Used to combat reduced production of erythropoietin of end-stage renal disease. Used as adjunct therapy in HIV-infected patients with anemia secondary to drug therapy.	Also used for patients with anemia secondary to chemotherapy and in chemotherapy and in rheumatoid arthritis patient who experience anemia from therapy. May be used to increase RBCs in anticipation of autologous blood transfusion before surgery.	May cause seizures. Monitor blood count closely; dosage may need to be reduced if hematocrit rises too rapidly. Monitor blood pressure closely, may cause rise. May cause pain in limbs and pelvis. Explain the purpose of the injections. Remind that the drug must be refrigerated; discard after 6 hours at room temperature.

monly prescribed for hematological and lymphatic disorders.

For *hemolytic* anemia, the underlying cause is found and corrected if possible, and then the blood volume is rebuilt with added iron and appropriate diet. If the anemia is severe, blood transfusion may be indicated.

Think about . . . Your patient who has suffered a blood loss and is now anemic complains that she is short of breath. Can you explain how blood loss might affect respiration?

Nursing Intervention Intervention begins with an understanding of the particular kind of anemia affecting the patient. Anemia from blood loss presents problems quite different from those related to chronic, and possibly incurable, anemia.

Actions are directed toward preventing complications for patients with anemias that interfere with

TABLE 17-10 ◆ *Nutrition Point: Common Foods That are High in Iron and Folic Acid*

Foods high in iron

Beef liver	Cooked shrimp	Prune juice
Blackstrap molasses	Dried apricots	Raisins
Chicken livers	Kidney beans	Spinach
Cooked oatmeal	Lean beef	Turkey
Cooked prunes	Lima beans	Whole grains

Adding raw spinach to dinner salads and snacking on raisins or dried apricots can quickly improve iron intake. Iron-enriched cereals and breads also can be added to the diet.

Foods high in folic acid

Asparagus	Legumes (Kidney beans, etc.)
Beef	Liver
Fish	Whole grains
Green leafy vegetables	

Note: Many of the foods high in iron also are high in folic acid.

clotting and tend to cause bleeding episodes. Assistance with ADLs is essential for any patient with anemia severe enough to cause fatigue. Planned rest periods must be provided for these patients.

Administering blood, iron, vitamin B_{12}, and folic acid and monitoring for desired effect are nursing functions. Patient education about needed dietary adjustments also is done. Table 17-10 provides suggestions for increasing iron and folic acid. **Patients should be taught that iron is absorbed more readily if vitamin C is present in the GI system at the same time.** Taking iron medication with orange juice provides the necessary vitamin C.

Elder Care Point... Many elderly persons have chronic conditions that require daily medication. Antacids and many other drugs interfere with iron absorption. Check all drugs a patient is receiving to determine whether drug interactions might interfere with iron absorption.

Analgesia for headache or joint pain is given as ordered, and the patient is monitored for adverse side effects. Table 17-6 identifies nursing diagnoses commonly associated with anemia and lists appropriate interventions.

◆ Aplastic Anemia

Aplastic anemia may develop after a viral infection, as a reaction to a drug, or because of an inherited tendency. **The disease is characterized by bone marrow depression. Red cells, white cells, and platelet levels are**

decreased. The toxic effects of certain substances can be responsible for aplastic anemia. Some of these agents include benzene; insecticides; drugs, such as chloramphenicol (Chloromycetin), phenylbutazone (Butazolidin), or sulfonamides; some anticonvulsants; gold compounds used to treat rheumatoid arthritis; or alkylating agents or antimetabolites used in chemotherapy. Many other drugs can potentially cause aplastic anemia, but this adverse effect is rare. Radiation exposure is another factor in the development of the disorder. See Figure 17-7 for the pathophysiology of aplastic anemia.

Signs and symptoms are the same as those of iron deficiency anemia, but also include ecchymosis, petechiae, and hemorrhage related to low platelet count. Infection may not cause an inflammatory response because of the very low leukocyte count.

Diagnosis is by blood count with differential, bone marrow biopsy, and by ruling out other disorders. **Aplastic anemia causes an emergency situation.**

Treatment must eliminate any identifiable underlying cause. Washed packed red cells and platelets are administered. Protective isolation is necessary to prevent infection in those with low leukocyte counts. Antibiotics are given for identified infection; oxygen is sometimes administered to those patients with low erythrocyte counts. Bone marrow transplant is the treatment of choice for those with severe bone marrow depression, but there must be an identical human leukocyte antigen (HLA) match.

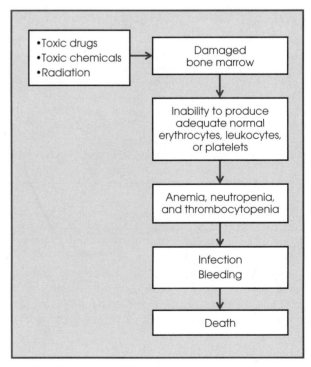

FIGURE 17-7   Pathophysiology of aplastic anemia.

Think about . . . What chemical products in your home or garage are capable of causing bone marrow depression?

Nursing Intervention Prevention of hemorrhage and of infection are top priorities. Psychological support of the patient and family is important when they are faced with this life-threatening condition. Nursing diagnoses might include "Activity intolerance," "Risk of injury," "Knowledge deficit," "Anxiety," "Risk of infection," and "Ineffective coping."

Another responsibility of the nurse is to monitor blood studies carefully for all patients who are receiving any drug that is potentially damaging to the bone marrow. All nurses should promote public education about the dangers of toxic agents. It is vitally important that people read and follow the label instructions on all cleaning agents, insecticides, and chemical compounds.

♦ Polycythemia Vera

Excessive production of red blood cells results in polycythemia vera. White cell numbers also increase. The cause of this disorder is unknown. The blood becomes thick from the increased numbers of cells, and there is a tendency to develop blood clots. Signs and symptoms include a reddish face with deep-red purplish lips, fatigue, weakness, dizziness, headache, and enlarged spleen (**splenomegaly**). Minor injury may result in excessive bleeding.

Treatment is aimed at reducing the number of blood cells. Antineoplastic agents, radiation therapy, and phlebotomy are all used. In phlebotomy, a blood vessel is pierced, and blood is drawn off. As much as 500 mL at a time may be withdrawn. Increased fluid intake is essential to decrease blood viscosity, and aspirin is used to decrease platelet clumping and clot formation.

♦ Thrombocytopenia

Thrombocytopenia occurs when the platelet count drops to less than 150,000/mm³. It can be a life-threatening condition. Causes include bone marrow depression from chemotherapy or radiation, autoimmune diseases, bacterial and viral infections, disseminated intravascular coagulation (DIC), and overfunction of the spleen. Certain drugs, such as nonsteroidal antiinflammatory drugs (NSAIDs), and thiazides also can result in platelet deficiency. Signs and symptoms include **purpura** (small areas of hemorrhage in the skin and mucous membranes) or large bruised areas called **ecchymoses**. Bleeding can occur in any part of the body.

Some patients recover spontaneously. Otherwise, transfusion of platelets is used to control hemorrhage.

Splenectomy is done when the cause of the thrombocytopenia is unknown and the patient does not respond to other therapy, with the hope that this will remove the cause of platelet destruction.

Nursing care is focused on prevention of bleeding by careful handling of the patient, close observation for signs of spontaneous bleeding, and quick intervention. Invasive procedures are used only when essential. Patients are taught to avoid activities that might induce bleeding, such as flossing the teeth, shaving with a safety razor, or engaging in contact sports.

♦ Sickle Cell Disease

Sickle cell disease is a genetic disorder in which the gene is inherited from both parents (homozygous). It is characterized by erythrocytes that contain more hemoglobin S than hemoglobin A. Sickle cell disease is found in 8-10% of African American newborns, but also affects some people whose ancestors were from the Mediterranean region, the Middle East, and India.

Sickle cell trait, in which only about 50% of an individual's total hemoglobin is affected, is present in about 10% of the black population of the United States. These people are carriers and can transmit the gene to their children. Therefore, genetic counseling and adequate screening for early detection of the disease are considered extremely important to control sickle cell anemia.

When the patient with sickle cell disease experiences lower oxygenation than normal, the defective hemoglobin forms clumps in the red cells, causing them to assume a sickle shape, blocking blood vessels, breaking apart, and forming thrombi that cause organ damage.

Sickle cell trait occurs in people who have only one gene, rather than a pair of genes, for sickle cell anemia. They usually do not have problems with sickling unless they experience severe deprivation of oxygenation. **The signs and symptoms are those that indicate lack of oxygen and blood flow, such as pallor, lethargy, and pain.**

Signs typical of anemia also occur after sickle cell crisis, as the abnormally shaped cells are very fragile and break easily. The RBC and hemoglobin count can drop very quickly during a crisis. There is no cure for sickle cell anemia; treatment is primarily symptomatic and preventive. The drug hydroxyurea has been found to reduce the frequency of sickling episodes. Patients on this drug have shown a 50% decrease in the number of hospitalizations for crisis. Should crisis occur, the patient is often treated at home with bedrest, adequate fluid intake, and analgesics. If his hemoglobin drops considerably or his condition suddenly deteriorates, he is hospitalized, given oxygen, and transfused with packed red cells. In addition, IV fluids are given, and narcotic analgesics may be needed to control pain. An attempt is made to mobilize the sickled cells and to prevent damage to major organs. Infection is treated with appropriate antibiotics. Sickle cell disease has been incurable, but international trials are showing that bone marrow transplant can possibly cure the disease in some people.

◆ Leukemia

The word *leukemia,* translated literally, means "white blood." Actually, the white blood cells would have to number 1,000,000/mm³ before the blood would have a milky white appearance, and, although leukemia is characterized by an increase in the number of leukocytes, their number rarely rises above 500,000/mm³. In addition to the increase in number, however, **the leukocytes of the patient with leukemia are abnormal cells that do not function as normal white cells do.** Malignant production of WBCs causes the disease.

Pathophysiology   An acute leukemia is one in which there are a lot of primitive cells, called blasts. In chronic leukemia, the predominant cells are more mature. Leukemias also are classified by the origin of the abnormal cells. *Myeloid leukemia* arises from the bone marrow, whereas *lymphoid leukemia* has its origin in the lymphatic system. There are four types of leukemia: acute myelogenous leukemia (AML), chronic myelogenous leukemia (CML), acute lymphocytic leukemia (ALL), and chronic lymphocytic leukemia (CLL).

About 27,600 people will develop this disorder in 1996. In acute leukemia there is a sudden, rapid growth of immature blast or stem cells, rapid progression of the disease, and a short survival if the disease is not treated.

Chronic forms of leukemia have a more gradual onset, slower disease progression, and a relatively longer survival time. **Chronic lymphocytic leukemia is common in men over age 50 and accounts for one-third of the new cases of leukemia annually.** Chronic myelogenous leukemia is most common in young and middle-aged adults. Over time it progresses to the acute form, and eventual death is common.

Causative Factors and Effects   As with other types of cancers, the exact cause of leukemia is not known. However, some factors are considered to be closely linked with the development of leukemia. **Exposure to ionizing radiation in relatively large doses is one such factor. Another is exposure to certain chemicals, such as benzene, that are toxic to bone marrow.** Benzene is an ingredient in lead-free gasoline and the incidence of leukemia has risen since lead-free gasoline has been in use. The amount of exposure to benzene and other chemicals that causes bone marrow suppression is unknown and possibly varies among individuals. The point is to be careful about breathing gasoline fumes

and using household chemicals and pesticides. The third factor is the retrovirus HTLV-1, which causes human T-cell leukemia. There has been a chromosomal link found for CML. About 90% of patients with CML have the Philadelphia chromosome.

> Leukemia has three major effects: (1) increased numbers of abnormal, immature leukocytes; (2) accumulations of these cells within the lymph nodes, spleen, and other organs; and (3) eventual infiltration of the malignant cells throughout the body.

The causes of symptoms produced by these pathological changes are presented in Table 17-11.

Diagnosis   Diagnosis is made by history, physical examination, complete CBC with differential, and bone marrow studies to rule out other disorders.

Treatment   Treatment is aimed at (1) slowing down the growth of the malignant blood cells; (2) maintaining a normal level of red cells, hemoglobin, and platelets; and (3) managing the symptoms and meeting the special needs of each patient. The patient with leukemia usually

TABLE 17-11 ◆ *Causes of Clinical Signs of Leukemia*	
Manifestations	**Causes**
Severe infections	Immature and abnormally functioning leukocytes, even though there is an increased number of them.
Symptoms of anemia	Rapidly proliferating white cells apparently "crowd out" developing red cells and platelets.
Enlarged spleen, liver, lymph nodes	Excess white cells accumulate within organs, causing distention of tissues.
Weakness, pallor, and weight loss due to elevated metabolic rate	Increased production of white cells requires large amounts of amino acids and vitamins. Increased destruction of cells leads to more metabolic wastes that must be disposed of by the body.
Renal pain, urinary stones and obstruction to flow of urine, and UTI	Large amounts of uric acid are released when white cells are destroyed by antileukemic drugs.
Headache, disorientation, and other central nervous system symptoms	Abnormal white cells infiltrate the central nervous system.

complains of fatigue and malaise and may have frequent infections.

Acute leukemia treatment consists primarily of chemotherapy with a combination of antineoplastic agents targeted at different phases of the cell cycle. The drug therapy is divided into three phases: induction, consolidation, and maintenance. *Induction* therapy is initiated at the time of diagnosis and consists of an intensive combination chemotherapy aimed to achieve a complete remission of symptoms. *Consolidation* therapy is another course of the same agents, or others, at a different dosage level and the goal is cure. Maintenance therapy is usually oral chemotherapy at lesser doses, is done to maintain remission, and is taken for 2 to 5 years.

Elder Care Point... Patients over the age of 65 require reduced doses of chemotherapeutic drugs to prevent toxicity because they have decreased kidney and liver function and the drugs are not metabolized as quickly as in a younger person.

> Before chemotherapy is started, the patient should be well hydrated and given allopurinol orally to prevent hyperuricemia and kidney stones.

Radiation therapy is used supplementally to increase the success of treatment. Cure is sometimes possible, as has been evidenced in children with ALL. Results in adults have not been as good. Bone marrow transplantation is a possibility for patients who have had an initial remission with chemotherapy. Eventually it is hoped that monoclonal antibody treatment can be combined with bone marrow transplant to provide lasting remission (see Treatment section in this chapter).

Chronic lymphocytic leukemia, the most common leukemia in the aged, is not treated until the patient experiences symptoms. At that time a combination of chemotherapy agents are used.

Chronic myelogenous leukemia is managed with oral alkylating agents, such as busulfan (Myleran) and hydroxyurea (Hydrea). Research with recombinant human alpha interferon to induce remission for CML is ongoing. **Leukapheresis** (extraction of WBCs) may be done to reduce the massive number of circulating leukocytes that clog organs and cause damage. A small percentage of patients are likely candidates for bone marrow transplantation.

Transfusions of blood components are prescribed to maintain a near-normal blood picture. Platelet transfusion during or after chemotherapy often is necessary. Antibiotics may be given prophylactically during chemotherapy and are started immediately upon signs of infection because the body's defense mechanisms are seriously compromised.

Nursing Intervention **Among the problems presented by a patient with leukemia are potential for infection, abnormal bleeding, anemia, nutritional alteration with severe anorexia and weight loss, altered urine elimination related to increased levels of uric acid in the urine and blood, and psychosocial problems related to the effects of the disease as well as the prescribed treatment.** Collaboration with the dietitian as well as the pharmacist is a key point in nursing care of the leukemic patient.

Infections from bacteria, viruses, and fungi are the most common cause of death in persons with leukemia. Infection is a threat to the patient with leukemia either because of abnormal function of bone marrow that is characteristic of the disease or because of suppression of bone marrow function as a result of therapy. Nursing measures to prevent infection are essential, as is vigilant assessment for early signs. Table 9-10 presents teaching guidelines for the patient at risk for infection due to the effects of chemotherapy or radiation.

Elder Care Point... The elderly patient with leukemia already has decreased immune system function. When leukemia develops, or is treated, this patient is at very high risk for infection. In addition, hemorrhage is not tolerated as well in the elderly and must be carefully guarded against. Other conditions also may affect appetite. Emphasis on an appropriate diet, supplements, and good nutritional status can make a marked difference in the quality of life of the elderly leukemia patient.

Abnormal bleeding as a result of a very low platelet count is the second most common and dangerous complication of leukemia. Observation of the patient, awareness of his current platelet count, and prevention of trauma to body tissues and blood vessels are primary concerns in the nursing management of leukemia. Table 9-11 presents guidelines for the patient prone to bleeding.

Anemia and its attendant problems of fatigue, hypoxia, gastrointestinal upsets, and cardiovascular complications, such as increased cardiac workload, is always a threat and in many cases a reality in patients with leukemia. The anemia can result from the disease itself, from excessive bleeding, or from the therapy administered. Nursing measures previously described for the patient with anemia are appropriate to the care of the patient with leukemia. Colony-stimulating factor drugs sometimes are used to counteract the anemia and neutropenia of treatment for leukemia. However, these drugs may stimulate the growth of abnormal cells, making the condition worse.

Nutritional problems arise from any of a number of conditions. **Extreme weight loss and emaciation are nearly always seen in patients with advanced cancer.**

Failure to eat sufficient amounts of nutritious foods is not the only reason this is so. As was explained in Chapter 9, metabolic changes that occur with the proliferation of malignant cells in the body also are responsible for weight loss and emaciation. If nursing measures to alleviate or minimize stomatitis, nausea, and vomiting are not effective, parenteral nutrition may be necessary.

The increased level of uric acid that results from rapid cell destruction during therapy often causes the uric acid crystals to settle out in the kidney structures, causing impaired renal function. Maintaining adequate hydration and administering drugs to decrease the production of uric acid are important nursing measures, as is close observation of fluid intake and urinary output.

The emotional impact of a diagnosis of cancer and the psychosocial needs of the cancer patient and his family are discussed in Chapter 9.

Think about . . . Why is it common for the leukemia patient to have frequent infections? What causes this problem? When caring for a leukemia patient, what would you need to assess to detect early signs of infection?

◆ Hemophilia

Hemophilia is an inherited disorder in which there is a deficiency of specific clotting factors. Classic hemophilia, also known as hemophilia A and factor VIII deficiency, affects more than 80% of all hemophiliacs. It is characterized by a delayed blood coagulation time that produces a prolonged period of bleeding after injury or surgery. This type of hemophilia almost always occurs in males and is transmitted through the female. Although the female does not have the disease herself, she and all her female descendants can transmit classic hemophilia to their offspring. Other types of hemophilia, similar to classic hemophilia, can affect both men and women.

Pathophysiology

In all types of hemophilia, there is a decrease in the amount of activity of one of the 11 different clotting factors normally present in blood and essential to the formation of clots.

Hemophilia A results from a deficiency in factor VIII. Hemophilia B, or Christmas disease, is the result of a deficiency of factor IX. In von Willebrand's disease, there is a decrease in the activity of factor VIII, even though the factor is present in normal amounts in the plasma. The blood of a hemophiliac forms a clot immediately after injury, but the clot breaks down and does not effectively stop bleeding.

There are varying degrees of severity in the types of hemophilia, depending on the amount of the factor present and the role of the factor in clot formation. For the patients with mild cases, who have 25% to 50% of the deficient factor present in the serum, symptoms may not appear at all until a severe injury or surgery is followed by prolonged bleeding and the hemophilia is thus discovered. In very severe cases, in which less than 1% of the factor is present, the affected individuals may bleed spontaneously without injury, and severe hemorrhage can develop very quickly whenever an injury does occur.

Signs and Symptoms
The most obvious symptom of hemophilia is, of course, bleeding. However, it is not surface bleeding that causes the most serious complications of hemophilia. Bleeding most often occurs internally, with leakage of blood into the joints, the intestinal wall or peritoneal cavity, and the deeper tissues of the body. **Hemarthrosis,** or bleeding into the joints, produces swelling, pain, warmth, and limitation of movement similar to that suffered by the patient with rheumatoid arthritis. If the bleeding occurs in the intracranial spaces and thereby increases intracranial pressure, the patient may experience convulsions and brain damage that can be fatal. Other serious complications from internal bleeding in the hemophiliac include obstruction of the airway as a result of hemorrhage into the neck or pharynx and intestinal obstruction resulting from bleeding into the intestinal wall or peritoneum.

Treatment
In the more common types of hemophilia transfusion with blood factors, fresh frozen plasma, or cryoprecipitate is used to replace the missing factors and prevent bleeding. These factor replacements include those needed to treat von Willebrand's disease, factor VIII deficiency (classic hemophilia), and factor IX deficiency (Christmas disease). The availability of these replacement factors has greatly improved the outlook for those with hemophilia and helped the hemophiliac person live a more normal life.

Many patients with hemophilia have been receiving blood products for a number of years. Unfortunately some patients have been infected with the human immunodeficiency virus (HIV) from contaminated plasma concentrates. Before the invention of an HIV-specific blood test, there was no way to tell whether blood donors carried the virus. This problem has created additional psychological stress for the patient with hemophilia.

Hemophilia is a complex disease requiring individual treatment and nursing care based on the needs of each patient. The hemophiliac should be encouraged to lead an active life insofar as he is able to avoid situations that predispose him to injury and illness. The parents of a child with hemophilia should avoid overprotecting him, because treating him as an invalid and sheltering him from normal childhood activities deny him the opportunity to develop into a healthy, well-adjusted person.

Nursing Intervention   In addition to administering the necessary clotting factors, interventions include elevating the injured body part, applying cold packs, controlling pain, observing for further bleeding, and providing psychological support for the patient and family. The nurse should also encourage genetic counseling for family members if this has not been done previously.

◆ Disseminated Intravascular Coagulation

Disseminated intravascular coagulation (DIC) is a complicated disorder that usually occurs in conjunction with tissue destruction. It accompanies serious problems, such as severe trauma, gram-negative sepsis, shock, respiratory distress syndrome, malignancy, or abruptio placenta. Damaged tissue liberates tissue thromboplastin, creating a state of excessive clotting. Hemorrhage follows when the blood's clotting factors are depleted. The condition is potentially life-threatening. The first signs are usually continued bleeding from an injection site, ecchymoses, and petechiae. There may be oral, vaginal, or rectal bleeding. Treatment consists of correcting the underlying problem. Fresh-frozen plasma and packed RBCs are administered to restore blood volume and replenish clotting factors.

DISORDERS OF THE LYMPHATIC SYSTEM

Disorders of the lymphatic system include malignant lymphomas, multiple myeloma, and other proliferative blood disorders; inflammation of the lymph nodes (lymphadenitis) and lymph vessels (lymphangitis); and obstruction to the flow of lymph, which results in swelling of the tissues served by the obstructed lymph vessels (lymphedema).

◆ Diagnostic Tests

Physical examination of the lymph nodes can reveal signs of infection, such as redness, swelling, hardness, and tenderness. Diagnostic tests including lymphangiogram, spleen sonogram, and spleen scan are presented in Table 17-4.

◆ Lymphangitis

Inflammation of the lymph vessels is usually diagnosed when red streaks and tenderness are noted along a part of the body near a site of infection. These red streaks follow the course of the infected and inflamed lymph vessel and extend from the site of infection to the nearest lymph nodes.

Treatment of lymphangitis is aimed at relieving the infection at the primary site with the use of antimicrobial agents. If these efforts fail, the infection spreads to the circulatory system, resulting in septicemia (called "blood poisoning" by many laypersons).

◆ Lymphedema

Swelling of the tissues drained by the lymphatic system occurs as a result of obstruction to the flow of lymph along the vessels. It is especially common in the lower extremities and other dependent organs. The obstruction may be the result of a congenital condition in which there is deficient growth of the lymphatic system in a lower extremity. This condition chiefly affects females and most often becomes apparent during the middle teens to early twenties.

Acquired lymphedema is the result of an obstruction caused by trauma to the lymph vessels and nodes, such as occurs during mastectomy when lymph nodes are removed. Other causes of obstruction include extensive soft-tissue injury and scar formation and, in tropical countries, parasites that enter lymph channels and block them.

Nursing Intervention   Lymphedema that involves an extremity often can be treated conservatively using simple nursing measures. Prevention and treatment of lymphedema of the arm and hand following mastectomy are covered in Chapter 26. In general, any lymphedema of an extremity responds to the following measures:

- ◆ Elevate the extremity to the level of the heart. This reduces hydrostatic pressure within the veins.
- ◆ Active exercise of the skeletal muscles. This promotes massage of the lymph vessels and the movement of lymph.
- ◆ Application of elasticized stockings or gloves. This increases pressure on vessels and encourages venous return.

◆ Lymphomas

Lymphomas are malignant neoplasms that affect the lymphoid tissue and lymph nodes. The two main types of lymphoma are Hodgkin's disease and non-Hodgkin's lymphoma. The most common sign of both is one or more enlarged lymph nodes.

Hodgkin's Disease   Hodgkin's disease primarily affects young adults, but also occurs in those over 50 years of age. Possible causes are viral infections and previous exposure to alkylating drugs for cancer treatment. The disorder often is discovered when swollen lymph nodes are found on a routine examination or an employment physical examination. Some patients experience remittent fever, itching, night sweats, or weight loss. The diagnosis is made by the presence of Reed-Sternberg cells in the blood. Lymphangiography is used to help determine the progression of the disease and appropriate therapy. Treatment depends on how far the disease has progressed. Table 17-12 presents the classification of stages for Hodgkin's disease. Remission and cure often are achieved with the use of radiation, chemotherapy, or both. Stage IA and IIA disease patients have a 90% 5-year remission/cure rate. Early Hodgkin's disease is one of the most curable types of cancer. Nursing care focuses on symptoms and the side effects of the therapy.

Non-Hodgkin's Lymphoma   Several similar cancers are classified as non-Hodgkin's lymphoma. The cause of lymphoma is unknown, but viruses, immunosuppression, and radiation are all thought to be possible

contributors. Since the 1970s, the incidence has increased in those over age 65. This type of lymphoma tends to have more widespread involvement of lymphoid tissue than found in Hodgkin's disease. Treatment is with chemotherapy or radiation, depending on the stage of disease and offers relief of symptoms. The survival rate has increased to 51% since the mid-1960s. Aggressive chemotherapy with a combination of drugs has been effective for some patients with advanced disease. An experimental vaccine is showing promise.

Nursing Intervention   Nursing care is directed toward supporting the patient through the diagnostic process and observing and treating the side effects of radiation and chemotherapy. Chapter 9 contains information on specific nursing diagnoses and interventions for the patient with cancer.

◆ Multiple Myeloma

Multiple myeloma is a condition in which abnormal plasma cells multiply out of control in the bone marrow. The abnormal plasma cells can migrate to the lymph nodes, liver, spleen, and kidneys, forming tumors there. The tumors disrupt normal bone marrow function and weaken the bone, predisposing the patient to frequent fractures. Average age at diagnosis is 60 years. The onset is gradual and symptoms appear when the skeletal system is heavily involved. Patients may experience backache, bone pain that is worse with movement, or pathological fractures and severe pain. Multiple myeloma is diagnosed by radiographic studies, bone marrow biopsy, and blood and urine tests. The appearance of light-chains from the abnormal immunoglobulin in the urine, Bence Jones protein, is a diagnostic sign.

When treatment is indicated, chemotherapy or palliative radiation is begun. Pain control is a primary concern. These patients often develop hypercalcemia and osteoporosis and must be monitored and treated for these complications. Measures to prevent pathological fractures are instituted.

THERAPIES FREQUENTLY USED IN THE MANAGEMENT OF HEMATOLOGICAL AND LYMPHATIC DISORDERS

◆ Transfusions

A blood transfusion is the administration of whole blood or one or more of its components. To minimize the risks of circulatory overload, hepatitis, transfusion reaction, and other problems related to the administration of whole blood, it usually is transfused only when there has been acute and massive blood loss or when there must be a total blood exchange in a newborn. For

TABLE 17-12 ◆ Ann Arbor Staging Classification for Hodgkin's Disease

Stage	Characteristics*
I	Involvement of a single lymph node region (I) or of a single extralymphatic organ or site (I$_E$).
II	Involvement of two or more lymph node regions on the same side of the diaphragm (II) or localized involvement of an extralymphatic organ or site and of one or more lymph node regions on the same side of the diaphragm (II$_E$).
III	Involvement of lymph node regions on both sides of the diaphragm (III), which may be accompanied by localized involvement of an extralymphatic organ or site (III$_E$), or by involvement of the spleen (III$_S$), or both (III$_{SE}$).
IV	Diffuse or disseminated involvement of one or more extralymphatic organs or tissues, with or without associated lymph node enlargement. Involvement of the liver or bone marrow is always considered Stage IV.

Source: Rakel, R., editor, (1994). *1994 Conn's Current Therapy*, Philadelphia: Saunders, p. 383.
*Unexplained increase in temperature (>38°C [100.5°F]), night sweats, and/or weight loss (>10% of body weight) in the 6 months preceding diagnosis are defined as systemic symptoms and denoted by the suffix letter B. Asymptomatic patients are denoted by the suffix letter A.

less extreme situations, packed red blood cells are administered.

Autologous (originating in one's self) blood transfusion is commonly used when the patient's own blood can be collected and reinfused. Blood is either collected during or after surgery, such as from chest drainage, or donated by the patient during the weeks prior to surgery for later use.

Laboratory procedures that separate the various components by centrifuge or other means allow for the administration of only the particular element of blood needed by a particular patient. Among the various blood components that can be given by transfusion are:

◆ Fresh plasma to expand blood volume.
◆ Platelet transfusion when platelet count is 20,000 mm^3 or less.
◆ Packed red cells for patients with anemia or those who need blood and cannot tolerate rapid shifts of blood volume.
◆ Granulocytes to help patients overcome progressive infections that are not responding well to antibiotics.
◆ Plasma albumin to expand blood volume.
◆ Coagulation factors VIII and IX or cryoprecipitate to help manage hemophilia.

A man-made substitute for human blood that eliminates the need for cross-matching is being tested. The blood substitute, polyethylene glycol (PEG) hemoglobin isn't seen by the body as a foreign substance as it is designed to fool the immune system.

A blood transfusion is initiated by two nurses who are certified to do so. A licensed practical nurse (LPN) who is not qualified to transfuse blood may be asked to help *monitor* the patient during the infusion. All blood bank and agency policies must be strictly followed to decrease the possibility of an adverse reaction or the administration of blood to the wrong patient.

When picking up a unit of blood from the blood bank, the nurse presents the proper forms, indicating the patient's name, identification number, and the type of blood component that is ordered. The nurse then checks the bag of blood product along with the blood bank personnel, comparing the label information with the log information and with the order form for the patient. **This should be done slowly and without distractions.** The blood bag should be handled very gently to prevent damage to the cells. When the nurse returns to the floor with the blood, she should immediately inform the nurse in charge of the patient that the blood is ready to be infused. Blood is normally administered through a Y-type infusion set with 250 mL of 0.9% saline on the other side of the "Y" (Figure 17-8). A special blood filter is included in the Y-type infusion set, and the drop factor is different from that of a regular IV tubing set. **A very slow infusion rate is begun initially so that there is time to observe the patient for an adverse reaction before a lot of blood is infused. Most reactions occur during the administration of the first 50 mL of the blood product.** After the first 15 to 20 minutes the rate may be increased to what the physician ordered if there are no signs of reaction. A unit of packed red blood cells can be administered to most patients in 1½ to 2 hours. The blood filter should not be used for more than one unit of blood. A blood warmer may be used to warm the chilled blood to prevent excessive chilling of the patient. Blood bags should never be heated in a microwave oven or placed in hot water.

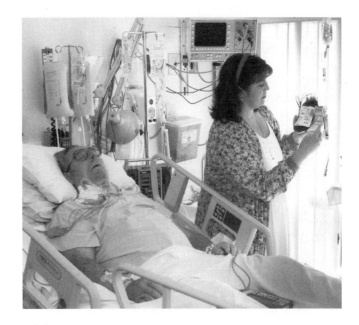

FIGURE 17-8   Nurse preparing to start infusion of a unit of blood. (Photo by Glen Derbyshire; courtesy of Goleta Valley Cottage Hospital, Goleta, CA.)

Blood should never be allowed to hang for more than 4 hours as it is an excellent medium for bacterial growth. Baseline vital signs are taken before the transfusion begins.

> The patient is observed for adverse reactions such as chills, fever, nausea, vomiting, rash, back pain, shortness of breath, sweating, tachycardia, or severe anxiety, such as a feeling of impending doom.

If any of these reactions occurs, the blood is stopped immediately, saline is started using fresh tubing, vital signs taken and the charge nurse notified. Diphenhydramine hydrochloride (Benadryl) may be ordered by injection if an allergic reaction is suspected.

> If no reaction is observed, vital signs are taken twice at 30-minute intervals and then each hour until the transfusion is complete. Should the patient's temperature rise above 100.4° F (38.0° C), the infusion is stopped, the saline started and the physician notified.

> No other solution or drug is ever administered through the same line or to the same site through which blood is infusing.

In general, prevention of reactions depends on properly matching donor and recipient; identifying patients who have an allergy, especially to transfused blood products; maintaining aseptic collection and administration techniques; and keeping the patient who is susceptible to febrile reaction covered and warm during a transfusion.

Think about . . . How might you know that your patient was experiencing a reaction to a blood transfusion? What would you do?

◆ Leukapheresis

This procedure is performed to clear excessive WBCs from the blood. It may be performed directly on the patient or on separated blood products. The patient is connected to a blood separator machine. Blood is drained a bit at a time from the patient, the white blood cells are washed out of the blood, and the red cells and plasma are returned to the patient. This treatment is used to lower the white blood cell counts in CML patients and also to treat certain immune disorders such as myasthenia gravis.

◆ Biological Response Modifiers— Colony Stimulating Factor Therapy

Drug research with DNA-recombinant techniques has developed drugs that stimulate the bone marrow to produce erythrocytes or neutrophils. Erythropoietin (Epogen) is given parenterally to patients who have

decreased erythropoietin resulting from end-stage renal disease or who have suppressed bone marrow from the toxicity of chemotherapy given for malignancy, rheumatoid arthritis, or the HIV virus.

Granulocyte-stimulating factor (G-CSF, Neupogen) is given parenterally to combat neutropenia. It is used for patients who have bone marrow suppression from chemotherapy, particularly in those with non-blood-related malignancies. Sometimes it is used in leukemia patients, but there is a danger of stimulating the growth of abnormal cells in these patients.

Granulocyte-macrophage colony-stimulating factor (GM-CSF, Leukine), accelerates the recovery of bone marrow after autologous bone marrow transplant in Hodgkin's disease, ALL, or non-Hodgkin's lymphoma patients who have undergone total destruction of the bone marrow during therapy. Drugs to increase platelet counts are being developed and, one hopes, will be released soon.

◆ Bone Marrow Transplantation

Bone marrow transplantation (BMT) is aimed at providing healthy bone marrow when the patient's own bone marrow is faulty or has been destroyed by chemotherapy and/or irradiation in an attempt to rid the body of leukemic or other cancer cells. The bone marrow used for transplantation can be **allogeneic** (from another person) or **autologous** (from the patient). If the transplant is to be autologous, it is taken from the patient during a period of remission of disease. Allogeneic bone marrow is harvested from a matched HLA person. The HLA match is determined by tissue typing. Finding a good HLA match is difficult and there is only a 25% chance of matching with the patient's own brother or sister.

Harvest bone marrow is done in the operating room, where multiple aspirations from the iliac crests are performed. About 500 to 1,000 mL of marrow is harvested. The marrow is filtered and may be purged to rid autologous marrow of cancer cells or to rid the allogeneic marrow of T-cells. Autologous marrow is then frozen. **Nursing care after harvest consists of monitoring the dressings for bleeding and medicating the donor for pain in the hip area. Nonaspirin analgesics often are sufficient to control pain.**

The patient undergoes a conditioning regimen to rid the body of malignancy or to obliterate the diseased bone marrow. This usually takes 5 to 10 days. The process involves intensive high-dose chemotherapy and often includes total body irradiation. The patient experiences all the side effects of these treatments: bone marrow suppression, diarrhea, stomatitis, severe nausea, and vomiting. The patient is at extreme risk for infection. Meticulous supportive and preventive nursing care is essential during and after this phase.

At least 2 days after the end of chemotherapy, the BMT infusion takes place through a central line over approximately 30 minutes. The process of engraftment begins as the cells find their way to the marrow-forming locations in the patient's bones and establish themselves there. Engraftment takes 2 to 5 weeks and is considered successful when the patient's erythrocyte, leukocyte, and platelet counts begin to rise. The patient is at dire risk of infection and hemorrhage until engraftment is complete. Other complications include failure of engraftment and graft-versus-host disease (GVHD), where the cells see the patient's tissues as foreign and mount an immune attack. Thrombosis and phlebitis in the liver also can occur and will cause liver damage if not resolved.

◆ Oxygen Therapy

The administration of low concentrations of oxygen may be employed to relieve severe dyspnea and hypoxia during the acute phase of a blood disorder. The treatment is purely symptomatic, but it does offer some relief if there is sufficient hemoglobin to carry the oxygen to the tissues. The care of a patient receiving oxygen therapy and the need for careful monitoring of blood gases are discussed in Chapter 16.

◆ Iron Therapy

Iron is one of the principal elements in the production and maturation of red blood cells. When the body lacks iron, the amount of hemoglobin is decreased in the red cells, making them very small and pale in color. In a simple iron deficiency anemia, the condition is relieved by administering iron salts. The iron preparations most often used are ferrous sulfate and ferrous gluconate.

Iron salts are irritating to the gastrointestinal tract when taken on an empty stomach. There will be fewer gastric upsets if this medication is given in divided doses and immediately after meals. The patient should be warned that taking iron salts by mouth produces greenish-black stools and that there is no cause for alarm if this change in the color of stools occurs. Because iron salts may form deposits on the teeth and gums, causing a discoloration, the liquid forms of this medication should be given through a straw. Following administration of each liquid dose, the teeth should be thoroughly cleansed and the mouth well rinsed.

Some patients suffer such severe gastric disturbances from the oral intake of iron salts that the medication must be given by another route. Patients who are anemic because of gastric or intestinal bleeding cannot take iron by mouth because the irritation aggravates their condition. The drug of choice in these cases is iron dextran (Imferon), an iron preparation that is injected into the muscle or given IV. Such IM injections must not exceed 2 mL at each site, and the sites of injection should be rotated to allow for proper absorption and to minimize the hazards of local inflammation. The "Z tract" technique for IM injection is recommended. Patients receiving an IV infusion of iron dextran must be watched closely for anaphylactic and other adverse reactions.

Vitamin C usually is given with iron because it enhances its absorption. If a pharmaceutical preparation of vitamin C is not prescribed, the patient can take the iron salts with orange juice or another juice that is a good source of the vitamin.

Think about . . . What would you teach a home care patient who is complaining that the iron medication is causing a mild nausea, stomach discomfort, and constipation?

◆ Vitamin B₁₂ Therapy

Vitamin B_{12} has two main functions in the body. First, it is needed for red blood cells to develop into mature, normally functioning cells; second, it is necessary for nerve cells to function normally. Another B-group vitamin, folic acid, also is needed for red blood cell maturation, but it has no effect on the nervous system. Vitamin B_{12} is used to treat pernicious anemia.

Injections of Vitamin B_{12} are given daily for the first few weeks and later may be spaced a week apart. As the patient improves, the injections may be necessary only once a month, but must continue for the duration of life.

In addition to administration of supplemental iron and vitamins, the patient with nutritional anemia should eat nutritionally balanced, high-protein meals. Hints for adding protein to the diet are shown in Table 17-13.

TABLE 17-13 ◆ *Nutrition Point: Hints for Adding Protein to the Diet*

Mix dry skim milk into the milk called for in recipes.
Provide between-meal shakes made with commercial protein powder available at the grocery or health food store.
Add dry skim milk to hot or cold cereal, scrambled eggs, soups, gravies, meal loaf or meat balls, casseroles, and to desserts.
Add diced or ground meat to soups and casseroles.
Drink commercial canned high-protein drinks between meals, available from pharmacies, or use instant breakfast drink mix.
Add cream cheese or peanut butter to breakfast breads.
Used cooked diced shrimp, tuna, crab, or ham with sliced boiled egg in cream sauce and eat over cooked rice, pasta, biscuits or toast.
Eat peanut butter on crackers, apple, celery, or toast for snacks.
Eat desserts made with eggs.
Eat commercial high-protein bars for snacks, available at the grocery, health food store, or sporting goods store.

◆ Splenectomy

Indications for surgical removal of the spleen include (1) severe trauma to and rupture of the spleen; (2) splenomegaly with rapid destruction of blood cells; and (3) splenomegaly from blood disorders, such as Hodgkin's disease.

Although the known functions of the spleen are important and other functions have not yet been identified, the spleen is not an essential organ. The other organs of the monocyte-macrophage system take over many of its chores once it has been removed. However, those persons who no longer have a functioning spleen, whether as a result of disease or surgical removal, are at a very high risk to develop life-threatening infections, especially those caused by pneumococci. It is recommended that these persons receive vaccination against 14 strains of pneumococcal bacteria with the Pneumovax vaccine. They are advised to consult a physician and take preventive antibiotics as prescribed when they experience even a seemingly trivial respiratory infection.

The patient with a ruptured or torn spleen is in immediate danger of hemorrhage and shock. Whenever an accidental blow, stab wound, or gunshot wound occurs in the vicinity of the spleen, the patient must be watched closely for signs of internal bleeding. After surgery, the patient is observed for early signs of infection, abdominal distention, and other more general complications of abdominal surgery.

COMMUNITY CARE

Patients with blood or lymphatic disorders are treated in many different places in the community. Patients undergoing chemotherapy may be attending an outpatient clinic to receive the doses of the drugs they need. Support groups for patients with the various disorders may be meeting in hospitals, clinics, churches, schools, or at other community locations. Patients with sickle cell disease or hemophilia may be attending ambulatory clinics.

Patients with blood disorders are frequently treated as home care patients. The elderly patient with pernicious anemia who is house-bound may need a nurse to give her vitamin B_{12} injections and draw lab specimens for periodic blood counts. The leukemia patient frequently is followed at home during chemotherapy and recovery periods. The patient with sickle cell problems is more likely to be treated in the home setting after the initial crisis period is over. In some instances blood products are administered at home. Some types of chemotherapy agents are given in the home setting, and the nurse must monitor the patient for all of the adverse effects that such therapy can cause.

The home care nurse must do considerable patient and family teaching about prevention of infection, prevention of and treatment of bleeding episodes, appropriate nutrition, and regulation of medication. The home care nurse manager will coordinate care for the patient with the physician, pharmacist, home infusion company, home health aide, and family.

CRITICAL THINKING EXERCISES

Clinical Case Problems

Read each clinical case problem and discuss the questions with your classmates.

1. You come upon an automobile accident and stop to help. The first victim has a bleeding wound on the forehead. What method would you use to stop the bleeding? The second victim has a gash in his thigh and blood is spurting at regular intervals from the wound. What method would you use to stop the bleeding?

2. Mrs. Thomas is a young mother who has three small children. She is admitted to the hospital with a severe anemia. Her hemoglobin is 7.5 g/dL, and her red cell count also is very low. Mrs. Thomas confides in you that she has never eaten as she should, especially when she was a teenager, and with the added strain of having the children to care for at home, she doesn't take the time to cook the meals she knows they should have because she is so tired all the time. Her husband makes a fairly good salary, but Mrs. Thomas is under the impression that an adequate diet would cost more than they can afford at present.

   a. How can you teach the patient the value of nutritious food and help her with shopping practices that would provide her family with food items that are not expensive?

   b. Which foods that are high in iron would you suggest she include in her diet?

   c. What practical suggestions could you make to help cope with fatigue?

   d. What points would your teaching plan include regarding her prescribed medications?

3. Mr. Ross is a 24 year old who has acute lymphocytic leukemia. He is receiving chemotherapy with cyclophosphamide, vincristine, prednisone, and daunorubicin and is experiencing many of the problems associated with a blood disorder, as well as the problems caused by the side effects of the potent drugs he is receiving.

   a. Describe the physiological problems Mr. Ross is likely to experience as a result of the disease and the therapy.

   b. Identify psychosocial concerns that Mr. Ross might have.

   c. Design a plan of nursing care that would help

alleviate or prevent each of the problems and concerns you have identified.

    d. If he goes into remission, he may be a candidate for a bone marrow transplant. What would you teach him about this procedure?

4. Mr. Harris, a 72-year-old white male, has just been diagnosed with chronic myeloid leukemia (CML). He has started chemotherapy with hydroxyurea and busulfan. If this is unsuccessful, he will begin treatment with interferon-alpha.

    a. What do you need to teach Mr. Harris about the drugs he is taking? Will he be on other drugs to control the side effects of this chemotherapy?

    b. What should Mr. Harris be taught about his general care?

    c. His wife asks whether he would be eligible for a bone marrow transplant. What should you answer?

BIBLIOGRAPHY

American Cancer Society. (1997). *Cancer Facts and Figures—1997*. Atlanta: Author.

Applegate, E. (1995). *The Anatomy and Physiology Learning System*. Philadelphia: Saunders.

Belcher, A. E. (1993). *Blood Disorders*. St. Louis, MO: Mosby.

Bennett, J. C., Plum, F., eds. (1996). *Cecil Textbook of Medicine*. Philadelphia: Saunders.

Black, J., Matassarin-Jacobs, E. (1997). *Medical-Surgical Nursing: Clinical Management for Continuity of Care*, 5th ed. Philadelphia: Saunders.

Bonnadona, G. (1994). Modern treatment of malignant lymphomas: a multidisciplinary approach. *Annals of Oncology*. 5(suppl 2):5–17.

Borton, D. (1996). WBC Count and Differential: Review the defensive roster. *Nursing 96*. 26(9):26–31.

Campbell, K. (1995). The causes and incidence of haematological malignancies. *Nursing Times*. 91(31):25–6.

Carrera, C., Savern, A., Piro, L. (1994). Purine metabolism of lymphocytes: targets for chemotherapy drug development. *Hematology/Oncology Clinics of North America*. 8(2):357–382.

Carrol, P. A. (1995). When a Johovah's Witness refuses a transfusion. *Nursing 95*. 25(8):60–61.

Chiocca, E. M. (1996). Sickle cell crisis. *American Journal of Nursing*. 96(9):49.

Copstead, L. (1995). *Perspectives on Pathophysiology*. Philadelphia: Saunders.

Cordisco, M. E. C. (1996). Fighting DIC. *RN*. 58(8):36–54.

deWit, S. C. (1994). *Rambo's Nursing Skills for Clinical Practice*, 4th ed. Philadelphia: Saunders.

Flavell, C. M. (1994). Combating hemorrhagic shock. *RN* 57(12):26–30.

Goldberg, K., et al., eds. (1988–1997). *Hematologic problems. Nurse Review, a Clinical Update System*. Springhouse, PA: Springhouse Corporation.

Guyton, A. C., Hall, J. E. (1996). *Textbook of Medical Physiology*, 9th ed. Philadelphia: Saunders.

Harovas, J., Anthony, H. H. (1993). Your guide to trouble-free transfusions. 26–35.

Hawley, K. (1996). Pernicious Anemia. *American Journal of Nursing*. 96(11):52–53.

Held, J. L. (1995). Cancer care: managing myelosuppression. *Nursing 95*. 25(8):74.

Huston, C. J. (1996). Hemolytic transfusion reaction. *American Journal of Nursing*. 96(3):47.

Ignatavicius, D., Workman, M., Mishler, M. (1995). *Medical-Surgical Nursing*, 2nd ed. Philadelphia: Saunders.

Jefferies, L. C. (1994). Transfusion therapy in autoimmune hemolytic anemia. *Hematology Oncology Clinics of North America*. (6):1087–1084.

Kajs, M. (1995). Thrombotic thrombocytopenic purpura: pathophysiology, treatment, and related nursing care. *Critical Care Nurse*. 15(6):44–51.

Kantarjian, H. M. (1994). Adult acute lymphocytic leukemia: critical review of current knowledge. *American Journal of Medicine*. 97(2):176–184.

Lammon, C. B., et al. (1995). *Clinical Nursing Skills*. Philadelphia: Saunders.

Matteson, M., McConnell, E. (1997). *Gerontological Nursing: Concepts and Practice*, 2nd ed. Philadelphia: Saunders.

McBrien, N. J. (1997). Thrombotic thrombocytopenia purpura. *American Journal of Nursing*. 97(2):28–29.

Norris, M. K. G. (1994). Disseminated intravascular coagulation. *Nursing 94*. 24(7):53.

Nursing 96. (1996). Blood transfusions: Playing it safe. Author. 26(4):50–52.

Purandare, L. (1995). Caring for patients with chronic leukemia. *Nursing Times*. 91(31):17–18.

Rakel, R. E., ed. (1997). *Conn's Current Therapy 1997*. Philadelphia: Saunders.

Rosenberg, S. A. (1994). The treatment of Hodgkin's disease. *Annals of Oncology*. 5(suppl 2):17–21.

Ross, E. C. (1994). Red cell transfusion therapy in chronic anemia. *Hematology Oncology Clinics of North America*. 8(6):1045–1052.

Russell, S. (1994). Hypovolemic shock. *Nursing 94*. 24(4):34–39.

Seymour, J. F., et al. (1994). Refractory chronic lymphocytic leukemia complicated by hypercalcemia treated with allogeneic bone marrow transplantation. *American Journal of Clinical Oncology*. 17(4):360–368.

Taptich, B., Iyer, P., Bernocchi-Losey, D. (1994). *Nursing Diagnosis and Care Planning*, 2nd ed. Philadelphia: Saunders.

Tenenbaum, L. (1994). *Cancer Chemotherapy and Biotherapy*, 2nd ed. Philadelphia: Saunders.

Ulrich, S., Canale, S., Wendell, S. (1994). *Nursing Care Planning Guides: A Nursing Diagnosis Approach*, 3rd ed. Philadelphia: Saunders.

Weber, M. (1994). Thrombocytopenia. *RN*. 57(11):46–47.

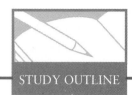

I. **Causes of Hematological and Lymphatic Disorder (see Table 17-3)**

  A. Genetic: hemophilia, sickle cell disease, some types of anemias.

  B. Trauma: accidental cutting of vessels or blunt trauma to spleen can cause major loss of blood.

  C. Chemicals or transfusion error leads to hemolysis of blood cells.

  D. Iatrogenic: some drugs, such as anticancer agents, cause bone marrow suppression, which causes decreased blood cell production.

  E. Nutritional deficiencies can interfere with RBC formation and normal cell function.

II. **Prevention**

  A. Prevention of excessive blood loss through hemorrhage often involves vigilant assessment of the patient by the nurse, such as after surgery or childbirth.

  B. Education about nutrition can help prevent anemia.

  C. Monitoring patients for side effects of drugs and blood transfusions often is a nursing responsibility.

III. **Diagnostic Tests and Procedures**

  A. Large quantity of information available from CBC count with differential.

  B. Cell counts, differential count of WBCs (see Table 17-4), study of shape and maturity of cells.

  C. Types and amount of hemoglobin.

  D. Hematocrit: ratio of cells to plasma.

  E. Bone marrow biopsy (sternal puncture).

  F. Schilling test for pernicious anemia.

  G. Sickle cell test; hemoglobin electrophoresis.

  H. Coagulation tests include prothrombin time, partial thromboplastin time, and bleeding time.

  I. Tests for problems in the lymphatic system include spleen scan or sonogram, and lymphangiogram.

IV. **Nursing Assessment of the Blood and Lymphatic Status**

  A. History: family history; history of abnormal bleeding, weakness, fatigue, pain, neurological symptoms, gastrointestinal problems; inability to tolerate cold; abnormal coloration of urine or stools; repeated infections, swollen lymph nodes may indicate abnormality.

  B. Physical assessment.

   1. Skin color: pallor, cyanosis, jaundice; bruises and petechiae; plethora.

   2. Mucous membranes; swollen, bleeding gums.

   3. Stools and urine for abnormal color.

   4. Swollen and painful joints.

   5. Lymph node involvement, red streaks.

   6. Mental state: depression, irritability.

   7. Activity intolerance.

  C. Planning.

   1. Goals

    a. Prevent infection.

    b. Conserve energy and prevent fatigue.

    c. Correct nutritional deficiencies.

    d. Provide treatment to correct or slow the disease process.

    e. Control pain or discomfort.

   2. Specific individual expected outcomes are written.

  D. Intervention.

   1. Handle gently to prevent bruising.

   2. Provide good skin care.

   3. Provide nutritional and other self-care teaching.

   4. Provide adequate pain control.

   5. Individualize nursing interventions to each patient.

  E. Evaluation.

   1. Determine whether expected outcomes are being met.

   2. Monitor laboratory values to determine effectiveness of treatment and to monitor adverse side effects.

V. **Common Nursing Diagnoses Related to Hematological and Lymphatic Disorders (see Table 17-6.)**

VI. **Disorders of the Hematological System**

  A. Anemia: a state in which there are not enough functioning red cells to meet the oxygen demands of the tissues.

   1. Classification.

    a. According to cause

     (1) Blood loss.

     (2) Failure to produce RBCs.

     (3) Excessive destruction of RBCs (hemolytic anemias).

b. According to laboratory findings in tests for size, shape, and hemoglobin content.

2. Signs, symptoms, and medical treatment.

   a. Hypovolemia: hypotension; decreased urine output; pallor; rapid, weak pulse; cool, damp skin; restlessness; stupor.

   b. Blood loss treated with blood transfusion and fluids.

   c. Other anemias: pallor, fatigue, dizziness, headache, weakness, shortness of breath with exertion.

   d. Treated with iron, vitamin B$_{12}$, folic acid, protein, and nutritious diet, depending on cause.

3. Nursing Interventions.

   a. Assess patient's status and determine nursing diagnosis.

   b. Set realistic goals.

   c. Intervention to prevent, minimize, or alleviate each problem (see Table 17-6).

B. Hemorrhagic or hypovolemic shock.

   1. Rapid, severe, bleeding leads to hypovolemia.

   2. A blood loss of 500 to 2,800 mL in an adult who had normal circulating volume may cause hypovolemic shock.

   3. The elderly develop hypovolemic shock more quickly.

   4. **Classic signs: falling blood pressure; rapid, weak pulse; cool, damp skin; thirst; decreased urine output; and restlessness progressing to decreased level of consciousness.**

   5. Treated by administering fluids, maintaining airway, and giving oxygen; positioning flat with legs straight and elevated 45 degrees; vasoconstrictors or vasodilators depending on situation.

   6. Nursing actions for hypovolemic shock (see Table 17-8).

C. Aplastic anemia.

   1. Various causes: virus, toxic substance, inherited tendency, radiation exposure.

   2. Signs and symptoms: same as other anemias, plus indications of bleeding.

   3. Susceptible to infection because of low leukocyte levels.

   4. Treatment: eliminate underlying cause; reverse isolation; packed cell and platelet transfusions; oxygen.

   5. Bone marrow transplant.

   6. Prevent infection and hemorrhage.

   7. Psychological support of patient and family.

   8. Educate patients and public about substances that can damage bone marrow.

D. Polycythemia vera.

   1. Excessive production of RBCs.

   2. Viscosity causes clotting.

   3. Signs and symptoms: ruddy complexion, fatigue, weakness, headache, enlarged spleen, bleeding tendency.

   4. Treatment primarily by phlebotomy; may use antineoplastic agents and radiation.

E. Thrombocytopenia.

   1. Disorder of decreased platelets.

   2. Signs include bleeding, purpura, and ecchymoses.

   3. Treated with blood transfusion; platelets; possibly splenectomy.

F. Sickle cell disease.

   1. Includes all genetic disorders in which there is abnormal hemoglobin and sickling of cells.

   2. Difference between sickle cell trait and sickle cell anemia.

   3. Sickle cell anemia is the most common type of sickle cell disease.

   4. In addition to the anemia there are complications arising from occlusion of blood vessels.

   5. Symptoms include those of oxygen deprivation and occlusion of blood vessels, such as pallor or pain.

   6. There is no cure for sickle cell anemia. Antisickling agents are currently under evaluation.

   7. Nursing care is supportive; medicate for pain, keep well hydrated; decrease stress; assess for complications.

G. Leukemia.

   1. A malignancy of white blood cells.

   2. Classification: acute and chronic; myeloid and lymphoid.

   3. Causative factors and effects.

      a. Exposure to the retrovirus, HTLV-1 seems to cause human T-cell leukemia.

      b. Exposure to ionizing radiation and toxic chemicals, such as benzene, are believed to contribute to development of leukemias.

      c. A chromosomal link for chronic myelogenous leukemia (CML) has been found in people who have the Philadelphia chromosome.

   4. Three major effects:

      a. Increased numbers of abnormal leukocytes.

      b. Accumulations of masses of white cells in the lymph nodes.

      c. Infiltration of malignant cells throughout the body.

   5. Symptoms of leukemia (see Table 17-11).

   6. Treatment: chemotherapy, radiation, transfusions, bone marrow transplant.

7. Nursing intervention.

   a. Susceptibility to infection (most common cause of death in leukemia patients).

   b. Abnormal bleeding. Second most common and threatening complication.

   c. Anemia: fatigue, hypoxia, gastrointestinal problems, cardiovascular complications.

8. Nutritional alteration; common to all malignancies.

9. Increased levels of uric acid.

10. Emotional impact and psychosocial needs.

H. **Hemophilia: an inherited disorder in which there is a deficiency of specific clotting factors**

   1. Classic hemophilia: factor VIII deficiency. Most common of all hemophilias.

   2. Three major types: classic hemophilia (hemophilia A), Christmas disease (hemophilia B), and von Willebrand's disease.

   3. Symptoms primarily caused by internal hemorrhage involving joints, muscles, and peritoneal and cranial cavities.

   4. Medical treatment and nursing intervention.

      a. Transfusions of replacement factors have improved prognosis.

      b. Overprotective attitudes should be avoided. Patient encouraged to live as normal a life as possible within limitations imposed by disease.

I. Disseminated intravascular coagulation (DIC).

   1. Occurs in conjunction with other disorders that cause tissue destruction, such as severe trauma, gram-negative sepsis, shock, respiratory distress syndrome, malignancy, or abruptio placenta.

   2. Causes massive clotting followed by hemorrhage when clotting factors in the blood are depleted.

   3. Treated by correcting the underlying problem; administer fresh-frozen plasma and packed RBCs.

VII. **Disorders of the Lymphatic System**

   A. Most disorders of the lymphatic system are not primary in origin.

   B. Diagnostic tests: lymphangiography and physical examination of lymph nodes; spleen scan, sonogram; urine for Bence-Jones protein.

   C. Lymphangitis: inflammation of lymph vessels.

      1. Red streaks and tenderness along lymphatic vessels.

      2. Treatment aimed at relieving infection at the primary site.

      3. Can lead to septicemia.

   D. Lymphedema: swelling of tissues drained by lymphatic vessels.

      1. Usually caused by obstruction to flow of lymph.

         a. Congenital hypoplasia of lymph vessel of lower extremities.

         b. Acquired lymphedema: surgical destruction of lymph nodes and vessels; extensive soft tissue injury; parasites.

      2. Nursing intervention.

         a. Elevate swollen extremity.

         b. Active exercise of skeletal muscles.

         c. Apply full-length elasticized stockings and gloves.

   E. Lymphomas.

      1. Malignancy of lymph tissue.

      2. Hodgkin's disease.

         a. Affects primarily young adults or those over 50.

         b. Signs: swollen lymph nodes, fever, night sweats, weight loss.

         c. Diagnosed by Reed-Sternberg cells in blood; lymphangiography.

         d. Treatment: chemotherapy, radiation, bone marrow transplant.

      3. Non-Hodgkin's lymphoma.

         a. Widespread involvement of lymph tissue.

         b. Treatment with chemotherapy and radiation.

      4. Multiple myeloma.

         a. Abnormal plasma cells multiply in the bone marrow.

         b. Most common symptom is bone pain.

         c. Diagnosed by bone marrow biopsy and serum and uric protein electrophoresis.

         d. Symptoms are controlled with radiation and chemotherapy.

VIII. **Therapies Frequently Used**

   A. Transfusions: whole blood, blood components.

      1. Plasma to expand blood volume.

      2. Packed red cells to avoid shifts in blood volume.

      3. Granulocytes for infections.

      4. Coagulation factors.

      5. Autologous transfusion.

      6. Preventing transfusion reactions.

         a. Signs: chills, fever, nausea, vomiting, rash, back pain, shortness of breath, sweating, tachycardia, severe anxiety, feeling of impending doom.

      7. Bone marrow transplants.

   B. Leukapheresis: remove leukocytes from the blood.

   C. Biological response modifiers: colony-stimulating factor (CSF) therapy.

1. Drugs made with DNA-recombinant technology.
2. Erythropoietin (Epogen) stimulates erythrocyte production.
3. Granulocyte stimulating factor (G-CSF, Neupogen) is given to combat neutropenia.
4. Granulocyte-macrophage colony-stimulating factor (GM-CSF, Leukine) hastens the recovery of bone marrow.

D. Bone marrow transplantation (BMT).
   1. Treatment option for leukemia and for patients whose marrow is completely destroyed by chemotherapy or radiation during treatment for a malignant condition.
   2. BMT requires an HLA identical match with a donor.
   3. Own bone marrow may be harvested for an autologous transplant before aggressive chemotherapy or radiation treatment.
   4. Patient is at high risk of infection after intensive radiation or chemotherapy that destroys the bone marrow.
   5. Bone marrow is transfused through a central line and the cells find their way to the bone marrow locations in the patient.
   6. Engraftment takes 2 to 5 weeks; the patient is at dire risk of infection and hemorrhage during this period.

E. Oxygen therapy: administration of low concentrations for relief of symptoms of hypoxemia.

F. Iron therapy for iron-deficiency anemia.
   1. Iron salts irritating to stomach mucosa. Give oral preparations after meals.
   2. Vitamin C enhances iron absorption.

G. Vitamin B_{12} injections given for pernicious anemia.

H. Splenectomy.
   1. Indicated when there is traumatic injury, degeneration of splenic tissue, and splenomegaly.
   2. Spleen is not indispensable.
   3. Patient is watched postoperatively for signs of infection, abdominal distention, and other problems related to abdominal surgery.
   4. Persons who have had a splenectomy are at higher risk for infections, particularly pneumonia.

IX. Community Care
   A. Patients are treated in hospitals, outpatient clinics, ambulatory clinics, doctor's offices, at home, and at many other locations in the community.
   B. Home care patients with blood and lymphatic disorders are numerous.
   C. Community care requires the collaboration of many health professionals, including physicians, nurses, pharmacists, dietitians, social workers, respiratory therapists, physical therapists, and home health aides . . . .

X. Elder Care Points
   A. Anemias in elderly mostly are a result of poor nutrition.
   B. The elderly frequently take many medications; some medications interfere with iron absorption.
   C. Patients over 65 require lower doses of chemotherapeutic drugs to prevent toxicity as both the liver and the kidney functions are decreased.
   D. The elderly patient has decreased immune system function; when leukemia develops, she is at even higher risk of infection.
   E. Hemorrhage is tolerated poorly in the elderly because compensatory mechanisms do not function as well.

CHAPTER 18

Care of Patients with Vascular Disorders

OBJECTIVES

Upon completing this chapter, the student should be able to:

1. Discuss the risk factors and incidence of vascular disease.
2. Describe the diagnostic tests, specific techniques, and procedures for assessing the vascular system.
3. Identify three likely nursing diagnoses for patients who have common problems of vascular disease and list the expected outcomes and appropriate nursing interventions for each.
4. Describe the complications that can occur as a consequence of hypertension.
5. Briefly describe the treatment program for mild, moderate, and severe hypertension.
6. Develop and implement a teaching plan for a patient who has hypertension.
7. List four factors that contribute to peripheral vascular disease.
8. Describe the points to be included in the teaching plan for the patient who has experienced thrombophlebitis and has vascular insufficiency.
9. List four nursing interventions for the patient undergoing anticoagulant therapy.
10. List types of surgery performed for problems of the peripheral vascular system.

In conjunction with the heart the vascular system provides the body with nutrients and oxygen needed for life. It also transports metabolic wastes that are excreted by the lungs and the kidneys. When a disorder of the vascular system occurs, homeostasis is upset. Many of the disorders that afflict the vascular system can be prevented or controlled. The nurse must act within the community to educate the public about the risk factors for the various peripheral vascular disorders and about lifestyle changes that may decrease those risks.

The peripheral blood vessels are those situated some distance from the heart. Disorders of the peripheral veins and arteries are almost always chronic, affect people in older age groups, and are associated with other diseases of the cardiovascular system. For example, atherosclerosis affects the aorta as well as the arteries branching from it. Diseases of the peripheral arteries invariably lead to **ischemia** (localized deficiency of blood) of the tissues. If the ischemia is not relieved, the ultimate outcome is tissue necrosis and gangrene.

Resistance to the flow of blood through the veins leads to increased pressure within the walls of the vessel. When blood is not moved out of the veins of the lower extremities, it accumulates there and provides a medium for the growth of bacteria and may contribute to the formation of leg ulcers.

OVERVIEW OF ANATOMY AND PHYSIOLOGY

How Does the Vascular System Function to Carry Blood Throughout the Body?

⅄ Three types of blood vessels make up the vascular system: arteries, veins, and capillaries; these vessels conduct the blood from the heart to the body tissues and back through the lungs to the heart.

⅄ Small veins, venules, and small arteries, arterioles, are connected by the capillaries.

⅄ The aorta is the largest artery in the body, and it receives blood from the heart.

⅄ The inferior and superior vena cava are the largest veins in the body and empty blood into the heart.

- Arteries are elastic and accommodate changes in blood flow by constricting or dilating.
- Three layers of tissue make up the artery wall; the outer layer, the *tunica adventitia*, is connective tissue; the middle layer, the *tunica media*, is smooth muscle; and the inner layer, the *tunica intima*, consists of endothelial cells.
- Veins have the same three layers but with less smooth muscle and connective tissue. The veins are thinner and less rigid, and for that reason the veins can hold more blood.
- The heart pumps blood through the arterial system with each contraction. (Figure 18-1).
- Skeletal muscle contraction, respiratory movements that change the pressures, and constriction of the veins propel blood back to the heart.
- Sets of valves in the medium and large veins open and close, keeping blood flowing toward the heart. Figure 18-2 shows the venous system.
- For blood to circulate the arteries must be unobstructed, and they must be able to dilate and constrict as necessary to regulate the blood flow. Veins also must be patent, their valves must function normally, and surrounding muscles must contract so that venous blood is continually being moved in the direction of the heart.

What Is Blood Pressure and What Affects It?

- Blood pressure is the force that the blood exerts against the walls of the vessels.
- Blood pressure equals the cardiac output multiplied by the peripheral vascular resistance.
- If the caliber of blood vessels becomes smaller because of atherosclerosis, blood pressure increases in an effort to force the blood through the smaller opening.
- If there is an increase in the volume of fluid in the blood vessels, the pressure within the vessels increases, and the heart must work harder to pump the increased volume of fluid through the vessels.
- Angiotensin acts directly on the blood vessels, causing them to constrict, and stimulates the adrenal gland to release aldosterone. Angiotensin increases resistance to blood flow in the peripheral vessels and causes sodium and water retention by the renal tubules through the influence of aldosterone.
- The retained sodium and water increase the blood volume, causing increased cardiac output and blood pressure elevation.
- Blood flow is affected by the amount of resistance in the vessels and by the viscosity of the blood.
- Vascular resistance is controlled by the nervous system, hormones, blood pH, and some ions that regulate the diameter of the vessels.
- **When the vessel diameter increases, resistance falls and blood flow increases. When vessel diameter decreases, resistance rises and blood flow decreases.**
- The sympathetic nervous system plays a major role in regulating vessel diameter as it prompts the release of the hormones norepinephrine and epinephrine that cause vasoconstriction.
- Blood viscosity is affected by the hydration status of the body. When dehydration occurs, blood viscosity increases; thicker blood causes an increase in blood pressure.

What Changes Occur in the Vascular System with Aging?

- Atherosclerosis is a natural part of the aging process and atherotic plaque begins to occur after age 20 (Figure 18-3).
- The arterial walls thicken and lose elasticity, making them less able to adjust to changes in volume and to comply with sympathetic stimulation.
- Varicose veins develop in the elderly as veins lose their elasticity, valve function lessens, and the leg muscles weaken and atrophy from decreased exercise.
- Platelet aggregation and increased coagulation potential lead to a greater incidence of thrombus formation, deep vein thrombosis, and thrombophlebitis in those of advanced age.
- Chronic health problems and failing eye sight often lead to less activity in the elderly, predisposing to vascular problems.

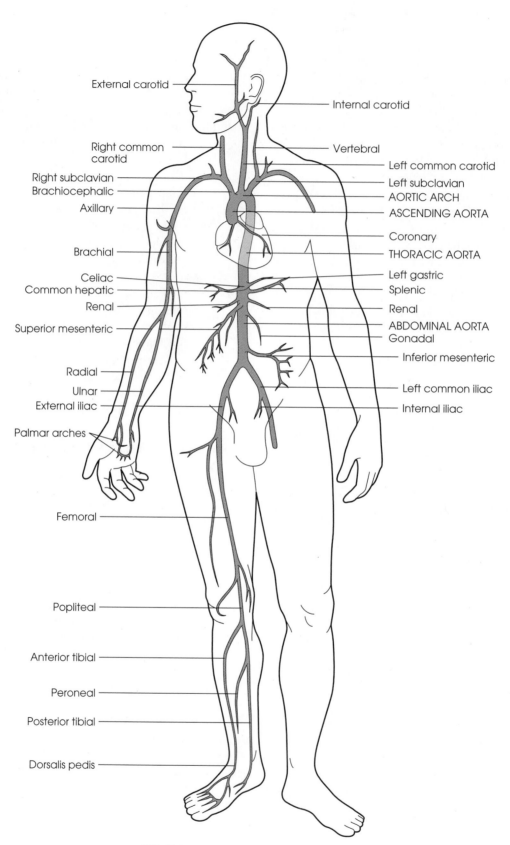

FIGURE 18-1   Major arteries in the body.

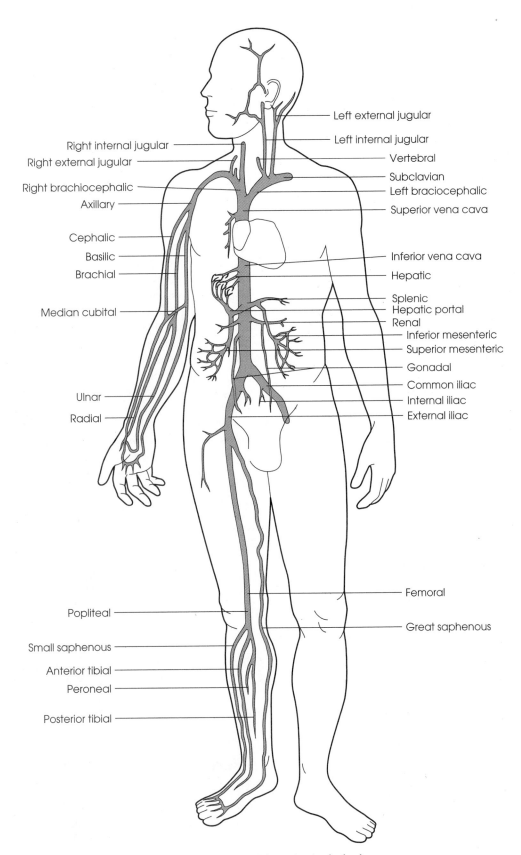

FIGURE 18-2   Major veins in the body.

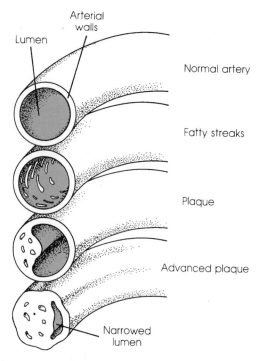

FIGURE 18-3   Cross section of an artery showing progressive narrowing of the diameter of the artery as a result of atherosclerosis and plaque formation.

Think about... Can you think of two physiological reasons why the elderly are more at risk for hypertension?

CAUSATIVE FACTORS AND PREVENTION OF VASCULAR DISORDERS

The arterial wall can be injured by several factors. **Hypertension** (persistently elevated blood pressure) causes a mechanical injury by applying increased pressure continuously on the arterial walls. Elevated levels of low-density lipoproteins and decreased levels of high-density lipoproteins predispose to the deposition of fatty deposits in the arterial walls, causing a narrowing of the vessels. Chemical toxins such as carbon monoxide present in the blood when a person smokes, and the toxins caused by renal failure, cause injury to the arterial walls. Physiological disorders such as diabetes mellitus directly cause physical changes in the vessel walls, leading to more rapid **arteriosclerosis** (loss of elasticity), possibly from elevated blood glucose levels, an increased rate of atherosclerosis, and an earlier onset of hypertension. Some inherited disorders, such as hyperlipidemia, contribute to atherosclerosis.

Obesity, a sedentary lifestyle, and stress are all directly related to the increased incidence of atherosclerosis and hypertension. Smoking and the changes it causes in the vessel walls is directly related to arteriosclerosis of the peripheral vessels and decreased circulation in the lower extremities. Long-term hypertension causes arteriosclerosis and is a direct factor in the development of aortic aneurysm in many patients.

Approximately 50 million Americans have high blood pressure. One out of four adults has high blood pressure. Between 2% and 6% of teenagers have persistent blood pressure elevation. Hypertension is more severe and more prevalent in blacks than in whites by an overall ratio of 2 to 1.

Essential hypertension cannot be prevented, but it can be managed with diligent therapy and cooperation of the patient. Controlling obesity, cigarette smoking, alcohol intake, blood lipid levels, and stress; improving dietary habits; and increasing the level of physical activity can help manage certain kinds of hypertension and prevent some of the more serious consequences. Through the efforts of the American Heart Association and the National Heart, Lung, and Blood Institute, the American public is becoming more aware of the risk factors of hypertension and the need to develop more sensible and wholesome habits of daily living.

A major component in the prevention and control of high blood pressure is education. Nurses can play a major role in teaching others about the disease and supporting their efforts to avoid hypertension and its long-term consequences.

Elder Care Point... Although systolic blood pressure rises as a natural process of aging, systolic hypertension should be treated in the elderly patient. Hypertension in the elderly is associated with an even higher risk of heart disease, stroke, and death from coronary thrombosis. Hypertension has been associated with more rapid memory loss and loss of cognitive function in some research studies.

Nurses can contribute to reducing the incidence of the harmful effects of hypertension by participating in community screening programs to detect hypertension in its early stages, confirm its presence, and initiate prompt treatment. In addition, nurses and other health care professionals have some obligation to serve as models for a healthy lifestyle.

♦ Peripheral Vascular Disorders

The most common cause of peripheral arterial disorders is atherosclerosis (Figure 18-3). Diabetes mellitus, particularly when uncontrolled, speeds the development of atherosclerosis and arteriosclerosis. Other causes of problems include spasm of the smooth muscles in the arterial walls, structural defects in the arteries, trauma, or embolus (blood clot or debris that travels and lodges in a blood vessel) that causes occlusion. Peripheral venous problems are caused by defective valvular function and formation of blood clots (venous thrombosis), which may be accompanied by inflammation (thrombophlebitis).

Prevention of peripheral vascular disease is focused on decreasing atherosclerosis and arteriosclerosis, controlling diabetes mellitus and preventing smoking. Hypertension greatly contributes to arteriosclerosis and its prevention or control will help decrease the incidence of peripheral vascular disease.

Prevention of arteriosclerosis and atherosclerosis focuses on maintaining a healthy lifestyle: a low-fat, healthy diet; regular exercise; normal weight; prevention of excessive stress; and control of diabetes mellitus.

◆ Venous Insufficiency and Varicose Veins

The cause of venous valve failure is unknown. Two things seem to increase the likelihood of occurrence of varicosities and consequent venous insufficiency: standing for long periods over years, and wearing very tight, constricting clothing, such as a tight girdle. People who must be on their feet a great deal are encouraged to wear support stockings to encourage venous return. Patients must be taught not to wear excessively constricting clothing; weight reduction is a better alternative than a girdle.

Think about . . . Can you identify two lifestyle changes you could personally make that would decrease your chances of a vascular disorder later in life?

DIAGNOSTIC TESTS AND PROCEDURES

Determining a vascular problem begins with a history and physical examination that includes a variety of tests for risk factors for vascular disorders.

A complete blood (CBC) count, urinalysis, blood lipid and cholesterol assessment, including high-density lipid (HDL) and low-density lipid (LDL), or sequential multiple analyzer (SMA) panel that screens liver and kidney function, electrolytes, and blood glucose are ordered. If blood pressure is elevated, tests of thyroid, adrenal glands, kidneys, and renal arteries are done to rule out the possibility of another disease that might cause secondary hypertension. Hyperthyroidism, Cushing's syndrome, pheochromocytoma, nephrosclerosis, and renal arterial stenosis all elevate blood pressure.

Doppler flow studies are performed to detect a thrombus when one is suspected and to assess the patency of the carotid arteries. Angiography may be performed to determine areas of narrowing in arteries or to detect a lodged embolus. Nuclear medicine scans are performed to detect emboli in the lungs.

The *retrograde filling test* is performed to assess the competency of the valves in the saphenous and communicating veins of the legs. Position the patient supine and raise the leg to 90 degrees to drain the venous blood. Place a tourniquet around the upper thigh to occlude the vessels. If the vein does not fill from below within 35 seconds, the valves are not functioning correctly. Release the tourniquet and observe vein filling. Normal valves slow the filling process; if valves are incompetent, filling occurs immediately.

The Trendelenburg test, another version of the retrograde filling test, is an assessment of the ability of the valves to prevent the backflow of blood in the veins. The patient is placed in a recumbent position with the affected leg elevated above the level of the heart. A tourniquet is applied below the knee to compress the superficial veins. The patient is then asked to stand up, and the tourniquet is removed. If the valves are incompetent, the veins will quickly become engorged with blood. Table 18-1 presents the diagnostic tests used to detect other problems in the vascular system. Serum cholesterol and lipids are discussed more fully in Chapter 19.

Think about . . . Can you identify four teaching points to be covered for the patient who is to undergo an arteriogram?

NURSING ASSESSMENT

◆ History Taking

Subjective information is gathered during history taking. The patient is questioned about personal and family history of disorders, injuries, and lifestyle that relate to vascular disease. Table 18-2 presents a guide for history taking. Other subjective data include questions regarding medications taken regularly, both prescription and nonprescription, as many drugs can cause vasoconstriction and elevate blood pressure. Cold remedies, decongestants, and diet pills are particularly noted for having this effect. A careful, specific diet history should be gathered. Fast food intake is significant because it is often high in fat and sodium. **Excessive alcohol intake is a factor in the development of hypertension.** Questions are asked that relate to changes from damage to the vascular system, such as congestive heart failure, angina, or kidney failure. *Intermittent claudication,* cramping pain in the muscles brought on by exercise and relieved by rest, is a common symptom of arterial insufficiency to the lower extremities. This pain most frequently occurs in the calves of the legs, but it also can affect the muscles of the thighs and buttocks.

TABLE 18-1 ◆ *Common Diagnostic Tests for the Vascular System*

Test	Purpose	Procedure	Nursing Implications
Ultrasound Doppler flow studies	Detect clot in vessel; determine degree of narrowing of vessel or detect arterial spasm. Most commonly performed on the lower extremities and the carotid vessels.	A gel is applied to the skin. An ultrasound wand is moved over the skin above the vessel; the skin should be clean and dry with no lotions or powders.	Explain the the test takes about 30 minutes.
Venogram	To detect thrombosis or narrowing of a vein	Requires a consent form as radiopaque substance is injected into the vessel and radiographs are taken.	Explain that the procedure is somewhat uncomfortable as the dye can be irritating to the vessels, causing a burning sensation.
Venous imaging B/mode	Ultrasound detection of deep vein thrombosis. B/mode shows a two-dimensional image.	Uses real-time duplex scanning. Patient is placed supine in reverse Trendelenburg position; the vessels are scanned. Then patient is placed prone for further vessel examination.	Explain positioning necessary and that the scan head will be moved down the leg to scan each venous segment.
Angiogram (arteriogram)	Determine areas of narrowing or structural changes, such as an aneurysm in an artery. Detect the presence of an embolus. Most frequently performed on vessels in the heart, lungs, or head.	Requires a consent form. A catheter is threaded into an artery and a radiopaque dye is injected. Radiographs are taken. Preoperative preparation is necessary. Postoperative care includes careful monitoring for bleeding from the catheter insertion site, and neurological signs and vital signs are taken frequently to monitor for the possibility of embolus or bleeding. Sensation distal to the catheter insertion site also is checked as internal bleeding can cause a hematoma that presses on nerves.	Preparation is similar to that for surgery. Explain that preoperative medication will be given. Increase fluids if a contrast medium was used to flush the dye through the kidneys. Consent form required.
Impedence plethysmography	Estimates blood flow in a limb based on electrical resistance present before and after inflating a pneumatic cuff placed around the limb. Used to detect deep vein thrombosis.	Measurements of electrical resistance are taken before and after a pneumatic cuff placed around the limb is inflated. Electrodes are placed on opposite sides of the limb.	Instruct to wear loose clothing. Explain that some discomfort may occur during inflation of the cuff. The patient is placed on an examination table and positioned supine in a relaxed comfortable position. The limb is properly positioned, and electrodes and the pneumatic cuff are applied.
Nuclear medicine scan	Detect blood clots, particularly pulmonary emboli.	A radioisotope is injected, and after a waiting period for uptake, a scintillation scanning camera is used to measure the amount of radioactivity present in the area in question.	Determine whether patient has an allergy to the dye. Posttest encourage large fluid intake to flush the dye through the kidneys.
C-T scan	Determine size and condition of aortic aneurysm.	Noninvasive, unless dye contrast used. Patient positioned on scanning table and moved under the scanner.	Instruct in necessity of holding still during scan.
Carotid duplex examination	Study blood flow in external carotid arteries.	Patient is positioned supine with neck extended. The probe is moved up and down each side of the neck over the external carotid arteries.	Explain that plaque in the arteries can be visualized in this manner. This test assists in determining need for endarterectomy surgery.

TABLE 18-2 ◆ *Assessment of Vascular Disease: Guide to History Taking*

Ask the patient the following questions to gather data:

◆ Have you or any member of your family ever been told that you have diabetes mellitus, cardiovascular, thyroid, or renal disease, arteriosclerosis, atherosclerosis, peripheral vascular disease, or an immune disorder such as lupus erythematosus?
◆ Have you ever had a bad injury to either leg?
◆ Have you ever had a deep vein thrombosis (DVT) or thrombophlebitis?
◆ What medications do you take that are prescribed by your doctor? What over-the-counter medications do you take?
◆ Do you ever take cold or allergy medications? Decongestants?
◆ Do you ever take diet pills?
◆ Do you smoke? Have you ever smoked? How much and for how long?
◆ Do you drink alcohol? What do you usually drink? How many drinks do you have? About how many times a week do you drink something alcoholic?
◆ What do you usually eat? Can you tell me what you generally eat for breakfast, lunch, and dinner? Do you have a mid-morning, mid-afternoon, or evening snack? What do you eat for a snack? Do you have fast food often? What type? What do you usually drink at meals? Do you take liquids between meals?
◆ Do you regularly add salt to your food?
◆ Have you experienced dizziness? headaches? blackouts? or vision changes?
◆ Do you have to get up at night to urinate?
◆ Are you ever short of breath? Do you ever have swelling of the feet and ankles? Do you ever have chest pain?
◆ Do you have pain in your legs or feet when you walk?
◆ Do you have leg pain at night?
◆ Have you ever had a sore on your foot or ankle that was slow to heal?

Often chronic occlusive arterial disease will cause pain described as burning and tingling, with numbness of the toes. It is most noticeable at night when the patient is in bed.

Think about... How would you phrase questions about alcohol intake so that the patient would not take offense and would answer the questions honestly?

◆ Physical Assessment

Pulses   Check the arterial pulses and determine the pulse rate, rhythm, and character (force) of the pulse. When performing a vascular assessment, the radial pulse should be assessed and compared with the apical pulse. The apical pulse should be counted for a full minute. The carotid, femoral, popliteal, and pedal pulses should also be palpated and compared bilaterally, noting quality and character. Figure 18-4 depicts the arterial pulse sites. The pulse may be described as

normal or absent, regular or irregular, strong, weak, or thready.

If pulsations are weak or undetectable, the nurse uses a Doppler device to check them. A Doppler device measures the velocity of blood flow through a vessel with ultrasound waves. It can sense weak pulsations even in severely narrowed arteries (Figure 18-5).

Think about... Can you recall the correct way to locate a pedal and posttibial pulse? Could you demonstrate the technique to a classmate?

Examine the abdomen with the patient lying supine for a visual abdominal pulsation from the aorta. This sometimes indicates the presence of an aneurysm.

Bruits   A whooshing or purring sound is made when blood passes through a partially obstructed artery. To detect bruits, listen with the bell of the stethoscope applied lightly over the skin of the carotid arteries, abdominal aorta, and femoral arteries.

Blood Pressure   For more accurate readings, be certain the patient has not had a cigarette or any caffeine

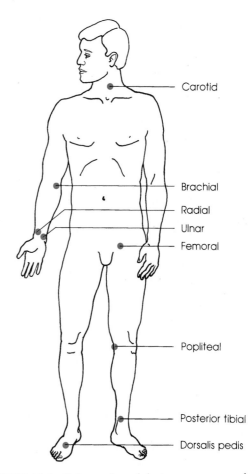

FIGURE 18-4   Pulses palpated during assessment of the arterial system.

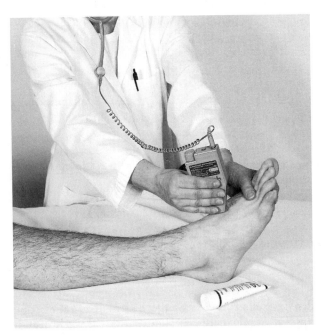

FIGURE 18-5 The Doppler stethoscope is used to detect a faint pulse. (*Source:* Jarvis, C. [1996]. *Physical Examination and Health Assessment,* 2nd ed. Philadelphia: Saunders, p. 588.)

for the past 30 minutes. Blood pressure should be carefully measured with the correct-size cuff. The cuff should fit the upper arm with the lower edge 2.5 cm (1 inch) above the antecubital space. If it is too narrow, the pressure will be erroneously elevated. The bladder must be centered over the brachial artery, and its length should cover at least 80% of the extremity's circumference when positioned correctly. The pressure should be taken sitting, lying supine, and standing for a thorough assessment. Standing blood pressure measurements also are important when a patient is started on a new medication, particularly an angiotensin-converting enzyme (ACE) inhibitor. Blood pressure should be measured on both arms. The patient's arm on which the cuff is placed should be placed at heart level. The patient should be resting quietly for 5 minutes before the measurement is taken. The equipment used should be calibrated, and the valve should open and close smoothly. The cuff should be deflated slowly and smoothly to obtain a correct diastolic reading.

Elder Care Point... The blood pressure of the elderly patient will be less right after a meal. For accurate readings, assess blood pressure between meals.

Skin   Tissues that are receiving an adequate supply of oxygenated blood appear pink and rosy, whereas those deprived of normal amounts of arterial blood appear pale and mottled. However, the environment must be taken into account. Pale and mottled skin also can indicate that the patient is just cold. Reddish-blue color can indicate venous insufficiency.

One way to assess arterial blood flow more accurately is by having the patient elevate the feet and legs above the level of the heart for 1 to 3 minutes until pallor occurs. Have the patient lower the legs to a dangling position while sitting. Compare both feet, noting the time necessary for pinkness to return (usually about 10 sec). Note the time it takes for the veins of the feet and ankles to fill (usually about 15 sec). For black persons, inspect the soles of the feet for color change and use a light shining at an angle to visualize vein filling.

Return of color to the lowered feet is delayed in arterial insufficiency. If there is severe ischemia, the dangling feet soon take on a dusky-red color (**rubor**). **This indicates permanent dilation of the vessels; they are no longer able to constrict as they should. In addition to being reddened, the feet and ankles may appear swollen and edematous.**

A cold environment and immobility will cause the extremities to feel cold to the touch. However, when a patient experiences persistent coldness of an extremity in a warm environment, arterial insufficiency should be suspected. When observing a patient for signs of arterial disease, the nurse should note differences in skin temperature in various areas of the same limb, as well as differences between limbs.

Skin that is chronically malnourished because of decreased blood supply has a characteristic appearance: it appears smooth, shiny, and thin, and there is little or no hair on its surface. The nails are thick with deposits of thick, corn-like material under them.

Elder Care Point... Hair loss is a natural occurrence with aging, as is thickening of fingernails and toenails. These signs are not reliable indicators of vascular problems of the extremities in the elderly.

If there is severe malnutrition of the tissues for several days, the tissues become necrotic. This causes the skin to assume a purple-black color. This is a deep cyanotic condition indicative of gangrene. Gangrene of the toes is not an uncommon complication in the diabetic patient who has poor circulation in the feet.

Chronic venous insufficiency is accompanied by chronic edema. This in turn leads to inflammation of the tissues (**cellulitis**) and eventually to the formation of ulcers. Increased pigmentation of the skin, dryness and scaling, and excoriations are objective signs of venous insufficiency.

The capillary refill test has traditionally been used to check peripheral circulation. A fingernail or a toenail is squeezed over the bed of the nail sufficiently to cause blanching; the pressure is removed and an observation of how quickly the color returns is made. Normally the color returns immediately, Although it is a good gross assessment of circulation to the extremity, this test is unreliable as many factors can cause a decrease in time for color to return. This test is most useful for determining whether circulation is occluded by constriction or thrombosus above the area. Table 18-3 presents a guide to physical assessment. Review Chapter 5 for the assessment and staging of edema.

♦ Nursing Diagnosis

Nursing diagnoses are chosen based on the assessment data that indicate problems for the patient. Common nursing diagnoses associated with vascular disorders are listed in Table 18-4. Nursing diagnoses may be added to the care plan for problems secondary to treatments, such as drug therapy or surgery. Other nursing diagnoses sometimes used include:

♦ Sleep pattern disturbance related to pain in the legs while at rest.

♦ Self-esteem disturbance related to inability to perform usual roles because of chronic leg ulcers.

♦ Planning

The nursing goals for the patient with a vascular disorder are to:

♦ Promote vascular integrity.

♦ Decrease risk factors for vascular disease.

♦ Maintain blood pressure within normal limits.

♦ Improve circulatory function.

TABLE 18-3 ♦ *Assessment: Guide to Focused Physical Assessment of the Vascular System*

Head and neck
Color of skin.
Appearance of neck veins; any distention?
Auscultate carotid arteries for presence of bruit.

Chest
Auscultate heart; any abnormal sounds? Rate, Rhythm.

Abdomen
Any visible abdominal pulsation over aorta?
Auscultate over aorta for presence of bruit.

Extremities
Assess brachial, femoral, popliteal, and pedal pulses; compare bilaterally.
Assess blood pressure on both arms, sitting and standing.
Assess skin for temperature, color, appearance, dryness, presence or absence of hair.
Presence of varicosities.
Assess capillary refill.
Assess feet for venous insufficiency; presence of rubor?
Presence of ulceration?
Presence of edema?

♦ Prevent thrombosis and embolism.

♦ Maintain or restore tissue integrity.

♦ Prevent the complications of leg ulcers and gangrene.

When a patient has a history of thrombosis, the nurse must plan measures to prevent recurrence regardless of what patient problem is currently the focus of treatment. If the patient has arterial insufficiency, the nurse should be alert to prescribed medications that may cause further vasoconstriction.

Appropriate exercise is important to treat vascular disease and the nurse collaborates with the physical therapist about activity, exercises, and the reinforcement of teaching. Collaboration with the dietitian is vital to the patient who has atherosclerosis and a high cholesterol count. Specific expected outcomes must be written on an individual basis. Examples are included in Table 18-4.

♦ Implementation

A large part of what the nurse does for the patient with a vascular disorder is to monitor the condition and determine whether treatment is effective. Considerable time is spent on teaching patients about the disease, self-care, and medications. Monitoring side effects or adverse effects of medication is very important. Specific interventions are discussed with the various disorders in this chapter and in the section Common Problems. Table 18-4 lists helpful interventions for the most common nursing diagnoses associated with problems of the vascular system.

♦ Evaluation

It is important to look at serial blood pressure readings to evaluate the effectiveness of treatment and of nursing interventions. Pressures that are consistently higher than normal in between medication doses indicate a need to change either the dosage schedule or the medication.

Carefully evaluating pulses and comparing them bilaterally is an important part of nursing care for patients with problems of the vascular system. Writing a good description of the quality and character of the pulses monitored in the nurse's notes will give co-workers an accurate assessment baseline on which to evaluate changes in the pulse.

It is important to determine if skin color and temperature have changed since the last assessment. Areas of discoloration should be accurately measured and documented in the nurse's notes. Ulcerated areas are monitored closely and are measured to determine whether healing is occurring. The color of the healing tissue and presence of exudate also are evaluated. If the

TABLE 18-4 ♦ *Common Nursing Diagnoses and Interventions for Patients with Vascular Disorders*

Nursing Diagnosis	Goals/Expected Outcomes	Intervention
Altered tissue perfusion related to: Vascular damage.	Patient's blood pressure will be within normal range within 3 months.	Assess blood pressure; determine effectiveness of therapy. Administer medications to lower blood pressure. Assess for side effects of medication. Discourage intake of caffeine and excess sodium. Discourage smoking. Teach to arise slowly and stabilize before walking to counteract postural hypotension effect from medication. Teach anxiety- and tension-reduction techniques to decrease blood pressure. Encourage regular rest, relaxation, and exercise program.
Obstructed blood flow.	Patient will not develop other deep vein thrombosis. Thrombosis will resolve within 10–14 days.	Assess for signs and symptoms of deep vein thrombosis and impaired blood flow. Maintain activity restrictions as ordered. Elevate affected extremity as ordered. Increase fluid intake to 3,000 mL/day unless contraindicated. Administer anticoagulants as ordered; monitor for side effects. Teach to prevent future episodes by encouraging not to sit with legs crossed, not to sit for long periods, and not to put pressure on the back of the knees. Apply elastic stockings or sequential pneumatic devices to promote venous return.
Surgical revascularization.	Patient will not develop thrombosis.	Check incisions for bleeding q 1 to 2 h × 24 h then q 4 h × 6, then q shift. Assess for internal hematoma by checking sensation below surgical area. Assess for adequate blood flow by checking pulses distal to incision on same schedule. Assess skin color and temperature above and below incision when checking for bleeding. Reinforce dressing as needed; change dressing per orders using strict aseptic technique.
Pain related to decreased blood flow and edema.	Patient will verbalize adequate pain control attained from analgesics and comfort measures provided.	Assess type and location of pain experienced. Handle gently and avoid jarring the bed. Use a bed cradle or footboard to prevent pressure from bed linens. Administer analgesics and antiinflammatory agents as ordered. Apply heat as ordered; monitor closely to prevent burns. Teach relaxation techniques, imagery, or distraction to decrease pain. Elevate edematous extremity. Apply elastic stockings or sequential pneumatic devices to encourage venous return and decrease edema. Medicate for sleep as ordered if discomfort is interfering with rest.
Activity intolerance related to pain in legs when walking.	Patient will develop own activity program within 3 weeks. Patient will exercise regularly according to devised program.	Collaborate with physical therapist to encourage prescribed exercises. Assist to plan walking, swimming, or cycling program.
Body image disturbance related to: Diagnosis of chronic illness. Edema and dilated veins in the legs. Loss of limb by amputation.	Patient will verbalize feelings regarding diagnosis, body changes, and needed lifestyle changes. Patient will identify personal strengths and coping mechanisms.	Allow to ventilate feelings about illness and disease process. Assist through the grief process. Assist to identify personal strengths. Reinforce coping mechanisms that have been helpful before. Be with patient for first dressing change. Clarify misconceptions about physical limitations after amputation.

TABLE 18-4 ◆ *Common Nursing Diagnoses and Interventions for Patients with Vascular Disorders* (Continued)

Nursing Diagnosis	Goals/Expected Outcomes	Intervention
	Patient will become as independent as possible in tasks of daily living (within 2 months).	Involve patient in care of the wound after initial period of adjustment. Foster independence in tasks of daily living. Assist to explore lifestyle changes. Encourage significant others in their support of the patient. Teach ways to decrease risk of further amputation.
Impaired skin integrity related to: Ulcer from decreased circulation. Surgical wound. (Risk for infection may be used here also.)	Patient will not develop a wound infection.	Use strict aseptic technique for wound care. Treat and dress wound per physician's orders. Promote adequate nutrition to promote healing. Administer medication as ordered to prevent infection. Position affected limb as ordered. Maintain correct body alignment.
Risk for impaired skin integrity related to bedrest and impaired circulation	Patient will not develop impaired skin integrity.	Inspect pressure points q 2 h. Turn at least every 2 hours. Maintain smooth linens on bed, provide appropriate padding to prevent pressure areas. Keep skin clean and dry. Refrain from raising the knee section of the bed. Encourage foot and ankle exercises every hour while patient is awake. Prevent shearing when patient is moving in bed by using a lift sheet and two people to turn the patient. If skin breakdown occurs, notify physician immediately and provide appropriate wound care.
Knowledge deficit related to inadequate information about disease process, medications, and self-care.	Patient will verbalize knowledge of disease process and ways to prevent further damage. Patient will verbalize how to take medications and side effects to report. Patient will demonstrate self-care techniques.	Explain what is happening in the body to cause the decreased blood flow. Allow time for questions. Instruct in ways to decrease risk factors. Teach self-care methods, including exercises, skin care, foot care, dietary changes, lifestyle changes. Teach about medications including: schedule of administration, action, side effects, what to report to the physician. Encourage regular visits to the doctor.
Noncompliance related to refusal to follow treatment regimen.	Patient will verbalize frustrations and problems in complying with treatment regimen and lifestyle changes. Patient will demonstrate compliance with treatment regimen.	Reinstruct about disease process. Explore problems with treatment regimen. Allow to express feelings about lifestyle changes. Explore ability to obtain and afford medications. Explore any difficulty in swallowing medications. Explain progression of disease and consequences of poor control; discuss complications and impact on lifestyle. Seek support system for compliance with treatment program. Give praise for each attempt at compliance. Respect the patient's right to make decisions about compliance.
Risk for injury related to: Embolus or bleeding from anticoagulant medication.	Coagulation times will remain within safe therapeutic range. Patient will have no signs of bleeding. Patient will have no signs of embolus.	Do not massage affected extremity. Encourage activity restrictions as ordered. Monitor laboratory values: PT or APTT and notify physician when values are outside of accepted therapeutic limits. Assess urine and stool for signs of blood. Assess patient for excessive bruising; bleeding gums, nosebleeds, bleeding at puncture sites. Check injectable anticoagulant dosages and IV admixtures with another nurse before administration to verify correct ordered dosage and rate of infusion.
Circulatory occlusion from embolus.		Assess for signs of embolus: chest pain, shortness of breath, change in level of consciousness, sudden headache, or other neurological signs.

wound is growing or not improving, the nursing actions or treatment must be changed.

Often the nurse must rely on subjective data from the patient to evaluate whether treatment and nursing actions are effective. Increases in peripheral circulation may be evident only by a decrease in pain or an ability to walk further without pain.

COMMON PROBLEMS AND THERAPIES AND THEIR NURSING IMPLICATIONS

◆ Altered Tissue Perfusion

In peripheral vascular disease, blood flow may be altered by constriction of the vessels or by sluggish blood flow. The smooth muscles of the arterial walls respond to temperature by constricting in the presence of cold and extreme heat and relaxing in the presence of warmth. Therefore the nurse's care plan should include (1) providing a warm environment for the patient; (2) covering the hospitalized patient with warm blankets; dressing him or her in warm clothing; and (3) instructing the patient to avoid extremes of cold and heat.

The constricting effect of extreme heat rules out the use of local applications in the form of hot water bottles. In addition to the danger of burning the patient because of decreased sensitivity to extremes of temperature, local heat increases metabolic activity in the tissues to which it is applied and therefore upsets even more the balance of supply and demand for blood flow to all of the tissues.

> The goal in application of additional warmth is even distribution throughout the body.

***Think about* . . .** What would you recommend to the elderly home care patient to keep his lower extremities warm during the winter? The patient does not have the funds to keep the house heated above 68° F.

A second consideration is that of *pressure* against the walls of the blood vessels. Constricting clothing is avoided, particularly circular garters and elastic materials in underclothing. Frequent position changes are essential; position must be changed at least every 2 hours.

> The patient with poor venous circulation can benefit from periodic elevation of the lower extremities to facilitate venous return of blood to the heart. Elevation above the level of the heart is preferred.

Even, well-distributed support of the vessels near the surface of the body will help improve venous

return. To provide this kind of support, the physician may prescribe an elastic bandage or fitted elastic stockings. The stockings or elastic bandage should be applied early in the morning, before the legs are placed in a dependent position, because the blood vessels are less congested after a prolonged rest. Bandages and hose should be applied by beginning at the feet and working upward to avoid trapping blood in the lower leg. The patient should have two pair of elastic hose and should wash them after each day's wearing. Elastic hose should be replaced every 6 months as they lose their elasticity. When stockings are removed, the heels should be checked for pressure areas. **Elastic stockings are not used for patients with arterial disorders.**

Exercise is especially beneficial to patients with decreased blood flow. Walking is ideal exercise for the ambulatory patient. Bed-ridden patients will need range of motion (ROM) exercises and the other kinds of muscular movements described in Chapter 11. Use of a treadmill for patients who cannot exercise by walking outside is very beneficial. An exercycle is another alternative.

In addition to mechanical factors, certain chemical factors affect the constriction of blood vessels. *Nicotine,* which is inhaled with tobacco smoke, has the effect of producing spasmodic narrowing of the peripheral arteries. Patients with arterial insufficiency are therefore encouraged to stop smoking. Used in conjunction with a community stop smoking support program, the booklet *You Can Quit Smoking,* available from the Agency for Health Care Policy and Research Publications Clearinghouse (P.O. Box 8547, Silver Spring, MD 20907), can be very helpful.

***Think about* . . .** Can you describe the specific actions you would take to help a patient recognize the need for and to establish a "quit smoking" program?

Alcohol is a mild vasodilator when taken in moderate amounts. Unless the patient has moral or religious convictions against its use, the physician may approve daily intake of a specific small amount of wine or liquor.

Drugs that are helpful to relieve vasoconstriction and improve blood flow are prescribed. These drugs are of value only when the arteries are still capable of dilating. Severely sclerosed vessels respond very poorly to therapy of this kind. Some think that vasodilators may actually be harmful because they shunt blood away from the zone of ischemia to well-perfused tissues.

Sympathectomy is a surgical technique that may be used to relieve vasoconstriction. Because this procedure severs sympathetic nerve fibers supplying the peripheral vessels, it is of benefit only to those patients who do not have advanced pathological changes in these vessels.

TABLE 18-5 ◆ *Patient Education: Information for Patients with Peripheral Vascular Disease*

- Keep warm; avoid extreme heat or cold. If the feet become cold, soak them in lukewarm water.
- Do not use tobacco in any form.
- Take great care that the foot and lower leg are not injured; avoid crowded places.
- Never go barefoot. Wear properly fitted shoes that are wide-toed and thick-soled with soft tops and that cause no pressure at any point.
- Use a mirror when dressing to check the bottom of the feet for areas of redness or broken skin.
- Wear only clean, cotton socks.
- Do not wear circular garters or trousers with legs that constrict when sitting.
- Do not sit for long periods; never cross legs at the knee. When on a trip, take a walk every 2 hours.
- If the weight of the bed linens is uncomfortable, use a pillow at the foot of the bed to hold them off the feet.
- Perform daily foot care by washing with mild soap and water. Inspect for cuts, blisters, ulcers, or infections. Dry thoroughly by blotting, not rubbing. If the feet are sweaty, lightly powder them with cornstarch. If the feet are dry and scaly, apply lanolin or a similar cream.
- Have nails trimmed by a doctor or podiatrist, and let him treat calluses and corns; never shave these yourself.
- For foot pain at night, elevate the head of the bed on 18- to 30-cm blocks to increase blood flow to the legs and feet.
- For exercise, walk 1 to 2 miles each day in short segments. Stop if leg pain develops, rest, and then continue.
- Drink the equivalent of 10 to 18 glasses of water every day, unless this is contraindicated.

◆ Impaired Skin Integrity

Tissues that have a diminished blood supply are subject to severe and permanent damage from the slightest injury, because the normal processes of healing and repair are impaired.

Arterial and venous stasis often lead to chronic leg ulcers.

These ulcers are particularly distressing to the patient because they heal very slowly and many never completely heal. Patients must be taught to avoid conditions that contribute to injury of the extremities and to report any injury, no matter how minor. The kind of information usually given to a patient is listed in Table 18-5.

Prevention of leg ulcers includes (1) wearing elastic bandages or support hose; (2) proper positioning and exercise; (3) avoiding injury to the feet and legs; and (4) avoiding extremes of heat and cold and other mechanical and chemical factors that contribute to obstruction of blood flow. Nursing interventions for selected problems in a patient with a venous stasis ulcer are summarized in Table 18-4 and in Nursing Care Plan 18-1 on page 528.

ARTERIAL DISORDERS

◆ Hypertension

Hypertension is defined as persistently high blood pressure. In adults, this means a systolic pressure that is equal to or greater than 140 mm Hg and a diastolic pressure that is equal to or greater than 90 mm Hg when taken at least twice and averaged on two different occasions 2 weeks apart. The diastolic pressure usually is the focus of treatment because it reflects the amount of pressure being exerted against the vessel walls while the heart is in its phase of relaxation and there is no added pressure from blood being forced out of the left ventricle and into the arteries. Table 18-6 presents ranges for the classification of hypertension.

Hypertensive individuals usually die from long-term damage to the so-called end organs or target organs; that is, the brain, heart, and kidney. Over half the deaths associated with persistent and unrelieved hypertension are caused by myocardial infarction. Immediate causes of death related to high blood pressure include cerebral hemorrhage and heart failure.

The cause of essential hypertension is not known. High blood pressure is a reflection of homeostatic mechanisms that (1) control the caliber of blood vessels and their responsiveness to various stimuli; (2) regulate fluid volume in the intravascular and extravascular compartments; and (3) control cardiac output.

There are two major types of hypertension: essential (primary or idiopathic) and secondary hypertension. About 90% of all cases of hypertension are classified as essential hypertension. The cause of hypertension is unknown, and the goals of treatment are (1) reduction of high blood pressure; and (2) long-term control to decrease the risk of stroke, heart attack, and kidney disease.

In the remaining 10% the hypertension is actually a symptom of another disorder; that is, the hypertension is secondary to another disease. If the primary disease can be detected and treated successfully, the problem of

TABLE 18-6 ◆ *Classification of Hypertension*

Systolic Pressure	Diastolic Pressure	Classification
<130	<85	Normal
130–139	85–89	High normal
140–159	90–99	Stage I: mild hypertension
160–179	100–109	Stage II: moderate hypertension
180–209	110–119	Stage III: severe hypertension
>210	>120	Stage IV: very severe hypertension

hypertension is eliminated. Examples of diseases that can produce secondary hypertension include renal vascular disease (for example, atherosclerosis of the renal artery), dysfunction of the adrenal cortex and medulla, atherosclerosis of the arteries of systemic circulation, and coarctation of the aorta.

Some major factors associated with essential hypertension are age, race, obesity, and sodium intake. Female hormone therapy, nicotine, and caffeine consumption appear to be contributing factors in some people. Persons with a family history of hypertension also are at greater risk for developing essential hypertension.

Blood pressure tends to rise with age. Average blood pressure readings for various age groups are shown in Table 18-7. An elevation above normal limits in either systolic or diastolic blood pressure at any age is not normal and increases the risk for illness and death from a cardiovascular disease.

Obesity is closely associated with an elevation of blood pressure. There is a correlation between an increase in body weight over a period of years and a simultaneous increase in blood pressure. **Many times a loss of excess weight alone can return a slightly elevated blood pressure to normal.**

Nicotine and caffeine can have immediate effects on the level of blood pressure. Smoking increases the chances of developing cardiovascular disease and also elevates the blood pressure significantly each time a cigarette is smoked.

There is evidence that salt intake also is a factor. Epidemiological studies have shown that many people who consume large amounts of salt have abnormal blood pressure; others are not affected by a high-sodium diet. A possible explanation is that sodium brings out an inherent susceptibility to hypertension in some people. At any rate, a moderate reduction of salt intake has been effective in lowering the blood pressure of some persons with mild or moderate hypertension.

Pathophysiology   Blood pressure equals the amount of blood pumped out by the heart (cardiac output) multiplied by the peripheral vascular resistance. If the caliber of blood vessels becomes smaller because of atherosclerosis or vasoconstriction, blood pressure increases in an effort to force the blood through the smaller opening. If there is an increase in the volume or viscosity of fluid in the blood vessels, the pressure within the vessels increases, and the heart must work harder to pump the increased volume of fluid through the vessels. A pathological response to stress can result in an elevation in blood pressure by stimulating the sympathetic nervous system and causing peripheral vasoconstriction and increased heart rate.

In some instances of hypertension an excess of renin is secreted by the kidneys. Renin acts on a substance called angiotensinogen, converting it to angiotensin I. Angiotensin I is converted to angiotensin II by another enzyme. Angiotensin II acts directly on the blood vessels, causing them to constrict, and also stimulates the adrenal gland to release aldosterone. Angiotensin thereby increases resistance to blood flow in the peripheral vessels and causes retention of sodium and water by the renal tubules through the influence of aldosterone. The retained sodium and water increase the blood volume, causing increased cardiac output and elevation of blood pressure. Figure 18-6 shows the pathophysiology of hypertension.

Elder Care Point . . .   The arteriosclerosis that causes blood vessel rigidity is a natural part of aging. Systolic blood pressure may be higher in the elderly person. The baroreceptors that normally help adjust blood pressure become less sensitive with age. The lack of elasticity of the vessels and the decreased sensitivity of the baroreceptors cause the elderly to be at risk for orthostatic (postural) hypotension when changing position.

Signs and Symptoms   Hypertension has been called the "silent killer," because in the early stages it does not usually cause discomfort or any other subjective signs and symptoms to indicate that it is present. About one-third of those who have hypertension are not aware of it. Signs may appear only in the later stages when damage has already been done to the target organs—that is, the kidney (renal ischemia), brain (arteriosclerosis and microaneurysms), aorta (aortic aneurysm), and heart (left ventricular hypertrophy and reduced cardiac output). **Patients with symptoms may complain**

TABLE 18-7 ◆ *Average Blood Pressure Readings for Various Age Groups*	
Age (Years)	**Average Reading**
4	98/60
6	105/60
10	112/64
11 to 16	120/75
20–30	124/78
30–40	126/80
40–50	130/82
50–60	138/84
60–70	140/82 (male)*
	152/84 (female)
70–80	142/80 (male)
	156/82 (female)
80+	142/78 (male)
	140/89 (female)

*Average blood pressure becomes higher in the female after age 60.

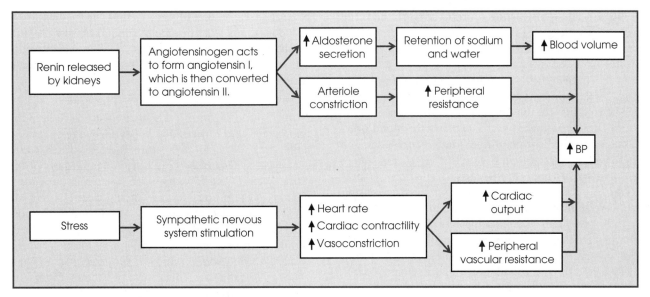

FIGURE 18-6   Pathophysiology of hypertension.

of headache, dizziness, blurred vision, blackouts, irritability, fatigue, or nervousness.

Hypertensive patients develop coronary heart disease at a rate two to three times greater than that of persons with normal blood pressure. If blood pressure is maintained at or below 140/90, the risk in patients with hypertension does not increase.

Malignant hypertension is a term describing rapidly progressive moderate to severe hypertension that is difficult to control. Diastolic pressure ranges from 140 to 170 mmHg, and unless effective intervention is found, the patient may suffer heart, kidney, and brain damage.

Hypertensive crisis is a life-threatening emergency in which the patient experiences severe headache, blurred vision, nausea, and possibly confusion. It may occur if a patient has stopped taking antihypertensive medication, or it may be secondary to another disease process. The patient is placed in the intensive care unit and treated with intravenous emergency drugs, such as IV sodium nitroprusside or nitroglycerin to bring the blood pressure down. Short-acting Nifedipine may be given orally.

Diagnosis and Treatment   If no underlying disease can be identified as elevating the patient's blood pressure, the patient is said to have essential hypertension. Examination of the blood vessels of the retina will reveal any damage to the retinal vessels. This assessment gives an indication about how much damage the high blood pressure has done to vessels throughout the body. If damage has occurred, it is an indication that the person's hypertension is moderate to severe. Electrocar-

diogram (EKG) and cardiac stress testing may be ordered to determine whether any damage has been done to the coronary arteries or heart muscle.

Treatment is directed at blood pressure control to prevent complications and death from cerebrovascular, cardiovascular, and renal damage. The target is to maintain a blood pressure of less than 140/90. Treatment is individualized, using a stepped-care approach. For mild hypertension, stopping smoking, weight control, sodium restriction, alcohol restriction, exercise, a low-fat diet, and stress control are tried first. Sodium should be kept to less than 2,300 mg/day. Alcohol intake should not exceed 2 oz of liquor, 8 oz of wine, or 24 oz of beer per day. Aerobic exercise of 30 to 45 minutes three to five times per week is recommended. If the blood pressure doesn't fall to within normal limits over a period of 6 months, the second step is initiated, and a thiazide diuretic or antihypertensive drug is usually prescribed and lifestyle modifications suggested.

Other drugs are added, if needed, to keep the blood pressure consistently within normal limits. Patients with more severe hypertension often require more than two drugs to attain control. The third step is to add such drugs. Other drug possibilities include ACE inhibitors, beta-blocking agents, calcium-channel blocking agents, and adrenergic inhibitors or vasodilators. The dose of each drug is increased as needed to achieve the desired blood pressure level unless side effects occur. In this event, another drug is substituted. A common combination used is a diuretic, a vasodilator, and an adrenergic inhibitor. Many of the newer blood pressure medications are very expensive, and there is an ongoing debate as to whether these drugs are really more effective than the older, less expensive medications.

If a potassium-wasting diuretic is prescribed, the patient is taught to increase his potassium intake. A potassium supplement is added to his treatment and electrolyte levels are monitored regularly.

The patient often is told to monitor his blood pressure at home and keep records of his readings. Periodic visits to the physician's office for regular examinations are necessary. **The better the blood pressure is controlled within normal limits, the less damage there will be to the target organs.**

Antihypertensive therapy. The drugs prescribed to reduce blood pressure work by decreasing blood volume, cardiac output, or peripheral resistance. *Diuretics* reduce circulating blood volume. Drugs that decrease cardiac output and also decrease peripheral resistance include the beta-adrenergic inhibitors (beta-blockers) and calcium-channel blockers. Adrenergic inhibitor medications decrease peripheral resistance. Vasodilators are most commonly used in combination with a beta-blocking agent and a diuretic. Angiotensin-converting enzyme inhibitors have been quite effective in patients with severe hypertension. They reduce peripheral resistance without lowering cardiac output. Tables 18-8 and 18-9 list examples of the drugs most commonly prescribed for hypertension and relevant nursing interventions. Table 18-10 lists safety measures for patients with orthostatic hypotension, a common side effect of many antihypertensive drugs.

Elder Care Point... The blood pressure of the elderly patient who is taking antihypertensive medication should be measured with the patient sitting and standing. Many of these medications can cause orthostatic hypotension; measuring blood pressure with the patient standing will reveal whether the medication is reducing the blood pressure too much. Assess patients receiving antihypertensives for dizziness, confusion, syncope, restlessness, and drowsiness, which may indicate hypotension.

Nursing Intervention   The nurse's job is to help the patient make the necessary lifestyle changes that will help control his blood pressure and slow further atherosclerosis. *Diet changes* are often the hardest for the patient. It is best to work with the patient's current dietary likes and dislikes, modifying methods of food preparation to decrease sodium and fat content. Sources of hidden sodium should be learned, and the patient should become a reader of food labels, looking for the words *salt* and *sodium* and the letters *NaCl*. Regular canned vegetables are a big source of added sodium, and it is better to use fresh or frozen vegetables or canned goods without sodium whenever possible. Smoked or preserved meats are other products that contain a lot of sodium and should be avoided. Table 18-11 presents guidelines for decreasing sodium in the diet. Patients who need to increase their potassium intake are taught to include citrus fruits and juices, beef and turkey, tomatoes, and potatoes in their diet. The person who does the shopping and food preparation must be included in the diet instruction process. **Weight loss is the most important lifestyle change in obese clients.** The goal is a weight that is within 15% of ideal body weight.

Working with patients from diverse cultures who have very different diets is a challenge. The nurse must work on fat and sodium restriction in the cultural diet of the patient. This requires working with the patient to discover the food preferences and food preparation patterns inherent in the family.

TABLE 18-8 ◆ *Drugs Commonly Used for Patients with Vascular Disorders*

Type of Drug	Action
Diuretics	
Thiazides and related drugs	These drugs increase the excretion of water, sodium, potassium, and chloride by blocking the reabsorption of sodium and chloride.
Chlorthalidone (*Hygroton*)	
Hydrocholorothiazide (*Esidrex, Hydrodiuril*)	
Metolazone (*Diulo, Zaroxolyn*)	
Indapamide (*Lozol*)	
Loop diuretics	These drugs work in the loop of Henle to block reabsorption of sodium and chloride. This prevents passive reabsorption of water and promotes its excretion. These drugs produce the greatest amount of diuresis.
Bumetanide (*Bumex*)	
Ethacrynic acid (*Edecrin*)	
Furosemide (*Lasix*)	
Torsemide (*Demadex*)	
Potassium-sparing diuretics	These drugs block the action of aldosterone in the distal nephron. This prevents the promotion of sodium uptake in exchange for potassium secretion usually caused by aldosterone and potassium is "spared" (not secreted) and sodium is excreted. These drugs cause very little diuresis.
Spironolactone (*Aldactone*)	
Amiloride (*Midamor*)	
Triamterene (*Dyrenium*)	

TABLE 18-8 ◆ *Drugs Commonly Used for Patients with Vascular Disorders* (*Continued*)	
Type of Drug	**Action**
Antihypertensives	
Adrenergic inhibitors	
Beta-blockers	It is not certain how these drugs work to reduce blood pressure. Blockade of the beta$_1$ receptors lowers cardiac output by decreasing heart rate and contractility. Action on the beta$_1$ receptors in the kidney decreases the release of renin, which is a factor in rising blood pressure.
atenolol (*Tenormin*)	
propanolol (*Inderal*)	
metoprolol (*Lopressor*)	
timolol (*Apo-timol*)	
pindolol (*Visken*)	
Bisoprolol (*Zebeta*)	
Carvedilol (*Coreg*)	
Celiprolol (*Selecor*)	
Alpha-blockers	These drugs block alpha$_1$ stimulation on arterioles and veins, preventing sympathetic vasoconstriction. This action results in vasodilation, reducing peripheral vascular resistance and venous return to the heart.
Doxazsoin (*Cardura*)	
Prazosin (*Minipress*)	
Terazosin (*Hytrin*)	
Alpha-beta-blocker	This drug blocks both alpha$_1$ and beta$_1$ receptors, producing decreased heart rate, contractility, peripheral vascular resistance, and venous return.
Labetalol (*Normodyne, Trandate*)	
Angiotensin-converting enzyme (ACE) inhibitors	These agents lower blood pressure by inhibiting the conversion of angiotensin I into angiotensin II, thereby preventing vasoconstriction. They also restrict volume expansion mediated by aldosterone. Losartan is an angiotensin II inhibitor.
Benazepril (*Lotensin*)	
Captopril (*Capoten*)	
Enalapril (*Vasotec*)	
Fosinopril (*Monopril*)	
Losartan (*Cozaar*)	
Lisinorpril (*Prinivil*)	
Moexipril (*Univasc*)	
Quinapril (*Accupril*)	
Ramipril (*Ramace*)	
Spirapril (*Renormax*)	
Perindoprol (*Aceon*)	
Cilazapril (*Inhibace*)	
Calcium channel blockers	These drugs reduce blood pressure by causing dilation of arterioles. Calcium channels are blocked, preventing the influx of calcium that promotes contraction.
Diltiazem (*Cardizem*)	
Felodipine (*Argon*)	
Nicardipine (*Cardene*)	
Nifedipine (*Procardia*)	
Verapamil (*Calan, Isoptin*)	
Nisoldipine (*Sular*)	
Central acting agents	These agents act within the brainstem to suppress sympathetic impulses to the heart and blood vessels. This action decreases the release of norepinephrine by sympathetic nerves, reducing activation of peripheral adrenergic receptors, and promotes vasodilation. The agents also decrease heart rate and cardiac output.
Clonidine (*Catapres*)	
Guanabenz (*Wytensin*)	
Guanfacine (*Tenex*)	
Methyldopa (*Aldomet*)	
Peripherally acting adrenergic blockers	These agents reduce blood pressure by blocking adrenergic receptors in the postganglionic sympathetic neurons and causing decreased sympathetic stimulation of the heart and blood vessels.
Guanadrel (*Hylorel*)	
Guanethidine (*Ismelin*)	
Reserpine (*Serpaline*)	Guanethidine inhibits release of norepinephrine. Reserpine promotes depletion of norepinephrine.
Direct acting vasodilators	These agents reduce blood pressure by promoting arteriole vasodilation.
Hydralazine (*Apresoline*)	
Minoxidin (*Loniten*)	

Note: Generic names are given first followed by trade names in parentheses. Many of the drugs used for chronic hypertension are combination drugs. The nurse must check the ingredients of each drug.

TABLE 18-9   ◆   *General Nursing Implications for the Administration of Diuretics and Antihypertensive Drugs*

DIURETICS

- ◆ Follow the "five rights" of medication administration to prevent errors and injury to the patient: right patient, right drug, right dose, right route, right time.
- ◆ Verify allergies with the patient before administering the drug. Thiazide and thiazide-like diuretics are related to sulfonamides. Patients allergic to sulfas may have adverse reactions.
- ◆ Monitor intake and output to determine amount of diuresis and the drug's effectiveness.
- ◆ Track the patient's weight to determine the drug's effectiveness.
- ◆ Evaluate for decreased edema.
- ◆ Check all drugs the patient is receiving for drug interactions with the diuretic drug to prevent toxicity or lack of absorption. **Several diuretics are ototoxic, and this adverse effect may be potentiated by other ototoxic drugs.**
- ◆ If possible, administer dose in the morning, and if a second dose is required give it mid-afternoon, to avoid sleep interference by need to urinate.
- ◆ Provide assistance with urination in a timely manner (answer call bell quickly).
- ◆ Assess for signs of dehydration and hypotension; take blood pressure on a set schedule. **The elderly are prone to excessive diuresis and can quickly become dehydrated.**
- ◆ Monitor diabetic patients for increased blood glucose levels when taking loop or thiazide diuretics, as these drugs may cause hyperglycemia.

Regarding possible side effects or adverse effects of the drug, the nurse should:

- ◆ Monitor potassium levels frequently if patient is taking a potassium-wasting diuretic; assess for signs of hypokalemia: weakness, tremor, muscle cramps, change in mental status, cardiac dysrhythmia.
- ◆ If the patient also is taking digoxin, consult the physician before administering the dose if the potassium level is below 3.5 mEq/L or if the patient exhibits signs of hypokalemia as hypokalemia increases risk of fatal cardiac dysrhythmia in patients taking digoxin.
- ◆ If patient is taking a potassium-sparing diuretic and potassium level is above 5 mEq/L, or if signs of hyperkalemia develop (abnormal cardiac rhythm), consult the physician before administering the dose.
- ◆ Monitor blood pressure. If it drops considerably, speak with the physician before giving another dose of the medication.
- ◆ Monitor the patient for signs of constipation as diuresis may cause this problem.
- ◆ Monitor patients with a history of deep vein thrombosis for recurrence as diuretics reduce circulating fluid volume.
- ◆ Monitor the patient for side effects or adverse effects of the particular drug taken. The most common general side effects are constipation, electrolyte disturbance, gastric upset, hypotension. Adverse effects are dehydration, ototoxicity, hyperglycemia, hyperuricemia.
- ◆ Monitor the patient for signs of allergic reaction, such as rash or itching.

The nurse should teach the patient taking a diuretic to:

- ◆ Expect frequent need to urinate and increased volume of urine.
- ◆ Report any new heart beat irregularity.
- ◆ Report any signs of ringing of the ears, roaring sounds, a feeling of fullness in the ears, or decreased hearing.
- ◆ Eat foods high in potassium, such as bananas, orange juice, cereals, meats, tomatoes, potatoes, and raisins, unless taking a potassium-sparing diuretic.
- ◆ If taking a potassium-sparing diuretic, restrict foods high in potassium.
- ◆ Take potassium supplement regularly if one is prescribed.
- ◆ Increase fiber in the diet if prone to constipation; consult physician if constipation occurs. **The elderly patient who is inactive is more prone to constipation.**
- ◆ Watch for signs of postural hypotension, such as dizziness or light-headedness when changing position. Encourage patient to arise slowly from a supine position and to sit a minute before standing. **(The elderly are particularly prone to this side effect.)**
- ◆ Avoid the sun or take precautions; do not use a sun lamp when taking a loop or thiazide diuretic as the medication may cause photosensitivity.
- ◆ Watch for signs of gout (tenderness or swelling of joints) when taking a loop or thiazide diuretic and notify the physician if these occur. Loop diuretics may cause an increase in uric acid levels.
- ◆ When taking spironolactone menstrual irregularities or impotence may occur; report these occurrences to the physician.

ANTIHYPERTENSIVE DRUGS

- ◆ Establish that the patient is not hypotensive before giving a dose of an antihypertensive drug. If the patient's blood pressure is below normal levels, consult the physician before giving the dose.
- ◆ Monitor the heart rate for bradycardia or tachycardia. Follow specific parameters for administration of the specific drug; some drugs may cause bradycardia, others may cause tachycardia.
- ◆ Follow the "five rights" of medication administration, and check the patient's ID band before *each* dose.

TABLE 18-9 ◆ *General Nursing Implications for the Administration of Diuretics and Antihypertensive Drugs (Continued)*

◆ Measure blood pressure standing and sitting to determine whether the patient is experiencing orthostatic hypotension; several antihypertensives may cause orthostatic hypotension.
◆ Note contraindications and precautions for each specific drug the patient is taking. Angiotensin-converting enzyme (ACE) inhibitors are contraindicated during pregnancy.
◆ Check all drugs the patient is receiving for drug interactions to prevent toxicity or increased severity of side effects. Many of the antihypertensive drugs have a depressant effect on the heart.
◆ Monitor blood pressure readings to evaluate effectiveness of the drug.

Regarding possible side effects or adverse effects of the drug, the nurse should:

◆ Monitor the patient for the side effects of each drug administered.
◆ Monitor serum glucose levels in diabetics who are taking a beta-blocker drug as the drug may mask hypoglycemia.
◆ Monitor lipid levels for changes in patients taking beta-blocker drugs as these drugs interfere with lipid metabolism.
◆ Observe for hypersensitivity reactions such as rash; ACE inhibitors may cause hypersensitivity.
◆ Monitor patients for signs of congestive heart failure, such as edema. Beta-blockers, calcium-channel blockers, and other drugs that decrease cardiac output may precipitate heart failure in patients with borderline cardiac function.
◆ Check the skin of the patient using a clonidine patch for signs of irritation, a potential side effect of the patch. Be certain the old patch is removed when applying a new one.
◆ Give the first dose of an ACE inhibitor at bedtime, as it often causes hypotension.
◆ Monitor the potassium level of the patient taking an ACE inhibitor. Because it suppresses the release of aldosterone, it increases potassium retention.
◆ Monitor liver function tests for patients taking centrally acting drugs, such as clonadine, as these drugs may cause liver damage in some patients.
◆ Monitor renal function tests in patients taking hydralazine, as this drug may cause renal impairment.

The nurse should teach the patient taking an antihypertensive to:

◆ Monitor blood pressure regularly and keep a log of the readings.
◆ Alter lifestyle factors that contribute to hypertension, such as smoking, excess weight, excessive stress, excessive alcohol ingestion, high-salt diet, and lack of exercise.
◆ Rise slowly from a lying position and stabilize before standing for a couple of minutes.
◆ Report alteration in sexual response, as some of the antihypertensive drugs may cause impotence.
◆ Report persistent side effects and any adverse effects of the drug.
◆ Monitor for weight gain from retention of sodium and water by weighing at least twice a week; report weight gain of more than 2 lb to the physician.
◆ Report signs of ankle edema, as several of the antihypertensive drugs can precipitate congestive heart failure.
◆ Be aware that methyldopa may cause dark urine for the first few weeks of therapy.
◆ Refrain from abruptly discontinuing centrally acting antihypertensives, such as clonidine, as rebound hypertension may occur.
◆ Check with the physician before taking over-the-counter drugs as many are contraindicated in hypertension.
◆ Comply with medication therapy even when blood pressure is normal as long-term compliance is the key to preventing the organ damage that hypertension can cause.
◆ Set own goals for lifestyle changes and medication therapy; a patient-directed program has a better chance of success.

If caffeine restriction is recommended, the patient should be told gradually to decrease his caffeine consumption so that he will not experience withdrawal symptoms such as headache and nervousness. The patient should be reminded that many types of soft drinks, as well as coffee and tea, contain caffeine.

Nicotine has a major impact on blood vessels and blood pressure, and stopping smoking can be a difficult task for many patients. Referral to a self-help program should be made.

An exercise program that fits the patient's personality, ability, and preference should be designed. Walking to work from a parking lot a few blocks away,

climbing stairs instead of using elevators, and a daily walk in the neighborhood often are sufficient. Other patients might prefer to use a stationary bicycle. The object is to work on something that the patient will continue to do for the rest of his life.

Weight loss will begin to occur if the patient is faithful to the prescribed diet and exercise program. As the weight decreases, the nurse can remind the patient of the direct effect his efforts have had on his blood pressure. **Even a moderate weight loss of 7 to 12 lb (3–5 kg) can reduce blood pressure.** Positive reinforcement should be given for even small amounts of weight loss.

TABLE 18-10 ◆ *Patient Education: Safety Measures for Orthostatic Hypotension*

If the patient suffers the side effect of orthostatic hypotension from medication, instruct to:

◆ Rise slowly from a lying to a sitting position; don't hold your breath as you arise. Sit for 1 minute before standing; stand slowly holding on to a stable object. Stand for 1 minute before walking.

◆ While seated, flex and rotate the feet several times before attempting to stand; have feet firmly planted on the floor before standing.

◆ When walking, do not turn your head or body abruptly.

◆ When feeling unsteady while standing, call for assistance before walking.

◆ Report lightheadedness or sudden dizziness.

◆ Use the bathroom before meals and try to avoid getting up for 30 to 60 minutes after meals.

TABLE 18-11 ◆ *Patient Education: Decreasing Sodium in the Diet*

For the patient who must reduce the sodium in the diet, instruct to:

◆ Use fresh or frozen fruits and vegetables rather than cheese as a snack.

◆ Stay away from "convenience" foods: ready-mixed sauces, frozen dinners, cured or smoked meats (including lunch meats), canned soups, and prepared salad dressings, unless the label truly indicates a low sodium content.

◆ Be aware that regular canned vegetables often contain a large amount of sodium; in some instances rinsing will greatly decrease the sodium content. Use fresh or frozen vegetables or those canned without sodium when possible.

◆ Check soft drink labels for sodium content; many contain a lot of sodium.

◆ Check cereal box labels for sodium content; switch to a lower-sodium cereal, such as shredded wheat.

◆ Use one-fourth to one-half the amount of salt that a recipe calls for.

◆ Leave the salt shaker off the table.

◆ Make a salt substitute seasoning of: ½ tsp garlic powder, mixed with one teaspoon each of basil, black pepper, marjoram, onion powder, parsley, sage, savory, and thyme, or use a product such as "Mrs. Dash" or Lemon Pepper instead of salt.

◆ When ordering at restaurants, ask which dishes are low in sodium; or ask that the cook refrain from salting your dishes.

◆ Ask fast food restaurants to supply you with a list of their available foods showing sodium content of each item.

◆ Do not eat preserved or commercially prepared smoked meats, such as bacon, hot dogs, salami, pastrami, ham, smoked turkey, or sausage.

◆ Read all labels on food containers looking for the words "sodium" or "NaCl."

◆ Check condiments for amount of sodium. Catsup, soy sauce, steak sauce, and others contain high quantities of sodium.

Stress reduction requires an evaluation of lifestyle. Meditation, yoga, leisure activities, or just saying "no" to extra obligations can all decrease stress. The nurse should help the patient determine where his stressors are and what can practically be done about them.

Lifetime compliance with the diet, exercise, stress reduction, and medication plan is the biggest problem for most patients. Many do not understand that it is up to them to control their disease. They do well for several months or a few years, but then, because they feel fine (while their blood pressure has been controlled), they stop taking their medication and gradually return to previous lifestyle patterns. By teaching them what high blood pressure does to the blood vessels and the heart, brain, eye, and kidneys, the nurse can do much to see that patients follow the treatment plan for life. Table 18-12 presents an outline for teaching patients about the complications of uncontrolled hypertension. Each patient needs continuing praise for maintaining control of his blood pressure. See Nursing Care Plan 2-1 in Chapter 2 for information on caring for a patient with hypertension.

There are many resources to help hypertensive patients manage their illness more effectively. The American Heart Association has booklets such as "How You Can Help Your Doctor Treat High Blood Pressure," and "About Your Heart and High Blood Pressure." Other resources include the National High Blood Pressure Education Program, Health and Human Services, Washington, DC, and the National High Blood Pressure Committee, National Institutes of Health, Bethesda, MD 20814, (301) 951-3260.

◆ Chronic Arterial Occlusive Disease (Atherosclerosis Obliterans)

Pathophysiology   A diminished flow of blood through the arteries is caused by atherosclerosis. Atherosclerotic changes can affect any large artery of the body, but when the peripheral arteries are involved,

TABLE 18-12 ◆ *Patient Education: Complications of Uncontrolled Hypertension*

◆ Hypertension can contribute to and accelerate atherosclerosis, placing an increased workload on the heart. This may cause: myocardial infarction, left ventricular hypertrophy, and congestive heart failure.

◆ Atherosclerosis of the vessels in the brain disrupts circulation and may lead to transient ischemic attacks (TIAs) and stroke.

◆ Hypertension may cause accelerated atherosclerosis and rigidity of the renal vessels and may lead to kidney failure.

◆ Hypertension damages the arteries of the eye, causing the formation of clots or occurrence of hemorrhages that may lead to blurred vision or blindness.

the arterial insufficiency usually affects the lower extremities. Smoking causes vasoconstriction, further narrowing the vessels and causing worsening of the condition. Although arterial perfusion can be impaired in both legs, one extremity is often more severely involved than the other.

Elder Care Point... The main cause of peripheral vascular disease in the elderly is atherosclerosis. Early recognition of decreased peripheral circulation, combined with teaching about proper self-care can prevent problems with ulceration, gangrene, and possibly amputation.

Signs and Symptoms   Signs and symptoms of peripheral arterial insufficiency of the lower extremities include intermittent claudication, pain at rest, and ischemic changes. Occlusion in the peripheral system produces the "5 Ps"—pain, pallor, pulselessness, paralysis, and paresthesia. There also is a temperature change distal to the occlusion. The severity of these symptoms depends on the extent of the lesion, degree of occlusion, and amount of collateral circulation that has been established. Table 18-13 shows the differences between arterial and venous insufficiency.

If severe ischemia occurs from occlusion of arterial blood flow, tissue distal to the occlusion blanches, becomes cold, hurts, and eventually becomes numb as necrosis occurs. Eventually the affected part becomes gangrenous, necessitating amputation.

Treatment   **The best treatment for arterial occlusive disease is regular exercise.** Walking vigorously for 20 minutes twice a day will encourage growth of collateral circulation and reduce the severity of claudication in the majority of patients. The exercise program is started slowly, working up to a faster pace and the full 20 minutes.

Pentoxifylline (Trental), a drug that reduces blood viscosity, may be prescribed for patients who have claudication but are not yet candidates for reconstructive surgery. Because the medication acts on the cell wall during its formation, it has to be taken for at least 4 months before its effect on all circulating red blood cells can be determined. It is not effective for patients with severe occlusion. Other types of vasodilators may still be prescribed, but research has shown they are of little, if any, benefit. The patient's best hope is to make lifestyle changes that decrease the rate of atherosclerosis.

Surgical treatment of peripheral arterial insufficiency is a palliative measure only. It does not cure the disease or halt the atherosclerotic process. It can, however, relieve ischemic pain, help avoid amputation, and add years to a patient's life. The purpose of vascular surgery is to revascularize and nourish cells in the affected area.

Laser angioplasty is now used more commonly to open up clogged arteries. This procedure is done in a fashion similar to percutaneous balloon angioplasty. The surgeon enters the artery with a catheter and uses the laser to destroy the plaque buildup that is occluding the artery.

Percutaneous transluminal angioplasty (PTA) may be done to open an occluded artery. A catheter is introduced into the artery, and when the proper spot is reached, a balloon is inflated multiple times to dilate the vessel, promoting better blood flow. A metal **stent** (tubular device to give support to a vessel interior) may be placed to prevent narrowing or closure of the artery.

An aorto-iliac bypass or a femoral-popliteal bypass is performed to correct arterial occlusion of the leg to prevent the need for amputation. A synthetic graft is placed to divert blood around the obstructed area, or

---

TABLE 18-13   ◆   *Differences in Signs and Symptoms of Arterial and Venous Disease*

Characteristic	Arterial Disease	Venous Disease
Pulses	Diminished, weak or absent.	Strong and symmetrical; may be difficult to palpate if edema is present.
Skin	Pallor, dependent rubor; thin, dry, shiny, cool.	Mottling with brown pigmentation at ankles, veins may be visible; legs and/or feet bluish when dependent; dermatitis; warm.
Edema	Absent or mild.	Present, particularly around ankle and in foot.
Ulceration	On toes or at pressure points on feet.	At bones of ankle.
Necrosis and gangrene	Likely.	Unlikely.
Pain	Intermittent claudication when walking; sharp, stabbing, gnawing; lessens when at rest.	Aching, cramping, particularly when dependent; may have nocturnal cramps.
Nails	Thick, brittle (normal in elderly).	Normal.
Hair	Hair loss distal to area of occlusion (hair loss normal in elderly).	Normal.

the occluded portion is dissected and replaced by a graft from the patient's saphenous or other vein. Figure 18-7 shows a clinical pathway for bypass graft surgery. Postoperative care is the same as for other operative procedures, but includes careful assessment of pulses distal to the graft to detect thrombus formation. As with any vascular surgery, extra attention is paid to assessment for signs of bleeding. An aorto-iliac bypass requires both an abdominal and a groin incision.

A hyperbaric oxygen chamber is sometimes used for patients with severely compromised circulation to a lower extremity to increase tissue oxygen and avoid amputation.

Nursing Intervention The nurse can encourage blood flow by keeping the patient and the environment warm. Constricting clothing is to be avoided, and the leg gatch on the bed should never be used, as it puts added pressure on the back of the knees and further occludes blood flow. The nurse should encourage the patient to change his position frequently while awake. The lower legs should be elevated at every opportunity.

Exercise is especially beneficial to patients with decreased blood flow. Walking regularly every day is best for the ambulatory patient. Swimming also is good, as it applies light pressure to the surface of the legs and requires muscle action that encourages venous return. Bedrest patients should be encouraged to do foot and leg exercises at least once an hour. The nurse can encourage those who watch television to do the exercises during each commercial.

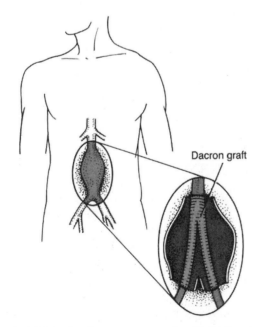

FIGURE 18-7 Aortic aneurysm repair with graft. (*Source:* Ignatavicius, D. D., Workman, M. L., Mishler, M. A. [1995]. *Medical–Surgical Nursing: A Nursing Process Approach,* 2nd ed. Philadelphia: Saunders, p. 950.)

Think about . . . Hugh, a 63-year-old male executive, is experiencing worsening intermittent claudication. Can you describe how you would interact with him to develop an exercise program that could lessen his symptoms?

The major nursing care goals following peripheral arterial surgery are (1) maintaining arterial blood flow to the lower extremities; (2) protecting tissues from further injury due to pressure and constriction of blood flow; and (3) preventing wound infection. Rehabilitation of the patient requires instruction and guidance in special exercises to increase collateral circulation to the legs. See Table 18-4 for common nursing diagnoses and interventions appropriate for patients with peripheral arterial occlusive disease.

◆ Thromboangiitis Obliterans

Thromboangiitis obliterans, or *Buerger's disease,* involves the small- and medium-size arteries. Inflammation, thickening of the arterial walls, and occlusion of the vessels occur. The disease occurs more often in men than women and is commonly found in people from Eastern countries, particularly those of Jewish descent. Smoking is directly linked to the progression of the disease. The signs and symptoms include numbness and tingling of the toes or fingers in cold weather, pain in the feet, and intermittent claudication that progressively becomes more severe. If ischemia causes gangrene, amputation is performed. **Cessation of smoking is the single most important treatment factor.** Exercise is used to increase leg circulation in the legs and feet.

◆ Raynaud's Disease

The cause of Raynaud's disease is unknown. Raynaud's disease is characterized by spasm of the arteries. The disease is seen more often in women than in men. It mostly affects the fingers and toes and can be a primary disorder or occur secondary to another disease such as lupus erythematosus. In the latter instance it is known as *Raynaud's phenomenon.* The arterial spasm occurs in response to emotional stress or exposure to cold. The affected body part changes color, ranging from white to red to blue. When the spasm stops, there often is burning pain and throbbing. In about 10% of those affected, the disease progresses to the point where ischemia from arterial spasm is so severe that gangrene occurs and amputation is necessary. Medical therapy consists of stress control, avoidance of exposure to cold, cessation of smoking, and the use of calcium-channel blockers to prevent arterial spasm.

◆ Aneurysm

Pathophysiology   An aneurysm can occur along any artery. It is an outpouching of the wall of the artery due to a structural defect in the layers of the arterial wall. Blood flow is stagnant along the wall of the aneurysm, and clots can form, causing either thrombosis or embolus. Once an aneurysm develops, it continues to grow larger. Aneurysms may eventually rupture if not repaired.

Congenital malformations predispose to many types of aneurysm. However, atherosclerosis and hypertension are thought to be the major factors in their development. Atherosclerotic plaque weakens the vessel wall, and hypertension puts extra pressure on the weakened walls. Diabetes mellitus and hyperlipidemia are two other conditions that contribute to the development of such vessel problems.

Signs and Symptoms   Aneurysm rupture is common in the cerebral vessels, causing intercerebral bleeding and stroke. Aortic aneurysms can occur along either the thoracic or the abdominal portion of the vessel. A ruptured aneurysm often leads to sudden death. Aneurysms often display no obvious symptoms, although cerebral aneurysms may bring about headaches or blurred vision and an aortic aneurysm may cause back pain or a feeling of pressure and may cause a visible pulsation of the abdomen. An aortic aneurysm in the thoracic area may cause substernal or tracheal pressure and difficulty with breathing.

Treatment   If an aortic aneurysm is detected early, it often can be surgically repaired before it ruptures. The patient is checked every few months by the physician and serial ultrasound measurements track the size of the aneurysm. The aneurysm is electively repaired when it reaches 6 to 7 cm in diameter. The surgical procedure and nursing care depend on the location of the aneurysm.

Cerebral aneurysm is treated by craniotomy; this is covered in Chapter 14. Aortic aneurysm is treated by thoracotomy or abdominal surgery depending on the location of the aneurysm, and the care is similar to that of other types of thoracic and abdominal surgery. The main difference is that the nurse must also carefully assess pulses and function distal to the repair site. The nurse closely monitors renal function to detect signs of acute renal failure postoperatively as blood flow to the kidneys is briefly cut off when the aorta is clamped for surgical repair.

The patient spends 24 to 48 hours in an intensive care unit postoperatively. A ventilator is used overnight, and thereafter the nurse assists the patient to deep-breathe and cough every 1 to 2 hours. Paralytic ileus occurs for a few days after abdominal surgery and a nasogastric tube will be in place. The nurse auscultates every shift for the return of bowel sounds.

The patient undergoing thoracic aortic aneurysm repair will undergo chest surgery with placement on the cardiopulmonary bypass machine. The care is the same as for other chest surgery patients. Chest tubes will be in place. This patient is especially at risk for atelectasis and pneumonia. Good pain control is necessary to promote adequate respiratory effort. The nurse also must monitor for the presence of cardiac dysrhythmias.

◆ Carotid Occlusion

When atherosclerosis has narrowed the carotid arteries leading to the brain, the signs and symptoms include carotid **bruit** (a purring sound heard with a stethoscope), confusion, visual abnormality in one eye, fainting, extremity weakness or paralysis, or other signs of decreased blood flow to the brain. The condition is treated by *carotid endarterectomy,* which surgically removes the atherosclerotic plaque, or by bypass surgery, which connects an artery from outside the cranium to an area on the cerebral artery beyond the obstruction. Both procedures are done to prevent the occurrence of stroke.

Specific postoperative care for endarterectomy includes assessing for signs of bleeding, for pressure from hematoma on the trachea (evidenced by increasing hoarseness), and for neurological problems caused by thrombosis or embolus. Neurological signs are monitored every 2 to 4 hours. If a carotid bypass is done, the patient must have a craniotomy; see Chapter 14 for nursing care of the craniotomy patient.

VENOUS DISORDERS

◆ Varicose Veins

Varicose veins are enlarged and tortuous veins that are distorted in shape by accumulations of pooled blood. Veins that develop varicosities have incompetent valves that allow reflux of blood from the deep to the superficial veins. The increased blood flow and resultant pressure on the vein walls cause the vessel to dilate and become tortuous. Heredity, standing for a long time, obesity, and pregnancy all contribute to the formation of varicose veins.

Elder Care Point... Varicose veins develop in the elderly as the veins lose their elasticity and the leg muscles weaken and atrophy from decreased exercise.

Signs and symptoms include dilated, twisted-appearing, superficial vessels on the legs. Swelling of the foot and ankle on the affected leg may occur by the end of the day and is often accompanied by aching.

Treatment includes the use of elastic support hose, exercising the legs and feet periodically throughout the day, and elevating the legs whenever possible. Prolonged standing, sitting, or crossing the legs are to be avoided. Weight reduction is recommended for obese patients. Exercises such as walking or swimming are beneficial because the muscle contraction encourages venous return to the heart.

Small varicosities can be treated by *scleropathy*, which involves injecting an agent that will sclerose the vessel, causing thrombosis, thereby preventing further blood from filling the area. Veins with multiple, severe varicosities (over 4 mm in diameter) are treated by *vein stripping*, done as an outpatient procedure. Generally there will be multiple incisions along the leg to ligate and strip out the vein. The legs are wrapped with elastic bandages postoperatively to decrease bleeding and hematoma formation. Bedrest and leg elevation the night after surgery are recommended. Range of motion exercise of the legs is done every hour to help prevent thrombosis. Prevention of infection after this procedure is essential.

◆ Venous Stasis Ulcers

Chronic venous insufficiency causes chronic skin and tissue lesions on the lower extremities, especially around the ankle. The diabetic patient with venous insufficiency is at high risk for this disorder because of compromised circulation in the extremities and a slow rate of healing. Blood flows into the area, but is not adequately returned to the heart because of valvular problems in the veins. The ulcers may extend deeply into the tissue and are very slow and difficult to heal because of tissue congestion and edema that prevents nutrients from reaching the cells. The ulcer may begin as a small, tender, inflamed area. With the slightest trauma, the skin breaks and the ulcer grows. Any skin trauma to the lower extremity may cause an ulcer to form, and it is imperative that the patient with venous insufficiency be taught the extreme importance of good foot and leg care. An inflamed area discovered by the nurse can be preventively treated with a clear occlusive dressing such as Tegaderm or OpSite.

Treatment for the hospitalized patient with an open ulcer consists of leg elevation, a dry or wet-to-dry saline dressing, and hydrotherapy. Dressings are changed several times a day, helping to debride the area (i.e., peel away dead tissue). Often the wound needs a graft to heal completely. Venous stasis ulcers can take weeks to months to heal. Ambulatory patients are treated with compression dressings. An Unna boot may also be applied; this consists of gauze saturated with zinc oxide and calamine lotion in a glycerine base. This is covered with outer gauze, and then an elastic bandage is applied from the foot to the knee. The "boot" becomes rigid. It is changed from every 2 to 3 days to every 2 weeks as needed.

Thorough teaching is done to alert the patient to proper self-care and to signs of beginning skin breakdown. The slightest injury to an ischemic area can take a very long time to heal and can easily become infected, as the blood supply is inadequate to provide the usual leukocyte defenses. Any injury to an affected extremity should be reported to the doctor immediately, no matter how minor it is.

The nurse can give the patient considerable support, as treatment is long, recurrent, and tedious. Patients with stasis ulcers frequently become depressed. Praise for compliance with instructions and for any small gain made toward healing can do much for their morale.

◆ Thrombosis and Embolism

Thrombosis is the formation, development, or presence of a clump of blood elements, particularly platelets and fibrin, that form a clot in a blood vessel and diminish or completely obstruct blood flow.

A thrombus can occur or develop as a result of injury to vascular endothelium, sluggish flow of blood, or changes in the number of blood elements (for example, an increase in the number of red blood cells or platelets). Immobility is a major factor in the formation of thrombi. Thrombosis can be present in either veins or arteries, but because the flow of blood is slower through the veins than through the arteries, venous thrombosis is more common. Venous thrombosis in which there is an inflammation of the vein wall is called **thrombophlebitis.**

The effects of thrombosis depend on (1) the location and size of the thrombus; (2) whether it completely or only partially blocks blood flow through a vessel; and (3) whether the body is able to establish collateral circulation to prevent ischemia in the area formerly served by the obstructed vessel.

An **embolism** is the sudden obstruction of an artery by a mass of foreign material that has been brought to the site by the blood current. The **embolus** usually is a blood clot that has broken off from a thrombus. However, it can be a globule of fat, air bubble, piece of tissue, clump of bacteria, or bolus of liquid that is not dissolved in the blood.

The effects of an embolism depend on the site at which it is lodged, and its size compared with the caliber of the blood vessel in which it is located.

Deep Vein Thrombosis   A clot in a deep vein, or deep vein thrombosis (DVT), most often occurs in the lower leg, although it can occur in any vein in the body. A great many factors contribute to the formation of a deep vein thrombosis. Immobility, trauma, sepsis, clotting problems, surgical procedures, dehydration, obesity, cancer, estrogen hormone therapy, or any condition that causes slowing of venous flow can cause a clot to form.

The main sign of a DVT is edema in one extremity. There may be pain in the calf of the leg when the foot is dorsiflexed (Homan's sign). The area over the thrombosis may feel warm. The nurse should never rub or vigorously palpate the area, as this can dislodge the clot and send it into the circulation, which can cause severe damage or death. Encouraging patients on bedrest to perform leg and ankle exercises each hour while awake can do much to decrease the incidence of deep vein thrombosis.

Elder Care Point... Factors that contribute to deep vein thrombosis include venous stasis, changes in the lining of the veins, and increased ease of clotting.

Elderly patients who have problems with mobility or stress incontinence tend to drink less fluid so that they don't have to visit the bathroom so often. This can lead to dehydration and more viscous blood, which in turn can predispose to thrombus formation in those susceptible to this disorder. Encourage high fluid intake and provide a means for convenient toileting for these patients. The occurrence of thrombophlebitis increases with advanced age.

Medical treatment usually consists of bedrest and IV heparin and then oral warfarin sodium (Coumadin) with good hydration. Anticoagulants will not dissolve the clot but will prevent it from growing larger. The body dissolves the clot on its own over time. Thrombolytic therapy may be used to dissolve the thrombus; streptokinase, urokinase, or tissue plasminogen activator (TPA) are the agents used.

There is a high risk of bleeding with these drugs. A thrombolytic agent is followed by a few additional days of heparin while the patient is started on warfarin.

Warfarin takes at least 3 days to build up to an effective blood level. Elastic hose are prescribed for continuous use thereafter. Nursing care of the patient with a deep vein thrombosis and thrombophlebitis is presented in Nursing Care Plan 18-2. Information and nursing care for the administration of anticoagulants are presented in Chapter 19.

Elastic stockings are usually prescribed to prevent recurrence of the thrombus. Support stockings, thromboembolic disease (TED) hose, or Jobst hose should be applied in the morning before the legs have been dependent. Hose must be properly fitted and should be checked and straightened frequently so that they do not bunch up and put pressure on the back of the knee.

Sequential compression (SCD) devices (Figure 18-8) often are applied postoperatively to the legs of patients who will be confined to bed and are at risk of deep vein thrombosis. These must be applied properly and checked for positioning frequently. They may be used along with elastic stockings.

A new anticoagulant, dalteparin (Fragmin), is used to prevent deep vein thrombosis in the high-risk patient undergoing abdominal surgery. Enoxaparin (Lovenox), a low-molecular-weight heparin, is given after hip replacement surgery to prevent deep vein thrombosis.

The patient with thrombosis is taught not to rub his extremity. The nurse encourages high fluid intake to reduce blood viscosity. Elastic hose are applied correctly, and the procedure for their use is explained to the patient. They must be kept smooth. They are removed only for bathing. The nurse administers anticoagulant therapy and monitors for adverse side effects, checking for bleeding and monitoring coagulation times. Specifically check for signs of bruising, petechiae, bleeding gums, and blood in the urine or stool. The patient receiving IV heparin should be placed on a Biofoam or similar pad before therapy begins to reduce bruising. The patient must be told to move cautiously, to avoid hitting the head or bumping into furniture, doors, or other objects. The IV site should be monitored closely,

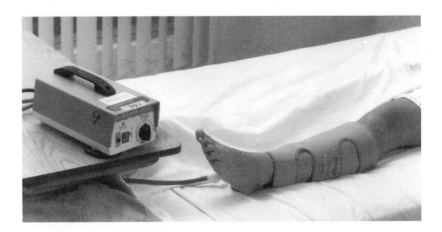

FIGURE 18-8 Patient using sequential compression devices to prevent thrombus formation after surgery. (Photo by Glen Derbyshire; courtesy of Goleta Valley Cottage Hospital, Goleta, CA.)

Nursing Care Plan 18-1

Selected nursing diagnoses, goals/expected outcomes, nursing interventions, and evaluations for a patient with a venous stasis ulcer

Situation: A male patient, age 52, with chronic peripheral vascular disease (PVD) has a large stasis ulcer on the inner aspect of the lower third of his left leg. His lower right leg shows some edema; dry, scaly skin; and brownish coloration. The ulcer is being treated with saline compresses and Elase ointment, bed rest, and elevation of the leg. Duoderm will be applied, beginning in another 3 days.

Nursing Diagnosis	Goals/Expected Outcome	Nursing Intevention	Evaluation
Impaired skin integrity related to decreased peripheral circulation and abrasion. SUPPORTING DATA Ulcer on anterior lower third of left leg 2½ cm × 4 cm; history of chronic PVD.	Ulcer will heal completely.	Apply wet compresses q 3 h. Apply Elase ointment b.i.d. Inspect for signs of infection: purulent drainage, elevated WBC count, increased size of wound.	Wet compress at 10:30 A.M. and 11:30 P.M.; Elase used on wound; serosanguinous drainage; edges less reddened; WBC count; 12,800; continue plan.
Noncompliance as evidenced by continued smoking. SUPPORTING DATA Quit smoking for 3 months; has resumed smoking ½ pack per day	Patient will quit smoking and not smoke again.	Obtain literature on the smoking cessation program from American Lung Association. Re-explain what smoking does to decrease peripheral circulation. Teach relaxation exercises.	Began teaching relaxation exercises; gave ALA literature on quitting smoking; dicussed smoking effects on vesels again; continue plan.
Knowledge deficit related to care of skin and ways to prevent ulceration. SUPPORTING DATA Has not been wearing support hose, obtaining little exercise; cannot verbalize points of proper self-care.	Patient will verbailze six points in proper self-care. Patient will not cross legs or ankles when sitting. Patient will wear support hose daily.	Explain how sluggish circulation contributes to breakdown of skin and tissues. Encourage active exercise: ankle rotation and leg bending while on bed rest; walking when ambulatory. Teach patient and wife how to apply elastic stocking before patient arises in A.M. Teach him to inspect feet and legs each day after bath; use lotion bid to decrease drying and scaling. Teach him to report any sign of reddening or break in skin to doctor immediately. Teach him not to cross ankles or legs at knee when sitting and to avoid prolonged standing. Teach patient to place wedge under foot of mattress at home to raise the legs above the level of the heart. Teach him to elevated legs when sitting.	Catches self when crosses legs while sitting; peforming foot and ankle exercises each day; demonstrated proper application of elastic stockings; legs elevated when not standing; continue plan.
Depression related to repeated leg ulceration; inability to work because of hospitalization. SUPPORTING DATA Third hospitalization for leg ulcers; works as a car salesman; acts withdrawn and is having difficulty sleeping; states he is depressed.	Patient will express that he is less depressed. Patient will be able to sleep all night. Patient will talk about taking charge of his own self-care and returning to work.	Establish trusting relationship. Encourage him to ventilate feelings. Assist him to set small goals for self. Assure him that condition can be improved with proper self-care. Give praise for each effort at self-care and for efforts to quit smoking.	Verbalizing discouragement about wound not healing and interference with work; encouraged to set small goals so he can see progress; planned to work on this together tomorrow; praise given for doing own foot care toady; continue plan.

Nursing Care Plan 18-2

Selected nursing diagnoses, goals/expected outcomes, nursing interventions, and evaluations for a patient with a deep vein thrombosis and thrombophlebitis

Situation: Mrs. Hanson, age 72, sustained multiple bruises and a concussion in an automobile accident. She has cardiac arrhythmias and was admitted 2 days ago for observation and recuperation. She has now developed pain in her right calf, and her lower leg is swollen, with a hot, tender area in the midcalf region. She has been placed on a continuous heparin drip.

Nursing Diagnosis	Goals/Expected Outcome	Nursing Intervention	Evaluation
Alteration in peripheral tissue perfusion related to deep vein thrombosis and thrombophlebitis. SUPPORTING DATA Thrombus in saphenous vein, right calf. Reddened, warm, tender area on midcalf. Temperature, 101.2° F.	Thrombus will resolve within 2 weeks as evidenced by Doppler flow studies. Thrombophlebitis will resolve by discharge as evidenced by normal temperature and no calf tenderness, redness, or swelling.	Maintain on bed rest with bathroom privileges; keep right lower leg elevated. Active ROM of left ankle, knee, and hip. Elastic stocking on left leg. Warm packs to right leg; handle right leg gently. Maintain heparin drip on IV pump at ordered rate; assess IV site q h for infiltration. Assess legs q shift for status of thrombus and development of other problems.	Heparin drip continuous; IV site without redness or swelling; right leg elevated; active ROM on left leg at 8, 10, 12, and 2; moist heating pad to right calf for 30 minutes each hour; swelling down slightly; continue plan.
Risk to injury related to heparin drip and to possibility of embolus. SUPPORTING DATA Heparin drip 50,000 U in 500 mL at 50 mL per hour. Deep vein thrombosis in right leg.	Patient will not experience embolus during hospitalization. No hemorrhage from heparin as evidenced by no sign of bleeding internally or externally.	Auscultate lung sounds q shift; be alert for signs of pulmonary emboli. Monitor level of consciousness (LOC) and neurologic status q shift. Observe for bleeding of gums, excessive bruising, blood in urine or stool, nosebleeds, and abdominal pain and rigidity. Monitor Hgb and hematocrit to detect blood loss. Monitor PTT and advise physician immediately if it rises above 2½ times the control value. Begin Coumadin therapy as ordered 3 days before heparin is stopped. Handle patient very gently.	Lung clear to auscultation; PEARL without headache, alert and oriented; PTT 2 × control value; no change in Hgb and hematocrit; no evidence of blood in urine or stool; bowel sounds present all 4 quadrants, abdomen soft; bruising from previous needle sticks; buttocks bruised from bed rest; continue plan.
Knowledge deficit related to precautions necessary when taking Coumadin. SUPPORTING DATA Will go home on Coumadin for at least 6 to 12 months; has never taken this medication.	Patient will verbalize danger signs to report to physician and proper dosage schedule before discharge. Patient will verbalize understanding of need for regular medical follow-up and periodic clotting times before discharge.	Teach the following: • Avoid foods high in vitamin K (give list). • Avoid over-the-counter medications and drugs that might extend clotting time or interfere with action of Coumadin (e.g., aspirin, etc.). • Move around carefully trying not to hit head on anything or bump into things, as internal hemorrhage is a threat. • Observe urine and stool for signs of bleeding. • Maintain good hydration by drinking at least 10 glasses of fluid a day. Instruct her to maintain close contact with physician to monitor clotting times, as many things can alter it when on Coumadin. Explain dosage schedule. Give written instruction sheet.	Began teaching regarding dangers of Coumadin; needs time to absorb information; will continue teaching tomorrow; gave written instruction sheet; continue plan.

as heparin can be irritating to the vessel in some people. At the first sign of inflammation, the IV site should be changed. Firm pressure should be applied to any needle stick for at least 5 minutes to prevent hematoma formation. The nurse must be alert for signs of pulmonary embolus (dyspnea, chest pain, hemoptysis, tachypnea, tachycardia).

The patient with deep vein thrombosis is taught to prevent venous stasis by exercising, keeping well hydrated, quitting smoking, avoiding substances that cause the blood to coagulate more easily (e.g., hormones), and avoiding sitting for long periods. The legs should never be crossed.

Arterial thrombosis is treated according to the severity of the symptoms it is causing. If total blockage of an artery is occurring, surgical thrombectomy may be necessary. If there is collateral circulation to provide nutrients for the tissues distal to the thrombus, intraarterial enzyme dissolution of the thrombus may be used. A catheter is threaded into the artery and one of the enzyme substances such as Urokinase or Streptokinase may be used to dissolve the clot over a 36- to 72-hour period. In other instances, IV heparin is used to prevent further clotting, and the patient is closely monitored while the body breaks down the thrombus.

Thrombophlebitis   Thrombophlebitis is inflammation of a superficial vein caused by a blood clot. It occurs from trauma, irritation to the vein, infection from an IV line, or dirty IV drug needles. Signs include swelling, redness, warmth, and considerable tenderness and pain upon touching.

Treatment includes discontinuing the source of irritation; applying warm, moist heat; elevating the extremity; and administering aspirin and antibiotics.

Think about... What teaching points would you cover for the 52-year-old female who is being discharged after a hospitalization for thrombophlebitis of the right leg? The woman is a waitress.

Embolism   Embolism may be caused when a portion of a deep vein thrombus in a leg breaks loose and travels to the lungs, heart, or brain. Cardiac arrhythmias also cause emboli. Release of fat droplets from a long-bone fracture and amniotic fluid introduced into a vein during the birthing process also can result in the formation of an embolus. Cancer patients often die from pulmonary embolus. The National Institutes of Health estimate that 50,000 people die as a result of pulmonary embolus each year.

Elder Care Point... Many elderly patients are being treated for cardiac dysrhythmias, such as atrial fibrillation, which can cause the formation of clots. When

---

pumped out of the heart these clots become emboli. These patients are usually taking an anticoagulant to prevent clot formation. The nurse must teach such patients the importance of continuing to take the anticoagulant if they have an irregular heart rate and not to discontinue it without the prescribing doctor's permission.

Signs and symptoms of pulmonary embolus are dyspnea, hemoptysis, tachypnea, tachycardia, chest pain, a feeling of impending doom, cyanosis, and possibly coughing and altered mental status. These signs indicate an emergency situation. Supportive treatment during diagnostic testing consists of providing a calm atmosphere, oxygen, and anticoagulants. Cardiac and ventilatory support often is necessary. Treatment may consist of thrombectomy (excision of the clot) or thrombolytic therapy with an enzyme substance.

If a patient is considered at risk for further embolus formation from deep vein thrombosis, a vena caval umbrella may be inserted to prevent damage from emboli. This is a strainer-like device positioned in the vena cava that catches the emboli, preventing them from traveling further. The umbrella is collapsed, and with the use of a special catheter, threaded into the vena cava. The umbrella catches the emboli and the body slowly dissolves and disposes of them.

The outcome of thrombosis or embolus can range from mild local congestion and edema to sudden death from occlusion of a major artery in the brain, lungs, or heart.

SURGICAL INTERVENTION FOR VASCULAR DISORDERS

Surgeries performed for the various vascular disorders include percutaneous transluminal angioplasty (PTA), endarterectomy, vein ligation and stripping, arterial bypass, aortic aneurysm repair, embolectomy, and thrombectomy. Preoperative care is similar to that of any major surgical procedure. A good baseline vascular assessment is essential. All pulses are evaluated and their quality noted; pedal pulse locations are marked with indelible ink for ease of postoperative assessment. Careful neurological assessment is important, too, to provide a baseline for postoperative neurological changes. There always is a danger of embolus whenever the vascular system is entered.

The patient undergoing PTA will usually have an IV heparin drip postoperatively. This must be closely monitored by the nurse, with assessment of clotting times, and evaluation for spontaneous bleeding. Other types of surgical patients may be receiving subcutaneous heparin injections.

If the aorta has been clamped during surgery, it is essential to monitor kidney function closely for signs of acute kidney failure. An output of less than 30 mL per hour should be reported to the physician. Measurement of abdominal girth is performed each shift to detect internal bleeding.

Careful vascular assessment postoperatively includes checking the pulses, sensation, skin color, and temperature and comparing bilaterally. Any decrease in sensation, or paresthesia, occurring postoperatively may indicate an internal hematoma that is pressing on the nerves. This should be reported immediately. Increasing pain or edema of the extremity may indicate internal bleeding and should be reported. Measuring the extremity's circumference daily, and marking where the measurement is taken may detect edema from thrombosis. However, this alone is not a reliable indicator.

Pain control will depend on the type of surgery and the patient's response to it. Patient-controlled analgesia with morphine or meperidine is common after major surgery. Whatever the method, the nurse must evaluate its effectiveness and seek order changes as needed.

Prophylactic antibiotics are commonly prescribed. Stool softeners are ordered for bypass graft patients and others in whom the Valsalva maneuver (which elevates blood pressure) might cause bleeding. In patients where thrombosis is a continued risk, gradual weaning from heparin to oral coumadin will begin.

Attention to respiratory effort is very important, and incentive spirometry may be ordered for patients with abdominal or chest incisions or for those who have a history of respiratory problems. Proper splinting of the incision during coughing should be taught to the patient to encourage compliance with the coughing routine.

Elastic hose, Ace wraps, or sequential compression devices will be utilized postoperatively. Proper positioning of the affected extremity is very important. The nurse should be careful to position pillows so that pressure is not placed on the back of the knee. Range of motion exercises should be performed on the nonaffected extremity, and progressive activity orders are followed for the affected limb.

All wounds are monitored for bleeding and for signs of infection. Dressing changes must follow strict aseptic technique to prevent complications for the patient. Good nutrition with attention to protein and vitamin C intake will aid in healing.

COMMUNITY CARE

Many patients with vascular disease are treated in outpatient clinics. Nonambulatory patients who have venous stasis ulcers are treated as home care patients. With early discharge after surgery, many patients re-ceive postoperative care in the home setting. Patients with arterial bypass may be referred for rehabilitation exercise programs at a rehabilitation center. The nurse's role in these settings is focused on ongoing assessment, coordination of care with other members of the health care team, monitoring progress and compliance with treatment, and patient education. Wound care and dressing changes are a daily function of the home care nurse. All nurses must constantly monitor for the presence of hypertension.

CRITICAL THINKING EXERCISES

Clinical Case Problems

Read each clinical case problem and discuss the questions with your classmates.

1. Mr. Dunn is being discharged from the hospital after being treated for arterial insufficiency in both lower extremities. His physician requests that Mr. Dunn receive instruction in the care of his feet and legs before he is permitted to leave.

    a. What are some problems you might expect Mr. Dunn to have because of his peripheral vascular disease?

    b. What kinds of information would Mr. Dunn need to alleviate these problems and prevent others?

2. Mrs. Harris is 83 years old and is hospitalized with congestive heart failure. She has a history of deep vein thrombosis (DVT) in the lower extremities.

    a. What techniques would you include in your assessment, considering her history?

    b. What would you include in the care plan to try to prevent further DVT?

BIBLIOGRAPHY

Allen, S. L. (1995). Perioperative nursing interventions for intravascular stent placements. *AORN Journal.* 61(4): 689–691, 693–698, 701–710.

American Heart Association. (1995). *Heart and Stroke Facts: 1995 Statistical Supplement.* Dallas: Author.

American Heart Association. (1996). *Heart and Stroke Facts.* Dallas: Author.

Anderson, F. D., and Maloney, J. P. (1994). Taking blood pressure correctly—it's no off-the-cuff matter. *Nursing 94.* 24(11):35–39.

Applegate, E. J. (1995). *The Anatomy and Physiology Learning System: Textbook.* Philadelphia: Saunders.

Barber, D. A., et al. (1995). Antiotensin II receptors and potassium channels: targets for new cardiovascular drugs. *Journal of Practical Nursing.* 45(1):32–42.

Baum, P. (1995). Vascular rehabilitation: preserving and empowering the nurse–patient relationship. *Journal of Vascular Nursing.* 13(1):24.

Bennett, J. C., Plum, F. (eds.) (1996). *Cecil Textbook of Medicine,* 20th ed. Philadelphia: Saunders.

Blondin, M. M., Titler, M. G. (1996). Deep vein thrombosis and pulmonary embolism prevention: What role do nurses play? *MEDSURG Nursing* 5(3): 205–208.

Brenner, Z. R. (1995). Vascular disease. *AACN Clinical Issues: Advanced Practice in Acute and Critical Care.* 6(4):503–676.

Bright, L. D. (1995). Clinical snapshot: deep vein thrombosis. *American Journal of Nursing.* 95(6):48–49.

Bright, L. D., and Georgi, S. (1995). Peripheral vascular disease: is it arterial or venous? *American Journal of Nursing.* 92(9):34–43, 45–47.

Bunt, T. J. (1995). Elder care: revascularization versus amputation for elderly patients. *AORN Journal.* 62(3):433–435.

Cahall, E., Spence, R. K. (1995). Practical nursing measures for vascular compromise in the lower leg. *Ostomy Wound Management.* 41(9):16–8, 20–26, 28–32.

Cantwell-Bab, K. (1996). Identifying chronic peripheral arterial disease. *American Journal of Nursing.* 96(7):40–46.

Catania, U. M. (1994). Monitoring coumadin therapy. *RN.* 57(2):29–34.

Cookingham, A. (1995). Peripheral vascular disease: educational concerns for patients with a chronic disease in a changing health-care environment. *AACN Clinical Issues: Advanced Practice in Acute and Critical Care.* 6(4):670–676.

Cuddy, R. P. (1995). Hypertension: keeping dangerous blood pressure down. *Nursing 95.* 25(8):34–43.

Eaton, L. E., Buck, E. A., Catanzaro, J. E. (1996). The nurse's role in facilitating compliance in clients with hypertension. *MEDSURG Nursing.* 5(5):339–345.

Fahey, V. A. (1994). *Vascular Nursing,* 2nd ed. Philadelphia: Saunders.

Fazio, A. (1995). Stepped-care to hypertension therapy. *Journal of Practical Nursing.* 45(2):44–55.

Fellows, E. (1995). Abdominal aortic aneurysm. *American Journal of Nursing.* 95(5):26–32.

Guyton, A. C., Hall, J. E. (1996). *Textbook of Medical Physiology,* 9th ed. Philadelphia: Saunders.

Harris, A. H., Brown-Etris, M., Troyer-Caudle, J. (1996). Managing vascular leg ulcers, Part 1: Assessment. *American Journal of Nursing.* 96(1):38–43.

Harris, A. H., Brown-Etris, M., Troyer-Caudle, J. (1996). Managing vascular leg ulcers, Part 2: Treatment. *American Journal of Nursing.* 96(2):41–46.

Hickey, A. (1995). DVT: clearing the record. *Nursing 95.* 25(1):4.

Hill, E. M. (1995). Perioperative management of patients with vascular disease. *AACN Clinical Issues: Advanced Practice in Acute and Critical Care.* 6(4): 547–561.

Holcomb, S. S. (1997). Understanding the ins and outs of diuretic therapy. *Nursing 97.* 27(2):34–40.

Ignatavicius, D. D., Hausman, K. A. (1995). *Clinical Pathways for Collaborative Practice.* Philadelphia: Saunders.

Ignatavicius, D. D., Workman, M. L., Mishler, M. A. (1995). *Medical-Surgical Nursing: A Nursing Process Approach,* 2nd ed. Philadelphia: Saunders.

Jarvis, C. (1996). *Physical Examination and Health Assessment.* 2nd ed. Philadelphia: Saunders.

Karch, A. M. (1995). Pain, pills, and possibilities: drug therapy in peripheral vascular disease. *AACN Clinical Issues: Advanced Practice in Acute and Critical Care.* 6(4):614–630.

Lacey, K. O., et al. (1995). Outcomes after major vascular surgery: the patients' perspective. *Journal of Vascular Nursing.* 13(1):8–13.

Lehne, R. A. (1994). *Pharmacology for Nursing Care,* 2nd ed. Philadelphia: Saunders.

Maldonado, K. (1996). Care of patients after aortic aneurysm repair. *Journal of Post Anesthesia Nursing.* 11(1):29–31.

Matteson, M. A., McConnell, E. S., Linton, A. D. (1997). *Gerontological Nursing: Concepts and Practice,* 2nd ed. Philadelphia: Saunders.

Matula, P. (1996). Aortic rupture! *RN.* 59(11):38–41.

McAbee, R. (1995). Hypertension: resources for client information. *AAOHN Journal.* 43(6):306–312.

McGrath, A. (1997). Raynaud's Syndrome. *American Journal of Nursing.* 97(1):34–35.

Monahan, F. D., Drake, T., Neighbors, M. (1994). *Nursing Care of Adults.* Philadelphia: Saunders.

Nunnelee, J. D. (1995). Minimize the risk of DVT. *RN.* 58(12):28–32.

Painter, L. M., et al. (1995). Abdominal aortic aneurysm pathway: outcome analysis. *Journal of Vascular Nursing.* 13(4):101–105.

Pettinicchi, T. (1996). Actionstat: Hypertensive crisis. *Nursing 96.* 26(8):25.

Porsche, R. (1995). Hypertension: diagnosis, acute antihypertension therapy, and long-term management. *AACN Clinical Issues: Advanced Practice in Acute and Critical Care.* 6(4):515–525.

Rakel, R. E., ed. (1997). *Conn's Current Therapy 1997.* Philadelphia: Saunders.

Redeker, N. S., Sadowski, A. V. (1995). Update on cardiovascular drugs and elders. *American Journal of Nursing.* 95(9):34–41.

Roper, M. (1996). Assessing orthostatic vital signs. *American Journal of Nursing.* 96(8):43–46.

Sandler, R. L. (1995). Clinical snapshot: abdominal aortic aneurysm. *American Journal of Nursing.* 95 (1):38.

Sansevero, A. C. (1996). Managing aortic dissections: A critical care challenge. *Critical Care Nurse.* 16(5):44–50.

Sieggreen, M. Y., Maklebust, J. (1996). Managing leg ulcers. *Nursing 96.* 26(12):41–47.

Solomon, J. (1994). Hypertension: New drug therapies. *RN.* 57(1):26–33.

Sparks, K. S. (1996). Are you up to date on weight-based heparin dosing? *American Journal of Nursing.* 96(4):33–36.

Springhouse Company. (1988–1997). *Nurse Review: Vascular Disease.* Springhouse, PA: Author.

Springhouse Corporation. (1996). *Nursing 96 Drug Handbook.* Springhouse, PA: author.

Stiesmeyer, J. K. (1994). Caring for the patient with peripheral arterial occlusive disease. *Nursing 94.* 24(5):32C–33C.

Weber, M., Neutel, J., Smith, D., Ceraettinger, W. (1994). Diagnosis of mild hypertension by ambulatory blood pressure monitoring. *Circulation.* 90(5):2291–2297.

Wills, E. M., Sloan, H. L. (1996). Assessing peripheral arterial disorders in the home. *Home Healthcare Nurse.* 14(9):669–680.

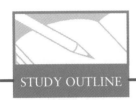

STUDY OUTLINE

I. Introduction
  A. The vascular system helps provide the body with nutrients and oxygen needed for life.
  B. Disorders of the vascular system upset homeostasis.
  C. Disorders of peripheral arteries invariably lead to ischemia.
  D. Disorders of peripheral veins lead to increased pressure within the vessel.

II. Causative Factors and Prevention of Vascular Disorders
  A. Arterial wall injury may be caused by hypertension, deposit of fatty plaque, chemical toxins, or diabetes mellitus.
  B. Obesity, stress, and sedentary lifestyle contribute to the incidence of atherosclerosis and hypertension.
  C. One out of four adults has hypertension, about 50 million Americans.
  D. Hypertension is more prevalent and more severe in blacks than in whites.
  E. Although it cannot be prevented, essential hypertension can be controlled.
  F. Education, public screening, and encouragement for compliance with treatment can decrease the incidence of damage from hypertension.
  G. Atherosclerosis is the most common cause of peripheral vascular disease (PVD).
  H. Quitting smoking, following a low-fat diet, controlling diabetes mellitus, and following an exercise program decreases the incidence of PVD.
  I. Standing for long periods of time over many years and wearing tight, constricting clothing are two factors that contribute to venous insufficiency and varicose veins.

III. Diagnostic Tests and Procedures (Table 18-1)

IV. Nursing Assessment of the Vascular System
  A. History taking (see Table 18-2).
  B. Physical assessment.
    1. Pulses: assess and compare bilaterally.
    2. Blood Pressure: lying, sitting, and standing.
    3. Bruits: whooshing or purring sound heard over partially occluded arteries.
    4. Skin.
      a. Have patient elevate feet and legs above level of heart for 2 to 3 minutes, then dangle legs.
      b. Delayed return of color to feet indicates arterial insufficiency.
      c. Pale, mottled appearance may indicate only that patient is cold.
      d. Reddish-blue color indicates severe ischemia.
      e. Skin temperature.
        (1) Note coldness of extremity when environment is warm.
        (2) Compare temperature of limbs.
      f. Trophic changes resulting from malnutrition of tissues.
        (1) Skin smooth, shiny, without hair.
        (2) Thick nails.
        (3) Necrosis and gangrene after prolonged malnutrition.
      g. Assessment of venous blood flow.
        (1) Edema and cellulitis: increased pigmentation, dry and scaly skin, excoriations, and ulcers.
        (2) Trendelenburg test.

V. Nursing Diagnosis (Table 18-4)
  A. Altered tissue perfusion.
  B. Pain related to decreased blood flow.

C. Activity intolerance related to pain in legs when walking.

D. Impaired skin integrity related to ulceration.

E. Sleep pattern disturbance related to pain in legs while at rest.

F. Body image disturbance related to edema and dilated veins on legs.

G. Body image disturbance related to loss of limb by amputation.

H. Knowledge deficit related to causes of peripheral vascular disease, treatment, and proper self-care.

I. Risk for injury related to potential for embolus or bleeding from anticoagulant medication.

J. Risk for infection related to impaired skin integrity.

K. Self-esteem disturbance related to inability to perform usual roles because of chronic leg ulcers.

VI. Planning

   A. Goals.

      1. Promote vascular integrity.

      2. Decrease risk factors for vascular disease.

      3. Maintain blood pressure within normal limits.

      4. Improve circulatory function.

      5. Prevent thrombosis and embolism.

      6. Maintain or restore tissue integrity.

      7. Prevent the complications of leg ulcers and gangrene.

   B. Collaboration with the dietitian and physical therapist is important to the success of a plan of care.

VII. Implementation

   A. Interventions are directed at monitoring the condition and determining whether treatment is effective.

   B. Patient education about knowledge of the disease process, self-care, and medication regimen is a large part of nursing care.

   C. Specific nursing interventions (see Table 18-4).

VIII. Evaluation

   A. Serial blood pressure readings are necessary to evaluate therapy for hypertension.

   B. Evaluation of pulse and comparison bilaterally.

   C. Skin color and temperature assessments.

   D. Subjective data from the patient are needed for evaluation.

IX. Common Problems and Therapies and Their Nursing Implications

   A. Altered tissue perfusion.

      1. Smooth muscles of arterial walls constrict in presence of cold and extreme heat and relax when warm.

      2. Pressure against vessel walls.

         a. Avoid constricting clothing.

         b. Change position frequently.

         c. Elevate extremities periodically to increase venous return.

         d. Wear support hose or elastic bandages.

         e. Walk and exercise.

      3. Vasoconstriction.

         a. Chemical factors: nicotine is a vasoconstrictor.

         b. Alcohol in moderate amounts is a vasodilator.

         c. Vasodilating drugs.

         d. Sympathectomy.

   B. Impaired skin integrity.

      1. Chronic leg ulcers.

      2. Gangrene.

      3. Patient education in care of feet and legs (Table 18-5).

X. Disorders of the Vascular System

   A. Hypertension: persistently high blood pressure.

      1. Causes damage to heart, brain, and kidney.

      2. Cause of essential hypertension is unknown.

      3. Secondary hypertension is caused by another disease.

      4. Factors associated with essential hypertension are age, race, obesity, and sodium intake.

      5. Contributing factors may be nicotine, female hormone therapy, caffeine, stress.

      6. Blood pressure tends to rise with age (see Table 18-7).

      7. A loss of excess weight may return slightly elevated blood pressure to normal.

      8. Pathophysiology.

         a. Blood pressure equals the amount of blood pumped out of the heart multiplied by the peripheral vascular resistance.

         b. When blood vessels constrict, blood pressure rises.

         c. An excess of renin secreted by the kidneys elevates blood pressure (Figure 18-6).

      9. Signs of hypertension.

         a. Absent other than elevated blood pressure readings in the early stages.

         b. Later signs and symptoms include headache, dizziness, blurred vision, blackouts, irritability, fatigue, or nervousness.

     10. Malignant hypertension is a progressive moderate to severe hypertension that is difficult to control.

     11. Hypertensive crisis is a life-threatening emergency in which pressure rises very high

and causes severe headache, blurred vision, nausea, and possibly confusion.

12. Diagnosis and medical treatment.

    a. Elevated readings taken twice and averaged on two different occasions at least 2 weeks apart.

    b. Treatment is individualized using a stepped-care approach.

        (1) First step: modification of lifestyle: stop smoking, weight control, sodium restriction, alcohol restriction, exercise, low-fat diet, and stress control.

        (2) Second step: one drug is prescribed; either a diuretic or an antihypertensive.

        (3) Subsequent steps involve adding medications in combination to achieve control.

        (4) Drugs work by decreasing blood volume, cardiac output, or peripheral resistance.

    c. Nursing care: counseling and education about lifestyle changes, diet, weight control, stress relief, and exercise.

B. Chronic arterial occlusive disease (atherosclerosis obliterans).

1. Pathophysiology: Caused by atherosclerosis of peripheral arteries; usually affects lower extremities.

2. Signs and symptoms include intermittent claudication, pain at rest, and ischemic changes. The "5 Ps" are pain, pallor, pulselessness, paralysis, and paresthesia.

3. Peripheral vasodilators and medication to decrease blood viscosity are given to improve blood flow.

4. The best treatment is exercise, specifically walking.

5. A hyperbaric oxygen chamber sometimes is used to increase oxygen in tissues and avoid amputation.

6. Surgical treatment helps relieve ischemic pain, avoid amputation, and add years to patient's life.

    a. Laser angioplasty.

    b. Percutaneous transluminal angioplasty (PTA).

    c. Bypass procedure with synthetic arterial graft.

    d. Aneurysm repair.

7. Nursing care.

    a. Maintain blood flow.

    b. Protect tissues from injury.

    c. Prevent wound infection.

    d. Promote rehabilitation through exercise.

C. Thromboangitis obliterans (Buerger's disease).

1. Involves small- and medium-sized arteries and is linked to smoking.

2. Cessation of smoking is the most important treatment factor.

3. Exercise is prescribed to increase circulation.

D. Raynaud's disease: spasm of small arteries; mostly affects fingers and toes.

E. Aneurysm.

1. Pathophysiology: common in cerebral vessels and aorta.

    a. Long-standing hypertension and atherosclerosis are factors in the development.

    b. Ruptured aneurysm often causes sudden death.

    c. May have no obvious symptoms; cerebral aneurysms may cause headaches or blurred vision.

    d. Aortic aneurysm may cause back pain or a feeling of pressure and visible pulsation in abdomen.

2. Medical treatment.

    a. Watched until 6 to 7 cm in diameter.

    b. Repaired by surgical resection and graft.

    c. Requires ICU care in immediate postoperative period.

F. Carotid occlusion.

1. Occlusion is signified by a carotid bruit, confusion, blackouts, extremity weakness or paralysis, visual abnormality in one eye, or other neurological symptoms.

2. Treated by carotid endarterectomy or bypass surgery.

G. Venous disorders.

1. Varicose veins: enlarged, tortuous veins engorged with pooled blood.

    a. Symptoms: fatigue, feeling of heaviness in legs after prolonged standing or sitting, pain, itching along course of blood vessel.

    b. Medical management: support hose, treatment of obesity, exercise.

    c. Surgical treatment: scleropathy, vein stripping, or ligation.

2. Venous stasis ulcers: skin lesion, usually on lower leg, from venous insufficiency.

    a. Occur with slightest trauma.

    b. Difficult to treat and slow to heal.

    c. Treatment: acute debridement and prevention of infection.

3. Thrombosis and embolism.

    a. Thrombosis: formation of clot within blood vessel.

(1) Effects depend on location and size of clot.

(2) Degree of obstruction to blood flow.

(3) Whether body can establish collateral circulation.

4. Deep vein thrombosis: clot in deep vein occluding blood flow.

   a. Causes: immobility, trauma, surgery, dehydration, abnormal clotting.

   b. Signs and symptoms: edema in one extremity, positive Homan's sign, warmth over area.

   c. Treatment: IV heparin, oral warfarin (Coumadin), and hydration; thrombolytic therapy may be used.

5. Thrombophlebitis: clot and inflammation of vessel.

   a. Symptoms: vein appears distended; tenderness; redness.

   b. Medical management: elevation of part, support hose, warm packs, aspirin, and sometimes antibiotics.

   c. Surgical treatment: vein ligation.

   d. Nursing care.

      (1) Instruct patient not to rub extremity.

      (2) Encourage increased fluid intake if permitted.

      (3) Apply elastic hose or inflatable pressure boots.

      (4) Monitor anticoagulant therapy: check clotting times; assess for bruising and bleeding.

6. Observe for signs of embolus.

7. Encourage exercise to decrease venous stasis in other leg.

H. Embolism: thrombus lodges in a vessel, blocking blood flow beyond it.

   a. Causes: DVT of lower leg the most common cause; fat droplets from fracture, clots formed from cardiac arrhythmias, and amniotic fluid also cause emboli.

   b. Signs and symptoms of pulmonary embolus: dyspnea, hemoptysis, feeling of impending doom, cyanosis, chest splinting.

   c. Treatment: oxygen, thrombolytic therapy, anticoagulants, or thrombectomy; vena caval umbrella insertion.

XI. Elder Care Points

A. Systolic pressure rises with age, but systolic hypertension should be treated in the elderly.

B. Measure the blood pressure of the elderly between meals as it will be less accurate after a meal.

C. Hair loss and nail thickening on the extremities are natural aspects of aging and do not necessarily indicate a vascular problem.

D. Because of arteriosclerosis and loss of elasticity of the vessels, plus the decreased sensitivity of the baroreceptors that help adjust blood pressure in the elderly, orthostatic hypotension often occurs when the patient is changing position.

E. Measure the blood pressure of the elderly patient who is taking antihypertensive medication both sitting and standing to detect orthostatic hypotension.

F. Atherosclerosis is main cause of PVD in elderly.

G. Varicose veins: vessels lose elasticity; muscles weaken.

H. Thrombophlebitis more frequent in elderly, who have altered coagulation, are quick to dehydrate, and are less mobile.

I. Lessened activity as a result of arthritis and other conditions predisposes patients to problems with PVD.

J. Many elderly are being treated for cardiac dysrhythmias such as atrial fibrillation that can cause the formation of clots. The nurse must be alert to signs of emboli in these patients and should encourage them not to discontinue their prescribed anticoagulant.

K. Nurse should encourage as much physical activity as possible within patient's limitations.

CHAPTER 19

Care of Patients with Heart Disorders

OBJECTIVES

Upon completing this chapter the student should be able to:

1. List the modifiable and uncontrollable risk factors for the development of heart disease.
2. State ways in which nurses can contribute to the prevention of heart disease.
3. Teach patients about the more common diagnostic tests and procedures used by doctors to diagnose and evaluate heart diseases.
4. Describe initial and ongoing nursing assessment to evaluate heart patients.
5. List common nursing diagnoses with nursing interventions for patients with angina pectoris, myocardial infarction, cardiac dysrhythmias, and congestive heart failure.
6. Describe the various ways in which inflammatory disorders contribute to heart problems.
7. Compare the signs and symptoms and treatment of mitral stenosis, mitral insufficiency, aortic stenosis, and aortic insufficiency.
8. State six nursing responsibilities in the administration of cardiac drugs, dietary control, and oxygen therapy for patients with cardiac disorders.
9. Describe pre- and postoperative problems and nursing care for patients undergoing heart surgery.
10. Discuss the nurse's role in caring for elderly patients with heart disorders in the long-term care facility or the home.

Heart disease affects about one in four people in the United States. Even though there has been a steady decline in the death rate from heart disease since 1979, it is still the leading cause of death. Approximately one million people die in the United States from heart problems each year. Preventing and controlling heart disease are major factors in the attempt to control health care costs. Heart disease is responsible for the largest portion of Medicare funds spent each year. Each nurse can be instrumental in educating the public and in promoting a heart-healthy lifestyle. To understand the various disorders of the heart it is necessary to recall the structure and normal functions of the heart.

OVERVIEW OF ANATOMY AND PHYSIOLOGY

What Are the Structures of the Heart and Their Functions?

⋏ The heart wall consists of three layers. The epicardium is the outer layer of tissue; the myocardium is the middle layer of muscle fibers that contract to pump blood, and the endocardium is the lining of the inner surface of the heart chambers.

⋏ A membranous sac, the pericardium, surrounds the heart.

⋏ The four chambers of the heart make up two coordinated pumps; the right-side pump is a low-pressure system, and the left-side one is a high-pressure system.

⋏ The right atrium and right ventricle receive blood from the vascular system and pump it through the lungs.

⋏ The left atrium and left ventricle receive oxygenated blood from the lungs and pump it through the systemic circulation.

⋏ A septum separates the atria and the ventricles.

⋏ The cardiac valves direct the flow of blood through the heart chambers.

⋏ Blood enters the right atrium via the superior vena cava and goes to the right ventricle through the tricuspid valve.

⋏ Blood leaves the right ventricle through the pulmonic valve and goes into the pulmonary artery to circulate in the lungs, exchanging carbon dioxide for oxygen.

⋏ The left atrium receives oxygenated blood from the pulmonary veins and the mitral valve controls the flow from the atrium into the left ventricle.

⋏ The left ventricle ejects the blood through the aortic valve into the aorta and the systemic circulation (Figure 19-1).

⋏ The coronary arteries branch from the aorta and supply the cardiac muscle with blood.

⋏ The left coronary artery divides into the anterior descending and the circumflex artery providing blood for the left atrium and the left ventricle.

⋏ The right coronary artery supplies the right atrium, right ventricle, and part of the posterior wall of the left ventricle as well as the atrioventricular node of the cardiac conduction system (see Figure 19-2).

⋏ The heart sits in the center of the chest within the thoracic cavity with the apex pointing downward and to the left.

⋏ The point of maximal impulse (PMI) can normally be felt between the fifth and sixth ribs on a line dividing the left clavicle in half. Listen to the apical heart rate at this location.

What Causes the Heart to Contract and Pump Blood?

⋏ The heart's pumping action is sparked by specialized pacemaker cells and conduction fibers that initiate spontaneous electrical activity, causing muscle contractions that result in a heart beat.

⋏ The conduction pathways are located in the myocardium and transmit the electrical impulse throughout the heart.

⋏ The sinoatrial (SA) node is located in the right atrium and is called the "pacemaker" of the heart because it normally initiates the electrical impulses.

⋏ The atrioventricular (AV) node is located in the lower part of the right atrium. It relays the impulse from the SA node to the bundle of His and throughout the ventricles via the Purkinje fibers (Figure 19-3).

⋏ The heart rate and rhythm also are influenced by the autonomic nervous system; factors affecting that system can speed up or slow down the heart rate.

What Is the Cardiac Cycle?

⋏ The cardiac cycle consists of contraction of the muscle (systole) and relaxation of the muscle (diastole).

⋏ The heart sends out about 5 L of blood every minute.

⋏ *The amount of cardiac output depends on the heart rate, the amount of blood returning to the heart (venous return), and the strength of contraction.*

What changes occur in the cardiovascular system with aging?

⋏ The aging heart becomes stiffer and contractile ability decreases resulting in decreased stroke volume in the elderly.

⋏ The coronary arteries become tortuous and dilated and have areas of calcification.

⋏ The cardiac valves become thickened, particularly the mitral and aortic valves which are subject to higher pressures. A systolic murmur is common in those over 80 years of age.

⋏ The SA node loses about 40 percent of the pacemaker cells over time predisposing to cardiac dysrhythmias or SA node failure.

⋏ The aorta becomes stiffer contributing to an increase in systolic blood pressure because the left ventricle must pump against greater resistance.

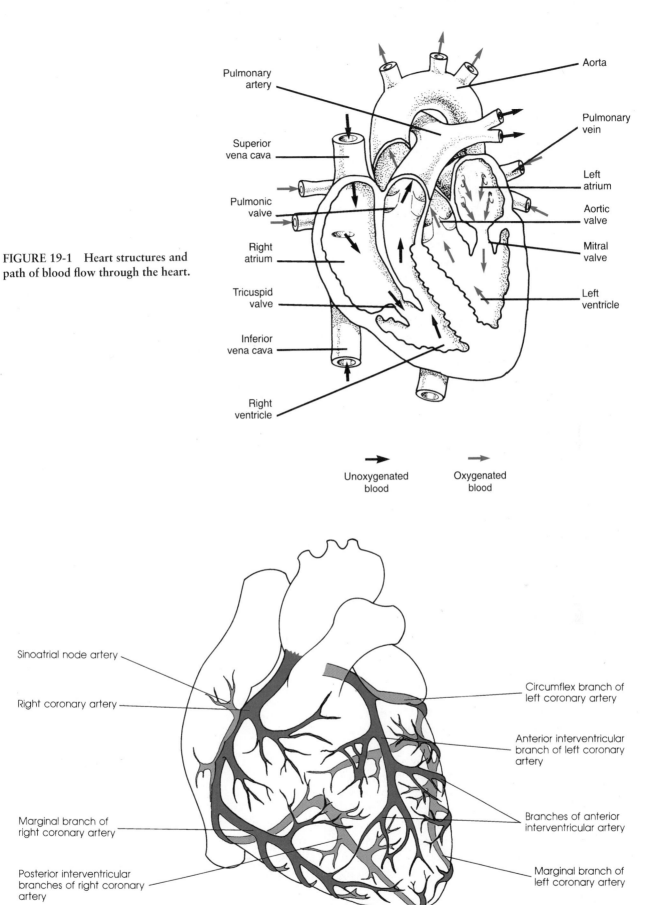

Pulmonary artery

Aorta

Superior vena cava

Pulmonary vein

Pulmonic valve

Left atrium

Right atrium

Aortic valve

Tricuspid valve

Mitral valve

Inferior vena cava

Left ventricle

Right ventricle

Unoxygenated blood

Oxygenated blood

FIGURE 19-1   Heart structures and path of blood flow through the heart.

Sinoatrial node artery

Circumflex branch of left coronary artery

Right coronary artery

Anterior interventricular branch of left coronary artery

Branches of anterior interventricular artery

Marginal branch of right coronary artery

Posterior interventricular branches of right coronary artery

Marginal branch of left coronary artery

The arteries serving the posterior aspect of the myocardium are shown here in a lighter shade.

FIGURE 19-2   A view of the coronary arterial system.

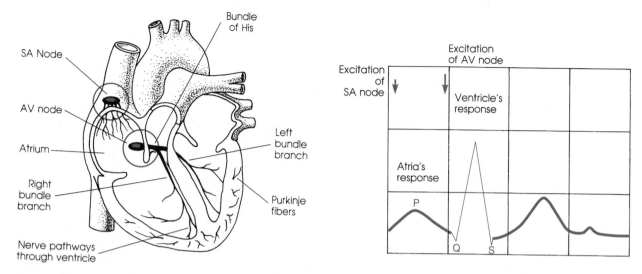

Electrical impulses that excite the heart muscle to contract originate in the sinoatrial (SA) node and spread through the atrium (P wave on the EKG). They then pass through the atrioventricular (AV) node (Q wave) to the bundle of His, which divides into a left and right branch. The impulses travel along these branches and excite the ventricle (S wave). The Smaller fibers that branch into the myocardium are called the *Purkinje fibers.*

FIGURE 19-3   Cardiac conduction system *(left)* and impulses it produces on electrocardiogram *(right).*

CAUSES OF HEART DISORDERS

Abnormal structure of the heart or vessels can be either congenital or acquired. Narrowing of the aorta *(coarctation),* holes in the septum, or abnormal formation of a cardiac valve can occur congenitally. Acquired defects include narrowing or hardening of the blood vessels from arteriosclerosis or atherosclerosis; aneurysms of the large vessels; alteration of the valve structure caused by inflammation, causing narrowing (**stenosis**) or incomplete closure (**insufficiency**); alteration of the myocardial muscle tissue by extra growth with thickening (**hypertrophy**) or fibrosis, lack of adequate blood supply (**ischemia**), or **infarct** (area of tissue that has died from lack of blood supply); deterioration of the pacemaker cells and conduction fibers; or inflammation of the various tissues.

Any disorder involving either the heart or the vessels through which it pumps blood can eventually weaken and damage the heart muscle and lead to a slowing down or congestion of blood flow. This condition, called *congestive heart failure,* is a complication of many cardiovascular diseases. Another complication that occurs when the heart is greatly stressed by various cardiovascular disorders or is damaged by a virus is **cardiomyopathy.** *Cardiomyopathy* causes the heart muscle to lose its ability to pump effectively, and heart failure occurs. The only cure for severe cardiomyopathy is a heart transplant.

Disturbances in any part of the heart's conduction system can result in an increase in heart rate (**tachycardia**), a slowing down of the heart rate (**bradycardia**), and disturbances in the rhythm of the heart beat (**dysrhythmias**).

Infection and inflammation also can take their toll on the structure and function of the heart. **Endocarditis,** inflammation within the lining and valves of the heart, and **pericarditis,** an inflammation of the sac surrounding the heart, can occur as primary diseases, but they are more often secondary to infection and inflammation elsewhere in the body. An example is rheumatic heart disease, which occurs after a streptococcal infection.

Substances in the blood such as excess carbon dioxide and certain drugs can affect the rate and rhythm of the heart through their effect on the autonomic nervous system. The heart also responds to physiological changes that indicate a need for more or less oxygen.

This chapter discusses the various disorders of the heart, how they occur, their diagnosis and treatment, and the nursing care and teaching involved in returning the patient to a high level of wellness.

PREVENTION OF HEART DISEASE

Cardiovascular diseases claim 925,000 lives annually in the United States. Heart disease remains the major cause of death in the United States. Cardiovascular diseases also account for a large percentage of the chronic illnesses that disable to some degree a large portion of the U.S. population.

Although the numbers for death and illness from cardiovascular diseases are high, it should be remembered that not all heart problems are either fatal or totally disabling. There are many kinds and degrees of

TABLE 19-1 ◆ *Warning Signs of Heart Attack (Myocardial Infarction)*

- Chest pain: a feeling of tightness or a crushing or squeezing pain. Pain may radiate to one or both arms, shoulder, back, neck, jaw, or the top of the stomach.
- Chest pain unrelieved by prescribed doses of nitroglycerin.
- Chest discomfort with lightheadedness, fainting, sweating, nausea, or shortness of breath.
- Difficulty breathing or shortness of breath.
- Rapid or irregular pulse along with any other symptom.

Call 911 or emergency number immediately—get help!

heart disease. Advances in medical science have made it possible either to cure or successfully manage a large number of cardiovascular problems. Reasons for the decline in deaths from heart disease since the mid-1980s include improved emergency treatment of persons experiencing a coronary occlusion or "heart attack," improved education of the public regarding ways to prevent heart disease, and teaching about the warning signs of a heart attack. Every nurse has a responsibility to

assist with public education about heart disease. See Table 19-1 for the warning signs of heart attack.

Table 19-2 presents the risk factors for heart disease. **Modifiable risk factors are the major focus for education to prevent heart disease.** Old habits are hard to change, but there is strong evidence that reducing these risk factors can greatly cut down the chance of developing heart disease and thereby improve the quality of an individual's life.

The increased use of cocaine has added to the problem of heart disease. Cocaine causes vasoconstriction and is thought to speed up the atherosclerosis process. Also, cocaine has been known to cause sudden cardiac death, or stroke, in susceptible individuals. Research is finding that the ingestion of both alcohol and cocaine greatly increases the chance of cardiac death. Cigarette smoking–related health problems are heavy contributors to heart disease, and smoking is a key factor in sudden cardiac death.

Uncontrollable risk factors cannot be prevented by an individual. However, control of diseases such as hypertension and diabetes mellitus, and the reduction

TABLE 19-2 ◆ *Risk Factors for Heart Disease*

Factor	Significance
Unavoidable risk factors	
Heredity	Children of parents with cardiovascular disease are more likely to develop the same problem.
Race	African Americans experience high blood pressure two to three times more frequently than whites. Consequently the risk of heart disease in this group is higher.
Sex	Males experience more heart attacks than females earlier in life. After age 65, the death rate from heart disease increases in women.
Age	Four out of five people who die of a heart attack are 65 or older. Increasing age increases the risk.
Diabetes mellitus	Diabetes seriously increases the risk of cardiovascular disease. Good control of the disease by keeping blood sugar within normal limits reduces the risk and/or onset of cardiovascular disease.
Hypertension	High blood pressure increases the workload of the heart and hastens the arteriosclerotic process in the blood vessels. Although most cases of hypertension cannot be prevented, control of blood pressure within normal limits can prevent the onset of heart problems.
Familial hypercholesterolemia	Genetic predisposition to high cholesterol levels cannot be prevented. Close attention to a strict diet and the use of cholesterol-lowering medication, plus exercise, can reduce the total blood cholesterol level, thereby lowering the risk of early heart problems.
Avoidable Risk Factors	
Obesity	Keep weight within normal limits by diet and exercise.
Cholesterol >200* mg/dL	Exercise and low-fat diet.
Lack of regular exercise	Exercise program of 30-minute sessions at least three times a week
High blood pressure*	Keep blood pressure <140/90; monitor blood pressure every year.
Cigarette smoking	Quit smoking.
Cocaine use	Do not use cocaine.
Excessive stress	Use stress-reduction techniques regularly, such as exercise, relaxation techniques; reduce hostility, maintain positive support system.
Excessive alcohol intake	Limit alcohol consumption to two mixed drinks, two 4-oz glasses of wine, or two 12-oz beers at any one time, no more than two to three times per week.

*Avoidable to some degree, although can be hereditary.

of high cholesterol, which are factors in the development of atherosclerosis, are possible and can help prevent the early onset of heart disease. It has been proven that, if a diabetic can keep the blood sugar consistently below 140 mg/dL, the risk of atherosclerosis is lessened.

Management of hypertension is one of the major tools for heart disease prevention (see Chapter 18).

Think about . . . Can you identify two risk factors that you can modify to decrease your risk of heart disease?

DIAGNOSTIC TESTS AND PROCEDURES

In addition to a routine physical examination and medical history, the physician has access to a number of both noninvasive and invasive procedures and tests to help diagnose heart disease. Because of the hazards and risks of invasive procedures that require entry into the cardiovascular system or the injection of substances into the circulating blood, noninvasive procedures usually are performed first.

Nuclear imaging often is combined with an exercise EKG—the stress test. Echocardiography also can be done now from inside the esophagus using a esophagogastroscope and special transducer. Digital subtraction angiography (DSA) is a form of computer-enhanced angiography that provides a clearer picture of the coronary arteries and their patency. Arterial ultrasound is a new test that may some day replace angiography. Specific diagnostic tests and their nursing implications are listed in Table 19-3. In women, a thallium exercise stress test is better than the standard treadmill test for detecting heart disease. A stress echocardiogram also is helpful.

TABLE 19-3 ◆ *Diagnostic Tests for Heart Disorders*

Test	Purpose	Description	Nursing Implications
Electrocardiography 12-Lead electro-cardiogram	Records electrical impulses of the heart to determine rate, rhythm of heart, site of pacemaker, and presence of injury at rest.	Small electrodes are placed on the chest and extremities, to show conduction patterns in different directions of electrical flow. Figure 19-3 shows a basic EKG tracing.	Inform patient that there is no discomfort with this test. Maintain electrical safety. Normal finding: normal EKG
Exercise EKG—stress test	Record electrical activity of the heart during exercise. Insufficient blood flow and oxygen show up in abnormal wave forms.	Small electrodes are placed on the chest, and a tracing is made while the patient exercises on a treadmill, bicycle or stairs. The degree of difficulty of the exercise is increased as the test continues to see how the heart reacts to increasing work demands. Vital signs are continuously recorded. May be combined with radionuclide imaging or echocardiography. Physician is present.	Requires a signed consent form. Have patient wear comfortable clothes and walking shoes. Light meal 2 to 3 hours prior, then NPO. Regular medications are given. Chest is shaved as needed for electrode placement. Inform patient that the test will be stopped if he experiences chest pain, severe fatigue or dyspnea. Test takes approximately 30 minutes. Normal finding: No ST segment depression with exercise and no angina.
Ambulatory EKG—Holter monitor	Correlate normal daily activity with electrical function of the heart to determine whether activity causes abnormalities.	Patient wears a small EKG recorder for 6, 12, or 24 hours while he goes about his usual tasks. He keeps a diary showing at what time he performs different activities and any symptoms experienced. The tape is analyzed to correlate any arrhythmia with the activity that caused it.	Remind patient that all activities must be recorded in the diary: brushing teeth, climbing stairs, seuxal intercourse, bowel movements, sleeping, etc. Caution him not to remove the electrodes and not to get the recorder or wires wet. Have patient wear a loose shirt during test.

TABLE 19-3 ◆ *Diagnostic Tests for Heart Disorders* *(Continued)*

Test	Purpose	Description	Nursing Implications
Echocardiography	Useful in evaluating size, shape, and position of structures and movement within the heart. Test of choice for valve problems.	A metal wand that emits sonar waves is guided over the chest wall while the patient is supine or turned on his left side. Takes 30 to 60 minutes. May be done in combination with the exercise (stress) test. Transesophageal echocardiography may be performed with a gastroscope to position the wand.	Inform patient that there is no discomfort, although conduction jelly may feel cool. Normal finding: No abnormalities of size or location of heart structures; normal wall movement. Used for very obese patients or those with a barrel chest. Positioning the gastroscope requires sedation.
Cardiac catheterization	Assesses pumping action of both sides of the heart. Measures pressure within the heart chambers. Measures cardiac output. Calculates differences in oxygen content of arterial and venous blood.	Requires a signed consent form, as it is not without risk. Catheter is inserted into vein or artery, depending on which side of the heart is to be tested. Femoral artery or brachial vein is often used. With local anesthetic, the catheter is threaded up into the heart, and pressure readings and oxygen saturation determinations are taken. Contrast media may be injected to visualize the size and shape of the chambers and structures. Takes 1½ to 3 hours. Fluoroscopy is used during the procedure.	Patient is NPO for 6 to 8 hours prior to test. Assess for allergy to iodine, shellfish, or contrast dye. Have patient void before giving preop medications. Record baseline vital signs and mark location of pedal pulses. Inform patient that he will be strapped to a table that tilts, will have an I.V. and that he must lie still during the test. EKG leads will be in place during the test. If dye is injected, patient will feel a hot flush for about a minute. He may be asked to cough during the procedure. He will be constantly monitored and emergency equipment is at hand. Posttest: vital signs q 15 min × 4, q 30 min × 4, then q 1 h × 4, or until stable. Assess peripheral pulses with vital signs, and question patient about numbness or tingling. Inspect insertion site for bleeding or sign of hematoma. Pressure dressing and sandbag weight are left in place for 1 to 3 hours. If femoral insertion site was used, keep patient flat and leg extended for 6 hours. If brachial site was used, immobilize arm for 3 hours. If dye was used, encourage fluids unless contraindicated.
Coronary angiography	Determines patency of coronary arteries and presence of collateral circulation.	Performed by dye injection during cardiac catheterizations. Video recording made during procedure for later review.	Same as for cardiac catheterization.

(Table 19-3 continued)

TABLE 19-3 ◆ *Diagnostic Tests for Heart Disorders* (*Continued*)

Test	Purpose	Description	Nursing Implications
Intravascular ultra-sound	Provide visual information about the interior of a coronary artery.	A flexible catheter with a miniature transducer at the tip is introduced into a peripheral vessel and advanced into a coronary artery. The transducer emits high-frequency sound waves which create a 2 or 3 dimensional image of the vessel lumen.	Consent form required. See cardiac catheterization for post-test care.
Electrophysiology studies	Measures and records electrical activity from within the heart to determine the area of origin of the arrhythmia and the effectiveness of the antiarrhythmic drug for the particular arrhythmia.	Three to six electrodes are placed in the heart through the venous system. They are attached to an oscilloscope that records the intracardiac and EKG waveforms simultaneously. After baseline tracings are taken, the cardiologist tries to trigger the arrhythmia that is to be studied by programmed electrical stimulation through the electrodes. Once the arrythmia is triggered, an antiarrhythmic drug is administered to determine its effectiveness in stopping the abnormal rhythm. Studies may take from 1½ to 4 hours; serial studies may be done on different days.	Provide psychological support for the patient, who is often scared of having arrhythmias induced. Antiarrhythmic drugs may be stopped 24 hours or more before the test to eliminate them from the patient's system. Assure the patient that he will be monitored constantly and that emergency equipment and staff will be on hand. Keep patient NPO after midnight. Patent IV line is maintained. Electrodes are placed using fluoroscopy. Patient will be supine on an x-ray table. Chest surface electrodes will be placed before the electrodes are threaded into the heart. The femoral vein is most commonly used; the groin is shaved, and local anethesia is used. Posttest care: much the same as for cardiac catheterization.
Nuclear imaging Thallium perfusion imaging	Evaluates blood flow in various parts of the heart; determines areas of infarction.	Thallium 201 is injected IV; radioactive uptake is counted over the heart by a gamma scintillation camera. May be done in conjunction with an exercise EKG stress test.	Explain that the radioactivity used is a very small amount and lasts only a few hours. Explain that a camera will be positioned over the heart. EKG electrodes are placed on the chest; scanning is done 10 to 15 minutes after injection; can be done as an outpatient procedure. May be done in 2 parts a few hours apart.

TABLE 19-3 ◆ *Diagnostic Tests for Heart Disorders (Continued)*			
Test	**Purpose**	**Description**	**Nursing Implications**
Persantine thallium stress test	Used for those who cannot exercise for an EKG stress test.	An EKG is done, and IV dypyridamole (Persantine) is given. Blood pressure and pulse are taken and recorded q 15 min while the drug takes effect by diverting blood flow from the coronary arteries, causing cardiac ischemia. Thallium is injected, and scanning images are taken over a period of about 40 minutes. Repeat scan is done several hours later. The patient is NPO during the test.	Mild nausea or headache may occur. Explain that patient will lie on his back for the imaging.
Technectium pyrophosphate scan and multiple gated acquisition (MUGA) scan	Determine area and extent of myocardial infarction. Assess left ventricular function.	Technectium Tc99m is injected IV and is taken up by areas of infarction, producing hot spots when scanned. Multiple serial images are obtained. Best results occur when done 1 to 6 days after a suspected MI.	Inform patient that scan is done 1½ to 2 hours after injection of the technectium. Explain that it will determine if he actually suffered damage from MI.
Laboratory tests Cardiac serum enzymes	Measures specific enzyme levels to determine what type of cells have been injured and to what extent.	Creatine kinase (CK) is found in the heart, skeletal muscle, and brain cells. It rises within 6 hours of MI and returns to normal within 48 to 72 hours. CK-MB is a fraction of the enzyme, or isoenzyme, that is specific to heart muscle cells. Lactic dehydrogenase (LDH) rises following MI but is not specific. LDH_1 and LDH_2 are the isoenzymes contained in heart muscle. If LDH_1/LDH_2 >1, it indicates MI has occurred. Aspartate aminotransferase (AST) rises 6 to 8 hours after MI, peaks within 24 to 48 hours, and returns to normal in 4 to 8 days but is not specific to heart damage. Cardiac enzymes are usually tested every 8 h × 3.	Explain purpose of lab work. Inform patient that blood will be drawn at intervals to check the rise and fall of enzyme levels.
CK	Normal values: Female: 5–35 mU/mL Male: 5–50 mU/mL		
CK-MB	<5% total CK		
LDH	150–450 U/mL		
LDH_1	17%–27%		
LDH_2	27%–37%		
AST	5–40 U/mL		
Serum protein troponin T	Quick test for acute MI.	Done by enzyme-linked immunosorbent assay. Provides results in 2 hours. Is very accurate from 10 to 120 hours after onset of MI symptoms.	Quicker and more accurate than other cardiac enzyme blood tests.

(Table 19-3 continued)

TABLE 19-3 ◆ *Diagnostic Tests for Heart Disorders* (Continued)

Test	Purpose	Description	Nursing Implications
Serum lipids	Determines level	Elevation of cholesterol is a risk factor for atherosclerotic heart disease.	Patient is NPO except for noncaloric liquids for 12 hours.
	Normal values:		
Cholesterol	150–200 mg/dL		
HDL	32–75 mg/dL		
LDL	73–200 mg/dL		
Triglycerides	50–250 mg/dL	Triglycerides contribute to arterial disease. As triglycerides rise, so do low-density lipoproteins, which are a factor in atherosclerosis. The lipoproteins (LDL, VLDL and HDL) are increased in hyperlipidemia. Lipoprotein fractions are determined by electrophoresis and are used to assign a "risk" factor in cardiovascular disease. High levels of HDL appear to protect against coronary artery disease and MI, whereas increased levels of LDL are associated with increased atherosclerosis and MI.	

See the following listed tables, or Appendix I, for information on:

Arterial Blood Gases (ABGs)	Table 16-1
Electrolytes	Tables 5-2, 5-3, 5-5
Coagulation Tests	Table 17-4

◆ Telemetry

Continuous monitoring of cardiac rate and rhythm often is done by telemetry. Disposable electrodes and wire leads from a bedside monitor or battery-operated transmitter unit (Figure 19-4) are applied to the patient. The wave pattern signals are sent to a monitor in a central station, where they are continually observed. This allows patients to walk around the nursing unit while being monitored. The wave may also be displayed on a bedside *oscilloscope*. An oscilloscope is a machine that shows a picture of electrical current and its variations. In this instance, the patient's movement is limited by the wire attachments. Modern computerized telemetry monitors can detect specific **dysrhythmias** (abnormal variations of heart rhythm), automatically store the wave pattern, and alert the nurse to the abnormality with sound. Telemetry monitoring is used for patients experiencing an acute cardiac disorder, following cardiac surgery, and after pacemaker insertion. Figure 19-5 shows proper placement for telemetry leads.

NURSING MANAGEMENT

◆ Assessment

History Taking   It is important to determine whether there are risk factors for heart disease. Important data include any family history of heart disease, diabetes mellitus, high blood pressure, stroke, gout, or kidney disease. It is helpful, too, to know about the patient's

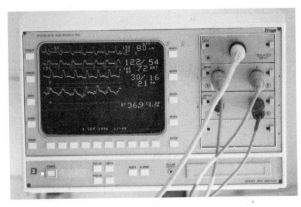

FIGURE 19-4   Bedside EKG monitoring. (Photo by Glen Derbyshire; courtesy of Goleta Valley Cottage Hospital, Goleta, CA.)

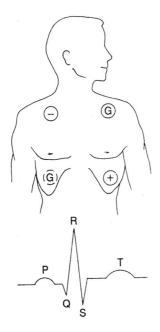

Placement of lead II electrodes.

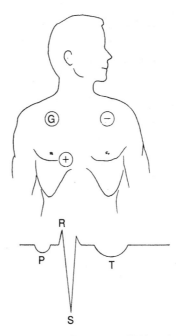

Placement of MCL₁ electrodes.

FIGURE 19-5   Placement of most commonly used telemetry leads. (*Source:* deWit, S. C. [1994]. *Rambo's Nursing Skills for Clinical Practice,* 4th ed. Philadelphia: Saunders, p. 1074.)

lifestyle, such as smoking, drinking, drug use, and eating habits; weight gains or losses; type and amount of daily exercise; occupation; and sources of stress.

Much of this information is obtained by the physician when he takes a medical history and by the nurse in a complete nursing assessment done at the time the patient is admitted to the hospital. There will be some additional information, however, that is gathered in less formal interactions when the patient becomes more relaxed and comfortable with the nurses who care for him.

Information concerning the patient's actual eating habits, such as snacking on "junk" food or daily consumption of several drinks containing caffeine, is more likely to be obtained during nursing care activities than during the initial assessment. Data concerning stressors in the patient's life and his response to them are more easily assessed while interacting over time.

> An understanding of the patient's perception of his disorder and overall health are necessary to plan appropriate teaching for him.

Important subjective data related to heart status include chest pain, fatigue, complaints of shortness of breath, cough, hemoptysis (bloody sputum), palpitations, and nocturia. Light-headedness, dizziness, or fainting also are associated with cardiovascular disease. The effectiveness of your communication with the patient will determine the quality of subjective data obtained. Table 19-4 provides a history taking guide.

Physical Assessment   Guidelines for physical assessment are presented in Table 19-5. Significant findings include abnormal or extra heart sounds; crackles in the lungs; orthopneic position (sitting up in bed

---

TABLE 19-4 ◆ *Assessment: Guidelines for History Taking*

When interviewing the patient who has a probable heart problem, ask the following questions:

◆ Where is the pain? What does it feel like? What, if anything, seems to bring it on? What makes it worse? How long does it last? Is it worse when you breathe in deeply? What gives relief? Does the pain radiate (spread) to other parts of the body, for example, down the arm, upward to the neck and jaws, to the upper abdomen? Is it localized, or does it cover a large area? On a scale of 1 to 10, with 10 being the worst and 1 being the least, how do you rate your pain?

◆ When do you notice shortness of breath? Do you sleep on more than one pillow? Is your shortness of breath worse after physical activity? What kind of activity? Walking up steps? Does it occur when you are at rest? Does resting relieve it? Do you wake up at night short of breath or feeling like you are suffocating? Does sitting up on the side of the bed or getting up give you relief?

◆ What kind of cough do you have—dry and hacking or wet and productive? What does the sputum look like? Is there ever any blood in your sputum?

◆ Do you notice your heart beating very fast or pounding in your chest? Does it skip a beat?

◆ Do you get up in the night to urinate? How many times do you get up each night?

◆ Do you ever feel lightheaded or faint?

TABLE 19-5 ◆ *Assessment: Guide to Physical Assessment of the Heart*

When assessing the heart, assess and check for:

- Skin color, temperature, and texture
- Facial expression; signs of pain or anxiety
- Vital signs
- Heart sounds, S_1, S_2, abnormal sounds, murmurs
- Apical pulse rate and rhythm; presence of pulse deficit
- Quality of peripheral pulses
- Breath sounds, presence of crackles in lung bases
- Shape of fingers; presence of clubbing
- Appearance of neck veins; presence of venous jugular distention
- Abdomen; presence of distention; abdominal pulsation
- Degree of body tension
- Ankles and feet; presence of edema and degree
- General body appearance; presence of edema
- Weight; gain of 2 lb or more over a few days

with two or three pillows behind the back) to ease breathing; placement of hand on chest, indicating pain; a bluish cast to skin, or pallor; diaphoresis (sweating); clubbing of the fingers; pitting edema of the feet, ankles, or sacral area; distended jugular veins; and abnormal rate or volume of pulses, or a pulse deficit. A pulse deficit is the difference between the apical and radial pulse rate when they are counted at the same time.

An apical pulse rate should be taken on all patients upon admission. Privacy should be provided before baring the chest and the room should be warm. Heart sounds are auscultated at least every 8 hours on all patients who have a known dysrhythmia or a potential for dysrhythmia, a valve problem, or heart failure. The diaphragm of the stethoscope is placed over the bare skin at the mitral area to listen to the apical pulse. S_1 (lub) and S_2 (dub) should be distinguished. **The pulse should be counted for a full minute.**

The bell of the stethoscope is used to listen for heart murmurs. **It must be placed lightly on the skin for the sounds to be heard.** Aortic valve sounds are heard in the second right intercostal space close to the sternum. The pulmonic valve is heard in the left second intercostal space close to the sternum. The tricuspid valve sounds are located at the left lower sternal border, and the mitral valve sounds are found in the apical area at the left fifth intercostal space at the midclavicular line. Figure 19-6 shows the locations for auscultation of heart sounds. As heart sounds often are very soft, ask the patient to refrain from talking, and turn off the television or radio while listening. (Just remember to turn it back on.) Having the patient roll to the left side or lean forward may make the sounds louder and clearer.

Elder Care Point . . . The thickening of valve leaflets with age may cause a systolic murmur commonly heard in persons over age 80.

◆Nursing Diagnosis

In addition to the individual nursing care plans in this chapter, Table 19-6 presents general nursing diagnoses and nursing interventions for patients experiencing problems with heart disease. Additional nursing diagnoses that also may apply include:

- Alteration in tissue perfusion related to decreased cardiac output (i.e., kidney failure related to decreased perfusion).
- Pain related to cardiac ischemia (e.g., deficiency of blood supply to a part of the heart).
- Risk for infection related to abnormality of lining of heart structures.
- Impairment of tissue integrity related to cardiac surgical incisions.
- Body image disturbance related to disease of heart, surgical scar, or inability to maintain former lifestyle.
- Anxiety related to life-threatening disease.

◆Planning

General nursing goals for care of patients with heart disease are:

- Prevent death and complications.
- Monitor for complications.
- Promote adequate oxygenation.
- Alleviate or control pain.
- Decrease fear and anxiety.

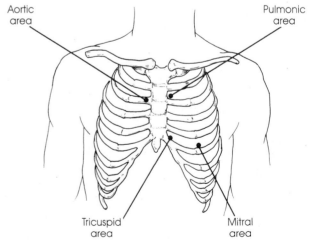

FIGURE 19-6   Sites for auscultation of heart sounds.

TABLE 19-6 ◆ *Common Nursing Diagnoses and Interventions for Patients with Heart Disorders**		
Nursing Diagnosis	**Goals/Expected Outcomes**	**Interventions**
Activity intolerance related to decreased perfusion.	Patient will not experience undue fatigue with activity as evidenced by changes in vital signs.	Space activities of daily living and nursing procedures to prevent undue fatigue. Encourage use of oxygen as ordered. Implement actions to promote rest.
Risk for injury related to dysrhythmia or complications of MI or CHF.	Patient will not experience myocardial infarction or congestive heart failure as a result of dysrhythmia.	Monitor EKG or telemetry tracings, observing for changes and life-threatening dysrhythmias. Assess for complications: ◆ Monitor lungs for crackles. ◆ Check for jugular venous distention. ◆ Auscultate for changes in heart sounds, extra sounds, changes in rhythm. ◆ Assess respirations for increasing dyspnea. ◆ Assess for signs of inflammation or infection; check temperature trend, WBCs. ◆ Assess for chest pain upon exertion or at rest. ◆ Monitor for central and peripheral edema. ◆ Assess trends in daily weight. ◆ Assess trends in 24-hour intake and output. ◆ Monitor vital signs.
Decreased cardiac output related to dysrhythmia or ineffective cardiac muscle.	Patient will demonstrate adequate cardiac output as evidenced by normal pulses, vital signs, skin color, and urine output.	Assess apical pulse q shift. Administer antiarrhythmic and cardiotonic medications as ordered. Observe for side effects of medications. Assess for adequate perfusion: ◆ Check peripheral pulses. ◆ Assess color of extremities and around mouth. ◆ Assess mentation. ◆ Monitor urine output (related to perfusion of kidneys). ◆ Auscultate lungs for crackles q shift. ◆ Assess level of fatigue. ◆ Treat impaired oxygenation and fluid imbalance.
Impaired gas exchange related to cardiac failure.	Patient will not experience impaired oxygenation; SaO$_2$ will be within normal limits; pO$_2$ between 80 and 100.	Place in high Fowler's position. Administer oxygen as ordered. Feed frequent small meals to decrease oxygen demand. Administer diuretics as ordered. Monitor intake and output. Enforce fluid restrictions. Assist with ADLs. Promote relief of anxiety. Give morphine as ordered to ease breathing and decrease anxiety. Monitor lung sounds, pulse oximetry, and blood gases. Assist to use incentive spirometer q 2 hours as ordered. Provide measures to drain pulmonary fluid as ordered; i.e., postural drainage, suction, nebulizer treatments.
Self-care deficit, bathing, toileting, grooming, and dressing related to fatigue, weakness, or dyspnea.	Patient will increase performance of own ADLs of 1 to 3 METs within 1 week. Patient will not experience constipation.	Assist with all ADLs as needed. Plan nursing treatments to provide rest periods. Encourage to do small tasks of ADLs as condition improves. Assist to turn in bed q 2 h. Assess skin q shift and when turning. Provide mouth care before meals to stimulate appetite. Give stool softeners and/or laxatives as ordered to prevent straining at stool (Valsalva maneuver).

(Table 19-6 continued)

TABLE 19-6 ◆ *Common Nursing Diagnoses and Interventions for Patients with Heart Disorders* *(Continued)*		
Nursing Diagnosis	**Goals/Expected Outcomes**	**Interventions**
Fear related to life-threatening illness.	Patient will verbalize feelings and fears regarding life-threatening condition. Patient will identify own best coping mechanisms.	Perform a spiritual assessment. Determine usual coping style. Support in coping mechanisms. Obtain clergyman if patient desires contact. Provide privacy for prayer and devotions. Assist to ventilate fears to reduce anxiety. Keep informed of what is being done for treatment and what to expect. Inform of positive gains toward wellness. Allow state of denial in acute stage as denial may be protective. Provide time with loved ones. Provide therapeutic touch if patient is accepting. Assess cultural meanings of events to patient. Actively listen to the patient's fears and concerns. Offer realistic reassurance as appropriate.
Impaired home maintenance management related to fatigue, dyspnea, and activity intolerance.	Appropriate home services will be in place before discharge.	Refer for social services consult. Consider home health care services. Offer information on homemaker aide services. Consult with family regarding ongoing care of patient at home. Collaborate with patient regarding plans for home care.

*See Nursing Care Plans 19-1 and 19-2.

- ◆ Balance activity and rest to prevent fatigue and provide adequate tissue perfusion.
- ◆ Assist with activities of daily living (ADLs) until patient can resume self-care.
- ◆ Educate regarding disease, surgery, treatments, and self-care.
- ◆ Promote adjustment to condition.
- ◆ Promote rehabilitation and return to wellness.
- ◆ Obtain assistance with home maintenance as needed.

A goal of community nursing is the promotion of healthful living to prevent heart disease.

When planning care for cardiac patients, it is important to schedule nursing activities to conserve the strength of the patient and prevent excessive fatigue. Patients undergoing telemetry monitoring should not be disconnected from their monitor for any extended time. The nurse should check to see whether it is all right to disconnect the device before the patient showers. **Reconnect the leads immediately afterward.**

Planning the timing of medication administration is necessary because many patients prefer to take cardiac medications with food in their stomach. If medications are due when a meal is not scheduled, plan to take some juice to the room with the medications. Always check to see that the medication can be taken with food before administering with juice or milk.

Collaboration Cardiac patients often are being treated by the physical therapist, dietitian, and respiratory therapist as well as the physician and nurse. It is important that the nurse consult with the other health professionals involved in the patient's care. Early collaboration with the discharge planner is important to provide continuity of care after discharge. The nurse's work will go more smoothly if it is possible to plan when other health professionals see the patient. Providing others on the health care team with information useful to them promotes a good working relationship.

◆ Implementation

Remember that any patient experiencing fatigue or weakness takes longer to accomplish the tasks of daily living. Space nursing actions appropriately. Place patients in an upright position to administer oral medications. It is especially important that the elderly patient be upright to aid swallowing; have the patient take a sip of water to wet the throat and then give the medication.

Watch the patient receiving cardiac drugs for postural hypotension; have the patient hold onto the bedrail and steady himself for a couple of minutes after arising before beginning to walk. This will help prevent falls.

Appropriate nursing interventions are discussed with the various disorders in this chapter. Specific nursing interventions for common nursing diagnoses related to heart conditions also are found in the nursing care plans and in Table 19-6.

♦ Evaluation

Evaluation involves both subjective and objective data. This means that good communication skills must be used to ask the right questions and gather the required information from the patient. Ask the patient to describe any "different" feelings he has experienced. Inquire about changes in appetite and bowel movements that could indicate possible medication toxicity. Check laboratory values for therapeutic drug levels before giving doses of medication, and note the latest blood levels of electrolytes. **Assess for signs and symptoms of toxicity and fluid or electrolyte imbalance.** Ask yourself whether the patient is showing signs indicating that the medication you are giving is effective. The nursing care plan should be checked daily to evaluate whether each nursing action is effective or not. If an action is ineffective over time, it should be deleted and a new action should be devised to resolve the problem.

DISORDERS OF THE HEART

♦ Coronary Artery Disease

When a sudden obstruction to blood flow through one or more major coronary arteries (coronary occlusion) occurs, cutting off oxygen and nutrients to the cardiac cells, the result is commonly known as a heart attack. If tissue death results from the lack of blood flow to the heart muscle, the patient suffers a myocardial infarction (MI). Obstruction to blood flow usually is caused by atherosclerosis and thrombus formation, but can also result from embolus or arterial spasm.

> Coronary heart disease (CHD) is the leading cause of death in the United States and caused 487,490 deaths in 1994.

♦ Atherosclerosis

The term *atherosclerosis* refers to a disease process within the arteries. It can affect the cerebral vessels and the aorta and arteries other than the coronaries. It is one form of arteriosclerosis.

Pathophysiology   The process of atherosclerosis begins during childhood, when streaks or islands of fatty material are laid down on the inner walls of the arteries. Later, fibrinous plaques are formed as a result of inflammation and healing. The plaque area protrudes into the artery, decreasing the vessel's size.

Narrowing of the coronary arteries causes coronary insufficiency (decreased or insufficient blood flow). Obstruction occurs from this process and from thrombosis. The plaque areas eventually rupture, causing platelet clumping and clotting (thrombosis). Spasm of the artery may contribute to occlusion and consequent heart muscle damage.

Elder Care Point... Coronary blood flow in a 60-year-old is about 35% of the amount of flow in a 25-year-old.

Causative Factors   Experts do not agree completely on the reasons for the development of atherosclerosis and coronary artery disease. Atherosclerosis occurs from childhood on and affects all people to some degree. **There is a proven link between high serum cholesterol or high levels of low-density lipoproteins and coronary artery disease (CAD).** There also seem to be many environmental and genetic factors involved. Patients with diabetes and hypertension appear to develop arteriosclerosis more rapidly.

Environmental factors that are most strongly suspected of contributing to atherosclerosis include emotional stress, heavy smoking, obesity or a diet high in saturated fats, and lack of physical exercise. Genetic factors include such familial diseases as diabetes, hypertension, and abnormal fat metabolism (hyperlipidemia). Those who have had one or more immediate family members die of coronary artery disease during their middle years are considered to be at high risk for the disorder.

Atherosclerosis is indirectly diagnosed by blood lipid levels and by x-rays of the arteries. If elevated cholesterol and triglyceride levels cannot be lowered by a low-fat diet and exercise, then drugs that have been found to lower blood lipids are prescribed. Examples include cholestyramine (Questran), gemfibrozil (Lopid), lovastatin (Mevocor), and fenofibrate (Lipidol). The new anticholesterol drug simvastatin (Zocor) has proven effectiveness in prolonging the life of patients with heart disease.

♦ Angina Pectoris

The American Heart Association estimates that more than 7,120,000 people in the United States have angina pectoris and that approximately 350,000 new cases occur each year.

Pathophysiology   The decreased blood flow that occurs with coronary insufficiency causes pain in the heart muscle, known as *angina pectoris,* or "strangling pain in the chest." Decreased blood flow is caused by atherosclerotic plaque narrowing the artery or arterial spasm. **Any activity that increases the heart's workload increases its need for oxygen.** When the occluded coronary arteries cannot deliver adequate amounts of blood to meet these needs, the patient experiences an angina attack. Attacks can be brought on by physical exertion, emotional excitement, eating a heavy meal, or exposure to cold.

When the patient's angina is no longer adequately controlled by medication and his attacks become more frequent or severe, surgery is indicated to prevent a life-threatening myocardial infarction (MI).

Symptoms and Diagnosis   **The type of pain or discomfort may vary in individuals, but in most cases it is described as a dull pain or tightness under the sternum or pain that goes up into the neck and jaw. It may or may not radiate down one or both arms. It most commonly radiates down the right arm. Sometimes the patient experiences dyspnea, and there may be pallor or flushing of the face, profuse perspiration, and apprehension.** Angina pain is most often described as a dull ache and is seldom sharp or stabbing.

Medical diagnosis is established on the basis of history, clinical signs and symptoms, and whether rest and nitroglycerin provide relief during an acute attack. Response of the heart muscle to increased oxygen demands can be determined by exercise stress testing.

Treatment   The treatment of angina pectoris is mostly symptomatic, with emphasis on eliminating those factors that are known to precipitate an attack in the individual patient. With guidance and teaching, the patient may soon be able to correlate certain activities with an attack and thereby learn to avoid them whenever possible. Medications commonly used for patients with angina are presented in Table 19-7. Nitroglycerin, nitrates, calcium antagonists, and beta-blockers are used in combination with drugs to lower cholesterol and prevent platelet aggregation. A low daily dose of aspirin, or one baby aspirin, has been added to the treatment of CAD. Aspirin helps prevent clotting and may prevent a thrombosis that could cause an MI. New forms of nitroglycerin administration include a nitrolingual aerosol, which the patient sprays on or under his tongue, and a buccal tablet, Nitrogard, which is placed between the upper lip and gum. It dissolves slowly over a 3- to 5-hour period.

Effects of the Cold   When the body is exposed to cold, the blood vessels constrict. The patient with angina pectoris is already suffering from a narrowing of the arteries, and thus he must avoid exposure to cold, which will further aggravate the condition. He should be instructed to wear warm clothing and stay indoors when the weather is extremely cold. Guidelines for teaching patients who experience anginal attacks are in Table 19-8. Nursing interventions for selected problems in a patient with angina pectoris are summarized in Nursing Care Plan 19-1.

◆ Acute Myocardial Infarction (Acute MI)

About 1,500,000 Americans suffer an MI annually. Although male victims outnumber females almost 2 to 1, females die more frequently after an MI. At least 250,000 people a year die of heart attack within 1 hour of the onset of symptoms and never reach a hospital.

Pathophysiology   An **infarction** is an area of coagulation in tissue caused by an obstruction to the flow of blood to that area for a prolonged period (Figure 19-7). *Myocardial* means "pertaining to the heart muscle." Thus in a myocardial infarction, there is an area of **necrosis** (cell death) in the heart muscle. Dead tissue does not return to normal, scar tissue forms and interferes with normal function. Obstruction of blood flow in the coronary arteries may be caused by thrombosis, embolus, or severe arterial spasm. Most cases are related to obstruction from atherosclerosis.

The prognosis of the patient who suffers an acute myocardial infarction depends on the size of the artery plugged by an obstruction and the amount of heart tissue that the artery had formerly supplied with blood. If a large area of the heart is affected, instant death may occur. Smaller areas may heal if treated promptly and effectively. Most MIs occur in the left ventricle, the main "pump." Cardiopulmonary resuscitation of an acute MI victim is discussed in Chapter 30.

Symptoms and Diagnosis   The clinical picture presented by the patient with an acute MI is one that most people recognize as a "heart attack." There is a sudden, severe pain in the chest, usually described as crushing or burning, that is not relieved by nitrates or rest. Sometimes the pain is mistaken for a symptom of acute indigestion or anginal pain the patient has experienced before. Denial is a real factor in seeking treatment. The patient also shows symptoms of shock, with pallor, profuse sweating, anxiety, and often nausea and vomiting. The heart rate may be very fast (**tachycardia**) or very slow (**bradycardia**). In women and the elderly, the attack may present as an uncomfortable pressure, fullness, squeezing or pain in the center of the chest that lasts more than a few minutes or goes away and comes back.

Think about . . . How could you possibly determine whether a patient is suffering an anginal attack or an MI?

TABLE 19-7 ◆ *Medications Commonly Prescribed for Heart Problems*

Classification and Action	Examples*	Nursing Implications	Patient Teaching

Cardiotonics (Cardiac Glycosides)
Use:
CHF, atrial fibrillation, atrial flutter, tachycardia.
Action:
Strengthen contractions, providing more blood to body tissues and decrease the heart rate by slowing conduction of the cardiac impluse through the AV node.
	Digoxin (Lanoxin)
	digitoxin
		Before administration: take apical pulse for 1 full minute, listening for bradycardia and new irregular rhythm; verify the serum digoxin or digitoxin level.
		  Normal values are:
		  Digoxin 0.5–2.0 ng/mL
		  Digitoxin <35 ng/mL
		Verify that serum potassium is within normal limits of 3.5 to 5.3 mEq/L.; assess for signs and symptoms of digitalis toxicity: anorexia, nausea, vomiting, visual disturbances, headache, malaise, bradycardia, dysrhythmias. If abnormalities are found, consult physician before giving the drug.
			Instruct how to take own pulse rate; ask to record rate daily. Notify physician if rate is below 60 bpm or newly irregular. Ask to eat foods high in potassium, such as fresh and dried fruits, citrus fruit juices, avocados, and vegetables. Stress importance of compliance to dosage schedule.

Use: short-term treatment of CHF. **Action:** peripheral vasodilation that reduces preload and afterload.	Amrinone lactate (Inocor) Milrinone (Primacor)	Monitor for hypotension; watch hydration status. Assess lungs for decreasing crackles in bases. May decrease platelet count.	
Antianginals—Nitrates **Use:** angina pectoris, conditions helped by increased blood flow. **Action:** relaxes and dilates the vessels and lowers cardiac workload by decreasing venous return to the heart.	Nitroglycerin (Nitrostat) Nitroprusside (Nipride) Nitro-Bid (Isosorbide dinitrate (Isordil) Pentaerythritol (Peritrate) Transderm Nitro Nitroglycerin lingual spray (Nitrolingual) Nitroglycerine buccal tablets (Nitroguard) Nitroglycerin transdermal patch (Nitrdur II)	Take baseline blood pressure before administering sublingual form. Take blood pressure again at 5 minutes and at 10 minutes. If blood pressure continues to rise, call physician. Observe for possible hypotension. Use gloves to apply ointment; wash hands afterward. Check transdermal patch q shift to see that it is intact.	Teach to wet sublingual tablet with saliva and place it under the tongue. Warn it may cause headache. May repeat dose every 5 minutes up to three tablets. If pain persists, call emergency number. For patch: remove old patch when applying a new one. Take oral tablets on an empty stomach either ½ hour before meals or 1–2 hours after meals. Store tablets in cool place in light-proof container. Carry tablets at all times. Replace supply every 3 months.
Antianginals: Beta Blockers **Use:** angina pectoris, MI, some dysrhythmias. **Action:** Slow the heart rate and decrease strength of cardiac contraction, thereby decreasing cardiac workload.	Propranolol (Inderal) Atenolol (Tenormin) Metoprolol (Lopressor) Celiprolol (Selecor) Nadolol (Corgard)	Contraindicated in patients with asthma (may cause bronchoconstriction) or diabetes mellitus (masks signs of hypoglycemia). Check apical pulse rate before administering. Notify anesthesiologist before surgery that patient is taking a beta-blocker. Elderly may experience prolonged drug action; watch for toxic effects. Monitor blood pressure and potassium levels regularly. Elderly may experience prolonged drug action.	Take medication with meals. Do not stop taking the drug abruptly. Do not break, crush, or chew this medication. Protect capsules from direct sunlight.

(Table 19-7 continued)

TABLE 19-7 ◆ *Medications Commonly Prescribed for Heart Problems* (*Continued*)

Classification and Action	Examples*	Nursing Implications	Patient Teaching
Calcium Channel Blockers (antagonist) **Use:** angina pectoris, hypertension, some dysrhythmias, treat vasospasm post-MI. **Action:** Decreases cardiac contractility and may slow pulse, thereby decreasing cardiac workload; dilates coronary arteries.	Verapamil (Calan) Nifedipine (Procardia) Diltiazem (Cardizem) Nicardipine (Cardene) Amlopidine (Norvasc) Bepridil (Vascor)	**See information under Class II and Class III antidysrhythmics** Monitor drug serum level for therapeutic range. Monitor pulse and blood pressure for new dysrhythmia, bradycardia, or hypotension before administering drug. Assess for side effects, such as nausea, vomiting, diarrhea, urinary retention, or confusion. Assess for side effects particular to specific drug. Check for drug interactions with other drugs the patient is receiving.	Instruct to report side effects and adverse reactions. Stress drug dosage schedule compliance. Advise to avoid caffeine, alcohol, and smoking. Warn about hypotension and encourage to change from lying to sitting position to standing slowly.
Antidysrhythmics (antiarrhythmics) Class I **Use:** Atrial and ventricular dysrhythmias. **Action:** Slow the sodium channel, prolong time of depolarization, and increase refractory period.	Quinidine sulfate Procainamide (Pronestyl, Procan) Disopyramide (Norpace) Lidocaine (Xylocaine) Phenytoin (Dilantin) Tocainide (Tonocard) Mexiletine (Mexitil) Encainide (Enkaid)	Quinidine: monitor for cinchonism: tinnitus, headache, nausea, vertigo, and disturbed vision. Observe for changes in EKG pattern. If patient is taking digitalis, monitor for digitalis toxicity as quinidine can double digoxin levels. Cimetidine increases effects of quinidine. Quinidine may enhance action of anticoagulants. Monitor for diarrhea. Monitor drug level. With procainamide monitor for systemic lupus erythematosus–like syndrome: joint pain, hepatomegaly; unexplained fever, soreness of the mouth, throat, or gums. Discontinue medication if this occurs. Observe for side effects or adverse effects of particular drug administered. Monitor electrolyte levels; watch for postural hypotension, especially if patient is taking antihypertensives.	Instruct to report signs of adverse effects of the drug. Report noticable changes in cardiac rhythm to the physician. Advise to take quinidine with meals to prevent gastrointestinal (GI) upset. Advise to minimize citrus fruit intake as it changes the urine pH and decreases excretion of quinidine. Procainamide is absorbed best on an empty stomach; if GI upset occurs take immediately after a meal.
Class II (Beta Blockers) **Use:** atrial and ventricular dysrhythmias. **Action:** slow sinoatrial nodal impulses.	Propanolol (Inderal) Acebutolol (Sectral) Atenolol (Tenormin) Nadolol (Corgard) Timolol (Apo-Timol) Metroprolol (Lopressor) Pindolol (Visken) Esmolol (Brevibloc)	Monitor for signs of CHF; monitor pulse and blood pressure watching for bradycardia and hypotension. Monitor electrolytes. Monitor blood sugar in diabetics carefully.	Instruct not to discontinue the medication abruptly. Nofity physician if skin rash, confusion, fever, sore throat, or unusual bleeding or bruising occur. Monitor weight and report gain of more than 2 lb in 1 week. Report edema or shortness of breath.
Class III **Use:** control supraventricular and ventricular dysrhythmias. **Action:** increase the refractory period and action potential duration.	Amiodarone (Cordarone) Bretylium (Bretylol) Sotalol (Sotacort) Ibutilide (Corvert)	Check for drug interactions and for side or adverse effects of specific drug administered. Monitor heart rhythm, blood pressure, and pulse. Monitor renal function.	Instruct to report adverse reactions to specific drug being taken. Advise of need for physician supervision. Report any new heart rhythm irregularities.

TABLE 19-7 ◆ *Medications Commonly Prescribed for Heart Problems* (Continued)

Classification and Action	Examples*	Nursing Implications	Patient Teaching
Class IV (calcium-channel blockers) **Use:** paroxysmal supraventricular tachycardia (PSVT) **Action:** Converts PSVT to normal sinus rhythm by slowing conduction time through the nodes.	Verapamil (Calan, Isoptin, Verelan)	Monitor heart rate and rhythm; watch for signs of CHF. Observe for hypotension and edema. Use very cautiously with beta-blockers.	Instruct to report signs of edema, shortness of breath, or weight gain of more than 2 lb in 1 week. Notify physician of new changes in heart rhythm.
Diuretics—Thiazides and related drugs **Use:** edema and hypertension. **Action:** block tubular reabsorption of water, sodium, and chloride; promote excretion of potassium.	Chlorothiazide (Diuril) Chlortalidone (Hygroton) Hydrochlorothiazide (Esidrix) Indapamide (Lozol) Metolazone (Zaroxolyn)	Observe for side effects of thiazide diuretics, such as electrolyte imbalances, elevated blood sugar, and elevated uric acid levels. Hyperlipidemia also may occur. Potassium supplementation is frequently necessary. Patients also should be monitored for constipation.	Ask patient to monitor weight to determine effectiveness of diuretic. Instruct to eat foods high in potassium or take prescribed potassium supplement as ordered. Increase fiber and exercise to decrease potential for constipation.
Diuretics—Loop diuretics **Use:** edema, hypertension, CHF. **Action:** inhibits reabsorption of sodium in the loop of Henle; promotes water and sodium excretion; potassium also is excreted.	Ethacrynic acid (Edecrin) Furosemide (Lasix) Bumetanide (Bumex) Torsemide (Demadex)	Patients with a history of thrombophlebitis who are taking a diuretic should be monitored closely for recurrence. Given once a day doses in the A.M. to promote diuresis before bedtime. Loop diuretics are potent drugs. Side effects and nursing implications are much the same as for the thiazide diuretics except that loop diuretics promote calcium excretion and can be ototoxic (hearing loss). Monitor for changes in monitoring.	Instruct in the signs of hypokalemia and the importance of taking in sufficient potassium while taking a loop diuretic. Ask to keep a daily weight chart and report any weight gain of more than 2 lb over 1 week without any alteration in diet or exercise.
Potassium-sparing drugs **Use:** edema, hypertension. **Action:** act on distal renal tubules, promoting water and sodium excretion and inhibiting potassium excretion.	Spironolactone (Aldactone) Amiloride (Moduretic) Triamterene (Dyazide, Maxide)	Potassium intake should not be increased. Observe for signs of sodium depletion. **Electrolyte levels should be checked periodically for all patients receiving daily diuretics.**	**Patients receiving diuretics should all be taught: (1) the purpose and desired effects of the drug; (2) the importance of taking the medication exactly as prescribed; (3) that signs of side effects and toxicity should be reported to the physician; (4) symptoms of potassium and sodium depletion.**
Anticoagulants **Use:** prevent clot and emboli formation. **Action:** heparin blocks the conversion of prothrombin to thrombin and fibrinogen to fibrin. Warfarin sodium inhibits the synthesis of vitamin K needed to form clotting factors.	Heparin warfarin sodium (Coumadin) Dicumarol Enoxaparin (Lovenox) Dalteparin (Fragmin)	Observe for signs of abnormal bleeding by: periodically checking vital signs; monitoring urine and stool for signs of internal bleeding; inspect skin for bruises and petechiae; ask about bleeding of gums with tooth brushing. For patients on IV heparin drips, place extra foam mattress on bed to prevent bruising of thighs and buttocks. Monitor for interactions with other drugs the patient is receiving as drug interactions can enhance or counter-	Explain the rationale for the administration of heparin. For patients receiving oral anticoagulants, instruct about the drug being administered; the hazards of hemorrhage; the reason for frequent blood tests, safety precautions, foods that affect clotting, and not to take over-the-counter medications without consulting the physician as they may alter the drug's effect. Warn specifically not to take aspirin or other salicylates.

(Table 19-7 continued)

TABLE 19-7 ◆ *Medications Commonly Prescribed for Heart Problems* (*Continued*)			
Classification and Action	**Examples***	**Nursing Implications**	**Patient Teaching**
		act the effect of coumarin. Aspirin and other salicyliates are contraindicated when the patient is receiving an anticoagulant. Patients on oral anticoagulants may experience fatigue. Monitor clotting times. For heparin: APPT or PPT should be 1½ to 2 times the control value. Consult physician if APPT or PT is approaching 70 sec. For coumadin: PT should be 2 to 2½ times the control or if reported as international normalized ratio (INR) should be between 1 and 2.5; hold the medication and report values greater than this to the physician immediately.	

*Generic drugs are listed first, followed by brand name in parentheses.

TABLE 19-8 ◆ *Patient Education: Guidelines for the Patient with Angina*

Patients who experience anginal attacks are taught to:

- Avoid eating heavy meals.
- Avoid physical activity for an hour after meals to prevent excessive oxygen demands.
- Take nitroglycerin before heavy physical activity that is known to cause an attack, such as intercourse or sports activities.
- Avoid exposure to cold; do not walk into a cold wind.
- Decrease controllable risk factors, such as lifestyle stress, obesity, hypertension, and improper diet.
- Adopt a regular, graduated exercise program.
- Stop smoking.
- Learn meditation or other deep relaxation techniques.
- Take a sublingual nitroglycerin tablet and lie down at the beginning of an anginal attack. Nitroglycerin may be repeated twice more at 5-minute intervals for a total of three tablets if the pain persists. If the pain has not eased within 15 minutes, notify the physician and have someone drive the patient to the emergency department.
- Check pulse rate once daily if taking a calcium-channel blocker or a beta-adrenergic blocker. These drugs should never be stopped abruptly; call doctor if heart rate drops below 60 beats per minute.
- Rise slowly from a supine or sitting position because of potential postural hypotension.
- Cleanse area of previous application of nitroglycerin paste when applying a new dose.
- Keep appointments for regular checkups.
- Obtain sufficient rest daily.
- Avoid high environmental temperatures and high humidity; stay in air-conditioned areas when such conditions occur as they increase cardiac workload.
- Nitrates may initially cause a headache and hypotension.

Although these symptoms are usually present in an acute MI, they are not always severe, and in some cases patients have described their pain as mild. Sometimes the patient only experiences left-arm, jaw, or back pain. The electrocardiogram (EKG) may or may not show evidence of an MI initially. For this reason EKGs are repeated serially every 8 to 12 hours for three times or on a daily basis for 3 days. Changes slowly evolve and are evident on the EKG. The severity of the symptoms will depend on the size of the area of ischemia or infarction. Some researchers claim that chewing an aspirin when signs of an MI occur may decrease or prevent heart damage.

Whenever there is necrotic tissue anywhere in the body, the white cell count increases and the sedimentation rate rises. Within 24 hours of an acute attack, the temperature of the patient with MI rises slightly, and mild leukocytosis appears.

In addition to the clinical manifestations, EKG changes, and other diagnostic tests, laboratory determinations of specific enzymes are used to establish a diagnosis of MI and evaluate the extent of damage done to the heart muscle. Creatine kinase (CK) isoenzymes, aspartate transaminase (AST, SGOT), lactic dehydrogenase (LDH), and LDH isoenzyme levels are observed over a 72-hour period. New tests, serum troponin T and troponin I, are accurate within a few hours. These enzymes are measured by enzyme-linked immunosorbent assay (ELISA). They are 100% accurate from 10 to 120 hours after symptom onset. (See Table 19-3 for information on diagnostic tests.) The level of CK-MB bond rises in 4 to 8 hours and begins to decline in 12 to 24 hours; LDH level increases 24 to 48 hours after an

Nursing Care Plan 19-1

Selected nursing diagnoses, goals/expected outcomes, nursing interventions, and evaluations for a patient with angina pectoris (coronary insufficiency)

Situation: Patient is a 63-year-old female with a history of chest pains and dyspnea brought on by physical or emotional exertion. She is 55 pounds overweight and has smoked "about two packs" of cigarettes each day since she was 17 years old. She is admitted for diagnostic tests to evaluate the presence and extent of coronary atherosclerosis.

Nursing Diagnosis	Goals/Expected Outcome	Nursing Intervention	Evaluation
Pain related to cardiac ischemia SUPPORTING DATA Clutching hand to center of chest, states "I'm having chest pain."	Pain will be relieved within 15 minutes by sublingual nitroglycerin. Patient will identify any precipitating cause for pain.	Teach to lie down and rest when pain appears. Assess pulse, blood pressure, and respirations and administer sublingual nitroglycerin. Assess vital signs in 5 minutes; assess degree of continuing pain; administer another nitroglyercin tablet after 5 minutes if needed × 2. When pain has subsided and patient is stable and calm, explore possible causes of onset of pain.	Chest pain at 11:30 relieved after two nitroglycerin tablets; son had just visited; became upset over financial problem; continue plan.
Anxiety related to diagnostic tests and recurrent chest pain. SUPPORTING DATA "I don't want to die. Isn't a cardiac catheterization dangerous?"	Patient will verbalize understanding of procedure in event of anginal attack to help diagnose cause of pain. Patient will verbalize that anxiety has decreased within 12 hours.	Explain that EKG is to be done each time she has severe chest pain. Ask patient to report onset of pain promptly so that medication can be given and EKG can be done. Establish trusting relationship and allow patient to ventilate fears and concerns. Assure her that she will be monitored closely. Prepare her for stress test and cardiac catheterization and have other patients who have had these tests talk with her. Answer her questions and help her prepare a list of questions she wishes to ask her physician.	Teaching for diagnostic tests done; spoke with patient who had had cardiac catheterization; states she is less anxious about it; continue plan.
Lack of knowledge about low-fat, low-calorie diet and exercise program. SUPPORTING DATA Cannot describe ways to cut fat in diet and is unaware of calorie content of various foods. Does not exercise regularly.	Within 1 week patient will be able to verbalize ways to cut amount of fat in diet. Patient will express commitment to low-calorie diet and desire to lose 55 pounds over the next 6 months by discharge. Patient will design regular exercise program before discharge. Patient will stick to exercise and diet program at end of 2 months. Patient will reach and maintain normal weight. Cholesterol will be within normal limits at end of 6 months.	Perform a dietary assessment with 24-hour food intake history of usual diet. Provide consult with dietician. Provide materials from American Heart Association and telephone numbers for local support groups such as Weight Watchers, Overeaters Anonymous, or TOPS. Provide emotional support for patient and praise all efforts to learn about needed lifestyle changes. Help her to design an exercise program that fits into lifestyle and that she will be willing to continue.	Met with dietician; states that a neighbor goes to Weight Watchers and that she will consider that; she could walk in the evenings with her husband; is considering options; continue plan.
Risk of injury related to cigarette smoking. SUPPORTING DATA Has smoked 2 packs of cigarettes per day for 46 years; is craving cigarettes constantly.	Patient will state desire to quit smoking by discharge. Patient will stop smoking within 3 weeks.	Explain that nicotine causes vasoconstriction, which further compromises oxygen supply to the heart; explain danger of coronary occlusion. Allow patient to ventilate her anxiety and concerns over trying to quit smoking. Obtain American Lung Association and American Cancer Society literature for her on quitting smoking. Help her design realistic plan for quitting smoking, including support from significant others.	Discussed action of nicotine in body; given AHA literature on quitting smoking; cut back to 1 pack yesterday, ¾ pack today; continue plan.

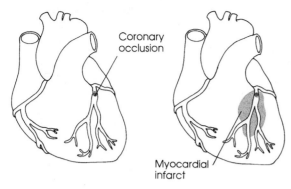

FIGURE 19-7 Occlusion of a major coronary artery in left leads to an area of infarct right, resulting from ischemia.

MI and stays high for up to 2 weeks. A flipped ratio of LDH-1 to LDH-2 occurs in the presence of an MI. A new CK-MB bond assay test may be able to diagnose an MI within 2 hours of onset of chest pain.

Think about . . . How would you prepare the patient who has experienced a probable MI for the diagnostic tests he will most likely undergo? What teaching is required?

Treatment   **As soon as a patient with an acute MI is brought to the emergency room, measures are taken to relieve pain, decrease ischemia, and prevent further circulatory collapse and shock.** In many large cities and some rural areas of the United States, there are specially designed and equipped mobile units staffed with trained personnel to give immediate care to the patient who has had a heart attack. This care is given while the patient is in transit to the hospital.

> Emergency care and cardiopulmonary resuscitation (CPR) are of critical importance in preventing death from an MI. Outside the hospital a trained emergency squad should be called immediately. If the patient shows signs of cardiac or respiratory arrest, help should be called and CPR with defibrillation, if indicated, should be started immediately.

Sublingual nitroglycerine is given unless contraindicated. Oral aspirin is administered in a dose of 160–325 mg. Drugs administered to control pain in a patient with acute MI are morphine sulfate, meperidine hydrochloride (Demerol), and hydromorphone hydrochloride (Dilaudid). One of these is given IV to provide immediate relief; morphine is the drug of choice. A nitrate infusion also may be started. Antiarrhythmia drugs are given as needed in the form or beta-blockers or lidocaine. Antianxiety agents, such as diazepam (Valium), are administered to relieve anxiety. Intrave-

nous fluids are started, oxygen is administered, and the patient's condition is stabilized.

> Close assessment of respiration is essential, as these drugs can depress respiration at a time when the heart needs all the oxygen it can get. Pain medication given IV has a shorter duration and doses must be repeated more frequently to keep the patient comfortable.

Acute care.   If the physician believes that damage is not extensive, the patient is admitted to a telemetry unit. If damage is considered extensive, admission to the coronary care unit (CCU) is the rule. Generally the patient is kept in the CCU for 1 to 2 days, then on a step-down telemetry unit for 2 to 4 days unless damage is very extensive. The patient is placed in bed and kept on bedrest with bedside commode privileges for 12 to 24 hours. Physical activity is gradually increased according to the patient's individual condition and response to therapy. An IV line or a PRN IV cannula is inserted to provide a route for administration of emergency drugs to control blood pressure and dysrhythmias.

Vital signs are continuously monitored by electronic means and are assessed by the nurse every 15 minutes to 2 hours. An automatic machine may be used electronically to read blood pressure, track heart rate and systolic and diastolic pressure, and calculate mean arterial pressure, which is an indicator of changes in heart function. A *pulse oximeter* is used to monitor oxygenation. This is an electronic device that, with the use of light and a sensor, measures oxygen saturation in the blood. The sensor is placed on the fingertip or ear lobe. Abnormal values are rechecked by arterial blood gas measurements, which are more accurate. Continuous EKG (cardiac telemetry monitoring) is essential to provide an accurate evaluation of the status of the heart. Death occurs most frequently within the first 2 hours and is due to ventricular fibrillation. Many complications can occur, and the nurse must be vigilant for the onset of signs and symptoms (Table 19-9).

The very critically ill patient will have more sophisticated monitoring done in the CCU. A pulmonary artery flow-directed catheter (Swan-Ganz type) may be inserted to read central venous pressure (CVP), pulmonary artery pressure (PAP), and pulmonary capillary wedge pressure (PCWP), which give a better picture of the injured heart's ability to pump. Noninvasive monitoring of cardiac output may be done with electrodes and computer software. The computerized impedance cardiograph is used externally to obtain data on cardiac output, cardiac index, and systemic vascular resistance. Thoracic electrical bioimpedance monitoring is new, and equipment is not available everywhere.

A liquid diet is ordered for the first 24 hours and then a low-sodium, low-fat diet is ordered when the patient's vital signs have stabilized. A stool softener is given to decrease the risk of bradycardia, which can be caused by straining. Potassium and magnesium are monitored closely as imbalances can cause dysrhythmias. Medication to correct dysrhythmia is ordered as needed. Measures to correct acid–base imbalance are begun. A beta-adrenergic blocker such as propranolol (Inderal) may be ordered to ease the heart's workload.

Continuous oxygen via mask or nasal cannula is begun at a rate of 2 to 5 L/minute. Various IV drugs may be used to regulate blood pressure or to control dysrhythmias; these include nitroglycerin (Nipride) to lower blood pressure and dopamine (Intropin) to raise blood pressure.

If the patient's heart rate drops below 40 and stays there, or if he experiences complete heart block where the electrical impulse does not go through the atrioventricular (AV) node to the ventricles and the ventricles are not signaled to contract, a temporary pacemaker may be inserted. (See "Disorders of the Heart's Conduction System" for information on pacemaker insertion.)

If the patient sought immediate medical attention upon experiencing the symptoms of MI, he may be given thrombolytic agents in an attempt to dissolve a clot obstructing the coronary artery. Thrombolytic therapy must be started within 2 to 6 hours to prevent necrosis of the myocardium and is indicated when the EKG shows ST segment elevation. Agents used IV to dissolve the clot include tissue plasminogen activator (t-PA), streptokinase, urokinase, and anistreplase (APSAC). These drugs are contraindicated in patients who have severe, uncontrolled hypertension, or a history of a hemorrhagic stroke, gastrointestinal (GI) bleed, intracranial or intraspinal surgery within the past 2 months, a brain tumor, arteriovenous malformation, or aneurysm. After one of these agents is infused, a heparin drip is started to prevent reocclusion. Heparin is continued for 3 to 4 days until the patient is stabilized on warfarin sodium (Coumadin), an oral anticoagulant. When a patient is not a candidate for thrombolytic therapy, heparin and low-dose aspirin may be administered to prevent further thrombosis.

When the patient is stabilized, further testing will be done. If a positron emmision tomography (PET) machine is available, an MRI, or PET scan may be ordered to assess the amount of cardiac damage present and determine which treatment is advisable. Otherwise coronary angiography via cardiac catheterization may be done. If only a few areas of stenosis are identified, the patient may have a percutaneous transluminal coronary angioplasty (PTCA) rather than coronary artery bypass graft surgery (CABG) to improve blood flow. The first, PTCA, is a nonsurgical technique to open blocked coronary arteries. It is performed in the cardiac catheterization laboratory using fluoroscopy. A catheter with a balloon attachment is threaded into the blocked artery, and when the narrowed area is reached, the balloon is inflated repeatedly, flattening the plaque and widening the interior of the artery. A stent may be left in place to help maintain the opening. A stent is made of stainless steel and acts as a brace for the artery wall. When a stent is left in place, the patient must take anticoagulants for a month afterward. Experimentation is under way with a new procedure using a laser to vaporize and extract the plaque from the artery. This is done with a similar-type catheter to avoid open-heart surgery. A new drug called ReoPro may be used to help prevent the formation of blood clots post PCTA. Another procedure called rotoablation, uses a similar catheter and a rotating device that shaves away plaque and extracts it to clear the artery. This is sometimes used when a patient has reocclusion after CABG and PTCA. CABG surgery is covered in the section on cardiac surgery.

Studies are ongoing to determine whether a regimen consisting of a very-low-fat diet, regular exercise, reduction of stress, and practice of relaxation techniques can reverse CAD without surgery. These methods have been effective in people who can maintain the discipline to stick to the program.

If the left ventricle is badly damaged, cardiogenic shock may occur and the intraaortic balloon pump

---

TABLE 19-9 ◆ *Signs and Symptoms of Complications after Myocardial Infarction*

Complication	Signs and Symptoms
Dysrhythmia	Irregular pulse; abnormal EKG pattern. Report more than three PVCs per minute, heart rate of more than 120 or less than 40 bpm.
CHF	Dyspnea, pedal edema, sacral edema, crackles in lung bases, distended neck veins, enlarged tender liver, weight gain of more than 2 lb in 24 hours.
Pulmonary edema	Crackles throughout lungs, severe dyspnea and orthopnea, frothy sputum, high anxiety, feeling that something terrible is wrong.
Cardiogenic shock	Significant drop in systolic blood pressure (>20 points), diaphoresis, rapid pulse, cold clammy skin, gray skin color, and restlessness.
Pericarditis	Pericardial friction rub upon auscultation, chest pain aggravated by movement and lessened by sitting up and leaning forward.

(IABP) may be used to ease the heart's workload while it begins to heal. This device is a highly technical machine using a balloon catheter positioned in the aorta that inflates during diastole and deflates during systole, effectively decreasing the workload of the heart and increasing blood flow through the coronary arteries.

Nursing Assessment and Intervention   All patients with heart disease should be taught the signs of MI and advised that the best survival rate is directly related to obtaining medical attention as early as possible (see Table 19-1).

Nursing care is directed at promoting rest, administering ordered medical therapy and observing for side effects, assisting with ADLs and ambulation, constantly monitoring physical status by performing a good cardiovascular assessment every 4 to 8 hours, and monitoring vital signs every 2 to 4 hours. Daily weight is recorded and compared with previous weight. Intake and output are accurately recorded and compared with previous amounts and urine output is closely monitored. A patent IV access is maintained at all times. Visitors are limited and the heart rate is monitored closely during visits. The nurse closely watches for signs of complications of MI, such as dysrhythmia, congestive heart failure, pulmonary edema, pericarditis, cardiogenic shock, or cardiac arrest. Table 19-9 presents hallmark signs and symptoms of these complications.

> It is vitally important that the nurse assess for signs of complications in the patient who has had a myocardial infarction. Quick identification and treatment of complications is lifesaving and greatly reduces the cost of treatment during recovery.

A very important nursing measure is to decrease anxiety and stress for the patient. It is helpful to explain the function of all equipment and tests in simple terms and to explain the routine of frequent assessment and tests so the patient will know what to expect. Visitors are restricted to immediate family for the first few days, and no phone calls are allowed. The nurse will need to help decrease the family's anxiety by reinforcing what the physician has told them about the patient's condition and treatment.

Through its local chapters, the American Heart Association provides an abundance of written material designed for the person recovering from an MI. Patients and their families should know about this valuable source of information and support as they work toward the goals of rehabilitation.

Intermediate care.   As the patient recovers from the acute phase of her illness, she is quickly weaned away from intensive care. When the physicians feel that very frequent assessment is no longer essential and that the patient is able to participate in his own personal hygiene activities without detrimental effects on the healing heart tissues, he is transferred out of the CCU into a telemetry or "step-down," medical unit. For some patients, this move is frightening, because they know they will no longer have a nurse in constant attention. Every effort is made to assure the patient that he is making progress toward recovery and no longer needs intensive care. While the patient is on the telemetry unit, physical activities are gradually increased according to ability to tolerate exercise, as evidenced by stable heart rate, blood pressure, and respiratory rate. **There is close monitoring for subjective and objective symptoms of excessive strain on the heart, such as dysrhythmia or dyspnea, or the development of complications.**

If there is stenosis in one or two locations in one of the main coronary arteries, a PTCA may be performed. These measures may minimize damage from an MI, but the patient still has CAD, requires treatment, and must lower her risk factors.

Rehabilitation.   As the patient gains an understanding of his illness and ways in which he can help himself toward recovery, he should become more confident and optimistic about his condition. Realization that one has suffered a serious heart attack is a frightening experience. The patient and his family will need much help and support as they work to make the necessary adjustments. Many hospitals offer an outpatient cardiac rehabilitation program to help the patient make lifestyle changes to reduce the future risk of heart problems. The program provides counseling on dietary changes for a healthy heart diet, stress-reduction techniques, reduction of risk factors, such as avoiding tobacco use, controlling hypertension and diabetes, and a supervised exercise program with continuous EKG monitoring for 4 to 6 weeks. Progressive, supervised exercise is continued for an additional 6 to 8 weeks, and then a maintenance program is devised that the patients can do on their own.

One area of major concern is sexuality. The patient may be fearful of resuming intercourse, thinking that it may cause a heart attack. The spouse, too, often has these fears. Both partners need reassurance that resumption of normal sexual activities will be possible. The patient may need to take a more passive role during intercourse, at least for a while, using alternate positions that cause less strain and less oxygen demand. The patient should be told that the workload of intercourse with a known partner is equal to climbing a flight of stairs. If he can climb a flight of stairs without much change in heart rate, respirations, or blood pressure, intercourse should not cause harm. The physician should cover this area with the patient and his spouse, but if he does not, the nurse should see that the patient gets the proper information. Sexual dysfunction may occur at first, but with patience on the part of both partners, it usually passes.

Patients need to be taught to plan sexual activity for times when they are well rested and to avoid an environment that is too hot or too cold. It is best to space such activity at least 2 hours after eating a meal or drinking any alcohol. Nitroglycerin should be used prophylactically if intercourse causes angina symptoms. If angina does occur, the patient should cease activity, place a nitroglycerin tablet under his tongue, lie down, and rest. Intercourse may be resumed 3 to 6 weeks after an MI and 6 to 8 weeks after open-heart surgery, depending on the patient's exercise tolerance as determined by stress testing. The target heart rate for exercise is aimed at 70% of that which the patient could safely achieve during graded exercise testing without an ischemic heart response or significant dysrhythmia.

Levels of physical activity are designated through metabolic equivalent (MET) units. One MET is the amount of oxygen needed by the body at rest. The patient's rehabilitation program slowly progresses stepwise to higher energy expenditures over a period of months. Table 19-10 shows examples of activities and their MET expenditures.

> Rehabilitation involves three major aspects: (1) a program of increasing activity based on the patient's individual progress and needs; (2) instruction of the patient and her family about the nature of her illness and the rationale for every aspect of its management; and (3) assistance to the patient and her family as they work toward the goal of accepting the limitations imposed and the changes in lifestyle that may be required.

In spite of all efforts to educate the post–MI patient about her illness and the need to continue her exercise program and modify her lifestyle, long-term continued compliance with the prescribed regimen is not as high as desired. The main purpose of instruction is to provide the patient with the information she needs to avoid the problems and complications that can occur once she leaves the structured program.

The patient's perception of her own situation greatly influences whether she will comply with the instructions she has received for continued treatment and preventive therapy. She may not follow instructions if she does not see herself as particularly susceptible to a condition—that is, if she doesn't think she is at risk for complications or further damage. She must also understand the rationale for the therapy and necessary lifestyle changes.

The patient is taught to:

- Recognize the signs of recurrent MI and to seek immediate medical attention should they occur. These are chest pain, diaphoresis, nausea, and anxiety.

TABLE 19-10 ◆ *Examples of Energy Expenditure (in METs)*
Activities of 1–3 METs
Eating
Conversing
Washing hands and face
Sewing by hand
Watching television
Shaving
Brushing teeth
Making bed
Cooking
Driving a car
Sewing with a machine
Typing
Activities of 3–6 METs
Showering
Using a bedpan
Walking up to 3.75 mph
Ironing, standing
Mopping floor
Bowling
Golfing
Dancing
Cycling on level ground up to 5.5 mph
Sexual intercourse
Light gardening
Activities of 6–8 METs
Ascending a flight of stairs
Mowing lawn by hand
Playing tennis singles
Walking at 5 mph
Horseback riding at a trot
Shoveling snow
Splitting wood
Waterskiing
Light downhill skiing
Playing basketball

- Adopt a lifetime regular, graduated exercise program.
- Alter controllable risk factors: reach and maintain a normal weight; cease smoking; keep alcohol consumption at a moderate level (no more than 1.5 oz per day); keep cholesterol within normal limits; control hypertension.
- Reduce stress and learn relaxation techniques.
- Observe for complications, such as irregular pulse rate, dyspnea and fatigue, chest pain, and fever.
- Continue on a low-fat, low-sodium diet individualized to taste.
- Take medications as ordered and monitor for side effects.

It is important to stress to the patient that she has control over her rehabilitation and prognosis. She and her physician and other health professionals are partners in fighting the disease that has caused her problem. She alone has full control over her lifestyle changes and the treatment program. She needs to know that she is the master of her own destiny. When the patient feels that she, rather than the physician, is in control, she is much more likely to stick to the treatment program.

◆ Congestive Heart Failure

Congestive heart failure (CHF) is actually a complication of other cardiovascular conditions, rather than a disease in itself. About 400,000 new CHF cases are diagnosed each year. About three million Americans have CHF. The numbers are increasing every year as more of the population reaches age 65. Congestive heart failure can occur any time the muscular strength of the heart weakens, causing it to fail as a pump and a circulator of blood. **This weakness can be caused by infection of the muscle, dilation from blood backup behind stenosed valves, poor pump action due to damaged myocardial tissue from an MI, and a number of other factors.**

According to the American Heart Association, the incidence of CHF has more than doubled since 1982, accounting for 874,000 hospitalizations in 1994 and 39,000 deaths. Ironically, the rise is a consequence of better treatment for MI so that people live long enough to develop CHF. This disorder is the leader in spending of Medicare dollars.

Pathophysiology   The key to understanding CHF is the word *congestion*. **Congestion develops because the heart is unable to move blood as quickly as it should.** This may occur because the heart muscle itself is too weak or because the blood vessels throughout the body are narrowed and constricted and cannot accommodate a normal supply of blood, causing the heart muscle to become exhausted trying to overcome the resistance. Poorly functioning valves may cause the chambers to dilate from blood backup, thinning the myocardium, decreasing pumping ability, and increasing the workload.

Normally, the ventricles of the heart contract, whereas the atria are relaxing, allowing for the filling and emptying of each chamber. If the muscle wall of the left ventricle cannot contract well, some of the blood is left in the ventricle. This prevents part of the blood in the left atrium from progressing into the ventricle. In turn, the blood backs up into the pulmonary vessels, pressure within those vessels increases, and fluid leaks into the lung tissue, producing congestion and, eventually, pulmonary edema. If not corrected, left-sided failure, because of the backup of blood, will soon lead to failure of the right side of the heart. This condition is called *congestive heart failure*. It does not mean that the heart has stopped functioning altogether (that, of course, would be fatal). **Instead, heart failure from congestion means that the heart is failing to meet the oxygen needs of the tissues of the body.**

If the right ventricle does not contract as strongly as it should, it cannot completely empty itself and it becomes engorged with blood. The blood flow is slowed down, preventing movement of blood out of the atrium. As it backs up, it prevents normal movement of blood flow out of the vena cava, thus increasing the pressure in the vena cava, the neck veins, and all other veins of the body.

As the rate of blood flow slows down, the body fluids in the intravascular fluid compartment begin to leak into the interstitial compartment. This produces retention of fluid and edema. **When the right side of the heart fails, the edema is first evident in the lower extremities** *(dependent edema)*. There is also an accumulation of fluid in the liver and abdominal organs as the portal circulation becomes involved. Congestion of blood flow to and from the kidneys may lead to impaired renal function, preventing normal excretion of urine and causing more accumulation of body fluids. Inadequate circulation to and from the brain may cause mental confusion and irritability, which sometimes progresses to delirium and coma.

The systemic backup of blood that occurs in right-sided heart failure may eventually lead to left-sided heart failure, as the heart will have to pump against increasing pressure in the aorta and systemic circulation. The circulatory system is exactly that: a *system*. Failure of one component affects the entire system. Figure 19-8 shows the pathophysiology of heart failure resulting from MI.

Think about . . . Can you explain to a patient in simple terms what happens in the body when heart failure occurs?

Symptoms and Diagnosis   The diagnosis of CHF is based on the patient's history of cardiovascular disease and the symptoms he presents. Table 19-11 presents the signs and symptoms of heart failure. Diagnosis is made on the basis of signs and symptoms, chest x-ray, EKG, and cardiac enzyme levels.

Treatment   Treatment of the underlying cause is carried out when possible. Surgical correction of valve or septal abnormalities may reverse heart failure. Medical treatment is largely symptomatic. Drugs and other therapies are used to reduce or eliminate the symptoms and complications of CHF, but they control only the condition; they do not cure it. Efforts are made to reduce the demand for oxygen and the workload of the heart, strengthen the heart's pumping action, relieve venous congestion in the lungs, and minimize sodium and water

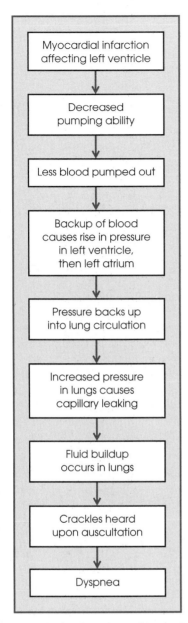

FIGURE 19-8 Pathophysiology of CHF after an MI.

MI or open-heart surgery is accomplished with the intraaortic balloon pump (IABP). Continuous ambulatory peritoneal dialysis (CAPD) is sometimes used to decrease circulating volume and lower the heart's workload.

To accomplish the goals of medical intervention, the following may be prescribed:

◆ Limited physical activity or bedrest in semi-Fowler's or high Fowler's position.

◆ Reduction of emotional stress.

◆ Oxygen therapy.

◆ Digitalization. Digitalis is an agent that increases the force of heart contraction (i.e., an inotropic agent) and slows the rate, thereby increasing cardiac output. Several large doses of the drug are given, followed by a lower, regular-maintenance dose. Other inotropic drugs, such as amrione (Inocor) and milrinone (Corotrope), which are new, may also be used. These two drugs are phophodiesterase (PDE) inhibitors; they boost cardiac contractility while producing peripheral vasodilation.

◆ Administration of "unloading" agents, which help the cardiovascular system to handle (or "unload") higher volumes of blood. Unloading agents include venous vasodilators such as isosorbide dinitrate (Isordil) and nitroglycerin (NTG), which relax and enlarge the veins, allowing them to accommodate larger percentages of the total blood volume. Beta-adrenergic blockers or calcium-channel blockers are sometimes used to slow the heart rate if tachycardia is causing the heart failure, thereby decreasing the oxygen demand. Beta-blockers are used cautiously as they can also cause heart failure. Diuretics are given to reduce fluid and decrease blood volume. Measures are taken to prevent electrolyte imbal-

retention in the tissues. Research is ongoing for the use of assistive pump devices, "artificial hearts," for severe CHF. An experimental surgery to reduce the size of an enlarged heart may change current treatment for advanced heart failure. The operation improves the pumping function of the failing heart by cutting out a big piece from the left ventricle, thereby improving contractility. The only life-saving treatment for those patients with end-stage heart failure until now is a heart transplant. Dobutamine therapy may be used to relieve symptoms and increase contractility while sustaining blood pressure. The drug is only used for long-term therapy for those who are waiting for a heart transplant or to lengthen life as it can cause serious complications. Short-term treatment for CHF after an

TABLE 19-11 ◆ *Signs and Symptoms of Heart Failure*
A few or many of the following signs and symptoms may be exhibited in the patient experiencing heart failure. Monitor especially closely for those marked with an asterisk.

Abdominal distention; ascites	Gastric distress, nausea, anorexia
Cool, dry, skin	
Cough	Increased central venous
Crackles in lungs*	pressure (CVP)
Cyanosis of lips	Jugular vein distention*
Decreased urine output*	Mental confusion
Dyspnea; nocturnal dyspnea*	Orthopnea
Elevated pulmonary artery	Pitting edema (ankles,
wedge pressure (PAWP)	sacrum, pretibial areas)*
Enlarged liver	Tachycardia
Fatigue; weakness	Weight gain*
Gallop heart sounds (extra sounds)*	

TABLE 19-12 ◆ *Patient Education: Ways to Prevent Hypokalemia*

Teach the patient who is at risk for potassium loss due to medications to consume foods from the following list daily:

Apricots (3)	Orange juice (½ cup)
Avocado (½)	Pinto beans (½ cup)
Baked potato with skin	Prune juice (½ cup)
Banana (1 medium)	Tomato juice (½ cup)

ances from the use of these drugs. (See Table 19-12 for ways to prevent hypokalemia.)

◆ Angiotensin-converting enzyme (ACE) inhibitors, such as captopril (Capoten) are used in severe CHF to increase renal blood flow and prolong life.

◆ Morphine is prescribed if pulmonary edema is present to relieve anxiety and make breathing easier.

◆ Limitation of sodium intake to 2 to 4 gm and, in severe cases, restriction of fluid intake (see Table 19-13).

◆ Phlebotomy of 100 to 500 mL of blood to decrease volume may be done if other treatment is not effective.

◆ Treatment of infection, which places an increased demand on the heart because of increased metabolic rate, or other underlying cause CHF.

TABLE 19-13 ◆ *Nutrition Tips: Assisting with Fluid Restriction*

Check with the physician to be certain that there are no contraindications before offering these suggestions.

◆ Encourage gum chewing to promote a feeling of moisture in the mouth.
◆ Provide mouth care every 2 hours while awake; brush teeth or encourage rinsing of the mouth.
◆ Provide ice chips rather than water; they stay in the mouth longer.
◆ Try to give all medications together when not contraindicated so that less fluid is used to take medications.
◆ Encourage use of margarine on bread, if permitted, to decrease need to "wash down" the bread.
◆ Collaborate with client on time schedule for fluids; divide fluid allotment evenly over the waking hours.
◆ Eliminate salty foods that cause thirst.
◆ Keep the lips lubricated.
◆ Observe for signs of dehydration.
◆ Remember that foods that turn liquid at room temperature are considered liquids (i.e., jello, ice cream, custard).
◆ Assist client to sit upright for meals so that fluid is not needed to assist swallowing.
◆ Encourage meal choices that are "moist" so that little fluid is needed at meal time.

Assessment   The effects of CHF can range from very mild to extremely serious. **A thorough nursing assessment can help not only identify specific patient care problems but also guide the physician in her evaluation of the patient's response to medical treatment and her decisions to continue or change prescribed drugs and other therapies.** The symptoms displayed by a patient with CHF are for the most part indications of changes taking place in tissues at some distance from the heart. For example, edema in the lower extremities, diminished flow of urine, with anorexia and a bloated feeling reflect involvement of the peripheral circulation, the kidney, and the circulation of blood to and from the liver and intestines and result from right-sided heart failure. It is important to ask the patient if his clothes, rings, or shoes fit more tightly than previously. Feelings of breathlessness or having to catch the breath in mid-sentence may indicate fluid in the lungs and left-sided heart failure.

Elder Care Point . . .   Elderly patients who have little cardiac reserve can be nudged into CHF by any condition that increases the body's demand for blood or oxygen. Generalized infection, pneumonia, severe trauma, and other conditions that increase the metabolic rate and demand for oxygen can be the precipitating factor. Watch elderly patients in your care with other conditions for signs of CHF.

Significant findings that may indicate heart failure in patients with conditions that predispose to CHF include the following:

◆ Increasing fatigue as a result of tissue hypoxia and shortness of breath, which may be caused by left ventricular failure and resultant fluid in the lungs.
◆ Cough.
◆ Feeling "bloated" and a loss of appetite due to diminished venous return from abdominal organs, liver enlargement resulting from increased pressure in the portal veins, edema in the intestines, and accumulations of fluid in the abdominal cavity.
◆ Jugular venous distention; visible jugular vein pulsation more than 4.5 cm above the clavicle when patient is in semi-Fowler's position. These signs are related to right ventricular failure.
◆ Complaint of feeling "warm" when others are comfortably cool because of vasoconstriction and poor circulation, which prevents removal of body heat.
◆ Feelings of anxiety, irritability, or depression, and difficulty concentrating and remembering due to diminished blood flow to brain.
◆ Pale, cool, and dry skin, which are signs of poor peripheral circulation; mottling of skin.

◆ Cyanosis of nail beds, indicating oxygen deficit.

◆ Dependent, pitting edema (check feet and ankles in ambulatory patient or one sitting up most of the time; check thighs and sacral region in patient confined to bed, due to congestion of the venous system and increased capillary pressure, which forces fluid out of the intravascular fluid compartment and into the tissue spaces.

◆ Fleeting or absent peripheral pulses.

◆ Gradually increasing heart rate, even when the patient is at rest, which is caused by attempts by the heart to remove blood from a distended ventricle.

◆ Reduced urinary output, which reflects the kidney's response to poor perfusion by retaining sodium and water.

◆ Crackles heard in lungs.

◆ Extra heart sound (S₃).

Think about... What signs detected during your beginning-of-shift assessment of the patient recovering from an MI might indicate CHF?

Nursing Intervention   Those who have mild CHF will not be hospitalized, but require instruction in self-care. This includes balancing rest with physical activity, limiting sodium intake and following other dietary restrictions, self-administration of medications with awareness of adverse side effects that must be reported, and the dangers of drug-to-drug interaction when taking nonprescription drugs, modification of lifestyle as indicated (diet, smoking, physical activity), and knowledge of symptoms that should be reported to the physician if they become worse or appear for the first time.

Elder Care Point... The elderly patient who is experiencing CHF often is taking many medications. It is especially important to look for drug interactions and to monitor for signs and symptoms of toxicity. It is of vital importance to monitor these patients for electrolyte imbalances, especially imbalance of sodium or potassium. Electrolyte imbalances may cause serious dysrhythmias.

Patients with moderate chronic CHF will need instruction in self-care and encouragement to follow the prescribed regimen. If treatment does not stop the progress of the disease, the patient may be admitted to the hospital for reevaluation and a change in therapies. Sometimes the patient's heart continues to fail in spite of aggressive therapy, and such complications as pulmonary edema and liver and renal failure occur.

Partial or full assistance with ADLs will decrease oxygen demand. **Scheduling all activities to promote as much rest as possible is a high priority. Activity is** alternated with rest throughout the day. Several pillows may be required to achieve a comfortable position. Accurate recording of intake and output is very important. Daily weight is recorded at the same time each day, preferably before breakfast. Careful attention to turning and skin care is essential, as edematous tissue breaks down easily. Bedrest causes venous pooling, and active or passive leg exercises should be performed every 1 to 2 hours to help prevent thrombosis. Elastic stockings or sequential compression devices to prevent venous pooling may be ordered. Observation for side effects of medications is another major responsibility (see Common Therapies). Careful ongoing physical assessment is essential.

Acute *pulmonary edema*, a complication of CHF, is a medical emergency that must be treated promptly to avoid death caused by the patient's "drowning" in his own body fluids. The patient with this condition has severe dyspnea; a cough productive of frothy, pink-tinged sputum; tachycardia; and moist, bubbling respirations with cyanosis.

Nursing intervention for acute pulmonary edema includes placing the patient in an orthopneic position to relieve the dyspnea; administering oxygen, diuretics, morphine, and other prescribed drugs; limiting and monitoring activity; and assessing cardiopulmonary status. Nursing interventions for selected problems in a patient with congestive heart failure are summarized in Nursing Care Plan 19-2.

◆ Disorders of the Heart's Conduction System

A normal heart is capable of generating tiny electrical impulses that are essential to normal contraction of the heart's ventricles and atria. The impulses originate in the sinoatrial (SA) node and the AV node. These are neuromuscular structures and are sometimes called the *heart's natural pacemakers.* The SA node is located in the wall of the right atrium between the openings for the inferior and superior vena cava. It stimulates contraction of the atria. The AV node is located in the septum between the atria and transmits impulses via the *bundle of His* and the *Purkinje fibers* to the ventricles, causing them to contract (Figure 19-3 on p. 540). The healthy heart beats in normal sinus rhythm (NSR) at 60 to 100 beats per minute (bpm). Figure 19-9 shows the EKG pattern of normal sinus rhythm, and Table 19-14 provides the procedure for evaluating an EKG strip. **The goal for the beginning nurse is to be able to determine when the tracing is *not* normal sinus rhythm.** Approximately 4,462,000 Americans experienced a disorder of cardiac rhythm in 1992.

Pathophysiology   The SA node generates impulses 70 to 100 times per minute. Each impulse travels

Nursing Care Plan 19-2

Selected nursing diagnoses, goals/expected outcomes, nursing interventions, and evaluations for a patient with congestive heart failure

Situation: Mrs. Brown, age 78, was admitted to the hospital with a diagnosis of chronic CHF associated with long-term atherosclerotic heart disease. For the first week of her hospitalization she was on bedrest with bathroom privileges only, received oxygen prn for dyspnea, and was given digoxin in divided doses for digitalization. She is now receiving a maintenance dose of digoxin (Lanoxin) 0.25 mg PO daily after breakfast. She is receiving furosemide (Lasix) 20 mg twice daily to manage edema. Her present symptoms include mild dyspnea, dependent edema, and fatigue. She is anxious about the chest pain and dyspnea associated with physical activity and is afraid she will "be an invalid and a burden" for the rest of her life.

Nursing Diagnosis	Goals/Expected Outcome	Nursing Intervention	Evaluation
Fluid volume excess related to poor pumping action of heart. SUPPORTING DATA Dyspnea on exertion, 2+ ankle edema, weight 6 lb above normal.	Normal fluid balance by discharge as evidenced by return to normal weight and absence of edema.	Balance rest with mild exercise to tolerance level. Administer digoxin and Lasix as ordered; take apical pulse before giving digoxin, check potassium levels, and observe for signs of hypokalemia: weakness, muscle cramps, numbness, and tingling in extremities. Administer potassium supplement as ordered. Monitor intake and output. Weigh daily and record. Encourage adherence to low-sodium diet. Elevate patient's feet when sitting or lying down. Monitor respiratory rate, breath sounds, and heart sounds.	Intake, 1,500 mL; output, 2,750 mL; weight down 2 lb today; complying with diet; less dyspnea when walking in room; ankle edema 1+; continue plan.
Risk for injury related to possible digitalis toxicity. SUPPORTING DATA Newly digitalized; on Lanoxin 0.25 mg PO.	Patient will not show signs of digitalis toxicity.	Observe for signs of digitalis toxicity before each dose: anorexia, nausea, vomiting, diarrhea, excessively slow pulse, new arrythmia, or yellow-green halos around objects. Check digitalis laboratory levels for values within normal range. Assess for signs of hypokalemia, which predisposes to digitalis toxicity.	No nausea, anorexia, diarrhea, or visual changes; pulse, 78 and regular; digitalis level, 1.2 ng/mL; K+, 3.8 mEq/L.
Anxiety related to misinformation about prognosis. SUPPORTING DATA States she is afraid that she will be an invalid for the rest of her life.	Patient will verbalize understanding of potential for normal life when disease is under control with medication, diet, and exercise. Patient will display less anxiety by assuming more responsibility for self-care. By time of discharge patient will verbalize optimism about the future.	Establish trusting relationship. Explain expected outcomes of therapy; set mutual goals for assuming self-care and increasing physical activity. Give praise for all efforts at self-care and increased physical activity. Encourage her to verbalize concerns.	Assisting with grooming and eating; verbalizing concerns; states she is "still so weak"; goals set for self-care before discharge; continue plan.
Knowledge deficit related to disease and various therapies. SUPPORTING DATA "Doesn't heart failure mean that my heart is worn out and going to quit?" What do these medicines do?	By time of discharge patient will verbalize simple explanation of CHF. By time of discharge patient will verbalize purpose of each medicine, how to take it, and side effects to watch for.	Teach what happens in CHF. Teach patient, husband, and daughter how to measure pulse rate and rhythm; symptoms of digitalis toxicity; purpose of watching for symptoms of hypokalemia; foods high in potassium content; purpose of low-sodium diet; importance of daily weight record; importance of keeping appointments for follow-up; symptoms that indicate a worsening of heart failure and the need to seek medical help promptly.	Teaching session no. 2 completed; can verbalize simple explanation of heart failure; measures own pulse accurately; can pick foods high in potassium from list; recording daily weight in notebook; continue plan. Meeting goals.

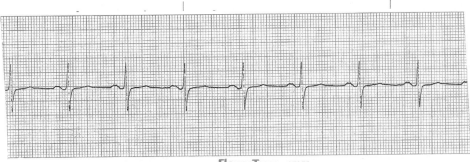

ELECTROTRACE   9705A

1. Rate between 60–100 bpm and regular.
2. P wave precedes each QRS complex; PR interval between 0.12–0.20 seconds. (3–5 small squares.)
3. QRS duration between 0.04–0.12 seconds (1–3 small squares.)
4. QRS complexes have essentially the same shape.

FIGURE 19-9   EKG tracing of normal sinus rhythm.

through the atria to the AV node, which relays the impulse via the bundle of His and the Purkinje fibers to the ventricles, causing them to contract (see Figure 19-3 on p. 540). If the SA node fails to produce an electrical impulse, the AV node will initiate an impulse at 40 to 60 beats per minute. If neither the SA nor the AV node is functioning, the ventricles will initiate an impulse at a slower rate. When there is disruption of the normal electrical conduction in the heart, irregular heart rhythm occurs. This is called an **arrhythmia** or a **dysrhythmia**. A pulse below 60 indicates bradycardia, one type of dysrhythmia. Bradycardia may drop cardiac output enough to cause symptoms of decreased blood flow to occur in the patient.

TABLE 19-14 ◆ *Evaluating an EKG Rhythm Strip*

- Obtain a strip with at least 10 large graph squares.
- Calculate the rate. Count the number of 0.2-sec divisions between two consecutive QRS complexes and divide this into 300 to determine the rate. For irregular rhythms, count the number of cycles or complexes in 6 sec and multiply by 10.
- Measure the distance between the P waves. Is the distance the same? If so, the rate is regular. Calculate the atrial rate by counting the number of small boxes between the P waves and dividing that number into 1,500. If the atrial rate is irregular, are there premature atrial beats?
- Measure the P-R interval. Is it normal (0.12–0.20 sec)? Does it vary?
- Measure the QRS duration. Is it normal (0.04–0.12 sec)? Measure with calipers from R wave to R wave throughout the tracing to determine whether the rate is regular. Are there premature QRS complexes? Do all the QRS complexes look the same? Calculate the ventricular rate by counting the number of small squares between R waves and dividing that number into 1500. Is the atrial and ventricular rate the same? A rough calculation can be made by counting the number of complexes in a 6-sec tracing and multiplying by 10.

If the heart rate rises above 100 to 120 beats per minute, the patient has a dysrhythmia known as **tachycardia. When the heart beats this fast, the ventricles do not have adequate time to fill with blood and therefore cannot pump out their usual amount. As a result, cardiac output falls.**

When the heart's electrical conduction system fails, the normal contractions of the heart that are necessary for its pumping action do not occur, and adequate blood is not pumped out to the body. Symptoms the patient may experience include dizziness, **palpitations** (abnormally rapid throbbing or fluttering of the heart), fatigue, chest pain, loss of consciousness, and possibly death. The severity of the symptoms depends on whether the abnormal rhythm is atrial or ventricular in origin, on the amount of cardiac output, and whether the dysrhythmia is persistent.

Other common cardiac dysrhythmias include:

- *Atrial fibrillation.* The atria quiver rather than contract many times a minute, with only some impulses being conducted to the ventricles; this causes a drop in cardiac output because not as much blood goes to the ventricles to be pumped out to the body, and it predisposes to clot formation in the atria.
- *Ventricular tachycardia.* The impulse is generated from one or more focal points in the ventricle at a very fast rate and travels through the bundle of His. The atria do not have a chance to contract and push blood into the ventricles. The ventricles contract too fast to allow time for adequate filling with blood; **cardiac output falls drastically, and death may occur. A pulse cannot be felt.**
- *Ventricular fibrillation.* **The ventricles quiver rather than contract; there is no effective cardiac output, and without CPR, death will occur.**

◆ *Premature ventricular contractions* (PVC). The ventricular impulse causes ventricular contraction before impulse and contraction of atria is complete. Blood is not received from the atria to be pumped out to body. A few PVCs are not abnormal, but when there are more than six to seven in a minute, cardiac output may fall. This dysrhythmia also makes the heart more likely to develop ventricular tachycardia or ventricular fibrillation.

◆ *Complete heart block* (third-degree heart block). Separate impulses cause contraction in the atria and in the ventricles; **contraction is uncoordinated, and blood is not received normally from the atria, which decreases the amount of blood available to be pumped out to the body; cardiac output falls drastically. This is a life-threatening dysrhythmia.**

There are many other types of cardiac dysrhythmias. Nurses assigned to a coronary care unit take a special course in dysrhythmias to learn the patterns, significance, and treatment of each type. Figure 19-10 shows EKG patterns of life-threatening dysrhythmias.

Elder Care Point . . . With age the left ventricle and cardiac valves thicken and the amount of fibrous tissue and fat in the SA node increases, which decreases the number of pacemaker cells it contains. These changes make those over 75 more prone to cardiac dysrhythmias as changes occur in the conduction system. Failure of the SA node and the need for a pacemaker occur fairly frequently.

Use of oxygen by the heart is less efficient with increasing years, and the heart does not tolerate tachy-

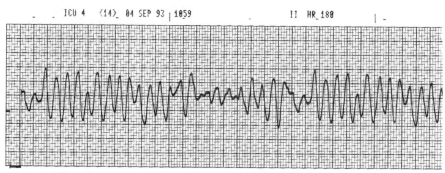

Ventricular Tachycardia

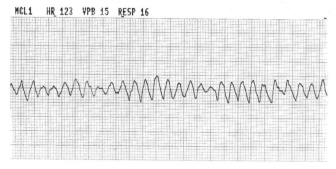

Ventricular Fibrillation

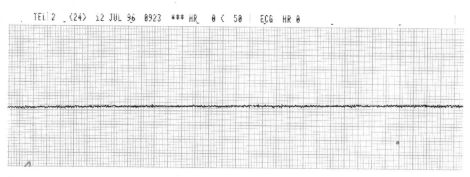

Asystole

FIGURE 19-10   EKG patterns of life-threatening dysrhythmias.

cardia well. **Tachycardia brought about by fever from infection can give rise to heart failure rather quickly in the older adult who has heart disease.**

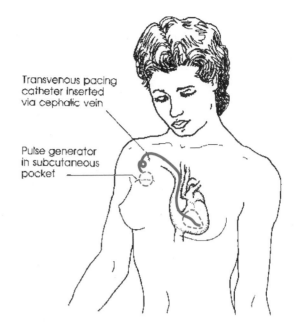

FIGURE 19-11   Thoracic placement of permanent pacemaker and transvenous pacing catheter.

Diagnosis and Treatment   Disorders of the cardiac conduction system are diagnosed by a 12-lead EKG, continuous EKG monitoring (Holter monitoring), patient history, and electrophysiology tests, which can be performed during cardiac catheterization.

Drug therapy is effective in correcting or controlling dysrhythmias in many cases. A variety of antiarrhythmic agents may be used alone or in combination to regulate the heart beat (Table 19-7 on p. 553).

When drug therapy does not control a life-threatening dysrhythmia, surgical destruction (**ablation**) of the tissue initiating the abnormal impulse can sometimes correct the problem if such an area can be located during electrophysiology testing.

Artificial cardiac pacing can be a temporary measure if the problem is an emergency, as in a transient condition such as drug toxicity. An external pacemaker often is used in the emergency room. A temporary transvenous pacemaker is placed if transient complete heart block (i.e., no impulse travels from the atria to the ventricles) develops after an MI. Pacemaker wires are often placed during cardiac surgery for quick use should the patient need to be "paced" in the postoperative period. When the need for the wires is past, the surgeon will pull them out.

A permanent pacemaker is indicated if the cardiac dysrhythmia is the result of an irreversible disorder, as in failure of the SA node. Other conditions in which a permanent pacemaker is inserted include pathological complete heart block, secondary AV block, supraventricular tachycardia, and bradytachycardia, in which the SA node alternates between firing too slowly and firing too rapidly.

Transvenous pacemakers are inserted by fluoroscopy with local anesthesia. Patient consent is required, and a sedative is given to the patient before the procedure. A permanent pacemaker is inserted in the operating room or cardiac catheterization laboratory to ensure an aseptic environment, even though the procedure is relatively minor (Figure 19-11).

The newer types of pacemakers can sense and pace in both the atrium and the ventricle, thus making the heart function in a more natural way and giving the patient better cardiac output. Another type of pacemaker is so sophisticated that it can speed up and slow down the heart rate according to the patient's activity needs, much as a normal heart does. Set rate pacemakers are still used in patients with atrial fibrillation as sensors have a problem reading what is going on in the atrium with this disorder.

Patients who experience supraventricular tachycardia or atrial fibrillation that does not respond to drug therapy may be treated with *cardioversion*. A mild electrical shock is delivered to the heart at a specific time in the cardiac cycle to interrupt the abnormal rhythm and begin a new, normal rhythm of electrical impulse and contraction. The patient is given a sedative prior to the procedure. Signed consent is required. The procedure may be performed in the cardiac catheterization laboratory or the emergency room by the physician. Resuscitation equipment must be at hand.

Frequent PVCs (more than 6 to 7 per minute) and ventricular tachycardia that are symptomatic (signs of decreased cardiac output occur) are treated with IV lidocaine. If ventricular tachycardia is not responsive to lidocaine, cardioversion is performed to restore a more normal rhythm. Ventricular fibrillation is treated by starting CPR and performing defibrillation as soon as possible. **Defibrillation** means to "get the heart to stop fibrillating." This procedure is covered in Chapter 31.

Automatic implantable cardiac defibrillators (AICD) are used for patients who have repeated episodes of life-threatening ventricular fibrillation or cardiac asystole (arrest). The defibrillator is implanted in the operating room. This device has saved many lives by monitoring the heart beat and providing an electrical shock similar to that delivered in cardiac defibrillation when a life-threatening rhythm is detected. The patient is warned not to go through airport metal detecting systems since the defibrillator is turned on and off by a magnet. The patient needs to carry a letter from the physician with this information when traveling.

Nursing Assessment and Intervention   If inserting a pacemaker is not an emergency procedure, the nurse will have opportunities to assess the patient's knowledge of and feelings about having a pacemaker regulate her heart beat. While the physician is responsible for explaining the purpose of the pacemaker and its benefits to the patient, these explanations can raise more questions and possibly create fears and anxiety. The nurse should assess the patient's learning needs and seek to identify the source of her fear and the level of her anxiety.

Both the American Heart Association and the manufacturers of pacemakers provide illustrated booklets to help patients learn more about their cardiac pacers. The nurse can go over these booklets with the patient and perhaps show him a demonstration model and explain how it works to his advantage.

Care of the patient who has a temporary pacemaker includes checking the connections of the lead wires to the pulse generator, keeping the device and wires dry, checking the control settings, and protecting the patient from electrical shock and infection. For protection the pulse generator and exposed wires are placed in a rubber glove, and contact is avoided with all electrical apparatus (e.g., unplug bed; do not use an electric razor). Other care is identical to that for the patient receiving a permanent pacemaker.

Postoperative nursing care for the permanent pacemaker patient includes continuous monitoring of heart rate and rhythm, dressing changes, and care of the insertion site according to the protocol of the nursing care unit. Vital signs, peripheral pulses distal to the insertion site, and level of consciousness are checked frequently during the immediate postoperative period.

Discharge instruction for the patient with a permanent pacemaker should include amount of physical activity allowed until healing occurs and the electrode is securely in place. This usually takes no more than 6 weeks, after which time the patient can be as physically active as he wishes, although he is warned not to engage in contact sports or other activities that may result in injury to the chest.

Although the newer pacemakers have a shield to protect them from electromagnetic signals from machinery, the patient should be cautioned not to expose his pacemaker unnecessarily to high-voltage equipment. Faulty microwave ovens, lawn mower motors, and other sources of electromagnetic signals can "confuse" a pacemaker with impulses that could cause it to malfunction. Should this occur, function will return to normal as soon as the patient moves away from the source of electromagnetic signals. The battery in a pacemaker should last 15 to 30 years, depending on the type, but it could weaken prematurely. Weakening results in a drop in pulse rate, which should be reported to the physician immediately.

The patient will need to know how to take his pulse so that he can regularly evaluate the performance of his pacemaker. He should take his pulse for 1 full minute every day while he is in a resting position.

A patient with a pacer should wear some form of identification such as a bracelet or necklace at all times and carry an identification card stating that he has a pacemaker. Follow-up care is an essential part of the life of every person with a pacemaker. He must understand the importance of periodic evaluations of his condition for the rest of his life. Some types of pacemakers have a telephone monitoring device that allows the patient to call a monitoring station and have his pacemaker checked. Instructions for the use of the pacemaker and monitoring device are included in the owner's manual.

Because of the sensors planted in the chambers of the heart, this patient is at risk for infection of the lining of the heart (endocarditis). He should be given prophylactic antibiotics before any invasive medical or dental procedure.

Elder Care Point... Older patients who have SA node disease and resulting cardiac dysrhythmias can achieve a far better quality of life with an implanted pacemaker. Many patients are fearful of the surgery required and can benefit from talking to another patient who has had a successful pacemaker implantation.

Think about... What would you include in a teaching plan for the patient who has received a pacemaker? How would the teaching differ for a temporary pacemaker versus a permanent pacemaker?

◆ Inflammatory Diseases of the Heart

The tissues of the heart are subject to the same inflammatory conditions that affect other parts of the body. The inflammation may be present in the inner lining (endocarditis), the heart muscle (myocarditis), or the sac surrounding the heart (pericarditis). The process also may involve the valves between the heart chambers or those located at the base of the major vessels leading from the heart. About 22,000 people were hospitalized with bacterial endocarditis in 1994.

Pathophysiology   Infection of the heart can result from an acute infection elsewhere in the body. The infection may be caused by staphylococci, pneumococci, gonococci, bacilli, or fungi. This condition is called *infective endocarditis* (IE), *bacterial endocarditis* (BE), or *subacute bacterial endocarditis* (SBE) depending on the cause. In adults the introduction of bacteria during dental or invasive diagnostic procedures is a frequent cause of endocarditis. Subacute bacterial endocarditis occurs most frequently in people who have a congenitally damaged heart or a prosthetic valve. Intravenous drug injection with unclean needles is another cause of endocarditis.

In the past, the most common cause of heart inflammation was damage resulting from rheumatic fever. Although antibiotics, particularly penicillin, have decreased the incidence of rheumatic fever, the danger is still present. Today, untreated strep throat is the most common cause of cardiac inflammation in children who do not have congenital cardiac abnormalities. Strep throat is a common disease of childhood caused by group A streptococcus. If the streptococcal infection is treated early with antibiotics, inflammation in the heart can be avoided. Rheumatic fever is much less common in adults. In adults circulating microorganisms in the bloodstream may attack the endocardium.

Elder Care Point . . . In the elderly systemic infections of the respiratory, urinary, or gastrointestinal tract, or skin often are the cause of endocarditis. Diagnosis is difficult because symptoms are frequently vague. The aortic valve is most often affected.

The invading microorganisms attack the heart valves or areas of the endocardium that are congenitally abnormal, causing small deposits on the valve called vegetation. (See Color Figure 5.) Vegetation decreases the effectiveness of the valve and is frequently the reason for valve replacement. The mitral valve is the most frequent location of infection. Mortality is 20% to 30% and rises as high as 70% in the elderly. Valve involvement is diagnosed by echocardiography.

A viral infection can cause myocarditis and *cardiomyopathy.* The virus attacks the muscle tissue, causing inflammation and resultant fibrosis. *Cardiomyopathy* is a term for cardiac degeneration from a source other than CAD, hypertension, cardiac structural disorders, or pulmonary disease. **The heart enlarges and becomes an inefficient pump.** Other causes of cardiomyopathy include alcoholism, drug toxicity, crack cocaine use, pregnancy, immune disorders, and nutritional deficiencies. The major problems exhibited by patients with cardiomyopathy are CHF and dysrhythmias. Severe cardiomyopathy is rapidly fatal. These patients are possible candidates for a heart transplant.

Pericarditis can be bacterial or viral in origin or can result from the inflammation in tissue damaged from myocardial infarction. If the inflammation causes an excess of the usual 50 mL of fluid contained in the pericardial sac, a *pericardial effusion* occurs. Should the fluid become excessive, *cardiac tamponade* may occur as the fluid restricts the filling and pumping of the heart. If unresolved, cardiac tamponade is soon fatal because the heart cannot supply the body with needed oxygen and nutrients.

Signs and Symptoms The signs and symptoms of infective endocarditis vary considerably. The sedimentation rate and leukocyte count are elevated, and signs of low-grade intermittent fever are evident. The spleen becomes enlarged. Splinter hemorrhages (thin black lines) can occur under the nails, and there may be petechiae inside the mouth. Cardiac inflammation (endocarditis) may be recurring. Each instance of endocarditis further damages the heart valves. The scar tissue that occurs as the inflammation subsides may cause the valve to leak, resulting in insufficiency (lack of closure), or the valve leaflets may become thickened and calcified, causing narrowing or stenosis. **An existing cardiac murmur may worsen, or a new murmur may appear as a valve is damaged.** The mitral and aortic valves are most often affected. When mitral or aortic stenosis or insufficiency cause symptoms sufficient to interfere with the patient's usual lifestyle, surgery becomes necessary (see section on cardiac surgery.) Both stenosis and insufficiency of cardiac valves may eventually cause congestive heart failure.

Elder Care Point . . . The valve leaflets thicken with age; this gives rise to the common systolic murmur heard in persons over age 80.

Pericarditis symptoms include chest pain eased by sitting up and leaning forward, dyspnea, and a pericardial friction rub. The rub is a high-pitched scratchy sound heard with the diaphragm of the stethoscope placed at the lower left sternal border of the chest. Symptoms of cardiac tamponade are muffled heart sounds, tachycardia, restlessness, anxiety and confusion, distended neck veins, and *pulsus paradoxus,* a drop in systolic BP upon inspiration greater than 10 mm Hg.

Diagnosis and Treatment Diagnosis is made by history and physical and confirmed by echocardiogram and blood cultures. Inflammatory conditions are primarily treated with rest of the affected part, and the same is true of inflammatory diseases of the heart. Treatment consists of measures intended to decrease the workload of the heart. The patient is placed on bedrest with bathroom privileges during the acute stage of the infection.

Medications. Specific medications for the treatment of inflammatory conditions of the heart include the antiinflammatories used for pericarditis and antiinflammatories plus antiinfectives used for infective endocarditis. Choice of drug is determined by blood culture for the particular organism responsible for the infection and sensitivity testing for the drug that kills the organism quickly. Generally a combination of at least two antibiotics is given IV through a central line for 4 to 6 weeks, with further oral therapy thereafter. The drugs most effective for BE may cause hearing loss, and hearing must be tested frequently during therapy. After the initiation of therapy and stabilization, the patient often is discharged home, usually within 7 to 10 days, and the medications are administered by visiting nurses, the patient or the family.

Surgery. Pericarditis may be surgically treated by *pericardiotomy* or *pericardiocentesis* (opening of the pericardium and removal of fluid). Repair of congenital cardiac problems, such as atrial or ventricular septal defect may be done. *Balloon valvuloplasty* is a relatively new procedure that is sometimes used to open stenosed valves. It is performed with a balloon-tipped catheter much like the one used for PTCA. However, it is questionable whether the valve will just close again with time. *Valve replacement* is an open-heart surgical procedure in which the valve is replaced with either a porcine (pork), bovine (beef), or synthetic valve (see section on specific cardiac surgeries). When a synthetic valve is used, the patient must be on anticoagulant therapy for the rest of his life, as the synthetic material tends to cause breakup of blood cells and clumping of platelets, which in turn cause clots and emboli. Prophylactic antibiotics are necessary prior to any invasive procedure (dental, endoscopy, etc.).

Think about . . . Can you list four diagnostic procedures prior to which a patient with an artificial or defective heart valve should take prophylactic antibiotics?

♦ Cardiac Valve Disorders

Besides congenital abnormalities, rheumatic fever, and bacterial endocarditis, long-term hypertension also can cause cardiac valve disorders. **Problems most commonly occur in the mitral valve between the left atrium and ventricle.** The aortic valve is the second most commonly diseased valve. **Valve disorders are of two types: stenosis or insufficiency.** In valvular stenosis a narrowing of the valve opening occurs and causes an obstruction to normal blood flow. **When stenosis occurs, the chamber that pumps the blood through the valve must do more work to force the blood through the valve. With valvular insufficiency (also called incompetency or regurgitation), the diseased valve is unable to close properly and blood flows back into the chamber after contraction, causing an overfilling.**

Mitral stenosis causes the left atrium to work harder to pump blood through the narrowed valve into the left ventricle. Mitral insufficiency results in blood flow back into the left atrium with every contraction of the left ventricle. This makes more work for the left atrium. With both conditions, the left atrium dilates and thickens in response to the increased workload. The increasing pressure of the extra blood in the left atrium causes a backward increase in pressure in the pulmonary circulation and the eventual development of CHF. As the atrial tissue dilates, the conduction system may be disrupted and dysrhythmias, particularly atrial fibrillation, may occur.

> When atrial fibrillation occurs, clots may form in the atria and be pumped out into the circulation as emboli, lodging in the coronary vessels, the brain, or elsewhere in the body. An MI or stroke may result.

Signs, symptoms, and treatment   **Signs and symptoms of mitral valve disorders include a cardiac murmur, progressive fatigue, exertional dyspnea, irregular heart rate, and the gradual onset of CHF.** Confirmation of a suspected valve disorder is made by echocardiogram or cardiac catheterization.

Treatment of mitral valve disorders is aimed at controlling atrial fibrillation and CHF with digitalis, diuretics, and antiarrhythmic medications, and prophylactic anticoagulants to prevent clot formation and emboli. Valve surgery is performed on the dysfunctional valve when the person's lifestyle is restricted by cardiac failure. See the following section on cardiac surgery.

Aortic stenosis causes the left ventricle to work harder to force blood through the valve into the aorta. Aortic insufficiency allows blood to backflow into the ventricle after it is pumped into the aorta. With these conditions the left ventricle dilates and thickens in an effort to handle the extra pressure and volume of blood in the ventricle. Eventually, left ventricular failure occurs.

Signs and symptoms of aortic valve disorders include cardiac murmur, syncope (fainting), angina, dysrhythmia, dyspnea, and signs of CHF. Aortic insufficiency causes a widened pulse pressure. Diagnosis is by echocardiogram or cardiac catheterization. Treatment is essentially the same as for mitral valve disorders except that different antiarrhythmic medication is used for ventricular dysrhythmia. There is a greater danger of sudden death with aortic stenosis due to decreased blood flow to the coronary arteries. For all types of valve disorders the patient is encouraged to attain and maintain a normal weight to minimize the workload of the heart.

Elder Care Point . . . Elderly people with long-term hypertension are at risk for aortic stenosis because of increased arteriosclerosis and stiffening of the aorta. Carefully assess aortic valve sounds of the elderly patient, especially if hypertension is not well controlled.

Nursing Management   The primary nursing goals for patients with cardiac valve disease are to maintain homeostasis, control dysrhythmias, and prevent or control CHF.

Think about . . . Can you list four findings from assessment of a patient that might indicate the presence of a valve disorder?

◆ Cardiac Trauma

Blunt chest trauma often causes myocardial contusion (bruising), but it also can cause tears in the great vessels and massive bleeding. Contusion may result in cardiac dysrhythmia, therefore, the patient's cardiac rhythm is monitored closely. Penetrating trauma usually causes a hemothorax. The condition called *cardiac tamponade* can occur from either type of wound if bleeding into the pericardial sac occurs. The fluid compresses the heart and restricts blood flow in and out of the ventricles. Cardiac output falls and venous pressure rises; the arterial blood pressure falls and there is a narrowing of pulse pressure accompanied by tachycardia. Shock and death will result if the bleeding is not stopped and the fluid removed. Pericardiocentesis may be performed to remove the fluid from the pericardial sac. Every effort is made to restore normal cardiac output.

◆ Cardiogenic Shock

Cardiogenic shock may occur as a result of hypovolemia or cardiac tamponade caused by trauma. It also may occur from serious dysrhythmias, cardiac arrest, myocardial degeneration, and as a complication of myocardial infarction or cardiac surgery. It results from circulatory failure due to the failure of the heart to pump sufficient blood. Signs and symptoms are those that accompany decreased cardiac output, such as confusion, restlessness, diaphoresis, rapid, thready pulse, increased respiratory rate, cold, clammy skin, and diminishing urinary output to less than 20 mL/hour. If cardiogenic shock is stemming from a mechanical defect, use of the intraaortic balloon pump until surgical repair can correct the defect may stabilize the patient. The best position for the patient is when the head of the bed is up 45 degrees to help breathing and oxygenation. The patient is cared for in the intensive care unit where a variety of drugs aimed at improving cardiac output may be administered.

COMMON PROBLEMS RELATED TO CARDIAC DISEASE

◆ Fatigue and Dyspnea

In the early stages of heart disease, the patient may be only slightly aware of his inability to do as much

physical work as he formerly could. If he lets the problem go too long, he will find that his physical activities will become increasingly restricted, because he will lack the energy to perform the simplest of tasks and becomes short of breath after the slightest exertion.

> When the coronary arteries fail to supply adequate oxygen to the cells of the heart muscle, the heart is unable to perform as it should when extra demands are placed on it. The result is a general hypoxia of the tissues throughout the body, which causes fatigue and dyspnea on exertion.

Nursing Assessment and Intervention   Traditionally, prolonged bedrest was prescribed for every patient with a heart condition. Currently, bedrest with bedside commode privileges is ordered for the first 24 to 72 hours for MI and severe CHF. The patient may feed himself and assist with his sponge bath. He is cautioned against any isometric activity, such as pushing himself up in bed. Stool softeners are given to prevent straining at stool (Valsalva maneuver), which causes a sudden increase in cardiac workload. Straining while coughing or repositioning in bed can cause the Valsalva as well and is to be avoided. Activity progresses to chair sitting, ambulating to the bathroom, and then down the hall. Patients are monitored by telemetry units to watch for dysrhythmias or excessive heart rate changes during ambulation. The amount of energy used in activity is expressed in *metabolic equivalents* (METs). The patient is guided from 1 to 3 METs before discharge. Sitting, eating, washing hands and face, and conversing are 1 to 3 MET activities. Table 19-10 on p. 561 shows the metabolic equivalents for various activities.

Criteria used to determine whether the patient is tolerating the activity include the following:

- ◆ The heart rate does not rise more than 20 beats per minute.
- ◆ Systolic blood pressure does not drop.
- ◆ There is no complaint of chest pain, dyspnea, or severe fatigue.
- ◆ There is no abnormal heart rate or rhythm.

Activity progression often is jointly supervised by a physical therapist and a nurse. More information on cardiac rehabilitation is presented in Chapter 12.

◆ Fluid Overload: Edema

Edema is an accumulation of fluid in the interstitial fluid compartment. It becomes a problem in heart disease when the blood flow into or out of the heart is inhibited, causing a slowing down of the normal movement of body fluids and their eventual excretion.

Nursing Assessment and Intervention The nurse continually assesses the fluid balance of a patient with cardiac disease by looking for signs of abnormal collections of fluid in the body tissues. Daily weight change is considered the best indicator of fluid buildup. The feet and ankles of ambulatory patients are checked for signs of dependent edema, and bedrest patients are watched for signs of swelling in the area of the sacrum, buttocks, and thighs. The patient is observed for progressive signs of shortness of breath, and lung fields are auscultated each shift to detect crackles, a sign of beginning pulmonary congestion.

Nursing responsibilities include recording the patient's weight daily before breakfast, supervising fluid restriction, accurately measuring intake and output, and assessing for signs of both fluid deficit and fluid overload. Elderly patients on fluid restriction and diuretics can easily become dehydrated.

Therapeutic measures to control edema include the administration of diuretics and restriction of sodium and possibly fluid. The nurse must observe for adverse effects of medication, such as electrolyte imbalance and postural hypotension. Potassium supplementation may be ordered for patient who is experiencing hypokalemia.

> Electrolyte imbalance alert: Look for the following signs of hypokalemia: fatigue, muscle weakness, muscle cramps, drowsiness, confusion, new onset of bradycardia or postural hypotension.

◆ Pain

Severe pain is most often associated with heart disease of an acute nature (e.g., MI). The analgesic drugs used most often are morphine sulfate and meperidine hydrochloride (Demerol). These are given IV initially for quick pain relief. As the acute phase and severe pain subside, these drugs may be replaced with oral dosages or milder sedatives that promote relaxation and freedom from anxiety.

Anginal pain can interfere with the patient's lifestyle, as well as cause discomfort. Medications that dilate coronary arteries to promote better blood flow and decrease ischemia are used to control anginal pain.

Nursing Assessment and Intervention The patient's pain may be increased because of nervousness and anxiety, and the nurse can do much to help relieve pain by providing a restful environment, interacting therapeutically with "active listening," and balancing rest with prescribed physical activity.

Each episode of pain is carefully assessed by noting when it started, the location and radiation pattern, degree on a scale, activity prior to onset, associated symptoms such as nausea, diaphoresis, or palpitations, and vital signs.

Sleep deprivation and fatigue can increase the pain. Turning, administration of medications, visiting, exercise, and other procedures should be coordinated so that the patient is not disturbed more than necessary.

Acute anginal pain is treated with nitroglycerin, oral nitrates, reassurance, and careful monitoring for relief. Determining those factors that seem to trigger an attack can identify stressors that the patient may be able to avoid.

Relaxation and other noninvasive techniques to manage pain are discussed in Chapter 10. Table 19-6 on p. 549 presents specific nursing diagnoses and nursing interventions related to heart disease.

COMMON THERAPIES AND THEIR NURSING IMPLICATIONS

The medical treatments most commonly used to manage heart disease include (1) pharmacological agents; (2) dietary controls; and (3) oxygen therapy. Patient education and rehabilitation of the cardiac patient also must be included.

Surgical treatment of cardiac conditions most often is employed to correct structural defects of the heart and great vessels and to bypass or enlarge the lumen of occluded coronary arteries to give the heart muscle a more reliable supply of blood.

◆ Pharmacological Agents

Many types of drugs are used to treat heart disorders. The most commonly administered drugs are listed in Table 19-7. Digitalis in its various forms is a widely prescribed drug in the United States. However, it is a potent drug that can produce serious toxicity. It can be very effective in treating certain kinds of cardiac disorders, but its therapeutic range is quite narrow. A therapeutic dose is only about one third less than the dose that will induce toxicity. Moreover, physiological changes resulting from age, electrolyte imbalances (particularly hypokalemia or hypercalcemia), renal impairment, metabolic disturbances, and certain heart conditions can predispose a patient to digitalis toxicity. Other drugs given simultaneously, including erythromycin, also can alter the effects of digitalis and make it more toxic. It should be remembered that digitoxin has a slower and more prolonged action and is 10 times more potent than digoxin. **For this reason, digitoxin and digoxin, are not interchangeable.**

It should be noted that most physicians do not want nurses to hold a dose of digitalis if the patient's pulse rate is below 60 bpm *as long as there are no signs of digitalis toxicity.* When the pulse rate is less than 60 bpm, the nurse should consider the other drugs the patient is taking. Both beta-blockers and calcium-channel blockers will lower the heart rate. Learn each physician's guidelines regarding a pulse rate lower than 60 bpm and check the nursing unit protocols.

When life-threatening complications arise from digitalis toxicity, Digoxin Immune Fab is given to counteract the excess digitalis. This drug is used cautiously as side effects include hypotension, hypokalemia, worsening of CHF, and rapid ventricular rates if the patient is experiencing atrial fibrillation.

Anticoagulants are prescribed to inhibit the formation of clots within blood vessels. Anticoagulants do not dissolve clots that have already formed, but they can prevent existing ones from growing larger and also interfere with the development of new clots. Heparin in some institutions is beginning to be administered in doses calculated by the patient's weight as well as by clotting times, which provides a more consistent level of the heparin in the right amount to prevent clot formation.

Think about . . . Can you list four signs and symptoms that might indicate that your patient is suffering from digitalis toxicity?

◆ Dietary Control

Contrary to popular opinion, obesity itself is not a direct cause of heart disease. However, the National Heart, Lung and Blood Institute lists obesity as a risk factor for cardiac disorders. When obesity is present in conjunction with other factors such as hypertension, diabetes mellitus, smoking, and family history of heart disease, the likelihood of cardiovascular problems is increased.

Prevent heart disease and moderate the factors that predispose one to cardiovascular disease, the American Heart Association recommends the following "prudent" measures:

◆ A caloric intake to achieve or maintain ideal body weight.

◆ Ingestion of a 2 to 1 ratio of polyunsaturated to saturated fat, up to about 10% of the total calories.

◆ A reduction in total fat calories from 45% (the national daily average for Americans) to no more than 30% of total calories.

◆ A reduction in dietary cholesterol to 300 mg per day.

◆ An increase in complex dietary carbohydrates, particularly those with fiber (*not* simple sugars), to replace calories from fats.

◆ Reduction of refined sugar intake to about 10% of total calories.

◆ Limitation of sodium intake to no more than 5 gm per day.

◆ Consumption of alcohol in moderation.

Table 19-15 presents guidelines for a heart-healthy diet.

One Harvard study has indicated the great benefit of adding fiber to the diet to cut cholesterol levels. Increased fiber will lower cholesterol even without cutting down on dietary fat. Adults should consume about 25 g of fiber per day; the national average consumption is about 12 gs. Increasing fiber in the diet also lowers the risk of cancer. Another study indicates that regular margarine may be as harmful as butter in raising cholesterol levels because of the trans-fatty acids it contains. A tub, soft-style, margarine that lists water or liquid vegetable oil as its first ingredient contains less trans-fatty acids than other types.

There are excellent resources for information and support for patients who have a cardiovascular disease and are attempting to follow a dietary regimen as part of their overall treatment plan. Many community hospitals sponsor weight management programs. Local chapters of the American Heart Association provide pamphlets and other sources of information about diet.

TABLE 19-15 ◆ *Nutrition Point: Guidelines for a Heart-Healthy Diet*

◆ Limit meat intake to no more than 6 oz of cooked lean meat, fish, and skinless poultry (singly or in combination) per day. Fix main dishes with pasta, rice, beans, and/or vegetables mixed with small amounts of lean meat, poultry, or fish to create "low-meat" dishes. Restrict intake of organ meats, such as liver, brains, chitterlings, kidney, gizzards, and sweetbreads, as they are very high in cholesterol.

◆ Eat 5 to 6 servings of fruit and vegetables per day.

◆ Increase intake of fiber and carbohydrate by eating 6 or more servings of cereals, breads, or grains per day.

◆ Keep daily use of fats and oils to 5 to 8 teaspoons. This includes what is used in cooking, baking, in salad dressings, and spreads for bread.

◆ Cook using little or no fat; broil, bake, roast, poach, stir-fry, microwave, or steam foods rather than frying them.

◆ Eliminate as much fat as possible by trimming meat and skinning poultry before cooking. After browning meats, drain off all fat. Chill soups, stews, etc. after cooking and skim off fat before reheating to serve.

◆ Limit consumption of egg yolks to 3 to 4 per week, including those in baked or cooked items. Check store packages for listing of eggs or egg yolk as an ingredient.

◆ Use skim or 1% fat milk and nonfat or low-fat yogurt, cheeses, and ice creams.

---

*Note: The healthy heart diet is promoted by the American Heart Association.

Although some persons are more susceptible to hypertension than others, such as the obese person, a high intake of sodium is thought by some to contribute to the development of high blood pressure in susceptible individuals. Limiting sodium intake is an important part in preventing and treating hypertension. Teaching efforts should recognize the patient's willingness to change his eating habits and the support and encouragement he receives from his family. There are several cookbooks sponsored by the American Heart Association and others that make low-sodium, low-cholesterol meals easier to plan and prepare and more tasty. The fact that the tendency to develop cardiovascular disease runs in families gives the patient and the whole family good reason to develop good eating habits and to change to more wholesome foods.

Many health professionals consider the self-help groups to be most successful in assisting persons to lose pounds and then to keep their weight within normal range once the excess is lost. These groups include Weight Watchers, TOPS (Take Off Pounds Sensibly), and Overeaters Anonymous. Results of studies have shown that the behavior modification techniques employed by these groups are very successful.

Restriction of sodium, prescribed because of sodium's association with retention of water in the tissues, is discussed in Chapter 5. Patients who are on sodium-restricted diets require special encouragement and instruction in the ways to avoid an intake of sodium that would be harmful and contribute to their discomfort. Table 19-16 suggests ways to decrease sodium in the diet.

Traditionally iced drinks, hot drinks, and those containing caffeine were denied the MI patient. Today post-MI patients can safely drink up to five cups of coffee or iced beverages a day **if there are not changes in heart rate, rhythm, or blood pressure after drinking them.**

Dietary programs to reverse coronary heart disease have been introduced by Pritikin and by Ornish. Both men have shown that their programs work, but many find that the one designed by Dr. Ornish is easier to follow. Dr. Ornish claims that 90% of his patients who were told they needed a bypass or angioplasty have been able to control their disease and avoid surgery with changes in diet and lifestyle. The diet program is high in vegetables, fruits and grains, but oils and nuts are denied, as is caffeine. Fat is reduced to about 10% of total calories in this fashion. People who have had CABG or angioplasty benefit by preventing further advance of ASHD and more occlusions in coronary arteries. The program takes considerable personal motivation, is best if both spouses participate, and also emphasizes exercise and management of negative emotions. A definite advantage of the program is weight loss; people on the Ornish program become lean and

---

TABLE 19-16 ◆ *Nutrition Tips: Ways to Decrease Sodium in the Diet*

- Shift snacks from cheese to fresh or frozen fruits and vegetables.
- Stay away from "convenience" foods: ready-mixed sauces, frozen dinners, cured or smoked meats (including lunch meats), canned soups, and prepared salad dressings—unless the label truly indicates a low sodium content.
- Be aware that regular canned vegetables often contain a large amount of sodium; in some instances rinsing will greatly decrease the sodium content.
- Check soda pop labels for sodium content; many contain high sodium.
- Check cereal box labels for sodium content; switch to a lower-sodium cereal such as shredded wheat.
- Use ¼ to ½ the amount of salt that a recipe calls for.
- Leave the salt shaker off the table.
- Make a salt substitute seasoning of: ½ tsp garlic powder, mixed with 1 tsp each of basil, black pepper, marjoram, onion powder, parsley, sage, savory, and thyme, or use a product, such as "Mrs. Dash" or Lemon Pepper instead of salt.
- When ordering at restaurants, ask which dishes are low in sodium; or ask that the cook refrain from salting your dishes.
- Ask fast food restaurants to supply you with a list of their available foods showing sodium content of each item.

---

trim as the whole program is combined with daily exercise.

***Think about* . . .** How could you specifically change your diet in one way that would help you to follow a more "heart-healthy" diet?

◆ Oxygen Therapy

The administration of supplemental oxygen to relieve the dyspnea and hypoxemia of a cardiac patient is a routine therapeutic measure. Any patient experiencing chest pain is started on low-dose oxygen. This form of therapy is discussed earlier in this chapter and in Chapter 16. The responsibilities of the nurse in regard to oxygen therapy for a cardiac patient are primarily concerned with observation to determine a patient's need for supplemental oxygen, maintenance of the ordered flow rate, and the response to this form of therapy once it has been initiated.

As previously explained, cyanosis is a late symptom of hypoxemia and oxygen need. It is important, therefore, that the nurse be alert to earlier signs such as increase in pulse rate and symptoms of cerebral anoxia such as irritability, confusion, and disorientation.

The response of the patient to the administration of oxygen is best determined by pulse oximetry or blood gas analysis and pH determination.

◆ Cardiac Surgery

Until the 1950s, little could be done in the way of surgical procedures involving the heart itself because prolonged interruption of circulation meant certain death for the patient. However, with the introduction of the heart-lung machine and hypothermic techniques, surgeons can now repair or replace damaged valves, correct many congenital heart defects, and bypass clogged coronary arteries.

The heart-lung machine, which has many variations in design and appearance, functions as an artificial heart (pump) and lung (oxygenator). For this reason, it is sometimes called a *pump-oxygenator*. Because all of this is done outside the patient's body, the procedure is called *extracorporeal circulation*. The surgeon inserts large tubes in the vena cava and reroutes the unoxygenated venous blood through the heart-lung machine. There, the blood is exposed to an atmosphere of oxygen in which an exchange of gases takes place (carbon dioxide is released and oxygen is taken up), and the oxygenated blood is returned to the patient via the femoral artery. The blood may be cooled so that the patient's body temperature is lowered (hypothermia), thereby reducing the body's metabolic needs during surgery.

Specific Types of Cardiac Surgery Open-heart surgery is performed by extracorporeal circulation and hypothermia. Congenital heart defects, valve replacements, bypass of clogged coronary arteries, and heart transplant are accomplished by open-chest techniques.

Coronary artery bypass surgery. Coronary artery bypass graft (CABG) is done when angina cannot be controlled medically or to prevent more occlusions and consequent MI. The surgery bypasses the artery that is blocked, replacing it with sections of a vein or artery taken from another part of the patient's body. Usually the mammary artery is used or sections of saphenous vein are grafted. The transplanted vessel is sewn into the heart muscle and attached to an open portion of a coronary artery so that an adequate supply of blood will reach the heart muscle. Although the heart is not "opened," its activity often is stopped for the procedure. The CABG patient will have a midsternal incision and, if saphenous veins were used for the grafts, will have leg incisions as well. Figure 19-12 shows CABG procedures using vein grafts or the internal mammary artery.

A new drug, Aprotinin (Trasylol), reduces perioperative blood loss for patients undergoing repeat CABG. It greatly reduces the need for blood transfusion.

Elder Care Point... The elderly tolerate CABG surgery quite well, but the recovery period is longer because the slower healing rate and lessened ability of the body to handle such stress.

A new technique for some CABG procedures, minimally invasive direct coronary artery bypass (MID-CAB), does not require stopping the heart's activity and therefore does not require using the heart-lung machine. The procedure requires only a 3-inch incision, is performed with the use of drugs to slow or stop the heart

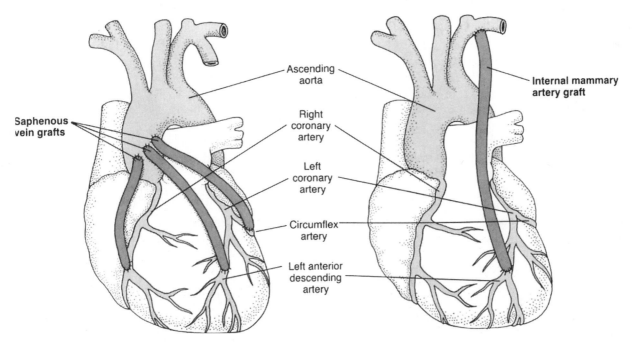

FIGURE 19-12 Two methods of coronary artery bypass grafting. (*Source:* Ignatavicius, D. D., Workman, M. L., Mishler, M. A. [1995]. *Medical–Surgical Nursing: A Nursing Process Approach,* 2nd ed. Philadelphia: Saunders, p. 1007.)

briefly and special instruments, takes approximately one-third the time to complete as traditional CABG, and patients go home in less than 36 hours. It is also only one-third the cost of CABG. However, only patients with one or two lesions in an easily accessible area of a major coronary artery are candidates for this simplified procedure.

Coronary bypass surgery is expensive, averaging $75,000 to $100,000 dollars for the surgery, anesthesia, and hospital costs. Anginal chest pain disappears in about 65% of patients, and another 25% show improvement. There is an average of a 10-year patency rate for CABG using the left internal mammary artery and even greater success rates when the right internal mammary artery is used. Some physicians still question the benefits of such surgery compared with the cost and effectiveness of more conservative medical therapies. Presently, many of those patients who had a coronary artery bypass in the 1980s are returning for a second operation because the new arteries have become occluded. A greater emphasis is being placed on the need for dietary and exercise therapy after the procedure.

Percutaneous transluminal coronary angioplasty (PTCA). Another treatment for occluded coronary arteries is PTCA. It is performed on patients with only one or two occlusions. The patient must be prepared to undergo CABG if the procedure is unsuccessful. A percentage of patients experience reocclusion about 6 months after PCTA and end up needing a CABG. The use of expandable stents implanted at the time of PCTA seems to be decreasing the incidence of reocclusion.

Transmyocardial laser revascularization. Patients who are critically ill are not candidates for PTCA or CABG, but transmyocardial laser revascularization is an option. A carbon dioxide laser is used to drill tiny holes in the heart's left ventricle. These channels heal on the outside of the heart, but remain open on the inside, allowing blood to flow into the myocardium where it was previously diminished because of blocked coronary arteries.

Cardiomyoplasty. Some patients with severe CHF who are not candidates for a heart transplant are undergoing dynamic cardiomyoplasty using the latissimus dorsi muscle. Part of the muscle is detached from its natural position and brought around to the front of the body. It is wrapped around the heart and a pacemaker is connected to the heart and the back muscle and implanted in the abdominal wall. The pacemaker makes the muscle contract in conjunction with the normal action of the heart and thereby boosts the heart's pumping power.

Valvuloplasty and valve replacement. For valve stenosis, balloon valvuloplasty may be performed in some cases. A balloon catheter is threaded via the circulatory system through the heart and into the valve and the balloon is inflated to break open the stenosed valve. Valve replacement surgery is more commonly done. Mitral or aortic valve replacement is scheduled when the patient's condition prevents him from going about his usual daily activities, whether the problem is stenosis or insufficiency. Replacement is done as an open-heart procedure using extracorporeal circulation with the heart-lung bypass machine and hypothermia. Preoperative and postoperative care are much the same as for CABG patients.

Open-heart surgeries usually take between 3 and 6 hours, depending on the amount of repair or replacement necessary. The patient returns to the cardiac surgical intensive care unit and remains on a ventilator for 8 to 24 hours. Patient care requires highly skilled nurses, as there are multiple tubes and lines for monitoring physiological status and for delivering drugs to control blood pressure and dysrhythmias. If the patient's recovery is uncomplicated, he will be transferred to a step-down telemetry unit 1 to 2 days after surgery. Ventricular aneurysm resulting from an MI or trauma may be surgically repaired, too.

Heart transplant. Heart transplants are performed for selected patients who have end-stage left ventricular failure resulting from **cardiomyopathy** (primary myocardial disease). Candidates must be under age 65, have end-stage cardiac disease with predicted survival of less than 6 months, no other systemic disease, have good renal function, and be psychologically stable. Other requirements are that the patient be within 20% of ideal weight and not an active tobacco user. A history of diabetes beginning more than 10 years ago or accompanying complications, or organ damage, is another contraindication. A good tissue match is essential for a transplant. Candidates for heart transplant undergo an extensive psychological evaluation and thorough physical assessment. Very few donor hearts are available, and the waiting lists are long. Patients who do receive a heart transplant face considerable financial burdens, a life of taking immunosuppressive drugs that have many serious side effects, and the constant threat of organ rejection. However, the benefits are considerable with a 1-year survival rate of 80% to 90% and a 3-year survival time of about 70%. Heart transplants are performed in highly specialized medical centers. A new drug, ketoconazole (Nizoral), may decrease the amount of cyclosporine needed to prevent rejection. Tissue matching for organ transplant and immunosuppression therapy for transplant patients is discussed in Chapter 7.

Preoperative care for cardiac surgery. Before cardiac surgery, the patient undergoes a series of diagnostic tests and examinations, mostly on an outpatient basis, such as those presented in Table 19-3 on p. 542. Once a decision is made to undergo surgery, measures are taken to ensure that the patient is in the best possible condition. All teaching and psychological preparation are done as an outpatient basis whenever possible. These are mostly the responsibilities of a nurse. There is considerable apprehension on the part of the patient and the family who are faced with open-heart surgery.

The patient is given information about the procedure, explaining what he can expect and the kind of equipment he will see. He is admitted early the morning of surgery for a scheduled procedure. If he has been on an oral anticoagulant, he is switched over to heparin by injection at least one day prior to surgery. Clinical Pathway 19-1 shows an example for CABG/valve surgery.

Postoperative Care   During the early postoperative period, the patient is kept in an intensive care unit (ICU), where specialized cardiac monitoring equipment is used and highly trained personnel are in constant attendance. Cardiac rate and rhythm are watched closely. Chest tubes for drainage and proper reexpansion of the lungs need special attention. The patient often continues to receive mechanical ventilation for several hours after surgery. Once consciousness has fully returned, weaning from the ventilator is begun if oxygenation is adequate. Autologous blood transfusion often is performed with blood drained from the chest cavity. Chest tubes are usually removed before the patient is moved out of the ICU. Temporary epicardial pacemaker leads will be in place and may or may not be hooked up to a pacemaker. There are usually at least two IV lines in place for medication delivery and fluid maintenance, as well as an arterial line for hemodynamic monitoring. If saphenous vein grafts were used rather than the mammary artery, there will be leg incisions to care for along with the chest incision. Urine output is monitored hourly initially and then every 2 hours to detect signs of decreased perfusion to the kidneys and cardiogenic shock.

After the first 24 to 48 hours, the surgeon will assess the patient's condition and decide whether he can be transferred to a step-down or general surgical unit. The patient will continue to need very special nursing care. His vital signs must be taken and recorded at frequent intervals. His urinary output must be measured and recorded hourly at first, then every 2 to 8 hours, and his fluid intake may be restricted for a period. Daily weight is monitored to assess fluid balance.

Coronary artery bypass surgery can produce many special problems related to physical and emotional disability and rehabilitation of the patient. Among the physiological symptoms that can persist into the home recovery period are fatigue and weakness, incisional discomfort, edema in the donor leg, dysrhythmias, loss of appetite, depression, and unusual physical sensations. There also is the possibility of closure of the graft and the reappearance of original symptoms. Sometimes the patient develops Dressler's syndrome, a type of pericarditis, which is treated with nonsteroidal antiinflammatory drugs (NSAIDs) such as indomethacin (Indocin).

Cardiac transplant patients are threatened by organ rejection, infection, development of CAD in the new heart, and development of a malignant tumor as a result of immunosuppressive therapy to prevent transplant rejection. Heart biopsies are performed regularly. Depression for weeks to months is not uncommon after heart surgery. Patients should be alerted to this possibility and referred for assistance if this occurs.

Most patients do not experience all of these problems during the home recovery period after coronary artery bypass surgery, and some have relatively trouble-free recovery periods. It is important, however, that health care professionals, as well as bypass surgery patients and their families, realize that it is not a cure for CAD. It is simply one form of therapy for a chronic condition that will require continued management to slow the disease process and reduce the incidence of life-threatening events in the person's life. Other specific postoperative care is directed at preventing infection, monitoring for complications, and promoting rehabilitation.

Usually after the first 48 hours, minimal medication is needed for pain. The patient often is quite fatigued and tends to have mood swings. With an uncomplicated recovery, the patient is usually discharged home within 3 to 7 days.

COMMUNITY CARE

With early discharge from the hospital after surgery, many patients have continuing care from home health nurses. Patients recovering from cardiac surgery, MI, atherosclerotic heart disease, angina, or valvular heart disease all may be referred to a cardiac rehabilitation program. The goal of such programs is to reduce risk of further heart problems or death. The program is directed toward restoring and maintaining optimal physiological function. Improving psychological outlook, maintaining ability to work, and social well-being are other components of the program. A supervised exercise program with cardiac monitoring for 6 to 8 weeks is combined with dietary counseling, classes on stress reduction, and the development of an individual action plan to reduce cardiac risk factors. A support group consisting of other individuals who have the same condition or have had similar surgery often is available. Most insurance coverage will pay for the program as it has been highly successful in helping people to develop and maintain a healthier lifestyle and to reduce risk factors.

Text continued on page 584

CLINICAL PATHWAY 19-1 • *Coronary Artery Bypass Graft or Valve Surgery*

University Hospitals of Cleveland

CARE PATH NAME: CABG/VALVE (Telemetry)
TOTAL ELOS: 6 Days
Expected Disposition: _____
Preop Weight: _____

Collaborative Problem List
1. Home maintenance-management
2. Potential for decreased cardiac output
3. Potential for fluid overload
4. Potential for activity intolerance
5.
6.

Focus	Postop-Day 1: Time of Transfer to 7:00 A.M.	Postop-Day 2	Postop-Day 3	Postop-Day 4	Postop-Day 5	Postop-Day 6
Laboratories/tests/procedures	• Dextrose stick q 6 h (diabetics) → • Pulse oximetry q 8 h and PRN → • Telemetry until discontinued • Full Disclosure until discontinued →	→ → → → • PT, PTT, q day (valve) • EKG • CBC, Chem 7	• Dextrose stick q 8 h (diabetics) → • Pulse oximetry (PRN) → → →	→ → → →	→ → → → CBC, Chem 23 Chest X-ray, EKG	⊤ ⊤ ⊤ ⊤ ⊤
Consults	• Cardiology • Respiratory SICU • Physical therapy consult for all patients ≥75 years old or in SICU >48 hrs. and for other pts. if ordered. • OT consult and evaluation if ordered.	• Social service consult		• Offer cardiac rehabilitation referral • Home care consult if applicable		
Physical assessment	• Nursing assessment q shift • Vital signs q 4 h • Assess need for arrhythmia management protocol • Input and output q shift, weight q day	→ →	Vial signs q shift → →	→ →	→ →	⊤ ⊤ ⊤
Activity	• Out of bed tid • BRP with assistance →	→ ⊤ ⊤	• Out of bed → chair all meals • Bathroom privileges, begin ambulation • Begin participation with ADL's	• Up ad lib → • Actively participates in ADLs →	→ →	↑ • Independently performs ADLs

Treatments

- Check isolated epicardial wires at time of transfer →
- Temporary pacemaker as ordered →
- Heparin lock/IVF →
- O$_2$ at ___ L/min by nasal canula. Wean as tolerated →
- Incentive spirometry q 1 h while awake →
- Encourage C + DB →
- Change CT, graft, epicardial wires DSGs →
- Maintain electrical isolation →
- D/C O$_2$ when room-air pulse oximeter ≥92% →
- Change CT and epicardial wires DSGs →
- Discontinue epicardial wires and apply band-aids
- Discontinue graft site sutures
- D/C temporary pacer
- D/C heparin lock

Diet

- Advance as tolerated to 2-3 Gm. sodium diet →
- Nutrition screen →

Medications

ECASA
Dipyridamole (DHV only)
Furosemide
KCl
Warfarin (valve)
Docusate
PRN:
- Flurazepam
- Acetaminophen 325 w/codeine 30
Other:
- Beta-blocker
- Consider preadmission medications

- Continue all medications as ordered →

CLINICAL PATHWAY 19-1 ♦ Coronary Artery Bypass Graft or Valve Surgery (Continued)

Focus	Postop-Day 1: Time of Transfer to 7:00 A.M.	Postop-Day 2	Postop-Day 3	Postop-Day 4	Postop-Day 5	Postop-Day 6
Discharge planning/teaching	Orient to Lerner Tower 3 at transfer ➤	◆ Assess home care needs ◆ Review meds while administering ◆ Intiate Gold Referral Form (GRF) if applicable	◆ Review medications, activity, incisional care, diet ◆ Offer videos, patient instruction sheets ➤	Initiate discharge folder: Medication schedule Medication cards PI sheets CT booklet ◆ Cardiac rehabilitation folder ◆ Follow-up appointments (if known)	Final review: ◆ Referral(s) to appropriate agencies ◆ Confirm arrangements for equipment (if applicable) ◆ Finalize GRF ◆ D/C folder ◆ Cardiac rehabilitation folder ◆ Follow-up appointments	Final review
Intermediate outcomes	◆ Hemodynamically stable ◆ Pain controlled ◆ Bowel sounds ×4 quads ◆ Able to ambulate 30 ft with pulse Ox ≥90%	◆ Hemodynamically stable ◆ Pain controlled ◆ Able to ambulate 60 ft and/or participate in ADLs with pulse Oximetry ≥90% ◆ Discharge plans discussed with pt/fam; pt discharge by 11 A.M. on Day 6 ◆ Patient and family assess home situation and determine appropriate home health services	◆ Hemodynamically stable ◆ Pain controlled ◆ Able to ambulate 60 ft and/or increasing ability to participate in ADLs ◆ No signs of hypoxia ◆ Discharge planning continuing	◆ Hemodynamically stable ◆ Pain controlled ◆ Able to ambulate 90 ft and/or increasing ability to participate in ADLs ◆ No arrhythmias ◆ No signs of hypoxia ◆ Bowel movement X l ◆ Discharge planning continuing	◆ Hemodynamically stable ◆ Pain controlled ◆ Able to ambulate 100 ft and/or increasing ability to participate in ADLs ◆ Discharge orders, prescriptions written by evening ◆ Patient not >24 ◆ Epicardial wires out day before discharge, no bleeding ◆ Graft site sutures discharge ◆ No arrhythmias ◆ No signs of hypoxia ◆ Discharge plans confirmed	See discharge outcomes.

Intermediate outcomes	☐ Met ☐ Not met (see notes)	☐ Met ☐ Not met (see notes)	☐ Met ☐ Not met (see notes)	☐ Met ☐ Not met (see notes)	☐ Met ☐ Not met (see notes)	See discharge outcomes
Date						
RN signature—days						
RN signature—evenings						
RN signature—nights						

Carepath review with patient or patient's family/guardian

Signature _____

Discharge outcomes	Met	Not Met	Comments	Date/Initials

Source: Courtesy of University Hospitals of Cleveland.

Note: University Hospitals' carepaths have been developed to assist clinicians in patient management and clinical decision-making. The carepaths are intended to meet the needs of patients in most circumstances. They are not intended to either replace a clinician's judgment or establish a protocol for all patients with this diagnosis.

Home care nurses have many patients who suffer from heart disease. The goal of home care is to monitor the patient's condition and to prevent complications, such as life-threatening dysrhythmias, MI, and CHF. Nurses supervise the medication regimen, monitor weight gain, draw blood for laboratory tests to determine drug levels and electrolyte status, and assess for beginning signs of complications. By catching complications early, patients can be treated at home rather than at the hospital, thereby decreasing costs of care.

The nurse working in the long-term care facility is dealing with heart patients every day as many of the elderly have a heart problem of one sort or another. Assessing changes in condition is a high priority. If changes can be found quickly, the severity of a complication can be reduced. The nurse in the long-term care facility and in the home setting acts as the "eyes and ears" of the physician.

CRITICAL THINKING EXERCISE

Clinical Case Problems

Read each clinical case problem and discuss the questions with your classmates.

1. Mrs. Weiber is admitted to the hospital with a medical diagnosis of CHF resulting from mitral stenosis. She has a history of atherosclerotic heart disease (ASHD) and angina pectoris. Her chief complaints on admission are dyspnea on exertion, fatigue, and palpitations.

   a. What disease processes probably led to the development of Mrs. Weiber's mitral stenosis and CHF?

   b. List three nursing diagnoses with interventions in your care plan for her.

   c. What should be included in the preoperative teaching plan for her mitral valve replacement surgery?

2. Mr. Nuñez, age 54, is admitted to the coronary care unit (CCU) after having suffered an acute MI while shoveling snow at his home.

   a. What disease processes probably led to Mr. Nuñez's MI?

   b. Describe the diagnostic tests that will most likely be ordered for Mr. Nuñez.

   c. After Mr. Nuñez is transferred from the CCU to the telemetry step-down unit, how would you go about assessing his status and identifying his specific problems and nursing care needs?

   d. Prepare a plan of care to help alleviate the problems you have identified and to avoid others that might develop.

   e. Make a discharge teaching plan for Mr. Nuñez that includes rehabilitation activities.

BIBLIOGRAPHY

Ahrens, S. G. (1995). Managing heart failure. *Nursing 95.* 25(12):26–31.

American Heart Association. (1995). *Heart and Stroke Facts.* Dallas: Author.

American Heart Association. (1997). *1997 Heart and Stroke: Statistical Update.* Dallas: Author.

Apple, S. (1996). New trends in thrombolytic therapy. *RN.* 59(1):30–34.

Applegate, E. (1995). *The Anatomy and Physiology Learning System.* Philadelphia: Saunders.

Arnold, S. E. (1997). Cardiac stress testing. *Nursing 97.* 27(1):58–61.

Ballard, J. C., Wood, L. L., Lansing, A. M. (1997). Transmyocardial revascularization: Criteria for selecting patients, treatment, and nursing care. *Critical Care Nurse.* 17(1): 42–59.

Bennett, J. C., Plum, F., eds. (1996). *Cecil Textbook of Medicine,* 20th ed. Philadelphia: Saunders.

Bernat, J. J. (1997). Smoothing the CABG patient's road to recovery. *American Journal of Nursing.* 97(2):23–27.

Black, J., Matassarin-Jacobs, E. (1997). *Medical-Surgical Nursing: Clinical Management for Continuity of Care,* 5th ed. Philadelphia: Saunders.

Boltz, M. (1994). Identifying cardiac rhythms. *Nursing 94.* 24(4):54–58.

Bosley, C. L. (1995). Assessing cardiac output: don't stop at the heart. *Nursing 95.* 25(9):43–45.

Bove, L. A. (1995). Now! Surgery for heart failure. *RN.* 95(5):26–30.

Bove, L. A., et al. (1995). Nursing care of patients undergoing dynamic cardiomyoplasty. *Critical Care Nurse.* 15(6): 96–100, 102–104.

Braun, A. (1994). A quick response to life-threatening arrythmias. *RN.* 57(1):54–62.

Carroll, P. (1996). Salvaging the blood from the chest. *RN.* 59(9):33–38.

Cerrato, P. L. (1997). New acute MI guidelines. *RN.* 60(1): 25–26.

Chase, S. (1997). Antiarrhythmics. *RN.* 60(5):41–48.

Chernecky, C. C., Berger, B. J. (1997). *Laboratory Tests and Diagnostic Procedures,* 2nd ed. Phildalphia: Saunders.

Copstead, L. C. (1995). *Perspectives on Pathophysiology.* Philadelphia: Saunders.

Cotran, R. S., Kumar, V., Robbins, S. L., Schoen, F. J., eds. (1994). *Robbins' Pathologic Basis of Disease,* 5th ed. Philadelphia: Saunders.

Crawford, M., ed. (1994). *Cardiology Clinics: Congestive Heart Failure.* Philadelphia: Saunders.

Cronin, S. N., Logsdon, C., Miracle, V. (1997). Psychosocial and functional outcomes in women after coronary artery bypass surgery. *Critical Care Nurse.* 17(2):19–21.

Crowley, A. (1997). Paroxysmal supraventricular tachycardia. *American Journal of Nursing.* 97(1):53.

Dambro, M. R. (1996). *Griffith's 5 Minute Clinical Consult.* Baltimore: Williams & Wilkins.

Damjanov, I. (1996). *Pathology for the Health Related Professions*. Philadelphia: Saunders.

Davis, J., Sherer, K. (1994). *Applied Nutrition and Diet Therapy for Nurses,* 2nd ed. Philadelphia: Saunders.

Dennison, R. D. (1994). Making sense of hemodynamic monitoring. *American Journal of Nursing,* 94(8):24–31.

Diamond, K. V., and Thornby, D. (1996). Mechanical circulatory support: What does the future hold? *American Journal of Nursing.* 96(5):32–35.

Dracup, K., Dunbar, S. B., Baker, D. W. (1995). Rethinking heart failure. *American Journal of Nursing.* 95(7):23–27.

Elder, A. N. (1994). Sinus bradycardia: elevating a slow heart rate. *Nursing 94.* 24(11):48–50.

Elder, A. N. (1994). Sinus tachycardia: lowering a high heart rate. *Nursing 94.* 24(12):62–64.

Fabius, D. (1994). Solving the mystery of heart murmurs. *Nursing 94.* 24(7):39–44.

Fabius, D., Stunkard, J. (1994). Uncovering the secrets of snaps, rubs, & clicks. *Nursing 94.* 24(7):45–55.

Forsha, B. (1997). Scaffolding the coronary arteries: Intracoronary stenting. *Home Healthcare Nurse.* 15(4):247–253.

Fowler, J. P. (1996). How to respond rapidly when chest pain strikes. *Nursing 96.* 26(4):42–43.

Fowler, J. P. (1995). When CHF turns deadly. *Nursing 95.* 25(1):54–55.

Garner, E., et al. (1996). Intracoronary stent update: focus on patient education. *Critical Care Nurse.* 16(2):65–68, 71–75.

Guyton, A. C., Hall, J. E. (1996). *Textbook of Medical Physiology,* 9th ed. Philadelphia: Saunders.

Hasemeier, C. S. (1996). Permanent pacemaker. *American Journal of Nursing.* 96(2):30–31.

Hayes, D. D. (1996). Understanding coronary atherectomy. *American Journal of Nursing.* 96(12):38–44.

Hicks, S. (1994). Standing guard against silent ischemia and infarction. *Nursing 94.* 24(1):34–39.

Hodgson, B., Kizior, R., Kingdon, R. (1997). *Nurse's Drug Handbook 1997.* Philadelphia: Saunders.

Ignatavicius, D. D., Hausman, K. A. (1995). *Clinical Pathways for Collaborative Practice.* Philadelphia: Saunders.

Ignatavicius, D. D., Workman, M. L., Mishler, M. A. (1995). *Medical–Surgical Nursing: A Nursing Process Approach,* 2nd ed. Philadelphia: Saunders.

Janowski, M. J. (1996). Managing heart failure. *RN.* 59(2):34–38.

Jarvis, C. (1996). *Physical Examination and Health Assessment,* 2nd ed. Philadelphia: Saunders.

Jensen, L., King, K. M. (1997). Women and heart disease: The issues. *Critical Care Nurse.* 17(2):45–52.

Kee, J., Hayes, E. (1993). *Pharmacology: A Nursing Process Approach.* Philadelphia: Saunders.

Keeys, M. (1994). Nuclear cardiology stress testing. *Nursing 94.* 24(10):63–64.

Kegel, L. M. (1996). Case management, critical pathways, and myocardial infarction. *Critical Care Nurse.* 16(2): 97–111.

Kirton, C. A. (1996). Assessing normal heart sounds. *Nursing 96.* 26(2):56–57.

Konick-McMahan, J. (1997). Discharged with dobutamine. *RN.* 60(4):24–29.

Lazzara, D., Sellergren, C. (1996). *Nursing 96.* 26(11):42–51.

Lehne, R. A. (1994). *Pharmacology for Nursing Care,* 2nd ed. Philadelphia: Saunders.

Lewandowski, D. M. (1995). Congestive heart failure. *American Journal of Nursing.* 95(5):36–37.

Lewis, S., Collier, I. (1995). *Medical-Surgical Nursing,* 4th ed. St. Louis, MO: Mosby Year Book.

Malarkey, L. M., McMorrow, M. E. (1996). *Nurse's Manual of Laboratory Tests and Diagnostic Procedures.* Philadelphia: Saunders.

Matteson, M., McConnell, E. (1997). *Gerontological Nursing: Concepts and Practice,* 2nd ed. Philadelphia: Saunders.

McGrath, D. (1997). Mitral valve prolapse. *American Journal of Nursing.* 97(5):40–44.

Merkley, K. (1994). Assessing chest pain. *RN.* 94(6):58–62.

Miracle, V., Sims, J. M. (1997). Atrial flutter. *Nursing 97.* 27(5):41.

Miracle, V., Sims, J. M. (1996). Normal sinus rhythm. *Nursing 96.* 26(5):50–51.

Miracle, V., Sims, J. M. (1996). Sinus bradycardia. *Nursing 96.* 26(7):43.

Monane, M., Boh, R., et al. (1994). Noncompliance with congestive heart failure. *Archives of Internal Medicine.* 154(4):433.

Moser, D. K. (1997). Correcting misconceptions about women and heart disease. *American Journal of Nursing.* 97(4):26–33.

Murphy, S. F., Nickerson, N. J., Kouchoukos, N. T. (1996). Functional outcome in the elderly after coronary artery surgery. *MEDSURG Nursing.* 5(2):107–110.

Newkirk, T., Leeper, B. (1996). Congestive heart failure: mapping the way to quality outcomes. *American Journal of Nursing.* 96(5):25–27.

Norman, C. H. (1997). Cardiac rehab: For spouses, too. *RN.* 60(2):17–20.

Ondrusek, R. S. (1996). Spotting an MI before it's an MI. *RN.* 26(4):26–29.

O'Donnell, L. (1996). Complications of MI: Beyond the acute stage. *American Journal of Nursing.* 96(9):25–30.

O'Neal, P. V. (1994). How to spot early signs of cardiogenic shock. *American Journal of Nursing.* 94(5):36–40.

O'Neill, P. A. (1995). Tachycardia: restoring a normal heart rate. *Nursing 95.* 25(6):33.

O'Toole, M., Waldman, A. R. (1995). A stable approach to unstable angina. *RN.* 58(7):29–32.

Owen, A. (1995). Tracking the rise and fall of cardiac enzymes. *Nursing 95.* 25(5):35–38.

Perez, A. (1996). Cardiac monitoring: Mastering the essentials. *RN.* 59(8):32–38.

Perez, A. (1996). EKG electrode placement: A refresher course. *RN.* 59(9):29–31.

Perra, B. M. (1995). Managing coronary atherectomy patients in a special procedure unit. *Critical Care Nurse.* 15(6): 57–59, 63–66.

Petrosky-Pacini, A. J. (1996). The automatic implantable cardioverter defibrillator in home care. *Home Healthcare Nurse.* 14(4):238–243.

Pool, N. (1994). Initiating temporary transvenous dual-chamber pacing. *Nursing 94.* 24(5):48–50.

Porterfield, L., Porterfield, J. (1993). Digitalis toxicity: a common occurrence. *Critical Care Nurse.* 13(12): 40–43.

Possanza, C. P. (1996). Coronary artery bypass graft surgery. *Nursing 96.* 26(2):48–50.

Rakel, R. E., ed. (1994). *Conn's Current Therapy 1994.* Philadelphia: Saunders.

Ramsey, P., Larson, E. (1993). *Medical Therapeutics,* 2nd ed. Philadelphia: Saunders.

Ray, G. L. (1994). Decision, decisions: which thrombolytic therapy is best for your patient? *American Journal of Nursing.* 94(11):11–15.

Riegel, B., Thomason, T., Carlson, B. (1995). Coronary precautions: fact or fiction? *Nursing 95.* 25(10):52–53.

Riley, M. C. (1997). Elective cardioversion: Who, when, and how. *RN.* 60(5):27–29.

Sandler, R. L. (1994). Atrial fibrillation. *American Journal of Nursing.* 94(12):26.

Shine, L., Howland-Gradman, J. (1996). Aortic stenosis in the elderly: valvuloplasty vs. surgery. *American Journal of Nursing.* 96(5):7–11.

Simko, L. C., Walker, J. H. (1996). Preoperative antioxidant and allopurinol therapy for reducing reperfusion-induced injury in patients undergoing cardiothoracic surgery. *Critical Care Nurse.* 16(6):69–73.

Sims, J. M., Miracle, V. (1997). Atrial fibrillation. *Nursing 97.* 27(4):55.

Sims, J. M., Miracle, V. (1996). Sinus tachycardia. *Nursing 96.* 26(6):49.

Stahl, L. (1995). How to manage common arrhythmias in medical patients. *American Journal of Nursing.* 95(3): 36–41.

Stamatis, S. J., Spadoni, S. M. (1997). Getting to the heart of IABP therapy. *RN.* 60(1):38–43.

Stovsky, B., Dehner, S. (1994). Patient education after valve surgery. *Critical Care Nurse.* 14(4):117–122.

Strimike, C. L. (1995). Caring for a patient with an intracoronary stent. *American Journal of Nursing.* 95(1): 40–45.

Strimike, C. (1996). Understanding intravascular ultrasound. *American Journal of Nursing.* 96(6):40–42.

Swearingen, P., ed. (1994). *Manual of Medical-Surgical Nursing Care,* 3rd ed. St. Louis, MO: Mosby.

Taptich, B., Iyer, P., Bernocchi-Losey, D. (1994). *Nursing Diagnosis and Care Planning,* 2nd ed. Philadelphia: Saunders.

Thompson, E. (1993). Transesophageal echocardiography: a new window on the heart and great vessels. *Critical Care Nurse.* 14(10):55–59.

Turner, D. M., Turner, L. A. (1995). Right ventricular myocardial infarction: detection, treatment, and nursing implications. *Critical Care Nurse.* 15(1):22–26.

Tsunoda, D. (1996). Clinical snapshot: acute myocardial infarction. *American Journal of Nursing.* 96(5):38–39.

Ulrich, S., Canale, S., Wendell, S. (1994). *Medical–Surgical Nursing Care Planning Guides,* 3rd ed. Philadelphia: Saunders.

Villaire, M. (1996). Early heart-attack care: the critical paradigm shift toward prevention. *Critical Care Nurse.* 16(1): 79–85.

Wallace, C. J. V. O. (1995). When digoxin harms instead of helps. *RN.* 58(9):26–29.

Weeks, S. M. (1996). Caring for patients with heart failure. *Nursing 96.* 26(3):52–53.

Weikart, C. (1994). New eye into the heart. *RN.* 57(10): 36–39.

White, E. (1994). Managing hyperlipidemia: new approaches to an old problem. *Nursing 94.* 24(8):66–69.

Yacone-Morton, L. A. (1995). Antiarrhythmics. *RN.* 58(4): 25–35.

Yacone-Morton, L. A. (1995). Inotropic agents and nitrates. *RN.* 58(3):22–28.

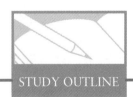

STUDY OUTLINE

I. Causes of Heart Disorders

A. Structural defects: congenital and acquired.

B. Coronary artery disease leading to myocardial ischemia.

C. Weakness of heart muscle and congestion of blood flow: congestive heart failure.

D. Infection and inflammation of heart structures.

E. Disturbances of heart conduction systems: dysrhythmias.

F. Cardiomyopathy.

II. Prevention of Heart Disease

A. Heart disease remains the leading cause of death in the United States.

B. Mortality rate for heart disease has declined, but the cost of heart disease has increased.

C. Risk factors: avoidable and unavoidable.

1. Avoidable (can be controlled or corrected): elevated blood lipids, obesity, habitual dietary excesses, lack of exercise, poor blood pressure control, cigarette smoking, cocaine use.

2. Unavoidable: age or aging, sex, race, ethnic origin, environment in early childhood, heredity, diabetes mellitus, hypertension.

3. Management of hypertension is a major tool to prevent heart disease.

III. Diagnostic Tests and Procedures (Table 19-3)

A. Telemetry—continuous monitoring of cardiac rhythm.

IV. Nursing Assessment of Cardiovascular Status

A. History taking: medical history of patient and his family; presence of known high-risk factors.

B. Subjective data: chest pain, fatigue, complaints of shortness of breath, cough, hemoptysis, palpitations of the heart, and nocturia.

C. Objective data: patient's posture in bed, color and temperature of skin, diaphoresis, pitting edema, abnormal breathing patterns, distended neck veins, heart sounds, apical pulse, and peripheral pulses.

V. Nursing Diagnosis and Nursing Interventions

A. Table 19-6 presents general nursing diagnoses and nursing interventions.

B. Nursing care plans in chapter provide examples of the complete nursing process.

C. Nursing care must be individualized for each patient.

VI. Planning

A. Nursing goals include preventing death and complications, educating the patient, assisting with care, and promoting a return to wellness.

B. A community goal is to promote healthful living to prevent heart disease.

C. Plan nursing care to prevent undue fatigue; be alert to medication interactions and side effects.

D. Collaboration with other health care professionals is essential in coordinating care for the patient with a heart disorder.

VII. Implementation

A. Work with the capabilities of the patient; monitor fatigue and oxygenation status.

B. Specific nursing interventions are listed in the nursing care plan, with the discussion of each disorder, and in Table 19-6.

C. Safety is a major consideration in caring for cardiac patients; monitor for electrolyte imbalances, medication toxicity, postural hypotension, and dysrhythmias.

VIII. Evaluation

A. Use subjective and objective data.

B. Determine whether nursing actions are effective.

C. Change nursing care plan as needed.

IX. Coronary Heart Disease (CHD), also Called Coronary Artery Disease (CAD)

A. Atherosclerosis: deposits of fibrous plaque on the inner lining of the arteries.

1. Pathophysiology: fatty material on artery walls, fibrinous plaque forms, vessel size decreased; coronary insufficiency occurs. If thrombosis occurs, blood flow stops and heart muscle dies.

2. Major forms: coronary insufficiency, angina pectoris, acute MI.

3. Causative factors:

a. Environmental: emotional stress, heavy cigarette smoking, high-fat diet, lack of physical exercise.

b. Genetic: familial tendency, diabetes mellitus, hypercholesteremia.

B. Angina pectoris: cardiac pain with effort or emotional excitement.

1. Pathophysiology: atherosclerotic narrowing of coronary arteries reduces blood flow; ischemia causes pain.

2. Medical diagnosis based on symptoms: chest pain, dyspnea, pallor or flushing of face, diaphoresis; exercise stress testing and coronary angiography aid diagnosis.

3. Medical treatment aimed at relief of symptoms, avoidance of factors that precipitate attacks.

a. Medications include vasodilators (e.g., nitroglycerin, calcium-channel blockers, and beta-adrenergic blockers, which block sympathetic impulses to heart).

b. Aspirin decreases platelet aggregation and helps prevent thrombosis.

c. Avoid or minimize effects of environmental cold.

4. Patient education is an important aspect of nursing care.

C. Acute MI.

1. Pathophysiology: severe narrowing or occlusion of a major coronary artery occurs from thrombosis, embolus, or spasm; area beyond the occlusion becomes ischemic; tissue dies.

2. Symptoms and medical diagnosis.
   a. Sudden, severe pain in the chest, arm, or jaw, sometimes mistaken for indigestion; pallor, symptoms of shock.
   b. Within 24 hours there is leukocytosis.
   c. Serum enzymes and isoenzymes elevated (AST, CK, CK-MB, LDH, LDH$_1$, LDH$_2$, troponin T/troponin I).
3. Medical treatment
   a. Pain relief: IV morphine or Demerol initially; then oral analgesia.
   b. Sedatives to reduce anxiety.
   c. Patent IV access for emergency drugs if needed.
   d. Oxygen therapy.
   e. Rest and gradual increase in physical activity.
   f. Avoidance of Valsalva maneuver.
   g. Intensive monitoring; hemodynamic monitoring with pulmonary artery flow-directed catheters for CVP, pulmonary artery pressure; pulmonary artery wedge pressure; arterial line; oximeter; cardiac output.
   h. Thrombolytic therapy if patient seeks help within 2 to 6 hours of onset of pain.
   i. Percutaneous transluminal coronary angioplasty (PTCA): nonsurgical method of improving coronary blood flow.
   j. Intraaortic balloon pump (IABP) may be used for seriously damaged left ventricle and low cardiac output.
   k. Liquids progressing to a low-sodium, low-fat diet; treatment of dysrhythmias.
4. Nursing intervention and patient teaching.
   a. Promote rest, relieve pain, decrease stress and anxiety.
   b. Monitor for dysrhythmias and complications: CHF, pericarditis, cardiogenic shock.
   c. Constant, thorough assessment.
   d. Record daily weight and intake and output; check for edema.
   e. Supervise progressive activity.
   f. Educate patient about disease, diet, medications, activity.
5. Rehabilitation.
   a. Teach patient about nature of disease and rationale for prescribed regimen.
   b. Attention to psychosocial concerns; issues of sexuality.
   c. Put patient in control of her disease and prognosis.
   d. Referral to community agencies such as American Heart Association.

X. **Congestive Heart Failure (CHF)**
   A. Chief complication in 70% of all cardiac patients.
   B. Pathophysiology: heart fails to pump as it should, and flow of blood becomes sluggish, backing up into lungs and/or systemic circulation. Fluid moves from intravascular compartment to tissue spaces, producing generalized or localized edema and lung congestion.
   C. Symptoms depend on whether the left or right side of the heart fails.
      1. Left-sided symptoms: dyspnea, cough, decreased urinary output, weight gain.
      2. Right-sided symptoms: pitting peripheral edema, abdominal distention, weight gain.
   D. Medical treatment.
      1. Bedrest or limited physical activity.
      2. Oxygen therapy.
      3. Digitalization.
      4. Administration of "unloading" agents; morphine.
      5. Limitation of sodium and fluid intake.
      6. Diuretic therapy and "unloading" agents.
   E. Nursing assessment.
      1. Subjective data: increasing fatigue, shortness of breath; feeling bloated, loss of appetite, complaints of feeling warm, anxiety and depression, difficulty in concentrating or remembering.
      2. Objective data: pale, cool, dry skin; cyanosis; dependent, pitting edema; fleeting or absent peripheral pulses; crackles in lung fields; distended neck veins; extra heart sound; increased heart rate; reduced urinary output.
   F. Nursing intervention: planned according to specific problems identified and whether patient is in mild, moderate, or acute congestive failure with pulmonary edema.
      1. Careful, thorough ongoing assessment.
      2. Administer oxygen; assist with ADLs.
      3. Promote rest; position patient upright with pillows behind back to ease breathing.
      4. Record daily weight and intake and output.
      5. Careful skin care to prevent breakdown.
      6. Prevent deep vein thrombosis with elastic stockings and leg exercises.
      7. Observe for side effects of medications.
      8. Discharge and self-care teaching.

XI. **Disorders of the Heart's Conduction System**
   A. Normal impulse originates in SA node at the rate of 60 to 100 bpm.
   B. Pathophysiology: disruption of normal SA node conduction, dysrhythmia occurs; lack of normal regular contraction decreases cardiac output.

1. Life-threatening dysrhythmias: ventricular tachycardia, ventricular fibrillation, asystole.
2. Dysrhythmias causing decreased cardiac output: severe bradycardia, atrial fibrillation, complete heart block, frequent premature ventricular contractions.

C. Diagnosis and medical treatment.
   1. Twelve-lead EKG, continuous EKG monitoring, patient history, and electrophysiology testing.
   2. Heart's natural pacemaker fails, must be replaced by artificial pacemaker.
      a. Artificial pacing can be temporary or permanent, external, transvenous, or internal.
      b. Indications for insertion of permanent pacemaker include sinus bradycardia, atrial fibrillation, complete heart block, secondary AV block, and bradytachycardia.
      c. Cardioversion: treatment for atrial fibrillation uncontrolled by medication.
   3. Antiarrhythmic drugs used for control of conduction disorders (Table 19-7).
   4. CPR and defibrillation (Chapter 31).
   5. Automatic implantable cardiac defibrillators (AICDs) used in patients with repeated episodes of ventricular tachycardia, ventricular fibrillation, or asystole.

D. Nursing assessment and intervention.
   1. Preoperative care includes teaching patient about pacemaker, its purpose and benefits.
   2. Postoperative care: continuous heart monitoring; dressing changes and care of wound site; peripheral pulses and vital signs; safety precautions.
   3. Discharge instruction to help patient live with his pacemaker or AICD.

XII. **Inflammatory Diseases of the Heart: Myocarditis, Endocarditis, Pericarditis.**
   A. Inflammation may occur as endocarditis, myocarditis, or pericarditis.
   B. Pathophysiology: infection causes inflammation and scarring of cardiac tissue; inflammation may cause exudate and fluid to form; fibrous tissue cannot function normally.
   C. Symptoms vary according to site of inflammation: Symptoms of infective endocarditis: intermittent fever, spleen enlargement, splinter hemorrhages under the nails, heart murmur, or petechiae inside the mouth.
   D. Medical treatment includes rest to reduce workload of heart; antiinfectives to control infection; surgery to replace or repair valves damaged by the inflammatory process; severe cardiomyopathy is treated by heart transplant.

XIII. **Cardiac Valve Disorders**
   A. Pathophysiology: caused by congenital defect, rheumatic fever, endocarditis, or long-term hypertension.
   B. Mitral valve most commonly affected; aortic valve second most frequently damaged.
      1. Stenosis: valve will not open fully; chamber has to pump harder to get blood through the opening.
      2. Insufficiency: valve does not close completely and blood leaks back into the chamber it was pumped from.
      3. Changes in pressures cause the heart chamber to dilate and thicken.
      4. Congestive heart failure is the final consequence of progressive, untreated, valve disease.
      5. Cardiac dysrhythmias are a complication of valve disease.
   C. Signs and symptoms are those of CHF and dysrhythmia plus the presence of a cardiac murmur; aortic stenosis may cause syncope.
   D. Treatment is symptomatic, with activity adjustments and medications to control CHF and dysrhythmias; when lifestyle becomes severely compromised, surgery is indicated.

XIV. **Common Problems Related to Cardiac Disease**
   A. Fatigue and dyspnea.
      1. Program of rest and exercise.
      2. Stool softeners; prevent Valsalva maneuver.
      3. Telemetry monitoring.
      4. Progressive activity measured by metabolic equivalents (METs).
      5. Outpatient rehabilitation programs.
      6. Psychological support important.
   B. Edema.
      1. Weigh daily.
      2. Measure fluid intake and output.
      3. Limit sodium intake.
      4. Watch for skin breakdown in dependent areas of body.
      5. Be alert for early signs of pulmonary edema.
   C. Pain.
      1. Administer analgesic or vasodilator.
      2. Provide restful environment.
      3. Relieve anxiety.
      4. Teach patient noninvasive relaxation techniques.

XV. **Common Therapies and Nursing Implications**
   A. Medical treatment with drugs, dietary control, and oxygen to combat hypoxemia.
   B. Pharmacological agents.

1. Cardiotonics slow and strengthen heart beat.
   a. Digitalis preparations: patient must be watched for signs of toxicity. Therapeutic dose is only about one third less than toxic dose. Apical pulse must be counted for 1 full minute before each dose. Patient education must prepare patient to administer his own medication safely at home.
   b. Signs of digitalis toxicity: fatigue, anorexia, nausea, diarrhea, blurred vision or yellow-green halos around objects, new dysrhythmia.
   c. Hypokalemia can cause digitalis toxicity.
2. Antiarrhythmic agents restore rhythmic movements of heart to normal or near normal. Overdosage can cause severe dysrhythmias and cardiac arrest.
3. Diuretics to increase water and sodium loss and correct edema; potassium may be lost; watch for hypokalemia.
4. Anticoagulants to treat abnormal clot formation. Patient monitored by laboratory tests to evaluate effective dose. Patient education important for safe self-administration of anticoagulants.
5. Vasodilators dilate or enlarge blood vessels to improve circulation of blood to heart muscle.
   a. Nitroglycerin: administered sublingually, topically, or by nasal spray.
   b. Long-acting nitrates (e.g., Isordil).
6. Calcium-channel blockers increase flow of blood through coronary arteries by relaxing smooth muscle in vessels and decreasing resistance to blood flow. Not intended to replace other modes of therapy, but to complement them.
7. Analgesics: morphine or meperidine for acute pain associated with coronary occlusion and ischemic heart disease.

C. Dietary control to restore or maintain normal body weight, reduce intake of fats, limit sodium intake. Healthy heart diet recommended by American Heart Association can be beneficial to family members as well as patient.
D. Oxygen therapy. Observe patient for early signs of hypoxemia and oxygen lack.
E. Cardiac surgery.
   1. Correct structural defects.
   2. Replace defective valves.
   3. Coronary artery bypass surgery.
   4. Heart transplant.
   5. Preoperative care:
      a. Support during diagnostic testing.
      b. Teaching for preoperative measures and postoperative care: what to expect; ventilator and other equipment; frequent monitoring; alarm sounds.
   6. Postoperative care: ICU then telemetry stepdown unit.
      a. Prevent infection.
      b. Promote balanced rest and activity.
      c. Monitor for complications.
      d. Psychosocial support and preparation for discharge.

XVI. Community Care
   A. Surgical patients who are discharged early may receive home health care.
   B. Cardiac rehabilitation programs are very important to reduce the risk of further heart problems in patients with heart disease or who have undergone heart surgery.
   C. Nurses in long-term care and in home health are the "eyes and ears" of the physician and assess for changes in condition that may indicate early signs of complications such as dysrhythmias, electrolyte imbalances, and CHF.

CHAPTER 20

Care of Patients with Digestive Tract Disorders

OBJECTIVES

Upon completing this chapter the student should be able to:
1. Identify three major causative factors and preventive measures in the development of disorders of the digestive system.
2. List nursing responsibilities in the pre- and posttest care of patients undergoing diagnostic tests for disorders of the intestinal tract.
3. Perform an assessment of gastrointestinal status.
4. Describe the pathophysiology, means of medical diagnosis, and treatment for stomatitis, gastritis, ulcerative colitis, appendicitis, and peritonitis.
5. Devise a nursing care plan for the patient with a peptic ulcer.
6. Write a nursing care plan for the patient with cancer of the colon and intestinal obstruction.
7. List nursing interventions for the patient with ulcerative colitis or irritable bowel syndrome.
8. Devise a nursing care plan for the patient having surgery of the lower intestine and rectum.
9. Formulate a nursing care plan for each type of intestinal ostomy, considering the type of stoma and the effluent it produces.
10. List four interventions for helping the patient psychologically adjust to his or her ostomy.

The central role of the intestinal tract and accessory organs of digestion is the intake, absorption, and assimilation of food to provide nourishment for the body. As food is processed in the stomach, acids, enzymes, and mucus are added to help with the breakdown of the food into specific nutrients. As the food moves down the intestinal tract, more enzymes and bile are added to it further to breakdown the components for absorption. As the large intestine is reached, the fluid is extracted and the residue becomes more solid and ends up as feces eliminated via the rectum and anus.

The transfer of nutrients from the intestine into the blood is referred to as **absorption.** Food substances are moved along the intestinal tract by wavelike motions of involuntary muscles within the walls of the organs. This rhythmic squeezing action is called **peristalsis. Metabolism** is the sum of all the many physical and chemical processes concerned with the disposition of nutrients absorbed into the bloodstream after digestion has taken place. Metabolic activities involve the synthesis of substances needed to build, maintain, and repair body tissues (**anabolism**) and the breakdown of larger molecules into smaller molecules so that energy is available (**catabolism**).

Disorders that affect ingestion, digestion, absorption, or elimination may lead to malnutrition and a weakening of the body's defenses from lack of energy. Inadequate nutrition accompanying any other disease or disorder brings a greater degree of illness and a higher mortality.

To understand the various problems of the gastrointestinal system, recollection of the normal anatomy and functions of the system is necessary. The accessory organs of the gastrointestinal system are discussed in the next chapter.

OVERVIEW OF ANATOMY AND PHYSIOLOGY

What Are the Organs and Structures Of the Gastrointestinal System?

⊿ Organs of the gastrointestinal (G.I.) system are the mouth, pharynx, esophagus, stomach, small intestine, large intestine, rectum, and anus. The accessory organs are the liver, gallbladder, and pancreas (Figure 20-1).

⊿ The gastroesophageal sphincter (cardiac sphincter) controls the opening from the esophagus into the stomach; it prevents reflux from the stomach into the esophagus.

⊿ The stomach lies in the upper left portion of the abdominal cavity. (Figure 20-2).

⊿ The pyloric sphincter controls release of food substances into the small intestine.

⊿ The small intestine is divided into the duodenum, jejunum, and ilium and is about 6 m long.

⊿ The ileocecal valve controls the progress of substances into the large intestine.

⊿ The large intestine is divided into the cecum, colon, rectum, and anal canal; the colon is about 1.5 m long.

⊿ The colon has four portions: the ascending, transverse, descending, and sigmoid colon.

⊿ The appendix is attached to the cecum and has no known function in the digestive process.

⊿ The small intestine is approximately 2 m long, extending from the pyloric sphincter to the ileocecal valve. There are three segments: the duodenum, jejunum, and ileum.

⊿ The walls of the digestive tract have four layers: mucosa, submucosa, muscular layer, and a serous layer called serosa.

⊿ The peritoneum is a serous sac that lines the abdominal cavity and encloses the intestines, stomach, liver, and spleen and partially encloses the uterus and uterine tubes.

What Are the Functions of the Gastrointestinal Tract?

⊿ The teeth and tongue are instrumental in the chewing (mastication) process, and they help break down food into smaller pieces that can be acted upon by various enzymes.

⊿ Food moves from the mouth through the pharynx down the esophagus to the stomach, where mixing movements occur.

⊿ Mucus, hydrochloric acid (HCl), intrinsic factor, pepsinogen, and gastrin are secreted into the stomach from cells within its walls and are mixed into the food to break down further the particles for absorption. The mixture produced is called chyme.

⊿ The small intestine receives the chyme from the stomach, adds more digestive enzymes and fluids, receives bile and pancreatic enzymes from the common duct, and further digests the chyme into a more liquid state.

⊿ Digested food particles are absorbed into the bloodstream from the villi on the walls of the small intestine.

⊿ The large intestine reabsorbs water and electrolytes and eliminates waste products. (Figure 20-3)

⊿ The large intestine is populated with bacteria that aid in the breakdown of the waste products.

⊿ The rectum stores fecal material until it is eliminated through the anus.

⊿ The internal anal sphincter at the top of the anal canal is under involuntary control; the external anal sphincter at the end of the anal canal is under voluntary control.

⊿ The gastrocolic reflex initiates elimination; it is stimulated by the ingestion of food. By tightening the voluntary anal sphincter, the reflex emptying of the rectum can be stopped.

What Effects Does Aging Have on the Gastrointestinal System?

⊿ After the age of 70, the parietal cells in the stomach decrease their secretion of hydrochloric acid.

⊿ The mucosa of the small intestine becomes less absorptive and the large intestine may develop diminished motility.

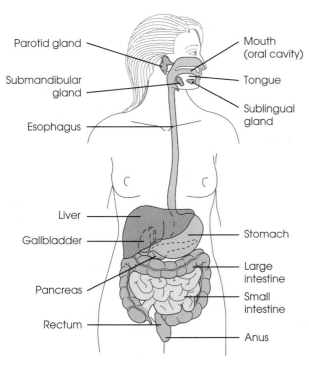

FIGURE 20-1   Organs of the digestive system.

CAUSES OF GASTROINTESTINAL DISORDERS

As with all other tissues of the body, those of the digestive tract are subject to infection, inflammation, physical and chemical trauma, and structural defects. Factors that contribute to these pathological conditions include the more obvious physical ones, such as exposure to infectious agents (as in food poisoning), and less apparent psychosocial factors.

Mechanical obstruction to the movement of food through the intestinal tract (as in intestinal obstruction) or to the flow of digestive juices and enzymes (as in blockage of the bile ducts) can give rise to serious disorders of digestion and absorption and can be life-threatening. Continued irritation and inflammation of the gastrointestinal mucosa can lead to intestinal bleeding and to increased peristalsis and inadequate absorption of nutrients.

Preventing intestinal disorders associated with stress and tension is difficult because usually other factors are involved. Stress is not necessarily harmful; and its effects are not always manifested in only one organ or even one system in the body. Teaching patients ways to relax and to cope with undue stress can be helpful, but it does not guarantee freedom from disorders that usually have multiple causes. Psychological and emotional stresses greatly influence appetite and motility of the stomach and intestines. The secretion of digestive juices in amounts sufficient for the breakdown of food is regulated in part by the emotions. Excessive stimulation of digestive acid and enzymes can cause a breakdown in the integrity of the mucous membrane lining the digestive tract and can bring about such disorders as gastric and duodenal ulcers and chronic colitis.

Some disorders, such as Crohn's disease and ulcerative colitis, are correlated with a genetic predisposition. Both disorders also have an ethnic correlation as they are more common among the Jewish population.

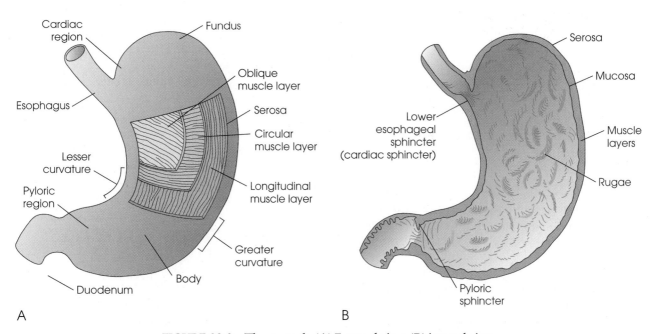

A   B

FIGURE 20-2   The stomach. (A) External view; (B) internal view.

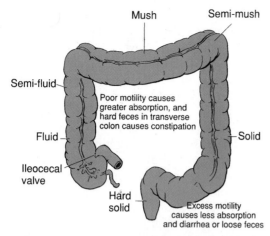

FIGURE 20-3   **Absorptive and storage functions of the large intestine.** (*Source:* Guyton, A. C., Hall, J. E. [1996]. *Textbook of Medical Physiology,* 9th Ed. Philadelphia: Saunders, p. 811.)

Certain forms of colon cancer have been identified as having a genetic link and definitely show a familial tendency for occurrence. Esophageal and stomach cancer are loosely linked to consumption of foods that have been charred or cooked to the point of carbonization. Certain types of fungi in the oriental diet also are linked to esophageal and stomach cancer. Decreasing the consumption of these types of food helps lower the incidence of cancer of the GI tract.

Autoimmune diseases often affect the GI system, causing inflammation or fibrosis of organs. Treatments such as drug and radiation therapy may cause GI problems as a side effect. Some people who have undergone chemotherapy for cancer develop a mechanical form of sprue, a malabsorption problem, that remains even after chemotherapy is complete. Lactose intolerance, which is not uncommon in the older adult, may cause continuous diarrhea and malabsorption.

Think about . . . Can you identify any GI problems that seem to run in your family?

PREVENTION OF GASTROINTESTINAL PROBLEMS

There are many ways to help prevent GI problems. Eating a normal, well-balanced diet, aids digestion. Consuming sufficient bulk in the diet helps maintain a healthy colon by enhancing timely passage of waste through the colon. A diet lacking in fiber is one factor in the development of diverticulosis, in which pockets form along the colon where waste material can lodge. Drinking at least eight glasses of fluid a day prevents constipation by helping to keep the stool moist.

Heeding the need to defecate promptly aids in keeping the gastrocolic reflex functioning well and prevents constipation and hemorrhoids. Straining at stool contributes to hemorrhoids. When defecation must be initiated by straining, intraabdominal pressure rises, causing the hemorrhoidal vessels to engorge. **Obtaining sufficient daily exercise maintains abdominal muscle tone and contributes to peristalsis and the ability to defecate normally.** Defecating at more or less the same time each day aids the process and helps promote continued ability to control defecation.

Elder Care Point . . . Mobility and exercise greatly influence digestion. Decreased mobility in the elderly patient often leads to digestive problems. Increasing mobility in any way possible helps the digestive process.

Maintaining one's body weight within normal limits helps prevent hiatal hernia and esophageal reflux. Developing healthy coping mechanisms and keeping stress within acceptable limits helps prevent ulcers and chronic irritability of the bowel.

Mechanical and chemical irritants that produce inflammation often can be identified by elimination diets to determine the foods that cause GI upsets. Once the offending foods are identified, efforts are made to help the patient both avoid these foods and maintain adequate nutrition.

Preventing infections of the intestinal tract is similar to preventing infections elsewhere in the body. Washing the hands before eating, care when cleaning cooking and eating utensils, and following general rules of good hygiene and sanitation can prevent many infectious GI upsets. Food poisoning can be prevented by adequate refrigeration and proper canning, freezing, and food-handling methods. Meats and foods containing mayonnaise or dairy products should be kept chilled. When not in the refrigerator, food should be kept covered. Refraining from eating gathered mushrooms, unless correctly identified as edible by a qualified botanist, prevents poisoning.

Think about . . . Can you teach your family and friends about ways to decrease the risk of colon cancer? What would you recommend to your parents regarding screening for colorectal cancer?

DIAGNOSTIC TESTS, PROCEDURES, AND NURSING IMPLICATIONS

Diagnostic tests for disorders of the intestinal tract consist of x-rays, ultrasound studies, endoscopy, complete blood cell (CBC) count, tests of gastric secretions, and stool studies.

The patient often is scheduled for a series of tests, some of which use a contrast medium. It is important that GI tests be done in the correct order so that the contrast media do not interfere with other tests. For example, if the patient is scheduled for an upper-GI series, a gallbladder sonogram, and a barium enema, he should have them done in this order: sonogram, barium enema, and then the upper GI series.

Soon a new test, virtual colonoscopy, may be available for colon cancer screening. The procedure combines images from a high-tech spiral CT scan to create a computer-generated three-dimensional picture of the colon. The procedure is being evaluated at the National Cancer Institute, is less costly than standard colonoscopy, and requires no sedation.

The nurse should include instructions to promote comfort when teaching about the preparation phase for a diagnostic test. Many of the studies require cleansing of the GI tract. When laxatives are administered in liquid form, the patient can drink them more easily if they are chilled or poured over ice. If a patient has trouble with nausea, sucking on an ice cube first and then using a straw to drink the solution helps as it decreases taste sensation.

Frequent, loose bowel movements cause rectal irritation. Instructing to apply a lubricant such as A&D ointment or petroleum jelly (Vaseline) before the laxatives act can protect this area and make the patient much more comfortable.

For many GI tests, the patient is kept NPO the night before. In the hospital, mouth care should be offered in the morning, and the door of the room should be kept closed so that food odors do not enter and increase hunger. A food tray should be obtained immediately upon return to the floor, as long as NPO status is no longer in effect. The nurse can provide juices and coffee or tea while waiting for the meal tray to be delivered.

Frequent assessment for signs of dehydration is necessary, as cleansing enemas and lack of oral intake can quickly dehydrate a patient who has already been ill with nausea, vomiting, or diarrhea. The purpose, description, and nursing implications for the diagnostic tests of the GI system are listed in Table 20-1.

Elder Care Point... The older patient is especially at risk for problems of electrolyte imbalance and dehydration when undergoing preparation for diagnostic tests that require a fasting state and/or cleansing enemas. Frequent assessment for these problems is essential.

TABLE 20-1 ◆ *Diagnostic Tests for Gastrointestinal Problems*

Test	Purpose	Description	Nursing Implications
Radiological exams Upper GI series (UGI)	X-ray examination with fluoroscopy to locate obstruction, ulceration, or growths in the esophagus, stomach, and duodenum.	Patient drinks a contrast medium and is placed in various positions on the x-ray table.	Keep patient NPO for 8 to 12 hours prior to the test. Explain what happens during test. After radiographs, increase fluids and give ordered laxatives to clear GI tract of contrast medium and prevent impaction. Stool may be white up to 3 days after test.
Barium enema (BE)	X-ray examination of the colon using fluoroscopy to locate tumors, obstruction, and ulceration.	A radiopaque substance is instilled into the colon by enema. After evacuation of this substance, air may be instilled for contrast studies (Figure 20-4).	Keep patient NPO for 8 hours prior to test. Give ordered laxatives and enemas. Bowel must be clear of stool. Explain what will happen during the test. Posttest care is same as for UGI.
Endoscopic studies Esophagogastroduodenoscopy	Visualizes the esophagus, stomach, and duodenum with a lighted tube (endoscope) to detect tumor, ulceration, or obstruction. Separate study of esophagus, stomach, or stomach and duodenum may be done.	Patient is given preoperative sedation. IV sedation may be used for the test. A local spray or gargle may be used to anesthetize the throat. The patient lies on a table, with head extended, and the endoscope is introduced through the mouth (Figure 20-5).	Keep patient NPO for 8 hours. Obtain signed consent. Explain what he will experience during the test. Give preoperative medication. After procedure, keep patient NPO until gag reflex has returned. Take vital signs q 15 to 30 minutes as ordered. Watch for signs of perforation: rising temperature, pain, changes in vital signs.

(Table 20-1 continued)

TABLE 20-1 ♦ *Diagnostic Tests for Gastrointestinal Problems* (Continued)

Test	Purpose	Description	Nursing Implications
Proctoscopy and sigmoidoscopy	Examination of the lining of the rectum and sigmoid colon to detect polyps, tumor, obstruction, or ulceration.	The patient is placed in the knee-chest position, often on a special table. A sigmoidoscope is introduced through the anus. Biopsies can be taken of suspicious areas; polyps can be removed. The patient will experience some cramping during the procedure.	Give laxatives and enemas the evening before as ordered. Give clear liquids for dinner the night before, then keep patient NPO until after exam. Explain what he will experience. Encourage use of deep breathing and relaxation techniques to decrease cramping. Observe for rectal bleeding after biopsy or polyp removal.
Colonoscopy	Direct visualization of the lining of the colon with a flexible endoscope.	Patient is moderately sedated for this procedure, which takes about 1½ to 2 hours. Polyps can be removed or biopsies taken.	Give clear liquid diet 1 to 3 days prior to test. Patient is NPO for 8 hours prior. Give laxatives for 1 to 3 days prior to test and enemas the night before. Explain procedure and what he will experience. Obtain signed consent. Give preoperative sedation. After procedure, observe for rectal bleeding and signs of perforation: abdominal distention, pain, elevated temperature.
Gastric analysis	Determines the rate of secretion of gastric juices and degree of acidity.	A nasogastric tube is inserted, the stomach contents are aspirated. A substance may be given to stimulate the flow of gastric secretions, and another sample is aspirated in 30 minutes. Increased secretion can indicate peptic ulcer or pancreatic tumor. A low degree of acidity may indicate gastric ulcer. An absence of acid can accompany cancer of the stomach or pernicious anemia.	Withhold drugs affecting gastric secretion for 24 to 48 hours prior to test. No smoking the morning of test (nicotine stimulates secretions). Keep patient NPO for 8 hours prior to test. Explain use of NG tube and procedure.
Tubeless gastric analysis	Determination of presence or absence of hydrochloric acid in the stomach secretions.	The patient is given special granules in 240 mL of water. Urine specimens are collected at specific intervals. If HCl is present in the stomach, the urine will be blue; if none is present, the urine will be normal color.	Explain test and procedure to patient.
Fecal analysis (stool exam)	Analysis for presence of mucus, elevated fat content, blood (guaiac), bacteria, or parasites.	Stool specimen is obtained in bed pan or container in commode. Small smear is made on special paper and tested with special solution for guaiac or Hemoccult test. Specimen is placed in container and sent to laboratory for testing.	Explain test to patient. Provide means for collection of stool. Promptly retrieve stool, obtain sample for guaiac test, place specimen in lab container, and dispatch to lab *immediately*. (Bacteria can multiply if specimen is left at room temperature for extended period; parasites may disintegrate). Patient must have red meat–free diet for at least 3 days before a stool guaiac test can be considered accurate.

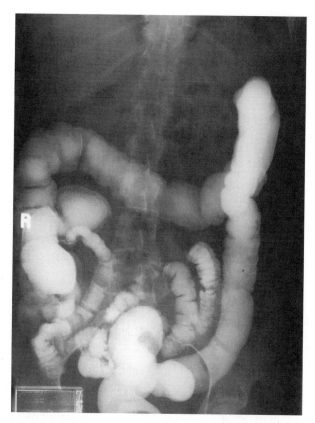

FIGURE 20-4   Barium enema x-ray.   (*Source:* Haubrich, W. S., Schaffner, F., Berk, J. E. [1995]. *Bockus Gastroenterology,* 5th ed. Philadelphia: Saunders, p. 195.)

Think about... How would you assess an elderly patient for signs of fluid and electrolyte problems resulting from diagnostic tests on the GI system?

NURSING MANAGEMENT

◆ Assessment

A focused assessment of the GI system includes the collection of both objective and subjective data. Although assessment for particular problems is covered later in the chapter, a general guide for history taking is presented in Table 20-2.

TABLE 20-2 ◆ Assessment: Guide to History Taking for the Gastrointestinal System

When gathering data, ask the following questions:

- ◆ Do you have any difficulty chewing or swallowing?
- ◆ When was your last dental exam?
- ◆ Have you been experiencing any abdominal pain or nausea and vomiting? Do you experience any regurgitation or reflux?
- ◆ When was your last bowel movement? How often do you normally have a bowel movement? Have you noticed any changes in your bowel pattern or in the appearance of your stool? Do you often experience diarrhea? Are you ever constipated? Do you use a laxative, suppositories, or enemas to stimulate a bowel movement?
- ◆ Have you traveled recently? Where did you go? (Especially pertinent if the patient has diarrhea.)
- ◆ Do you have a problem with hemorrhoids? Have you ever noticed blood in the stool, black stool, or blood on the tissue when wiping?
- ◆ How is your appetite? Has it changed in any way?
- ◆ Have you lost weight recently, and if so over what period of time?
- ◆ Do you ever experience indigestion? Do certain foods disagree with you?
- ◆ Have any members of your family had colon cancer? Do you have regular examinations for colon and rectal cancer?
- ◆ Is there a history of stomach or intestinal problems in your family?
- ◆ Can you describe your usual diet? How much of each item do you eat? (Ask for what is eaten at each meal typically, and then ask about in-between meal snacks and drinks.)
- ◆ What drugs do you take on a regular basis (aspirin, NSAIDs, and corticosteroids are particularly important)?
- ◆ Do you drink alcohol? About how often do you drink? How many drinks do you average?
- ◆ Are you able to shop and prepare meals? Is there any problem with obtaining sufficient food (if patient is known to have economic constraints).
- ◆ How do you handle stress? Blow off steam?
- ◆ How do you relax?

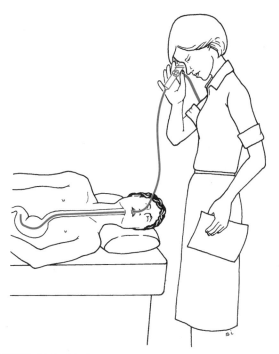

FIGURE 20-5   Endoscope inserted through patient's mouth for gastroscopy.

◆ Physical Assessment

Physical assessment includes inspection, auscultation of bowel sounds, palpation, and percussion. The teeth, gums, and oral mucosa are inspected for obvious problems. The skin is inspected for color, lesions, and any discolorations on the abdomen are noted. The presence of edema and **ascites** (fluid in the abdominal cavity) is checked by observing for marked abdominal distention and taut, glistening skin. The contour of the abdomen is checked, and any outpouchings indicating a hernia are noted.

Auscultation of bowel sounds is performed for each quadrant of the abdomen using the diaphragm of the stethoscope (Figure 20-6). **Bowel sounds are caused by air and fluid moving through the intestinal tract and are heard as soft gurgles and clicks every 5 to 15 seconds.** The normal range of frequency for these sounds is about 5 to 30 in 1 minute. Both the character and frequency of sounds are noted. Loud, frequent sounds occur when there is excessive motility in the bowel. **Auscultation is done before palpation or percussion.**

Light palpation is performed over each quadrant of the abdomen to detect areas of tenderness and any masses that might be present. It is important to watch the patient's face during palpation to detect signs of discomfort.

Percussion is performed by placing the middle finger of one hand on the abdomen and striking the finger lightly below the knuckle and listening for the pitch of sound produced. A resonant sound is heard

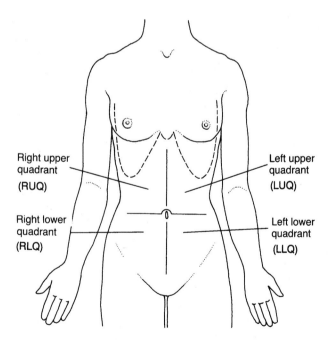

FIGURE 20-6   Division of the abdomen into quadrants.
(*Source:* Ignatavicius, D. D., Workman, M. L., Mishler, M. A. [1995]. *Medical–Surgical Nursing: A Nursing Process Approach,* 2nd ed. Philadelphia: Saunders, p. 1500.)

Right upper quadrant (RUQ)

Left upper quadrant (LUQ)

Right lower quadrant (RLQ)

Left lower quadrant (LLQ)

TABLE 20-3 ◆ *Assessment: Guide to Physical Assessment of the Gastrointestinal System*

Assess the following:

- Inspect the skin for color and areas of discoloration.
- Inspect the contour of the abdomen.
- Auscultate for bowel sounds in all four quadrants.
- Lightly palpate each quadrant of the abdomen.
- Percuss each quadrant of the abdomen if there seems to be a problem with intestinal irritation or inflammation.
- If there is evidence of ascites, measure abdominal girth.
- Inspect stool, if available, for characteristics; test for occult blood if need is indicated.
- Inspect anus for presence of external hemorrhoids.
- If vomiting has occurred, inspect vomitus for characteristics; test vomitus for blood if data gathered indicate need.

over areas filled with air and a dull, thudding sound is heard over solid organs. **Percussion detects excessive air in the intestinal tract, which occurs with irritation and inflammation.**

If there is a question of whether ascites is present, abdominal girth is measured. A tape measure is placed around the fullest part of the abdomen, usually at the umbilicus. Small ink marks are placed at the sides of the tape on the axillary lines so that future measurements may be taken at the same place for comparison. If ascites is present and continuing to be produced, the abdominal girth will increase with subsequent measurements. Table 20-3 presents an outline guide for physical assessment.

***Elder Care Point*...** Recording all the medications the elderly patient is taking, both prescription and over-the-counter drugs, is very important when assessing the digestive system. Many drugs affect digestion, bowel motility, and appetite in these patients.

◆ Nursing Diagnosis

Nursing diagnoses commonly used for problems of the GI tract are:

- Pain related to stomach or intestinal irritation or obstruction.
- Fluid volume deficit related to nausea and vomiting or persistent diarrhea.
- Alteration in nutrition, less than body requirements, related to inability to eat or retain food.
- Diarrhea related to intestinal irritation.
- Constipation related to improper diet, medications, or other factors.
- Bowel incontinence related to lack of anal sphincter control.

◆ Ineffective individual coping related to inability to handle excessive stress.

◆ Knowledge deficit related to disease or disorder process and treatment.

Other nursing diagnoses secondary to the GI problem, such as sleep pattern disturbance, fatigue, risk of impaired skin integrity, anxiety, noncompliance, and self-care deficit may be pertinent.

◆ Planning

The planning of nursing care is based on data collection and collaboration with the patient and other health team members. General goals for the patient with GI problems are:

◆ Control of nausea and vomiting.
◆ Control of diarrhea.
◆ Promotion of normal, continent, bowel movements.
◆ Control of abdominal pain.
◆ Promotion of adequate nutritional status.
◆ Assimilation of knowledge for self-care.
◆ Prevention of GI bleeding.
◆ Control or elimination of GI cancer.

Planning care for the patient who has diarrhea or is incontinent of feces requires considering the time it takes for toileting and cleaning up after loose bowel movements and the patience, teaching, and attention that a bowel retraining program takes in the shift schedule. Administering enemas can be quite time-consuming as well.

◆ Implementation

All nurses must ask each patient each day about bowel movements to prevent constipation and possible impaction in ill or hospitalized patients. Nursing actions for patients with the various disorders are discussed later in the chapter. Extensive nursing actions are presented in the nursing care plans in this chapter and in the section on specific problems related to ingestion, digestion, and bowel elimination. Nursing actions for other common nursing diagnoses are presented in Table 20-4.

◆ Evaluation

Evaluation involves reassessment to determine the effectiveness of nursing interventions and progress toward expected outcomes. Evaluation also involves considering data to determine whether complications are occurring. The nurse constantly evaluates whether the patient is experiencing adverse side effects of therapy and whether the therapy is achieving the desired result. When evaluation indicates that expected outcomes are not being met, the plan of care is revised and different nursing measures are tried.

COMMON PROBLEMS RELATED TO THE GASTROINTESTINAL TRACT

◆ Anorexia

Anorexia is the absence of appetite. Enjoying food partially depends on having an appetite. Physical causes for a diminished interest in eating include poorly fitting dentures, stomatitis, decaying teeth, halitosis, and a bad taste in the mouth.

Psychosocial factors have a significant impact on one's desire for food. Appetite depends on complex mental processes having to do with memory and mental associations that can be pleasant or extremely unpleasant. Appetite is stimulated by the sight, smell, and thought of food; hence it is influenced by the physical and social environment in which a person is eating. The enjoyment of eating can be inhibited by unattractive or unfamiliar food, surroundings, or company, and by emotional states such as anxiety, anger, and fear. Mental depression also can be a cause of anorexia.

Elder Care Point . . . Both taste and smell sensation diminishes with age. Teeth may be lost because of gingival or dental disease, making eating more difficult. Many elderly patients take a variety of medications for various conditions. The combination of these medications may greatly affect appetite and digestion. "Polypharmacy" (taking many medications) is a frequent cause of anorexia in the elderly patient.

If weight loss and loss of appetite occur in an elderly patient without evidence of any specific cause, the possibility of depression should be investigated. The depressed elderly patient may give up hope and just stop eating much.

Because of the complex nature of anorexia, it may be necessary for the nurse to talk with the patient, family, and significant others to learn why appetite has been lost. Consulting the patient's chart may reveal some physiological, social, or psychological reason why a patient does not eat normally. Once the apparent cause of anorexia is discovered, nursing intervention is aimed at minimizing or alleviating those factors that inhibit appetite.

Nursing Intervention   Loss of appetite is to be expected when a person becomes ill. However, persistent anorexia must be dealt with to avoid the consequences of inadequate nutrition. Nursing interventions include mouth care before each meal to eliminate or minimize physical causes of poor appetite.

TABLE 20-4 ◆ Common Nursing Diagnoses, Expected Outcomes, and Interventions for Patients with Gastrointestinal Problems

Nursing Diagnosis	Expected Outcomes	Nursing Interventions
Fluid volume deficit related to nausea and vomiting or diarrhea.	Vomiting will be controlled within 24 hours; diarrhea will be controlled within 24 hours. Fluid volume will be within normal limits within 48 hours as evidenced by adequate skin turgor and urine output >50 mL/hour.	Assess urine output for signs of fluid deficit. Provide mouth care after vomiting to decrease nausea. Medicate for nausea and vomiting as ordered. Provide quiet environment and rest. Medicate for diarrhea as ordered; keep patient clean and dry. Give only small sips of clear liquids by mouth until vomiting subsides. Continue clear-liquid diet until diarrhea is controlled.
Diarrhea related to intestinal infection or inflammation.	Infection or inflammation episode will resolve within 72 hours. Diarrhea will be controlled to prevent fluid imbalance within 24 hours.	Medicate with antibiotics, antiinflammatories, and antidiarrheals as ordered. Rest bowel with clear-liquid diet or bland diet as ordered. Protect anal mucosa with barrier ointment. Keep anal area clean and dry. Provide warm sitz bath to sooth anal tissues as needed. Medicate for discomfort from abdominal cramping as ordered. Provide restful environment.
Constipation related to side effects of medication, loss of ability to initiate defecation, or other cause.	Patient will have normal bowel movements regularly within 2 weeks.	Increase fluid intake to 2,500 mL/day unless contraindicated. Add fruit juices to diet. Increase fiber in diet; add slowly to prevent excessive gas formation. Increase exercise on a daily basis. Encourage patient to heed gastrocolic reflex and not delay defecation. Administer stool softener or bulk laxative as ordered. Monitor for fecal impaction.
Bowel incontinence related to lack of sphincter control.	Patient will use bowel training program. Continence will be achieved within 2 months.	Institute bowel training program. Provide toileting opportunity after each meal. Provide privacy and comfort for attempts at defecation. Adjust diet to provide optimal fiber in diet. Keep patient clean, dry, and odor free.
Ineffective individual coping related to inability to handle excessive stress.	Patient will identify desired ways of coping within 3 weeks. Patient will learn new coping techniques within 2 months.	Assist to identify present coping mechanisms. Assist to identify stressors. Instruct in ways to develop more effective coping mechanisms, such as relaxation techniques, alterations in perspective, exercise, or imagery. Refer for counseling as needed.

If psychosocial factors are involved, the nurse might try offering preferred foods whenever this is possible and not detrimental to health. Meals that are planned to include a variety of colors, textures, and tastes are more appealing and enjoyable than those that are monotonous and bland. The patient should be given ample time to eat and encouraged to eat slowly and enjoy the meal. If it is necessary to feed the patient, this should be done cheerfully and in a manner in which the nurse would eat a meal.

Eating is a social event, and very few people get as much pleasure eating alone as they would in the company of someone else. The nurse, a family member, or a friend can provide companionship while a patient eats. If there is a patient cafeteria or gathering place for patients to eat together, and the patient is able to go there for meals, this can sometimes alleviate or minimize a problem of anorexia.

Elder Care Point . . . Many elderly patients have dental problems that interfere with eating. This possibility should be explored. Some elderly are embarrassed by physical limitations that cause them to be awkward with eating and will eat very little in the company of others. Others who have difficulty swallowing and are afraid of choking are afraid to eat alone but embarrassed when eating with others. It is essential to explore the causes of anorexia and feelings about eating for each patient.

Food from home often is a welcome addition to institutional fare. The person bringing the meal will need to be advised of any restrictions on the patient's dietary intake and the importance of adhering to dietary limitations.

◆ Nausea and Vomiting

Interference with comfort and nutrition occur when nausea and vomiting are persistent. Nausea and vomiting may be related to illness, effects of cancer treatment, or stress and can interfere with nutrition. A transient problem is not treated, but when the disorder persists, medication with antiemetics, GI intubation, and administration of IV fluids are necessary. Nursing interventions for the patient with nausea and vomiting are discussed in Chapter 5.

◆ Accumulation of Gas

Surgical intervention, mechanical obstruction, and accidental injury to the intestinal tract can cause disturbances in the passage of material through the intestinal tract, leading to the accumulation of fluids and gases that causes mild to considerable discomfort for the patient.

Whenever ingested material cannot pass through the intestinal tract as it should, it accumulates in the stomach and the intestines, creating problems of pressure and distention. This can occur when peristalsis is decreased or the flow of chyme is inhibited by an obstruction. Gases are formed by the action of digestive juices and bacteria on the ingested material.

Assisting the patient to walk a lot has traditionally been the nursing intervention for this problem. This works for some patients, but others continue to have discomfort. If the physician will permit it, a slight Trendelenburg position can be useful in speeding the expulsion of gas. Placing the buttocks and legs higher than the trunk and head, causes gas to rise toward the rectum, making it easier to expel. Massaging the abdomen gently, working up the right side, across, and down over the left colon to move gas toward the rectum is also helpful. Use both hands, placing the left hand behind the right after moving the gas along the bowel before lifting the right hand. This helps prevent gas from moving backward.

The patient is advised to avoid chilled or hot drinks as these may create more gas. Antigas medications that contain simethicone, such as Phazyme, are helpful if the patient is not NPO. The physician may order the insertion of a rectal tube or a rectal suppository to help the patient move the gas out of the intestine.

Think about . . . Can you teach a patient three ways to prevent the occurrence of excessive gas postoperatively?

◆ Constipation

Signs and Symptoms   When constipation occurs, the stool is hard, dry, and difficult to pass. There may be a bloated feeling and pain may be experienced when the patient attempts to defecate. Consistency of stool is greatly influenced by the type of food eaten and the quantity of liquid consumed. A diet low in fiber predisposes to constipation, as does inadequate fluid intake. Physical inactivity, ignoring the gastrocolic reflex, stress, and neurological disorders also may contribute to constipation.

Elder Care Point . . . Constipation is a problem among many people over age 60. Decreased GI motility, lack of exercise, limited fluid intake, constipating medications taken for various conditions all contribute. In the very elderly, difficulty getting to the bathroom and suppression of the defecation urge may contribute to the problem. Reliance on laxatives is common among the elderly and is to be discouraged. Counsel with individual patients about ways to increase fiber in the diet that is to their liking and encourage fluid intake of at least 2,500 mL/day.

The first step is to identify the cause of constipation. Initial treatment may include a rectal suppository or enema to induce evacuation or the administration of a laxative. A stool softener may be prescribed. Fiber and liquids are increased in the diet. If this does not resolve the problem, the patient is placed on one of the bulk-forming laxatives to be used daily, such as Metamucil. If the patient has become impacted with stool, digital extraction may be needed. In this event, the nurse applies a lubricant, such as K-Y jelly or the anesthetic lubricant xylocaine jelly, into the rectum and around the anus and using a gloved finger, breaks up and removes the feces. An oil retention enema usually is given prior to this procedure. The patient may be medicated with a mild analgesic 30 to 60 minutes prior to impaction removal to decrease the discomfort of the procedure.

The nurse counsels the patient to add lots of raw fruits and vegetables to the diet; to eat more whole grain cereals and breads, add bran to the diet, and drink lots of fluids. Fruit juices are particularly helpful as they contain fructose, which is a natural laxative. The patient is helped to design an acceptable exercise program, such as walking, biking, running, swimming, or active sports participation. The patient is advised to heed the urge to defecate quickly and not to put it off.

Think about . . . Can you list six foods high in fiber that a patient might add to the diet to combat constipation?

◆ Diarrhea

The frequent passage of liquid or semi-liquid stool is called diarrhea. It occurs with a variety of illnesses, food poisoning, excessive stress, and with inflammation of the bowel. Mild diarrhea is not treated, but if it persists for more than 24 to 48 hours or the number of stools is so excessive that great quantities of fluid are lost, treatment should begin.

Antidiarrheal agents such as diphenoxylate hydrochloride (Lomotil), loperamide hydrochloride (Imodium), tincture of opium (Paregoric), or a combination product, such as Kaopectate, are administered. See Table 20-5 for nursing implications. If the diarrhea is severe, nothing is given by mouth until it subsides. If it is moderate, only clear liquids are permitted by mouth. Severe, long-term diarrhea may require the use of total parenteral nutrition. Because diarrhea depletes the natural bacterial flora in the intestine, taking tablets, capsules or granules containing *lactobacillus acidophilus* helps replace the flora. When diarrhea is caused by infection, antibiotics are prescribed. Stool cultures may be necessary. As the condition improves, the diet is advanced.

Nursing Intervention   The nurse monitors intake and output and assesses the amount of fluid lost in the stool, measuring it if needed. Medications are administered and fluids are replaced. The patient is monitored for electrolyte imbalances and watched for signs of dehydration, such as decreased skin turgor, thick oral secretions, and decreased urine output. Taking small amounts of an electrolyte replacement solution, or

---

TABLE 20-5 ◆ *Commonly Prescribed Drugs for Gastrointestinal Problems*

Classification*	Action	Nursing Implications	Patient Teaching
Antidiarrheals			
Diphenoxylate hydrocholoride (Lomotil)	Decreases motility, propulsion, and secretions.	Observe for effectiveness; should be effective within 48 hours.	Warn that medication will cause dry mouth. Instruct not to take more than rec-
Loperamide (Imodium)			ommended dosage as toxic-
Opium tincture (Paregoric)		Observe for signs of constipa-	ity can occur.
Kaolin-pectin combinations (Kaopectate)	Decreases fluid in stool.	tion.	With Lomotil warn not to oper-
		Use cautiously in patients with prostatic enlargement as may cause urinary retention.	ate machinery until effect on central nervous system (CNS) is known.
Bismuth subgallate (Pepto-Bismol)	Binds water; coats mucosa, absorbs toxins.	Warn that this drug will make stool black.	Advise to contact physician if acute diarrhea does not abate within 2 days.
Antiflatulents			
Simethicone (Phazyme, Mylicon, Di-Gel)	Defoaming action disperses gas.	Warn that the drug does not prevent gas formation, but will decrease bloating and discomfort.	Instruct to chew tablets before swallowing.
		Gas is expelled via belching or flatus.	
Laxatives			
Bulk-forming	Act like fiber, absorbing water in the bowel and hastening transit time through the bowel.	None specific; monitor effec- tiveness.	Instruct to take with an 8-oz glass of water to prevent esophageal obstruction.
Methylcellulose (Citracel)			
Psyllium (Metamucil, Konsyl)			
Surfactants	Facilitates absorption of water by stool by decreasing the surface tension. Enhances secretion of fluid and elec- trolytes in the bowel.	Contraindicated for patients with signs of intestinal ob- struction.	Instruct to take with a full glass of water. Not to be used for more than 1 week without physician's knowl- edge.
Docusate sodium (Surfak, Colace)		Act in 24 to 48 hours.	
Docusate potassium (Dialose)		Used to prevent constipation rather than treat it.	

TABLE 20-5 ◆ *Commonly Prescribed Drugs for Gastrointestinal Problems* (Continued)

Classification*	Action	Nursing Implications	Patient Teaching
Laxatives *(continued)*			
Contact laxatives Biscodyl (Ducolax) Phenolphthalein (Feen-a-Mint, Ex-Lax, Modane) Cascara sagadra and senna (Senokot, Fletcher's Castoria) Castor oil	Act on intestinal wall to increase secretion of fluid and electrolytes into the intestine.	Most act with 6–12 hours to produce a semi-fluid stool. Bisacodyl is available as a rectal suppository as well as an oral tablet. Phenophthalein may turn the urine pink. Cascara sagadra and senna may cause a brownish-yellow or pink tinge to the urine. Castor oil acts within 2–6 hours. Castor oil should not be used routinely to treat constipation. The unpleasant taste of castor oil can be decreased by chilling or pouring over ice or mixing in chilled fruit juice.	Contact laxatives should be used for only occasional treatment of constipation. They are habit-forming, decreasing the natural mechanisms for evacuation. Tablets should not be chewed. Take tablets with a full glass of water. Do not exceed recommended dosage. Take bisacodyl 1 hour after taking antacids or milk. Suppository form may cause burning sensation in the rectum.
Histamine receptor antagonist			
Cimetidine (Tagamet) Famotidine (Pepcid) Nizatidine (Axid) Rantidine (Zantac)	Suppress acid secretion by blocking H_2 receptors on parietal cells.	Cimetidine may interact with many other drugs; check drug interactions for other drugs patient is receiving. Cimetidine may cause confusion and other CNS effects. Separate administration of these drugs and antacids by 1 hour. Monitor for decreased abdominal pain and ulcer symptoms.	These drugs should be taken with meals and at bedtime. Once-a-day dose should be taken at bedtime. Advise to avoid cigarettes, aspirin, and other NSAIDs. Advise to avoid alcohol or only consume it in moderation and only in conjunction with food. Advise to utilize stress-reduction techniques.
Antacids			
Gelusil, Maalox, Mylanta-II, Riopan, Di-Gel, etc. There are four antacid families consisting of compounds of aluminum, magnesium, calcium, and sodium.	Neutralize stomach acid.	Aluminum hydroxide compounds promote constipation, whereas magnesium hydroxide compounds promote diarrhea. Sodium compounds may adversely affect hypertension and heart failure. All antacids may adversely affect the dissolution and absorption of other drugs. One hour should be allowed between antacid administration and administration of another drug. Magnesium compounds are used cautiously in patients with renal insufficiency.	Antacids should be taken seven times a day: 1 hour after meals, 3 hours after meals, and at bedtime. Shake liquid preparations well before pouring from container. Chew antacid tablets thoroughly, and follow with a glass of water or milk. Report problems of constipation or diarrhea to the physician. Take even after pain has disappearred; consult physician.
Antiulcer medications (miscellaneous)			
Sucralfate (Carafate)	Sucralfate provides protective coating barrier over ulcer crater.	Monitor for constipation.	Take only as directed. Wait 30 minutes before taking any other drug.

(Table 20-5 continued)

TABLE 20-5 ◆ *Commonly Prescribed Drugs for Gastrointestinal Problems* (Continued)			
Classification*	Action	Nursing Implications	Patient Teaching
Antiulcer medications (miscellaneous) *(continued)*			
Omeprazole (Prilosec) Lansoprazole (Prevacid)	Omeprazole and lansoprazole are proton pump inhibitors that suppress secretion of gastric acid	May cause headache, nausea, vomiting, or diarrhea. Use is preferably limited to 4–8 weeks.	Follow regimen of diet and stress reduction for ulcer healing.
Misoprostol (Cytotec)	Misoprostol prevents gastric ulcers caused by long-term therapy with NSAIDs.	May cause diarrhea or abdominal pain. Not safe during pregnancy.	
Antispasmodics			
Dicyclomine hydrochloride (Bentyl, Antispas) Probantheline bromide (Probanthine) Oxyphencyclmine hydrochloride (Daricon)	Block acetylcholine, thereby decreasing smooth-muscle spasm and GI motility and inhibiting gastric acid secretion.	These drugs interact with many other drugs; check each drug patient is taking for interactions. Most of theses drugs are contraindicated in glaucoma, prostatic hypertrophy, myasthenia gravis, and other conditions; consult information on each drug individually. May predispose to drug-induced heat stroke. Monitor vital signs and urine output carefully.	Take 30–60 minutes before meal. Patient can suck on hard candy to relieve mouth dryness unless contraindicated. Drink 2,500–3,000 mL of fluid to prevent constipation. Avoid driving and hazardous activities if drug causes dizziness, sleepiness, or blurred vision. Report rash or skin eruption to physician.
Drugs for inflammatory bowel disease (IBD)			
Sulfasalazine (Azullfidine) Mesalamine (5-ASA) Osalazine (Dipentum)	Sulfasalazine is a sulfonamide antibiotic. Mesalamine is the active agent in sulfasalazine. Osalazine contains two molecules of 5-ASA. These drugs reduce inflammation in the bowel by suppressing prostaglandin synthesis and the migration of inflammatory cells into the affected area.	May cause muscle aches, nausea, fever, or rash. Complete blood counts needed periodically as the drugs can cause agranulocytosis and anemia. Determine whether allergy to sulfonamides exists before administration.	Caution to avoid direct sunlight and ultraviolet light to prevent photosensitivity reaction. Advise to use other form of contraception than oral contraceptives as these drugs interfere with their effectiveness. Warn that when used with oral hypoglycemics an increased hypoglycemic effect may occur. Advise that urine may be tinted orange. GI upset may be minimized by taking drug after meals. Instruct to report rash or sensitivity reaction to physician promptly.

*Names of generic drugs are listed first, followed by the the names of brand drugs in parentheses.

Gatorade, helps prevent imbalances. Avoiding coffee or tea helps as they are gastric stimulants and increase peristalsis. Thorough handwashing is essential when caring for the patient, and *Standard Precautions* are followed. When infection is the cause of the diarrhea Contact Precautions to prevent spread of the infection are followed; gloves are donned when entering the room.

The anus and rectal mucosa must be protected from excoriation. The use of barrier ointment or cream helps protect the area. Warm sitz baths may relieve soreness and discomfort in the tissues as well as help cleanse the area without excessive wiping. Keeping the patient clean and dry is a high priority. Relieving odor in the room may be done with a deodorizing spray and by emptying and cleaning bedpans and commodes quickly.

◆ Bowel Incontinence

Severe illness, trauma, neurological damage, or prolonged bedrest may bring about bowel incontinence. This is very embarrassing for the alert patient. The nurse must be kind and gentle and must make every effort to keep the patient clean and dry. Tracking the time of incontinent movements and offering toileting after each meal may help eliminate the problem. Should incontinence be persistent, the cause should be identified and then a bowel training program instituted. See Chapter 14 for information on the bowel training program.

◆ Gastrointestinal Bleeding

Signs and Symptoms   Bleeding from the intestinal tract can be acute and profuse or chronic and gradual. Gastrointestinal bleeding is usually referred to as either *upper GI bleeding* or *lower intestinal bleeding,* depending on the source. The most common causes of upper GI bleeding are gastric and duodenal ulcers, varicose veins of the esophagus (esophageal varices), and erosive gastritis. Patients most at risk for blood loss resulting from gastritis are those who have ingested drugs (for example, large doses of aspirin or non-steroidal anti-inflammatory agents, NSAIDs) or who have consumed excessive amounts of alcohol. Tumors, trauma, and foreign bodies also can lead to bleeding anywhere in the GI tract.

Bleeding from a source in the lower intestinal tract usually is more chronic and gradual in nature. Possible causes include tumors and polyps in the lower intestines, chronic colitis, and diverticulosis. Hemorrhoids also can break down and bleed, in which case bright red blood is noticed in the stools.

> Subjective signs of acute GI bleeding include complaints of weakness and feeling faint, nausea and vomiting, restlessness, thirst, and mental confusion. Objective signs include the presence of bright red blood in either the emesis or stool; "coffee ground" emesis (hematemesis) or maroon or tarry stools (melena); diarrhea (blood acts as a cathartic); and decreased blood pressure, rapid pulse, and other signs of hypovolemic shock.

If bleeding from the upper GI system is profuse, maroon or bright red blood may be noted in the stools because of the rapid transit of the blood through the intestinal tract. Black stools almost always indicate the presence of digested blood, which means that the source of bleeding is in the upper GI tract. It is well to remember that iron salts can cause the stool to be black and that the ingestion of beets can cause the stool to be bright red.

Estimates of blood loss from the GI tract are based in part on blood pressure readings and pulse rates.

Hence blood pressure and pulse rate should be monitored every 15 to 30 minutes when there is evidence of extensive GI hemorrhage. Central venous pressure readings also are helpful in determining the amount of blood lost, especially in hypertensive patients, whose blood pressure may not reflect hypovolemia.

> Changes in the vital signs that signal hypovolemic shook do not appear until after the patient has lost 20% or more of the blood volume.

Additional data useful in determining the status of patients with GI bleeding include hematocrit and hemoglobin levels. These levels can be normal or even slightly elevated at the beginning of a bleeding episode, because it takes 4 to 6 hours for the body to shift fluids from other compartments to the intravascular compartment and thereby change the ratio of formed elements to fluids in the blood.

The white cell count may be elevated in massive GI bleeding, probably because of the body's response to injury or hypovolemia. An elevated level of blood urea nitrogen (BUN) can indicate digestion of large amounts of blood.

Treatment   The major concerns in the treatment of acute GI hemorrhage are replacement of the blood and fluids lost and stoppage of the bleeding. If there is major blood loss, transfusions of whole blood, packed cells, or fresh frozen plasma may be necessary. Normal saline, Plasmanate (plasma protein fraction), and Ringer's solution may be administered until blood is available. Maintenance of fluid balance is of extreme importance. Intake and output must be measured and recorded accurately. Oxygen therapy is started to maximize tissue oxygenation.

Once the patient's condition is sufficiently stabilized, diagnostic procedures are done to locate the source of bleeding. These procedures include endoscopic examination of the esophagus, stomach, and small intestine. Barium studies also may be ordered.

Treatment of gastric bleeding is begun by inserting a large-bore nasogastric (NG) tube and using a normal saline lavage to monitor the quantity of bleeding and evacuate the blood, clots, and stomach contents. This allows the stomach to constrict, halting the blood flow. Antacids are given via the tube to neutralize pepsin and help stop the bleeding. An H_2-receptor antagonist, such as Cimetadine (Tagamet), ranitidine (Zantac), or famotidine (Pepcid), is given IV to decrease stomach acid secretion (see Table 20-5). Eighty percent of GI bleeding will stop with these treatments.

Once the patient has stabilized, diagnostic procedures are done to locate the source of bleeding. Electrocauterization or laser photocoagulation of a vessel can be done through the endoscope. If endoscopy and barium radiographs are unsuccessful in locating the area of bleeding, angiography of the vessels supplying the intestinal tract are performed and embolization is done to stop the bleeding. Surgery may be required if the bleeding cannot be stopped by any other means.

Bleeding from esophageal varices, usually caused by cirrhosis of the liver, is controlled by injecting vasopressin (Pitressin) directly in the bleeding artery to stimulate contraction of the vessel or subcutaneous injection of octreotide and by using a Sengstaken-Blackmore tube, which compresses the vessels by inflating balloons (Figure 20-7). The tube has three lumens: one for the esophageal balloon, one for the gastric balloon, and one through which saline can be instilled and blood and stomach secretions can be evacuated. Endoscopic injection scleropathy is utilized for patients who have repeated hemorrhagic episodes despite medical management.

Nursing intervention for GI bleeding must include consideration for the patient's fear and anxiety. Many times these patients are afraid they are going to die. The sight of so much blood loss is frightening to the patient, to whom it usually appears more profuse than it actually is. Whatever procedures are used, the patient and family deserve an explanation and reassurance that everything is being done to control the hemorrhage.

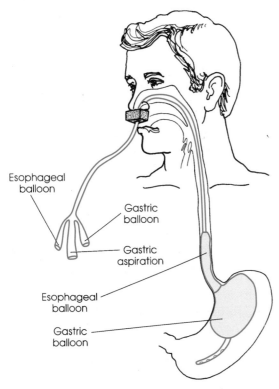

Esophageal balloon

Gastric balloon

Gastric aspiration

Esophageal balloon

Gastric balloon

If the bleeding site is in the esophagus, as from esophageal varices, the esophageal balloon is inflated. If the bleeding site is in the stomach, the gastric balloon is inflated. Inflation of the balloon creates pressure against bleeding vessels.

FIGURE 20-7   Sengstaken-Blackmore tube.

After the bleeding has apparently stopped and the patient's vital signs have stabilized, there must be continuous monitoring for signs of persistent or renewed bleeding. Blood pressure and pulse rate are measured regularly; skin color, diaphoresis, thirst, and other signs of continued blood loss and impending hypovolemic shock must be watched for; intake and output are measured and the character of vomitus, aspirated gastric fluid, and stools noted; and the patient's daily weight is taken and recorded.

PROBLEMS RELATED TO INGESTION

◆ Eating Disorders

Anorexia Nervosa   **Anorexia nervosa is a disorder in which the patient is preoccupied with eating but has a morbid fear of becoming fat.** Excessive exercise is commonly used by these patients as another means of staying thin. The patient refuses to eat adequate quantities of food. The cause is unknown, but it is thought to be an inappropriate coping mechanism in response to excessive expectations and controls imposed on the patient by parents or others. It most commonly is seen in females from early teens to 30 years old, although it also occurs in males.

Anorexia nervosa is a dangerous disorder because the patient can literally starve to death. Although it is a psychiatric disorder, the patient may be admitted to the medical floor for treatment of malnutrition by parenteral therapy. Behavior modification is the focus of treatment.

Bulimia   **Bulimia is the practice of inducing vomiting after binge eating.** Laxatives also may be taken to purge the system after an eating binge. The patient consumes large quantities of food and then gets rid of it so that weight is not gained. Some patients with anorexia nervosa also are bulimic.

Some individuals practice bulimia occasionally without harm. When it is practiced frequently, it can lead to severe fluid and electrolyte imbalances, starvation, and death. Treatment of bulimia includes psychotherapy and behavior modification. Both bulimia and anorexia nervosa are difficult to cure.

Obesity   People overeat for a variety of reasons. For some it is a reaction to stress; for others it is a substitute for absent pleasures. For many, overeating simply is habit. **A person is considered obese if he weighs more than 20% above the ideal weight for his height, age, and body type.**

Obese patients should be counseled by the nurse to lose weight to avoid developing one or more of the many diseases in which obesity is a contributing factor.

Diabetes and hypertension are particularly correlated to obesity.

The patient should have a physical examination with testing for thyroid abnormality and other problems before beginning a weight-reduction diet. Physician supervision is the best and safest way to treat obesity. Usually a lower-calorie diet and exercise are prescribed, and the patient is taught ways to change his thinking about food and his weight. Weight that is lost slowly is more likely not to be regained.

The nurse can offer considerable support for the patient who is dieting by being available to talk about the positive aspects and frustrations of staying on the diet. The nurse should discourage fad diets and emphasize the importance of a well-balanced, nutritious, low-calorie diet. Commercial programs are available to assist patients with weight reduction.

Weight Watchers is the only commercial program to date that has shown good results with safe weight loss and maintenance of normal weight over the years.

◆ Dysphagia

Dysphagia means difficulty in swallowing. It is the most common symptom of disorders of the esophagus and varies from a mild sensation that something is sticking in the throat to complete inability to swallow solids or liquids.

The nurse can help diagnose the specific cause of dysphagia by observing carefully the kinds of food the patient can tolerate and the conditions under which difficulties are experienced. Knowing the consistency and temperature of the foods most easily ingested by the patient is helpful. Some patients may strangle on liquids, tolerate soft and semi-solid foods, and have the feeling that high-fiber foods are not moving past a certain point in the esophagus.

Nursing Intervention   Measures that may be helpful in relieving dysphagia include instructing the patient to chew his food more thoroughly, to eat semi-soft foods, to drink liquids throughout the meal (if liquids do not cause choking), and to sit upright with the head forward and the neck flexed. Other factors may be related to the physical and social environment in which meals are eaten. Meals should be served in a relaxing atmosphere, with pleasant surroundings and relief from emotional stress. Further discussion of dysphagia is found in the chapter on neurological disorders.

Patients with chronic dysphagia are subject to respiratory problems resulting from the aspiration of food into the respiratory tree. Both acute and chronic dysphagia are likely to produce nutritional deficiencies and electrolyte imbalances. If the dysphagia is such that the patient cannot swallow sufficient amounts of food for adequate nutrition, tube feeding may be indicated.

This sometimes is necessary when the dysphagia is the result of cerebral damage, as in cerebrovascular accident (CVA).

If the patient cannot swallow anything because of a neurological condition, or if the esophagus is obstructed and cannot be corrected surgically, then the patient must have a gastrostomy. An opening in the wall of the stomach is created, and a permanent feeding tube is sutured in place.

Nursing interventions for the patient with a gastrostomy tube include aspirating for residual contents before each feeding, keeping the skin clean and dry around the tube, flushing the tube after each feeding, and changing the dressing every 24 hours or PRN until the site is healed.

◆ Hiatal Hernia (Diaphragmatic Hernia)

Hiatal hernia is the result of a defect in the wall of the diaphragm where the esophagus passes through. A hiatal hernia is formed by the protrusion of part of the stomach or the lower part of the esophagus up into the thoracic cavity; it is a common disorder in older people, especially women. Loss of muscle strength and tone, factors that cause increased intraabdominal pressure (such as obesity or multiple pregnancies), and congenital defects contribute to the formation of the hernia.

Signs and symptoms include indigestion, belching, and substernal or epigastric pain or feelings of pressure after eating caused by reflux of gastric fluid into the esophagus. The symptoms are more severe when the patient lies down. The problem can be visualized on an upper GI series.

Treatment includes weight reduction, avoidance of tight-fitting clothes around the abdomen, administration of antacids, H_2-receptor antagonists, and elevation of the head of the bed on 6-inch to 8-inch blocks. The patient is instructed not to eat within several hours of going to bed. Intake of alcohol, chocolate, and fatty food is limited and smoking should be avoided. If nighttime gastroesophageal reflux continues to be a problem, a new drug, cisapride (Propulsid), that prevents reflux may be effective.

Occasionally a patient with reflux esophagitis, which is caused by the hernia, may bleed extensively. If bleeding or discomfort cannot be controlled, surgical correction of the hernia is required.

INFLAMMATORY DISORDERS OF THE INTESTINAL TRACT

◆ Stomatitis

Stomatitis is a generalized inflammation of the mucous membranes of the mouth. Causes include trauma from ill-fitting dentures or malocclusions of the teeth, poor oral hygiene, nutritional deficiencies, excessive smoking, excessive drinking of alcohol, pathogenic microorganisms, radiation therapy, and drugs (especially those used in chemotherapy for malignancies).

Common symptoms of stomatitis include pain and swelling of the oral mucosa, increased salivation or excessive dryness, severe halitosis, and sometimes fever and small, crater-like ulcers in the mouth.

Treatment of stomatitis is chiefly symptomatic, unless a specific infectious causative agent is identified. Nursing measures to control the symptoms of stomatitis, including special mouth care, artificial saliva, and diet, are discussed in Chapter 9.

◆ Gastritis

Gastritis is an inflammation of the mucous membrane lining the stomach and may be acute or chronic in nature. *Atrophic* gastritis involves all layers of the stomach and is seen in association with gastric ulcer and malignancies of the stomach. Gastritis associated with uremia is common in the patient with kidney failure. Chronic gastritis frequently progresses to ulcer formation and upper-GI hemorrhage.

> The main causes of acute gastritis are drinking excessive amounts of alcohol, eating contaminated food, and ingestion of drugs, such as aspirin, ibuprofen, corticosteroids, or nonsteroidal antiinflammatory agents (NSAIDs).

In both acute and chronic gastritis, the main symptoms are nausea, vomiting, pain and tenderness in the stomach region, and sometimes diarrhea. The patient with chronic gastritis also may have massive hemorrhage from the stomach.

Medical Treatment and Nursing Intervention

Acute gastritis usually is of very short duration. Treatment consists of withholding all foods by mouth and administering drugs that slow down the peristaltic action of the gastrointestinal tract. If severe dehydration or nausea and vomiting occur, fluids may be given IV.

> The patient with gastritis must be watched closely for signs of fluid and electrolyte imbalance.

Chronic gastritis is not as easily treated as acute gastritis. Diet therapy is of primary importance in chronic gastritis because the patient frequently admits to indiscretion in his dietary and drinking habits and finds it difficult to change. The diet for these patients is devoid of those foods known to produce attacks in an individual patient. Treatment consists of antispasmod-

ics to decrease the pain of stomach spasms, antacids, and an H_2-receptor antagonist, such as ranitidine, to decrease acid secretions and change pH.

It is always difficult to change eating habits of long standing, and the nurse must use tact and patience in encouraging the patient to follow the prescribed diet faithfully.

◆ Ulcerative Colitis and Crohn's Disease

Ulcerative colitis is an inflammation, with the formation of ulcers, of the mucosa of the colon. It often is a chronic disease, and the patient usually is free from symptoms between acute flareups.

The exact cause of ulcerative colitis is not known. Infections and emotional tension frequently bring about acute attacks. It is more common among those of Jewish descent, and people with the disorder have a 40% higher incidence of some type of arthritis than the general public.

Ulcerative colitis and regional ileitis (Crohn's disease) share many of the same characteristics. One difference is that the inflammatory changes in ulcerative colitis are nonspecific, whereas those in Crohn's disease are granulomatous. Another very important difference is that the patient with long-standing chronic ulcerative colitis is at 10 to 20 times greater risk for developing cancer of the colon than one with Crohn's disease. Crohn's disease can affect any area of the intestine, although it more frequently affects the ascending colon and can affect the small intestine (Figure 20-8). Ulcerative colitis most often affects the rectosigmoid and left colon. Ulcerative colitis changes tend to be continuous along the affected portion of the bowel whereas those of Crohn's disease are segmental, leaving healthy sections of bowel in between diseased portions.

There is a growing tendency to include both disorders under the title of inflammatory bowel disease (IBD). It is suspected that ulcerative colitis and Crohn's disease are immunological responses to the same as-yet-unknown etiological agent.

Signs and Symptoms

The patient with IBD suffers from attacks of bloody, mucoid diarrhea, abdominal pain with cramping, malaise, fever, and weight loss. The bouts often are precipitated by events that cause undue physical or emotional stress. An acute attack can last for days, weeks, or even months, followed by periods of remission extending from a few weeks to several decades. A few patients experience only one attack and then remain free of symptoms for the rest of their lives. Others suffer such profound disturbances during the first attack that their lives are in danger if they do not receive prompt treatment to stop intestinal hemorrhage and correct fluid and electrolyte imbalances.

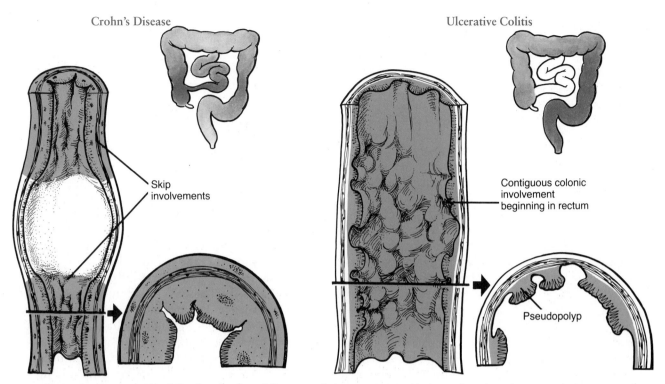

FIGURE 20-8 Comparison of the distribution of disease and characteristics of lesions of Crohn's disease and ulcerative colitis. (*Source:* Cotran, R. S., Kumar, V., Robbins, S. L., Schoen, F. J., eds. [1994]. *Robbins-Pathologic Basis of Disease,* 5th ed. Philadelphia: Saunders, p. 804.)

Medical diagnosis usually is based on the patient's medical history and presenting symptoms. Colonoscopy, barium enema, and stool analysis may be used to confirm the diagnosis.

Treatment Treatment for either ulcerative colitis or Crohn's disease varies according to severity of symptoms and whether the condition becomes chronic. Conservative approaches to medical treatment include administration of antidiarrheal drugs, long-term sulfasalazine therapy, medications to relieve abdominal cramps, and a diet of low-fat, low-fiber foods that have a high protein and caloric content. Small frequent feedings are best. Lactose avoidance helps some patients. Corticosteroids are used for moderate to severe cases. During acute attacks fluid replacement may be necessary. Oral 5-aminosalicylic acid (5-ASA) derivatives, such as osalazine sodium (Dipentium), have recently been found to be useful for those patients who cannot tolerate sulfasalazine. Patients with advanced disease who are not surgical candidates may be given azathioprine, 6-metacaptopurine, methotrexate, levamisole, or cyclosporine to help control the disease. Supplements containing 400 to 1,000 mcg of folic acid have been found to reduce the incidence of colon cancer in patients taking sulfasalazine.

A drug called anti-TNF, a monoclonal antibody, is undergoing clinical trials and has shown promise in the treatment of Crohn's disease. A single infusion produced a dramatic reduction of symptoms in 65% of patients treated in the trials at 18 medical centers in the United States and Europe.

Surgical intervention is an alternative treatment for some patients. The surgical procedure usually involves removing the affected portion of the bowel, often by proctocolectomy, and creating an ileostomy. Today a patient with ulcerative colitis may be a candidate for a Kock pouch or an ileoanal anastomosis rather than a standard ileostomy. Both of these new procedures allow the patient control over the discharge of wastes from the reservoir, and consequently a collection pouch is not necessary. The patient uses a catheter to empty the reservoir after the Kock procedure and retains control over the anal sphincter with voluntary defecation when an ileoanal anastomosis is performed. These procedures are not performed often for Crohn's disease because as the disease progresses, the area of the reservoir is involved.

Nursing Assessment and Intervention The nursing care plan for a patient experiencing an acute attack of IDB should include such observations as number and character of stools, periodic auscultation of bowel sounds, measurement of intake and output, daily weighings, checking for signs of internal bleeding and anemia, and monitoring laboratory data for evidence of electrolyte imbalances.

Long-term goals may be concerned with helping the patient adhere to the prescribed regimen, encouraging effective coping mechanisms, and instruction and encouragement in relaxation techniques. The frequent bouts of diarrhea and abdominal cramping can be embarrassing and depressing for the patient. The fatigue and malaise that often accompany these bouts makes performing usual daily tasks difficult; rest periods are necessary. There is a need for emotional support, empathetic listening, and encouragement to take part in cooperative planning of care. Family and significant others are included in the planning of care whenever possible.

◆ Appendicitis

Symptoms and Diagnosis   Appendicitis is an inflammation of the vermiform appendix (called *vermiform* because it is wormlike and *appendix* because it is an appendage of the cecum). The appendix is a blind pouch and is therefore easily infected by bacteria passing through the intestinal tract.

Pain in the lower right side, halfway between the umbilicus and the crest of the ileum, is the best-known symptom of appendicitis. However, the location of the pain may, and often does, vary among individuals. **An elevated temperature, nausea and vomiting, and an increase in the white cell count also are characteristic of appendicitis.**

Elder Care Point . . . Peritoneal inflammation does not necessarily cause abdominal rigidity in the elderly patient. These patients often present with only diffuse abdominal pain, malaise, and weakness. Confusion may be present.

A new test, focused appendix computed tomography (FACT), may eliminate unnecessary appendectomies.

Treatment   Appendicitis is treated by surgically removing the appendix *(appendectomy).* This procedure may be performed laparoscopically. Before surgery, the patient is allowed nothing by mouth, and an ice bag may be placed on the abdomen to slow down the inflammation and thus avoid rupture of the swollen and inflamed appendix.

Under no circumstances should laxatives be given when appendicitis is suspected. Heat applications to relieve abdominal pain are contraindicated.

The patient is usually allowed out of bed within several hours of surgery if there are no complications. The convalescent period is most often uneventful, and the patient may return to his former activities within 1 to 3 weeks.

◆ Peritonitis

Signs and Symptoms   Peritonitis is an inflammation of the peritoneum. It usually occurs when one of the organs it encloses ruptures or is perforated so that the organ's contents (including bacteria) are spilled into the abdominal cavity. **Examples of common causes of peritonitis are ruptured appendix, perforated duodenal or gastric ulcer, ruptured ectopic (tubal) pregnancy, and traumatic rupture of the spleen or liver.**

As the peritoneum becomes inflamed, there is local redness and swelling of the membrane and production of serous fluid that becomes more and more purulent as the bacteria multiply. Normal peristaltic action of the intestines slows or ceases altogether, and the symptoms of intestinal obstruction occur. The patient experiences nausea, vomiting, severe abdominal pain and distention, fever, chills, tachycardia, pallor, and other symptoms of shock. **Unless the condition is treated promptly and successfully, peritonitis can be fatal.**

Treatment   Broad-spectrum antibiotics are given in massive doses to combat infection, fluids and electrolytes are administered to restore a normal balance, and gastric or intestinal suction is initiated to relieve distention. Surgical procedures needed to repair a ruptured organ are done as soon as the patient's condition will permit.

Nursing Intervention   Nursing care is primarily concerned with frequent assessment of the patient and prompt and accurate reporting of unexpected changes in his condition. The patient is usually placed in the semi-Fowler's position to facilitate breathing, prevent respiratory complications, and aid in localizing the purulent material in the lower abdomen or pelvis. Vital signs are taken and recorded every 4 hours during the critical stage. If vomiting occurs, the characteristics and amount of vomitus are noted. The emesis of fecal material indicates complete intestinal obstruction.

A common complication of peritonitis is paralytic ileus. The nurse must auscultate at least once a shift for the return of bowel sounds. If the patient passes flatus or feces rectally, this should be recorded on the chart, as it indicates return of peristalsis.

Because of the high fever and toxicity that accompany peritonitis, the patient may be delirious or disoriented and must be protected from self-injury. This includes putting siderails on the bed and having someone at the bedside at all times. The patient should be turned *very gently* and moved in the bed with care because of extreme tenderness in the abdominal region. A high fever and the presence of the gastric tube demand frequent mouth care to protect the lips, prevent halitosis, and cleanse the mouth.

◆ Peptic Ulcer

A peptic ulcer is an ulceration with loss of tissue of the upper GI tract. The term includes both duodenal and gastric ulcers (Figure 20-9). Ulcers develop when the mucosa cannot protect itself from corrosive substances, such as gastric acid, pepsinogen, alcohol, bile salts, and irritating food substances. The most common site for development of a peptic ulcer is in the first few centimeters of the duodenum, just beyond the pyloric muscle. There are approximately 200,000 to 400,000 new cases of duodenal ulcers annually and about 87,000 new cases of gastric ulcers. Normally, the upper GI mucosa can resist corrosion. When gastric substances are out of balance, problems arise. Excessive stress is another cause of peptic ulcers. Severe illness, burns, or severe trauma can all predispose the patient to developing a *stress ulcer,* a result of increased gastric acid secretion.

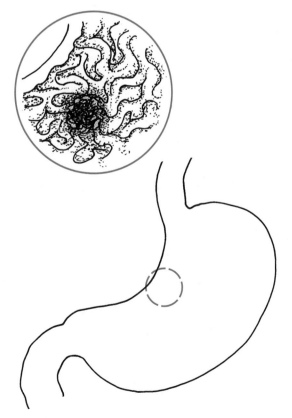

The ulcer has penetrated deeply into the stomach wall.

FIGURE 20-9   Ulcer of the gastric mucosa.

For some unknown reason the incidence of peptic ulcer has been gradually decreasing in the past few decades. It is more common in males than in females.

Causative Factors   It was thought that the usual cause of peptic ulcer was the presence of too much gastric juice *in relation to the degree of protection* normally afforded by the GI mucosa and the small intestine, which secrete mucus and other substances that neutralize gastric acid. Normally, all areas exposed to the hydrochloric acid and pepsin in gastric juice have an ample supply of mucous glands that secrete a protective alkaline mucus. However, the chief cause may be a bacterium called *Helicobacter pylori.* This bacterium is rich in an enzyme that may cause corrosion of the upper GI mucosa by damaging its mucous coating, making it more susceptible to damage from gastric acid and pepsinogen.

Because it is known that gastric acid and pepsin are responsible for ulcer formation, this would explain why mucosal resistance to them could become impaired. Duodenal ulcers and some prepyloric ulcers are associated with an increased amount or hyperacidity of the gastric juice and are 70% associated with *H. pylori.* Gastric ulcers, on the other hand, are characterized by normal or abnormally low levels of hydrochloric acid, but 90% are associated with *H. pylori.* It is likely that gastric ulcers develop because of the reduced resistance of the gastric mucosa to digestion by gastric juice. *Helicobacter pylori* is implicated in the development of gastric cancer as well.

Elder Care Point . . . By age 60, approximately 60% of the population in the United States of America is infected with the *H. pylori* bacterium. However, most people never have symptoms of gastritis, and few develop ulcers.

Theories about genetic and environmental causes of peptic ulcer abound. Both gastric and duodenal ulcers tend to occur in families. Relatives of persons with gastric or duodenal ulcers have three times the expected rate for ulcer formation, and a genetic link has been found for this.

Neither hot spicy foods nor caffeine have been proven to be a risk factor for ulcers, but these substances make symptoms worse in many people. Gastric ulcers do occur in those who are poorly nourished because of poverty or of poor eating habits. Despite the stereotype of the hard-driving executive suffering from an ulcer and gulping antacid tablets, there is a greater incidence of ulcers in blue-collar workers and in laborers.

Stress does have a bearing on the development of peptic ulcer, however. Tension, anxiety, and prolonged stress do alter gastric function. Prolonged psychological or physiological stress produces what is known as a *stress ulcer*, which is believed to be the result of unrelieved stimulation of the vagus nerves. A stress ulcer is pathologically and clinically different from a chronic peptic ulcer. It is more acute and more likely to produce hemorrhage; perforation occurs occasionally, and pain is rare. Stress ulcers are an "occupational hazard" of patients who are severely ill and in intensive care units for prolonged periods. Such patients often receive medication to prevent stress ulcers.

Drug-induced ulcers are most often caused by aspirin, nonsteroidal antiinflammatory drugs (NSAIDs), alcohol, and glucocorticoids. Cigarette smoking is known to be a causative factor in peptic ulcer, particularly if over one-half pack a day is smoked.

The technique most commonly used to diagnose peptic ulcer is an upper-GI series *(barium swallow)*. Endoscopy can help locate the site of ulceration and bleeding and differentiate between benign and malignant ulcerations and between esophageal ulcer and diverticulum (pouching of the intestinal wall).

A gastric analysis to measure the level of hydrochloric acid in gastric juice may be helpful in some cases, but there is a good bit of variation in gastric acid levels among patients with peptic ulcer. Serum tests for *H. pylori* detect antibodies indicating active or recent infection. The urea breath test involves the measurement of gas released in the breath following ingestion of a radiolabeled urea isotope. When *H. pylori* is present the test is positive.

Signs and Symptoms   Subjective symptoms of uncomplicated ulcer include epigastric pain that might be described as burning, gnawing, cramping, or aching and usually comes in waves that last several minutes. The daily pattern of pain is associated with the secretion of gastric juice in relation to the presence of food, which can act as a buffer. **For example, the pain is diminished in the morning when secretion is low and after meals when food is in the stomach and most severe before meals and at bedtime.** Discomfort often appears for several days or weeks and then subsides, only to reappear weeks or months later.

Other subjective symptoms include nausea, loss of appetite, and sometimes weight loss. Spontaneous vomiting usually accompanies duodenal ulcer more often than gastric ulcer.

Elder Care Point... The elderly patient may not display the typical symptoms. Pain is less typical and may be poorly localized, or it may be described as lower-chest discomfort or left-sided pain. Anorexia, weight loss, general weakness, anemia, nausea, and painless vomiting may occur; peptic ulcer is difficult to diagnose in this population.

Complications.   The three major complications of peptic ulcer are hemorrhage, perforation, and obstruction. Hemorrhage has been discussed earlier in this chapter under Gastrointestinal Bleeding. Perforation is erosion of the ulcer through all walls of the intestine and a spilling of the contents of the GI tract into the peritoneal cavity. It constitutes a surgical emergency because of the danger of hemorrhage and peritonitis.

Perforation is characterized by a sudden and severe pain in the upper abdomen that persists and increases in intensity and sometimes is referred to the shoulders. The abdomen is rigid and board-like and extremely tender. In a short time the patient shows signs of shock. Obstruction occurs as a result of scarring and loss of musculature at the pylorus. It is manifested chiefly by persistent vomiting.

Think about... How does the pain of a peptic ulcer differ from the pain of IBD?

Treatment   Peptic ulcer is treated conservatively at first to avoid surgery. The goals of treatment are to alleviate symptoms, promote healing, prevent complications, and educate the patient so that recurrence can be avoided.

Relief of symptoms.   Medications to relieve pain from local irritation of the intestinal mucosa include the antacids, which reduce the pain of ulcer by neutralizing gastric acid. Examples of antacids include aluminum hydroxide (Amphojel), aluminum hydroxide–magnesium trisilicate (Gaviscon), and aluminum hydroxide–magnesium hydroxide–simethicone (Gelusil). Antacids effective for antiflatulence include aluminum hydroxide–magnesium hydroxide–simethicone (Gelusil-M, Maalox Plus, and Mylanta).

If the presence of *H. pylori* has been identified, treatment consists of the administration of clarithromycin (Biaxin) and omeprazole (Prilosec). Sucralfate (Carafate) tablets may be used for short-term (up to 8 weeks) treatment of duodenal ulcer. It has negligible acid-neutralizing capacity. The action of this drug is local, and its benefits probably derive from its adherence to the ulcer site and protection from further damage by gastric juices. A proton-inhibitor drug, lansoprazole (Prevacid), that inhibits the enzyme system responsible for secreting acids into the stomach is now available to treat duodenal ulcers. Misorostol (Cytotec) is used to replace gastric prostaglandins depleted by NSAID therapy and thereby prevent ulcer formation caused by NSAIDs. Sedatives are sometimes prescribed for the peptic ulcer patient to help reduce anxiety and relieve tension.

Cimetidine (Tagamet) is specific for the treatment of peptic ulcer. It inhibits the effect of histamine on H_2-receptors, blocking the secretion of gastric acid.

Cimetidine relieves pain, reduces the need for antacids, and promotes healing. However, it interacts with many other medications. Ranitidine (Zantac) is a histamine inhibitor. It is used for short-term treatment, usually 4 weeks, of peptic ulcers. It does not have to be given at a particular time in relation to food and does not interact with as many other medications as does cimetidine. It should be given 1 hour before an antacid.

Diet. In the past, diet was a major part of treatment of ulcers. Today, most authorities believe that it is best to restrict only those foods that the patient identifies with the onset of symptoms. Exceptions are alcohol and caffeine, both of which can induce gastritis and aggravate erosion of the gastric mucosa.

It is generally agreed that the kind of food eaten by an ulcer patient is not as important as when the food is eaten. Food should be eaten at frequent and regular intervals throughout the day, rather than in two or three large meals. Meals should not be skipped and the patient should try to keep some food in the stomach at all times.

Patient education. Before a peptic ulcer can be successfully controlled, the patient must understand how and why the ulcer developed in the first place. Once the predisposing factors are understood, it is easier to avoid them. Unless the patient can cooperate fully with the physician and nurses, there is a strong possibility that ulcers will develop again despite medical or even surgical treatment. Nursing interventions for selected problems in a patient with a bleeding peptic ulcer are summarized in Nursing Care Plan 20-1. Table 20-6 presents guidelines for patient teaching.

Surgical treatment a of peptic ulcer. Surgical treatment becomes necessary when a chronic ulcer fails to respond to medical treatment; when complications such as perforation, obstruction, or hemorrhage occur; or malignancy is present.

In *pyloroplasty with truncal or proximal gastric vagotomy,* the pylorus, which has been narrowed by scarring, is widened. The branches of the vagus (Xth cranial) nerve that stimulate acid secretion in the stomach are selectively severed (vagotomy) so that the stomach does not receive impulses from the brain and therefore does not secrete hydrochloric acid. A vagotomy is often done at the same time a gastric resection is performed.

Subtotal gastrectomy (gastric resection) consists of removing a part of the stomach and then joining the remaining portion to the small intestine by *anastomosis* (Figure 20-10A). *Anastomosis* is the joining of two hollow organs by suturing the open ends together so that they become one continuous tube.

An *antrectomy,* in which the gastrin-producing portion of the stomach (the antrum) is removed, may be done in conjunction with a truncal vagotomy. When the fundus of the stomach is anastomosed to the duodenum, the procedure is known as a *Billroth I.* In the *Billroth II* procedure, the duodenum is closed and the fundus of the stomach is anastamosed to the jejunum. *Total gastrectomy* is the surgical removal of all of the stomach. The esophagus is anastomosed to the small intestine (Figure 20-10B).

◆Nursing Care of the Patient Undergoing Gastric Surgery

Preoperative Care The diet of the patient is restricted to liquids during the 24 hours before surgery. In case of obstruction, the patient is NPO, a nasogastric tube is inserted, and gastric suction is begun to remove all stomach contents before surgery.

The patient receives routine preparations necessary for all major abdominal surgery. These include enemas so that the colon is emptied of fecal material. If the patient has had a barium enema, the nurse should look for and report returns that contain whitish material. This is barium, and it will become hardened if left in the colon, thus presenting the possibility of a fecal impaction later on.

Postoperative Care Care of the patient having gastric surgery is routine, with the following exceptions. Following surgery in which part of the stomach has been removed, care must be taken in handling the nasogastric tube to avoid injury to the sutures and prevent introduction of infectious agents. The surgeon will have written specific orders about irrigating fluids allowed and movement of the gastric tube.

After the tube is removed, the patient is given small amounts of liquid to determine tolerance. These liquids are gradually increased according to the patient's ability to take them without nausea, vomiting, or abdominal distress. If the liquids are well tolerated, the patient progresses to small, frequent feedings. Within 6 months, most patients are able to take three regular meals a day as the remaining portion of the stomach stretches to accommodate more and more food. Patients who have had a *total* gastrectomy are usually restricted to small, frequent feedings of easily digested semi-solids for the rest of their lives. When the patient is to be dismissed from the hospital, the hospital dietitian usually is called to help the patient and his family learn about the special diet that the patient must follow after undergoing gastric surgery.

◆Dumping Syndrome

Some patients who have had a gastrectomy experience a complication known as the "dumping syndrome." **The patient has nausea, weakness, abdominal pain, and diarrhea and may feel faint and perspire profusely or experience palpitations after eating.** These sensations

Nursing Care Plan 20-1

Selected nursing diagnoses, goals/expected outcomes, nursing interventions, and evaluations for a patient with a bleeding peptic ulcer

Situation: Mr. Lee is a 47-year-old long-distance truck driver who is admitted to the hospital with a tentative diagnosis of bleeding peptic ulcer. He has had recurrent bouts of epigastric pain that is more pronounced before meals and at bedtime. Mr. Lee states that he eats "whenever I can grab a bite." He eats mostly fried and spicy foods and he smokes two packs of cigarettes a day. He went to the doctor because of fatigue and discomfort that seemed to be getting progressively worse in spite of antacid use. He also admits to having some vomiting episodes with blood in the secretions. Mr. Lee is the sole support of his wife and four children and is very concerned about the expense of hospitalization and the time away from work. He is scheduled for an endoscopic exam of the esophagus, stomach, and duodenum.

Nursing Diagnosis	Goals/Expected Outcomes	Nursing Intervention	Evaluation
Anxiety related to expenses, time off work, and worry about what is wrong with him. SUPPORTING DATA Sole support of family; expresses worry over hospital expenses; worried about blood in vomitus.	Patient will verbalize reduction in anxiety before discharge. Patient will devise plan to cover hospital expenses so as to decrease anxiety. Patient will verbalize understanding of diagnosis and treatment of his condition.	Encourage verbalization of concerns and fears. Ask for financial consultant collaboration regarding handling of hospital expenses. Explain all diagnostic procedures and medications. Assess usual coping techniques and teach new ways to cope as necessary. Reinforce wife's assurances that they can manage expenses at home. Encourage relaxation techniques.	Appointment with social worker; taught relaxation exercise and encouraged to practice it; wife says he tends to be a "worry wart"; encouraged him to talk about fears; is afraid of being off work; continue plan.
Pain related to irritation and possible ulceration of gastric mucosa. SUPPORTING DATA Recurrent bouts of epigastric pain more pronounced before meals; blood-tinged vomitus; stressful occupation.	Patient will verbalize relief of pain. Patient will verbalize ways to prevent gastric pain.	Assess location and severity of pain q shift. Administer ordered antacids, antispasmodics, and H$_2$ inhibitors. Give caffeine-free diet. Encourage him to quit smoking. Give frequent feedings to neutralize gastric acid. Provide quiet, relaxed environment.	Pain is epigastric; now occurring between meals; taking meds as ordered; no caffeine drinks; encouraged him to quit smoking; said he would think about it; continue plan.
Alteration in tissue perfusion related to loss of blood from gastric mucosa. SUPPORTING DATA Blood-streaked vomitus; history suggestive of peptic ulcer; increasing fatigue; pale conjunctiva.	No signs of intestinal blood loss by discharge. Hemoglobin and hematocrit will be within normal levels within 30 days.	Monitor CBC count for evidence of continued bleeding. Assess vomitus for blood. Check stool for occult blood as ordered. Monitor vital signs and assess for continued or rapid blood loss as ordered. Teach about foods high in iron content to correct anemia. Administer iron supplements as ordered.	Stool positive for occult blood × 2; taught him about foods high in iron; continue plan.

Mr. Lee's physician found a duodenal ulcer on endoscopic examination. He has prescribed sulcrafate (Carafate), 1 g PO qid 1 h ac and hs, ranitidine (Zantac), 300 mg HS, and Mylanta II, 30 mL 30 min PC, in hopes of healing the ulcer and preventing surgery.

Nursing Diagnosis	Goals/Expected Outcomes	Nursing Intervention	Evaluation
Knowledge deficit related to factors that contribute to peptic ulcer and information about medications. SUPPORTING DATA Was unaware that cigarette smoking contributed to ulcers; never has heard of the medications prescribed for him, except for the antacid.	Patient will verbalize factors that contribute to ulcer formation. Patient will attempt to quit smoking within 2 weeks. Patient will verbalize reason for each medication, dosage schedule, and side effects.	Instruct in contributing factors of ulcer formation. Assist him to learn new ways to cope with stress. Instruct him in food substances to avoid, including caffeine and alcohol. Discuss ways to manage proper eating when on the road. Teach action, dosage, and side effects of each medication. Obtain feedback for material taught.	States that he will quit eating foods that cause pain (i.e., spicy foods); has cut smoking down to ½ pack per day, states he will try to quit; verbalizes side effects of medications and proper dosage schedule; will begin exercise program for stress reduction.

*Can be used as outcome criteria to evaluate patient's progress.

TABLE 20-6 ◆ *Patient Education: Healing a Peptic Ulcer*

The patient must be taught to:

◆ Regulate the types of foods eaten and the schedule for eating. Mealtimes should be unhurried, relaxed, and spaced at regular intervals.

◆ Control stress and develop healthy coping techniques; avoid extremely stressful situations; fit regular relaxation into the lifestyle.

◆ Drink a lot of water. Because water dilutes the gastric juices and thereby makes them less corrosive, the patient should develop the habit of taking several swallows of water at least every hour during the day.

◆ Refrain from smoking. If the patient is unable to discontinue smoking altogether, he should moderate his smoking habits.

◆ Cooperate with the physician and remain under medical supervision for as long as the physician deems advisable. Report regularly for periodic assessment to determine progress.

◆ Report side effects of antacids should they occur, such as constipation or diarrhea, flatulence, and signs of edema resulting from sodium retention.

◆ Check with the pharmacist about possible drug interactions among all the drugs being taken.

◆ Unless otherwise ordered, take antacids 1 hour after meals. If antacid tablets are used in preference to liquid preparations, the tablet must be chewed thoroughly and followed by a full glass of water.

◆ Avoid aspirin and NSAIDs. There are more than 300 prescription and nonprescription medications that contain aspirin. The patient should develop the habit of reading carefully the labels of any medications before taking it. Tell all health care professionals involved in care that aspirin is contraindicated.

probably are caused by the rapid passage of large amounts of food and liquid through the remaining portion of the stomach (if any) and into the jejunum. This occurs because part or all of the stomach and duodenum has been surgically removed and is no longer present to slow down the progress of the intestinal contents through the upper portion of the GI tract. When a patient experiences dumping syndrome, instruction is given to avoid eating large meals and to drink a minimum of fluids during the meal. Fluids may be taken in small amounts later, between meals. If sweet foods and liquids seem to aggravate the condition, and they sometimes do, the patient should try to avoid them. It also may be helpful for the patient to lie down flat in bed for 30 minutes after a meal.

CANCER OF THE COLON

Cancer of the large intestine, also called colorectal cancer, is the third most common malignancy in the United States. The American Cancer Society estimates that 133,500 new cases of colon and rectal cancer will be treated in 1996. Colorectal cancer is the most curable of all cancers if it is found in the early stages and mortality rates have fallen over the last 30 years as detection has become easier.

The disease mainly occurs in persons over the age of 40 and is slightly more prevalent in males than in females. Persons most at risk include those with disorders of the intestinal tract, especially ulcerative colitis and familial polyposis. Other risk factors are lack of dietary fiber and a diet that includes large amounts of animal fat. **Hence preventive measures include a diet that is high in fiber and low in animal fat. Nutrients that offer protection against colon cancer are fiber, calcium carbonate, selenium, and vitamin C.** Recent studies have indicated that NSAIDs such as aspirin may reduce the risk of colorectal cancer. Nursing intervention is directed at public education. Table 20-7 presents prevention guidelines.

Diagnosis   In the early stages symptoms are typically mild and vague and depend on the location of the tumor and the function of the affected area. Weight loss may be the first sign. Later signs of colorectal cancer are the result of obstruction of the bowel and, eventually, extension of the growth to adjacent structures. **Any change in bowel habits, either diarrhea or constipation, could be a sign of colon cancer.**

Other symptoms include red blood in the stool, black, tarry stools, and anemia resulting from intestinal bleeding. Abdominal pain and a sensation of pressure in the lower abdomen or rectum frequently are present. Digital examination may reveal a mass in the anus. Tumors of the rectum or lower sigmoid colon are seen by proctosigmoidoscopy.

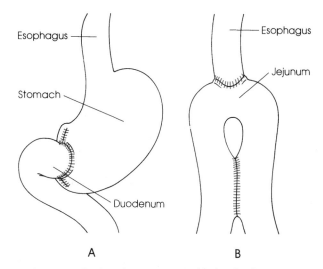

A, One type of subtotal gastrectomy, with the duodenum attached to remaining portion of stomach. B, Total gastrectomy. The jejunum is attached directly to the esophagus; the duodenum is closed.

FIGURE 20-10   Subtotal and total gastrectomy.

TABLE 20-7 ◆ *Patient Education: Prevention and Screening for Colorectal Cancer*

Patients should be taught the following information:

◆ A change in bowel patterns or rectal bleeding should be brought to a doctor's attention immediately.
◆ Everyone over 40 should have a digital rectal examination every year.
◆ A stool blood test should be done every year after age 50.
◆ A proctosigmoidoscopy examination and barium enema should be done every 3 to 5 years starting at age 50, assuming that the first examination is negative. If the examination locates suspected lesions, biopsy and/or surgery is performed.
◆ The nurse should listen closely when doing admission interviews and carefully question patients over the age of 40 about changes in bowel patterns and abdominal discomfort or fullness.

Diagnostic tests include a stool guaiac test, endoscopic examinations and barium x-ray, and an IV pyelogram to detect any displacement of the kidneys, ureters, or bladder. Transrectal ultrasound may be utilized to determine the extent of a small rectal lesion.

Treatment   Treatment of colorectal cancer usually involves surgical removal of the affected portion of the intestine with anastamosis of the remaining portions if the lesion is small and localized (hemicolectomy). Larger tumors are treated by excising the affected portion of the colon providing for elimination of fecal matter via a surgically created opening on the abdomen (**colostomy**). Cancer of the rectum may require an abdominoperineal resection and colostomy. Ostomy surgery and care is presented later in this chapter.

At the Cleveland Clinic Foundation trials are currently under way with laparoscopic bowel resection for colon cancer patients. Since the incisions are so much smaller, recovery time is quicker, and less pain is experienced. Patients are able to return to normal activities in 3 rather than 6 weeks.

Preoperative, intraoperative, or postoperative radiation and chemotherapy may be given for cancer of the rectum. Use of radiation or chemotherapy for colon cancer depends on the stage of the tumor and the presence of metastases. When metastasis is present, the patient is usually treated with 5-fluorouracil. Intraperitoneal chemotherapy may be given through a Tenckhoff catheter or a peritoneal Port-A-Cath. A new drug, irinotecan (Camptosar), is now available to treat recurrent colon cancer. See Chapter 9 for care of the patient with cancer. See Nursing Care Plan 20-2 for postoperative care of the patient who has had abdominal surgery with a colectomy.

INTESTINAL OBSTRUCTION

Intestinal obstruction is a blockage of the intestinal tract that prevents the normal passage of GI contents through the intestines. The condition may occur suddenly or progress gradually.

Causative Factors   Obstruction of the bowel may be mechanical, resulting from blockage of the lumen of the bowel, or *nonmechanical,* resulting from the absence of peristalsis. Mechanical obstructions include tumors, adhesions, strangulated hernia, twisting of the bowel (**volvulus**), telescoping of one part of the bowel into another (**intussusception**), gallstones, barium impaction, and intestinal parasites (Figure 20-11). Abdominal adhesions are a common cause of intestinal obstruction. Adhesions form when inflammation from abdominal trauma or surgery has occurred and fibrous bands of scar tissue hold two segments of bowel together that are normally separated.

Elder Care Point... The elderly are more prone to the occurrence of volvulus and consequent intestinal obstruction, partially because of decreased muscle tone. Suspect this disorder when the patient complains of sudden abdominal pain with vomiting, has abdominal distension with a palpable mass, has increased bowel sounds on auscultation, and exhibits signs of dehydration.

Nonmechanical obstructions may occur as a result of paralytic ileus following abdominal surgery or as a consequence of hypokalemia, or they may be secondary to intestinal thrombus. Infections can occur in some pelvic inflammatory diseases or peritonitis, in uremia, and in heavy-metal poisoning. All of these conditions can interfere with normal peristaltic action and produce a nonmechanical obstruction.

Symptoms   The symptoms of intestinal obstruction vary according to the location of the obstruction. Obstructions occurring high in the intestinal tract are characterized by sharp, brief pains in the upper abdomen that are coordinated with increased bowel sounds in the area of peristaltic contractions above the point of obstruction. Other symptoms include vomiting with rapid dehydration and only slight abdominal distention.

Obstructions of the colon are characterized by a more gradual onset with marked abdominal distention as the bowel fills, infrequent vomiting (which occurs late in the process if at all), and **pains that last several minutes or longer and correspond to peristaltic waves.** Bowel sounds above the point of obstruction are low in pitch.

Nursing Care Plan 20-2

Selected nursing diagnoses, goals/expected outcomes, nursing interventions, and evaluations for a patient undergoing colectomy for colon cancer

Situation: Mrs. Simpson, age 58, just returned from surgery. She had a colectomy because of a malignant lesion in the upper portion of the sigmoid colon. She is very frightened, because her father died with colon cancer. She has a family history of polyposis of the colon. Mrs. Simpson is a loan officer with a national bank, is very busy, and had put off having a physical and sigmoidoscopy until this month, when she noticed some blood in a loose stool. She had had some bouts of loose stools but thought these were a result of the stress she was experiencing on her job.

Nursing Diagnosis	Goals/Expected Outcomes	Nursing Intervention	Evaluation
Pain related to abdominal surgery. SUPPORTING DATA Colectomy; abdominal incision with wound drain.	Pain will be controlled with analgesia. Pain will be controlled by oral medication at discharge. Patient will use relaxation techniques to decrease pain.	Assess for pain q 3 to 4 h and document location and characteristics. Teach relaxation techniques to decrease anxiety and lessen pain. Provide comfort measures to decrease pain.	Requesting pain medication q 2 h; resp., 24; attempted to teach relaxation techniques; plan: seek order for PCA pump or increased dosage of analgesic.
Alteration in nutrition related to NPO status and nasogastric tube. SUPPORTING DATA Will be NPO for 3 to 5 days with an NG tube in place; IV fluid therapy.	Patient will not develop fluid or electrolyte imbalance as evidenced by good skin turgor, moist mucous membranes, and electrolyte studies within normal range. Patient will not develop complications of IV therapy.	Maintain patency of NG tube with irrigations of 30 mL normal saline every 2 h as ordered. Keep tube above level of stomach; loop with tape and pin to gown; maintain on low suction. Assess amount and character of stomach secretions q shift and document. Maintain intake and output record.	IV site without redness or swelling; mucous membranes moist, skin turgor normal; electrolytes within normal limits; NG tube draining well. Meeting goals.
Risk for infection related to colectomy and abdominal incision. SUPPORTING DATA Colectomy with abdominal incision and wound drain.	Patient will not experience wound infection as evidenced by temperature and WBC count within normal range at discharge, wound clean and dry without redness, pain, or purulent drainage.	Auscultate for bowel sounds q shift; assess for abdominal distention. Assess IV site q shift for redness, leaking, pain, and patency; document. Check for adequate urine output before hanging IV solution containing potassium. Assess IV site before administering each antibiotic IV piggyback medication. Maintain IV flow at ordered rate; check q 30 min. Reinforce dressings prn; change q 24 h or prn when ordered. Use strict aseptic technique for dressing changes. Clean skin around incision with hydrogen peroxide or povidone-iodine (Betadine) as ordered. Maintain patency of drain. Monitor temperature and WBCs. Administer prophylactic antibiotics as ordered.	Incision clean with slight serosanguineous drainage; cleaned with Betadine; drain patent; temp., 99.6° F; WBCs, 12,200. Antibiotics administered as ordered; continue plan.
Risk for alteration in tissue perfusion related to possible bleeding at surgical site. SUPPORTING DATA Fresh colectomy.	Patient will maintain adequate tissue perfusion as evidenced by stable vital signs and adequate urine output.	Assess vital signs per postop routine: q ½ h for 2 h; q 1 h for 2 h; q 2 h for 4 h; then q 4 h if stable. Notify physician of tachycardia with increased respirations that is not relieved by pain medication, or blood pressure 15 to 20 points below preoperative baseline level.	Vital signs stable; dressing clean and dry; abdomen soft; urine output >30 mL/h; continue plan.

Box continued on following page

Nursing Care Plan 20-2 (Continued)

Nursing Diagnosis	Goals/Expected Outcomes	Nursing Intervention	Evaluation
		Report urine output that falls below 30 mL/hour for 2 consecutive hours. Assess dressings for bleeding; check underneath patient. Monitor for internal bleeding with each set of vital signs for first 24 h: assess abdomen for increasing girth or rigidity.	
Risk of ineffective breathing pattern related to anesthesia, analgesia, and postoperative pain. SUPPORTING DATA Underwent general anesthesia; requiring morphine q 3 h for pain. Does not wish to cough.	Patient will not develop atelectasis as evidenced by normal breath sounds in all lobes of lungs. Patient will not develop respiratory infection from retained secretions.	Assist patient to turn, cough effectively, and deep breathe (TCDB) at least q 2 h; assist to side of bed for TCDB first postoperative day. Auscultate lungs q shift and document. Encourage use of incentive spirometer if ordered. Monitor temperature; assess characteristics of sputum.	TCDB sitting on side of bed at 8, 10, 12, and 2; bilateral breath sounds clear; using incentive spirometer correctly; no signs of infection; continue plan.
Anxiety related to fear of cancer and treatment and possible death. SUPPORTING DATA Father died of colon cancer; expresses fear of cancer and death; dreads chemotherapy.	Patient will openly discuss fears and concerns with nurse, family, and physician. Patient will verbalize positive outlook on chances for survival by discharge.	Establish trusting relationship with patient by active listening and attentive caring. Encourage "labeling" fears; talk through each one. Provide patient with positive statistics regarding colon cancer treated in early stages. Encourage patient to view cancer as a challenge rather than a defeat. Explain that she has a lot of control over her body and immune system and assist her with relaxation and imagery exercises. Help patient to express positive things about herself.	Withdrawn and quiet; doesn't wish to discuss situation until pathology report is back; sat with patient for 15 minutes; continue plan.

Treatment   Diagnostic x-rays will be ordered to determine where the obstruction is located. Surgery is indicated for obstruction caused by adhesions, volvulus, hernia, or tumor.

The physician may first try to relieve the obstruction by using a Canter tube, which is a long intestinal tube inserted via the nose. It has a mercury bag on the distal end that is carried through the intestine by peristalsis. In some patients this treatment can resolve the problem without the trauma of surgery.

Nursing Intervention   The patient with acute intestinal obstruction is very seriously ill. He often has respiratory difficulty because of the pressure of the distended abdomen against the diaphragm. Placing the patient in Fowler's position helps relieve this pressure and also aids in removing gas and intestinal contents through the intestinal tube. This tube is inserted before the patient goes to surgery and offers some relief of the symptoms of intestinal obstruction until surgery can be performed. If the obstruction cannot be resolved, surgical correction must be done. **Lysis** (breaking apart) of adhesions may be all that is necessary, or a more extensive procedure, such as a partial colectomy or colostomy, may be needed.

ABDOMINAL HERNIA

The internal organs of the body are contained within their respective cavities by the outside walls of the cavity. In the abdomen, the wall is *muscular*. If there is a defect in this muscular wall, the contents of the abdominal cavity may break through the defect. This protrusion is called a **hernia** or simply a *rupture*.

The most common locations for a hernia are in areas where the abdominal wall is normally weaker and more likely to allow a segment of intestine to protrude

(Figure 20-12). These include the center of the abdomen at the site of the umbilicus and the lower abdomen at the points where the inguinal ring and the femoral canal begin. **The most common contributing factors in the development of a hernia are straining to lift heavy objects, chronic cough, straining to void, straining at stool, and ascites.**

Hernias are classified as *reducible*, which means the protruding organ can be returned to its proper place by pressing on the organ, and *irreducible*, which means that the protruding part of the organ is tightly wedged outside the cavity and cannot be pushed back through the opening. Another name for an irreducible hernia is *incarcerated* hernia. If the protruding part of the organ is not replaced and its blood supply is cut off, the hernia is said to be *strangulated*.

Diagnosis   There is a "lump" or local swelling at the site of the hernia. **The most common sites are the umbilicus, groin, or along a healed abdominal incision.** When pressure on the abdominal wall is removed by

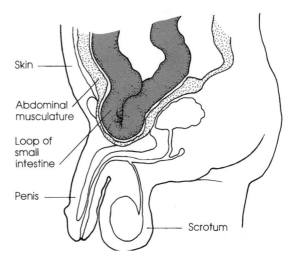

A loop of small intestine passes through the inguinal ring, a weak point in the abdominal musculature.

FIGURE 20-12   Inguinal hernia.

lying down, the swelling disappears. Lifting of heavy objects, coughing, or any activity that puts a strain on the abdominal muscles may force the organ back through the opening, and the swelling reappears. Pain occurs when the peritoneum becomes irritated or when the hernia is incarcerated or strangulated. **The flow of intestinal contents becomes blocked by an incarcerated hernia, and the patient has symptoms of intestinal obstruction.**

IRRITABLE BOWEL DISEASE (IBD)

Irritable bowel disease (IBD) is a group of symptoms that together represent the most common disorder presented by patients who consult gastroenterologists. The three characteristics typical of this disorder are (1) alteration in bowel elimination, either constipation or diarrhea or both; (2) abdominal pain; and (3) the absence of detectable organic disease. Although the pattern of bowel dysfunction varies from case to case, each patient seems to have a unique pattern.

Diagnosis   The cause of IBD is not known. Diagnosis is based on clinical manifestations and ruling out (by barium enema and other tests) the presence of organic bowel disease.

Treatment   Treatment of IBD is inevitably long and, because of the psychological factors involved, often includes such modes of therapy as psychotherapy, biofeedback training, and instruction in relaxation techniques. It is important to reassure the patient that there is no relationship between his disorder and a malignancy of the bowel.

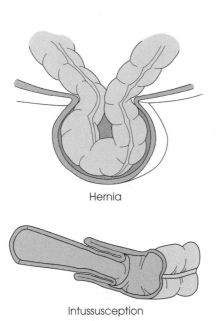

Hernia

Intussusception

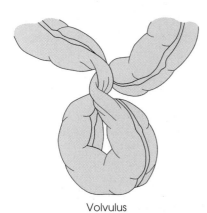

Volvulus

FIGURE 20-11   Intestinal obstructions.

Medications are prescribed according to each patient's need. Drugs that have been used include bulk-forming agents, antidiarrheals, antispasmodics, antidepressants, anticholinergic/sedatives, and mild analgesics to relieve discomfort. A diet high in bran and fiber also may be prescribed. Metamucil or other bulk stool softeners are very beneficial. Gas-forming foods such as the legumes and those in the cabbage family should be avoided. In some patients the intake of milk is restricted if they have shown evidence of intolerance to it. Lactase tablets may be used.

Nursing Intervention The more common nursing diagnoses and interventions for patients with IBD are essentially the same as for any patient with alteration in bowel elimination, either diarrhea or constipation. Instructing the patient about the nature of his disease can help diminish unwarranted fears.

Ineffective coping patterns in response to stress are likely to be present in these patients. Consultation with a psychiatric nursing specialist can help the staff nurse develop more realistic goals and effective nursing interventions to improve the patient's coping skills.

DIVERTICULA

The term **diverticula** refers to small, blind pouches resulting from a protrusion of the mucous membranes of a hollow organ through weakened areas of the organ's muscular wall. Diverticula occur most often in the intestinal tract, especially in the esophagus and colon. They are most prevalent in the older individual. When they are present, the patient is said to have *diverticulosis*. If the diverticula become inflamed or infected, the condition is referred to as *diverticulitis*. Increases in intraabdominal pressure from constipation and straining to defecate are thought to be factors in the development of colon diverticulum.

Diverticulitis occurs when food caught in the diverticulum mixes with bacteria. The intestinal wall becomes irritated and infected, and if it is not treated, perforation and peritonitis may occur.

Symptoms A person may have diverticulosis and remain unaware of his condition for quite a while because it often presents no symptoms. Eventually, however, the diverticula may fill with some material passing through the intestinal tract and become inflamed or infected, causing symptoms. If the diverticulitis is in the esophagus, the patient may have difficulty in swallowing, foul breath, and emesis of food that was eaten several days prior to the vomiting. **Diverticulitis of the intestine produces symptoms of diarrhea or constipation, abdominal pain, fever, and rectal bleeding. The**

TABLE 20-8 ◆ *Nutrition Point: Diet Modifications for Diverticular Disease*

To promote bowel regularity, the following foods should be added to or increased in the diet:

- Apples, (fresh, peeled)
- Bananas
- Bran cereals
- Brown rice
- Carrots (fresh)
- Cornbread
- Dried figs or apricots
- Lettuce
- Oatmeal
- Peaches (fresh)
- Peas
- Seedless grapes
- Whole-wheat bread

Add foods to the diet slowly and in small amounts, increasing as tolerance occurs. Liquids should be increased to ten 8-oz glasses a day. *During periods of inflammation, a low-fiber diet should be followed until the acute phase of the illness has passed.*

To prevent irritation of the bowel and prevent diverticular obstruction, eliminate the following foods from the diet:

Alcohol	Nuts
Apple Skin	Popcorn
Caffeine	Seeds of any type
Celery	Strawberries
Corn	Tomatoes (fresh)
Cucumbers	

Source: adapted from Ignatavicius, D., Bayne, M. (1991). *Medical–Surgical Nursing: A Nursing Process Approach.* Philadelphia: Saunders.

condition may be complicated by intestinal obstruction or by peritonitis if the intestinal wall ruptures.

Treatment Treatment is with parenteral antibiotics, withholding solid food, and hydration with IV fluids as necessary. If the patient experiences recurrent episodes of diverticulitis, or if perforation and peritonitis occur, surgical removal of that part of the colon is performed.

The symptoms of the patient will to some extent govern the treatment necessary. Esophageal diverticulitis, if severe, usually is treated by surgical removal of the sacs and repair of the muscular wall. Intestinal diverticulosis often can be managed conservatively with a high-residue diet and antidiarrheic medications or stool softeners to control constipation. Table 20-8 presents guidelines for diet modifications.

HEMORRHOIDS

Hemorrhoids are varicosities of the veins of the rectum. They may be *internal* (inside the sphincter muscles of the anus) or *external* (outside the sphincter muscles) (Figure 20-13).

Signs and Symptoms Local pain and itching are the most common symptoms of hemorrhoids. Bleeding from the rectum at the time of defecation may also

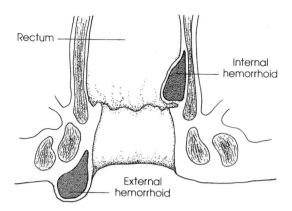

FIGURE 20-13   Internal and external hemorrhoids.

occur. External hemorrhoids are less likely to bleed, but they are more evident to the person examining the patient, because they appear as tumor-like projections around the rectum.

Constipation, prolonged standing or sitting, and pregnancy are predisposing causes of hemorrhoids. The habit of sitting on the toilet and straining at the stool for long periods is one of the primary factors responsible for many cases of hemorrhoids.

Treatment   The symptoms of hemorrhoids may be relieved by correcting constipation, local applications of heat or cold, sitz baths, and the use of ointments that contain a local anesthetic. The patient also should be instructed to wash the anal region with warm water and soap after each bowel movement.

Hemorrhoids can be treated by **scleropathy** (injection of a solution that causes the vessel to dry up and disintegrate), **cryotherapy** (freezing), **photocoagulation** (burning), or hemorrhoidectomy using a laser or standard surgical procedure. Another treatment method is rubber band ligation, in which a rubber band is slipped around the hemorrhoidal vessel, cutting off the blood supply. This causes the hemorrhoid to shrivel and disintegrate. All of these methods are most often done as an outpatient treatment. Hemorrhoidectomy may occasionally be done as an inpatient procedure.

Nursing Intervention   Thorough discharge teaching is done, and written instructions are sent home with the patient. A prescription for analgesics will also be sent home, as these patients experience quite a bit of pain. Cold or warm compresses and warm sitz baths using a rubber or air-filled ring to support the buttocks also help relieve pain. Mild, wet dressings that are commercially prepared also may be used on the surgical site. These dressings have a glycerin base and contain a mild astringent that reduces swelling and relieves pain. The ring may be used while the patient is lying down to remove pressure from the rectal area. Sitz baths are usually ordered twice a day.

Most patients dread the first bowel movement after a hemorrhoidectomy. There is no doubt that it will cause some pain, and the usual procedure is to administer a stool softener to make defecation less traumatic. The patient and family should be warned that the patient may become faint, and someone should stay close by.

A high-fiber diet is started right away, as it is best if formed stool is passed regularly. A sitz bath after each bowel movement will offer relief and also cleanses the affected area, keeping it free from irritation. The patient should continue to make a practice of sitting in a tub of warm water after bowel movements until healing is complete.

MALABSORPTION

Many disorders interfere with the normal absorption of nutrients, water, and vitamins from the intestine. Adult celiac disease (sprue), in which the patient cannot properly metabolize gluten (a protein found in all wheat products, barley, and rye) is one cause. Pancreatic disease with interference in secretion of pancreatic digestive enzymes also causes malabsorption. Some patients who have undergone chemotherapy for treatment of cancer experience alteration of the intestinal mucosa that causes malabsorption. **Whatever the cause, malabsorption creates a nutritional deficiency.**

A key sign of malabsorption is passage of stool that is bulky, frothy, and foul smelling and usually floats in the toilet. Other signs and symptoms include weight loss, weakness, and various signs of vitamin deficiency depending on the type of malabsorption the patient is experiencing.

Treatment is directed at the underlying cause. Pancreatic insufficiency can be treated by administering pancreatic enzymes with meals. Celiac disease is treated by omitting gluten from the diet.

PILONIDAL SINUS (PILONIDAL CYST)

The word *pilonidal* means "having a nest of hair." A pilonidal sinus is a lesion located in the cleft of the buttocks at the sacrococcygeal region. It is sometimes called a *pilonidal cyst,* but it is believed to be a subcutaneous canal (sinus) with one or more openings into the skin (rather than a true cyst or fluid-filled sac). The condition occurs when the stiff hairs in the sacrococcygeal region irritate and eventually penetrate the soft skin in the cleft of the buttocks. Factors that can lead to development of such a sinus include local injury, improper cleaning of the area, and obesity. People who have more than the usual amount of body hair are particularly susceptible.

A pilonidal sinus may cause no trouble until it becomes infected, and then the patient experiences pain in the area, with swelling and a purulent drainage. When this occurs, the area must be incised surgically and the connecting canals opened and drained. Hairs and necrotic tissue must be removed so the area can heal. This is usually done as an outpatient surgical procedure.

Postoperative care includes changing of dressings and measures to avoid contamination of the wound. A stool softener and an oil retention enema usually are given before the first bowel movement to avoid strain on the sutures. Antibiotics may be given to control infection.

ABDOMINAL TRAUMA

Abdominal injuries resulting from improperly worn seat belts, penetrating objects, blunt instruments and sharp cutting edges are all potential sources of hemorrhage and damage to internal organs. **A bluish tinge around the umbilicus may indicate abdominal hemorrhage.** If internal hemorrhage is suspected, the victim should be observed closely for symptoms of shock and handled very gently when being moved.

Peritoneal lavage is performed to diagnose intraabdominal bleeding. A lavage catheter is inserted into the peritoneal space and the contents of the cavity are aspirated with a large syringe. If no blood is aspirated, a liter of warmed saline solution is infused, allowed to remain in place for a time, and then drained by gravity flow from the cavity. The drainage is evaluated for the presence of blood.

External wounds with evisceration are covered with a piece of nonadhering material such as plastic wrap or aluminum foil until the patient can be treated in an emergency facility. This will keep the protruding intestinal contents moist and relatively free of contamination. After the occlusive covering is applied, a clean folded towel or sheet is placed over it to retain body heat in the protruding organs. No attempt should be made to replace the abdominal organs through the wound. The victim is transported to a medical facility as quickly as possible.

COMMON THERAPIES FOR DISORDERS OF THE GASTROINTESTINAL SYSTEM

◆ Gastrointestinal Decompression

Abdominal distention with increased pressure within the abdominal cavity is very uncomfortable. Excess fluids and gases also interfere with ventilation of the lungs and normal function of other nearby organs.

Measures to relieve distention include inserting a rectal tube, suppositories, and enemas to stimulate peristalsis and evacuation of the bowel. If these measures cannot be used or are ineffective, the physician may choose to use GI intubation and remove the intestinal contents by suction. Intubation and decompression also are used as preventive measures following abdominal surgery.

Gastrointestinal tubes vary in length, design, and purpose. The Levin tube and gastric sump tube are shorter because they are intended to reach only as far as the stomach (Figure 20-14). The Miller-Abbott, Cantor, and Harris tubes are longer tubes that are directed past the stomach and into the small intestine (Figure 20-15).

Nursing Intervention   During GI decompression the patient is observed for signs of abdominal distention, which would indicate that excess fluids and gases are not being removed as intended. **Nausea, vomiting, complaints of feeling full or bloated, increasing shortness of breath, and increase in the girth of the abdomen are signs that the stomach and intestines are not being decompressed adequately.**

Applying too much suction can pull the gastric mucosa into the drainage openings, or "eyes," of the tube, causing damage to the mucosa and traumatic ulceration. Using a gastric sump tube (Salem, Ventral) that has an air vent can help prevent this problem. Sump tubes are usually attached to continuous "low" suction; Levin tubes function best with intermittent suction.

Unless ordered otherwise, the low setting is used for suction. The tubing should be kept above the level of the

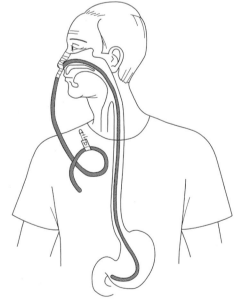

A nasogastric tube is used to aspirate gastric contents or to deliver liquids to the stomach.

FIGURE 20-14   Nasogastric tube in place.

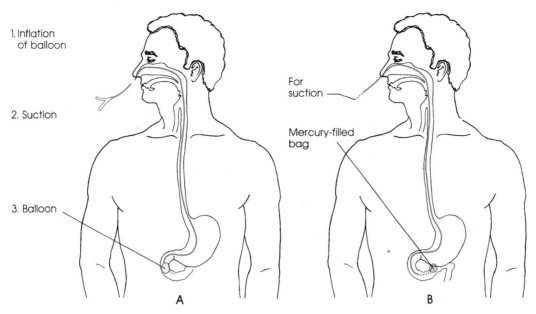

A, Miller-Abbott tube in place. It is advanced through the intestines to the prescribed point. The Miller-Abbott tube has a double lumen. 1, Portion of the metal tip leading to the balloon. 2, Portion of the metal tip leading to the lumen that can be suctioned. 3, Balloon inflated with air. *B*, Cantor tube in place. Intestinal tubes are not taped in place until they have advanced fully.

FIGURE 20-15   Intestinal tubes used for decompression.

stomach. The connecting tubing leading to the suction machine works best if it is kept above the height of entry into the drainage container.

Irrigations with normal saline are usually ordered to keep the tube patent. The amount instilled should be added to the patient's intake count, and the amount of drainage is recorded as output for each shift. If the patient has had surgery on the intestinal tract, the irrigation procedure should be done with aseptic technique rather than clean technique.

The characteristics of the drainage are charted each shift. **If the nurse notices coffee ground–like material in the tube, the drainage should be tested for presence of blood, as blood that has been in contact with gastric juices has this appearance.** If blood unexpectedly appears in the drainage, the physician should be notified. Fluid and electrolyte imbalance problems that can be caused by continuous suction and irrigation are discussed in Chapter 5.

An NG tube is uncomfortable for the patient. The nostril must be checked for signs of pressure, and the tube may need to be repositioned to relieve the problem. Common complaints are sore throat, dry mouth, earache (from congestion of the eustachian tube), and dry lips and nasal mucosa. Frequent mouth care and application of a lubricant to the lips and nostril will help. A room humidifier can also be helpful, but this requires a doctor's order. The physician may allow the patient to have limited amounts of ice chips, hard candy, or chewing gum to decrease the problem.

After the tube is removed, the patient is monitored for further nausea and vomiting and for abdominal distention. Sometimes it is necessary to insert the tube again.

◆ Enteral Nutrition

If a patient has long-term difficulty taking in food orally, as when in a coma, enteral feeding is indicated. Current practice calls for a nasoduodenal tube, frequently the Dobhoff or similar weighted-tip tube (Figure 20-16), to deliver special formula liquid feedings to the GI system. These tubes are inserted by the physician or a registered nurse certified in the procedure. The feedings can be given at specified times throughout the day or on a continuous basis. If continuous tube feedings are ordered, they frequently are administered with a feeding pump. Nursing Procedure 20-1 covers the steps involved in giving intermittent or continuous tube feedings.

The patient requiring long-term nutritional support for problems such as inability to swallow may undergo percutaneous endoscopic gastrostomy (PEG). A feeding gastrostomy tube is placed endoscopically through the abdominal wall. The patient then receives enteral feedings via the gastrostomy tube. The tube is marked with indelible ink at the point of exit so that correct placement can be checked daily. The area is observed for signs of infection and cleansed daily with soap and water until healing is complete. A 4 × 4 gauze dressing is used over

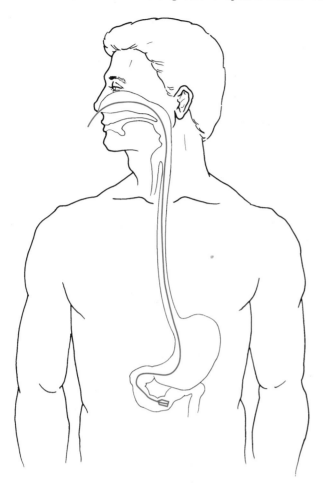

FIGURE 20-16   Placement of Dobhoff-nasoduodenal feeding tube.

physician may choose a direct central line into the vena cava, or he may use the jugular vein. Lipids also may be given via a peripheral vein. Further information about TPN and the principles for administration are found in Chapter 5.

Care of the patient must be a team effort on the part of physicians, pharmacists, dietitians, and nurses. Nursing care includes assisting with the insertion of the IV central line, changing the tubing with each new bag or bottle, changing the dressing, and removing the tubing when TPN therapy is discontinued. Some institutions have specially prepared TPN nurses to give direct care to these patients and supervise that given by general-duty nurses. However, day-to-day care, including monitoring vital signs and fluid and electrolyte balance, daily weighings, frequent mouth care, and dressing changes and observation of the insertion site, is the responsibility of the staff nurse to whom the patient has been assigned.

Sometimes the feeding tube is placed in the jejunum via a jejunostomy. If this is the case, the tube is sutured in place, and the spot where the tube enters the abdominal skin is marked. The mark and suture are checked before beginning a feeding to make certain that the tube has not been dislodged. It is difficult to aspirate anything from a jejunostomy. If the tube has moved or the suture is broken, no feeding should be given. The tube must be replaced by the physician.

SURGERY OF THE LOWER INTESTINAL TRACT

◆ Types of Surgical Procedures

Herniorrhaphy   Hernias are best treated by surgery. If surgery is not possible because of age or poor surgical risk, the patient may be fitted with an appliance called a *truss*. The truss is put on each morning before the patient gets out of bed, because the hernia is more likely to be reduced at that time. A truss simply reinforces the weakened cavity wall and prevents protrusion of the intestines. It is only a symptomatic measure and does not cure the hernia.

The surgical procedure used in the treatment of a hernia is called a *herniorrhaphy,* which means a surgical repair of a hernia. The defect is closed with sutures. If the area of weakness is very large, a *hernioplasty* is done. In this procedure, some type of strong synthetic material is sewn over the defect to reinforce the area. The procedure is now done on an outpatient basis.

Careful discharge instructions are given to the patient to prevent respiratory problems because the patient should not cough in the immediate postoperative period. Guidelines on signs and symptoms of complications are sent home with the patient, along

the outside bumper until healing has taken place. Change the dressing as needed.

When, for any reason, a patient cannot ingest foods and liquids normally, has a problem with malabsorption, or continues to have weight loss and a negative nitrogen balance, *total parenteral nutrition* (TPN) is indicated. Conditions that could warrant TPN include severe trauma to the intestinal tract, as in a gunshot wound, and chronic inflammatory conditions, such as regional ileitis that prevent absorption of nutrients. Other conditions not related to the intestinal tract but nevertheless capable of seriously interfering with normal nutrition over a time include prolonged sepsis, fever, extensive burns, and cancer.

◆ Total Parenteral Nutrition

Total parenteral nutrition is essentially a form of IV feeding. However, because the amounts and kinds of nutrients needed for long-term nutritional maintenance usually cannot be handled as well by peripheral veins, the nutrient mix is given into a larger central vein such as the superior vena cava. To accomplish this the

Nursing Procedure 20-1

Giving an Intermittent or Continuous Tube Feeding Nurses in a variety of settings give tube feedings. Home care nurses instruct in-home caregivers in the procedure. Tube feedings may be a temporary measure, or they may be given for the remainder of the patient's life. Tube feedings are administered via a nasogastric, nasoduodenal, gastrostomy, or jejunostomy tube. The "five rights" are followed before beginning a tube feeding; and *Standard Precautions* are observed. Gloves are used.

Steps	Rationale
General precautions:	
1. Elevate the head of the bed 30–45 degrees.	Elevation allows gravity to help the flow of the formula into the stomach and thus helps prevent reflux. The position should be maintained for at least ½ hour after the feeding. For the very elderly, keep the head of bed elevated for 1 hour as gastric motility is decreased.
2. Put on gloves.	Possible contact with body fluids requires the use of gloves.
3. Pinch off the tube and remove the plug, cap, or clamp.	Pinching the tube prevents fluid leaking from the tube.
4. Attach the syringe and verify tube placement within the stomach or duodenum. (For jejunostomy, check that sutures are intact and that mark on tube is still at entrance site.) For NG tube, aspirate small amount of stomach contents (5–10 mL); if no fluid is obtained, check the tube placement by introducing air through the tube and listening to the left of the xiphoid process with the stethoscope for a "swoosh"; for a small-bore feeding tube, verify that placement has been checked by radiograph; check that mark at nose entrance is still at that place on the tube. Reinstill aspirated fluid.	Obtaining gastric or intestinal contents is the best evidence of proper tube placement. Small-bore tubes frequently will collapse when aspiration is attempted and nothing can be obtained; in the home setting, checking for the "swoosh" of air in the stomach, gently attempting aspiration, and verifying that initial placement was assessed by x-ray are the best that can be done. Stomach or intestinal contents are high in electrolyte content and reinstilling them helps prevent electrolyte imbalance. When more than 150 mL of residual formula are obtained, the physician should be notified because it is an indication that the feeding is not well tolerated.
For intermittent feedings:	
5. If a gavage bag is used, fill it with the prescribed amount of formula and regulate it to run in slowly over 30 minutes. If a syringe is used, pinch off the tube, attach the syringe, and pour the formula into the barrel of the syringe, keeping it no more than 18 inches above the level of entry into the stomach or intestine. Pour down the side of the barrel to force air back out rather than into the tube. Unpinch the tube to start the flow.	The formula should be given over 20 to 30 minutes; gravity pull will draw it in. Flow can be regulated by raising and lowering the receptacle. Intermittent tube feedings should be used for stomach tubes only.
6. Add formula to keep the neck of the receptacle filled. Continue adding formula to the syringe until the prescribed amount is given.	If the formula level falls below the neck of the syringe, air will enter the tubing and the intestinal tract, causing great discomfort as a result of distention.
For continuous tube feeding:	
7. Fill the feeding bag with the prescribed amount of formula, clear the tubing of air, and attach it to an IV pole or feeding pump and set the correct rate.	Feeding can be hung at room temperature for 4 hours within the hospital environment. A feeding pump delivers a controlled flow of formula. Some gavage bags have a pocket in which to place ice; this type of bag can allow the formula to hang somewhat longer, up to 6 hours when ice is present.
8. Verify enteral, gastrostomy, or jejunostomy tube placement.	The jejunostomy tube should be sutured in place. Aspirating usually will not produce fluid from the jejunum; air cannot be easily detected when instilled into the jejunum. If the tube is not in place, the feeding could spill into the abdominal cavity, causing chemical peritonitis.
9. Check the amount of residual from previous feeding for gastrostomy tube by aspirating with a syringe; reinstall the fluid.	Residual should be checked every 4 hours for continuous gastrostomy tube feedings.
10. Attach the tubing from feeding bag to enteral, gastrostomy, or jejunostomy tube using an adaptor as needed. Turn on the pump and check the drip rate; begin feeding.	Drip rate should be checked frequently. Patient tolerance of the feeding should be assessed every hour while the patient is awake. Increasing abdominal distention, nausea, or pain indicate a problem.

Continued on following page.

Nursing Procedure 20-1 *(Continued)*

Steps	Rationale
For both intermittent and continuous tube feeding:	
11. Follow the formula with 1 to 2 oz water to clear the tube. Keep the liquid level about the neck of the syringe or bag to prevent air bubbles from collecting in the system or in the patient's intestinal tract until feeding is finished.	Water helps clear the tubing and prevents clogging.
12. Remove the syringe or connecting tubing, and clamp the tube by inserting the plug covering with a cap protector or with a 2 × 2 gauze secured with a rubber band; a clamp may also be used (for intermittent feedings).	This prevents backflow of the formula or stomach fluid.
13. Wash the bag and tubing or other equipment with soap and water every 8 hours; change the bag and tubing or syringe every 24 hours.	In the home setting, equipment is washed with soap and water every 8 hours but may be used for 3 to 7 days. Equipment is rinsed thoroughly after each feeding in the hospital and in the home.
14. Remove gloves and make a note of the amount given, including water intake.	It is important to tract the nutritional intake of the patient. Official charting should contain type of formula given, amount, verification of tube placement or securing sutures, amount of residual if obtained, and any signs of intolerance of the feeding.

with a written list of activities to avoid until healing is complete.

Colectomy or Hemicolectomy   Colectomy simply is the removal of the diseased portion of the colon. The remaining ends of the colon are reattached. Hemicolectomy is removal of one half of the colon.

Abdominoperineal Resection   Abdominal resection is a very extensive surgical procedure in which part of the colon and the entire rectum, anus, and regional lymph nodes are removed. Both an abdominal and a perineal incision are necessary for this procedure. Because of the nature of the surgery, a permanent colostomy is necessary. Because of the high lithotomy position used during surgery, these patients are at increased risk for phlebitis postoperatively.

Colostomy   In this procedure, an abdominal incision is made, and the colon is brought to the outside to drain fecal material. A colostomy is usually done after a colectomy. The colostomy may be permanent or temporary. If it is a temporary colostomy, the patient must return to surgery later for anastomosis of the open ends.

◆ Types of Ostomies

There are three basic types of ostomy surgery, and the stomas thus created are called (1) *loop ostomy;* (2) *single-barreled* or *end colostomy;* and (3) *double-barreled ostomy.*

Loop Colostomy   As the name implies, a loop of the colon is brought through an abdominal incision and onto the surface of the body. Some kind of bridge is placed under the loop to prevent it from slipping back into the abdominal cavity (Figure 20-17). The loop is formed and secured in place while the patient is in the operating room. About 2 days later, the surgeon will open the colostomy at the patient's bedside. This may be done with an electric cauterizing instrument, a scalpel, or surgical scissors and does not require anesthesia because the bowel has no sensory nerve endings.

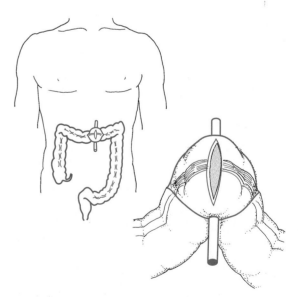

A segment of transverse colon that is brought out through the abdominal wall and supported by a bridge. A slit in the bowel allows feces to drain from proximal colon. Support is removed 5 to 7 days after surgery or when the bowel adheres to the abdominal wall.

FIGURE 20-17   A loop transverse colostomy.

Once the surgeon has made the opening in the wall of the intestine, fecal material passes through the opening (stoma) in the loop of the intestine. An appliance for collection of fecal material should be on hand before the intestine is opened so that it can be attached immediately after the stoma has been created. The pouch that collects feces fits over the stoma made by the slit in the loop of intestine. After about 5 to 7 days, the surgeon may remove the bridge if the stoma has adhered to the abdominal wall.

Double-Barreled Colostomy In a double-barreled colostomy, there are two separate stomas. The loop of intestine is completely severed, creating a *proximal stoma* and a *distal stoma*. The proximal stoma is the one closer to the small intestine, and so fecal material passes through it to the outside. The distal stoma leads to the rectum and should discharge only small amounts of mucus. The distance between the stomas varies; if they are too close together, it is difficult to get a good seal for the collection device around each one. Eventually the colon ends will be reattached.

Single-Barreled or End Colostomy There is only one stoma in a single-barreled colostomy. It is located on the lower left quadrant of the abdomen and is the proximal end of the sigmoid colon, that is, the end nearest the small intestine. The end is brought to the abdominal surface, *effaced* (cuffed over itself), and sutured to the skin, making what is called a *surgically mature stoma*.

If the colostomy is temporary, the remaining portion of bowel and rectum are left intact. If the colostomy is permanent, an abdominal perineal resection (APR) is done to remove the freed bowel, anus, and rectum.

◆ Colostomy Locations

An ascending colostomy is one in which either one end or a loop of a portion of the ascending colon is brought to the surface of the abdomen to form a stoma. The stool from an ascending colostomy is thus watery and unformed.

An ascending colostomy usually is temporary and is done to allow the bowel distal to the ostomy to rest and heal. This is sometimes necessary for the patient with IBD, to reconstruct an intestinal birth defect, or for the patient who has experienced an intestinal tear from trauma. After the rest and healing period, the surgeon will replace and reattach the intestine ends, and fecal material can be defecated normally.

A *transverse colostomy* is situated toward the middle of the abdomen, which is where the transverse colon is located (Figure 20-18A). This kind of colostomy usually also is temporary. The stool from a

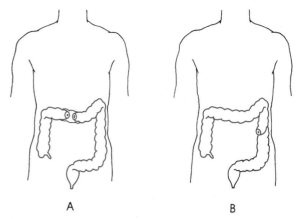

A, Transverse colostomy. Note two stomas. B, Descending colostomy (sigmoid colostomy).

FIGURE 20-18   Locations for colostomy.

transverse colostomy is semi-liquid and is discharged unpredictably.

A *sigmoid (descending) colostomy* is located on the surface of the lower quadrant of the abdomen (Figure 20-18B). It is the most common type of permanent colostomy and usually is done to treat cancer of the rectum. The stool from a sigmoid colostomy is more solid and well formed and may be discharged no more often than once a day or every 2 days. It is therefore much easier to establish a pattern of evacuation to control the flow of fecal material through a sigmoid colostomy.

◆ Ileostomy

An ileostomy is performed to drain fecal material from the ileum. It is indicated when disease, congenital defects, or trauma require bypassing the entire colon. The most common indications for ileostomy are chronic IBD, such as ulcerative colitis and Crohn's disease (regional ileitis), malignancy, and the presence of many polyps in the colon *(multiple polyposis)*. The last disease is hereditary, and the polyps have a high potential for malignancy.

The site for the stoma of an ileostomy must be carefully selected so that it is not near any bony prominences, folds of skin, or scars and is in a place where the patient can see it and care for it (Figure 20-19). The stool from an ileostomy is liquid, and even though digestion is completed by the time the fecal material reaches the stoma, it still contains digestive enzymes that are highly irritating to the skin.

Surgeons may use a newer technique to create an ileostomy. The *pouch ileostomy* or *continent ileostomy* frees the ileostomy patient from the need to wear a collection device. A small segment of the ileum is looped back on itself to form a pouch, and a nipple effect is created. Pressure from the accumulating feces closes the

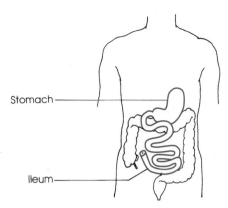

FIGURE 20-19   Location of ileostomy.

nipple valve, preventing constant drainage through the stoma. The patient empties the pouch every 3 to 4 hours during the day by inserting a catheter into the stoma.

Not every patient can be treated by this surgical technique. It has some disadvantages and must be performed by a surgeon skilled in the procedure. Among those who are not good candidates for a continent ileostomy are patients with chronic inflammatory disease that tends to recur. If they develop inflammation within the pouch itself, the pouch must be removed. Another contraindication has to do with the patient's potential for self-care. Because a catheter must be inserted for periodic drainage of the pouch, the patient must be mature enough and sufficiently able to comprehend instructions in self-care and be able to carry them out. The third contraindication is related to previous surgery. Patients who have had a conventional ileostomy cannot have a continent ileostomy done if they have less than 30 mm of terminal ileum remaining. This much is needed to construct the nipple valve.

Although not every patient needing an ileostomy can have a continent ileostomy, it is a safe and effective procedure for many. It eliminates the need for an external appliance, is a more natural way to handle waste, greatly reduces fear of embarrassment from leakage of gas and feces, and minimizes periostomal skin problems.

◆ Preoperative Care

Before surgery of the large intestine, efforts are made to remove as much fecal material from the colon as possible. To accomplish this, the patient is usually placed on a low-residue diet as early as 7 to 10 days before surgery. The last 24 to 72 hours before surgery, the diet is changed to liquids only. Vitamins and minerals may be given to supplement these restricted diets. Antibiotics such as neomycin and sulfasuxidine are given as prophylaxis against infection of the operative site.

In addition to the dietary preparation, laxatives and enemas are administered to cleanse the lower bowel further. The contents of the stomach are removed by inserting an NG tube and connecting it to a suction apparatus the morning of surgery. If it is necessary to remove the contents of the small intestine, a specially designed tube that passes through the stomach and into the duodenum is inserted. This tube is called a Miller-Abbott tube (see Figure 20-15). It is attached to the suction apparatus and given the same care as a gastric tube. The tube is usually left in place after surgery to remove accumulations of mucus and gas that may cause distention and strain on the sutures.

◆ Postoperative Care

The immediate postoperative care for the intestinal surgery patient is the same as for other patients having major abdominal surgery. Standard operations on the large intestine are usually of long duration. A retention catheter is usually inserted into the bladder and attached to a drainage bag while the patient is in the operating room.

> The prolonged period of anesthesia and exposure of the body, with loss of essential fluids, leaves the patient susceptible to shock. Therefore the patient must be watched closely for signs of shock during the immediate postoperative period.

The gastric or intestinal tube is connected to an electrical suction device as soon as the patient is returned to his room. The patient is NPO for the first 48 hours after surgery. Peristalsis usually becomes active after this period of time, the NG tube can be removed, and the patient will then be able to take liquids by mouth.

> The passing of gas, liquids, or solids through the rectum is an indication of active peristalsis.

It is the nurse's responsibility to observe these patients carefully for evidence of the return of peristalsis and to chart it in the nurse's notes.

The postsurgical goals for the patient with a new ostomy include promoting healing, preventing complications, maintaining bowel function, maintaining adequate nutrition, and promoting comfort. The IV site, fluids, and electrolyte levels are monitored very carefully, as the patient is especially prone to fluid and electrolyte imbalances. Pain assessment is ongoing, and the nurse should be certain to reassess the effectiveness of analgesia after administering pain medication.

Think about . . . How does the effluent from a transverse colostomy, a sigmoid colostomy, and an ileostomy differ?

Observation of the Stoma   The stoma is inspected for a normal pink or red color, which indicates adequate blood supply. It should look like healthy mucous membrane such as that inside the mouth. Later, the stoma will shrink in size and may be less highly colored. There may be slight bleeding around the stoma and its stem, but any more bleeding than this should be reported. Most collection devices are transparent so that checking for color and bleeding does not require removal of the appliance. The skin around the stoma is assessed for irritation or signs of breakdown.

> A noticeable lightening or blanching of the stoma may indicate inadequate blood flow through the tissues of the stoma itself. A deepening of color to a purplish hue may indicate blood flow obstruction to the stoma.

The stoma also is observed for signs of edema. However, in the early postoperative period, the stoma will be slightly edematous and larger than after complete healing has taken place. Stoma edema can be caused by a collection device that has an opening too narrow to accommodate the stoma.

> The opening of the collection device should be at least 1/8 inch larger than the circumference of the stoma.

Fecal output from the colostomy stoma does not occur for 2 to 4 days, as the patient has been NPO for surgery. If there is a perineal wound, the appearance, amount, and character of drainage are assessed and charted. Careful inspection for signs of infection is done. Such a wound may be left open to heal by secondary intention, in which case it may be 3 months before it is completely healed. A few days of antibiotic therapy is usually given postoperatively to prevent infection.

Psychosocial assessment postoperatively focuses on the patient's perception of his altered body image, the meaning of the altered body part, his usual and current coping skills, emotional state, support systems, presurgery lifestyle, and his perception of physical prognosis and its impact on his life.

Nursing Intervention   The patient who has undergone surgery for an external ostomy will require the same basic postoperative care as any patient who has had abdominal surgery. The nurse's attitude toward the patient, the stoma, and care has a major impact on the attitude the patient develops about body image changes and self-care. Disposing of body waste is not a pleasant nursing task, but response to the sight and smells can be controlled. A matter-of-fact, efficient approach to caring for the stoma, effluent, and drainage device is best. Nursing Care Plan 20-3 is a sample care plan for a patient with an ostomy.

Elder Care Point... Elderly patients may require assistance with ostomy care because of poor vision or severe arthritis in the hands. In this case a family member or significant other must be taught the techniques of care. The elderly patient needs easy-to-follow, large-print instructions for care. For the elderly patient, the focus of care is on improving the quality of life and ways to remain independent.

A surgical dressing is never placed over an ileal stoma. If there is a significant decrease in ileal output accompanied by stomach cramping, the ileum may be obstructed. Such symptoms should be reported to the surgeon immediately. If the condition is not relieved, perforation or rupture of the intestine eventually may occur.

Measurement of intake and output.   Accurate recording of intake and output is especially important in the care of an ostomy patient. Total output of fecal material is calculated every 8 hours. If the stool is liquid, the accuracy of measurement is very important. When the patient's condition is stable, ostomy output is regular, and the patient's nutrition and hydration status are normal, intake and output recording is discontinued.

> The ileostomy patient must always be watched for signs of dehydration and fluid imbalance.

This is especially important during the immediate postoperative period but remains a concern as long as the patient has the ileostomy. To prevent dehydration, fluid intake should be sufficient to compensate for the loss of fluid through the feces.

Evacuation and irrigation.   Once the patient is eating again, ileostomy drainage is usually emptied every 2 or 3 hours. The pouch should be emptied when it is half full. The patient sits on the toilet, unclamps the drainage device, and allows the effluent to drain into the bowl and the clamp is then closed. The outside of the bag is cleansed of any debris. Ileostomies are not usually irrigated unless there is blockage by large particles of undigested food.

A continent ileostomy has a tube attached to suction in the immediate postoperative period to prevent distention and allow the pouch to heal. In about 2 weeks, the patient is taught to insert a catheter into the pouch to drain the contents. As the pouch matures and its capacity increases, the time between drainings will lengthen. The pouch is irrigated occasionally to remove fecal residue.

A sigmoid colostomy will usually drain formed stool on a relatively regular schedule. Irrigation of the colostomy gives the patient some control over when elimination takes place. The procedure is done daily or every other day at about the same time and takes close

Nursing Care Plan 20-3

Selected nursing diagnoses, goals/expected outcomes, nursing interventions, and evaluations for a patient with an ostomy

Situation: A 22-year-old female patient has a long history of ulcerative colitis that has not responded to conservative therapy. A permanent ileostomy was performed 3 days ago.

Nursing Diagnosis	Goals/Expected Outcomes	Nursing Intervention	Evaluation
Risk for alteration in fluid and electrolyte balance; deficit related to loss of fluid and electrolytes via ileostomy. SUPPORTING DATA New ileostomy; recovering from surgery; beginning solid foods.	Fluid and electrolyte balance will be maintained as evidenced by sodium and potassium levels within normal range and normal skin turgor, stable weight, and balanced intake and output.	Monitor for signs of fluid volume deficit; weigh daily; check electrolyte values. Observe for signs of hypokalemia and hyponatremia. Accurately record intake and output and assess pattern. Instruct patient to avoid foods that may cause diarrhea: whole milk, raw fruits, iced or hot fluids; administer antidiarrheal agents as ordered.	Input, 2,800; output, 2,300; skin turgor normal; electrolytes within normal limits; weight stable; continue plan.
Risk for impaired skin integrity related to irritation of ileostomy drainage. SUPPORTING DATA Ileostomy drainage containing enzymes and bile salts; unfamiliarity with caring for ileostomy stoma and skin.	No evidence of skin irritation or breakdown at discharge. Skin integrity will be maintained.	Inspect skin with each appliance change; document status. Wash skin with mild soap and water; dry very thoroughly; apply skin barrier before applying appliance. Maintain an intact appliance. Treat beginning irritation immediately.	Stoma cherry red and moist; skin intact and without signs of irritation; continue plan.
Anxiety related to self-care of ostomy and impact on lifestyle. SUPPORTING DATA "I'm afraid it will smell," "I'm not sure I can handle this." "How will I work?" "Can I still exercise?"	Anxiety will be decreased by discharge as evidenced by expressed confidence in ability to handle problems of odor, appliance change, application of skin barrier, and work schedule. Within 6 months patient will have adjusted lifestyle and be able to participate in usual activites without problems.	Establish trusting relationship; allow her to verbalize concerns and fears freely. Answer questions honestly. Assist her to identify potential problems and ways to solve them. Encourage learning of self-care; give praise for efforts and accomplishments. Enlist aid of enterostomal therapist for suggestions of how to handle ileostomy during exercise class and at work. Obtain referral to local ostomy support group; have well-adjusted visitor establish contact and answer questions.	Enterostomal therapist in; watched appliance change and asked questions today; ostomate visitor scheduled for tomorrow; continue plan.
Knowledge deficit related to care of ileostomy and self-care. SUPPORTING DATA States she has never seen an ostomy stoma. Doesn't know anything about ostomy care; unaware of diet restrictions and precautions.	Patient will demonstrate ability to empty appliance, clean skin, apply skin barrier, and reattach a clean appliance by discharge. Patient will verbalize ways to prevent odor, protect skin, and prevent problems of fluid and electrolyte imbalance.	Encourage patient to look at stoma; utilize consistent teaching plan for care of stoma, appliance, and skin. Demonstrate care of ileostomy step by step; leave written instructions with patient. Have patient begin by doing one part of care and increasing the tasks each day. Instruct her in dietary precautions, signs and symptoms of fluid and electrolyte imbalance and what to do should they occur. Show various ways to prevent odor; instruct in foods to avoid because they cause offensive odor; have enterostomal therapist work with patient.	First teaching session on ostomy care; able to hold supplies and watch procedure; asked questions; taught dietary restrictions; will obtain feedback in 2 days; continue plan.

Nursing Care Plan 20-3 (Continued)

Nursing Diagnosis	Goals/Expected Outcomes	Nursing Intervention	Evaluation
Self-esteem disturbance related to altered method of elimination. SUPPORTING DATA States she feels that she will not be attractive to any man now that she has an ileostomy.	Will begin acceptance of ileostomy before discharge as evidenced by looking at stoma, applying own appliance, and cleaning equipment. Within 6 months will be comfortable with new body image.	Assist her to list reasons the ileostomy was necessary; list the positive benefits of having the ileostomy versus the way things were before the surgery. Encourage discussion of male–female relationships for ostomates with ostomy group visitor and enterostomal therapist. Assist her to look at positive strengths of the person she still is.	Assisting with ostomy care; will see fellow ostomate tomorrow; continue plan.

to an hour. A catheter with a cone tip is attached to a bag, which is filled with 500 to 1,000 mL of warm (not hot) tap water. The bag is positioned 18 to 20 inches above the height of the stoma. The colostomy appliance is removed and an irrigating sleeve attached to direct the drainage into the toilet. The cone tip is lubricated and inserted gently into the ostomy stoma, and the water is slowly infused to prevent cramping and distention. The cone tip is removed, and the drainage flows through the sleeve into the toilet. When drainage is complete, the sleeve is removed, skin care is performed, and a clean appliance is secured in place. If the patient is fortunate enough to have a regular evacuation pattern, irrigation is not necessary.

The major reason for irrigating a colostomy is to establish a pattern of predictable bowel movements at the convenience of the colostomate.

If the patient prefers not to irrigate, suppositories can be used to stimulate evacuation. The patient does need to wear a drainable pouch if he does not irrigate, as evacuation can be unpredictable.

Periostomal skin care   The area of skin around the stoma must be kept clean and protected from fecal material seeping around the opening of the collection device and pooling on the skin. Drainage from an ileostomy contains enzymes and bile salts that are very damaging to the skin. In the immediate postoperative period, the pouch should not be changed any more than is necessary to avoid trauma to the skin.

The two major principles to follow to protect the skin are cleanliness and the provision of a protective barrier to prevent contact between the skin and the discharge from the stoma. If there is a proper seal to prevent seepage of either feces or urine around the stoma, irritation and breakdown of the skin occur much less frequently.

When the appliance is changed, it should be removed carefully and the skin washed gently with soap and water so that it is not damaged by vigorous rubbing and scrubbing. The area should be rinsed thoroughly and dried by patting, not rubbing, the skin. In humid weather, a hair dryer on the low setting may be used to dry the skin. Possible causes of skin problems are allergic reactions, yeast infections, or irritation from changing the face plate too frequently. A protective skin barrier paste, which serves to prevent contact between the skin and the waste being discharged through the stoma, is applied after cleansing. This may or may not be used for a sigmoid colostomy stoma.

Protective barriers are available in a number of forms and types. The enterostomal therapist or surgeon will indicate which type of barrier is most effective for the individual patient. Should the skin become highly irritated in spite of efforts to protect it, the physician will prescribe topical medications (Figure 20-20).

Gauze packing of a perineal wound is changed regularly. Prophylactic antibiotics are given to prevent infection.

Changing the collection device. There are essentially two kinds of pouches or appliances: the temporary, or disposable, pouch and the permanent, or reusable, pouch. Both types are either drainable or closed-ended. Each is attached to a face plate that is secured to the skin around the stoma with special adhesive. Drainable pouches are used when regulation of the flow of waste cannot be established and the contents must be emptied frequently throughout the day. Closed-end pouches are used only for security once bowel movements have been regulated.

Psychosocial concerns. The ostomy patient will go through the stages of grief and loss (see Chapter 13). The nurse provides active listening, emotional support, and understanding. It is essential that a trusting nurse–patient relationship be established to assist the patient with his psychosocial concerns. Only then will the patient respond to encouragement to share feelings openly.

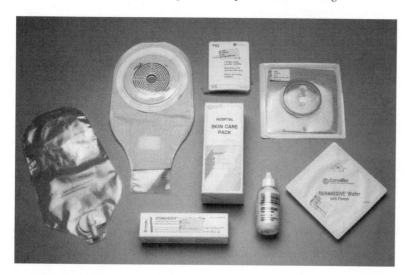

FIGURE 20-20   Pouches and equipment for ostomies. (Photo by Glen Derbyshire; courtesy of Goleta Valley Cottage Hospital, Goleta, CA.)

Social interaction with others is encouraged, and contact with available support groups should be initiated. **As soon as postoperative pain is well controlled, it is best if the ostomate can talk with another who has fully adjusted to his ostomy and is living a full and active life.** A series of visits is best to provide time to formulate and answer questions. Such visits do require an order by the physician.

The ostomate should be treated warmly and acceptingly by the nurse. The patient should be guided to express his specific concerns about physical, sexual, and social problems he might encounter as a result of his ostomy. Most patients have concerns about odor, leakage, and noise from the passing of flatus. The nurse encourages joint exploration of necessary changes in lifestyle and suggests realistic alternatives.

The nurse should indicate to the patient that he might have some concerns about sexual function, thereby cueing him that it is acceptable to talk about this area of his life. Concerns should be addressed matter-of-factly, and his sexual partner should be included in discussions. The enterostomal therapist is a wonderful resource for specific information and suggestions in this area as well.

When the patient continues with dysfunctional grieving too long, becomes clinically depressed, or cannot accept his altered body image, the nurse should seek referral for professional counseling for him. See Nursing Care Plan 20-3 for an example of an individualized care plan for an ostomy patient.

Patient Education. After teaching the patient about the physiology of his ostomy and the steps involved in taking care of the stoma and skin, the nurse teaches the patient how to control odor. Good basic hygiene is essential. Another measure used to control odor is to eliminate from the diet certain foods known to cause problems with odor or gas. Such foods include eggs, fish, garlic, raw onions, sauerkraut, corn, broccoli, cabbage, cauliflower, beans and other legumes, and spicy foods. Eating too quickly and not chewing food well can cause gas. Carbonated beverages also contribute to the problem.

Gas entering the pouch from the stoma will accumulate there until the pouch is opened and the gas released. This can be done by opening the lower end of the pouch and gently pressing against its sides to remove the gas. If not released, the gas may cause enough pressure to make the device separate from the stoma. Newer pouches have a charcoal-filtered valve that allows gas to escape. Reusable pouches are washed with soap and water and rinsed with cool vinegar solution.

Dietary guidelines are taught to prevent problems with diarrhea, constipation, and blockage. Blockage of the ileostomy is fairly common. The major offenders in the case of blockage are foods that absorb water, such as for example, dried fruits, corn (including popcorn), hard nuts, and those foods that are high in fiber. Particles from these foods are not small enough to pass through the ostomy stoma, thereby causing abdominal cramping, vomiting, and decreased flow from the ileostomy. Treatment for this condition consists of oral administration of enzymes to encourage digestion, gentle lavage, and massage of the abdomen to encourage passage of the obstructing food particles. As a last resort, surgical intervention may be necessary. *Laxatives are never given, as they will only add to the problem.* Of course, there is odor when the drainage pouch is changed or emptied, just as there is with normal bowel movements.

Other pointers that ostomates are taught include the following:

◆ Ileostomy patients should not take time-release capsules and enteric-coated tablets, as there is not enough time for adequate absorption before the medication is expelled through the stoma.

◆ Suppositories may be inserted into a colostomy stoma. If it is a double-barreled colostomy, which stoma the suppository is placed into depends on the action of the drug. Glycerin suppositories to stimulate evacuation are inserted in the proximal stoma; a drug that is to be absorbed from the intestine, as for relief of vomiting, should be inserted into the distal stoma, where it will not be expelled. Adequate intake of fluids is important for all ostomates to prevent dehydration and electrolyte imbalance.

Many sources of information are available to the ostomate. These include the local branches of the American Cancer Society, ostomate clubs, enterostomal therapists, and other members of the health care team who have expertise in managing a stoma. Information about local ostomate clubs and groups can be obtained from the United Ostomy Association, Inc., 36 Executive Park, Suite 120, Irvine, CA 92714. A directory of enterostomal therapists to contact for local consultation can be obtained from the Wound Ostomy and Continence Nurses Society (WOCN), 2755 Bristol St., Suite 110, Costa Mesa, CA 92626.

COMMUNITY CARE

Nurses in the community are in a position to do considerable teaching to promote healthy function of the GI system. Promoting a healthy diet with appropriate quantities of fiber and fluid, counseling regarding exercise programs, and teaching about the warning signs of colon cancer are all appropriate nursing interventions to be used whenever possible. Nurses can provide a good example to the public by maintaining weight within normal limits and following a healthy diet and exercise program themselves.

Nurses who work in long-term care facilities and in the home setting must use constant assessment to spot problems of the GI system. Monitoring nutritional and bowel status is standard practice for every patient. It is important to assess on a continuing basis bowel changes that might indicate colon cancer. Remembering that patients who are under care for other disorders still need to have regular cancer screenings and speaking to the patient and physician about this can help detect early colon cancer.

Questioning patients about digestive problems, watching for undue fatigue that could be caused by anemia from intestinal bleeding, and monitoring for signs of peptic ulcer are other ways community nurses can promote health in the GI system.

CRITICAL THINKING EXERCISES

Clinical Case Problems

Read each clinical case problem and discuss the questions with your classmates.

1. Mr. Post, age 42, is admitted to the hospital because he has epigastric pain, is vomiting blood, and has a suspected gastric ulcer.
   a. What tests might be done to establish a diagnosis for Mr. Post?
   b. What kind of information will help Mr. Post avoid difficulty with his diet after he is discharged?
   c. What would Mr. Post need to know to keep his ulcer under control and eventually cure it?

2. Mrs. Blein, age 29, has had frequent bouts of diarrhea associated with physical and emotional stress since her early teens. She is admitted to the hospital with a diagnosis of possible ulcerative colitis. Her admitting physician, a gastroenterologist, feels certain that she has ulcerative colitis and that she will benefit from an ileostomy, as previous efforts on the part of several other physicians have brought no lasting relief from Mrs. Blein's symptoms. She is admitted to the hospital to establish a definitive diagnosis.

   Mrs. Blein is 40 pounds underweight and currently is suffering from severe diarrhea and fluid deficit.
   a. What questions would be relevant when taking Mrs. Blein's nursing history?
   b. What should be included on Mrs. Blein's nursing care plan regarding observations, measurements, and nursing interventions?
   c. Discuss some benefits of an ileostomy over the alternative of continued bouts of severe diarrhea.

3. Mr. Huang, age 52, was found to have occult blood in his stool when he underwent a physical examination for a new insurance policy. Fiberoptic flexible sigmoidoscopy revealed a small lesion in the sigmoid colon; the biopsy result was positive for malignancy. He is scheduled for a hemicolectomy.
   a. What are the probable postoperative nursing diagnoses that should be on Mr. Huang's care plan?
   b. What are the psychosocial concerns that need to be addressed for this patient? What would be appropriate nursing interventions?
   c. What further treatment will be necessary for Mr. Huang?

4. Your home care patient, Ms. Tobin, is under care for congestive heart failure, cardiac dysrhythmias, and arthritis. She has hemiparesis from a stroke.

Her weight has dropped 5 pounds over the past month, and she says she just "isn't hungry" any more.

a. How could her other illnesses affect her appetite?

b. What assessments would you make to try to determine the cause of her anorexia?

BIBLIOGRAPHY

Allison, O. C., Porter, M. E., Briggs. G. C. (1994) . Chronic constipation: assessment and management in the elderly. *Journal of the American Academy of Nurse Practitioners.* 6(7):311–317.

Amara, A., Cerrato, P. L. (1996). Eating disorders—still a threat. *RN.* 59(6):30–34.

American Cancer Society. (1996). *Cancer Facts and Figures—1996.* Atlanta: Author.

Anastasi, J. K., Capili, B. (1997). Cryptosporidium. *Home Healthcare Nurse.* 15(5):307–315.

Applegate, E. J. (1995). *The Anatomy and Physiology Learning System: Textbook.* Philadelphia: Saunders.

Barnie, D. C., Currier, J. (1995). What's that GI tube being used for? *RN.* 58(8):45–48.

Beitz, J. M. (1994). The ileoanal reservoir: an alternative to ileostomy. *Journal of Wound, Ostomy and Continence Nursing.* 21(3):120–125.

Bennett, J. C., Plum, F., (eds.) (1996). *Cecil Textbook of Medicine,* 20th ed. Philadelphia: Saunders.

Black, J. M., Matassarin-Jacobs, E. (1997). *Medical-Surgical Nursing: Clinical Management for Continuity of Care,* Philadelphia: Saunders.

Bockus, S. (1996). When your patient needs tube feeding: Making the right decisions. *C. E. Test Handbook,* Vol. 7. 48–56.

Bosley, C. L. (1995). Applying perianal pouches with confidence. *Nursing. 95.* 25(6):58–61.

Brozenec, S. A. (1996). Ulcer therapy update. *RN.* 59(9): 48–53.

Cole-Arvin, C., Notich, L., Underhill, A. (1994). Identifying and managing dysphagia. *Nursing 94.* 24(1): 48–49.

Copstead, L. C. (1995). *Perspectives on Pathophysiology.* Philadelphia: Saunders.

Costello, M. C. (1996). Home health nutrition. *MEDSURG Nursing.* 5(4):229–237.

Dambro, M. R. (1996). *Griffith's 5 Minute Clinical Consult.* Baltimore: Williams & Wilkins.

Davidhizar, R., Dunn, C. (1996). Malnutrition in the elderly. *Home Healthcare Nurse.* 14(12):948–955.

Davis, J., Sherer, K. (1994). *Applied Nutrition and Diet Therapy for Nurses, 2nd ed.* Philadelphia: Saunders.

deWit, S. C. (1994). *Rambo's Nursing Skills for Clinical Practice, 4th ed.* Philadelphia: Saunders.

Dollar, B. M., Lawson, G. C. (1994). Protocol for nursing assessment and management of stomatitis. *Home Healthcare Nurse.* 12(2):25–27.

Doughty, D. B. (1994). What you need to know about inflammatory bowel disease. *American Journal of Nursing.* 94(7):24–30.

Eckler, J. A. L. (1996). Combating infection: defending against diarrhea: ways to avoid an outbreak. *Nursing 96.* 26(3):22–23.

Eisenberg, P. G. (1994). Gastrostomy and jejunostomy tubes. *RN.* 57(11): 54–60.

Epps, C. K. (1996). The delicate business of ostomy care. *RN.* 59(11):32–37.

Erstad, B. L. (1994). Fluid replacement therapy. *Journal of Practical Nursing.* 44(3):24–33.

Fruto, L. V. (1994). Current concepts: Management of diarrhea in acute care. *Journal of Wound, Ostomy and Continence Nursing.* 21(5):199–205.

Fulton, J. S. (1994). Chemotherapeutic treatment of colorectal cancer: rationale, trends and nursing care. *Journal of Wound, Ostomy and Continence Nursing.* 21(1):12–21.

Gianino, S., Seltzer, R., and Eisenberg, P. (1996). The ABCs of TPN. *RN.* 59(2):42–47.

Goff, K. L. (1997). The nuts and bolts of enteral infusion pumps. *MEDSURG Nursing.* 6(1):9–15.

Gonzales-Cortes, S. B., and Procuniar, C. E. (1994). Home study program. Laparoscopic inguinal herniorrhaphy. *AORN Journal.* 60(3):417, 419, 421–426, 429–430, 432, 434–436.

Guyton, A. C., Hall, J. E. (1996). *Textbook of Medical Physiology,* 9th ed. Philadelphia: Saunders.

Hammerhofer-Jereb, K. (1996). Laparoscopic bowel resection? *RN.* 59(3):22–25.

Handerhan, B. (1994). Investigating peritoneal irritation. *American Journal of Nursing.* 94(4):71–73.

Heslin, J. M. (1997). Peptic ulcer disease. *Nursing 97.* 27(1):34–39.

Huber, D., Hemstrom, M. (1994). GI nursing: the community health aspect. *Gastroenterology Nursing.* 16(5):219–223.

Huston, C. J. (1996). Ruptured esophageal varices. *American Journal of Nursing.* 96(4):43.

Ideno, K. T. (1996). Enteral nutrition formulas: An overview. *Medsurg Nursing.* 5(4):264–268.

Ignatavicius, D. D., Workman, M. L., Mishler, M. A. (1995). *Medical–Surgical Nursing: A Nursing Process Approach,* 2nd ed. Philadelphia: Saunders.

Jones, S. A., Guenter, P. (1997). Automatic flush feeding pumps. *Nursing 97.* 27(2):56–58.

Keithley, J. K., Keller, A., Vazquez, M. G. (1996). *MEDSURG Nursing.* Promoting good nutrition: Using the food guide pyramid in clinical practice. *MEDSURG Nursing.* 5(6):397–403.

Killen, J. M. (1996). Understanding dysphagia: interventions for care. *MEDSURG Nursing.* 5(2):99–105.

Kinsey, G. C. (1995). Combating infection: Preventing contamination during enteral feedings. *Nursing 95.* 25(3):20.

Kirton, C. A. (1997). Assessing bowel sounds. *Nursing 97.* 27(3):64.

Krzywda, E. A. (1996). Administering TPN safely. *Nursing 96.* 26(9):61–62.

Lord, L. M., Lipp, J. Stull, S. (1996). Adult tube feeding formulas. *MEDSURG Nursing.* 5(6):407–418.

Masoorli, S. (1997). Central lines: Controversies in care. *Nursing 97.* 27(3):72.

Matteson, M. A., McConnell, E. S. (1996). *Gerontological Nursing: Concepts and Practice,* 2nd ed. Philadelphia: Saunders.

McConnell, E. A. (1994). Clinical do's and don'ts: managing a nasoenteric-decompression tube. *Nursing 94.* 24(3):18.

McConnell, E. A. (1995). Clinical do's and don'ts: testing stool for occult blood. *Nursing 95.* 25(6):26.

McConnell, E. A. (1994). Loosening the grip of intestinal obstructions. *Nursing 94.* 24(3):34–41.

McConnell, E. A. (1996). Maintaining a feeding tube exit site. *Nursing 96.* 26(12):61.

McConnell, E. A. (1995). Myths & facts . . . about hemorrhoids. *Nursing 95.* 25(4):17.

Mehler, E. L. (1994). Colorectal cancer: early detection is your priority. *American Journal of Nursing.* 94(8):16A–B, 16D, 16F.

Meissner, J. E. (1994). Caring for patients with ulcerative colitis. *Nursing 94.* 24(7):54–55.

Nursing 94. (1994). Caring for a gastrostomy: guidelines and trouble shooting tips. *Nursing 94.* 24(8):48–50.

Peterson, K. J., Solie, C. J. (1994). Caring for the patient with intestinal obstruction. *American Journal of Nursing.* 94(10):48A–48B.

Phaneuf, C. (1996). Screening elders for nutritional deficits. *American Journal of Nursing.* 96(3):58–60.

Price, A. L., Rubio, P. A. (1994). Laparoscopic colorectal surgery: a challenge for ET nurses. *Journal of Wound, Ostomy and Continence Nursing.* 21(5):179–182.

Quayle, B. K. (1994). Making positive choices: body image and the new ostomy patient. *Ostomy Wound Management.* 40(4):16–18, 20–21.

Rieger, P. T. (1994). Biotherapy for colon cancer: promise or progress? *Journal of Wound, Ostomy and Continence Nursing.* 21(3):111–119.

Rush, C. (1995). Gastrointestinal bleeding. *Nursing 95.* 25(8):33.

Sauderlin, G. (1994). Celiac disease: a review. *Gastroenterology Nursing.* 17(3):100–105.

Seaman, S. (1996). Basic ostomy management: assessment and pouching. *Home Healthcare Nurse.* 14(5): 335–343.

Spiro, C. M., Grant, E. G., Gilley, M. T. (1994). Home study program. Diverticular disease: surgical options, patient management. *AORN Journal.* 59(3):623, 625, 627–629, 632–637, 639–640.

Thompson, L. (1995). Taking a closer look at percutaneous endoscopic gastrostomy. *Nursing 95.* 25(4):62–63.

Town, J. (1997). Bringing acute abdomen into focus. *Nursing 97.* 27(5):52–57.

Viall, C. D. (1996). Location, location, location: When your patient has an NG tube what's the most important thing? *Nursing 96.* 26(9):43–45.

Viall, C. (1995). Taking the mystery out of TPN (part one). *Nursing 95.* 25(4):34–41.

Viall, C. (1995). Taking the mystery out of TPN (part two). *Nursing 95.* 25(5):57–59.

Warmkessel, J. H. (1997). Caring for a patient with colon cancer. *Nursing 97.* 27(4):34–39.

Weant, C. A. (1995). Easing the pain of esophageal surgery. *RN.* 95(8):26–30.

Wells, J. A., Doughty, D. B. (1994). Pouching principles and products. *Ostomy Wound Management.* 40(6):50–52, 54–58, 60–63.

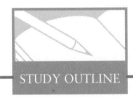

STUDY OUTLINE

I. Introduction

A. The role of intestinal tract and accessory organs is the intake, absorption, and assimilation of food to provide nourishment for the body.

B. Enzymes, acid, and mucus help break down food into nutrients.

C. Absorption is the transfer of nutrients from the intestine into the blood.

D. Peristalsis, wave-like action of smooth muscle, moves substances along the intestinal tract.

E. Metabolism is the sum of all physical and chemical processes concerned with the disposition of nutrients.

F. Pathological conditions of the digestive tract and accessory organs of digestion affect metabolism, the health of the organism, and repair and healing of injury and illness.

II. Causes of Gastrointestinal Disorders

A. Inflammation and infection.

B. Chemical and physical trauma.

C. Structural defects such as congenital defects.

D. Infectious agents.

E. Genetic predisposition.

F. Stress and emotions.

G. Autoimmune disease.

III. **Prevention of Gastrointestinal Problems**

  A. Eating a normal, well-balanced diet aids digestion.

  B. Consuming sufficient fiber prevents constipation and helps prevent diverticulosis.

  C. Drinking at least eight glasses of fluid a day prevents constipation.

  D. Heeding the need to defecate helps prevent constipation.

  E. Maintaining body weight within normal limits helps prevent the formation of a hiatal hernia and helps limit esophageal reflux.

  F. Avoiding foods and spices that cause GI discomfort helps prevent inflammation.

  G. Preventing infection from contaminated food and drink, washing the hands, and thoroughly cleaning utensils and food-preparation areas are important.

  H. Proper food storage and food handling help prevent food poisoning.

  I. Cautious use of aspirin and nonsteroidal anti-inflammatory drugs (NSAIDs) helps prevent ulcer formation.

IV. **Diagnostic Tests and Procedures and Nursing Implications**

  A. Radiological examinations: upper- and lower-GI series (barium swallow and barium enema) (Table 20-1).

  B. Endoscopic examination of the interior of the esophagus (esophagoscopy), stomach (gastroscopy), and small intestine (esophagogastroduodenoscopy).

    1. Patient is usually kept NPO, explained procedure, and mildly sedated.

    2. If local anesthetic used, food and liquids are withheld after procedure until reflexes return.

    3. Patient is watched for signs of perforation, bleeding.

  C. Proctoscopy, sigmoidoscopy, and colonoscopy: examination of interior of rectum and colon.

  D. Gastric analysis to determine level of HCl in stomach contents.

  E. Tubeless gastric analysis to find out whether there is any HCl in stomach.

  F. Stool examination for infectious organisms, blood, cysts, ova, and parasites.

V. **Nursing Management**

  A. Assessment.

    1. History taking (Table 20-2).

    2. Physical assessment (Table 20-3).

      a. Inspection.

      b. Auscultation.

      c. Palpation.

      d. Percussion.

  B. Nursing diagnosis.

    1. Pain.

    2. Fluid volume deficit.

    3. Alteration in nutrition.

    4. Diarrhea.

    5. Constipation.

    6. Bowel incontinence.

    7. Ineffective individual coping.

    8. Knowledge deficit.

    9. Additional pertinent secondary nursing diagnoses.

  C. Planning.

    1. Goals.

      a. Control of nausea and vomiting.

      b. Control of diarrhea.

      c. Control of abdominal pain.

      d. Promotion of normal, continent, bowel movements.

      e. Promotion of adequate nutrition status.

      f. Assimilation of knowledge for self-care.

      g. Prevention of GI bleeding.

      h. Control or elimination of GI cancer.

    2. Specific expected outcomes are written to the needs of individual patients.

  D. Implementation.

    1. Monitor every patient for bowel movements.

    2. See nursing care plans and Table 20-4 for specific interventions.

  E. Evaluation.

    1. Reassess to determine effectiveness of actions.

    2. Determine whether expected outcomes are being met.

VI. **Common Problems Related to the GI Tract**

  A. Anorexia: absence of appetite.

    1. Assessment to identify cause, if possible.

      a. Physical causes: poorly fitting dentures, stomatitis, decaying teeth, halitosis.

      b. Psychological factors: unattractive or unfamiliar foods, unpleasant surroundings, company, emotional state.

    2. Nursing interventions.

      a. Mouth care.

      b. Cater to patient's preference whenever possible.

      c. Plan meals with variety of foods.

      d. Feed patient slowly and as nurse would eat the meal.

      e. Provide companionship.

f. Allow foods from home to supplement meals.

B. Eating disorders: see VII, Problems Related to Ingestion.

C. Nausea and vomiting interfere with nutrition (see Chapter 5).

D. Accumulation of gas.
1. Gas accumulation causes distention and discomfort.
2. Walking a lot helps dispel gas.
3. Abdominal massage may help evacuate gas.
4. Trendelenburg position, when permitted, is effective.
5. Avoid hot or iced drinks and drinking through straws.
6. Antigas medications, such as Phazyme, Milicon, or Di-Gel, may help.
7. A rectal suppository or a rectal tube may assist with the passage of gas.

E. Constipation.
1. Stool is hard, dry, and difficult to pass.
2. Diet and fluid consumption affect consistency of stool.
3. Physical inactivity contributes to constipation.
4. Ignoring the gastrocolic reflex and delaying defecation contributes to constipation.
5. Increase fiber and fluid in the diet.
6. Observe for impaction.
7. Use of laxatives, suppositories, or enemas may be necessary initially.
8. Adding raw fruits and vegetables to the diet is important.

F. Diarrhea.
1. Frequent passage of liquid or semi-liquid stool.
2. May accompany inflammation of the bowel.
3. Antidiarrheal agents used to slow the number of stools.
4. Nothing by mouth or only clear liquids allows bowel to rest.
5. Replacing normal flora in the bowel with acidophilus is helpful.
6. Monitor intake and output; observe for signs of dehydration.
7. Replace fluids as necessary.
8. *Standard Precautions* plus contact precautions are necessary when diarrhea is of infectious origin.
9. Protect the anal mucosa from excoriation with proper cleansing and barrier ointment or cream.
10. Keep the patient clean and dry.

G. Bowel incontinence.
1. Illness, trauma, neurological damage, or prolonged bedrest may contribute to bowel incontinence.
2. Patient must be kept clean and dry.
3. Toileting after each meal may help.
4. Bowel training program should be instituted.
5. Bowel training takes a great deal of time and patience.

H. Gastrointestinal bleeding.
1. Common causes: gastric and duodenal ulcer, esophageal varices, gastritis, tumors, and polyps in lower-GI tract, ulcerative colitis, diverticula.
2. Nursing assessment.
   a. Obtain history to identify patients likely to have GI bleeding: history of anemia, weakness, reported change in color of stools or in pattern of elimination, nausea, chronic indigestion or heartburn.
   b. Subjective data: feeling faint, nausea and vomiting of old or new blood, restlessness, thirst, confusion.
   c. Objective data: maroon or bright red blood in emesis or stools; black stools; change in vital signs, central venous pressure readings; hematocrit and hemoglobin levels; white cell count.
3. Medical and nursing intervention.
   a. Replacement of blood by transfusion of whole blood, packed cells, or fresh frozen plasma; normal saline, Plasmanate, or Ringer's lactate if blood not available.
   b. Gastric bleeding may be treated with saline lavage.
   c. Antacids and H_2-receptor antagonists are given to decrease acid secretion.
   d. Measure and record intake and output.
   e. Oxygen often is administered.
   f. After condition is stabilized, diagnostic procedures to locate source of bleeding.
   g. Surgery when indicated.
   h. Injections of vasopressin directly into bleeding artery for esophageal varices; by subcutaneous injections of octreotide; insertion of Sengstaken-Blackmore tube to apply pressure and cold; injection of embolus; endoscopic scleropathy.
   i. Reassurance of patient to allay fears and anxiety; continuous monitoring for signs of continued bleeding, hypovolemic shock; daily weighings; measure intake and output, note characteristics of body fluids excreted or aspirated.

VII. **Problems Related to Ingestion**

  A. Eating Disorders.

    1. Anorexia nervosa: preoccupation with food coupled with fear of being fat; patient often exercises excessively.

    2. Bulimia: binging and induced vomiting; use of laxatives.

    3. Obesity: more than 20% over ideal body weight.

    4. Treatment for eating disorders focuses on behavior modification and psychological counseling along with appropriate diet.

  B. Dysphagia: difficult swallowing. Most common symptom of disorders of the esophagus.

    1. Nursing intervention.

      a. Observe patient for foods he cannot tolerate and conditions under which he experiences difficulty.

      b. Instruct patient to chew food thoroughly, eat semi-solid foods, drink liquids throughout meal (if liquids do not cause choking), assume more erect posture when eating.

      c. Sit upright with head forward and neck flexed to swallow.

      d. Provide pleasant surroundings and relaxed atmosphere.

      e. Tube feeding may be necessary for severe dysphagia.

      f. Inability to swallow might require gastrostomy feeding.

  C. Hiatal hernia: esophagus passes through defect in diaphragm.

    1. Signs and symptoms: indigestion; substernal pain, especially after eating.

    2. Treatment: elevation of head of bed, antacids, H_2-receptor antagonists, cispride (Propulsid), weight loss; surgery occasionally necessary.

    3. Avoid smoking, alcohol, chocolate, and fatty food.

VIII. **Inflammatory Disorders of the Intestinal Tract**

  A. Stomatitis: inflammation of the oral mucosa.

    1. Causes: ill-fitting dentures or malocclusions of the teeth, poor oral hygiene; excessive smoking or drinking; physical trauma, nutritional deficiencies, radiation, and drugs.

    2. Assessment: pain and swelling of oral mucosa, bleeding gums, alteration in salivation, halitosis, small, crater-like ulcers.

    3. Intervention: frequent mouth care (see Chapter 9), correction of nutritional deficiency, avoidance of irritants.

  B. Gastritis: inflammation of gastric mucosa.

    1. Causes: overeating, alcohol abuse, or ingestion of contaminated food, poison, aspirin, or NSAIDs.

    2. Assessment: nausea, vomiting, heartburn, diarrhea.

    3. Medical treatment and nursing intervention: restriction of foods that cause pain, antacid medications, antispasmodics, H_2-receptor antagonists, antibiotics as needed for *H. pylori* bacterium.

  C. Ulcerative colitis: inflammation with ulceration of intestinal mucosa.

    1. Similar in symptoms to regional ileitis (Crohn's disease). Tendency is to include both under name of *inflammatory bowel disease (IBD)*. Major difference is that ulcerative colitis is more likely to develop into intestinal malignancy.

    2. Cause unknown. Immunological response and emotions play some role.

    3. Medical diagnosis based on medical history and presenting symptoms.

      a. Chief symptoms are attacks of bloody, mucoid diarrhea and cramping pain, usually precipitated by physical or emotional stress.

      b. Endoscopic and x-ray examination helps confirm diagnosis.

    4. Nursing assessment.

      a. Nursing diagnoses common to inflammatory bowel disease include potential or actual fluid volume deficit, diarrhea, sleep pattern disturbance, pain, ineffective individual coping, potential for impairment of skin integrity in anal region.

      b. Long-term problems include anxiety, disturbance in self-concept, and fear of malignancy.

    5. Medical treatment and nursing intervention.

      a. Conservative approach: antidiarrheals, long-term sulfasalazine, or 5-ASA therapy; analgesics; corticosteroids, low-residue, bland, high-protein, high-calorie diet.

      b. Surgical intervention: colectomy, colostomy, ileostomy.

      c. Nursing interventions include monitoring bowel elimination and bowel sounds, measuring intake and output and daily weight, watching for signs of intestinal bleeding, and encouraging stress-reduction techniques.

      d. Long-term goals related to patient education and psychological support.

D. Appendicitis: inflammation of vermiform appendix.

1. Assessment: pain in lower-right quadrant, elevated fever with white cell count, nausea, and vomiting.

2. Treatment: appendectomy.

3. Prior to surgery, patient should not be given laxative or have heat applied to abdomen.

E. Peritonitis: inflammation of peritoneum.

1. Common causes: ruptured appendix, perforated ulcer, ruptured ectopic pregnancy, infection of peritoneum, any condition in which contents of intestinal tract spill into the peritoneal cavity.

2. Assessment: vomiting, severe abdominal pain, fever, tachycardia, symptoms of shock, paralytic ileus.

3. Treatment: massive doses of antibiotics, IV fluid and electrolytes, intestinal decompression.

4. Nursing intervention: monitor vital signs, observe for signs of intestinal obstruction, check bowel sounds and other evidence of return of peristalsis, place patient in semi-Fowler's position.

IX. **Peptic Ulcer**

A. Loss of gastric mucosal tissue, ulceration involves loss of muscular coat. Incidence has decreased in recent decades.

B. Causative factors: the presence of too much acid in relation to degree of protection; presence of *H. pylori* bacterium.

1. Duodenal ulcers usually characterized by hyperacidity, gastric ulcers by normal or low level of HCl.

2. Genetic predisposition: relatives of persons with peptic ulcers have three times expected rate for development of ulcers.

3. Tension, anxiety, prolonged physical or emotional stress.

4. Diet not thought to be a cause, but ulceration is more prevalent in the undernourished.

5. Drugs: unbuffered aspirin, NSAIDs, alcohol, glucocorticoids.

6. Excessive smoking.

C. Diagnostic tests and procedures.

1. Barium swallow.

2. Esophagogastroduodenoscopy (endoscopy).

3. Gastric analysis.

4. Tests for the presence of *H. pylori.*

D. Nursing assessment.

1. Family history of peptic ulcer.

2. Patient's eating habits.

3. History of smoking and extent of alcohol use.

4. History of injuries or other stresses that could cause stress ulcer.

5. Subjective data: epigastric pain and pattern of discomfort in relation to presence of food in stomach, pattern of recurrence of pain; nausea, loss of appetite, weight loss; spontaneous vomiting.

E. Complications: GI hemorrhage, perforation, obstruction.

F. Medical management and nursing intervention.

1. Relief of symptoms: antacids and mild sedatives; H_2-receptor antagonists, and sulcrafate (Carafate) relieve pain, reduce the need for antacids, promote healing.

2. Diet: when patient eats is more important than what he eats. Patient instructed to avoid those foods he knows to cause symptoms, to restrict alcohol and caffeine, and to avoid skipping meals.

3. Patient education: see Table 20-6.

X. **Surgical Treatment of a Peptic Ulcer**

A. Surgery is indicated when medical treatment fails to heal the ulcer, when complications such as perforation, obstruction, or hemorrhage occur, or when malignancy is present.

B. Surgical procedures.

1. Pyloroplasty.

2. Total gastrectomy and subtotal gastrectomy: antrectomy; Billroth I or Billroth II.

3. Vagotomy.

C. Preoperative care: routine with exception of intubation and decompression.

D. Postoperative care: after decompression is discontinued, patient is given small amounts of liquid by mouth, and diet is gradually increased. "Dumping syndrome" may occur after gastrectomy.

XI. **Cancer of the Colon**

A. Relatively common; occurs mainly in persons over 40.

B. Persons most at risk are those with other disorders of the digestive tract, especially ulcerative colitis and familial polyposis. Diet low in fiber and high in refined carbohydrate and red meat is a contributing factor.

C. Symptoms and medical diagnosis.

1. In early stages mild symptoms. Later symptoms result in intestinal obstruction and spread to adjacent structures; may have alternating diarrhea and constipation; weight loss; diameter of stool may change.

2. Diagnostic tests include proctosigmoidoscopy, colonoscopy, barium studies, and stool guaiac.

D. Surgical treatment: colectomy and colostomy.

XII. Intestinal Obstruction

A. Causes: strangulated hernia, twisting or telescoping of the bowel, or interference with conduction of nerve impulses.

B. Symptoms vary according to the site of obstruction.

1. High obstruction characterized by sharp pain, vomiting, slight abdominal distention.

2. Low-bowel obstruction symptoms include marked distention, longer-lasting pain.

C. Treatment: intestinal decompression and surgical correction of obstruction.

XIII. Abdominal Hernia

A. An abdominal hernia is a protrusion of the intestines through a weakened area in the abdominal wall.

B. Most common sites are umbilical area and beginning of inguinal canal and femoral canal.

C. Reducible hernia: protruding organ can be replaced by pressing on the organ.

D. Incarcerated hernia: cannot be reduced.

E. Strangulated hernia: blood supply to organ has been obstructed.

F. Surgery most effective means for treating hernia (herniorrhaphy); often an outpatient procedure.

XIV. Irritable Bowel Disease (IBD)

A. Characterized by alteration in bowel elimination: constipation or diarrhea, abdominal pain, and absence of detectable organic disease.

B. Cause is not known. Diagnosis established after ruling out organic bowel disease.

C. Medical treatment and nursing intervention.

1. Therapy long-term and focused on psychological factors as well as medications to relieve discomfort and reduce spasms.

2. Nursing intervention essentially the same as for patients with diarrhea and constipation from other causes. In addition, patient will need help learning effective coping skills.

XV. Diverticula

A. Small, blind pouches of mucous membrane that have protruded through a weakened wall of a hollow organ.

B. Symptoms not apparent until inflammation (diverticulitis) or infection occurs.

1. Esophageal diverticulitis may produce foul breath, emesis, and difficulty in swallowing.

2. Intestinal diverticulitis produces abdominal pain, fever, diarrhea or constipation, and rectal bleeding.

C. Treatment for diverticulitis may be surgical removal of affected portion of organ or liquid diet, antibiotics, and bulk stool softeners.

D. Treatment for diverticulosis: high-fiber diet, increased fluids, bulk stool softeners.

XVI. Hemorrhoids

A. Hemorrhoids are varicose veins of the rectum.

B. Symptoms: local pain, itching, and bleeding at time of defecation.

C. Treatment by hemorrhoidectomy.

D. Postoperative care concerned with prevention of infection and relief of pain.

XVII. Malabsorption

A. Malabsorption interferes with nutritional status.

B. Has many causes: adult celiac disease, pancreatic disease, effects of chemotherapy.

C. Treatment: correct underlying cause, give pancreatic enzymes.

XVIII. Pilonidal Sinus (cyst)

A. Subcutaneous canal located in the cleft of the buttocks in the sacrococcygeal area.

B. Produces pain and purulent drainage.

C. Treatment: surgical incision of canal, drainage of purulent material, and removal of hairs and necrotic tissue; antibiotics given to control infection; often an outpatient surgical procedure.

XIX. Common Therapies for Disorders of the Gastrointestinal System

A. Gastrointestinal decompression.

1. Gastrointestinal intubation using short tube to stomach or longer tube to reach small intestine. Tube is attached to an electric suction apparatus.

2. Nursing assessment and intervention.

a. Monitor for nausea, vomiting, complaint of feeling full or bloated, increasing shortness of breath, and increase in girth of abdomen, signs that decompression is not taking place.

b. Hazards of decompression with electric suction: damage to gastric or intestinal mucosa, excessive removal of electrolytes, acid–base imbalance; **low setting is used for suction unless "high" is a written order.**

c. Tubes must be kept open and draining freely. Irrigation to remove clots or mucus plugs done by order.

d. Record amount, characteristics of drainage. Some bloody drainage may be expected following gastric surgery.

e. Frequent mouth care, lubrication of nares where tube is inserted, ice if allowed by surgeon, chewing gum, anesthetic spray and lozenges.

f. After tube is removed, observe for signs of distention, absence of peristalsis.

B. Enteral nutrition.

1. Nasoduodenal tube such as the Dobhoff to deliver special formula liquid feeding.

2. May be continuous or intermittent feeding.

3. Feeding pump may be used or may be given by gravity system.

4. See Nursing Procedure 20-1 for intermittent or continuous feeding.

5. Percutaneous endoscopic gastrostomy with insertion of a gastric feeding tube is performed for long-term therapy.

C. Parenteral nutrition.

1. Instituted for long-term and severe nutritional deficit.

2. A form of IV feeding. Must be a coordinated effort on part of all health team members.

a. Staff nurses responsible for monitoring vital signs and fluid and electrolyte balance and other routine interventions, changing dressings, and observing insertion site.

b. Weight is monitored closely; blood sugar is monitored closely during initiation of therapy.

c. TPN is covered more fully in Chapter 5.

D. Surgery of the lower intestinal tract.

1. Types of surgical procedures.

a. Herniorrhaphy: surgical repair of a hernia.

b. Colectomy (removal of the diseased portion of colon).

c. Abdominoperineal resection: removal of the affected portion of colon, the entire rectum, the anus, and regional lymph nodes; usually done for cancer.

d. Colostomy (creation of an artificial anus with bowel opening on the abdominal surface).

E. Types of ostomies.

1. Loop colostomy: loop of intestine is brought to the outside of the abdomen through an incision.

a. Bridge support is used to keep loop from sliding back through the incision.

b. Surgeon slits the intestine to create a stoma.

2. Double-barreled colostomy: the proximal stoma is closest to the small intestine; the distal stoma leads to the rectum.

3. Single-barrel or end colostomy: only one stoma on the surface of the body.

F. Colostomy location depends on whether stoma is from ascending, transverse, or sigmoid (descending) colon.

G. Ileostomy: stoma from the ileum, completely bypasses the colon.

1. Indications: ulcerative colitis, Crohn's disease (regional ileitis), and multiple polyposis.

2. Site for stoma must be carefully selected.

3. Continent or "pouch" ileostomy frees patient from need to wear external pouch; some patients are not good candidates for this procedure.

H. Preoperative care: low-residue diet, cleansing of the lower bowel, and intestinal decompression.

I. Postoperative care: observation for signs of shock, care of retention catheter, care of GI tube, and observation of drainage (watch for signs of returning peristalsis).

1. Assessment.

a. Goals include the following.

(1) Promote healing.

(2) Prevent complications.

(3) Maintain bowel function.

(4) Maintain adequate nutrition.

(5) Promote comfort.

b. Observation of the stoma.

(1) Color should be similar to that of mucous membrane inside the mouth.

(2) Will eventually become smaller as it heals.

(3) Check for excessive bleeding.

(4) Watch for increase or decrease in output from stoma.

(5) Prolapse is not necessarily an emergency.

(6) Stenosis is treated by progressive dilatation or surgery.

(7) Edema is usually caused by too narrow an opening on the collection device.

c. Accurate intake and output; monitor for dehydration and electrolyte imbalance.

d. Perineal wound, if present, is assessed.

e. Psychosocial assessment focuses on patient's perception of altered body image and self-esteem.

f. There are many possible appropriate nursing diagnoses for the patient with an ostomy.

2. Nursing intervention.

a. Postoperative care is essentially the same as for any abdominal surgery patient.

b. Nurse's attitude strongly influences patient's acceptance of stoma.

c. Measurement of intake and output is especially important for ostomy patient.

   (1) Includes flow of urine as well as feces.

   (2) Obstruction can be very dangerous.

   (3) Ileostomy patient must always guard against fluid and electrolyte imbalance.

d. Evacuation and irrigation.

   (1) Ileostomy drainage is emptied every 2 to 3 hours.

   (2) Continent ileostomy is allowed time to heal.

   (3) Sigmoid colostomy drains formed stool on a fairly regular schedule.

   (4) Irrigation of the colostomy allows control over elimination.

   (5) Irrigation is done with bag of 500 to 1,000 mL warm tap water, and a cone-tipped catheter.

   (6) Suppositories can be used to stimulate evacuation instead of irrigation.

   (7) Urine drainage is immediate when urinary diversion procedures are performed.

   (8) Continent urinary conduit is catheterized to drain the urine.

e. Periostomal skin care: cleanliness is very important.

   (1) Cleanse skin and use protective barrier.

   (2) Remove appliance gently.

   (3) Possible causes of skin problems are changing the faceplate too frequently, allergic reaction, yeast infections.

f. Changing the collection device.

   (1) Change face plate only as often as necessary.

   (2) Measure stoma to be sure opening is correct size.

   (3) There are disposable and nondisposable types of collection devices.

   (4) Reusable devices must be cleansed thoroughly and dried.

   (5) Pouches are designed so that drainage can be removed without disturbing the faceplate.

g. Perineal wound care.

   (1) Gauze packing is changed regularly.

   (2) Prophylactic antibiotics are given to prevent infection.

h. Psychosocial concerns.

   (1) Patient will go through stages of grief and loss.

   (2) Contact with ostomy support group is desirable.

   (3) Encourage verbalization of questions and concerns.

   (4) Enterostomal therapist is an excellent resource.

   (5) Encourage self-care by slowly increasing participation in care of stoma and collection device.

   (6) If clinical depression occurs, refer for counseling.

i. Patient teaching.

   (1) Physiology and care of ostomy.

   (2) Odor and gas control.

   (3) Dietary guidelines.

   (4) Helpful suggestions for ostomates.

   (5) Sources of information and support.

XX. Elder Care Points

A. After age 70, secretion of gastric HCl and pancreatic lipase decreases.

B. Peptic ulcer presents with atypical symptoms.

C. Anemia and vitamin deficiencies are common as a result of poor eating habits in many elderly.

D. Simplify steps in care of ostomy and provide easy-to-read printed instructions.

E. Focus on improving quality of life and ways to remain independent.

XXI. Community Care

A. Teach all patients about healthy diet and increasing fiber and fluids to promote healthy bowel function.

B. Promote regular exercise program.

C. Teach ways to decrease risk of colon cancer, warning signs, and recommended screening.

D. Assess for signs of GI problems in home care and long-term care patients diligently; elderly may not present with typical signs.

CHAPTER 21

Care of Patients with Gallbladder, Liver, and Pancreas Disorders

OBJECTIVES

Upon completing this chapter the student should be able to:

1. Discuss ways the nurse can be instrumental in preventing disorders of the gallbladder, liver, and pancreas.
2. Specify the nursing interventions for pre- and posttest care of patients undergoing tests of the liver, gallbladder, and pancreas.
3. Describe the assessment factors and care of the patient with cholecystitis and cholelithiasis.
4. Discuss the teaching necessary for the patient undergoing cholecystectomy.
5. State the care needed for the patient who is having a liver biopsy.
6. Specify the assessment factors to be considered for the patient with possible liver disease.
7. Create a nursing care plan, including psychosocial concerns, for the patient who has hepatitis and is jaundiced.
8. List the ways in which the various types of hepatitis can be transmitted.
9. Devise appropriate nursing interventions for the patient with cirrhosis.
10. Make a discharge teaching plan for the patient who has been in the hospital with a flareup of chronic pancreatitis.

The gallbladder, liver, and pancreas are considered the accessory organs of the digestive system. They lie outside the gastrointestinal tract but are directly concerned with digestion. Although the gallbladder can be removed without harm to the individual, the liver is essential to life. If the pancreas is removed or nonfunctional, the patient must take many enzymes plus insulin for life. To understand the disorders of the accessory organs, the structure and location of the organs as well as their functions must be clear.

OVERVIEW OF ANATOMY AND PHYSIOLOGY

What Are the Structure and Location of the Accessory Organs?

⅄ The *gallbladder* is a small sac attached to the lower portion of the liver.

⅄ The *liver* is a large reddish-brown organ located in the upper right quadrant of the abdominal cavity under the diaphragm and is protected by the rib cage.

⅄ The portal vein transports venous blood and nutrients absorbed from the small intestine to the liver.

⅄ The *pancreas* is an elongated, flat organ that sits behind the stomach and consists of a "head" and a "tail" (Figure 21-1).

⅄ The gallbladder connects to the common bile duct that leads from the liver to the duodenum.

⅄ The pancreatic duct extends the length of the pancreas, connects with the common bile duct, conducting its secretions into the duodenum.

What Are the Functions of the Gallbladder, Liver, and Pancreas?

⅄ The gallbladder stores bile produced in the liver and delivers it as needed to the small intestine; it can store up to 50 mL of bile.

⅄ The liver manufactures and secretes bile and bile salts necessary to digest fat.

⅄ The liver synthesizes albumin, fibrinogen, globulins, and clotting factors.

⅄ The liver is a storage area for glucose in the form of glycogen, vitamins A, D, E, K, and B_{12}, and iron.

⅄ The liver detoxifies and breaks down many compounds and drugs, preparing them for excretion; it alters ammonia, a by-product of protein metabolism, so that it does not harm the body.

⅄ The liver helps break down and excrete hormones, drugs, cholesterol, and hemoglobin from worn-out red blood cells.

⅄ The liver plays a major role in glucose metabolism, removing excess glucose from the blood, converting it to glycogen, and then, as glucose is needed, converting glycogen back to glucose.

⅄ The liver plays key roles in lipid metabolism, breaking down fatty acids, synthesizing cholesterol and phospholipids, and in converting excess carbohydrates and proteins into fats.

⅄ The liver is instrumental in protein metabolism, converting certain amino acids into different ones as needed for protein synthesis.

⅄ The liver is a large filter containing phagocytic Kupffer cells that remove bacteria, damaged red blood cells, and other toxic materials from the blood.

⅄ The liver may store between 200 and 400 mL of blood.

⅄ The liver synthesizes the prothrombin needed for normal blood clotting.

⅄ The pancreas islets of Langerhans secrete the hormones insulin and glucagon into the blood; insulin is essential to the metabolism of carbohydrates.

⅄ The pancreatic acinar cells secrete digestive enzymes into ducts that connect with the pancreatic duct.

⅄ The major pancreatic enzymes are amylase, trypsin, and lipase; these enzymes are essential to the digestion and absorption of nutrients from the small intestine.

⅄ Secretion of pancreatic enzymes is controlled by secretin and cholecystokinin, two substances secreted by the intestinal mucosa.

How Does Aging Affect the Accessory Organs of Digestion?

⅄ Gallbladder function becomes more sluggish in the older person, and consequently gallstones increase in incidence.

⅄ Secretion of lipase from the pancreas decreases, altering fat digestion, and may contribute to a depressed nutritional state in the elderly.

DIAGNOSTIC TESTS

Sonography, x-rays, laboratory tests, CT scans, nuclear medicine scans, magnetic resonance imaging (MRI), and biopsy are used to diagnose problems of the gallbladder, liver, and pancreas. The nurse is responsible for teaching the patient about each of these tests. Patient allergies are always checked to make certain that a particular contrast medium or injectable marker is not contraindicated. Psychological care of the patient should not be overlooked. What seems to be a routine test to the nurse can have very different meaning to the patient. It is best to assess what fears the patient might have before beginning teaching about the test. The purpose, description, and nursing implications for the tests of the gallbladder, liver, and pancreas are listed in Table 21-1.

Think about . . . What would you need to teach a patient who is scheduled to have an endoscopic retrograde cholangiopancreatography (ERCP)?

CAUSES AND PREVENTION OF DISORDERS OF THE ACCESSORY ORGANS

The formation of stones within the gallbladder can cause irritation and areas susceptible to inflammation and infection from organisms in the bloodstream. They

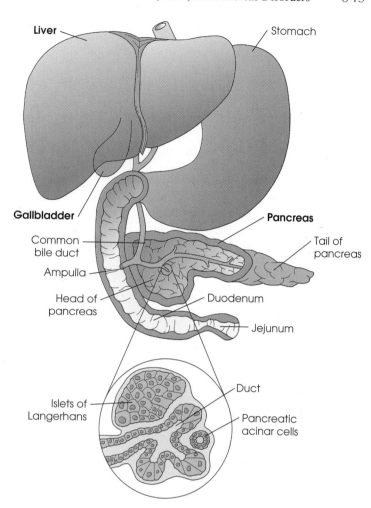

FIGURE 21-1   Accessory organs of the digestive system.

can lodge in the common duct, causing obstruction to the flow of bile. Scientists do not know why gallstones form in some persons and not in others. It is known, however, that when bile is saturated with cholesterol, a precipitate settles out and the nucleus of a stone is formed. The stone grows as layers of cholesterol, calcium, or pigment accumulate over the nucleus.

Persons at risk for developing gallstones are those who have hemolytic disease, have had extensive resection of the bowel to treat Crohn's disease, are obese, or have diabetes mellitus. Multiple pregnancies and use of oral contraceptives increase the chance for gallstone formation. Rapid weight loss sometimes predisposes to gallstone problems.

The liver filters out many toxic substances and is constantly exposed to any infectious organisms circulating in the bloodstream. Many parasites migrate to the liver and can cause problems when cysts or abscesses develop. The hepatitis virus in particular attacks the liver, causing inflammation and damage to the tissue.

Many drugs are toxic to the liver, and the nurse should always be aware of the drugs a patient is taking that may cause liver damage. Acetaminophen, isoniazid

(INH), phenytoin (Dilantin), methyldopa, oxacillin, allopurinol, and amiodarone are just a few common drugs that can be responsible for liver problems. **Exposure to the chemicals carbon tetrachloride or to vinyl chloride can cause liver disorders.** The pancreas is subject to inflammation from various drugs as well.

Cancer can affect any of the accessory organs, but is more prevalent in the liver and pancreas than in the gallbladder. Cancer in these organs may be primary, or may be secondary to metastasis from a site elsewhere in the intestinal tract.

Trauma to the liver is not uncommon because of automobile accidents. Liver lacerations may cause massive internal hemorrhage. However, the liver is a resilient organ and, if repair is performed quickly and part of the liver is functional, it will regenerate.

Alcohol and other toxic substances are major factors in the development of cirrhosis of the liver. Parasites also may cause cirrhosis, but this is not a usual cause of the disorder in the North American continent.

Avoiding contact with parasites can prevent the problems that they can cause. Most parasites that damage the liver enter the body when people wade or swim in contaminated water in tropical countries.

TABLE 21-1 ◆ *Diagnostic Tests for Gallbladder, Liver, and Pancreas Problems*

Test Purpose	Description	Nursing Implications
Ultrasonography Obtains images of soft tissue that indicate density changes. Commonly used for the liver, biliary system, gallbladder, pancreas, and spleen.	Sonograms are produced with high-frequency sound waves that pass through the body. Echoes vary with tissue density. Used to diagnose gallstones, tumor, cysts, abscess, etc.	Patient NPO after midnight. Explain procedure: will be supine on table, lubricant will be applied to the skin surface, and a handheld metal probe is passed back and forth with light pressure. It takes about 30 minutes. Patient needs to remain still.
X-ray studies Cholecystography/Cholangiography Locates obstructions and structural defects in the gallbladder and biliary ducts.	Radiopaque contrast medium is given orally or IV. Serial x-rays are taken at intervals to visualize the gallbladder and the biliary and common ducts. For the cholecystogram, the patient may be asked to drink a substance that contains fat after the first series to cause the gallbladder to contract; more x-rays are then taken to see whether the gallbladder functions properly.	For oral cholecystogram, administer the required tablets at 8 P.M. the evening prior to the test. A low-fat dinner is best, and no fats are to be eaten for breakfast. Requirements vary per x-ray department and contrast medium used. There should be no barium in the intestinal tract.
Computed tomography Visualizes soft tissue and density changes when sonography is inconclusive.	X-rays are combined with computer techniques to provide a series of sectional pictures of the gallbladder.	Patient NPO for 3 to 4 hours. May require a consent form. Assess for allergy to iodine or shellfish. Explain to patient that she will be in a supine position on a special narrow table with her body in the circular opening of the scanner. She will have a strap over her waist to secure her to the table. Clicking noises will be heard from the scanner. The test takes about 1½ hours. A contrast agent, which causes a transitory warm feeling, may be given IV to enhance images. She will be asked to hold her breath at certain points in the test. The machine uses narrow x-ray beams.
Endoscopic retrograde cholangiopancreatography (ERCP) Performed when common radiological studies do not reveal the cause of the problem. Used to identify obstruction and other pathological conditions in the biliary and common ducts.	An endoscope is passed through the mouth into the duodenum with the use of fluoroscopy. A cannula is positioned in the common bile duct, and a contrast medium is injected. X-rays are then taken.	Obtain a signed consent for procedure. Patient NPO after midnight. Explain the procedure to the patient (same as for esophagogastroendoscopy). A pretest sedative may be ordered. Posttest care is same as for esophagogastroendoscopy. (See Chapter 20).
Liver biopsy Removal of a tissue sample for microscopic exam and diagnosis of various liver disorders.	Under local or general anesthesia, a biopsy needle is inserted into the desired area of the liver, and a tissue sample is aspirated.	Explain the procedure to the patient and obtain signed consent. She will have to remain very still during biopsy if local anesthetic is used. She will feel pain similar to a punch in the shoulder, lasting only a minute or so. Keep patient NPO for 4 to 6 hours prior to biopsy. Assess for allergy to local anesthetics. Have patient empty bladder right before procedure. Take baseline vital signs. Check coagulation studies for abnormalities that contraindicate procedure. Following test, position patient on right side with support to provide pressure over biopsy site. Observe for bleeding: monitor vital signs q 15 min for 1 h; then q 30 min for 4 hr; then q 4 h for 24 h; assess for tenderness at biopsy site. Observe for respiratory problems indicative of pneumothorax.

TABLE 21-1 ◆ *Diagnostic Tests for Gallbladder, Liver, and Pancreas Problems* (Continued)

Test Purpose	Description	Nursing Implications
Liver-spleen scan		
Determines size, shape, and location of abnormal tissue in the liver.	A radioactive isotope is given by IV infusion. The liver is scanned for areas of concentrated radioactivity.	Explain the procedure to the patient. An IV catheter will be inserted for administration of the radioisotope. The small amount of radioactivity is not harmful to the patient or others. Patient needs to hold very still while the scanner is crossing back and forth over his body. The machine makes a soft clicking noise.
Laboratory tests for liver disorders		
Serum bilirubin	Elevated in all types of jaundice; aids in determining cause.	Total: 0.1–1.2 mg/dL Conjugated: up to 0.3 mg/dL Unconjugated: 0.1–1 mg/dL
Alanine aminotransferase (ALT; formerly SGPT)	Elevated 30 to 50 times normal in toxic hepatitis; 20 times normal in infectious mononucleosis.	1–21 U/L
Aspartate aminotransferase (AST; formerly SGOT)	Elevated within 8 to 12 hours of damage to parenchymal cells; aids in determining degree of problem.	7–27 U/L
Alkaline phosphatase (ALP)	Elevated with metastatic lesions, abscess, cirrhosis, active liver cell damage.	13–39 U/L
Plasma ammonia	Elevated in presence of severe liver damage, as it cannot be detoxified.	12–55 µmol/L
Prothrombin time (PT) Partial thromboplastin time (PTT)	Elevated with liver dysfunction that interferes with production of coagulation factors that are vitamin K—dependent. Prolonged PT is associated with abnormal bleeding.	PT: 25–38 sec PTT: 11–12.5 sec INR 2.0–3.0
Protein Albumin	Total protein and albumin are decreased in liver failure, as albumin-rich fluid seeps into the peritoneal cavity. Altered protein metabolism also lowers these values.	6.8–8.0 g/dL 3.5–5.0 g/dL
Laboratory tests for pancreatic disorders		
Serum amylase	Elevated with acute pancreatitis	4–25 U/mL
Serum lipase	Elevated with acute pancreatitis	2 U/mL or less
Urine amylase	Elevated with acute pancreatitis	24–76 U/mL

Practicing good hygiene and avoiding contact with substances that transmit the hepatitis virus are preventive measures. Obtaining immunization against hepatitis A and hepatitis B prevents these diseases. A vaccine against hepatitis C is under study at present. Using *Standard Precautions* when handling body fluids, particularly blood, greatly reduces the risk of infection with hepatitis B and C. Refraining from eating raw oysters and shellfish from contaminated waters may prevent infection with hepatitis A.

Refraining from consuming excessive amounts of alcohol cuts down the risk of developing cirrhosis of the liver and inflammation of the pancreas (**pancreatitis**). Avoiding exposure to known toxic or carcinogenic chemicals helps prevent liver damage and liver cancer.

NURSING MANAGEMENT

◆ Assessment

Assessment for problems of the accessory organs of the digestive system begins during history taking. Questions regarding family history, diet, dietary intolerances, presence of pain, and problems with blood clotting are asked. Immunization status is verified. Because of the many functions of the liver, assessment of the patient with liver disease must include all systems of the body. A comprehensive history of illnesses and exposure to toxic agents, both chemical and infectious, is part of a thorough evaluation. Some major areas for history taking include:

- Exposure to toxins; (1) inhalation of agents toxic to the liver (for example, cleaning agents containing carbon tetrachloride or anesthetics, such as halothane); (2) ingestion of alcohol, (how much and how often?); and (3) drugs: what medications is the patient taking? How long has patient been on each medication? Does the patient use recreational (illegal) drugs?
- Exposure to infectious organisms: contact with person who has hepatitis; ingestion of contaminated shellfish; blood transfusions.
- Trauma: accidental injury or surgery of the liver, pancreas, or spleen.

Physical assessment includes general techniques for assessing the abdomen (See Chapter 20). Laboratory values for blood glucose, serum amylase, cholesterol, lipids, prothrombin, bilirubin, and the complete blood count (CBC) are checked. The urine is evaluated for presence of bilirubin, which makes the urine dark or the brown color of tea. The stool is assessed for presence of fat and urobilinogen. If undigested fat is present, the stool will float in the toilet bowl. If bile is not reaching the intestine, the stool appears clay-colored or whitish.

◆ Nursing Diagnosis

Nursing care focuses on problems of discomfort, nausea and vomiting, appropriate diet, maintenance of fluid and electrolyte balance, and adequate nutrition. Nursing diagnoses often chosen for patients with gallbladder, liver, or pancreatic problems are:

- Pain related to inflammation and contraction of the gallbladder or to inflammation of the pancreas.
- Fluid volume deficit from persistent vomiting and inability to eat.
- Noncompliance with a low-fat or low-protein diet.
- Fluid volume excess related to ascites.
- Risk for alteration in tissue perfusion related to danger of hemorrhage from esophageal varices and decreased clotting factors.
- Risk for infection related to decreased resistance.
- Alteration in nutrition, less than body requirements, related (1) to nausea, vomiting, anorexia, and inability of liver to metabolize nutrients or (2) to lack of enzymes to digest fat.
- Diarrhea related to decreased tolerance to fatty acids because of diminished bile production.
- Altered thought processes related to increased levels of circulating ammonia.
- Risk for impairment of skin integrity related to edema and itching from increased levels of ammonia.
- Self-care deficit related to fatigue, ascites, and nausea.
- Risk for impaired gas exchange from pressure of ascites on the diaphragm.

◆ Planning

General goals for patients with gallbladder, liver, and pancreas disorders are:

- Organ will return to normal function (obstruction or inflammation will be relieved).
- Further damage to the organ will be prevented.
- Pain will be alleviated and/or eliminated.
- Digestion and absorption will return to normal.
- Patient's physiological safety will be maintained during period of malfunction of organ (prevention of complications).

Expected outcomes are written for individual nursing diagnoses pertinent to the patient's problems. Goals are aimed at regaining or maintaining normal gallbladder, liver, and pancreas function. Maintenance of adequate nutritional status is a major goal. *Standard Precautions* must be followed whenever a patient has hepatitis. Diapered or incontinent patients are treated with Contact Precautions also.

◆ Implementation

Nursing interventions to control and eliminate pain, maintain fluid and electrolyte balance, promote adequate nutrition and rest and healing, and prevent complications are instituted. Specific nursing interventions are discussed with the various disorders, in the Nursing Care Plan for the cirrhosis patient, and are shown in Table 21-2.

◆ Evaluation

Reassessment is performed to determine the effectiveness of the nursing interventions and medical treatment. Data are gathered to determine whether the expected outcomes are being met. Laboratory values are analyzed to see whether problems are resolving with treatment. Urine and stool are observed to see whether the blockage of bile from the liver and gallbladder has resolved. If so, the urine and stool will be of normal color again.

DISORDERS OF THE GALLBLADDER

◆ Cholelithiasis

Cholelithiasis is the presence of gallstones within the gallbladder itself or in the biliary tract. The stones may

TABLE 21-2 ◆ *Common Nursing Diagnoses, Expected Outcomes, and Nursing Interventions for Patients with Disorders of the Gallbladder, Liver, and Pancreas*

Nursing Diagnosis	Expected Outcomes	Nursing Interventions
Fluid volume deficit, related to nausea and vomiting.	Vomiting will be controlled within 24 hours. Fluid volume will be restored within 24 hours as evidenced by moist mucous membranes and good skin turgor.	Administer antiemetics as ordered. Monitor IV infusion site and fluid rate. Encourage clear oral fluids as tolerated. Monitor electrolyte levels for imbalances. Provide mouth care q 2 h while awake.
Alteration in nutrition, less than body requirements, related to anorexia, nausea, and vomiting.	Patient will ingest a 1,200-calorie diet per day within 7 days after subsidence of acute vomiting. No further weight loss will occur.	Initiate IV fluids as ordered if dehydration occurs. Keep door of room closed to keep odors out. Offer mouth care before meal time Provide six small meals a day plus small, high-calorie snacks between meals. Weigh q 3 days and record. Keep hard candy at bedside for snacking.
Pain or discomfort, related to jaundice and bile pigments in skin, causing itching.	As verbalized by patient, pain or itching will be minimized by nursing measures.	Assist patient to bathe with tepid water three times a day. Apply lotion q 2 h. Provide activities to keep mind off of itching. Teach patient relaxation exercises.
Knowledge deficit, related to ways in which hepatitis B is transmitted, impact of hepatitis on the body, self-care measures, and measures to prevent transmission to others.	Before discharge, patient will verbalize ways hepatitis B is transmitted, impact on body, self-care measures, and measures to prevent transmission to others.	Teach ways in which hepatitis B is transmitted: parenteral routes, sexual contact. Give explanation in understandable terms of what hepatits B does to the body. Reinforce teaching regarding self-care measures: hygiene, diet, rest, follow-up. Teach importance of not sharing personal articles, especially razor, toothbrush, etc., with others. Instruct to inform health care workers of the presence of the virus until tests for it are negative. Inform that sexual partner(s) will need injection of special immune globulin for protection.
Body image disturbance, related to yellow skin color from jaundice.	Patient will accept present body image by allowing visitors within 3 days.	Assure patient that jaundice is not permanent. Allow to ventilate feelings about the illness and present appearance. Encourage verbalization of positive aspects about self. Increase fluid intake to help flush bilirubin from blood during recovery.
Pain related to irritation of gallstones or pancreatic inflammation.	Pain will be controlled within 8 hours	Medicate with analgesic as ordered. Instruct in use of patient-controlled analgesia (PCA) pump if ordered. Encourage relaxation techniques to decrease discomfort. Assess q 4 h for adequate pain relief.

vary in size, from very small "gravel" to stones as large as a golf ball. It is usually the smaller ones that cause the most trouble, because they pass into the bile ducts, where they become lodged and obstruct bile flow (Figure 21-2).

Gallstones are relatively common in persons over the age of 40 and affect women four times more often than men. They do not always cause symptoms and go undetected in anywhere from 60% to 80% of the population. The use of oral contraceptives by young adults has brought about an increase in gallstones in 20- to 30-year-old women.

Elder Care Point . . . Symptoms of gallstones may be atypical in the elderly. Cholelithiasis should be considered a possibility in any elderly patient presenting with abdominal pain when another cause cannot be found.

Diagnosis **Symptoms of gallstones vary from none at all to severe and unbearable pain (biliary colic), depending on the degree of obstruction to bile flow and extent of inflammation of the gallbladder. Early signs include indigestion, nausea after eating, and some discomfort in the gallbladder region.**

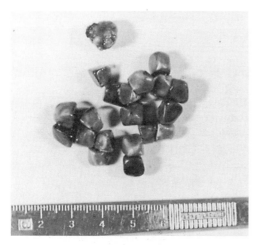

FIGURE 21-2   Gallstones.

If a stone becomes lodged in the common bile duct, it prevents the flow of bile into the small intestine. The bile accumulates in the blood, causing jaundice. The absence of bile in the intestine results in clay-colored stools that float as a result of undigested fat content. If unrelieved, this condition can cause cholecystitis, which can progress to liver damage.

Gallstones usually can be diagnosed with sonography or computed tomography (CT) of the gallbladder and biliary tract. If the patient is jaundiced, endoscopic retrograde cholangiopancreatography (ERCP) may be done.

Treatment   If the patient does not respond to treatment with a low-fat diet and loss of excessive body weight or symptoms indicate bile obstruction, surgical correction of the obstructed biliary tract is indicated.

The surgical procedure of choice is cholecystectomy. When stones are thought to be in the common bile duct, it is explored during surgery, and a T tube is inserted to keep the duct open and drain bile during healing. Sometimes small stones may be removed during (ERCP), where the common duct can be visualized.

◆ Cholecystitis

Cholecystitis is an inflammation of the gallbladder and is most often associated with gallstones. Other causes include typhoid fever and obstructive tumors of the biliary tract. A systemic streptococcal infection also can cause cholecystitis, but in most cases the infection is secondary to biliary obstruction rather than a primary factor.

Signs, Symptoms, and Diagnosis   **The symptom most often presented in chronic cholecystitis is biliary colic. The pain sometimes is referred to the back at the level of the shoulder blade.** Attacks can occur as frequently as daily or may not appear but once every year or so. Vomiting may accompany acute flareups, and the person may experience chills and fever. If the inflammation is not corrected or if there is an infection, the gallbladder can become filled with pus and will eventually rupture, spilling its contents into the abdominal cavity and causing peritonitis.

The diagnosis of cholecystitis is aided by abdominal sonogram, cholecystogram, IV cholangiography, and endoscopic examination. Laboratory tests helpful to diagnose gallbladder and biliary tract disease include evaluation of direct bilirubin and alkaline phosphatase; levels of both are elevated in biliary obstruction.

Think about . . . What questions would you ask when assessing a patient who may have cholecystitis?

Treatment   The preferred treatment of cholecystitis with gallstones is surgical removal of the gallbladder (*cholecystectomy*). If surgery is contraindicated, the symptoms might be controlled to some degree by a low-fat diet, restriction of alcohol intake, and spacing of meals so that no large amounts of food are put into the intestinal tract at any one time to avoid overly stimulating gallbladder activity.

An alternative for patients who are not candidates for surgery or for elderly patients with mild symptoms is bile acid therapy. A drug, either chenodiol (CDCA) or ursodiol (UDCA), is given orally to reduce small cholesterol stones. The drug is expensive and may take up to 2 years to dissolve the stones. Often stones appear again after the patient stops the therapy. Only a small percentage of people qualify for this procedure, and the stones tend to recur after treatment. The procedure may be done on an outpatient basis.

Lithotripsy, or "shock wave" therapy, is undergoing trials at some major medical centers. The procedure involves using sound waves directed through the body to break up the stones. The procedure takes 1 to 1 1/2 hours, and the debris is then carried by the bile into the intestine. There must be no more than three cholesterol gallstones, each smaller than 1 1/2 inches.

A less traumatic surgical procedure is laparascopic cholecystectomy. The gallbladder is removed by dissection through an endoscope, often with the use of a laser. This requires only three or four puncture wounds in the abdomen through which the equipment is introduced, rather than the large upper abdominal incision of the standard cholecystectomy. Not all patients are candidates for this procedure. One advantage is that the hospitalization period is shorter and the patient usually can return to work within 1 week. In some locales this procedure is done as outpatient surgery.

During history taking the nurse should be alert for patients at risk for developing gallstones and record on the patient's chart the risk factors identified. In addition, the patient is assessed for subjective and objective signs and symptoms of gallbladder disease and liver involvement.

The patient scheduled for surgery has needs similar to those of any patient having abdominal surgery. Teaching depends to some degree on whether or not the surgery is a standard procedure or a laparoscopic procedure.

Nursing Care of Patients Having Surgery of the Gallbladder

Preoperative Care. Preoperatively the patient may have a nasogastric (NG) tube to relieve nausea and vomiting. Meperidine may be ordered to decrease pain, and antiemetics are given for nausea. IV fluids are begun to prevent dehydration if the patient is experiencing symptoms. Coagulation times are monitored if jaundice is present, and vitamin K, if needed, is administered prior to surgery to improve clotting ability of the blood.

Postoperative Care. Because the surgical incision is in the upper section of the abdomen, the patient is placed in the semi-Fowler's position after he recovers from anesthesia when a standard cholecystectomy has been performed. Aside from being more comfortable and having less strain on the sutures, the patient will also be able to take deep breaths and cough more easily in this position.

One of the most confusing aspects of nursing a patient who has had gallbladder surgery is proper care of the drains or tubes that may be in place when the patient returns from the operating room.

In many cases, the surgery has been performed to relieve an obstruction to the flow of bile through the bile ducts or to drain purulent material to the outside. If the patient has had an infection of the gallbladder, the drainage is absorbed by the dressings over the surgical wound. These must be changed often and should be checked quite frequently for signs of fresh bleeding. The drain is left in as long as necessary and is then removed by the surgeon.

When an obstruction of the common bile duct has occurred because of stones or tumors, the surgeon may insert a small T-shaped tube (T tube) directly into the common bile duct (Figure 21-3). This tube must be kept open at all times and is connected to a bedside drainage bag. The length of time the T tube is left in place depends on the condition of the patient. Even though the tube is in the common bile duct, no bile will be going to the duodenum as it normally would. Precautions must be taken so that no tension is put on tubes or drains that have been inserted in the surgical wound (Figure 21-4). **T tubes are sutured in place, and if they are accidentally pulled out, the patient must be returned to the operating room and the incision reopened to replace the tube.**

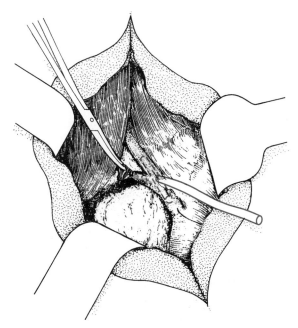

A hemostat *(left)* holds the end of the cystic duct, which has been cut and tied. The T tube is brought to the outside and attached to a drainage bag.

FIGURE 21-3   T tube inserted into the common bile duct and sutured in place.

Dressings must be changed with careful handling of the tube or drain. There usually is so much drainage that the dressings must be changed often, and Montgomery straps are best for holding the dressings in place. The sight of so much greenish-yellow discharge (bile) on the dressings may upset the patient unless he is told that this is to be expected.

Because the surgeon will be concerned with whether bile is beginning to flow through the duct and

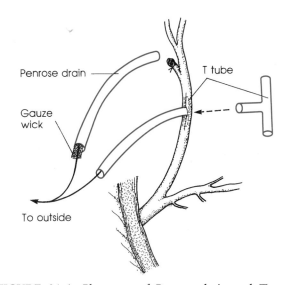

FIGURE 21-4   Placement of Penrose drain and T tube after cholecystectomy.

into the duodenum as it normally should, the nurse must carefully observe the color of the patient's stools. A return of the characteristic brown color to the stools is an indication that bile is entering the small intestine. If the bile duct is still obstructed, the patient will show signs of jaundice.

The standard cholecystectomy patient is reluctant to deep-breathe and cough because of considerable pain in the operative area. She should be assisted with these exercises, and her lung sounds should be auscultated every shift to discover quickly any signs of extra secretions or atelectasis. Using a patient-controlled anesthesia (PCA) pump for analgesia as ordered will help the patient cooperate with turning, coughing, and ambulating and thus prevent complications.

For the laparoscopic cholecystectomy, the patient will have dressings over the three or four small incisions on the abdomen. It is especially important to monitor this patient closely for internal bleeding. The nurse and family watch for signs of increasing abdominal rigidity and pain and for changes in vital signs. The patient is discharged after recovering from the anesthesia, or 1 to 2 days postoperatively, depending on her age and condition and must have careful discharge teaching about signs of complications. Her temperature is monitored daily and stools are watched for changes in color. **Increasing pain or abdominal distention should be reported to the surgeon.**

There is no specific diet recommended for the patient who has had surgery of the gallbladder, although it is wise to avoid excessive amounts of fatty foods.

> Light-colored stools, dark urine, or the early appearance of a yellowish cast to the skin must be reported as soon as one of these is noticed during the recovery period. These signs indicate obstruction of bile.

Think about... Can you outline the points to be covered for teaching the patient who is about to undergo a cholecystectomy?

LIVER DISORDERS

Subjective symptoms of liver disease include fatigue, weakness, headache, anorexia, abdominal pain, nausea, and vomiting. Objective symptoms include skin rashes, itching, fever, urine that is darker than normal because of the presence of bile, stools that are gray or clay-colored, thigh and leg edema, palmar erythema (redness of the palms that blanches with pressure), clubbed fingers, and bluish varicose veins radiating from the umbilicus (indicating portal hypertension). Bleeding and bruising also are associated with liver

disease because of deficiencies in vitamin K, thrombin, or prothrombin necessary for clot formation. Jaundice also can be a sign of damage to the liver cells.

◆ Jaundice

Jaundice is a symptom, not a disease. It indicates excessively high levels of bile pigment (bilirubin) in the blood. The pigment is deposited in the skin, mucous membranes, and body fluids, causing a change in color ranging from pale yellow to golden-orange. The first signs of jaundice are usually seen in the sclera of the eye, which takes on a yellow tint. There are three main types of jaundice: obstructive, hepatic, and hemolytic (breakdown of red blood cells).

Obstructive jaundice is caused by a blockage to the flow of bile in the bile ducts. The pigment in the dammed-up bile enters the bloodstream and causes the yellowing typical of jaundice. It can occur as a result of inflammation, stones, and tumors in the liver, gallbladder and biliary ducts, or pancreas. If the obstruction is not relieved, congestion eventually will lead to ischemia and destruction of liver cells.

Hepatic jaundice occurs as a result of the inability of the liver either to process bilirubin or to transport it to the bile ducts for excretion via the intestines. It can be caused by inflammation of the liver, cirrhosis, liver congestion, or liver cell malignancy.

Jaundice is not always a sign of liver damage. In *hemolytic jaundice* there may be an increased level of bilirubin as a result of excessive destruction of RBCs, with resultant release of the pigment into the bloodstream. Liver function can be normal in hemolytic jaundice, and the liver may actually speed up its function of processing bilirubin.

Some causes of hemolytic jaundice are transfusion reactions, sickle cell and hemolytic anemias, septicemia, and erythroblastosis fetalis caused by Rh-factor incompatibility between fetal and maternal blood.

The patient who is severely jaundiced experiences a drastic change in body image. She knows her skin color attracts attention and that she looks sick. The nurse needs to provide time for sharing of feelings and affirmation of her self-worth.

Think about... Can you list the assessments you would make in checking a patient for signs of jaundice?

◆ Hepatitis

There are five types of viral hepatitis: type A, type B (also called serum hepatitis), type C, type D, or delta hepatitis, and type E. Hepatitis A (HAV) and hepatitis E (HEV) are transmitted primarily by the oral-fecal route and are responsible for the epidemic forms of viral hepatitis.

Hepatitis E is primarily seen in less developed countries and is transmitted through fecal contamination of water.

Hepatitis B (HBV) is transmitted mainly by parenteral routes and is present in all body fluids and stool of carriers. Sexual partners of patients who are carriers of HBV are at high risk for contracting the virus. Hepatitis D (HDV) coexists with hepatitis B, is transmitted in the same ways, and is present only as long as hepatitis B is in the body. **Hepatitis B is one of the most serious forms, often progressing to chronic hepatitis, cirrhosis, liver cancer, and death.**

Hepatitis C is largely transmitted by parenteral routes. It has been the main cause of posttransfusion hepatitis, largely because there were no known diagnostic markers for this virus (meaning that donor blood could not be screened for this type of hepatitis). A new enzyme-linked immunosorbent assay (ELISA) test is expected to reduce the number of transfusion-related cases. **Intravenous drug use is a major cause of hepatitis C.** Hepatitis C also occurs in hemodialysis patients. Hepatitis C often progresses to chronic hepatitis, cirrhosis, and death.

Elder Care Point... Elderly patients who have had several major surgeries and blood transfusions during their lives are at higher risk for developing hepatitis B and hepatitis C as blood was not screened for the viruses before transfusion. These patients may be carriers of these viruses.

The incubation period, clinical manifestations, major route of transmission, and other characteristics differ among the five types of viral hepatitis. A comparison of these characteristics is shown in Table 21-3.

Signs and Symptoms   The clinical signs and symptoms of type A hepatitis, type E hepatitis, and type B hepatitis are similar, except that the onset of type A is acute, whereas in types B, C, and D the onset is slower and more insidious. In these types the patient can be virtually without symptoms and unaware that she is ill. When symptoms do occur, they include such vague and nonspecific manifestations as malaise, fever, loss of appetite, nausea, fatigue, and abdominal discomfort. The liver becomes tender and enlarged. The patient might think she has a mild case of influenza because the symptoms are so similar.

Hepatitis D sometimes causes massive death of liver cells, causing liver failure and death of the patient. Hepatitis B and D can become chronic in about 10% of infected patients. The patient is then a constant carrier of the virus.

A more specific group of symptoms are related to jaundice and include gray or clay-colored stools and dark, foamy urine. Viral hepatitis without jaundice is two to three times more common than viral hepatitis with jaundice.

The medical diagnosis is established by serological testing for immunoglobulins, specifically the presence of IgM-specific antibodies in the serum to distinguish current infection from past infection. There are more sophisticated tests for HBV and HDV components, but most laboratories test only for surface antigens and antibody to the surface antigen. The majority of patients are treated on an outpatient basis.

Preventive Measures   Both feces and blood of patients with hepatitis A contain virus during the *prodromal* (infected but without symptoms) stage and early symptomatic stage. Good hygiene, with handwashing after contact and careful handling and disposal of clothing and eating utensils, is necessary. The strict use of *Standard Precautions* is essential. Close contacts of patients with hepatitis A should be given immune serum globulin as soon as possible.

The greatest risk for transmission of HBV is from commercially prepared clotting concentrates derived from the plasma of paid donors. Serological testing for the presence of hepatitis B surface antigen (HBsAg) in whole blood has significantly decreased the incidence of transfusion-related hepatitis B.

Hepatitis B and D are rarely transmitted by the fecal-oral route, but it is best to be very careful when disposing of a patient's stool. *Standard Precaution* guidelines must be carefully followed for handling and disposing of equipment contaminated with blood. **These viruses are transmitted by sexual contact, and homosexual men in particular are at risk.** About 10% of patients with these forms of hepatitis become carriers. Carriers of HBV are at risk for chronic hepatitis, cirrhosis, and carcinoma of the liver. A carrier of HBV has a 300 times greater risk of liver cancer than someone in the general population.

Hepatitis B carriers are counseled to adhere to strict hygienic principles. They should not share personal items, such as razors, likely to be contaminated with their blood. Dentists, physicians, nurses, and other health care workers must be informed of their carrier status.

Hepatitis C is transmitted by blood and body fluids; other modes of transmission are unknown at present. *Standard Precautions* and careful handling of all body fluids are recommended. Various drugs, toxic agents, and other viruses also occasionally cause hepatitis.

Elder Care Point... The elderly patient is at higher risk for drug-induced hepatitis if she has chronic conditions that require the administration of various drugs over a long time.

TABLE 21-3 ◆ Guide to the Five Types of Viral Hepatitis

	Hepatitis A virus (HAV)	Hepatitis B virus (HBV)	Hepatitic C virus (HCV)	Hepatitis D virus (HDV)	Hepatitis E virus (HEV)
Mode of transmission	Fecal-to-oral route primarily; poor sanitation and contaminated water contribute to the risk; many outbreaks are traced to infected food handlers; intimate contact within households; sexual contact.	Sexual contact; blood-to-blood contact; perinatal (at birth); contaminated blood products; occupational risks from needlesticks and other blood exposures.	Blood-to-blood contact; contaminated blood products; risks not well defined for sexual or perinatal transmission; occupational risks to health care professionals are similar to that for HBV.	Can cause infection only together with HBV; routes of transmission the same as for HBV.	Fecal-to-oral route; contaminated water and poor sanitation contribute to risks as with HAV; seen in Asia, Africa, and Mexico but not common in the United States.
Incubation period	15 to 50 days (average: 28 days).	45 to 180 days (average: 60 to 90 days).	14 to 180 days (average: 40 to 60 days).	Not firmly established in humans; HBV infection must precede HDV; chronic carriers of HBV are at risk throughout their carrier state.	15 to 64 days (average: 26 to 42 days in different epidemics).
Infectiousness	Most infectious during 2 weeks before onset of illness; in most cases, unlikely to be infectious after first week of jaundice.	Begins before symptoms appear and persists for 4 to 6 months after acute illness; persists for the lifetime of chronic carriers.	Begins 1 to 2 weeks before symptoms appear; continues throughout clinical course and indefinitely in chronic carriers.	Blood is potentially infectious during all phases of active HDV infection; although HDV may fall rapidly to undetectable levels, it may be present in the blood of chronic HBV carriers for an extended period.	Not known; may be similar to HAV.
Laboratory tests (Note: All tests are done on blood serum.)	Anti-HAV IgM (indicates current infection). Anti-HAV IgG (indicates past, resolved infection).	HbsAg (indicates current or chronic infection). HBeAg (a marker for increased infectivity). Anti-HBc (a marker for infection at some time). Anti-HBe (a marker for decreased infectivity). Anti-HBs (a marker for immunity and the antibody produced in response to the HBV vaccine).	Anti-HCV (a marker for infection with HCV virus).	Anti-HDV IgM (indicates current infection). Anti-HDV IgG (indicates past infection).	Serological tests are currently under development.

Postexposure management	Immune globulin within 2 weeks of exposure; if given early in incubation period, it has 80% to 90% effectiveness.	In the unimmunized person exposed, give HBV vaccine and high-titer immune globulin (HBIG) to reduce the risk of HBV infection.	The value of immune globulin is unclear; no other treatment is presently available.	Focus of management is to prevent HBV; HBIG, immune globulin, and HBV; vaccines don't protect HBV carriers from HDV infection.	Exposures unlikely in the United States and immune globulin available in United States isn't likely to contain protective antibodies.
Complications	Rare, but can be fatal if fulminant hepatitis develops; protracted cholestasis can occur.	With acute HBV infection, death from fulminant hepatitis is possible; up to 10% become chronic carriers and may be at risk for cirrhosis, liver cancer, and death; anyone with HBV is at risk for HDV infection.	Chronic carrier state in as many as 50% of those infected via blood transfusions or IV drug abuse; chronic liver disease; cirrhosis; liver cancer; death.	Those with HBV and HDV have greater risk of serious morbidity or mortality.	Similar to HAV.
Prognosis	Good, generally full recovery; no chronic carrier state.	Good, generally full recovery, except for chronic carriers.	Chronic carrier rate high; generally a full recovery in others.	Infection may be acute and short-lived or become chronic; HDV should always be suspected in patients with fulminant HBV or when chronic HBV carriers have sudden exacerbations.	Good; full recovery likely; no chronic carrier state.
Prevention	Handwashing prior to food preparation; proper personal hygiene; environmental sanitation measures; food and water sanitation; immune globulin for travelers into areas where HAV is common; HAV vaccine (not yet licensed in the U.S.).	HBV vaccine for all infants, health care professionals, and others at risk; condom use; screening donated blood; devices to minimize risk to health care professionals (such as needleless IV access devices); personal protective devices for health care professionals (such as aprons, eye and mucous membrane protection, gloves, gowns).	Screening donated blood; avoidance of blood-to-blood exposure for at-risk individuals and health care professionals with the same measures as for HBV. (*Note:* There is no HCV vaccine.)	HBV vaccine for all at risk will also prevent HDV infection; other prevention measures same as for HBV. (*Note:* HDV infection isn't possible without HBV infection.)	Handwashing; food and water sanitation measures; improved personal hygiene; other measures as for HAV. (*Note:* It's unlikely that immune globulin from U.S. donors would provide protection.)

Source: Jackson, M. M., Rymer, T. E. (1994). Guide to the five types of viral hepatitis, *American Journal of Nursing*, 94(1):47. Reprinted by permission of Lippincott-Raven Publishers, 227 E. Washington Square, Philadelphia, PA 19106-3780.

Diagnosis   Hepatitis A, E, and B are diagnosed by history, physical examination, elevations in liver function tests (LFTs), and laboratory tests for the presence of the serological markers HAsAg (hepatitis A surface antigen) or HBsAg. Hepatitis D is identified by the presence of the delta antigen or a rise in the anti-HDV titer. Hepatitis C is diagnosed by anti-HCV. Liver function tests include bilirubin, alkaline phosphatase, alanine aminotransferase (ALT), and aspartate aminotransferase (AST). Chronic hepatitis is determined by liver biopsy.

Treatment   No specific treatment or drug can kill the hepatitis viruses. Interferon alfa-2b recombinant and ribavirin (Virazole) have been successful in inducing remission to HBV and HCV in a percentage of patients. The new drug Lamivudine (Epivir) may help control the disease in patients who do not respond to interferon. Medical treatment is directed at supportive care to enhance the patient's natural defenses and promote regeneration and healing of the liver. Hydration, sufficient rest, and adequate nutrition are the goals of treatment. Medication for nausea may be prescribed to encourage adequate nutrition. Because the patient tends to be anorexic, small, high-calorie meals several times a day are received better than three normal meals. Sucking on hard candy is recommended and adds to caloric intake.

Vaccines are available to provide active immunity against HBV and HAV for persons at high risk for infection. The vaccines produce immunity in about 95% of vaccinated individuals.

Passive immunity to type A hepatitis can be conferred by the administration of immune globulin (IG). There also is a high-titer immune globulin for type B hepatitis (HBIG). Both IG and HBIG are recommended for those who have been exposed to persons infected with HBV and have not been immunized against this virus. A vaccine is under development for hepatitis C.

Hepatitis is an occupational hazard for all persons who have direct contact with patients. The first line of defense is scrupulous handwashing, wearing rubber gloves when handling plasma-containing body fluids from a patient, and extreme care when handling used needles, syringes, and IV tubing. One does not have to be stuck with a contaminated needle or have an open wound to contract hepatitis B. The mucous membranes of the eye, nose, and mouth also can serve as ports of entry. All health care personnel should be immunized with the hepatitis B vaccine.

Nursing Assessment and Intervention   The nursing assessment of a patient with hepatitis should include a nursing history of previous contacts at home and at work and whether the contacts have been reported and the persons immunized. Viral hepatitis must, by law, be reported to the Department of Public Health. This necessitates filling out papers for patients being treated at home. When a patient with viral hepatitis has been admitted to the hospital, the infection control officer must be notified as soon as possible and no later than 48 hours after admission. Infection with type A hepatitis in a person who handles food on the job must be reported promptly so that a follow-up can be done by the health department.

Because the liver detoxifies many chemicals and metabolizes certain drugs, the nurse must have a complete list of medications the patient has recently taken or is currently receiving. It may be necessary to discontinue some drugs that are particularly toxic to the liver. Examples include acetaminophen, aspirin, chlorpromazine, and tetracycline. Sedatives can have a profound effect on patients with hepatitis and must be given with caution because a diseased liver cannot detoxify them very well. Alcohol is particularly damaging to the liver and is best avoided for 4 months following recovery from hepatitis.

During assessment the nurse will look for data that indicate a need for rest and any potential or actual nutritional deficit, or fluid imbalance. The patient and his family probably will need instruction in special precautions to prevent the spread of the infectious agent. This may include properly handling of body secretions, proper handwashing, and limiting contact with others.

Assessment of hospitalized patients also should include data that would be helpful in identifying problems related to silent gastrointestinal bleeding, respiratory distress, and neurological dysfunction, especially mental confusion and coma associated with portal systemic encephalopathy. Nursing interventions include monitoring the patient's progress by reviewing reports of serum enzyme levels and serum bilirubin values.

Preventing the spread of infection is a major concern in the nursing care of patients with viral hepatitis. In addition to knowledge of the type of hepatitis a patient has, the nurse also should know what stage the disease process has reached. For example, the greatest danger of infection with type A hepatitis is during the incubation period and early prodromal phase of the disease. As the infection progresses and jaundice and other symptoms appear, the shedding of viruses declines rapidly, and there is far less danger of contamination. In hepatitis B and C the virus lingers in the body and remains a threat for a much longer time.

The Centers for Disease Control and Prevention (CDC) have published guidelines for the care of patients hospitalized with hepatitis. These same guidelines can be modified for home care to prevent the spread of the infection.

The convalescence of the hepatitis patient is slow and long. Psychological support from the nurse during this period can help prevent depression. A variety of diversional activities that are not physically taxing should be planned. Perhaps this is the time for the patient to take up a new hobby or learn a new skill.

In a small percentage of cases the patient can develop massive necrosis of liver cells (fulminant hepatitis). Death occurs in about 75% of these cases. **Symptoms of fulminant hepatitis include mental confusion, disorientation, and drowsiness. These symptoms indicate portal systemic encephalopathy. Ascites and edema, which usually are present, indicate liver failure.**

Nursing interventions for selected nursing diagnoses relevant to the patient with hepatitis are found in Table 21-2. Nursing assessment and interventions for problems associated with severe liver damage are discussed in the following section on cirrhosis.

◆ Cirrhosis of the Liver

In cirrhosis of the liver destruction of normal hepatic structures and their replacement with necrotic parenchymal tissue occur. Fibrous bands of connective tissue develop in the organ and eventually constrict and partition it into irregular nodules. The scarring of liver tissue is generally considered irreversible and often is progressive. The outcome of cirrhosis of the liver is failure of its cells (liver failure) and the development of portal hypertension.

The disease process of cirrhosis is lengthy and ultimately leads to the appearance of symptoms. There probably is no one specific cause of cirrhosis. Although its incidence is high among known alcoholics, this does not mean that all those who have cirrhosis have a history of alcohol abuse. Between 30% and 60% of all cases of cirrhosis are associated with alcohol abuse.

Cirrhosis that is associated with alcoholism is called *Laennec's cirrhosis* or *portal cirrhosis. Postnecrotic* cirrhosis is caused by viral hepatitis, toxic substances, or infection. Biliary disease and some cardiac disorders, such as heart failure or cor pulmonale, also can lead to cirrhosis.

Cirrhosis is a common disorder. It is the fifth most frequent cause of death in the United States and the third most common cause of death in persons between 25 and 65 years of age.

Signs and Symptoms   The liver often is enlarged and "knobby" and is palpable below the level of the right rib cage. Elevations in ALT and AST levels usually do not occur until 65% of liver function is gone. The disease usually progresses without symptoms until severe liver damage is present. The patient may not seek medical attention until she develops ascites, gastrointestinal (GI) bleeding from esophageal varices (dilated, distorted blood veins), or neurological symptoms associated with hepatic encephalopathy, also known as

portal systemic encephalopathy (PSE). (Encephalopathy is any dysfunction of the brain.) These complications are directly related to liver failure. Other problems occur because the liver no longer performs its normal functions.

A definitive diagnosis of cirrhosis of the liver is made by liver biopsy. Laboratory testing may show hypoalbuminemia and elevated prothrombin time as well as elevated AST, ALT, and lactate dehydrogenase (LDH) values.

Treatment   The major goals of treatment are to (1) stop further degeneration of liver tissue; (2) minimize further trauma to liver cells by hepatotoxins; (3) reinforce the body's natural defenses and ability to heal itself; and (4) manage disabling symptoms.

Accomplishing these goals requires a coordinated effort on the part of the physician, nurse, and patient. The intake of alcohol and administration of drugs toxic to the liver must be restricted completely. Sedatives and opiates are either avoided or given with great caution. Rest may be prescribed to aid healing. The degree of rest and activity is dictated by the patient's stage of illness. Jaundice occurs either because the liver cannot metabolize bilirubin or because bile flow is obstructed.

The liver normally provides protection against infectious organisms. When the liver cells fail to function as they should, the patient is at great risk for infection. The patient should be protected from exposure to infectious agents, and antibiotics should be given quickly when infection occurs.

The management of symptoms usually focuses on the effects of pathological changes that occur as a result of degeneration of liver cells. When liver cells begin to degenerate, the blood vessels within the liver also fail to function normally. This causes an obstruction to the flow of blood through the portal circulatory system, causing portal systemic hypertension. This in turn leads to altered vessel permeability and fluid leakage into the abdomen, resulting in ascites.

Ascites is an abnormal accumulation of serous fluid within the peritoneal cavity. As pressure increases in the hepatic veins, there is a shift of protein-rich plasma filtrate into the lymphatic ducts. Some of the fluid enters the thoracic duct, but if the pressure is high enough, the excess fluid will ooze from the surface of the liver into the peritoneal cavity. Since the fluid has a high colloidal pressure because of its high protein content, it is not readily reabsorbed and therefore accumulates in the cavity, causing increased abdominal girth.

Medical treatment of ascites includes restriction of fluid and sodium intake and administration of diuretics. Management of ascites was at one time entirely limited to abdominal paracentesis to remove accumulated fluid. This is, however, only a temporary measure that poses problems of rapid fluid shift, loss of protein, and the potential for introducing infectious organisms into the peritoneum. In years past a procedure involving the shunting of ascitic fluid into the venous system has been used. The procedure is called a peritoneal-venous shunt (LeVeen or Denver shunt). Currently, a transjugular intrahepatic portosystemic shunt (TIPS) may be used to decrease pressure between portal and hepatic veins in the liver.

Symptoms of bleeding from the upper GI tract may indicate *esophageal varices*. These are engorged veins (similar to varicose veins) that line the esophagus. They, too, are the result of portal congestion and hypertension. In advanced cirrhosis, blood that normally flows from the intestines to the portal vein and on through the liver is shunted to other veins, including the veins of the upper stomach and lower esophagus. The added load of blood causes congestion of these veins and can lead to massive bleeding when the vein walls rupture from increased pressure or esophageal irritation. Another factor in hemorrhage is that the liver is no longer able to make vitamin K, which is an essential factor in the production of clotting factors in the blood. Lack of clotting factors can lead to hemorrhage. The patient is given vitamin K by injection. The treatment of hemorrhage of the upper GI tract resulting from esophageal varices was discussed in the previous chapter in the section on GI bleeding.

A third group of symptoms has to do with damage to the brain cells by abnormally high levels of ammonia in the blood. The liver is responsible for removing ammonia, a product of protein metabolism, from the blood and using it to form urea so it can be excreted by the kidneys. When the liver is diseased and can no longer handle it, ammonia accumulates in the blood. Excessively high levels of ammonia in the blood are a primary cause of the neurological changes that constitute portal systemic *encephalopathy* and produce such symptoms as delirium, convulsions, and coma.

An important aspect of treatment of patients with this condition is limitation of dietary protein intake. Dietary protein is limited to 40 to 60 g per day in an effort to lower ammonia levels. Thiamine and multiple vitamins are given to counteract vitamin deficiency. Neomycin is given orally or by enema to decrease the colonic bacteria that break down protein; this prevents formation of ammonia. The bowel is cleansed by enemas to decrease ammonia production further. Lactulose, an exchange resin, is given orally or by a feeding tube to induce diarrhea and prevent diffusion of ammonia out of the intestinal tract. The excessive ammonia levels can cause persistent itching of the skin. Kidney failure sometimes accompanies liver failure, further complicating the care of the patient.

Ascites, bleeding esophageal varices, and portal systemic encephalopathy are the most dangerous complications of cirrhosis and the most frequent causes of death. Of these three, esophageal varices can be the most deadly because of massive rapid hemorrhage. About half of the patients suffering from bleeding esophageal varices do not survive. Treatment options are to put pressure via balloon tamponade with a Blakemore-Sengstaken tube, administration of parenteral vasopressin (Pitressin) to lower portal pressure, injection scleropathy or ligation of the bleeding vessels, embolization of the left gastric vein or emergency portacaval shunt surgery.

A new option for treating liver failure is the Hepatix Extracorporeal Liver-Assist Device. It is a hollow fiber cartridge similar to hemodialysis cartridges used in kidney failure, but it contains cultured human hepatoblastoma (C3A) cells. These cells secrete liver-specific proteins and clotting factors. Liver "dialysis" may provide an alternative to liver transplant for the chronic liver failure patient.

Nursing Intervention   In view of the many functions of the liver, it is obvious that a patient with cirrhosis will require a thorough assessment to determine her status and identify specific patient care problems related to abnormal liver function. Nursing measures to help prevent, minimize, or alleviate the many problems associated with cirrhosis of the liver are planned according to the specific conditions presented by the patient. Interventions for selected problems in a patient with cirrhosis of the liver are summarized in Nursing Care Plan 21-1. Other nursing diagnoses and nursing interventions are provided in the section on nursing management and in Table 21-2.

Think about . . . Can you identify seven signs and symptoms that you might find when assessing a patient with advanced cirrhosis of the liver?

◆ Cancer of the Liver

Metastatic liver cancer is 20 times more prevalent than primary liver cancer, but the end result is the same. Liver cancer may be triggered by aflatoxin, a mold that grows on food, and possibly by estrogens and androgens. Cirrhosis and the hepatitis B virus increase the risk of developing liver cancer.

Symptoms may be upper-right quadrant pain, fatigue, anorexia, weight loss, weakness, or fever plus signs of poor liver function. Liver cancer is usually, but not always, fatal within 6 months of diagnosis. If the tumor is primary and has not metastasized, liver transplantation is an option. Treatment is combined radiation and chemotherapy. Care of the cancer patient is presented in Chapter 9. Additional care is directed at the problems of liver failure, such as ascites and encephalopathy.

Nursing Care Plan 21-1

Selected nursing diagnoses, goals/expected outcomes, nursing interventions, and evaluations for a patient with cirrhosis of the liver

Situation: Joe, a 59-year-old male with a 20-year history of alcoholism, is admitted with progressive alcoholic cirrhosis. His complaints include extreme fatigue, a swollen abdomen, edema of the feet and ankles, jaundice, itching, nausea and indigestion, drowsiness, and slight confusion.

Nursing Diagnosis	Goals/Expected Outcomes	Nursing Intervention	Evaluation
Risk for injury related to alteration in thought processes. SUPPORTING DATA Very drowsy; smokes; disoriented as to time and place.	Patient will not experience injury while hospitalized.	Keep long siderails raised and call bell within reach. Monitor mental status q 4 h. Supervise smoking.	Siderails up continuously; call bell in reach; confused; continue plan.
Risk for alteration in tissue perfusion related to possible hemorrhage from esophageal varices and decreased clotting factors. SUPPORTING DATA Elevated liver function tests; known cirrhosis; signs of liver failure and portal systemic hypertension; prolonged PT and PTT.	Patient will not experience death from hemorrhage.	Feed only soft foods to decrease mechanical irritation of esophagus. Give vitamin K as ordered. Monitor stool and vomitus for blood. Monitor vital signs every 2 to 4 h as ordered. Observe for increasing restlessness and confusion that might indicate hypoxia from bleeding. Monitor PT and PTT.	Vitamin K injection given; PT and PTT still prolonged; arms bruised from lab sticks; no signs of hemorrhage; continue plan.
Alteration in thought processes related to increased ammonia levels caused by liver failure. SUPPORTING DATA Elevated serum ammonia, confusion and drowsiness.	Serum ammonia levels will not increase further. Serum ammonia levels will return to normal.	Low-protein diet as ordered. Neomycin enemas as ordered. Administer lactulose as ordered to decrease absorption of ammonia; provide protective lubricant for anal region to decrease irritation from diarrhea. Monitor serum ammonia levels.	Lactulose given; profuse diarrhea; serum ammonia unchanged; continue plan.
Fluid volume excess related to ascites and edema from portal systemic hypertension. SUPPORTING DATA Ascites, edema of feet and ankles, 6 lb weight gain in 2 days.	Patient will have no further increase in ascites as evidenced by abdominal girth measurement. Patient will return to normal fluid balance as evidenced by normal weight and absence of edema.	Measure abdominal girth q shift and record. Administer diuretics as ordered. Maintain intake and output. Maintain fluid restriction as ordered. Weigh daily and record. Turn at least q 2 h. Provide good skin care.	Abdominal girth down ¼ inch; weight down ½ lb; intake, 500 mL; output, 1,200 mL; turned 8, 10, 12, and 2; continue plan.
Self-care deficit related to fatigue, drowsiness, and ascites. SUPPORTING DATA Cannot perform ADLs; very drowsy; ascites.	Patient will be able to assist with ADLs within 6 weeks. Patient will be able to perform ADLs independently.	Perform ADLs for patient while in liver failure. Bathe with tepid water and baking soda q shift to decrease itching. Offer mouth care q 2 h. Apply lotion to skin prn. Offer fluids as permitted. Assist with meals.	ADLs done; mouth care 8, 10, 12 and 2; continue plan.
Fear related to possibility of death from liver failure. SUPPORTING DATA States he is afraid he is going to die.	Patient will verbalize fears openly within 3 days. Patient will seek spiritual support.	Establish trusting relationship by attentive, caring attitude. Encourage verbalization of fears; actively listen. Encourage contact with minister or hospital chaplain or use of other spiritual supports.	Does not wish to see minister or chaplain; talks about fear of death; continue plan.

◆ Liver Transplantation

Liver transplantation is considered for patients with progressive and advanced liver disease that does not respond to treatment. It is most commonly done for nonalcoholic cirrhosis, chronic active hepatitis, sclerosing cholangitis, metabolic disorders, and biliary atresia in children. Some recovered alcoholics with cirrhosis are candidates. Seventy to eighty percent of liver transplant patients survive at least 3 years with good quality of life. Discussion of organ transplantation, tissue matching, and measures to prevent organ rejection are discussed in Chapter 7. If the patient has encephalopathy preoperatively, an epidural sensor is placed to monitor intracranial pressure (ICP). Every attempt is made to keep ICP within normal as increased ICP levels are correlated with decreased survival rates after transplantation.

After surgery there will be a T tube and Jackson-Pratt drains in place. The patient is placed on cyclosporine and prednisone for life to prevent rejection of the new liver. Strict measures are taken to prevent infection and the patient is monitored closely for signs of hemorrhage or hypovolemia. Liver functions, serum potassium, serum glucose, and coagulation factors are monitored closely. Right-quadrant or flank pain, increasing jaundice, fever, and changes in stool and urine color may indicate organ rejection.

DISORDERS OF THE PANCREAS

◆ Pancreatitis

Pancreatitis is an inflammation of the pancreas. It may be acute or chronic in nature and frequently accompanies obstruction of the pancreatic duct resulting from gallstones or the backflow of bile into the pancreatic duct.

Most cases of pancreatitis are related to alcoholism or biliary disease. Viral infections, trauma from certain types of surgery, ERCP, penetrating ulcers, drug toxicities, metabolic disorders, scorpion stings, and a variety of other factors also can cause pancreatitis. Men tend to develop pancreatitis related to alcohol; in women, it is seen more frequently with cholelithiasis.

In some types of pancreatitis, the severe inflammation and damage are caused by escape of pancreatic digestive enzymes, which act directly on the tissue, causing hemorrhage, autodigestion, and necrosis.

Signs and Symptoms   Pancreatitis causes abdominal pain that is usually acute, but this can vary among individuals. The pain is steady and is localized to the epigastrium or left upper quadrant. As it progresses, it spreads and radiates to the back and flank. **Eating** makes the pain worse. Nausea and vomiting often accompany pain.

Think about . . . What assessment data might tell you that your patient's pain is from cholelithiasis rather than pancreatitis?

Treatment and Nursing Intervention   Diagnosis is based on the presenting symptoms plus risk factors and results of tests performed to rule out other disorders. An abdominal sonogram, CT scan, and serum and urine amylase studies are usually ordered. Amylase levels are elevated, and the pancreas is enlarged in patients with pancreatitis.

Treatment is supportive and consists of pain control, fluid replacement, nasogastric decompression, and treatment of complications such as diabetes mellitus. Intravenous meperidine via PCA pump may be needed to control pain. The patient is allowed nothing by mouth during the acute phase so as to prevent stimulation of the pancreas and further aggravation of the inflammation. Fluids are given IV until the edema of the pancreas and the pancreatic duct has subsided and the digestive juices from the pancreas can once again flow into the duodenum. Most patients with acute pancreatitis recover after receiving this type of treatment. Pancreatic enzymes are given supplementally when an oral diet is resumed. When a powdered form of the enzymes must be taken, it should be mixed in nonprotein food, such as applesauce. Care must be taken not to let any of the medication remain on the lips or skin as it will cause irritation. If pancreatitis becomes chronic, some of the cells of the pancreas are destroyed and the pancreatic duct becomes fibrotic.

Chronic pancreatitis most frequently is seen in men who have been drinking alcohol for many years. Long-term pain control presents problems. The patient is started on non-narcotic pain medications to try to prevent addiction, but these often are not sufficient for pain control. Pancreatic enzymes are prescribed to be taken with meals, which should be low in fat. No alcohol is to be consumed. **Chronic pancreatitis greatly interferes with the patient's usual lifestyle and often is accompanied by depression requiring psychiatric intervention.**

◆ Cancer of the Pancreas

There will be about 26,300 new cases of cancer of the pancreas in the United States in 1996. It occurs in blacks more than in whites. **This cancer occurs twice as frequently among smokers than it does among non-smokers.** Cancer of the pancreas is almost always fatal. It is usually in a very advanced state when discovered, as the patient is asymptomatic in the early stages. Epigastric pain and weight loss are the main symptoms. The patient may develop a dislike for red meat.

Elder Care Point . . . Pancreatic cancer is most prevalent in the over-70 age group; it is more common in men than in women.

Diagnosis is made by ultrasonography, imaging techniques, and fine-needle biopsy. The tumor marker CA 19-9 may provide a means of earlier diagnosis and treatment, thereby setting the stage for a more positive outcome.

Surgical treatment has not been highly successful and is used mainly to relieve symptoms of obstructive jaundice or other complications. A Whipple procedure, or radical pancreaticoduodenectomy, may be done for cancer of the head of the pancreas. The head of the pancreas, gallbladder, duodenum, part of the jejunum, and all or part of the stomach are removed. Remaining structures are anastamosed to the jejunum. Another option is total pancreatectomy. Nursing care is the same as for any abdominal surgery. The patient will need enteral feedings, perhaps for life.

A new drug, gemcitabine (Gemzar) has been released for the treatment of non-resectable or metastatic tumors. It was considerably more effective than 5-flurouracil formerly used. Only time will provide sufficient data to determine this drug's success.

COMMUNITY CARE

Nurses in long-term care facilities should be alert to signs of jaundice in patients. Cancer and gallstones are both more prevalent in the elderly, and when abdominal pain occurs these disorders must be considered.

Nurses in the community should promote immunization against hepatitis B in all persons at risk. Teenagers and adults should be counseled about the possibility of transmission of hepatitis B by sexual contact and advised of measures for protection. The hepatitis A vaccine should be recommended for those traveling in areas where this disorder is prevalent.

Home care nurses must be particularly alert to the possibility of liver or pancreatic problems due to medications the patient is taking. Encouraging regular lab work, as recommended by the physician, when the patient is taking a drug known to be potentially damaging to the liver is a nursing function.

CRITICAL THINKING EXERCISES

Clinical Case Problems

Read each clinical situation and discuss the questions with your classmates.

1. Mr. Moser is admitted to the hospital with a diagnosis of cirrhosis of the liver. He is 59 years of age and has been hospitalized several times for his condition. He suffers from shortness of breath as a result of a swollen and enlarged abdomen, is anemic because of minimal, but constant, esophageal bleeding, and appears jaundiced. He has severe abrasions on his arms, legs, and abdomen from repeated scratching to relieve his pruritus.

   Mr. Moser is very depressed and will not converse with you when you enter his room with his breakfast tray the first morning you are assigned to his care. He refuses to eat and indicates his attitude by pushing the tray away and turning on his side, face to the wall.

   a. What nursing measures might help relieve some of Mr. Moser's problems?

   b. Why do you think he is mentally depressed?

   c. How would you go about helping him emotionally?

   d. What special observations must you make while caring for Mr. Moser?

   e. How would you explain a paracentesis to Mr. Moser if one were ordered for him?

2. Mrs. Lincoln, age 46, is admitted to the hospital for a standard cholecystectomy. She is extremely obese and enjoys eating rich, fatty foods, even though she knows this will add to her obesity and precipitate attacks of cholecystitis. You are assigned to care for Mrs. Lincoln when she returns from surgery.

   a. How will you position this patient?

   b. If she has a large amount of drainage from the surgical incision, how will you take care of this problem?

   c. When you get this patient out of bed the next day, how are you going to manage the dressings and prevent strain on the sutures?

   d. What other problems might you anticipate?

BIBLIOGRAPHY

Ambrose, M. S., Dreher, H. M. (1996). Pancreatitis: managing a flare-up. *Nursing 96.* 26(4):33–39.

American Cancer Society. (1996) *Cancer Facts and Figures—1996.* New York: Author.

Andreoli, T. E., et al. (1993). *Cecil Essentials of Medicine,* 3rd ed. Philadelphia: Saunders.

Angelucci, P. (1995). T.I.P.S. for controlling bleeding. *Nursing 95.* 25(7):43.

Applegate, E. J. (1995). *The Anatomy and Physiology Learning System: Textbook.* Philadelphia: Saunders.

Bennett, J. C., Plum, F., eds. (1996). *Cecil Textbook of Medicine,* 20th ed. Philadelphia: Saunders.

Bouley, G., et al. (1996). Transjugular intrahepatic portosystemic shunt: an alternative. *Critical Care Nurse.* 16(2):23–29.

Butler, R. W. (1994). Managing the complications of cirrhosis. *American Journal of Nursing.* 94(3):46–49.

Copstead, L. C. (1995). *Perspectives on Pathophysiology.* Philadelphia: Saunders.

Cotran, R. S., Kumar, V., Robbins, S. L., Schoen, F. J., eds. (1994). *Robbins Pathologic Basis of Disease,* 5th ed. Philadelphia: Saunders.

Dambro, M. R. (1996). *Griffith's 5 Minute Clinical Consult.* Baltimore: Williams & Wilkins.

Guyton, A. C., Hall, J. E. (1996). *Textbook of Medical Physiology,* 9th ed. Philadelphia: Saunders.

Ignatavicius, D. D., Workman, M. L., Mishler, M. A. (1995). *Medical–Surgical Nursing: A Nursing Process Approach,* 2nd ed. Philadelphia: Saunders.

Jackson, M. M., Rymer, T. E. (1994). Viral hepatitis: anatomy of a diagnosis. *American Journal of Nursing.* 94(1):43–48.

Kirton, C. A. (1996). Assessing for ascites. *Nursing 96.* 26(4):53.

Lisanti, P., Talotta, D. (1994). An overview of viral hepatitis: A through E. *AORN Journal.* 59(5):997–998, 1000–1005.

Marx, J. F. (1993). Viral hepatitis: unscrambling the alphabet. *Nursing 93.* 23(1):34–41.

Matteson, M. A., McConnell, E. S. (1996). *Gerontological Nursing: Concepts and Practice,* 2nd ed. Philadelphia: Saunders.

McConnell, E. A. (1994). What's wrong with this patient? Assessing upper abdominal pain. *Nursing 94.* 24(10):81–82.

McCorkle, R., Grant, M., Frank-Stromborg, M., and Baird, S. B. (1996). *Cancer Nursing: A comprehensive Textbook.* Philadelphia: Saunders.

McGinnis, C., Matson, S. W. (1994). How to manage patients with a Roux-en-Y jejunostomy. *American Journal of Nursing.* 94(2):43–45.

Meissner, J. E. (1996). Caring for patients with liver cancer. *Nursing 96.* 26(1):52–53.

Monahan, F. D., Drake, T., Neighbors, M. (1994). *Nursing Care of Adults.* Philadelphia: Saunders.

Murphy, D., Berry, D. (1994). Mechanical lithotripsy. *Gastroenterology Nursing.* 16(5):204–209.

Noone, J. (1995). Acute pancreatitis: an Orem approach to nursing assessment and care. *Critical Care Nurse.* 15(8):27–35.

Nursing 95. (1995). Liver disease: new options. *Nursing 95.* 25(6):56.

O'Hanlon-Nichols, T. (1995). Portal hypertension. *American Journal of Nursing.* 95(11):38.

Ondrusek, R. S. (1993). Cholecystectomy: an update. *RN.* 56(1):28–32.

Peterson, K. J., Solie, C. J. (1994). Interpreting lab values in pancreatitis. *American Journal of Nursing.* 94(11):56A–56B, 56F.

Reishtein, J. (1993). Liver failure: case study of a complex problem. *Critical Care Nurse.* 13(10):36–44.

Ruth-Sahd, L. A. (1996). Acute pancreatitis. *American Journal of Nursing.* 96(6):38–39.

Siconolfi, L. A. (1995). Clarifying the complexity of liver function tests. 25(5):39–44.

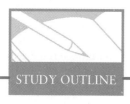

STUDY OUTLINE

I. Introduction

   A. The accessory organs for the digestive system are the gallbladder, liver, and pancreas.

   B. The gallbladder can be removed without a problem, but the liver is essential to life; if the pancreas is removed, pancreatic enzymes and insulin must be taken for life.

II. Diagnostic Tests

   A. Purpose, description, and nursing interventions are included in Table 21-1.

III. Causes and Prevention of Disorders of the Accessory Organs

   A. Gallstones cause irritation and predispose to infection of the gallbladder; they can obstruct the common duct, preventing bile from reaching the intestine.

   B. Excessive cholesterol may contribute to gallstone formation.

   C. Because the liver filters toxic substances, it is susceptible to infection; parasites often lodge in the liver.

   D. Many drugs may damage the liver; chemical substances also are harmful.

   E. Alcohol may cause cirrhosis of the liver.

F. Trauma may cause laceration or hematoma of the liver.

G. Avoiding substances harmful to the liver helps prevent liver disorders.

H. Immunization against hepatitis B and hepatitis A decreases the incidence of hepatitis.

I. Following *Standard Precautions* when dealing with all patients helps prevent transmission of the hepatitis B and C virus.

J. Good handwashing, hygienic food preparation practices, and avoiding eating raw shellfish help prevent hepatitis A.

K. Avoiding excessive alcohol intake helps prevent cirrhosis and pancreatitis.

IV. **Nursing Management**
   A. Assessment.
      1. Full physical assessment is essential to detect liver problems.
      2. Assessment includes questions regarding exposure to toxins or infectious organisms, trauma, and drugs regularly taken.
      3. Thorough abdominal assessment is essential.
      4. The appearance of the urine and stool is important.
   B. Nursing diagnosis.
      1. There are many appropriate nursing diagnoses for problems of these organs.
      2. See Nursing Care Plan 21-1 and Table 21-2.
   C. Planning.
      1. Expected outcomes are individualized.
      2. Goals are geared toward comfort, nutrition, prevention of complications, and return to normal function.
   D. Implementation.
      1. Interventions are geared to pain control, maintenance of fluid balance, promotion of adequate nutrition, and prevention of complications.
      2. See Nursing Care Plan 21-1 and Table 21-2.
   E. Evaluation.
      1. Reassessment is essential to gather data.
      2. Data are analyzed to determine whether expected outcomes are being met.

V. **Disorders of the Gallbladder**
   A. Cholelithiasis: gallstones in gallbladder or biliary tract.
      1. Relatively common in persons over 40. Does not always cause symptoms.
      2. Causative factors.
         a. Specific cause not known.
         b. Persons at risk are those who have hemolytic disease, who have had extensive bowel resection for treatment of Crohn's disease, or who are obese.
         c. Multiple pregnancies and oral contraceptives also contribute to stone formation.
      3. Medical diagnosis confirmed by sonography. ERCP ordered if patient is jaundiced.
         a. Severity of symptoms depends on location of stone and degree of inflammation.
         b. Obstructive jaundice can be present. Cirrhosis is a possibility if obstruction of bile goes unrelieved.
      4. Medical and surgical treatment.
         a. Low-fat diet and weight loss.
         b. Cholecystectomy, with or without insertion of T tube; standard or laparoscopic procedure may be performed.
      5. Nursing assessment and intervention.
         a. Nursing history of persons at risk for gallstones.
         b. Common nursing diagnoses: pain, fluid volume deficit, and noncompliance with low-fat diet.
   B. Cholecystitis: inflammation of gallbladder. Most often caused by gallstones. Other causes include tumor, infection, and typhoid fever.
      1. Medical diagnosis.
         a. Clinical signs: indigestion, pain, and tenderness in the upper right quadrant, malaise, low-grade fever. Indigestion and pain most noticeable after ingestion of a fatty meal.
         b. Can lead to rupture of gallbladder, resulting in peritonitis.
         c. Diagnosis confirmed by sonography and x-ray studies.
         d. Laboratory data show elevated levels of direct bilirubin and alkaline phosphatase.
      2. Medical and surgical treatment.
         a. Conservative treatment with low-fat diet, restriction of alcohol intake, spacing of meals.
         b. Cholecystectomy is preferred treatment.
         c. Drug to dissolve the stone (cholelithiasis).
         d. Laparoscopic cholecystectomy.

VI. **Nursing Care of Patients Undergoing Gallbladder Surgery**
   A. Preoperative care.
      1. NG tube to relieve nausea and vomiting.
      2. Pain control.
      3. Medication of nausea.
      4. Maintenance of hydration.
      5. Treatment of infection.
   B. Postoperative care.
      1. Place in semi-Fowler's position.
      2. Monitor tubes for drainage.
      3. Frequent dressing changes.

4. Medication for pain.

5. Careful observation of stools for signs of return of bile to intestinal tract.

6. Close attention to respiratory care to prevent complications such as atelectasis or pneumonia.

VII. Liver Disorders

A. Jaundice—a symptom.

   1. Indicates very high levels of bile pigment (bilirubin) in the blood.

   2. First appears in sclera of eye.

   3. Mucous membranes and skin become yellow.

   4. Urine turns tea colored or brownish.

   5. Three main types: obstructive, hepatic, and hemolytic.

      a. Obstructive jaundice: caused by blockage of bile flow.

      b. Hepatic: inability of liver to process bilirubin due to internal inflammation, tumor, or cirrhosis.

      c. Hemolytic: excessive destruction of RBCs with release of pigment into the bloodstream.

B. Hepatitis: inflammation of the liver.

   1. Caused by one of five strains of virus: hepatitis A virus (HAV), hepatitis B virus (HBV), hepatitis C, hepatitis D, and hepatitis E.

   2. Comparison of clinical manifestations of each is shown in Table 21-3.

   3. Medical diagnosis based on clinical signs and symptoms and serological testing for immunoglobulins: surface antigens and antibodies to surface antigens.

   4. Preventive measures.

      a. Measures to prevent cross-infection and spread of disease; *Standard Precautions.*

      b. Immunization for active immunity against HBV.

      c. Passive immunity: serum immune globulin for hepatitis A and immune globulin for hepatitis.

      d. Serological testing on whole blood prior to transfusion.

   5. Medical treatment: treatment is supportive and symptomatic. Majority of patients not hospitalized.

      a. Interferon alfa-2b recombinant, ribavirin, and lamivudine may help control hepatitis B and hepatitis C.

   6. Nursing assessment and intervention.

      a. Identify learning needs of patient and family to protect themselves and others.

      b. History of previous contacts.

      c. Prompt reporting of hepatitis to health department.

      d. Seek data to identify needs for rest, adequate nutrition and hydration, potential for cirrhosis and its complications.

C. Cirrhosis of the liver: diffuse fibrosis of liver cells and formation of nodular malfunctioning compartments in liver tissues. Scarring progressive and irreversible.

   1. Types.

      a. Laennec's cirrhosis: associated with alcoholism (30% to 60% of all cases).

      b. Posthepatitis or toxin-induced cirrhosis; postnecrotic cirrhosis.

      c. Biliary cirrhosis from obstruction to bile flow.

   2. Medical diagnosis.

      a. Often not made until disease has progressed to serious stage.

      b. Definitive diagnosis made by liver biopsy.

      c. Elevated serum enzymes, abnormal liver scan, hypoalbuminemia, and elevated PTT also indicate cirrhosis.

   3. Medical treatment.

      a. Major goals are to stop further degeneration of liver tissues, minimize further hepatotoxic damage, manage disabling symptoms.

      b. Restrict alcohol intake.

      c. Stop administration of all hepatotoxic drugs.

      d. Avoid sedatives and opiates.

      e. Prescribe rest to aid healing.

      f. Antibiotics as indicated to prevent infection.

      g. Manage ascites: restrict sodium and fluids; give diuretics to remove excess fluid in peritoneal cavity; insert transjugular intrahepatic portosystemic shunt (TIPS).

      h. Control bleeding from esophageal varices: pitressin infusion; scleropathy; Blakemore-Sengstaken tube with saline lavage; fresh frozen plasma infusion.

      i. Portal-caval shunt to divert blood flow and reduce portal systemic pressure sometimes done.

      j. Manage portal systemic encephalopathy: limit protein intake; administer lactulose; neomycin enemas.

   4. Nursing assessment and intervention: see Table 21-2 and Nursing Care Plan 21-1.

D. Cancer of the liver.

   1. Metastatic tumors 20 times more common than primary.

   2. Cirrhosis and hepatitis B virus increase risk.

   3. Symptoms: right upper-quadrant pain, fatigue, anorexia, weight loss, weakness, fever, signs of poor liver function.

4. Often fatal within 6 months.

5. Treatment is combined radiation and chemotherapy; liver transplant is an option if there is no metastasis.

VIII. Liver Transplantation

A. **Liver transplantation is performed for biliary atresia, cirrhosis, chronic active hepatitis, sclerosing cholangitis, metabolic disorders, and cancer.**

B. Seventy to eighty percent of transplant patients survive at least 3 years.

C. Postoperative care to prevent infection and rejection.

D. Patient must take cyclosporine and prednisone for life.

E. Right-quadrant or flank pain, increasing jaundice, fever, and changes in stool and urine color may indicate rejection.

IX. Pancreatitis: Inflammation of the Pancreas

A. Usually caused by long-term alcoholism or by biliary disease.

B. Symptoms: acute attack similar to acute indigestion; severe pain that radiates to the back.

C. Diagnosis: elevated amylase levels; abnormal abdominal sonogram and CT scan.

D. Treatment and nursing care: medications to relieve pain, restriction of foods and fluids, IV feedings (TPN).

E. Chronic pancreatitis treated with pain medication, restriction of fat, pancreatic enzymes, and abstinence from alcohol.

X. Cancer of the Pancreas

A. Insidious disease; discovered when well advanced; usually fatal.

B. Symptoms: epigastric pain and weight loss.

C. Diagnosis by ultrasound, imaging techniques, and fine-needle biopsy; CA 19-9 tumor marker.

D. Surgery to decrease tumor bulk: Whipple procedure; pancreatectomy is another option.

XI. Elder Care Points

A. Symptoms of gallstones may be atypical.

B. Elderly patients who have had several surgeries and blood transfusions are at greater risk for developing hepatitis B and C.

C. Elderly patients who have chronic conditions that have required the administration of multiple drugs over a long time are at greater risk for a drug-induced hepatitis.

XII. Community Care

A. Nurses in long-term care facilities should be alert to signs of jaundice.

B. Cancer and gallstones are more prevalent in the elderly.

C. Nurses in the community should promote immunization against hepatitis B for all, and against hepatitis A for those traveling in areas where it is prevalent.

D. Home care nurses must be alert to the possibility of liver or pancreatic problems from drug administration.

CHAPTER 22

Care of Patients with Musculoskeletal System Disorders

OBJECTIVES

Upon completing this chapter the student should be able to:
1. Teach a patient about the following diagnostic tests: bone scan, arthroscopy, electromyography.
2. Describe the steps included in a nursing assessment of the musculoskeletal system.
3. State the factors to be assessed for the patient who has an immobilization device.
4. Identify the "do's and don'ts" of cast care.
5. Describe nursing assessment and intervention for the patient in traction.
6. Identify the special problems of patients with arthritis and specific nursing interventions that can be helpful.
7. Compare the preoperative and postoperative care of a patient with a total knee replacement with that of a patient with a total hip replacement.
8. Explain the process by which osteoporosis occurs, ways to slow the process, and how the disorder is treated.
9. Identify important postoperative observations and nursing interventions in the care of the patient who has undergone an amputation.
10. List ways in which the elderly can increase musculoskeletal strength and protect bones.

The special branch of medical science concerned with the preservation and restoration of the functions of the skeletal system is called *orthopedics*. The principles of orthopedic nursing are applicable to the nursing care of all patients and most especially to those with limited mobility.

The three main functions of the musculoskeletal system are motion, support, and protection. Preservation of motion is probably the most important consideration to prevent orthopedic disabilities resulting from immobility.

The bony tissues of the infant differ greatly from those of the adult because bone cells do not all follow the same pattern of development from the embryonic stage to full maturity. *There are two distinct groups of bone cells.* The cells in the first group are designed so that they are immediately transformed into mature cells. The normal infant will have this type of firm bone cells in his skull and shoulder bones. In the second group, the bone cells form cartilage first and then are gradually replaced by mature bone cells as the person grows older. *Ossification*, or replacement of cartilage by more solid bony tissue, is not completed throughout the body until 20 to 25 years of age.

Because the bony structures of infants and young children are softer and more pliable than those of adults, there is less danger of breaking bones during the time of life when they are learning to walk and run and are therefore more likely to have frequent falls. If a fracture does occur, it will heal more rapidly in a very young person because growth is still taking place within the bone.

Trauma and disease cause dysfunction of the musculoskeletal system. Exercise and correct diet help preserve function. To understand thoroughly the problems that can occur in the musculoskeletal system, it is necessary to recall the structures of the system and their functions.

OVERVIEW OF ANATOMY AND PHYSIOLOGY

What Are the Structures of the Musculoskeletal System?

⅄ The musculoskeletal system consists of the bones, joints, cartilage, ligaments, tendons, and muscles.

⅄ A total of 206 bones make up the human skeleton (Figure 22-1).

⅄ Bone is either compact or spongy. Spongy bone contains red bone marrow (Figure 22-2).

⅄ Bones are classified as long, short, flat, or irregular.

⅄ Each bone has markings on its surface that make it unique (Table 22-1).

⅄ A canal system (haversian system) runs through the bone and contains the blood and lymph vessels.

⅄ A joint is the articulation point between two or more bones of the skeleton. There are immovable, slightly movable, and freely movable joints.

⅄ Ligaments join the bones of a joint together.

⅄ Tendons are connective tissue that provide joint movement.

⅄ Cartilage is a type of connective tissue in which fibers and cells are embedded in a semi-solid gel material. Cartilage acts as a cushion. The meniscus in the knee joint is a type of cartilage.

⅄ A bursa is a fluid-filled sac that provides cushioning at friction points in a freely movable joint.

⅄ Skeletal muscle is made up of hundreds of muscle fibers bundled together surrounded by a connective tissue sheath.

⅄ Fascia is a connective tissue that surrounds and separates the muscles.

⅄ The muscle coverings contain blood vessels and nerves.

⅄ Muscle has properties that allow it to be electrically excited, cause it to contract, extend, or stretch, and provide elasticity.

⅄ Skeletal muscles are attached to bones by tendons.

What Are the Functions of the Bones?

⅄ Bones provide shape to the body.

⅄ The skeleton provides a rigid framework that supports the internal organs and the skin.

⅄ The skeleton protects the internal organs of the body.

⅄ The skeleton provides attachments for tendons and ligaments and contributes to movement of the body.

⅄ The red bone marrow in the spongy bones forms red blood cells, white blood cells, and platelets.

⅄ The bones store and release minerals such as calcium and phosphorus.

⅄ The blood and lymph vessels in the canals transport nutrients to the bone cells and remove wastes.

⅄ Bone is maintained by remodeling: existing bone is resorbed into the body and new bone is built by osteoblasts to replace it.

What Are the Functions of the Muscles?

⅄ Contraction of skeletal muscles is produced by synchronized contraction of many muscle fibers.

⅄ Skeletal muscles contract, thereby providing movement, and joint stability, maintaining posture, and producing body heat.

⅄ By shortening and stretching, opposing muscle groups provide movement of the joints.

What Changes Occur in the Musculoskeletal System with Aging?

⅄ Bone density decreases because of the resorption of minerals.

⅄ The loss of bone mass, osteoporosis, occurs with aging, and is more severe in women.

⅄ The bones of elderly people are brittle and less compact; thus they break easily.

⅄ When a fracture occurs, elderly bones do not heal readily because the physiological exchange of minerals has decreased with advancing age, making the process of repair much slower.

⅄ Thinning of the intervertebral cartilage and collapse of the vertebra result in kyphosis (dowager's hump). This is responsible for the decrease in height the elderly experience.

⅄ Joint cartilage thins and erodes from years of use and results in stiffness and **crepitation** (a sound like that of hair rubbed between the fingers) of the joints.

⅄ Joint motion may decrease, limiting mobility; swelling may occur.

⅄ Ligaments become calcified and lose their elasticity.

⅄ Muscles decrease in mass and do not have the strength or endurance of the muscles in the younger person. Muscle cells decrease in number and the muscles atrophy.

⅄ Tendons shrink and become sclerotic, slowing muscle movement.

⅄ Muscle cramping, especially at night, increases because of impaired circulation and accumulation of metabolic wastes.

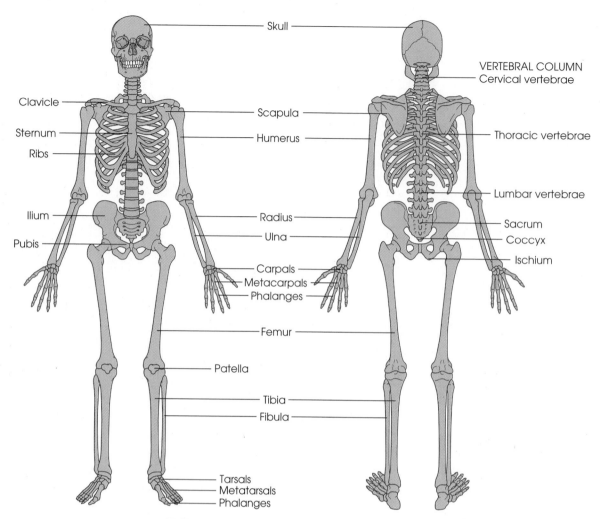

FIGURE 22-1   Major bones of the human skeleton.

CAUSES AND PREVENTION OF MUSCULOSKELETAL DISORDERS

Disease, trauma, malnutrition, and aging all contribute to musculoskeletal problems. Trauma may cause bruising, strain, sprain, or fracture. Poor nutrition may deprive the body of sufficient calcium and phosphorus to build strong bones. Inadequate protein intake can cause muscle wasting. Malignant tumors place a large nutritional demand on the body and nutritional imbalances may occur that cause muscle wasting. Tumor may invade bone as a primary tumor or as a metastatic tumor.

The decrease in estrogen production after menopause in women is thought to be a contributing factor to the occurrence of osteoporosis. It is hoped that the use of hormone replacement therapy after menopause will decrease the incidence of osteoporosis in women.

Diagnosing and treating cancer in other parts of the body early can prevent the occurrence of metastases to the bone. Refraining from using steroids on a long-term basis can help prevent osteoporosis and fractures.

Weight training and exercise throughout life can decrease the incidence of osteoporosis and increase muscle strength, mass, agility, balance, and coordination, thereby preventing falls and consequent fractures. Weight-bearing exercise is needed to maintain bone mass.

Learning to lift and move objects correctly by using large muscle groups can help prevent muscle strain and sprains. Using seat belts when riding in an automobile can reduce the incidence of trauma to bone and muscle during accidents. Wearing bicycle, motorcycle, and sports helmets will reduce the incidence of skull fractures. Consuming recommended amounts of calcium throughout the lifespan, obtaining sufficient vitamin D through sunshine, and maintaining adequate protein intake all helps build healthy bone and muscle.

Think about... What could you do now to promote healthy bones during your elderly years?

DIAGNOSTIC TESTS AND PROCEDURES AND NURSING IMPLICATIONS

Specific diagnostic tests of the musculoskeletal system are listed in Table 22-2. Blood counts, blood cultures, and various tests for problems of the immune system may also be performed to detect rheumatoid arthritis or other connective tissue diseases. These tests include an erythrocyte sedimentation rate (ESR), serum protein electrophoresis, and tests to determine the levels of serum complement and immunoglobulins (See Chapter 7).

Range of motion (ROM) testing involves both active and passive maneuvers. In active testing, the part being measured must be moved by the patient himself. In passive testing, the evaluator moves the body part while the patient is relaxed.

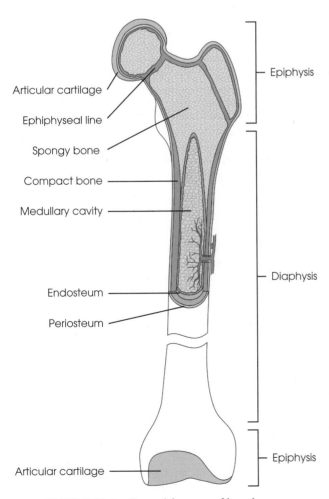

Articular cartilage

Ephiphyseal line

Spongy bone

Compact bone

Medullary cavity

Epiphysis

Diaphysis

Endosteum

Periosteum

Epiphysis

Articular cartilage

FIGURE 22-2   General features of long bones.

The measurement of ROM in a joint is called *goniometry.* One system of measurement that is commonly used is based on a full circle of 360 degrees. Each joint is evaluated in terms of the number of degrees it can be moved from the zero-degree position.

Muscle strength can be measured on the basis of the ability of a muscle to move the part to which it is attached, working against the force of gravity. A grading system is used, ranging from grade 5 (normal strength) to grade 0 (complete paralysis).

Other techniques used to evaluate musculoskeletal function include inspection, palpation, and tests for stability of a joint under stress.

Think about... What would you tell a patient who is to have an MRI of a knee when asked what the experience will be like?

NURSING MANAGEMENT

♦ Assessment

History Taking   When reviewing the patient's past history the nurse should keep in mind the significance of disorders that primarily affect other systems but secondarily affect the bones and muscles. For example, diabetes mellitus can predispose a patient to degenerative joint disease; sickle cell disease and hemophilia can cause bleeding into the joints and muscles, and psoriasis is sometimes the first sign of psoriatic arthritis. Nutritional deficiencies can affect the mineral composition of bone and muscle, making them more susceptible to trauma and loss of function.

Family history also can be significant, as there are some bone and muscle disorders that either are inherited or have a familial tendency. For example, muscular dystrophy is inherited, and about 30% of those who have psoriatic arthritis have a family history of psoriasis. Table 22-3 provides a guide to history taking.

Physical Assessment   Observe the patient for signs of joint pain, such as limping, poor posture, awkward gait, difficulty in arising or walking, and wincing upon movement. Much can be learned about the musculoskeletal system by just watching the patient, noting problems of movement and changes in facial expression as the routines of bathing and grooming occur:

♦ Is any supportive device being used, such as a cane, brace, splint, or elastic bandage.

♦ Pressure from swelling or deformity can injure adjacent nerve endings and produce sensory changes and loss of feeling. Ask whether the patient has experienced any sensory changes, when they were first noticed, and what they feel like.

TABLE 22-1 ◆ *Terms Related to Bone Markings*

Term	Description	Examples
Projections for articulation		
Condyle (KON-dial)	Smooth, rounded articular surface.	Occipital condyle on the occipital bone; lateral and medial condyles on the femur.
Facet (FASS-et)	Smooth, nearly flat articular surface.	Facets on thoracic vertebrae for articulation with ribs.
Head (HED)	Enlarged, often rounded, end of bone.	Head of the humerus; head of the femur.
Projections for muscle attachment		
Crest (KREST)	Narrow ridge of bone.	Iliac crest on the ilium.
Epicondyle (ep-ih-KON-dial)	Bony bulge adjacent to or above a condyle.	Lateral and medial epicondyles of the femur.
Process (PRAH-sess)	Any projection on a bone; often pointed and sharp.	Styloid process on the temporal bone.
Spine (SPYN)	Sharp, slender projection.	Spine of the scapula.
Trochanter (tro-KAN-turr)	Large, blunt, irregularly shaped projection.	Greater and lesser trochanters on the femur.
Tubercle (TOO-burr-kul)	Small, rounded, knoblike projection.	Greater tubercle of the humerus.
Tuberosity (too-burr-AHS-ih-tee)	Similar to a tubercle, but usually larger.	Tibial tuberosity on the tibia.
Depressions, openings, and cavities		
Fissure (FISH-ur)	Narrow cleft or slit; usually for passage of blood vessels and nerves.	Superior orbital fissure.
Foramen (foh-RAY-men)	Opening through a bone; usually for passage of blood vessels and nerves.	Foramen magnum in the occipital bone.
Fossa (FAW-sah)	A smooth, shallow depression.	Mandibular fossa on the temporal bone; olecranon ossa on the humerus.
Fovea (FOH-vee-ah)	A small pit or depression.	Fovea capitis femoris on the head of the femur.
Meatus (mee-ATE-us)	A tubelike passageway; tunnel.	External auditory meatus in the temporal bone.
Sinus (SYE-nus)	A cavity or hollow space in a bone.	Frontal sinus in the frontal bone.

Source: Applegate, E.J. (1995). *The Autonomy and Physiology Learning System: Textbook.* Philadelphia: Saunders, p. 99.

◆ If the patient is admitted with a fracture, obtain a history of the precipitating event so that an assessment can be made of other areas that may have been injured.

◆ An assessment of the patient's ability to perform activities of daily living (ADLs) should be made. Sometimes it is necessary to consult family members or someone who lives with the patient about this area. **A self-care deficit is one of the primary problems for patients who suffer a problem of immobility.**

◆ Note the patient's posture; is there evidence of **kyphosis** such as a rounded upper back that is called a "dowager's hump"? Are the knuckles swollen or deformed, indicating arthritis?

◆ Does the patient seem to be strong or weak? Is there difficulty opening the items on the food tray or other containers? If the patient can make a fist and place each finger in sequence to the thumb without undue pain, hand movement is not seriously affected. Is muscle strength sufficient to arise normally from a seated position?

Table 22-4 provides a guide to physical assessment of the musculoskeletal system.

Think about . . . How would you gather data about an elderly patient's ability to perform self-care activities at home before the patient is discharged? Can you trust the patient's statement of "I can shop, cook, clean, and do everything I need to do by myself"? Why not?

◆Nursing Diagnosis

Nursing diagnoses are chosen based on assessment findings. Diagnoses most commonly used for patients with musculoskeletal problems are:

◆ Impaired physical mobility
◆ Activity intolerance
◆ Pain
◆ Body image disturbance
◆ Self-care deficit in bathing, grooming, toileting, feeding

TABLE 22-2 ◆ *Diagnostic Tests for Musculoskeletal Problems*

Test	Purpose	Description	Nursing Implications
X-rays of the bones or joints	Detect fracture, avulsion, joint damage.	No preparation necessary. Part to be x-rayed is positioned by technician and x-rays are taken.	Explain the purpose, procedure, and possible sensations.
Tomography and xerography	Produces radiographic planes or slices; highlights contrast between structures.	Specialized equipment is used; xerography uses a higher amount of radiation than normal x-rays.	Explain that the tomography procedure takes longer as the machine takes a series of views.
Computed tomography (CT)	Detection of musculoskeletal problems, especially of the spine and skull.	A special machine is used and the patient is placed on a hard table. The procedure takes 30 to 60 minutes. Contrast material may or may not be used. Some patients experience claustrophobia from being encased by the machine. A computer enhances the radiographic findings.	Explain that lying perfectly still is required. The part under study is enclosed in the machine. There is a clicking sound as the machine rotates to take the next view.
Bone scan	Detects tumor, metastatic growths, bone injury, or degenerative bone disease. Can detect problems earlier than can x-rays.	An IV injection or oral dose of a radioisotope is given, and after an interval time for the substance to be taken up by the bone, the area is scanned by scintillation camera.	Explain the purpose and procedure. Check for allergies and pregnancy. Patient will be asked to lie quietly for 30 to 60 minutes during the scanning. All metal should be removed from the area to be scanned. Explain that the dose of radiation he will receive is lower than usual with radiographs. Assure him he will not be "radioactive." The isotope is eliminated from the body in 6 to 24 hours.
Gallium/thallium scans	Detect bone problems, especially tumor invasion.	The radioisotope gallium citrate GA 70 or thallium 201, is administered prior to the scan. A bone scan is then performed.	The addition of the radioisotope helps locate areas of rapid bone growth activity that might indicate tumor. Explain that the radioisotope is administered 1 to 2 days before scanning. The procedure takes 30 to 60 minutes, during which lying still is required; sedation may be given.
Magnetic resonance imaging (MRI)	Diagnose musculoskeletal disorders.	Is often preferred over bone scan. Magnetic fields and radiowaves are used to visualize tissue densities by the density of hydrogen ions. Computer enhancement depicts normal and abnormal tissue.	Instruct that there must be no metal on the body and no metal implants because of the strong magnetic fields used. The patient will need to lie still for 15 to 60 minutes. Older machines totally encase the patient; newer ones are more open.
Anthroscopy	Inspects the interior aspect of a joint, usually a knee, with a fiberoptic endoscope to diagnose problems of the patella, meniscus, and synovium. Also used to evaluate the progress of arthritis or effectiveness of treatment.	After injection of local anesthesia, an incision is made, and the arthroscope is introduced into the interior of the joint; instruments for tissue biopsy or surgical procedures may be passed through the arthroscope.	Explain the purpose and procedure. A preprocedure sedative may be administered. When the patient has recovered from any sedation he is allowed to walk but should not overuse or strain the joint for a few days. The area is observed for bleeding or swelling; ice packs may be used in the immediate postprocedure period, especially if biopsy or surgey was performed. Assessment for swelling, circulation, and sensation is done periodically to detect any complications.

(Table 22-2 continued)

TABLE 22-2 ♦ *Diagnostic Tests for Musculoskeletal Problems* (Continued)

Test	Purpose	Description	Nursing Implications
Arthrocentesis	Performed to extract synovial fluid for analysis or to reduce swelling.	A needle is inserted into the joint space, and synovial fluid is aspirated. Synovial fluid analysis may detect cells indicating infection, inflammation, rheumatoid arthritis, or lupus erythematosus. Corticosteroid may be injected after aspiration of fluid. If a large amount of fluid is aspirated, the joint is immobilized with an elastic bandage. Ice packs are applied to relieve pain and reduce swelling.	Explain the procedure. Have ice packs ready to apply afterward. Wrap with elastic bandage if ordered and show patient how to do this. It should be worn for 2 to 3 days. Instruct him not to overuse the joint until pain and swelling have subsided. Administer ordered analgesics if needed after corticosteroid injection, as this can be quite painful.
Biopsy	Bone biopsy done to detect tumor cells. Muscle biopsy done to obtain tissue for cellular analysis, which is helpful in differential diagnosis of several muscle disorders.	Under local anesthesia, a piece of bone or muscle is excised and sent for pathological analysis.	Offer emotional support during the procedure. Afterward, medicate for discomfort as needed, apply ice packs to decrease swelling, observe for bleeding; perform circulation and sensation checks distal to the area biopsied.
Culture of synovial fluid	Determine organism responsible for infection.	Explain purpose and procedure. See that specimen of fluid is transported to laboratory immediately.	Synovial fluid is aspirated and sent for culture and sensitivity to determine appropriate antibiotic for therapy. Results take 48 to 72 hours.
Electromyelography (EMG)	Detects abnormal nerve transmission to the muscle and abnormal muscle function. Determines rehabilitation progress.	Needle electrodes are inserted in affected muscles, and, as the muscles are stimulated, the electrical impulses generated by the muscle contractions are amplified and displayed on an oscilloscope; tracings also are made on graph paper.	Obtain a signed consent form. Caffeine-containing drinks and smoking are restricted 3 hours prior to the test. Muscle relaxants, anticholinergics, and cholinergic drugs should be withheld prior to the test; check with the physician. Explain that there may be slight discomfort when the electrodes are inserted. Explain that he will be asked to relax and contract his muscles. The test usually takes about an hour. If serum enzyme tests are ordered, draw the blood before the EMG.
Uric acid	Detects abnormally high levels of uric acid in the blood, which is a sign of gout.	Requires 5 to 10 mL of blood in a clot (red-top) tube. Normal range: female: 2.8–6.8 mg/dL; male: 3.5–7.8 mg/dl.	No food or fluid restrictions.
Rheumatoid factor	Detects antibodies, indicating possible rheumatoid arthritis, lupus, or scleroderma.	Requires 5 to 10 mL of blood in a clot (red-top) tube. Normal range: adult: <1:120 titer; >1:160 indicates rheumatoid arthritis	No food or fluid restrictions.
Antinuclear antibodies (ANA)	Assesses tissue antigen antibodies; useful for diagnosis of rheumatoid arthritis, lupus erythematosus, and other connective tissue disorders.	Requires 2 to 5 mL of blood in a clot (red-top) tube. Check drugs patient is receiving for interference with this test. Normal finding: negative.	No food or fluid restrictions.

TABLE 22-3 ◆ *Assessment: History Taking*

To obtain a history from the patient with a musculoskeletal problem, ask the following questions:

- Have you ever suffered an injury to a bone?
- Have you ever experienced a severe muscle strain or muscle problem?
- Do you have any joints that are stiff, swollen, or painful?
- When is the pain the worst? What seems to bring it on? What relieves it?
- Do you have any restriction of movement in any joint?
- Do you have trouble sleeping because of muscle or joint pain?
- Have you noticed any changes of sensation in your hands, feet, or elsewhere?
- Do you find that your fatigue level has increased?
- Do you have any problems with bathing, dressing, grooming, toileting, eating, ambulation, or going on social outings?
- Do you have any joint deformity? Bunion? Hammer toe? Knuckle?
- Do you have any pain in your wrists, elbows, or knees?
- Is there a history of osteoporosis or arthritis in your family?
- Do you have diabetes, sickle cell disease, psoriasis, systemic lupus erythematosus, or any other chronic metabolic disease?
- Are you taking any steroid medications regularly?
- How is your calcium intake? What do you eat or drink that contains calcium? How much of it do you eat or drink?
- Are you out in the sunshine very much?
- Do you exercise? What do you do? How often do you exercise?
- Can you tell me what you see as your problem?

Social history
- Is there any difficulty in obtaining the medications the doctor wants you to take?
- How do you get to the clinic/office for your appointments?
- Tell me about your work; is it very stressful?
- Is the environment you are in most of the day a comfortable temperature for you?
- Do you think you will have any difficulty in following your physician's recommendations for exercise, diet, rest, or medication?

TABLE 22-4 ◆ *Guide to Physical Assessment of the Musculoskeletal System*

Note the following points during physical assessment of the patient with a problem of the musculoskeletal system:

- Posture
- Gait
- Mobility without assistive devices
- Range of motion of the neck, shoulders.
- Spine; palpate the vertebrae to determine any tenderness
- Appearance of joints of elbows, hands, knees, ankles, and feet; presence of redness, warmth, deformity, or loss of motion.
- Skeletal muscle appearance in arms and legs; any atrophy.
- Ability to perform activities of daily living.

Review results of recent laboratory and diagnostic tests.

- Risk for disuse syndrome
- Impaired home maintenance

There may be several other secondary nursing diagnoses that are appropriate for patients who are highly immobile. Constipation, impaired tissue integrity, social isolation, and other problems caused by immobility may occur (see Chapter 11).

◆ Planning

Caring for immobile patients requires careful planning of time. Making beds for the bed-confined orthopedic patient is best done by two people. Bathing and grooming is more time-consuming when the patient has a limb immobilized or is in some sort of traction. The nurse may be a social contact for the patient as well as a care giver, and more time is spent in interaction to meet psychosocial needs. **Planning for toileting needs at regular intervals is important to the well-being of the patient who is unable to get out of bed to the toilet.** Neglecting such needs may cause incontinence and the time-consuming task of changing the bed and cleaning up the patient, besides causing a demoralizing episode for the patient.

General goals for patients with musculoskeletal disorders:

- Pain relief
- Prevention of infection
- Promotion of healing and rehabilitation
- Improved physical mobility
- Improved activity tolerance
- Promotion of effective coping
- Prevention of complications of immobility
- Proper use of therapeutic and assistive devices
- Improved body image

Specific individual expected outcomes are written for each nursing diagnosis. Outcomes are written in collaboration with the patient and other members of the health care team. **The physical therapist and occupational therapist are very important in this process.**

◆ Implementation

Nursing interventions are chosen based on the expected outcomes desired. Specific nursing interventions are found in Table 22-5, Clinical Pathway 22-1, and with the specific disorders discussed in the chapter.

Lifting and Turning the Patient   When working with the orthopedic patient, all movements must be *gentle* and *firm*. When moving or turning the patient, the nurse **should have sufficient help from adequately trained personnel. Each person involved, including the patient,**

TABLE 22-5 ◆ *Common Nursing Diagnoses, Expected Outcomes, and Interventions for Patients with Problems of the Musculoskeletal System*

Nursing Diagnosis	Goals/Expected Outcomes	Nursing Interventions
Impaired physical mobility related to immobilization, loss of limb, stiffness, pain, weakness, or inability to bear weight.	Range of motion (ROM) of unaffected joints will be maintained. No signs of joint contractures at discharge.	Active ROM at least tid for all unaffected joints while on bedrest. Passive ROM on affected joints *as ordered*. Ensure that joints are in correct alignment when at rest and after turning. Maintain traction and body in proper alignment. Assess immobilizer for correct fit and positioning q shift; assess for signs of complications due to pressure or pins. Supervise exercise to prepare muscles for ambulation. Instruct in use of ambulatory devices as appropriate; supervise practice; assess for proper "fit" of device. Encourage use of prosthesis for ambulation; assist with practice. Assess for signs of complications in stump and assess that prosthesis is attached correctly. Maintain abduction pillow between legs if one is ordered.
Activity intolerance related to stiffness, pain, impaired mobility, fatigue, etc.	Patient will space activities and rest to conserve energy. Patient will use assistive devices to conserve energy.	Determine factors that increase fatigue. Space activities with rest periods throughout the day. Assist to set goals for slow, steady increase in exercise and activity during periods of remission of arthritis symptoms. Use heat or cold treatments to decrease stiffness and discomfort. Perform exercises after heat treatments to decrease discomfort; apply in safe manner. Apply cold as needed after exercise for discomfort. Administer medications to decrease inflammation and pain, allowing greater level of activity. Advise of assistive devices that might make ADLs easier and conserve energy. Assist in obtaining needed devices. Supervise practice with assistive device.
Pain related to injury, surgery, or joint disorder.	Pain will be controlled as evidenced by patient verbalization. Pain will be decreased with medication.	Instruct in relaxation, distraction, and imagery techniques to decrease pain. Instruct in use of various heat and cold treatments to decrease pain. Administer analgesic, antiinflammatory and steroid medications as ordered to decrease pain. Instruct in use and side effects of each drug. Advise of alternative methods of pain control, such as transcutaneous electrical nerve stimulation (TENS). Monitor patient-controlled analgesia (PCA) use for effectiveness of pain control. Assess for factors contributing to pain level such as increased pressure, infection, positioning, or swelling. Assess pain in systematic, objective manner and track course of pain and effectiveness of pain control (see Chapter 10).
Risk for injury related to hemorrhage, fat embolus, thrombophlebitis, or dislocation of prosthesis.	Patient will not experience injury. No evidence of thrombophlebitis; no dislocation of hip joint.	Observe dressing for bleeding; monitor drainage in drainage device q 1 h for 8 h, then q 2 h for 24 h. Monitor vital signs q 4 h. Assess for signs of thrombophlebitis and possible emboli; apply antiembolic stockings as ordered; apply sequential compression devices as ordered; assess q 2 h for correct position and function of such devices. Use wedge pillow between legs for hip surgery patient as ordered; turn q 2 h to back or unaffected side *or per physician instructions*. Perform neurovascular checks q 1 h for 8 h, then q 2 h.

TABLE 22-5 ◆ *Common Nursing Diagnoses, Expected Outcomes, and Interventions for Patients with Problems of the Musculoskeletal System* (Continued)

Nursing Diagnosis	Goals/Expected Outcomes	Nursing Interventions
Risk for infection related to trauma or surgical incision.	No signs of infection as evidenced by normal WBC and normal temperature; wounds clean and dry.	Follow *Standard Precautions* and strict contact precautions when performing patient care, and use strict aseptic technique for wound or pin care. Assess for signs of infection q shift; assess wound for redness, swelling, and tenderness. Administer prophylactic antibiotics as ordered. Assess temperature trends and trend of WBC values for signs of infection. Assess patient for subjective signs of malaise. Sniff around cast for signs of foul odor indicating infection.
Risk for alteration in tissue perfusion related to swelling and pressure.	No evidence of seriously decreased circulation distal to site of trauma. No evidence of nerve compression from swelling.	Perform neurovascular assessment q 1 h for 8 h, then q 2 h for 48 h. Question patient regarding sensation distal to site of trauma or surgery. Apply cold to area of injury or surgery as ordered to reduce swelling; elevate extremity to slightly above heart level. Immediately report signs of compartment syndrome to physician and obtain order for measures to relieve pressure.
Self-care deficit in bathing, grooming, toileting, feeding related to immobilization.	Patient will receive assistance for all ADLs as needed.	Assess degree of inability to perform various self-care activities. Formulate plan to assist patient with ADLs. Answer calls for assistance with toileting promptly; do not leave on bedpan longer than necessary. Open food containers and cut food as needed for self-feeding with one hand. Do not serve extremely hot liquids to patients who have difficulty with coordination or with holding drinking containers or to immobilized patients. Provide assistive devices and help patient to be as self-sufficient as possible without incurring undue fatigue when performing ADLs. Caution patients about change in body's center of gravity when a limb is casted or amputated.
Body image disturbance related to change in appearance and/or loss of mobility or function.	Patient will begin adaptation to change in appearance or loss as evidenced by: verbalization of feelings of self-worth; maintenance of relationships with significant others; active interest in personal appearance; willingness to resume usual roles and participate in social activities; making plans to adapt lifestyle to meet restrictions imposed by loss.	Assess degree of body image disturbance, noting verbal or nonverbal clues to negative response to changes. Assist to verbalize feelings about effect of loss on usual roles and lifestyle. Be present and supportive during initial dressing changes on stump after an amputation. Assist patient to identify strengths and abilities and positive coping mechanisms. Clarify misconceptions about limitations on mobility and activity. Promote activities that require patient to confront the body changes that have occurred, such as bathing, ADLs, or dressing changes. Demonstrate acceptance of patient and encourage significant others to do the same with touch and affection. Encourage as much independence as possible; allow to do things for self. Assist patient to explore viable options for changes in lifestyle and career. Refer for vocational retraining if needed. Encourage maximum participation in planning of care and self-care to provide a sense of control over life. Encourage participation in social activities and in a support group. Refer for psychological counseling if adaptation does not occur within 6 months and patient is depressed or in denial.

(Table 22-5 continued)

TABLE 22-5 ◆ *Common Nursing Diagnoses, Expected Outcomes, and Interventions for Patients with Problems of the Musculoskeletal System* (Continued)

Nursing Diagnosis	Goals/Expected Outcomes	Nursing Interventions
Impaired home maintenance related to immobility or self-care deficits.	Patient will obtain needed assistance with home maintenance.	Assess degree of self-sufficiency and ability to perform ADLs before discharge. Contact social worker for coordination of home care if needed. Obtain bathing and homemaker assistance as needed. Assess continued need for in-home services weekly. Instruct in home adaptations that could aid in efforts at self-care, such as grab bars in bathroom, alterations in counter spaces for food preparation, transportation options for grocery shopping and appointments, or assistive devices for self-feeding and grooming. Assess degree of assistance significant other can provide for patient in home environment. Determine safety of home environment for patient.
Risk for disuse syndrome related to immobility or trauma.	Patient will not suffer permanent joint deformity or muscle atrophy.	Position joints as ordered; keep rest of body in correct alignment. Begin exercise of affected joint as soon as physician orders. Encourage active exercise of unaffected joints tid. Perform passive ROM as ordered tid. Assist with use of continuous passive motion (CPM) machine as ordered. Medicate regularly for pain while CPM machine is in use. Use heat and cold treatments before and after exercising stiff or deformed joints. Assess joints for contractures and muscles for atrophy q 24 hours. Encourage participation in ADLs to exercise joints.

should understand exactly what is going to be done and the steps to be taken in accomplishing the move. If the patient can help without damaging the diseased joint or limb, he should be encouraged to do so. If he is not able to help, the nurse explains the procedure to him and asks him to cooperate by relaxing completely during the procedure. Many times the patient is afraid that moving and turning will cause pain. Explanation as to the reason for moving and turning must be given so that confidence and cooperation is gained.

Nurses are sometimes tempted to allow their patient the privilege of assuming any position and remaining in that position as long as he is comfortable. They believe it is unkind and unnecessary to force the patient to move about when he is apparently resting and does not wish to be disturbed. **This is actually not a kindness and could be considered as nothing short of neglect when we know the terrible consequences of poor body posture and inactivity.** The nurse might also take the time to find a reason for the patient's assuming certain postures in bed. The patient may be curled up in a fetal position because he is trying to keep warm.

Elder Care Point . . . Older patients and those with poor circulation instinctively round their shoulders and tuck their limbs close to their bodies when they are chilly. Because of decreased subcutaneous fat and thin skin, the elderly often feel cooler than younger people in the same room. Feeling cold can increase feelings of pain and discomfort. Supply sufficient blankets, heat, socks, sweaters, and the like to keep the elderly person warm.

Orthopedic Bed Making   When traction is being applied to a patient's lower limb, or when he is in a large body cast, or external fixation device, it is not always convenient to arrange the bed linens in the conventional manner. (See the section on traction later in this chapter for information on safe handling.)

The nurse must improvise with the materials at hand. This requires some ingenuity and imagination, but it can be done. For example, two draw sheets may be used for the foundation of the bed in lieu of one large bottom sheet. This would be useful in instances in which the patient's lower limb is in a traction apparatus that uses a frame resting on the mattress, rather than one that hangs from an overhead frame. Obviously, there will be a good bit of disturbance of the frame and the traction if the large bottom sheet must be changed each time it becomes soiled. When two draw sheets are used, however, only the draw sheet under the patient's body need be changed often, and the frame will not be disturbed at all. When changing the bottom sheet for the patient in traction, the nurse begins on the side opposite the limb in traction. For example, if traction is on the left leg, work from right to left and from the foot of the bed toward the head. Top covers may be folded so that the limb in traction is not covered. If extra warmth is needed for the affected limb, it can be covered with a pillow case or towel.

> One important point to remember in changing the linen is to avoid pulling sheets from under the patient and causing friction against the skin.

Interventions to Prevent Disability   The formation of contractures (shortening of skeletal muscle tissue causing deformity), loss of muscle tone, and fixation of joints can be prevented in most cases by aggressive and consistent nursing intervention. The major components of the intervention are gradual mobilization, an exercise program, proper positioning, and instruction of the patient and family.

It is the responsibility of the nursing staff to initiate the necessary measures to prevent complications and to carry them out consistently. To wait for a physician's order for care that is within the domain of nursing is tantamount to negligence on the part of the nursing staff.

Within a matter of a few days the structures of immobilized muscles and joints begin to undergo changes. If no effort is made to prevent these changes the patient will become permanently disabled. The pathological changes most commonly associated with lack of motion include (1) contractures; (2) loss of muscle tone; and (3) **ankylosis** (permanent fixation of a joint).

Preventing contractures.   Joint motion is the result of a shortening and stretching of opposing muscles. For example, when the flexor muscles of the leg contract and shorten, the opposing extensor muscles relax and tighten. When skeletal muscles are not regularly stretched and contracted to their normal limits, they attempt to adapt themselves to this limited use by becoming shorter and less elastic. This "adaptive shortening" is called contracture. Contracture formation begins within 3 to 7 days after immobilization of a part, and the process usually is completed in 6 to 8 weeks. This means that there is no time to lose in planning and implementing nursing measures to prevent permanent and crippling disability. The most frequent contractures occurring in patients immobilized for long periods are "foot drop," knee and hip flexion contractures, "wrist drop," and contractures of the fingers and arms (Figure 22-3).

Loss of muscle tone.   *Muscle tone* is defined as the readiness of the muscle to go to work—to contract and relax as needed. If a muscle is not regularly

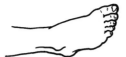
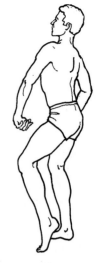

A. Foot drop, resulting from improper supoport of the feet while patient is confined to bed.

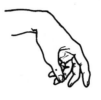

B. Wrist drop, resulting from improper support of the hand.

C. Flexion contracture of knee and hip force this patient to walk on tiptoe on the affected side. If both legs are involved, walking is impossible.

FIGURE 22-3   Joint contractures.

stimulated to action or if it is stretched beyond its normal limits for an extended time, it will lose its ability to contract and relax. For example, in foot drop, the calf muscles are shortened while the opposing flexor muscles are stretched. The result is loss of muscle tone and inability to produce motion.

Prevention of ankylosis.   Ankylosis is the result of injury or disease in which the tissues of the joint are replaced by a bony overgrowth that completely obliterates the joint. Sometimes it is extremely difficult to prevent this process (as, for example, in some types of arthritis). In these cases the physician may brace the joint in the position that will be most useful to the patient, even though there is no motion in the joint.

Gradual mobilization.   **The first step in nursing intervention to accomplish goals of progressive mobilization is assessment of the patient's ability to move his limbs, turn himself in bed, transfer himself from bed to chair and back again, and stand and walk.** These measurable signs of independent movement can represent various stages to which it is hoped the patient will gradually progress.

Setting goals for progressive mobilization must take into account the pathological condition causing immobility, any contraindications to movement of a body part, and the ability of the patient to understand and take part in carrying out the rehabilitation activities. In some cases passive exercises and positioning may be necessary until the patient is able to carry out exercises and positioning on his own. If the patient is to be cared for by family members once back at home, it is essential that they may be included in planning and setting goals of intervention to prevent disability and promote mobilization.

Exercise. Range of motion (ROM) exercises, both passive and active, are planned and carried out as soon as feasible after immobilization occurs as a result of disease, injury, or surgery. The exercises are done to maintain functional connective tissue within the joint and thereby ensure that every joint retains its function and mobility. **Range of motion exercises should be done three to four times a day.** Other kinds of exercises are planned according to each patient's needs and the amount of motion allowed by the physician.

Isometric exercises involve generating tension between two opposing sets of muscles. For example, trying to flex the lower arm while using the opposite hand to try to extend it. **Isometric exercise is used with caution in patients with hypertension, increased intracranial pressure, or congestive heart failure as there is a marked increase in blood pressure and heart rate during the exercise.**

Patients suffering from intense joint pain as a result of rheumatoid arthritis will need proper timing of exercises to follow administration of analgesic and antiinflammatory drugs. If at all possible, the schedule for drug administration should be adjusted so that the patient receives his first dose of medication in the morning *before* he begins his exercises.

Sometimes after joint surgery, especially after a total knee replacement, the surgeon will attach an apparatus to the affected limb that provides continuous passive motion (CPM) of the joint within the limits desired. The apparatus is driven by a motor and requires no effort on the part of the patient or nurse to move the limb (Figure 22-4). It usually is left on all day and is discontinued at night while the patient sleeps. When this kind of apparatus is used, the nursing care plan should include specific instructions regarding its proper use.

Exercises to recondition muscles for ambulation after injury or immobilization include quadriceps setting and gluteal setting. For *quadriceps setting* ask the patient to straighten the leg out while lying down and tense the leg muscles, straightening the knee, while raising the heel slightly. The contraction is held for a

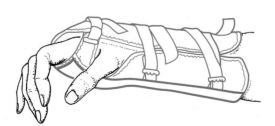

FIGURE 22-4   Wrist splint.

count of five and released for a count of 5. The exercise is done on each leg 10 to 15 times hourly while the patient is awake. Commercial breaks on television are a good reminder to do this. For gluteal setting, the buttocks are contracted and pinched together for a count of 4, and relaxed for a count of 5. This is also repeated 10 to 15 times hourly.

Positioning. Even though it is well understood by most nurses that turning a patient, changing his body position, and getting him up in a chair will prevent pressure ulcers, circulatory stasis, and respiratory and urinary complications, nurses may not realize that **changing body position does not necessarily guarantee freedom from orthopedic deformities. It also is necessary to change joint positions.**

Assessing a patient's need for proper positioning should include watching for early signs of muscle tightness and resistance to joint motion. This can be done during routine ROM exercises and could signal the need for positioning a body part so that the joint is extended and muscles are stretched to their normal capacity.

Patients with flaccid paralysis are not necessarily positioned in the same way as those with spastic paralysis. For example, a footboard is appropriate for proper positioning of the feet to prevent foot drop in a patient with flaccid paralysis. In contrast, putting the soles of the feet of a patient with spastic paralysis in contact with a footboard could trigger muscle contraction and aggravate the spasticity. Using a bed cradle to relieve pressure of the bed clothes can help prevent foot drop in these patients.

Some guiding principles for proper positioning are as follows:

◆ When the patient is lying on his back, place only one pillow under his head, and position it so that it also supports his neck and upper shoulders.

◆ *Don't* place two or three pillows under his head so that the neck is flexed and the chin is close to his chest.

◆ Place a folded towel under the achilles tendon to relieve pressure on the heels when the patient is lying on his back with the legs extended.

◆ *Don't* put a pillow under the knees or break the Gatch bed at the knees so that they are flexed.

◆ Use a trochanter roll and other supports along the leg and ankle to prevent abduction of the leg.

◆ *Don't* allow the patient to lie on his back with one leg flexed and rotated outward.

◆ Keep the arms extended and supported and the fingers extended or splinted with a hand splint.

◆ *Don't* allow the patient to keep his arms folded or flexed against his chest and his fingers curled into a fist.

Table 22-6 presents Positioning pointers for various types of fractures.

Special beds. A type of bed that often is used for patients in cervical traction is the Rotorest bed. This bed very slowly turns the patient about 300 times a day. It provides passive exercise and stimulates peristalsis without risk of injury to the patient. The bed has many other advantages, including several hatches that provide the nurse access to all of the common pressure points on the patient. There is a hatch for bowel and bladder care so that a bedpan can be placed without moving the patient. The back side of the patient can be bathed through the various hatches also. Once the nurse is familiar with the bed, it greatly simplifies care of the immobilized patient.

The FluidAir bed also is used for various types of immobilized patients. It is an air-fluidized bed and is very helpful in preventing pressure sores.

Use of slings and splints. A sling used to support the wrist or elbow should support both joints of the arm. The sling should be positioned so that the fastening at the neck area does not rub the neck or press on a neck vessel. When a splint is applied to an extremity, it should support the joint that is to be immobilized, fit properly without impeding circulation or slipping out of

place, and not cause increased pain (see Figure 22-4). If in doubt about how a particular splint is to be applied, seek help from another nurse or the physical therapist.

Teaching ambulation with assistive devices. For the convalescent patient or for one who may always need support while walking, crutches can mean the difference between freedom to move about and confinement to one location. Before attempting to walk with crutches, the patient should be instructed in their use and manipulation so that he can handle them safely and effectively.

The type of crutch to be used will depend on the extent of disability or paralysis and the patient's ability to bear weight and maintain balance. If the crutches are too short or too long, they can create problems of lifting and moving about for the patient. **Long crutches should be about 16 inches shorter than the patient's height. When in the standing position with axillary crutches, the axillary bar should be two finger breadths below the axilla. The elbow should be flexed at a 30-degree angle when the palms of the hands rest on the hand grip.** When walking, the patient should straighten the elbow and the wrist during weight bearing. One must bear in mind that the muscles of the arms, shoulders, back, and chest are all used in the manipulation of crutches. Because this is true, many physical therapists start the patient on special exercises to strengthen these muscles several weeks before the patient begins to use the crutches. Table 22-7 describes the gaits that can be used for crutch walking.

Although the physical therapist supervises the preparation and instruction of the patient before he starts to use crutches and then evaluates his ability to use them correctly, the nurse will sometimes be responsible for assisting a patient with crutch walking while he is in the hospital. **It is important that the patient not rest his body at the axilla on the top of the crutch; body weight should be borne by the arms on the hand rests of the crutches.** Table 22-8 presents steps for special maneuvers on crutches.

When teaching a patient to ambulate with a cane, be certain that the cane has a rubber tip. The cane is the right length if the hand grip is at hip level and the elbow is bent at a 30-degree angle when weight is placed on the cane. It should be used on the good side unless the physician orders otherwise. The tip of the cane should be placed 6 to 10 inches (15 to 25 cm) to the side and 6 inches (15 cm) in front of the near foot when walking. The patient should look straight ahead, rather than down, when ambulating. **The cane is advanced at the same time as the affected leg.** Advance the good leg first when going upstairs and the unaffected leg first going downstairs.

Walker height is correct when the person's elbow is bent at a 15- to 30-degree angle while standing upright

---

TABLE 22-6 ◆ *Positioning Patients with Fractures*	
Fracture	**Positioning**
Cervical spine	Before treatment—supine, immobilize neck with sandbags or Philadelphia collar. Turn with head well supported.
Thoracic spine	Position of comfort.
Lumbar spine	Avoid high sitting positions, logroll.
Pelvis	Stable fracture or after fixation—turn to side *opposite* fracture. Unstable—do not turn.
Hip	Before surgical treatment—turn *toward* fracture (avoid dislocation or further displacement of fragments) with pillows between legs. Postoperative—turn away from fracture until comfortable enough to turn on operative side, pillows between legs. Arthroplasty—maintain abduction at all time with abduction pillow or regular pillows between legs.
Shoulder/humerus	Elevate head of bed to comfort. Turn to side opposite fracture.
Forearm/foreleg	Elevate distal portion of extremity higher than heart.

Source: Maher, A. B., Salmond, S. W., Pellino, T. A. (1994). *Orthopaedic Nursing.* Philadelphia: Saunders, p. 751.

TABLE 22-7 ◆ *Crutch Gaits*

Gait	Description	Pattern
Four-point gait	Sequence 1. Advance left crutch. 2. Advance right foot. 3. Advance right crutch. 4. Advance left foot. Advantages: most stable crutch gait. Requirements: partial weight bearing on both legs.	
Three-point gait	Sequence 1. Advance both crutches forward with the affected leg and shift weight to crutches. 2. Advance unaffected leg and shift weight onto it. Advantages: allows the affected leg to be partially or completely free of weight bearing. Requirements: full weight bearing on one leg, balance, and upper-body strength.	
Two-point gait	Sequence 1. Advance left crutch and right foot. 2. Advance right crutch and left foot. Advantages: Faster version of the four-point gait, more normal walking pattern (arms and legs moving in opposition). Requirements: Partial weight bearing on both legs, balance.	

Source: deWit, S. C. (1994). *Rambo's Nursing Skills for Clinical Practice,* 4th ed. Philadelphia: Saunders, p. 536.

TABLE 22-8 ◆ *Special Maneuvers on Crutches*

Maneuver	Description
Walking upstairs	1. Stand at foot of stairs with weight on good leg and crutches. 2. Put weight on the crutch handles, and lift the good leg up on to the first step of the stairs (angels go up). 3. Put weight on the good leg, and lift other leg and the crutches up to that step. 4. Repeat for each stair step.
Walking downstairs	1. Stand at top of stairs with weight on good leg and crutches. 2. Shift weight completely on to the good leg, and put the crutches down on the next step. 3. Put weight on the crutch handles, and transfer injured leg down on the step with the crutches (devils go down). 4. Bring good leg down to that step. 5. Repeat for each stair step.
Sitting down	1. Crutch-walk to the chair. 2. Turn around slowly so that back is to the chair and the backs of the legs touch the seat of the chair. 3. Transfer both crutches to the side with the injured leg, and grasp both hand grips with that one hand. 4. As weight is supported on the crutches and good leg, reach back with free hand, and grasp the arm of the chair. 5. Lower slowly onto the chair seat, using the support of both the crutches and the chair. 6. Sit back in the chair, and elevate the leg, but not to an angle greater than 90 degrees at the hip. 7. Keep the knee slightly flexed when elevated because too much extension can decrease the circulation. 8. To get up, bring both crutches along the side of the injured leg, and grasp the hand grip firmly. Make sure the crutch tips are firmly on the floor. Place other hand on the arm of the chair, and push up. 9. After becoming upright, transfer one crutch to the other hand for walking.

Source: deWit, S. C. (1994). *Rambo's Nursing Skills for Clinical Practice,* 4th ed. Philadelphia: Saunders, p. 536.

and grasping the hand grips. The walker is lifted or rolled on its wheels slightly in front of the patient while leaning the body slightly forward. A step or two is taken into the walker, and then it is lifted and placed in front of the person again.

Elder Care Point... Many elderly patients are hospitalized with injuries they sustain from inability to maneuver crutches, cane, or walker. It is essential that elderly patients be taught proper methods of using assistive devices and that they receive supervised practice before they are discharged.

Psychosocial care. Unfortunately, many orthopedic conditions require prolonged periods of confinement to bed or, at best, immobilization of a part of the body and restricted physical activities. This leads to frustration and a feeling of hopelessness and despair on the part of the patient. When the patient is young and unaccustomed to depending on others for personal care, a reaction of anger and bitterness toward his plight may occur. If the patient is a wage earner or an active member of the family and one upon whom others are dependent, there is the additional burden of financial and social problems. Chapter 11 discusses psychosocial care of the immobile patient.

♦ Evaluation

Data are gathered through reassessment to determine whether expected outcomes are being met. Determining the effectiveness of interventions to treat pain is based mainly on subjective information given by the patient, but the nurse should also be alert to nuances of body language. Observation of the patient's ability to accomplish activities of daily living (ADLs) gives clues to improvement in mobility and activity tolerance.

Diagnostic test data, from x-rays and laboratory reports is used to determine the effectiveness of treatments. For example, x-rays show whether fractures are healing, laboratory reports help to determine how well rheumatoid arthritis is controlled.

Whenever expected outcomes are not being met, the plan of care must be revised. Collaboration among all health professionals working with the patient is vital to the creation of a realistic, workable, plan of care.

DISORDERS OF THE MUSCULOSKELETAL SYSTEM

♦ Soft Tissue Injuries

Sprains, strains, and dislocations are the kinds of injuries likely to occur when ligaments, muscles, and joints are subjected to undue stress, twisting, or a physical blow. A summary of strain, sprain, and dislocation is presented.

Sprain   A sprain is defined as a partial or complete tearing of the ligaments that hold various bones together to form a joint.

- **Most common sites:** ankle and knee.
- **Symptoms:** *grade 1* (mild)—tenderness at site; minimal swelling and loss of function; no abnormal motion.
- *Grade 2* (moderate)—more severe pain, especially with weight bearing; swelling and bleeding into joint; some loss of function.
- *Grade 3* (severe, complete tearing of fibers)—pain may be less severe, but swelling, loss of function, bleeding into joint, and loss of function are more marked.
- **Intervention:** RICE is the acronym used for treatment of sprains: **rest, ice, compression, and elevation.** Apply ice immediately after injury and for 24 to 72 hours. Apply the ice bag for 10 to 20 minutes every 1 to 2 hours during the day. Wrap with an elastic bandage snugly, being careful not to cut off circulation, and elevate the injured part. These measures can help minimize swelling and pain and stabilize the joint in proper alignment. The goal of treatment is to protect the ligament until it heals by scarring. Ligaments do not "grow" back together. An air cast, braces or supports are used only until a joint has been strengthened. If a joint is immobilized too long and muscles are not exercised, muscle atrophy, which begins in a matter of days, can cause permanent disability. In some cases surgical repair may be necessary. Grade III sprains often require a cast. Patients with Grade II or Grade III sprains need to rest the joint; crutches are needed for a lower-extremity sprain. Nonsteroidal antiinflammatory drugs (NSAIDs) should be prescribed on an around-the-clock basis for the first couple of days.

When cartilage in the knee or shoulder has been damaged, surgery is sometimes necessary as cartilage does not repair itself. Arthroscopy is performed and surgical repair can often be accomplished through the arthroscope. Experiments are under way using a procedure developed by Swedish researchers. Healthy cartilage cells are harvested from the patient and then cloned in the laboratory. The new cells are introduced into the damaged joint to regenerate healthy tissue after the damaged cartilage has been removed and the site has been prepared. The procedure can be used only on joints not affected by arthritis.

Strain   A strain is defined as a pulling or tearing of either muscle or tendon or both.

- **Most common sites:** hamstrings, quadriceps, and calf muscles.
- **Symptoms:** history of overexertion; soft-tissue swelling and pain; bleeding (ecchymosis, hemorrhagic spot) present if muscle is torn.
- **Intervention:** immediately apply ice and compression and rest the part. Surgical repair may be necessary.

Dislocation   A dislocation is defined as stretching and tearing of ligaments around a joint with complete displacement of a bone. *Subluxation* is a partial dislocation.

- **Most common sites:** shoulder, knee, temporomandibular joint.
- **Symptoms:** history of an outside force pushing from certain direction; severe pain aggravated by motion of joint; muscle spasm; abnormal appearance of joint. An x-ray will reveal displacement of bone.
- **Intervention:** reduction of displacement under anesthesia or manual or spontaneous reduction. Stabilization of joint and rehabilitation to minimize muscular atrophy and strengthen joint.

Bursitis   Bursitis may occur in any heavily used joint, but it most commonly occurs in the elbow, shoulder, or knee. Bursitis is an inflammation of a bursa, the sac-like structures that line freely movable joints. Symptoms are mild to moderate aching pain, localized to the joint, that is exacerbated by activity of the joint. Swelling may be present. There is localized tenderness to palpation.

Treatment is rest of the joint by altering activity that is aggravating it, antiinflammatory agents, ice massage, and a compression wrap if there is soft-tissue swelling. If these measures, plus time, do not relieve the symptoms, an injection of cortisone into the bursa is administered.

◆ Fractures

A fracture is a break or interruption in the continuity of a bone. The amount of injury to the neighboring tissues varies according to the type of fracture, but there is always some degree of tissue destruction, interference with the blood supply, and disturbance of muscle activity at the site of injury.

Elder Care Point . . . The elderly person is at risk of sustaining a fracture because of decreased reaction time, failing vision, lessened agility, and decreased muscle tone, all of which predispose to falls.

Types of Fractures   *Complete fracture* is when a bone breaks into two parts that are completely separated. An

incomplete fracture is when a bone breaks into two parts that are not completely separated.

- A *comminuted fracture* is one in which the bone is broken and shattered into more than two fragments.
- A *closed (simple) fracture* is one in which there is no break in the skin.
- An *open (compound) fracture* is one in which there is a break in the skin through which the fragments of broken bone protrude.
- A *greenstick fracture,* common in children, is one in which the bone is partially bent and partially broken.

Other types of fracture may be classified according to their x-ray appearance (Figure 22-5).

The primary aim in the treatment of fractures is to establish a sturdy union between the broken ends so that the bone can be restored to its former state of continuity. The healing and repair of a fracture begin immediately after the bone is broken and go through five stages:

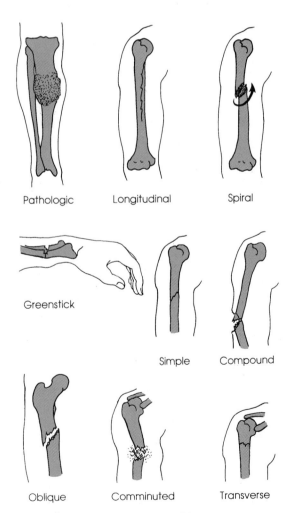

FIGURE 22-5   Types of fractures.

1. Blood oozes from the torn blood vessels in the area of the fracture, clots and begins to form a hematoma between the two broken ends of bone (1–3 days).

2. Other tissue cells enter the clot, and granulation tissue is formed. This tissue is interlaced with capillaries, and it gradually becomes firm and forms a bridge between the two ends of broken bone (3 days to 2 weeks).

3. Young bone cells enter the area and form a tissue called "callus." At this stage, the ends of the broken bone are beginning to "knit" together (2–6 weeks).

4. The immature bone cells are gradually replaced by mature bone cells (ossification), and the tissue takes on the characteristics of typical bone structure (3 weeks to 6 months).

5. Bone is resorbed and deposited depending on the lines of stress. The medullary canal is reconstructed. This is consolidation and remodeling (6 weeks to 1 year).

Nursing Assessment and Intervention Assessment of a suspected fracture includes noting pain, swelling, and discoloration, as well as a deformity in the contour of the bone. If there is a possibility of a fracture of an extremity, the affected limb is checked for pulse to determine whether circulation has been impaired. Nerve damage in a fractured leg is assessed by having the person flex and extend the foot and by touching a toe and asking the person which toe has been touched. To determine whether the nerve pathways have been damaged by a fracture in the arm, the person is asked to wave his hand, to identify fingers that have been touched by the examiner, and to grip the examiner's hand. Paralysis and total loss of sensation in the extremities may indicate damage to the spinal cord.

Pain is not always present when a fracture has occurred. Numbness and tingling also can accompany a fracture. **If there is some question as to whether or not a bone has been broken, it is best to treat the injury as if there were a fracture.** Proper first aid will be helpful and will prevent further trauma and pain regardless of the degree of injury to a bone.

The emergency treatment and nursing care of fractures consist of preventing shock and hemorrhage and the immediate immobilization of the part to avoid unnecessary damage to the soft tissue adjacent to the fracture.

The words *splint it as it lies* mean exactly that. An inexperienced person should never attempt to straighten or set a broken bone. **The injured part should be immobilized in the position in which it is found at the time of injury and should be supported firmly so that it will not be jarred when the victim is being moved.** If it is available, ice in a plastic bag can be applied to the fracture area to help minimize edema.

If the broken bone has pierced the skin and bleeding is severe, apply direct pressure over the wound or compress the appropriate pressure point. Cover the open area with a clean dressing. Try to avoid introducing infectious agents into the wound, and remember the need for the prevention and treatment of shock.

In the emergency room or clinic, the patient will be examined by a physician and an x-ray will be ordered if fracture is suspected. After an x-ray film of the injured part has been made and the type of fracture and extent of damage have been established, the physician will decide which method to use in reducing the fracture and providing immobilization.

Assessment for neurovascular status and infection is performed at least once each shift (Table 22-9). When a fracture is fresh, this assessment should be performed

---

TABLE 22-9 ◆ *Assessment of Neurovascular Status*	
This assessment format should be followed at least once each shift for any patient who has suffered a musculoskeletal injury.	
Skin color	Inspect the area around the injury and distal to the injury for increasing signs of discoloration that might indicate internal bleeding. Area may be pale if arterial flow is impeded.
Skin temperature	Feel the area distal to the injury with the back of the hand; if the skin is increasingly hot to the touch, report this to the physician.
Pulses	Palpate pulse sites distal to the injury; compare bilaterally. Report marked differences from one side to the other to the physician.
Movement	Ask the patient to move actively the affected area or the area distal to the injury. Note the amount of discomfort. If active movement is not possible, passively move the area distal to the injury. This checks for swelling and potential nerve damage.
Sensation	Ask whether numbness or tingling is present (paraesthesia). Touch the area distal to the injury gently with the end of a paper clip in a manner so that the patient cannot see where you are touching. Ask what this feels like and where it is felt. Loss of sensation may indicate nerve damage.
Pain	Ask the patient to evaluate the pain by location, nature, and intesity. Note whether pain is increasing; evaluate whether pain-control measures are effective.
Capillary refill	Press down on a nail bed distal to the injury with the side of a clip of a pen until blanching occurs; let up, and count the time it takes for color to return. Usual color should return in 3 to 5 sec.

every 2 to 4 hours. The cast should be inspected for problems, such as flattened areas, soft spots, cracking, and crumbling. Traction devices must be assessed to see that they are in correct position and that the weights are hanging free. The patient's body position should be assessed for proper alignment.

Every immobilized patient should be consciously assessed for the various problems of immobility. **The most commonly found problems include skin breakdown, urinary tract infection or stones, and constipation.**

Elder Care Point . . . When the elderly person has to be immobilized because of trauma and fractures, the complications of immobility are much more likely to occur than in a younger person. Aggressive nursing care and careful assessment for signs of complications are very important. Respiratory problems can be prevented by scheduled, supervised deep-breathing and coughing or the use of an incentive spirometer.

Attention to pain control is important, especially when the patient is adjusting to traction or a new cast. It is essential to try to keep the patient's mind occupied, as boredom can greatly increase discomfort.

A patient with a fracture sometimes is immobilized for an extended period, which interferes with his usual roles. The patient may be very worried about usual responsibilities and about employment and finances. Allowing ventilation of concerns and fears and then assisting with solving problems can often bring some peace of mind.

Treatment   To facilitate the process of repair and ensure proper healing of the bone without deformity or loss of function, the surgeon must bring the two broken ends together in proper alignment and then immobilize the affected part until healing is complete. The procedure for bringing the two fragments of bone into proper alignment is called *reduction of the fracture.*

Trials are under way to test a new way of repairing fractured bones by using a liquid bone-like paste that can be injected directly into the fracture. The substance hardens in 10 minutes and within 12 hours is as strong as the natural bone—or stronger. The body seems to treat it as real bone and over time transforms it into natural bone.

Reduction, Surgery, and Stabilization   Four methods of reducing a fracture are (1) closed reduction; (2) open reduction; (3) internal fixation; and (4) external fixation.

In *closed reduction* the bone is manipulated into alignment; no surgical incision is made. A general anesthetic may be given before the fracture is reduced.

An *open reduction* is done after a surgical incision is made through the skin and down to the bone at the site of the fracture. In cases of open (compound) fractures and comminuted fractures, an open reduction has always been necessary so that the area can be adequately cleansed and bone fragments removed.

When a fracture cannot be properly reduced by either open or closed reduction and it is impossible to guarantee adequate union of the bone fragments, the physician must perform a procedure called *internal fixation* of the bone. This means that pins, nails, screws, or metal plates must be used to stabilize the position of the two broken ends. Internal fixation is particularly useful in treating fractures in elderly patients whose bones are brittle and may not heal properly (Figure 22-6).

One of the most common internal fixation procedures is performed on a fractured hip: open reduction and internal fixation (ORIF). An incision is made, the fracture is realigned, and the bone is secured with pins, screws, nails, or plates. A drain will be in place for at least 2 days. If a prosthesis is implanted, there will be more blood loss and the patient will be receiving autotransfusion of salvaged blood after surgery. Administration of IV antibiotics to reduce the risk of infection is standard. Care includes maintaining good alignment of the affected leg, preventing complications of immobility, and keeping the patient comfortable with pain-control measures.

External fixation of fractures involves the use of a device composed of a sturdy external frame to which are attached pins that have been drilled into the bone fragments. Figure 22-7 shows a fixator that is applied by inserting heavy pins on either side of the fracture and then reducing the fracture by tightening nuts attached to the connecting rods.

External fixation is indicated when (1) there are massive open fractures with extensive soft-tissue damage; (2) infected fractures do not heal properly; and when there is (3) multiple trauma with one or more fractures and other injuries such as burns, chest injury, or head injury. External fixators are commonly used for fractures of an extremity or of the pelvis. The fixator frame is large and bulky and may cause the patient a body image disturbance. If there is tissue damage and dressings are used around the pins, consideration for patient comfort during dressing changes is necessary. Medication 30 minutes ahead of time, being well organized with supplies and actions, and using a gentle touch will be appreciated.

Because the pin sites are left open to the air during convalescence, special daily care is necessary to prevent infection. Pins must be kept clean and dry. As soon as it is feasible, the patient is taught to care for the pin sites and to report any signs of infection. Physician preferences for pin care varies, so follow doctor's orders for cleansing or check the agency's policy. Most frequently, hydrogen peroxide is utilized. *Standard Precautions* must be followed when providing pin care.

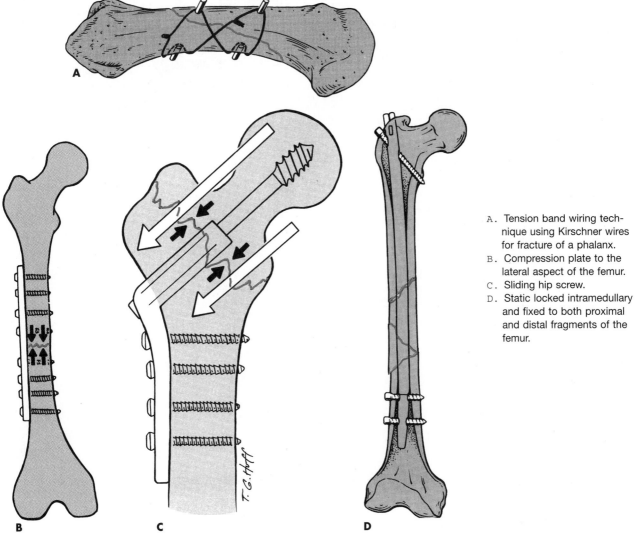

A. Tension band wiring technique using Kirschner wires
   for fracture of a phalanx.
B. Compression plate to the
   lateral aspect of the femur.
C. Sliding hip screw.
D. Static locked intramedullary
   and fixed to both proximal
   and distal fragments of the
   femur.

FIGURE 22-6   Examples of internal fixation. (From Browner, B. D., et al. [1992]. *Skeletal Trauma,* Philadelphia: Saunders, pp. 253, 254, 942, 1551. Reprinted with permission.)

External fixation has the advantage of allowing more freedom of movement than traction or casting and usually is more comfortable. With good stability there is no need for restricting the patient to bed. In some cases it is possible for the patient to bear weight on his affected limb, but even if this is not allowed, he is free to move about on his own, perform physical therapy exercises, and avoid many of the problems of immobility. External fixation is preferred over treatment by casting or traction whenever possible.

Nonunion of a fracture can be treated by an electrical bone growth–stimulating device, which may be an external electromagnetic device, a percutaneous stimulator with electrodes placed at the fracture site, or an implanted direct current stimulator whose current stimulates osteogenesis (growth of bone cells). Using such a device can prevent further surgery and bone grafting. This treatment is based on the fact that bone has inherent electrical properties used in healing. Elec-

trical coils or electrodes are used to induce weak electrical current in the bone.

In elderly patients who have suffered a fracture of the head of the femur, the surgeon may choose to take out the broken head fragments. He replaces the fragments with a prosthesis designed with a ball to replace the head of the femur and is shaped so that it can be fitted into or onto the shaft of the femur in such a way that the patient can bear weight on it. Although a prosthesis is not as good as a normal hip joint, many patients who have such a prosthesis are able to walk again and use the limb effectively. Total hip replacement (THR) for osteoarthritis is discussed later in this chapter.

Think about . . . If you are in the park and you observe a child fall from a tree and obviously suffer a broken forearm, what steps would you take to assist?

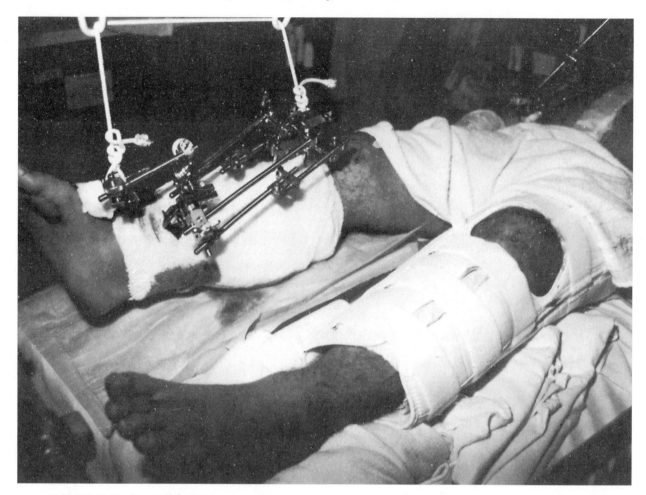

FIGURE 22-7   **External fixation.** (*Source:* Cardona, V. D. [1994]. *Trauma Nursing,* 2nd ed. Philadelphia: Saunders, p. 574.)

Casts   Casts are used to hold bone fragments in place after reduction. A cast is rigid and immobilizes the body part that is mending while allowing movement of other body parts. Casts are made from a variety of materials. Fiber glass and polyester-cotton knit casts are used more frequently than the traditional plaster of Paris casts now. The newer materials are lighter weight, dry quickly, and can bear weight within 30 minutes of application. Some physicians still use plaster of Paris casts for lower extremities because these can bear more weight and will stay intact longer with weight bearing than the lighter-weight casts.

There are four main groups of casts: arm casts, leg casts, cast braces, and body or spica casts. Leg and arm casts may cover all or part of the limb (Figure 22-8). These are called *long-leg* or *short-leg* casts, depending on how much leg they cover. A *cast shoe* is a canvas sandal with a thick sole for weight bearing that fits over the bottom of the leg cast. A *spica* cast covers the trunk of the body and one or two extremities. There are long-leg and short-leg spicas that cover one or both legs and shoulder spicas that include the trunk and one arm.

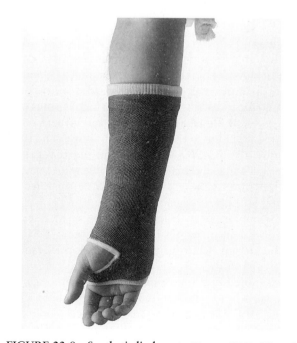

FIGURE 22-8   **Synthetic limb cast.** (*Source:* 3M Healthcare.)

Each type of cast presents unique problems of mobility and self-care activities.

Before a cast is applied, the patient's skin is thoroughly cleansed with soap and water, and any breaks in the skin are reported to the doctor if she is not aware of them. Shaving is not done unless surgery is to be performed before applying the cast. In this case, a special orthopedic surgical cleanser prepared according to hospital procedure is used.

In emergencies, a thorough explanation of what is going to be done is not always possible. In all other cases, however, it is best if the patient is prepared for the type of cast that will be applied, the precautions that must be taken while the cast is drying, and any special devices that may be put on his bed to help him turn and move about in the bed. An example is the trapeze bar attached to an overhead frame, which allows the patient to lift himself and turn without strain on the affected part.

Although fiber glass and polyester-cotton knit casts dry very quickly, the newly applied plaster cast is usually not dry for about 48 hours. While the plaster is damp, its shape can be changed by careless handling or improper support. It follows, therefore, that extreme care must be used in moving the patient or the cast during this time. **During the first 24 to 48 hours after any cast has been applied to an extremity, the extremity should be elevated to minimize swelling.**

Ice bags can be used to help control swelling. Because the weight of an ice bag could make an indentation in a wet plaster cast, the ice bags should be only about half full, and they should be laid against the cast and propped in position, rather than set on top of it.

When the patient is transferred from the stretcher to the bed, there must be enough help available so that the patient is not "tumbled" into bed. Pillows for support should be placed on the bed *before* moving the patient on to them. Pillows are used to support the curves of large casts so that there will be no cracking or flattening of the cast by the weight of the body.

The patient in a body cast or spica is more comfortable if pillows are not put under the head and shoulders because they push the chest and abdomen against the front of the cast, causing an uncomfortable crushing sensation and dyspnea.

Turnbuckles or bars between the legs of a cast are never to be used as handles for lifting and turning the patient. Even after the cast is dry, these braces may be dislocated or pulled out of the cast.

An effort should be made to use only the palms of the hands or the flat surface of the extended fingers when moving a wet plaster cast because fingertips can sink into the damp plaster and make impressions through the thickness of the cast, thus pressing mounds of plaster against the tissues under the cast. These can harden and in time lead to pressure sores. A plaster cast generates heat as it dries and assessments must be made frequently of the amount of heat generated and the sensation under the cast that the patient feels; burns can occur. A dry plaster cast is white, has a shiny surface, and will resound when tapped. A wet plaster cast is grayish and dull in appearance and will give a dull thud when tapped.

Any body part encased in a cast is in danger of pressure against nerves and blood vessels and resultant nerve damage or serious obstruction to blood flow. Periodic assessment of the patient's neurovascular status is an essential part of the nursing care plan for a patient in a cast (see Table 22-9). Failure to notice the early signs of pressure on nerves or blood vessels and to initiate preventive measures can cause an avoidable paralysis and possibly gangrene.

A thorough assessment of a patient in a cast should include the following:

♦ *Listen to the patient's complaints.* He may report numbness, a tingling sensation, increased pain with motion of his fingers or toes, or sharp localized pain; any of these symptoms could be caused by pressure from a tight cast. Do not attempt to judge whether his complaints are justified. **If elevating the limb does not relieve the patient's complaints within 30 minutes, notify the physician.**

♦ Check frequently to see whether the cast is properly supported or if there is undue pressure on any part of the body. A sharp, localized, burning pain could mean the beginning of a pressure sore. This should be reported so that the surgeon or orthopedic technician can cut a "window" in the cast to relieve pressure.

♦ Lean down and smell at the edges of the cast to detect any foul odor that might indicate the presence of infection.

Daily care. After the cast is thoroughly dry and the initial swelling under the cast has subsided, the nurse must concern herself with the cleanliness of the patient and the cast. The problems involved will vary according to the type of cast and the area it covers. All parts of the body not included in the cast should be bathed daily, using care not to wet a plaster cast. Patients may have permission to shower with a synthetic cast; a plastic covering is secured over the cast and taped to the skin and the patient is asked not to place the casted area directly under the stream of water.

The skin around the edges of the cast should receive special attention, including massage with lotion and close observation for signs of pressure or breaks in the skin. The edges of plaster casts tend to crumble, with bits of plaster dropping down inside the cast and causing the patient discomfort and skin irritation. This can be avoided by covering the rims of the cast with stockinette or tape.

When a bedpan is used by the patient in a spica, there is the possibility of a backward flow of urine under the cast unless the head of the bed is slightly elevated. Because the patient cannot bend at the hips to sit up on the pan, the head of the bed should be elevated on shock blocks or some other device and the lumbar area of the cast supported to prevent cracking.

Itching is a common complaint. Patients must be instructed not to use sharp objects such as pencils or rulers to scratch under the cast. These can, of course, tear the skin, leaving an open break for the entrance of bacteria. An experienced orthopedic nurse has found that forceful injection of air, using a 50-mL bulb syringe or one with a plunger and directing the air under the cast, can relieve intense itching. A hair dryer on the low setting that blows air into the cast also may relieve itching.

When a cast is removed, the underlying skin is usually dry and scaly. Cleansing of these areas should be done in consultation with the physician, because the type of care to be given will depend on whether another cast is to be applied. In any case, overenthusiastic scrubbing of the area must be avoided to prevent damage to the deeper layers of skin. Nursing interventions for selected problems of a patient in a cast are summarized in Table 22-5.

Synthetic casts. In addition to their advantage of setting quickly, synthetic casts are not as heavy as plaster casts and therefore allow more freedom of movement. They also are less bulky, do not crumble as easily, and are less likely to be damaged by wetting.

In spite of all their advantages, synthetic casts do have limited use. They cost three to seven times more than plaster casts. They are less easily molded to a body part and are not suitable for immobilizing the fragments of severely displaced bones or for stabilizing serious fractures. Their rough exterior surfaces can damage the skin and tend to snag clothing and other soft materials. They are used mostly for upper-extremity fractures.

Think about . . . Your patient has an arm cast in place and is complaining of severe itching inside the cast. What could you do to help relieve the problem?

The cast brace or cast shoe permits early ambulation and weight bearing in patients who have a fracture in the shaft of the femur. It is applied 2 to 6 weeks after the fracture has been reduced, during which time skeletal traction has been used to hold the fragments in alignment during healing.

As soon as the cast brace is dry, the patient is allowed to get out of bed. His gradual progression from standing to partial weight bearing, full weight bearing, and walking is supervised by the physical therapist.

Traction   Traction is the application of a mechanical *pull* to a part of the body for the purpose of extending and holding that part in a certain position during immobilization. Through a system of ropes and pulleys, weights are attached to a fixed point below the area of injury or disease. The apparatus is rigged so that the weights on one end and the weight of the patient's body on the other will pull the affected part in opposite directions, thus straightening and holding that part in the desired position. There are several ways to accomplish this.

The two general types of traction are *skeletal* and *skin*. In skeletal traction, the surgeon inserts pins, wires, or tongs directly through the bone at a point distal to the fracture so that the force of pull from the weights is exerted directly on the bone. With skin traction, a bandage such as moleskin or ace-adherent is applied to the limb below the site of fracture and the pull is exerted on the limb in this manner.

Traction may be continuous, as in the alignment and resultant immobility of fractured bones, or it may be intermittent, as in traction on the spinal column to relieve the symptoms of a slipped disc or muscle spasms.

The system of ropes, pulleys, and weights used to provide the various kinds of traction can be very confusing at first, but the principles on which traction is based are actually quite simple. Some types of traction are named for the orthopedic surgeons who first designed them. Figure 22-9 illustrates some of the different types of traction.

- *Bryant's traction* for small children with fracture of the femur uses the weight of the child's lower body to pull the bone fragments of the fractured leg into alignment. To accomplish this, the child's buttocks should just clear the mattress and his legs should be at a 90-degree angle to his trunk.

- *Buck's extension* is a simple skin traction that is used to treat muscle spasms from fractures of the hip or femur preoperatively and for dislocation of the hip.

- *Russell's traction* uses a knee sling to provide support of the affected leg. It is commonly used to treat fractures of the end of the tibia in the leg.

- *Balanced suspension* with the *Thomas splint* and *Pearson attachment* is used to treat fractures of the femur and pelvis. The Thomas splint supports the thigh and knee and provides countertraction. The Pearson attachment supports the lower leg.

- *Cervical traction* can be provided through the use of tongs inserted into the skull or by using a halo device (see Chapter 14).

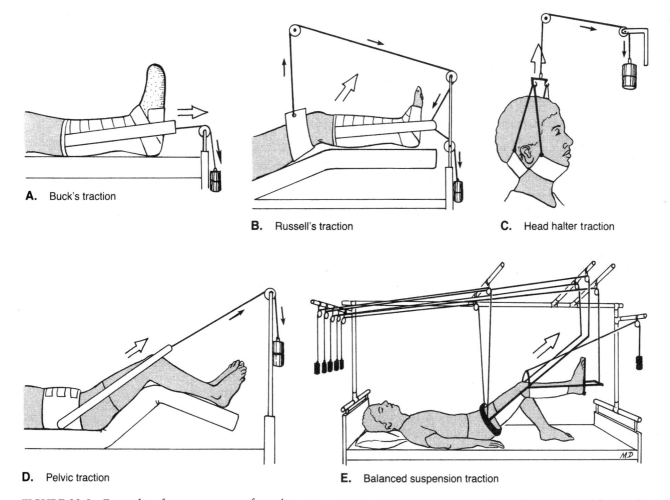

A. Buck's traction

B. Russell's traction

C. Head halter traction

D. Pelvic traction

E. Balanced suspension traction

FIGURE 22-9   Examples of common types of traction. (*Sources:* Black, J. M., Matassarin-Jacobs, E. [1993]. *Luckmann and Sorensen's Medical-Surgical Nursing: A Psychophysiologic Approach,* 4th ed. Philadelphia: Saunders, p. 1885.)

- *Sidearm traction* is indicated when stabilization is needed to treat fractures and dislocations of the arm and shoulder.
- *Pelvic traction* with a pelvic belt or sling is indicated for pelvic fractures and other pelvic injuries.

Care of patients with injury to the spinal column and spinal cord is covered in Chapter 14. The chapter also includes care of the patient with cervical tongs, halo traction, laminectomy, and spinal fusion.

Nursing Assessment and Intervention   Most patients in traction for the treatment of fractures and other orthopedic conditions requiring a continuous pull on a part of the body must lie on their backs, with only a limited amount of turning permitted. This is not an excuse for neglecting care of the patient's body. He must still be kept clean and comfortable and free of pressure sores.

If the physician does not permit turning the patient far enough to allow for adequate back care, the patient may use a trapeze bar to lift himself so that back care can be given and the bottom sheet changed or tightened. The patient should be instructed to lift himself straight up so that the amount of pull exerted on the limb in traction will not be altered. This same maneuver can be used when the patient is placed on a bedpan. A small, "fracture" bedpan should be used and the lower back supported by a small pillow or folded blanket.

Frequent observations of both the patient and the traction apparatus are necessary to protect the patient and ensure that the traction is effective. Table 22-10 presents points of care.

Think about... Your patient is in balanced leg traction. Can you list the points you should check before leaving the room to ensure that the traction is working properly and the patient's safety is protected?

Complications of Fractures   The healing of a fracture can be impeded by improper alignment and inadequate immobilization of the bone. Poor alignment almost inevitably leads to some permanent deformity. Inadequate immobilization of the bone allows continued twisting, shearing, and abnormal stresses that

TABLE 22-10 ◆ Points of Care for the Patient in Traction

- Keep the patient in the center of the bed in a supine position.
- Keep the body part in traction in a straight line with the trunk. **Misalignment causes pain.**
- *Be sure the weights are hanging free.* If the weights are resting on or against any support, such as the foot of the bed or the floor, the purpose of the traction is defeated. Be careful not to bump against the weights when walking around the foot of the bed. This can be painful to the patient and may cause damage to the healing bone. It is not necessary to lift the weights when pulling the patient up in bed. The amount of pull on the limb will remain the same as long as the weights are hanging free. Also check that the ropes run over the midline of the pulley without interference. Keep knots away from the pulleys, and arrange bedding so that it doesn't interfere with the ropes and pulleys.
- *Check the position of the patient, making sure his body weight is counteracting the pull of the weights.* Should the patient slip down in bed so that his feet are resting against the footboard, there will be a loss of force exerted on the limb.
- Observe all bony prominences for signs of impaired circulation and pressure or tissue necrosis.
- To prevent pressure sores, be sure slings and ropes are not pressing against or cutting into an area of the extremity.
- When a patient has skeletal traction, observe the sites of entry of pins, tongs, etc., for signs of infection.
- Devise a systematic routine for observing the patient and the apparatus at specified times during the day so that no aspect of the assessment will be overlooked.

prohibit a strong bony union. Notify the physician if the patient states that she can feel the bone fragments grating against each other (**crepitation**).

Infection.   Infection of the tissue at the fracture site is probably the most serious impediment to healing. It is of special concern in open comminuted fractures. Systemic infections, inadequate levels of serum calcium and phosphorus, vitamin deficiency, and generalized atherosclerosis—which deprives the healing site of adequate blood supply—also can complicate a fracture by delaying healing. It is important to monitor the patient's temperature and white blood cell (WBC) count for elevations and to monitor the appearance of the area carefully for redness, swelling, heat, or purulent drainage.

Osteomyelitis.   Osteomyelitis is a bacterial infection of the bone. The causative organism is most often *Staphylococcus aureus*, which enters the bloodstream from a distant focus of infection, such as a boil or furuncle, or from an open wound, as in an open (compound) fracture. It occurs most often in older adults and is usually found in the tibia or fibula, vertebrae, or at the site of a prosthesis, but it can also occur in other patients at any age.

Osteomyelitis has a sudden onset with severe pain and marked tenderness at the site, high fever with chills, swelling of adjacent soft parts, headache, and malaise.

Diagnosis of osteomyelitis is made on the basis of (1) laboratory findings indicating an acute infection, for example, high sedimentation rate and white cell count; (2) x-rays, which may show bone destruction 7 to 10 days after onset of the disease; (3) history of injury to the part, open fracture, boils, furuncles, or other infections; and (4) biopsy, in which the bone sample exhibits signs of necrosis.

The earlier the condition is diagnosed and treatment is begun, the better the prognosis for the patient with osteomyelitis, as it can be difficult to eradicate. Specific treatment includes elimination of the infection through the use of antibiotics for 4 to 6 weeks and immobilization of the affected limb for complete rest. Surgical incision for drainage of the abscess and removal of dead bone and debris from the site of infection is necessary. Sometimes amputation is the only cure. The care of a patient with an infection is presented in Chapter 6.

Fat embolism.   Fat embolism can be one of the most serious complications of a fracture of a bone that has an abundance of marrow fat (e.g., the long bones, pelvis, and ribs). A high percentage of patients with multiple fractures resulting from severe trauma die from this complication. It occurs at any age, but is most commonly seen in young men age 20 to 40 and in older persons between 70 and 80 years of age. Not all fat emboli are fatal. To be life-threatening, the fat globules released when a bone is fractured must be large enough or sufficient in number to occlude a blood vessel partially or completely. The fat embolism arises from injury of the fat-bearing bone marrow and rupture of small venules in the area, thus permitting the entrance of fat globules into the circulation. **Embolism, if it occurs, happens within 48 hours of fracture.**

> The first sign of fat embolism is usually a change in mental status followed by respiratory distress, tachypnea, rapid pulse, fever, and petechiae (a measles-like rash over the chest, neck, upper arms, or abdomen). Signs must be reported immediately, as there is about an 80% mortality rate from this complication.

Crackles and wheezes will be heard when auscultating the lungs if emboli are present.

The nurse should stay with the patient; put him in a high Fowler's position, if possible, to ease the dyspnea; remain calm; begin oxygen administration at 2 to 3 L/minute if it is available; and summon the doctor immediately. Hydration with IV fluids is usually ordered.

Elder Care Point... The elderly patient with a fractured hip is at high risk for fat embolism. Be especially vigilant in assessing for signs and symptoms of this complication.

Compartment syndrome. Compartment syndrome occurs in one or more muscle compartments of the extremities. It is caused by external or internal pressure and seriously restricts circulation to the area. External pressure can occur from dressings or casts that are too tight. Internal pressure occurs from excessive IV fluid infusion, inflammation, and edema (a shifting of fluid from the vascular spaces to the intercellular spaces). The increased fluid puts pressure on the tissues, nerves, and blood vessels, thereby decreasing blood flow. Considerable pain results.

> Signs and symptoms of compartment syndrome include edema, pain, pallor, tingling, paresthesia, numbness, weak pulse, cyanosis, paresis, and severe pain. The pressure can cause permanent tissue and nerve damage if unrelieved. The physician should be notified immediately if this complication is suspected as permanent loss of function will result if the problem is not relieved.

If a cast is in place, the front of it will need to be split through all layers of the material. Dressings will be cut or replaced. Surgical fasciotomy (linear incisions in the fascia down the extremity) may be necessary to relieve the pressure on the nerves and blood vessels if other measures do not relieve the problem.

◆ Carpal Tunnel Syndrome

Carpal tunnel syndrome is a nerve problem that occurs when the median nerve is compressed as it passes through the carpal tunnel in the wrist. It produces pain, numbness and tingling of the hand, particularly at night. Repetitive movements of the hands and wrists, such as occurs in certain types of assembly factory work and in computer keyboarding, sometimes is a cause.

Treatment by rest, splinting, changing the angle of the wrist during repetitive movements, or steroid injection may solve the problem. If the symptoms are of long duration, there is muscle atrophy, or sensory loss in the fingers and hands is progressive, surgery is indicated. Surgical decompression of the medial nerve by transection of the carpal ligament is performed, usually as an outpatient procedure.

◆ Bunion (Hallux Valgus)

A bunion is the most common foot problem. A bunion is a painful swelling of the bursa that occurs when the great toe deviates laterally at the metatarsophalangeal joint. It may be congenital, or it may occur from ill-fitting shoes. Bunions are more common in females than in males.

Wearing open-toed shoes of soft leather or athletic shoes that are wider in the toe area helps reduce pain. Metatarsal pads can relieve some of the pressure. Corticosteroid injections are placed in the joint if active bursitis is present. Analgesics are used for discomfort. Bone resection of the first metatarsal on the big toe that removes bony overgrowth and bursa (the bunion) is performed when walking becomes too painful.

◆ Inflammatory Disorders: Arthritis

The word *arthritis*, translated literally, means inflammation of a joint. Most laypersons use the term to cover any kind of joint disease; however, specialists in the treatment of arthritis limit its meaning to diseases of the joint that are the result of inflammatory changes. There are approximately 100 different types of arthritis, ranging from hereditary disorders such as hemophilic arthritis to the more common types in which the exact cause is known.

In adults, the two most prevalent forms of arthritis are osteoarthritis and rheumatoid arthritis. A comparison of these two types of arthritis is shown in Table 22-11. All forms of arthritis are capable of producing joint pain and disability. Medical management, surgical procedures, and nursing interventions are intended to minimize the problems associated with inflammatory changes in the joint, deformities and limitation of motion, and the systemic reactions to these pathological changes.

Osteoarthritis Osteoarthritis is a noninflammatory degenerative joint disease that can affect any weight-bearing joint. It usually occurs after age 40 and most commonly presents between age of 50 to 60. Recently scientists identified a faulty gene that causes one form of osteoarthritis. Causes of other types are unknown. In people with osteoarthritis there seems to be lessened production of the collagen material that strengthens the cartilage that covers and protects joints in the body. With time and use, the joint becomes thickened and withstands weight bearing poorly, with consequent damage to the cartilage. The synovial cells then release enzymes that cause further cartilage degeneration. **Osteoarthritis occurs asymmetrically and typically affects only one or two joints.** Aching pain with joint movement and stiffness with limitation of mobility are the chief complaints. On assessment, joint deformity and the presence of nodules may be found.

Treatment consists of pain management, exercise, weight reduction if the patient is overweight, and maintenance of joint function. Salicylates, acetaminophen, or NSAIDs may be used.

TABLE 22-11 ◆ *Comparison of Rheumatoid Arthritis and Osteoarthritis*		
Characteristic	**Rheumatoid Arthritis**	**Osteoarthritis**
Definition	A systemic disease, but pathological changes and disability result from chronic inflammation of the joints.	A progressive degenerative joint disease.
Pathology	Chronic inflammation of synovial membranes and formation of chronic granulation tissue (pannus) in the joint. Pannus capable of eroding cartilage in joints and spreading to bone, ligaments, and tendons.	Microscopic changes in the cartilage in the joint. Eventually there is loss of cartilage, bony enlargement, and malalignment of joints.
Etiology	Unknown. Evidence that the pathological changes are immunological.	Unknown. May be caused by "wear and tear" of aging.
Rheumatoid factors (autoantibodies)	Usually present.	Usually absent.
Age at onset	30 to 40 years.	50 to 60 years; rarely before 40.
Weight	Normal or underweight.	Usually overweight.
General state of health	Usually anemic, "chronically ill." Low-grade fever and slight leukocytosis.	Well nourished.
Appearance of joints	Early; soft-tissue swelling. Late: ankylosis: extreme deformity. Joint involvement usually symmetric and generalized.	Early: slight joint enlargement. Late: enlargement more pronounced, slight limitation of motion. Joints usually involved are weight bearing; spine, hips, and knees.
Muscles	Pronounced muscular atrophy, particularly in later stages.	Usually not affected.
Other	Morning stiffness, pain on motion, swelling and tenderness of joints. Subcutaneous nodules. Typical rheumatoid changes seen on radiograph.	Stiffness, relieved by moderate motion; joint malalignment. Symptoms increase in cold, wet weather.

Elder Care Point . . . NSAIDs are not recommended for use in all elderly because of their side effects and interactions with other drugs an elderly patient may be taking. NSAIDs decrease the effectiveness of ACE inhibitors used for hypertension and heart failure and increase the effects of anticoagulants.

Corticosteroid injection into the joint is performed if oral medication does not control the problem. Exercises for joint mobility are encouraged. Surgery or joint replacement may be done to relieve severe pain and improve mobility. The hip and knee are the most common sites for joint replacement.

Nursing interventions for osteoarthritis include teaching the patient to balance exercise and rest, moist heat application, the use of imagery and diversion to reduce pain, and encouragement to maintain weight within normal limits to decrease joint stress. Quadriceps-strengthening exercises may relieve pain and disability of the knee.

Rheumatoid Arthritis   Rheumatoid arthritis is an inflammatory disease of the joints. It most frequently begins between the age of 30 and 60. There is a familial tendency. The cause is not known, but it is thougt that it is the result of an autoimmune defect or an infectious agent.

The signs and symptoms of rheumatoid arthritis are joint pain, warmth, edema, limitation of motion, and multiple joint stiffness in the morning lasting more than 1 hour. The joints of the hands, wrists, and feet are the most commonly affected, and involvement is usually symmetrical. Subcutaneous nodules may appear over bony prominences. Systemic symptoms of low-grade fever, weight loss, and malaise also are present. Considerable joint deformity and consequent dysfunction can occur.

Elder Care Point . . . Pain or immobility of joints interferes with self-care activities. The elderly patient may not be able to maintain locomotion or may not be able to perform ADLs necessary to lead an independent lifestyle. Maintaining mobility and controlling pain with the least amount of side effects are the goals for the elderly patient.

Treatment   Treatment is aimed at relieving pain, minimizing joint destruction, and promoting joint function. Rest and exercise, medication, immobilization with splints and other supportive devices during periods of severe inflammation, and hot and cold treatments are stanard. Medications include salicylates, NSAIDs, corticosteroids, antimalarial drugs, methotrexate, gold compounds, sulfasalazine, D-penicillamine, and immunosuppressants (Table 22-12). Surgical joint repair or replacement can be done to reduce pain and improve mobility.

Medications. There is a wide selection of drugs from which the physician can choose to treat the various forms of arthritis. No drug will cure the disease, however, and medication is but one part of the overall regimen of treatment. Usually NSAIDs are the first kind of agents used for arthritis. Of these, aspirin is the drug of choice if the patient can tolerate it. The amount of aspirin prescribed is quite large and ranges from 15 to 25 tablets a day. Table 22-12 presents examples of drugs prescribed to treat arthritis.

The greatest disadvantage of these drugs is that they can cause serious gastrointestinal (GI) irritation, ulceration, and bleeding. Some of the NSAIDs are combined with other agents or are specially coated to minimize adverse GI side effects. These agents include aspirin compounded with antacids (Ascriptin), enteric-coated aspirin (Ecotrin), and choline salicylate (Trilisate). Although these agents are associated with a lower incidence of GI bleeding and heartburn, they are more expensive than plain aspirin.

TABLE 22-12 ◆ *Pharmacological Management of Arthritis*

Classification	Examples	Nursing Implications
Salicylates	Aspirin, plain or buffered; Ecotrin	Give with food, milk, or antacid. Do not crush enteric-coated tablets and do not give them with milk. Teach patients to report black tarry stools and tinnitus.
Nonsteroidal antiinflammatories (NSAIDs)	Motrin, Indocin, Voltaren, Lodine, Naprosyn, Nalfon, Advil, Nuprin, Orudis, Meclomen, Daypro, Butazolidin, Feldene, Tolectin, Clinoril, Relafen	May take 2 weeks to obtain response. Give with milk, food, or a full glass of water, but some NSAIDs are best given 30 minutes before a meal or 2 hours afterward. Teach patients to report heartburn, dyspepsia, nausea, vomiting, diarrhea, or abdominal pain. Monitor hematological, renal, liver, auditory, and ophthalmic functions. Teach patient to avoid alcohol because of increased risk of GI irritation. Ask patient to report any changes in vision. Dosage in elderly may need to be reduced by ½. Monitor weight gain and peripheral edema; report weight increase of 5 lb in 1 week.
Antimalarials	Plaquenil, Aralen	May take 6 months to obtain effect desired. Give with food or milk to decrease GI irritation. Instruct patient about need for eye examinations and a blood count every 3 months when on plaquenil. Aralen may cause urine to be rusty yellow or brown. Caution about driving until response to drug is known.
Antirheumatic agents Gold compounds	Myochrysine, Solganal, Ridaura	Baseline and periodic blood counts and urinalyses are necessary. Instruct patient to report signs of toxicity: rash, pruritus, stomatitis, metallic taste. Inject Myochrysine deep into gluteus muscle and have patient remain flat for 30 minutes to decrease dizziness, sweating, and flushing. Ridaura should be administered with food or fluids. Instruct to use added fiber or antidiarrheal agent as necessary. Inform that benefits may not be seen for 3–4 months. Instruct to avoid the sun to decrease pruritus and dermatitis.
D-penicillamine	Cuprimine, Depen	Monitor CBC, liver function, urine, and platelets weekly for 8–10 weeks, then monthly. Give 30 minutes before meals or 2 hours afterward. Instruct to report fever, sore throat, chills, bruising, or bleeding.
Antimetabolites	Methotrexate	Instruct to refrain from drinking alcohol as it increases hepatotoxicity. Monitor liver and renal function weekly. Teach patient to report mouth sores or inflamed gums.
Immunosuppressants	Imuran	Give in divided doses to decrease GI irritation. Advise women to use contraceptives as drug is highly toxic to the fetus. Instruct to report signs of infection and avoid persons with colds. Monitor blood and urine weekly. Therapeutic effect may take 6–8 weeks.
Corticosteroids	Hydrocortisone, prednisolone, and prednisone	Instruct to take daily dose between 6:00 and 8:00 A.M. when natural steroids are released. Instruct not to stop taking the drug abruptly. Taper dosage downward as soon as symptoms improve. Monitor elderly closely for fluid retention, elevated blood pressure, and peripheral edema. Handle patients gently to prevent bruising; avoid using tape on skin.

Although the major difficulty with NSAIDs is GI intolerance, all of these agents can be toxic to the liver, kidney, and central nervous system. Blood dyscrasias, tinnitus, and hearing loss may occur. Only a small percentage of patients suffer toxicity to NSAIDs, but the side effects can be serious and sometimes permanent. If early signs of toxicity appear, they should be reported promptly to the physician.

In selected cases of rheumatoid arthritis that do not respond to other forms of drug therapy, more potent drugs may be prescribed. Although these medications provide periods of remission, they also have some serious side effects in most patients. Agents included in this group of drugs include gold, D-penicillamine (Depen, Cuprimine), hydroxychloroquine (Plaquenil), sulfasalazine, and methotrexate.

Systemic corticosteroids have a profound antiinflammatory effect on arthritis. They were once thought to be "miracle drugs" to treat arthritis, but their use is now questioned by many authorities. Their antiinflammatory action tends to diminish over time, thus requiring higher doses to obtain the same results. In addition, long-term steroid therapy exposes the patient to some rather severe side effects. These include diabetes mellitus, osteoporosis, hypertension, acne, and weight gain. Because of these and other problems associated with steroid therapy, long-term oral steroid preparations are reserved for patients who cannot find relief from other drugs.

The injection of steroids directly into a joint (intraarticular administration) has been used successfully in treating painful flareups, shortening the period of inflammation, and relieving pain and other symptoms. When intraarticular steroid therapy is used, it is recommended that not more than three or four doses be injected into any joint within 1 year's time.

Immunosuppressive therapy is limited to patients who do not respond to other, less dangerous forms of therapy. Azathioprine (Imuran) is used for this purpose. Experimental drugs and modalities of therapy continue to be tried in an effort to find some form of treatment in which the benefits far outweigh the risks (Table 22-12).

Studies are under way on gammalinolenic acid, a fatty acid found in the seeds of evening primrose and borage plants. The substance was found to give relief to a group of rheumatoid arthritis sufferers and may one day be an accepted treatment. Some patients find that they have fewer symptoms if they eat fish such as salmon or mackerel that are high in omega fatty acids at least twice a week. Other patients experience decreased pain and swelling if they take an omega-3 fatty acid capsule once a day. These substances do not seem to help all patients, however.

As with many other chronic and incurable diseases, arthritis victims are particularly vulnerable to unproven claims for a cure and to outright quackery. Because rheumatoid arthritis sometimes goes into spontaneous remission, many patients who undergo an unorthodox treatment at the same time their disease is in remission give credit for their improvement to the treatment.

Elder Care Point... Elderly patients experience side effects of drugs more often and more quickly than younger people. These patients must be taught to watch for side effects and to report them to the physician or nurse promptly and to refrain from taking another dose until the effects have been reported. Dizziness may be experienced when taking analgesics for arthritis pain, particularly if the medication contains codeine. This predisposes the elderly patient to falls. The elderly should be cautioned to arise slowly, hold on to furniture until stable on their feet, and to wait until dizziness has cleared to ambulate. An assistive device for ambulation is of benefit to help prevent falls.

Surgical Intervention and Orthopedic Devices   In the past, surgical intervention was reserved for patients who already had suffered severe joint deformity and loss of motion. There is now a trend toward the use of surgery in the early stages of the disease to prevent or at least modify deformities and mechanical abnormalities.

One such surgical procedure is *synovectomy,* which is the excision of the synovial membrane of a joint. The goal of synovectomy is to interrupt the destructive inflammatory process that eventually leads to ankylosis and invasion of surrounding cartilage and bone tissues.

Researchers at MIT are performing a procedure called neutron capture synovectomy using an accelerator that bombards the affected joints with subatomic particles. The technique is 10 times cheaper than standard surgery and requires little, if any, hospitalization. Although experimental, this procedure may one day be a treatment of choice.

Surgical repair of a hip joint (arthroplasty) is performed when there is extensive damage and ambulation is not possible. The purpose of joint repair is to restore, improve, or maintain joint function. In cases in which it is not possible to repair the damaged hip joint, total hip replacement may be done. A similar operation can be done on the knee joint.

Casts or braces and splints (orthoses) sometimes are used to immobilize an affected part so that it can rest during an active phase of the disease. Devices that immobilize the affected joint should allow for motion of adjacent muscles, thereby improving muscle strength and permitting more independence on the part of the patient. Braces also work to prevent deformities by maintaining optimal functional position of the joints.

Joint replacement. An arthroplasty (joint replacement) may be done for a knee, shoulder, elbow, finger, ankle, or hip. The hip is the most frequently

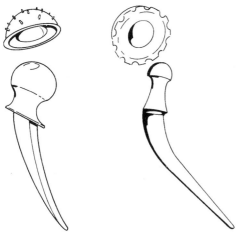

A. The McKee-Farrar procedure involves replacement of the femoral head and acetabulum with a metal prosthesis.

B The Charnley prosthesis involves total prosthetic replacement of the hip joint.

FIGURE 22-10   Hip prostheses.

replaced joint. Noncemented press fit prostheses are often used now for young, heavier, and very active patients. The cement used for bone prostheses only has a life-span of about 10 years; it may cause damage to the bone marrow from the heat generated during its initial "curing." A press fit prosthesis is custom-sized by computer-aided design (CAD) for each patient. The outer coating is porous metal that allows new bone to "grow into" the device over a period of a few months.

Total Hip Replacement   A hip joint may be replaced with either a low-friction polyurethane socket for the acetabulum with a metallic replacement for the head of the femur or with synthetic materials combined with a porous bone implant (Figure 22-10). Partial weight bearing is permitted very soon after surgery. The porous

bone implant requires 6 weeks of healing before weight bearing. Cemented prostheses patients refrain from full weight bearing for 4 to 6 weeks. Full weight bearing is avoided for 3 to 6 months. Crutches or a walker are used for ambulation depending on the ability of the patient.

There are several kinds of prostheses to replace the hip, and the surgeon chooses the appropriate one according to an individual patient's needs (Figure 22-10).

The primary purpose of total hip replacement (THR) is to relieve chronic pain. The greatest dangers to successful replacement are infection, dislocation, and failure to function. Rehabilitation of the patient is a team effort involving the patient himself, the surgeon, nurse, and physical therapist.

Preoperative care.   Preoperatively the patient is given specific instructions about the kind of surgery to be performed, the prosthesis to be used, the procedures to be followed after surgery, and what is expected of him to help achieve the goals of rehabilitation. He is given instructions in postoperative exercises and in the use of ambulation equipment such as a walker, crutches, or canes.

A surgical bacteriostatic scrub solution is usually prescribed for use during the daily shower for several days prior to hip replacement to lessen the chance of infection. The patient is told he will be placed in an orthopedic bed with an overhead trapeze bar attached after surgery and often is transported to and from the operating room on the bed if he is hospitalized prior to surgery. The triangular abductor pillow is shown to the patient, and its use between the legs for turning postoperatively is explained. Other care is much the same as for other types of major surgery.

Postoperative care.   It is imperative that all concerned with the patient's care after surgery understand what is necessary to ensure successful hip replacement and rehabilitation and to prevent dislocation of the prosthesis. Immediately after surgery, nursing inter-

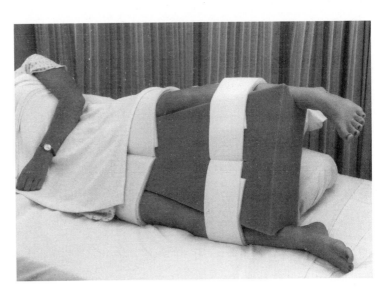

FIGURE 22-11   Abduction wedge in place to prevent dislocation of hip prosthesis. (Photo by Glen Derbyshire; courtesy of Goleta Valley Cottage Hospital, Goleta, Ca.)

vention includes all the measures required to avoid respiratory and circulatory complications. However, extreme care must be exercised in positioning and repositioning the patient. **To prevent dislocation, an abduction wedge is secured between the legs (usually in the operating room) and left in place until the surgeon requests its removal** (Figure 22-11). The wedge is positioned with the narrower end between the thighs, and the straps should not go over an incision, bony prominence, or drain. Circulation should be checked after each application of the wedge to be certain that the straps are not too tight.

A common complication of joint replacement has been deep vein thrombosis (DVT). A new low-molecular-weight heparin, enoxaparin (Lovenox), has been recently approved by the FDA to prevent this problem. It works more quickly than sodium heparin and causes less incidence of hemorrhage because it doesn't prevent platelets from aggregating at bleeding injury sites. Daily coagulation studies are not needed with this drug as its anticoagulant action is very predictable and stable. It is usually given in a 30-mg dose by SC injection into the abdomen twice a day.

In most cases the patient is allowed to stand at the bedside on the first postoperative day, supported by a walker and two persons. Weight bearing on the operated joint is sometimes allowed, but there should be a

---

TABLE 22-13 ◆ *Patient Education: Total Hip Replacement*

Before he is discharged, the patient who has undergone hip surgery should be given instructions so he can care for himself at home. These include:

- It is all right to lie on your operated side.
- For 3 months you should not cross your legs. You should put a pillow between your legs when you roll over on your abdomen or lie on your side in bed.
- It is all right to bend your hip, but not beyond a right (90-degree) angle (demonstrate).
- Continue your daily exercise program at home in the same way you did the exercises at the hospital.

---

specific written order from the physician saying it is all right to permit weight bearing on the joint. The patient will need instruction in transferring himself from bed to chair, wheelchair, and toilet. **Whenever he sits down, the chair seat should be raised so that the hips are not flexed beyond a 90-degree angle.** Table 22-13 shows the points to cover in discharge teaching. In addition to these instructions, the patient may be referred for outpatient or in-home physical therapy. Nursing interventions for selected problems of a patient with a total hip replacement (THR) are summarized in Clinical Pathway 22-1.

CLINICAL PATHWAY 22-1 ◆ *Home Care Clinical Pathway for Total Joint Replacement*

Program Description: Total Joint Replacement

Description

This program provides teaching, in-home safety evaluation, and management of patient care from the initial preoperative visit through hospitalization and continues through home care with transition to outpatient therapy when appropriate. This program is appropriate for patients receiving an elective orthopedic surgery, including, but not limited to, total hip arthroplasty and total knee arthroplasty.

Goals

Patient/caregiver will demonstrate understanding of disease process and rationale for surgery.

Patient/caregiver will be physically and emotionally prepared for surgery.

Patient/caregiver will have apporparite discharge plan prior to surgery.

Patient/caregiver will be able to verbalize understanding of medication regime and demonstrate compliance.

Patient/caregiver will be able to verbalize and demonstrate pain-management strategies.

Patient will demonstrate optimal self-care, activities of daily living, and mobility.

Patient/caregiver will be able to verbalize postsurgical complications and prior intervention.

Patient will transition smoothly through the continuum of care: from home to hospital, return home, and on to outpatient as appropriate.

Resources

VNS Standard Patient Education Manual

7.11	Nonsteroidal antiinflammatory medications
8.01	Arthritis
8.03	Range of motion
8.05	Total hip replacement precautions
13.03	Care of patient confined to bed
13.06	Helping a patient to sit up/stand
13.08	Pivot transfer bed to wheelchair and wheelchair to bed
14.17	Fractures

CLINICAL PATHWAY 22-1 ◆ *Home Care Clinical Pathway for Total Joint Replacement* (*Continued*)

Potential referral criteria

Patient's medical condition is appropriate for safe management at home. Home environment is a safe place in which to provide care. Any patient with a diagnosis of total joint replacement with:

* Any patient having an elective orthopedic surgery.
* Knowledge deficit regarding care.

Patient outcome

Visit #	Patient Outcome
1	States definition/reason for surgical procedure.
1–2	States understanding of the following teaching instructions: hospital course, anesthesia, pain management, pre-, intra-, and post-surgery, postsurgical precautions, bowel management, signs and symptoms (S & S) infection/complications and need to notify MD.
1	Actions/side effects of medication, including pain medication.
1–2	Demonstrates correctly: pre-/postsurgical exercises, precautions, turn, cough, and deep-breath (TCDB).
1–2	Demonstrates good skin care to potential pressure areas.
1–2	States signs/symptoms of skin breakdown and when to report.
1–3	Will have personal care needs met.
6–10	Will have ADL and mobility needs met.

Care pathway

Component of Care	Admission	Visits: 1–3	Visits: 4–7
Assess/monitor disease process	▶ RN Assessment 1–4 weeks before scheduled surgery. ▶ Full systems assessment with focus on muscular skeletal system. ▶ Assess: ▫ Vital signs. ▫ In-home safety evaluation. ▫ Mobility. ▫ Pain management and effectiveness. ▫ Knowledge deficit regarding surgical procedure. ▫ Risk for skin breakdown. ▫ Functional level, ability to perform ADLs. ▶ Establish frequency of visits needed and project possible post surgical needs.	▶ Continue to assess: ▫ S&S infection. ▫ S&S deep vein thrombosis. ▫ Family/patient coping. ▫ Need for home health aide. ▶ Monitor vital signs, medication, diet, skin, integrity, pain management. ▶ Review frequency of visits relative to achievement of goals; decrease if appropriate.	▶ Continue systems assessment. ▶ Modify care plan relative to assessment. ▶ Weekly team conferences with other disciplines. ▶ Assess homebound status weekly. ▶ Assess readiness for outpatient services.
Consults/evaluations	▶ Physical therapist (PT), occupational therapist (OT), evaluations per MD order. ▶ First visit within 72 hours. ▶ Discuss treatment plan with MD.	▶ MSW evaluation per MD order.	▶ Communicate with MD PRN regarding changed patient status, need for new orders.
Teaching/treatments	▶ Assess patient/caregiver teaching needs; preoperative teaching regarding disease process, hospital course, anesthesia, pain management, respiratory management, post-surgical precautions/complications, bowel management, strengthening exercises. ▶ Review advance directives, rights and responsibilities, admission forms. ▶ Instruct how to contact agency.	▶ Continue instruction in: ▫ Safety/household hazards. ▫ Mobility. ▫ Skin care. ▫ S&S infection. ▫ S&S complications. ▫ Need to notify MD.	▶ Remove staples as ordered (10–14 days).

Continued on following page

CLINICAL PATHWAY 22-1 ◆ *Home Care Clinical Pathway for Total Joint Replacement* (Continued)			
Component of Care	**Admission**	**Visits: 1–3**	**Visits: 4–7**
Teaching/treatments (Continued)	▶ Assess and teach regarding home safety, review of safety hazards. ▶ Assess and instruct in S&S of infection.		
Medication	▶ Review medications and continue as ordered. ▶ Assess patient/caregiver knowledge. ▶ Instruct on indication, dose, time, route, side effects. ▶ Instruct in use of pain medications, arthritis medication. ▶ Instruct in holding off blood thinners, NSAIDs prior to surgery per MD instructions.	▶ Assess effectiveness of pain medication. ▶ Update and review medication regime.	▶ Monitor response to medication. ▶ Continue medication instruction until patient/caregiver can state: indication, dose, time, action, route, side effects of each.
Nutrition/hydration	▶ Assess nutritional status. ▶ Assess patient/caregiver knowledge of diet and hydration.	▶ Monitor intake/hydration for adequate protein intake for healing, roughage for elimination. ▶ Consider dietician consult if indicated.	▶ Continue to monitor intake/hydration.
Functional/rehabilitation	▶ Evaluate strength, ROM, general physical status, pain, balance, mobility, signs of complications, cognitive level. ▶ Evaluate appropriateness of adaptive equipment. ▶ Instruct in gait training with walker. ▶ Instruct in proper weight bearing technique. ▶ Instruct in transfer training, bed mobility, transfers to/from chair while maintaining precautions. ▶ Begin home exercise program instruction.	▶ Continue gait training with walker on level surfaces. ▶ Encourage increased weight bearing as tolerated. ▶ Continue transfer training bed mobility, progress to shower if appropriate. ▶ Therapeutic exercises act/asst and active therapeutic exercises. ▶ Begin standing weight shift exercise. ▶ Continue home exercise program instructions with active exercise, increase intensity to tolerate. ▶ Inspect and adjust any new equipment. ▶ Instruct patient in proper use of acquired equipment.	▶ Continue gait training, begin gait on steps with assistant. ▶ Review proper transfer techniques while maintaining precautions, to/from car. ▶ Continue active exercise of involved extremity, begin resisted exercise of knee. ▶ Assess patient's ability to safely exit home to be transported to MD. ▶ Active exercise bilateral lower extremity for ROM and strength.
Tests Psychosocial/spiritual	▶ Lab tests as ordered by MD. ▶ Assess impact of condition on coping skills of patient/caregiver.	▶ Draw Protime if ordered. ▶ Assess patient's support systems and effectiveness. ▶ Assess living situation, financial needs, ability to care for patient at home. ▶ MSW consults as indicated.	▶ Lab tests as ordered by MD. ▶ Assess for need for additional community resources. ▶ Supportive counsel.
Continuing care needs	▶ Assess caregiver needs, ability to care for patient at home.	▶ Schedule MD appointment.	▶ Refer to outpatient therapy if appropriate. ▶ Instruct patient to schedule MD appointment.

CLINICAL PATHWAY 22-1 ◆ *Home Care Clinical Pathway for Total Joint Replacement (Continued)*

Recommended visits per discipline per week

Nursing: 1-2W2
Home health aide: 2W2
PT: 3W2
OT: Evaluation as necessary
MSW: Evaluation as necessary

Variables affecting frequency and intensity of care

These guidelines are outcome oriented. Each patient will be evaluated on an individual basis to establish an appropriate treatment program. Frequency and duration are dependent on variations in population base, severity of condition, level of cognitive functioning and presence or absence of other chronic or debilitating disease states.

Source: Courtesy of Visiting Nurse Association, Ventura, CA.

Knee Replacement   Chronic, uncontrollable pain is the main indication for knee arthroplasty. Either part or all of the knee joint may be replaced. For the best postoperative result emphasis is placed on exercise. A continuous passive motion (CPM) machine is used soon after surgery (Figure 11-2). The patient must be kept well medicated for pain to tolerate the exercise. Within 2 to 5 days, quadriceps-strengthening exercises and straight-leg raising are started. Exercises are taught by the physical therapist, and the nurse often assists the patient in performing them. The patient then progresses to ambulation with a walker or crutches. Other pre- and postoperative care is similar to that of the patient undergoing any major surgery. After early release from the hospital, the patient continues physical therapy in the outpatient setting.

Nursing Assessment and Intervention   The manifestations of arthritis are many and varied, particularly when the diagnosis is rheumatoid arthritis. Pain, limited motion, and the chronic and incurable nature of the illness have some impact on almost every aspect of the patient's life. To set realistic goals and plan for their accomplishment, the nurse will need to know about the patient's social history, her personal and family health history, current general health status, ability to do the things she wants to do, and her experience of pain and how she has been dealing with it.

Nursing interventions are aimed at providing a balance of rest and exercise, freedom from pain, minimizing emotional stress, preventing or correcting deformities, and maintaining or restoring function so that the patient can enjoy as much independence and mobility as possible.

Rest and exercise.   The amount of rest needed will depend on the extent of inflammation. The more inflamed a joint is, the more rest is needed; this includes rest of the whole body, as well as of the inflamed joint. **Fatigue is a common problem and usually requires that the patient change his lifestyle somewhat so that he has rest periods during the day before he becomes too** fatigued or exhausted. During periods of acute exacerbation of symptoms, the patient may need continuous bedrest.

During the time the patient is lying down he should maintain good body position and avoid pillows and other devices that support joints in a position of flexion. A firm mattress is recommended, with only one pillow under the head and neck.

The purpose of rest is to allow the body's natural defenses and healing powers to overcome the inflammatory process. It is necessary, however, even in the acute phase, to balance rest with exercise. The patient should sit to do tasks whenever possible. Activities should be paced and interspersed with rest. The exercise program is prescribed on the basis of assessment of each patient's status, the severity of inflammation, the particular joints affected, and the patient's tolerance for activity. Because anemia and other blood disorders can accompany arthritis, the fatigue experienced by a patient may be somewhat alleviated by correcting any underlying blood disorder.

In any exercise program it is necessary to enlist the patient's cooperation or compliance, as the exercises must be continued at home. The patient may need to be taught how to perform specific exercises so that they do not increase his pain. Each exercise should be done 3 to 10 times for each joint, with the lower number used on days when pain or fatigue is increased. **When joints are inflamed, exercises should not be done; rest is needed.** In many instances, doing the exercises in the right way can actually diminish discomfort. **If pain persists for hours after exercises have been done, the patient's status should be reassessed and the exercise program revised.** When a patient is performing routine physical activities at home, carrying out general exercise, or following a prescribed exercise program at home, precautions to avoid joint injury should be followed (Table 22-14).

Applications of heat and cold.   There is no hard-and-fast rule to follow in deciding whether heat or cold is best for treating arthritic joints. Either one may be suitable, depending on the patient's preference

TABLE 22-14 ◆ *Patient Education: Instructions for Joint Protection*

◆ Always stop an exercise at the point of real pain. Some discomfort can be expected, but it should be minimal. If your joints are still hurting 1 or 2 hours after exercise, you have done too much.

◆ Always use your biggest muscles and strongest joints. For example, push doors open with your arm instead of your hand; carry a shoulder bag instead of a hand purse.

◆ Try to do only those jobs that will allow you to stop and rest if you need to when pain develops. Learn to conserve your energy to do the things you really want to do.

◆ Exercise in a way that doesn't put strain on the joints. Exercising in water decreases joint strain.

◆ Slow down and move slowly and smoothly. Avoid rapid, jerky movements. Use the palms of the hands rather than the fingers to push up from a bed or chair when arising.

◆ Turn doorknobs counterclockwise to prevent extensive twisting of the elbow.

◆ Don't lift weights. Pick up heavier items with two hands.

◆ Let swollen, red, hot, and painful joints rest as much as possible. Don't use them any more than absolutely necessary.

◆ Change your body position frequently, alternating standing, sitting, and lying down.

◆ Set your own limits and compete with yourself, not with anyone else.

◆ Use assistive/adaptive devices, such as velcro closures and built-up utensil handles to protect joints of the hands. Use a long-handled hair brush.

and the effectiveness of each. The purpose of either hot or cold applications is to minimize pain, increase the joint's ROM, and improve exercise performance. **In general, heat is better for subacute or chronic joint inflammation and cold is more effective in the acute phase when joints are hot, red, and obviously inflamed.**

Various forms of heat therapy can be used, including moist or dry heat and superficial or deep heat. For dry heat a therapeutic infrared lamp is convenient and inexpensive for home use. For treatment of the hands, paraffin baths are effective. Wet heat can be applied by hot tub baths with the water temperature not exceeding 102°F (39°C) or by means of a towel dipped in hot water, wrung out, and applied to the joint. Whirlpool baths promote relaxation and motion with minimal pain, especially when prolonged treatment is indicated. However, immersing the whole body in warm water can cause physiological changes in respiration and pulse rate and may be contraindicated in debilitated or elderly patients.

Whatever method of heat or cold application is used at home, the patient will need specific instructions on how to avoid injury to the skin and other hazards. Information for teaching patients precautions for applications of heat and cold is summarized in Table 22-15.

Diet. No special diet will cure or relieve arthritis, in spite of many fraudulent claims to the contrary.

However, some patients find that eliminating foods from the "nightshade" family, such as tomatoes, decreases their joint pain. The patient should eat an average, well-balanced diet with no excess or limitations in amount or types of foods. **Obesity can contrib-**

TABLE 22-15 ◆ *Patient Education: Application of Heat and Cold*

For the safe application of heat or cold, follow these guidelines:

Applications of heat

◆ Recommended for chronic or subacute inflammation. Heat should be used for 20 to 30 minutes at a time; repeat the application every 1 to 2 hours while awake.

◆ Shower massager. Use shower massager for massage pulsation. Regulate water by turning on cold and adding hot water to desired temperature *before* entering the shower. Use a shower stool if balance is poor or fatigue is likely.

◆ Hot water bottle. Use a pad between the bottle and the skin to prevent burning.

◆ Heating pads. Use the type that provides moist heat; it will penetrate best. Do not go to sleep on the heating pad. Use the low settings. Heating pads often cause burns when turned up too high or used for too long.

◆ Reusable heat pack. Molds well to body part as it is pliable. Follow directions explicitly, and test temperature by feel of pack on skin before applying to area in need. Use a light pad or thin dishtowel between pack and skin. Heat in microwave oven. Reheat as needed. Does not retain heat long.

◆ Heat-producing ointments and gels. Gels containing menthol, camphor, or papain (extract from red peppers) may be applied to the sore muscle or joint as long as it doesn't produce skin irritation. Covering the area after application with saran or other plastic wrap helps hold the heat in longer. Wash hands thoroughly after application as these substances can cause eye irritation.

Applications of cold

◆ Recommended for acute phase of inflammation or acute pain. Do not apply to one area for more than 10-20 minutes at a time; apply no more than once an hour.

◆ Discontinue when numbness occurs.

◆ Not recommended for patients with impaired circulation.

◆ Dry skin well after treatment.

◆ Ice water bath. Useful for hand or foot. Extremity can be exercised during treatment.

◆ Ice pack. Can be made by partially filling double plastic bag with ice. Zip type closures work best. May use thin pad or dishtowel between pack and skin.

◆ Commercial cold pack can be refrozen in the freezer. Disposable chemical packs that are activated when needed also are available.

◆ Commercial cold packs mold to body part better than ice bag. Does not stay cold very long. Often takes two of these to finish 10-20-minute treatment. Return to freezer after use.

◆ Ice massage. Freeze ice in paper cup; peel back part of cup to use so that cup provides hand grip. Wear rubber glove or use pad to protect hand from ice. Rub ice over body part until skin feels numb, but no longer than 10–15 minutes at one time.

ute to additional stress on the weight-bearing joints and aggravate the arthritic condition. This should be explained to the patient who has a tendency to be overweight so he can be properly motivated and encouraged to lose weight and continue to keep his weight within normal limits.

Resources for patient and family education. It is very easy for the arthritis patient and his family to be overwhelmed with information about the illness and treatment. The Arthritis Foundation provides some excellent printed material written with the layperson in mind. *Rheumatoid Arthritis—Handbook for Patients* and *Arthritis—The Basic Facts* are available free of charge from the Arthritis Foundation, 1314 Spring Street, NW, Atlanta GA 30309.

The Self-Help Device Office of the World Rehabilitation Fund, 386 Park Avenue South, #500, New York, NY 10016, supplies information on specially designed self-help devices for arthritic patients. Another source of information is the Arthritis Information Clearinghouse, 1235 E. Cherokee Street, Springfield, MO 65804.

◆ Gout

Gout is arthritis of one joint caused by high serum levels of uric acid. Uric acid crystals precipitate from the body fluids and settle in joints and connective tissue. Gout affects men more than women and generally occurs during the middle years. It is more common among populations that consume a high-protein diet. Two factors seem to be implicated: (1) a genetic increase in purine metabolism; and (2) consumption of a high-purine diet or excessive alcohol. The big toe is the most common site, but many other joints can be affected. **Diuretic therapy sometimes causes a secondary gout because the loss of fluid increases the serum uric acid in the body.**

Typical signs and symptoms are elevated serum uric acid and tight, reddened skin over an inflamed, edematous joint, accompanied by elevated temperature and extreme pain in the joint.

Treatment during acute attacks consists of administration of NSAIDs for 2 to 5 days. Colchicine may be used if started within 24 hours of the beginning of the attack, but it is very toxic and its use is controversial. Allopurinol or probenecid may be prescribed to prevent further attacks. Dietary management includes weight control and restriction of high-purine foods, such as anchovies, sardines, sweetbreads, liver, kidney and meat extracts, or alcohol. Patients placed on allopurinol need periodic liver function testing as this drug can cause liver failure.

◆ Osteoporosis

Osteoporosis is a metabolic bone disorder that causes a decrease in bone mass and makes the person more susceptible to fractures. Fractures often are "atraumatic," meaning that they occur without being precipitated by trauma. Starting at age 35, most women lose bone mass at a rate of 1% a year; after menopause loss accelerates to 2% a year. Causative factors for osteoporosis include long-term calcium deficiency and estrogen deficiency in patients predisposed to the problem, particularly after menopause. Contributing factors are thought to be cigarette smoking, excessive caffeine ingestion, high salt intake, alcoholism, various medications, such as corticosteroids, endocrine disorders, prolonged bedrest, and liver disease, because these factors either have an effect on estrogen production or calcium metabolism. There is a familial tendency to osteoporosis in some patients. The risk of osteoporosis increases considerably in women after menopause because of the reduction of estrogen production.

Elder Care Point... Osteoporosis is a side effect of steroid treatment. Many elderly patients are taking steroids to treat chronic diseases such as arthritis. This makes the older person more susceptible to fractures. Kyphosis from compression fractures of the spinal column resulting from osteoporosis can restrict lung expansion and cause decreased respiratory reserve.

Signs and symptoms of osteoporosis are height loss, kyphosis, and back pain. Compression fractures of the spine may cause debilitating pain. Often osteoporosis is diagnosed after the patient sustains a fracture following little or no known trauma.

On x-rays the bone of the patient with osteoporosis appears porous. However, this aspect occurs late in the disease. The newest test to determine bone density is performed by dual energy x-ray absorptiometry (DXA or DEXA) and is used to assess loss of bone density in postmenopausal women to arrest and possibly correct the problem before it becomes severe. The test costs about $185. Studies are in progress to see whether a less expensive test using digitized, computerized analysis of hand x-rays can be used for tracking bone density loss. Testing should begin at age 50.

Treatment is aimed at stopping loss of bone density, increasing bone formation, and preventing fractures. Postmenopausal estrogen replacement therapy and adequate dietary or supplemental calcium **in combination with weight-bearing exercise** are the mainstays of treatment. Calcium supplementation of 1,000 mg is recommended for premenopausal women and 1,500 mg after menopause. Research at the Southwestern Medical School in Dallas has determined that many of the name brand calcium supplements do not dissolve very well. Citracal is one that was found to dissolve better than others tested. Some drug chains have generic brands that state on the package that they are guaranteed to dissolve properly so that the mineral can be absorbed.

Exposure to sufficient sunlight or vitamin D supplementation is necessary for the proper absorption and metabolism of the calcium. Daily weight-bearing exercise is thought greatly to decrease the incidence of osteoporosis. Walking downstairs seems to be especially helpful. Salicylates and NSAIDs are prescribed to control back pain. A back brace may be ordered for the patient who has suffered vertebral compression fractures.

A new drug, aldendronate (Fosamax), was approved in 1995. This drug is used to build up bones weakened by osteoporosis. It belongs to a new class of compounds called bisphosphonates, which are cousins to a bone resorption–inhibiting substance found naturally in the body. Fosamax must be taken first thing in the morning with a 6- to 8-oz. glass of natural water at least 30 minutes before breakfast as absorption is reduced by food, coffee, or orange juice. Miacalcin Nasal Spray, which contains calcitonin, slows the rate of bone loss. It is an alternative treatment for postmenopausal osteoporosis in women who cannot take estrogens. The spray is used with adequate calcium and vitamin D supplementation. FDA approval is being sought for a slow-release form of sodium fluoride to be used to increase bone strength and reduce the risk of fracture.

◆ Paget's Disease

Paget's disease is a problem of abnormal bone resorption followed by abnormal bone formation. The abnormal bone is weak and prone to fractures. The cause of Paget's disease is unknown, although it does occur in clusters in some families. Often the disease is found at the time a fracture occurs as x-rays reveal the abnormality of the bone. Diagnosis is by x-ray and laboratory testing. A 24-hour urine collection for hydroxyproline, which indicates osteoclastic activity, is performed. Serum alkaline phosphatase is elevated if the disease is active.

The main problem is pain, and that is the focus of treatment. Calcitonin, alendronate, and etidronate may be given to slow bone resorption. Mithramycin (Mithracin), a cytotoxin, may be used as well.

◆ Bone Tumors

Bone is subject to both benign and malignant tumors. They arise from several different types of tissue including cartilage (chondromas), bone (osteomas), and fibrous tissue (fibromas). Benign tumors often are found on x-ray or at the time of fracture.

Malignant bone tumors are either primary or secondary to metastatic disease. Primary malignant bone tumors are most often seen in people 10 to 20 years of age. The most common type is osteosarcoma or osteogenic sarcoma. More than half of the cases affect the knee area. However, the distal femur, humerus, and proximal tibia are other frequent sites of occurrence. Other types of primary malignant tumors include Ewing's sarcoma, chondrosarcoma, and fibrosarcoma.

Signs and symptoms of malignant bone tumor include pain, warmth, and swelling. Metastatic bone tumors greatly outnumber primary bone malignancies. Malignancies of the prostate, kidney, thyroid, breast, and lung commonly metastasize to bone. Sites of metastases are usually the vertebrae, pelvis, ribs, and femur.

Treatment for malignant bone tumors includes surgery, radiation, and chemotherapy. Osteosarcoma has a 60% to 80% cure rate when surgery and chemotherapy are combined for treatment. Chapter 9 covers care of the cancer patient.

◆ Amputation

About 80% of all limb amputations involve lower extremities. The most common reasons for amputation of a lower limb are related to peripheral vascular disease, often associated with diabetes mellitus, and resultant gangrene. Other conditions necessitating lower-limb amputation include severe trauma, malignancy, and congenital defects (Figure 22-12).

About 70% of upper-extremity amputations are brought on by crushing blows, thermal and electric burns, and severe lacerations. Vasospastic disease, malignancy, and infection also can necessitate amputation of an upper extremity.

Preoperative Care Unless the amputation of a limb is an emergency procedure, the patient is prepared physically and psychologically for the removal of all or part of the extremity. If at all possible, the patient should participate in the decision to amputate a limb. He should understand the need for the amputation and have opportunity to discuss realistic goals of rehabilitation with several members of the health care team.

Although the loss of a limb can be very difficult for the patient and his family to accept, they can find some consolation in knowing that the procedure is absolutely necessary and that every effort will be made to take full advantage of the patient's remaining resources. The patient may experience stages of denial, anger, and so on similar to those of the dying process as discussed in Chapter 13. In a sense, the patient must recognize the death of the former "self," work through the grief process, and move toward acceptance of a new body image.

A member of the rehabilitation team should discuss with the patient what can be expected postoperatively in regard to pain, immobility, and readjustment to self-care.

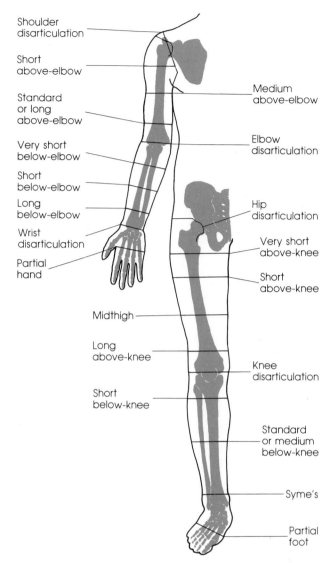

FIGURE 22-12 Levels of amputation of the upper and lower extremities.

"Phantom sensations" in the limb that has been removed are not unusual. There is no scientific explanation for these sensations, but they are nonetheless real to the amputee who experiences them.

If the patient is informed preoperatively that the sensations are not unusual, are not considered a psychiatric problem, and will be dealt with as the reality that they most certainly are, he will be less apprehensive about asking for help should the problem arise.

Physical preparation of the patient includes muscle-strengthening exercises in the hope that the patient can be active following amputation. These exercises are the first stages of the rehabilitation process, designed to help the patient achieve independence as rapidly as possible.

Immediate Postoperative Care   When the patient returns from the surgical suite, the two most immediate problems are hemorrhage and edema. To combat these problems, the stump is elevated for 24 to 48 hours. A lower extremity is not elevated for more than 24 hours because of the danger of hip contractures, which would prohibit rehabilitation efforts to achieve ambulation.

The stump is checked at frequent intervals to determine whether bleeding is excessive. Fresh bleeding on the dressing should be reported immediately.

Postoperative wound care is essentially the same as that discussed in Chapter 4. Wound drainage usually is handled with a Hemovac or similar wound-drainage system. The incision should be dry, intact, and only slightly reddened along the suture line.

Phantom limb sensations, mentioned earlier, may or may not be painful but are quite disconcerting if the patient has not been previously warned that they may occur. If the pain is severe, or persists, various methods are used to control it.

Three alternative modes for managing the stump after amputation are (1) soft dressing with delayed prosthetic fitting; (2) rigid plaster dressing and early prosthetic fitting; and (3) rigid plaster dressing and immediate prosthetic fitting.

Each method has its particular advantages and disadvantages. If a soft dressing is used, it is important that the stump be wrapped properly to control edema and ensure proper shrinkage of the stump for later fitting of a prosthesis.

Many complications can be avoided if the patient is able to get up and about early in the postoperative period. However, weight bearing before the stump is adequately healed can cause weakening of the suture line and rupturing of the operative wound. Patients with amputations below the knee are better able to begin early walking and weight bearing than are those whose limb has been amputated above the knee. The amputation of a limb displaces the body's center of gravity and interferes with the sense of balance. Adaptation to this change in the center of gravity occurs slowly, and the patient needs to be warned to move cautiously. When the prosthesis is off during the night, the patient may need assistance in turning until he adjusts to his new center of gravity.

The bedridden patient who has had a lower-extremity amputation should be encouraged to lie on the abdomen several hours each day. This will help prevent joint contractures. Proper positioning is required to prevent *abduction* contractures. Range of motion exercises are carried out with the amputee as with any patient who must be protected from the disabilities of immobility.

When a lower limb has been removed, the patient must learn how to balance on one leg, how to stoop and bend over without losing balance, and how to use his back muscles to maintain good posture while wearing an artificial limb. Teaching for self-care begins as soon as possible. Points for instruction in care of the stump and the prosthesis are presented in Table 22-16.

Rehabilitation   Usually both a physical therapist and occupational therapist work with the patient who has suffered an amputation to help regain mobility, confidence, and the ability to handle ADLs. The nurse then assists with practice at bathing, shaving, dressing, and so on. The nurse's attitude and encouragement can make a positive difference in the adjustment the patient makes to the situation.

Elderly and chronically ill amputees can benefit from a positive, yet realistic, approach to their problems. The nurse must, of course, avoid giving false hopes or unreal assurances that everything is going to be all right. The focus of attention should be on what the patient can do for himself and on what strengths

he has in his favor. By helping the patient find short-range goals that can be accomplished without great difficulty and that indicate progress toward independence, the nurse can be of real help to the amputee. For example, the nurse can guide the patient toward devising ways in which personal needs such as bathing and grooming can be met. Later, encouragment to sit up, exercise the other limbs, and assist with changing of the dressing can be given. Finally, the goal can be set for wearing a prosthesis successfully and walking without assistance. Types of lower-limb and upper-limb prostheses are shown in Figures 22-13 and 22-14. Rehabilitation issues are covered more fully in Chapter 12.

◆ Muscular Disorders

Most muscle disorders are neuromuscular; for this reason they are covered in Chapter 14.

Muscle Strain   The most common muscle strain occurs in the back muscles. Back problems are discussed in Chapter 14 as they often have a neurological component. Muscle strains do occur in other skeletal muscles and are treated the same as a joint strain with rest and applications of heat and cold. Antiinflammatory medications are used for discomfort, and, when spasm is present, a muscle relaxant may be prescribed. Time is the greatest healer. The patient is cautioned against reinjury and is taught proper ways to lift and move.

COMMUNITY CARE

Rehabilitation programs for amputees, arthritis patients, and others with musculoskeletal disorders exist in most large cities and are being introduced into more communities through agencies such as the YMCA. The arthritis foundation has been very instrumental in working with the "Ys" to bring programs for exercise to local neighborhoods.

Outpatient rehabilitation programs through clinics work with patients who are regaining mobility and ability to perform ADLs with a prosthesis. Rehabilitation is moving to a program "without walls," indicating a shift from an inpatient institute to rehabilitation in the home and community.

Home care nurses are particularly instrumental in preventing musculoskeletal injury in home care patients. The premises of the elderly patient are surveyed and recommendations are made to make it safer for the patient. Flat, nonglare surfaces for walking, well-lit walkways, absence of loose rugs, installation of grab bars in showers and bathrooms, and use of

---

TABLE 22-16 ◆ *Patient Education: Stump and Prosthesis Care*

The nurse should instruct the client in stump care as follows:

◆ Inspect the stump daily for redness, blistering, or abrasions.

◆ Use a mirror to examine all sides and aspects of the stump. Skin breakdown on the stump is extremely serious because it interferes with prosthesis training and may prolong hospitalization and recovery. Clients with diabetes mellitus are particularly susceptible to skin complications, because changes in sensation may obliterate the awareness of stump pain.

◆ Perform meticulous daily stump hygiene. Wash the stump with a mild soap, and then carefully rinse and dry it. Apply nothing to the stump after it is bathed. Alcohol dries and cracks the skin, whereas oils and creams soften the skin too much for safe prosthesis use.

◆ Wear woolen stump socks over the stump for cleanliness and comfort. To maintain the size and shape of woolen socks, wash them gently in cool water with mild soap and dry flat on a towel.

◆ Replace, do not mend, torn socks; mending creates wrinkles that irritate the skin.

◆ Put on the prosthesis immediately when arising and keep it on all day (once the wound has healed completely) to reduce stump swelling.

◆ Continue prescribed exercises to prevent weakness.

The nurse should instruct the client in prosthesis care as follows:

◆ Remove sweat and dirt from the prosthesis socket daily by wiping the inside of the socket with a damp, soapy cloth. To remove the soap, use a clean damp cloth. Dry the prosthesis socket thoroughly.

◆ Never attempt to adjust or mechanically alter the prosthesis. If problems develop, consult the prosthetist.

◆ Schedule a yearly appointment with the prosthetist.

Source: Polaski, A. L., Tatro, S. E. (1996). *Luckmann's Core Principles and Practice of Medical–Surgical Nursing.* Philadelphia: Saunders, p. 813.

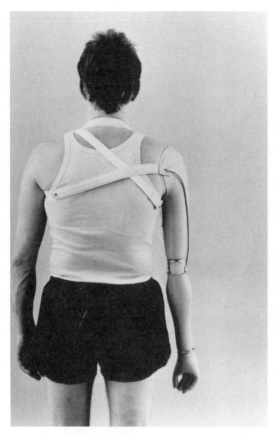
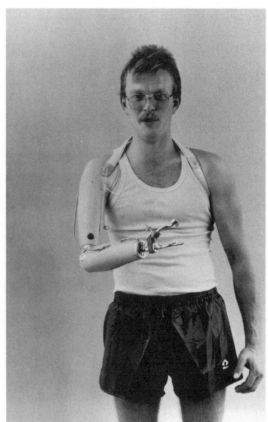

FIGURE 22-13   Upper-limb prostheses. (Courtesy of Otto Bock Orthopedic Industry, Inc.)

communication systems to summon help are some of the measures instituted to protect the elderly patient.

When a home care patient is on crutches, the nurse should assess the patient's ability to go up and down-stairs and to sit down and arise from the sitting position

safely. Table 22-8 presents the steps for performing these maneuvers correctly. Home care nurses must assess the capability and safety of elderly patients who are newly using assistive devices for ambulation and determine whether alterations in pathways in the home

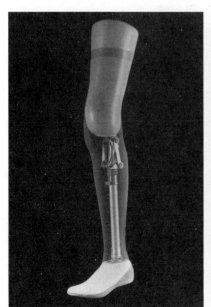
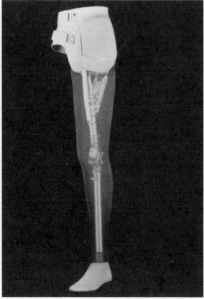
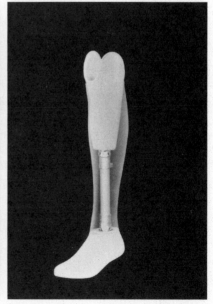

FIGURE 22-14   Lower-extremity prostheses. (Courtesy of Otto Bock Orthopedic Industry, Inc.)

need to be made. Scatter rugs should be removed, and furniture may need to be moved to provide a wide enough path for the patient to move from one area to another.

Long-term care facility nurses survey patient units and group spaces daily to check for obstacles to ambulation and potential safety hazards. Slowly our communities are becoming easier to navigate for the elderly, and public places are becoming more accessible for the handicapped and safer for the frail elderly.

Perhaps with the trend in America toward considerable exercise during the middle years, the next generation will have fewer musculoskeletal system problems. Also, with the emphasis that has been placed on calcium intake throughout life, the incidence of osteoporosis and fracture in the older age group should decrease.

CRITICAL THINKING EXERCISES

Clinical Case Problems

Read each clinical case problem and discuss the questions with your classmates.

1. Mrs. Wilson, age 38, weighs 210 pounds and has been admitted to the hospital with a diagnosis of fracture of the right tibia. You have been told that when the patient returns from surgery, she will have an external fixation device in place.

   a. How would you perform a neurovascular assessment?

   b. How can you support the affected extremity? What can you do to decrease swelling?

   c. List the observations you must make while the fixator is on Mrs. Wilson's leg.

   d. What complications might occur? What would be the signs or symptoms of such complications?

2. Mr. Moss, aged 33, has been injured in a fall from a building on which he was working. When you are assigned to the care of this patient, you are told that the tibia and fibula of the left leg are fractured. These fractures were reduced with the patient under anesthesia, after which pins were inserted for skeletal traction. The accident occurred 3 days ago, and now you are assigned to give morning care to this patient.

   a. What nursing problems will skeletal traction present?

   b. What subjective and objective symptoms would you look for when assessing Mr. Moss's condition?

3. Mrs. Cox, aged 50, is a moderately obese woman who comes to the orthopedic clinic for treatment of arthritis of the knees and ankles. She has great difficulty walking and would use a wheelchair if she could afford one. Her daughter states that she is becoming more and more inactive and, though her mother says she does not want to become an invalid, that she refuses to move about and do things for herself. Mrs. Cox lives alone and prefers not to live with her daughter because the grandchildren make her nervous. In fact, she prefers to be left alone because she feels that she cannot be of use to anyone. Her daughter feels that her mother could find many useful things to do in her neighborhood if she would only try.

   a. How does obesity interact with arthritis in causing immobility?

   b. What medications might decrease Mrs. Cox's pain?

   c. What sort of exercise would be best for this patient?

   d. How could you make Mrs. Cox feel more useful and motivate her to move about and get out of the house more?

4. Mr. Oliver is a 78-year-old male who is discharged home after a total hip replacement. You are assigned as his home care nurse to do wound care, assess for complications, and monitor rehabilitation.

   a. What teaching for self-care would you reinforce for Mr. Oliver on your first visit?

   b. How would you determine whether the home environment is safe for Mr. Oliver?

   c. Mr. Oliver is very depressed because he feels he will no longer be able to get out to go fishing and visit with his buddies. How would you approach the psychosocial aspects of his care?

BIBLIOGRAPHY

American Journal of Nursing. (1996). Alendronate (Fosamax): new treatment option for osteoporosis. *American Journal of Nursing.* 96(2):53–54.

Anonymous. (1995). Back pain: less is more. *Nursing 95.* 25(4):9.

Applegate, E. J. (1995). *The Anatomy and Physiology Learning System: Textbook.* Philadelphia: Saunders.

Barker, E. (1995). Don't dismiss whiplash. *RN.* 58(11):26–30.

Bennett, J. C., Plum, F., eds (1996). *Cecil Textbook of Medicine,* 20th ed. Philadelphia: Saunders.

Black, J. M., Matassarin-Jacobs, E. (1997). *Medical–Surgical Nursing: Clinical Management for Continuity of Care,* 5th ed. Philadelphia: Saunders.

Bradley, C. F., Kozak, C. (1995). Nursing care and management of the elderly hip fractured patient. *Journal of Gerontological Nursing.* 21(8):15–22.

Copstead, L. C. (1995). *Perspectives on Pathophysiology.* Philadelphia: Saunders.

Cotran, R. S., Kumar, V., Robbins, S. L., Schoen, F. J., eds. (1994). *Robbins Pathologic Basis of Disease,* 5th ed. Philadelphia: Saunders.

Dambro, M. R. (1996). *Griffith's 5 Minute Clinical Consult.* Baltimore: Williams & Wilkins.

Damjanov, I. (1996). *Pathology for the Health Related Professions.* Philadelphia: Saunders.

Davis, J., Sherer, K. (1994). *Applied Nutrition and Diet Therapy for Nurses,* 2nd ed. Philadelphia: Saunders.

Deutsch, N. (1995). Keeping current. Bacteria may trigger rheumatoid arthritis. *Canadian Nurse.* 91(8):20.

deWit, S. C. (1994). *Rambo's Nursing Skills for Clinical Practice,* 4th ed. Philadelphia: Saunders.

Fecht-Gramley, M. E. (1994). Recognizing compartment syndrome. *American Journal of Nursing.* 94(10):41.

Galindo-Coicon, D., Ciocon, J. O., Galindo, D. (1995). Functional impairment among elderly women with osteoporotic vertebral fractures. *Rehabilitation Nursing.* 20(2):79–83, 130.

Galsworthy, T. D., Wilson, P. L. (1996). Osteoporosis: It steals more than the bone. *American Journal of Nursing.* 96(6):27–33.

Gio-Fitman, J. (1996). The role of psychological stress in rheumatoid arthritis. *MEDSURG Nursing.* 5(6): 422–426.

Gupta, M. (1995). Pharmacist consult: seven steps for administering enoxaparin. *Nursing95.* 25(9):72.

Guyton, A. C., Hall, J. E. (1996). *Textbook of Medical Physiology,* 9th ed. Philadelphia: Saunders.

Halverson, P. B. (1995). Extraarticular manifestations of rheumatoid arthritis. *Orthopaedic Nursing.* 14(4): 47–50.

Ignatavicius, D. D., Hausman, K. A. (1995). *Clinical Pathways for Collaborative Practice.* Philadelphia: Saunders.

Ignatavicius, D. D., Workman, M. L., Mishler, M. A. (1995). *Medical–Surgical Nursing: A Nursing Process Approach,* 2nd ed. Philadelphia: Saunders.

Kelly, M. (1996). Understanding treatment for rheumatic diseases. *NURSEweek.* 9(1/8):14–15.

Lehne, R. A. (1994). *Pharmacology for Nursing Care,* 2nd ed. Philadelphia: Saunders.

Maher, A. B., Salmond, S. W., Pellino, T. A. (1994). *Orthopaedic Nursing.* Philadelphia: Saunders.

Malarkey, L. M., McMorrow, M. E. (1996). *Nurse's Manual of Laboratory Tests and Diagnostic Procedures.* Philadelphia: Saunders.

Matteson, M. A., McConnell, E. S., Linton, A. D. (1997). *Gerontological Nursing: Concepts and Practice,* edition 2. Philadelphia: Saunders.

McConnell, E. A. (1996). Myths & Facts . . . about acute compartment syndrome. *Nursing 96.* 26(2):30.

McConnell, E. A. (1997). Myths and Facts: About amputations. *Nursing 97.* 27(4):17.

McCorkle, R., Grant, M., Frank-Stromborg, M., Baird, S. B. (1996). *Cancer Nursing: a comprehensive Textbook.* Philadelphia: Saunders.

Miller, C. A. (1995). Drug consult: interventions for osteoporosis. *Geriatric Nursing.* 16(6):295.

Monahan, F. D., Drake, T., Neighbors, M. (1994). *Nursing Care of Adults.* Philadelphia: Saunders.

Neal, L. (1997). Basic musculoskeletal assessment: Tips for the home health nurse. *Home Healthcare Nurse.* 15(4):227–233.

Pellino, T. A. (1994). How to manage hip fractures. *American Journal of Nursing.* 94(4):46–50.

Polaski, A. L., Tatro, S. E. (1996). *Luckmann's Core Principles and Practice of Medical–Surgical Nursing.* Philadelphia: Saunders.

Springhouse Corporation. (1996). *Nursing96 Drug Handbook.* Springhouse, PA: author.

Rankin, J. A. (1995). Pathophysiology of the rheumatoid joint. *Orthopaedic Nursing.* 14(4):39–46.

Ryu, R. K. N., Proctor, C. S. (1996). New treatment for knee injuries. *St. Francis Medical Center News & Health.* Summer, 1996:5.

Ulrich, S. P., Canale, S. W., Wendell, S. A. (1994). *Medical–Surgical Nursing Care Planning Guides,* 3rd ed. Philadelphia: Saunders.

Webber-Jones, J. E., et al. (1994). Managing traction: do you know Carol P. Smith? *Nursing 94.* 24(7):66–70.

Whipple, B. (1995). Patient teaching: common questions about osteoporosis and menopause. *American Journal of Nursing.* 95(1):69–70.

Winslow, E. H. (1995). Research for practice. We need more calcium. *American Journal of Nursing.* 95(6):60–61.

Zavotsky, K. E., Banavage, A. (1995). Management of the patient with complex orthopaedic fractures. *Orthopaedic Nursing.* 14(5):53–54, 56–57.

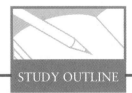

STUDY OUTLINE

I. Introduction

    A. Orthopedic nursing is not confined to primary diseases and disorders of the musculoskeletal system.

    B. The main functions of the musculoskeletal system are motion, support, and protection.

    C. Ossification, the replacement of cartilage by more solid bony tissue, is not completed throughout the body until 20 to 25 years of age.

D. Health of muscle and bones is essential to general well-being and continued mobility.

E. Trauma or disease can cause dysfunction of the musculoskeletal system.

II. Causes and Prevention of Musculoskeletal Disorders

A. Disease, trauma, malnutrition, and aging all contribute to musculoskeletal problems.

B. Decreased estrogen production after menopause is thought to contribute to the incidence of osteoporosis.

C. Weight training, weightbearing exercise, and general fitness exercise on a regular basis throughout life help maintain the integrity of the musculoskeletal system.

D. Using proper body movements when lifting and moving objects decreases the incidence of muscle strains and sprains.

E. Consuming recommended amounts of calcium throughout the lifespan and obtaining sufficient vitamin D through sunshine, plus adequate protein intake, help build and maintain healthy bones.

III. Diagnostic Tests and Procedures and Nursing Implications (Table 22-2).

A. Radiological studies: most often used. Help diagnose changes in the contour, size, and density of bone. No special preparation or postradiological care is needed.

B. Magnetic resonance imaging (MRI) is performed to detect tumors or joint problems.

C. Bone scan: use of radioactive tracer compound to locate areas of abnormal activity in bone.

D. Arthroscopy: endoscopic visualization of interior of a joint. Allows for collection of biopsy specimen; concurrent joint surgery.

1. Valuable in examining meniscus, patella, condyles, and synovia of knee and internal structures of other joints.

2. Patient watched for signs of infection, bleeding into joint, swelling, thrombophlebitis, and injury to and loss of joint motion.

E. Arthrocentesis (aspiration of synovial fluid) and analysis of synovial fluid. Also can be therapeutic. Synovial fluid analyzed for abnormalities; for example, white blood cells, bacteria, rheumatoid arthritis cells, and lupus erythematosus cells.

1. After arthroscopy the extremity is supported on pillows. Ice or cold packs are used to relieve pain and swelling.

2. Elastic bandage is applied to give joint stability after removal of large amount of fluid.

3. Patient cautioned not to overuse joint until after pain and swelling subside.

F. Cultures aid diagnosis of bone infection.

G. Biopsy aids in determining the type of tumor present.

H. Electromyography evaluates intrinsic electrical properties of muscle in response to stimulation. Helpful in diagnosing neuromuscular disease, location of site of muscle disorder.

I. Dual energy x-ray absorptiometry (DXA or DEXA) is used to assess loss of bone density in postmenopausal women.

J. Blood tests.

1. Uric acid: high levels indicate presence of gout.

2. Rheumatoid factor: detects antibodies that possibly indicate rheumatoid arthritis, lupus, or scleroderma.

3. Antinuclear antibodies (ANA): useful for diagnosis of lupus erythematosus, rheumatoid arthritis, and other connective tissue disorders.

K. Other testing procedures: ROM testing (goniometry), muscle strength, stability of joint under stress.

IV. Nursing Management

A. History taking: diseases that secondarily affect the musculoskeletal system; family history of bone and muscle disease, gout, psoriasis (Table 22-3).

B. Physical assessment (Table 22-4).

1. Pain and discomfort: location, description, factors that aggravate or relieve pain. Daily pattern of pain.

2. Signs of joint stiffness, daily pattern.

3. Signs of deformity; sensory changes; use of supports, such as cane, crutch, elastic bandage.

4. Signs of inflammatory changes or infection, sensory changes.

5. Assessment of ability to perform ADLs also are important.

C. Nursing diagnosis.

1. Common nursing diagnoses.

a. Impaired physical mobility.

b. Activity intolerance.

c. Pain.

d. Body image disturbance.

e. Self-care deficit in bathing, grooming, toileting, feeding.

f. Risk for disuse syndrome.

g. Impaired home maintenance.

2. Secondary nursing diagnoses may be appropriate for patients who are highly immobile, such as constipation, impaired tissue integ-

rity, social isolation, sleep pattern disturbance, or fatigue.

D. Planning.

1. Caring for orthopedic patients often takes more time than for someone who is mobile and agile.

2. The nurse may be one of the few social contacts the patient has while immobilized.

3. Scheduled toileting time at intervals is important to the patient who is immobilized.

4. Specific individual expected outcomes are written for each nursing diagnosis.

E. Implementation (see Table 22-5).

1. Avoidance of injury: lift, turn, and position carefully.

2. Orthopedic bedmaking: make bed with minimum of disturbance to limb in traction and damage to skin.

3. Prevention of disability.

   a. Goal is to prevent permanent disability and limitation of motion.

   b. Contractures: adaptive shortening of the muscles when they are not regularly contracted and stretched to their normal limits.

     (1) Process begins 3 to 7 days after immobilization of a part. Completed in 6 to 8 weeks.

     (2) Evident in foot drop, wrist drop, contractures of fingers and arms.

       (a) Loss of muscle tone from disuse.

       (b) Ankylosis: permanent fixation of a joint; little or no motion possible. If it cannot be avoided, joint is immobilized in position of optimum use or maximum function.

   c. Gradual mobilization: progressive improvement in motion and ability to perform self-care activities.

     (1) Must take into account cause of immobility.

     (2) Patient involved in goal setting.

     (3) Passive exercises and positioning until patient is able to do these on his own.

   d. Exercise.

     (1) ROM, both passive and active, should be done at least three to four times daily.

     (2) Isometric exercises to prepare for ambulation and wheelchair transfers; muscle setting exercises.

     (3) Daily exercises scheduled after pain medication is given.

     (4) Continuous passive motion (CPM) can be accomplished by motor-driven apparatus for knee joint and leg muscles.

   e. Positioning.

     (1) Changing body position does not necessarily change joint positions.

     (2) Patients with spastic paralysis and those with flaccid paralysis are not always positioned in same way.

     (3) Follow guidelines to avoid positioning problems.

   f. Special beds used to prevent hazards of immobility and make care of patient in cervical traction easier.

   g. Use of slings and splints for immobilization.

   h. Teaching ambulation with assistive devices.

     (1) Crutches must be adjusted to patient height.

     (2) Several gaits can be used for crutch walking.

     (3) Safety when using assistive devices is a primary concern.

     (4) A cane must be the correct height; patient must be taught to use the cane properly.

     (5) A walker is the correct height when the patient's elbow is bent at a 15- to 30-degree angle while standing upright and grasping the hand grips.

   i. Psychosocial care.

     (1) Consider impact of prolonged periods of immobility and dependence on others.

     (2) Involve patient in setting realistic and measurable goals for self-care to improve self-concept and promote better mental outlook.

F. Evaluation.

1. Data gathered through reassessment to determine whether expected outcomes are being met.

2. Observation of ability to accomplish ADLs gives clues to improvement in mobility and activity tolerance.

3. If expected outcomes are not being met, the plan must be revised; collaboration with all health team members, as well as the patient, is essential.

V. Disorders of the Musculoskeletal System

A. Soft tissue injuries.

1. Sprain: stretching or tearing of ligaments around a joint.

   a. Most common sites are ankle and knee.

    b. Symptoms vary from tenderness and minimal swelling (grade 1) to bleeding into joint and marked loss of function (grade 3).

    c. Intervention: apply ice immediately and for 10 to 20 minutes out of each hour for first 24 to 36 hours. Wrap tightly and elevate part. Surgical repair may be necessary in some cases.

  2. Strain: pulling and tearing of either muscle or tendon or both.

    a. Most common sites are hamstring, quadriceps, and calf muscles.

    b. Symptoms: soft-tissue swelling and pain. History of overexertion.

    c. Intervention: Apply ice and compression immediately; rest. Surgical repair may be necessary.

  3. Dislocation: stretching and tearing of ligaments with complete displacement of bones of the joint.

    a. Most common sites are shoulder, knee, temporomandibular joint.

    b. Symptoms: severe pain, muscle spasm, abnormal appearance of joint. History of outside force pushing against joint.

    c. Intervention: reduction of displacement. Stabilization of joint and rehabilitation to minimize muscle atrophy and strengthen joint.

  4. Bursitis: inflammation of the bursa in a joint causing moderate aching pain.

VI. Fractures

  A. A break in the continuity of bone.

  B. Types (Figure 22-5).

  C. Nursing assessment and intervention (Table 26-3).

    1. Assess for infection, sensation, circulation, and motor function each shift.

    2. Inspect casts for flattened areas, soft spots, cracking and crumbling; inspect skin at junction of cast; sniff for signs of infection inside of cast.

    3. Check traction devices for correct positioning and to see that weights are hanging free; check weights each time you enter the patient's room.

    4. Assess for problems of immobility: skin breakdown, urinary tract infection, constipation, respiratory problems.

    5. Pain control is important; prevent boredom, offer distraction.

    6. Attend to psychosocial concerns of long-term immobilization and disruption of usual roles.

  D. Surgical treatment and rationale.

    1. Purpose is to establish a sturdy union between broken ends of bone.

    2. Closed reduction done by manual manipulation without surgical incision.

    3. Open reduction: surgical incision made over fracture and exposed bone is aligned.

    4. Internal fixation: pins, plates, or screws may be used to stabilize position of the broken ends of bone.

    5. External fixation: pin sites need special care. Patient can be more mobile.

  E. Nonunion of bone can be treated with an electrical bone growth–stimulating device.

  F. Cast used to immobilize certain part of the body so that it is firmly supported and completely at rest; casts are made out of plaster or synthetic materials.

    1. Types of casts.

      a. Long-leg, short-leg, walking casts.

      b. Spica covers trunk and one or two extremities.

      c. Shoulder spica covers trunk and one arm.

    2. Cast care.

      a. Plaster cast: handle patient gently; takes a long time to dry.

        (1) Wet cast is handled only with the palms of the hands.

        (2) Supporting pillows should be waterproofed.

        (3) Turn patient frequently to avoid misshaping cast.

      b. Synthetic cast dries quickly.

      c. Ice bags may be used to control swelling.

    3. Nursing assessment.

      a. Listen to patient.

      b. Check neurovascular status (Table 22-9).

      c. Watch for signs of infection.

    4. Daily care.

      a. Protect plaster cast during bath or when patient uses bedpan.

      b. Observe condition of skin at edge of cast.

      c. Synthetic casts allow more freedom. Not suitable for serious fractures.

      d. Discharge with cast in place requires proper instructions for self-care.

    5. Cast brace or cast shoe.

      a. Combines stability of cast with mobility of brace.

      b. Used for patients with femoral shaft fracture.

      c. Ambulation with cast brace under supervision of physical therapist.

G. Types and uses of traction.

  1. Traction extends and holds part of the body in desired position by mechanical pull.

    a. Skeletal traction exerts pull on bone; skin traction exerts pull on the skin.

  2. Types include Bryant's traction, Buck's extension, balanced suspension, and side traction (Figure 22-10).

  3. Nursing intervention.

    a. Special and diligent back care.

    b. Bed is changed so that traction apparatus is disturbed as little as possible.

    c. Weights must be hanging free and patient positioned so that her body weight is counteracting the pull of weights.

    d. Check bony prominences frequently for signs of impaired circulation and pressure.

    e. Patient's body must be kept in good alignment.

H. Complications of fractures.

  1. Infection, especially in open fracture; danger of osteomyelitis.

  2. Osteomyelitis: bacterial infection of bone.

    a. Symptoms: sudden onset with severe pain and marked tenderness at site of infection, fever, swelling of adjacent parts.

    b. Treatment: rest, antibiotics, and measures to improve general health of patient. Surgical incision for drainage of abscess and debridement of infected bone if necessary.

  3. Delayed healing as a result of inadequate levels of serum calcium and phosphorus.

  4. Fat embolism: most common to fracture of long bones, pelvis, and ribs.

    a. Occurs within first 48 hours of fracture; high mortality rate.

    b. Signs and symptoms: respiratory distress, hypertension, tachypnea, fever, and petechiae over neck, upper arms, chest, or abdomen.

    c. Place patient in high Fowler's position to ease breathing; remain calm; begin oxygen administration at 2 to 3 L/minute if available; summon physician.

  5. Compartment syndrome: occurs in muscle compartments of the extremities.

    a. Caused by external or internal pressure; seriously restricts circulation.

    b. Causes considerable pain; signs and symptoms include edema, pallor, tingling, paresthesia, numbness, weak pulse, cyanosis, paresis, loss of function.

    c. Can cause permanent tissue and nerve damage if unrelieved.

    d. May be treated by surgical fasciotomy to relieve pressure.

VII. Carpal Tunnel Syndrome

A. Occurs when the median nerve is compressed as it passes through the carpal tunnel in the wrist.

B. Treatment is by rest, splinting, changing the angle of the wrist during repetitive movements, and steroid injection.

C. Surgical decompression may be necessary.

VIII. Bunion (Hallux Valgus)

A. Most common problem of the foot.

B. Painful swelling of the bursa with great toe deviation laterally.

C. When mobility is seriously affected, surgical resection is performed.

IX. Inflammatory Disorders

A. Arthritis: literally means inflammation of a joint.

  1. There are more than 100 different forms of arthritis; most common forms are osteoarthritis and rheumatoid arthritis.

    a. All forms produce joint pain and some degree of disability.

    b. Two forms most prevalent in adults are rheumatoid arthritis and osteoarthritis. Comparison of these two disorders in Table 22-11.

  2. Osteoarthritis: noninflammatory degenerative joint disease.

    a. Typically affects only a few joints.

    b. Occurs after age 35.

    c. Chief complaints are aching pain with joint movement and stiffness with limitation of mobility.

    d. Treatment: salicylates or NSAIDs; corticosteroid injection into joint if treatment does not control pain.

    e. Balance exercise and rest; exercise is encouraged.

    f. Nursing interventions: moist heat, imagery, and diversion to reduce pain; encourage weight control.

    g. Surgery may be done to relieve severe pain and improve mobility: joint replacement of hip or knee done frequently.

  3. Rheumatoid arthritis: inflammatory disease of the joints.

    a. Usually begins between age 25 and 55.

    b. Familial tendency, but is thought to be caused by autoimmune defect or an infectious agent.

c. Signs and symptoms: joint pain, warmth, edema, and limitation of movement and multiple joint stiffness in the morning.

d. Joints of hands, wrists, and feet are most commonly affected; involvement is usually bilateral and symmetric.

e. Systemic symptoms include low-grade fever, weight loss, and malaise.

f. Causes considerable joint deformity and dysfunction.

g. Treatment aimed at pain relief, minimization of joint destruction, and promotion of joint function.

h. Rest, exercise, medication, and immobilization with splints and supportive devices (orthoses) during periods of severe inflammation and heat or cold applications are all helpful.

i. Medications include salicylates, NSAIDs, corticosteroids, antimalarial drugs, sulfasalazine, methotrexate, gold compounds, penicillamine, and immunosuppressants (Table 22-12).

j. Surgical intervention and orthopedic devices.

   (1) Synovectomy and arthroplasty to prevent or modify deformities of joints.

   (2) Braces, splints, and casts to rest affected part during active flareups of symptoms.

4. Joint replacement

   a. Arthroplasty done for knee, shoulder, elbow, finger, ankle, or hip.

   b. Cemented or noncemented press-fit prosthesis used.

   c. Total hip replacement.

      (1) Joint replaced with combination of bone and synthetic joint parts or total synthetic joint.

      (2) Performed to relieve pain and provide mobility or to replace joint destroyed by trauma.

      (3) Preoperatively the patient is taught about the prosthesis and expected goals for rehabilitation after surgery.

      (4) Preoperative bacterial skin scrubs are usual for several days before surgery.

      (5) Postoperatively, proper positioning and exercise are essential to prevent complications and attain good mobility and joint function.

      (6) Discharge planning includes instruction of patient in ways to avoid injury to the artificial joint when he goes home.

   d. Knee replacement.

      (1) Chronic, uncontrollable pain is indication for knee replacement.

      (2) Emphasis on exercise postoperatively for best results; may use CPM machine soon after surgery.

      (3) Patient requires good analgesia to perform necessary exercises.

   e. Nursing intervention.

      (1) Rest and exercise.

         (a) Body in good alignment when patient is in bed.

         (b) Fatigue, muscle weakness, pain can inhibit exercise.

         (c) Patient instructed in proper way to engage in therapeutic exercises. Should take precautions not to injure joints.

      (2) Applications of heat and cold.

         (a) Either hot or cold may be suitable, depending on patient's preference and effectiveness of each.

         (b) In general, heat is better for subacute or chronic joint inflammation; cold for acute inflammation.

         (c) Safe methods for hot and cold applications shown in Table 22-15.

   f. Diet: no special diet other than that necessary to maintain normal body weight and avoid obesity.

   g. Resources for patient and family education: information available from local Arthritis Foundation, Arthritis Information Clearinghouse, and Self-Help Device Office of the Institute of Physical Medicine and Rehabilitation.

X. **Gout: Type of Arthritis Caused by High Serum Levels of Uric Acid**

   A. Uric acid crystals precipitate and settle in joints and connective tissue.

   B. Signs and symptoms: elevated serum uric acid; tight, reddened skin over an inflamed, edematous joint; temperature elevation; and extreme pain in the joint.

   C. Treatment: analgesics, allopurinol, probenecid or colchicine, NSAIDs; low-purine diet; restriction of alcohol; weight control.

XI. **Osteoporosis: Metabolic Bone Disorder Causing Decreased Bone Mass and Susceptibility to Fractures**

   A. Thought to be caused by long-term calcium deficit, estrogen deficiency, and inactivity.

   B. Contributing factors: cigarette smoking, excessive caffeine ingestion, and excessive alcohol intake.

C. Signs and symptoms: height loss, kyphosis, collapsed vertebrae and back pain, frequent fractures.

D. Dual energy x-ray absorptiometry (DXA or DEXA) used to assess bone loss.

E. Treatment aimed at prevention, with estrogen replacement therapy after menopause, calcium supplementation in midlife, regular weight-bearing exercise.

F. Calcium intake of 1,500 mg supplementally recommended after menopause.

G. Obtaining sufficient vitamin D through sunlight or vitamin supplements is essentially to bone growth.

H. Aldendronate (Fosamax) used to build up bones weakened by osteoporosis.

I. Micalcin nasal spray used to slow the rate of bone loss.

XII. **Paget's Disease: Abnormal Bone Resorption Followed by Abnormal Bone Formation.**

A. Abnormal bone is weak and prone to fractures.

B. Cause unknown.

C. Causes considerable pain from fractures.

D. Calcitonin, aldendronate, and etidronate given to slow bone resorption.

XIII. **Bone Tumors: Both Benign and Malignant**

A. Primary malignant tumors seen mostly between age 10 and 30; osteogenic sarcoma is the most common.

B. Metastatic bone tumors from cancer of the prostate, breast, kidney, thyroid, and lung are the most common and affect the pelvis, ribs, vertebrae, and femur.

C. Treatment includes surgery, radiation, and chemotherapy.

XIV. **Amputation**

A. Surgical removal of part or all of a limb because of severe physical trauma, malignancy, or gangrene. Eighty percent involve a lower extremity.

B. Preoperative care: prepare patient and family emotionally for loss of limb.

1. Help patient deal with sense of loss.

2. Prepare for "phantom sensations."

3. Team effort to plan rehabilitation with patient.

C. Postoperative care.

1. Observe for signs of hemorrhage.

2. Encourage lower-extremity amputee to lie on his stomach as much as possible, keeping the stump in good alignment to prevent flexion contractures.

3. Early ambulation to enhance recovery and rehabilitation.

4. Exercises done to keep joint mobile and prepare a limb for fitting of prosthesis.

D. Emotional aspects and rehabilitation:

1. Early ambulation and self-care to improve patient's morale and help achieve independence.

2. Nurse should have positive, hopeful attitude, help patient set short-range goals, and avoid giving false hope.

3. Focus on patient's strengths and what he is able to do.

4. Types of limb prostheses (Figures 22-13 and 22-14).

XV. **Muscle Disorders**

A. Most muscle disorders are neuromuscular; see Chapter 14 also.

B. Muscle strain most commonly occurs in the back muscles.

C. Other muscle strains often affect the joints. (See previous section under "strain.")

D. Treatment is rest, heat and cold application, antiinflammatory agents, and, if spasm is present, muscle relaxants.

E. Teaching the proper way to lift and move objects is important to prevent recurrence of back strain.

XVI. **Elder Care Points**

A. Greater risk of fracture due to decreased reaction time, failing vision, lessened agility, and decreased muscle tone.

B. Many chronic diseases require corticosteroids for treatment; these contribute to osteoporosis and fractures.

C. Arthritis occurs in 50% of population over 50 and increases in severity with aging.

D. Kyphosis from compression fractures of the spinal column can cause restricted lung expansion and predispose the patient to lung problems.

E. Hip fracture is common in people over 65 and is a major cause of morbidity and death from complications of immobility.

F. The elderly are more susceptible to problems of immobility.

G. The elderly have less subcutaneous fat and thin skin and get cold more easily than younger persons; take measures to keep the elderly patient warm as feeling cold increases pain and discomfort.

H. Elderly patients often are hospitalized for injuries sustained when improperly using ambulation devices; do thorough teaching and supervise practice before discharge.

I. Elderly patients with a fractured hip are at high risk for fat embolism; assess carefully for this complication.

J. NSAIDs are not recommended for all elderly patients as they cause so many side effects and may interact with other medications the person is taking for other chronic disorders.

K. The pain and immobility of arthritis can lead to a loss of independence; treatment is aimed at providing the greatest amount of relief of symptoms with the least amount of side effects.

L. Careful assessment for side effects of analgesics and other medications must be done for the elderly patient to prevent falls from dizziness.

XVII. Community Care

A. Rehabilitation programs for amputees, arthritis patients, and others with musculoskeletal disorders are available in many communities, often through the local YMCA.

B. Rehabilitation programs are shifting to "rehabilitation without walls," where the therapists go to the home of the patient or the patient attends an outpatient clinic.

C. Home care nurses are instrumental in preventing musculoskeletal injuries in home care patients. Safety assessment of the home and assessment of ability to use assistive devices for ambulation are performed.

D. Long-term care nurses constantly assess for hazards in the environment that might cause a fall and injury.

CHAPTER 23

Care of Patients with Urological Disorders

The kidneys and urinary tract are responsible for maintaining the proper balance of fluids, minerals, and organic substances necessary for life. In view of this, it is not surprising that a disease in any one system of the body may have a direct effect on the kidneys and urinary tract. Generalized diseases, such as atherosclerosis, other circulatory lesions, infections, or disturbances in the metabolic processes may very seriously impair the proper functioning of the kidneys. Similarly, problems in the heart, lungs, or circulatory system can arise from kidney failure.

Diseases do not always conveniently fit into clearly defined categories. The body functions as a whole and the systems are interdependent. This chapter will be concerned primarily with diseases of the urinary system; however, it should be remembered that the nurse frequently needs a good working knowledge of the basic principles of urological nursing in a wide variety of nursing care situations.

To understand how disorders of the urological system occur and how they affect the body, a review of the structure and function of the system is essential.

OVERVIEW OF ANATOMY AND PHYSIOLOGY

What Are the Structures of the Urological System and How Do They Interrelate?

⅄ The kidneys, ureters, urinary bladder, and urethra are the structures of the urinary system (Figure 23-1).

⅄ The kidneys are bean-shaped organs that lie on either side of the vertebral column at the level of the first lumbar vertebrae.

⅄ The kidney consists of the cortex, the outer layer, and the medulla; the cortex contains blood vessels and nephrons; the medulla contains the collecting tubules (Figure 23-2).

⅄ The nephron is the functional unit of the kidney; there are about 1 million nephrons.

⅄ The nephron consists of the glomerulus, which is a network of capillaries encased in a thin-walled sac called Bowman's capsule, and the tubular system.

⊿ The tubular system of the nephron consists of the proximal convoluted tubule, the loop of Henle, the distal convoluted tubule, and the collecting duct (Figure 23-3).

⊿ Urine is carried by peristaltic action from the kidney to the bladder by the ureters.

⊿ The bladder, a hollow muscular organ, serves as a reservoir for urine; the inner lining of the bladder is a mucous membrane.

⊿ The urine passes from the bladder down the urethra to the outside. The internal, involuntary, urethral sphincter is controlled by the detrusor muscle that is in the wall of the bladder.

⊿ The urethra is approximately 3 to 5 cm long in women and 20 cm in men. The external urethral sphincter controls release of urine to the outside. It is a voluntarily controlled sphincter.

⊿ Blood is brought to the kidney by the renal arteries, which branch off of the aorta. Blood is returned by veins to the inferior vena cava.

What Are the Functions of the Kidney?

⊿ The kidneys function to:

Eliminate metabolic wastes by filtration.

Regulate fluid volume by filtration, reabsorption, and excretion.

Regulate serum electrolytes by filtration and reabsorption.

Assist in maintaining acid–base balance by secreting H^+ ions into the urine.

Regulate blood pressure by secreting the enzyme renin.

Regulate red blood cell production by secreting erythropoietin.

⊿ The kidneys filter about one-fourth of the body's blood at any one time.

⊿ Each nephron filters blood plasma from the bloodstream through the semipermeable glomerular membrane; large protein molecules do not usually pass through the membrane. The glomerular filtration rate (GFR) is the amount of blood filtered by the glomeruli in a given time. The GFR is about 125 mL/minute normally.

⊿ Unwanted substances, such as urea, creatinine, uric acid, and other wastes, are retained in the tubules along with some water.

⊿ Most of the water and some of the electrolytes are reabsorbed into the bloodstream in the descending and distal convoluted tubules.

⊿ Approximately 200 L of liquid are filtered in a 24-hour period; 1.5 to 2 L are excreted as urine.

⊿ Three hormones that circulate in the blood influence urine volume and concentration: aldosterone, antidiuretic hormone (ADH), and atrial natriuretic hormone.

What Are the Functions of the Ureters, Bladder, and Urethra?

⊿ Each ureter is a small tube about 25 cm long that carries urine collected in the renal pelvis to the bladder.

⊿ The bladder holds the urine; initial urges to void occur when it contains 150 to 200 mL of urine; when it is distended with about 400 mL of urine a feeling of bladder fullness occurs and a signal to void (empty the bladder) is sent to the sacral area of the spinal cord. The **micturition** (voiding) reflex is then initiated and transmitted to the bladder.

⊿ Bladder capacity varies from about 1,000 to 1,800 mL.

⊿ The urethra carries urine from the bladder to the outside. The flow of urine is controlled by the internal urethral sphincter and the external urethral sphincter.

What Changes Occur with Aging?

⊿ Kidney function begins to lessen after age 45, and renal blood flow and GFR gradually decrease to about half the rate of a young adult.

⊿ In the male the prostate gland hypertrophies with age and causes varying degrees of obstruction to the normal flow of urine.

⊿ Degenerative changes in the bladder muscles lead to incomplete emptying and constant residual urine, which predisposes to infection.

⊿ Bladder capacity decreases, sometimes to as little as 200 mL, creating a need for more frequent emptying.

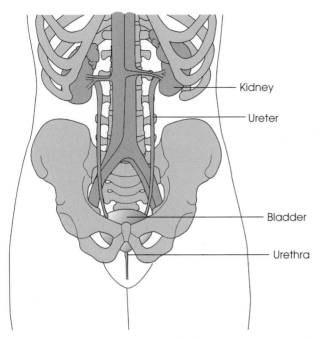

FIGURE 23-1   Structures of the urinary system.

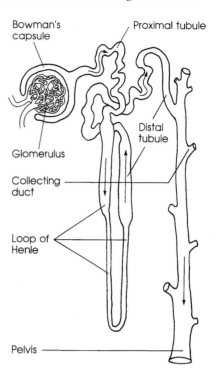

FIGURE 23-3   The nephron.

CAUSES AND PREVENTION OF DISORDERS OF THE UROLOGICAL SYSTEM

Many types of problems can affect the urological system. Bacterial infections, immunological disorders, metabolic disorders such as diabetes mellitus, and circulatory disorders can all cause dysfunction.

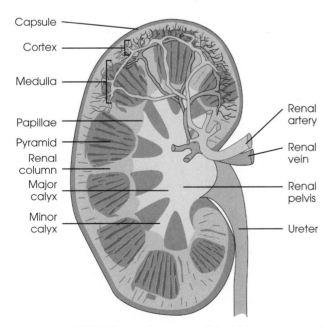

FIGURE 23-2   Structures of the kidney.

Circulatory shock or heart failure can bring about reduced blood circulation to the kidney. This in turn decreases the kidneys' ability to function in ridding the body of wastes.

Once urine is formed, the urinary system must be patent for urine to be excreted. Stones in the kidney or ureters may obstruct the flow of urine. An enlarged prostate may impede the ability to move urine from the bladder through the urethra in the male. Tubular necrosis due to bacterial or chemical destruction of cells affects the functional ability of the nephron and decreases kidney function. Many drugs can be toxic to the kidney, and heavy metals such as mercury can cause considerable damage. A lack of oxygen also causes tubular necrosis. The kidney is very sensitive to a lack of oxygen.

The urinary tract is very vulnerable to bacterial infection. In the high volume of blood that is filtered by the kidney there are some bacteria. These bacteria can colonize the kidney, causing an infection. Also, bacteria can easily enter the urinary tract through the urethra, which opens to the outside of the body.

Elder Care Point . . . Elderly females sometimes have a urethra that becomes displaced, opening into the vaginal outlet. This occurs from relaxed musculature and atrophy of surrounding structures. These women are more prone to develop urinary tract infections.

When an immune reaction occurs in the body, the glomeruli that filter the blood are exposed to antibodies and antigen–antibody complexes contained in that blood. These antibodies and antigen–antibody complexes can cause an autoimmune inflammatory reaction known as *glomerulonephritis* that interferes with normal kidney function.

Because so much of the kidney's function is directly related to the capillaries and arterioles, any disorder that systemically affects the blood vessels can affect the kidneys. Atherosclerosis and diabetes mellitus both affect the capillaries and arterioles. When these vessels become sclerosed, blood flow through the kidney is decreased and kidney function diminishes.

Tumors may form in the bladder, ureters, or kidney and interfere with normal function by altering cell structure or causing obstruction to urine flow. Tumors most often occur in the bladder. It is thought that, because urine contains excreted carcinogenic chemicals that sit in the bladder while urine is stored, this contact may be a cause of bladder tumors.

One of the best ways to prevent disorders of the urological system is to drink plenty of water. A fluid intake of 2,000 to 2,500 mL minimum per day is recommended to initiate good flow through the system. Adequate flow of fluid through the kidney helps prevent the formation of kidney stones. **Emptying the bladder regularly prevents stasis of urine, preventing substances contained in it from maintaining contact with the bladder wall for long periods.**

Elder Care Point . . . Many elderly people purposely restrict fluid intake to decrease the incidence of incontinence. Others restrict fluids to help control heart failure, renal failure, or other disorders that cause fluid retention. Restricting fluid intake decreases urine flow and makes the person more susceptible to urinary tract infection.

Practicing good hygiene, bathing regularly, and keeping the area around the urinary meatus clean help prevent bacteria from traveling up the urethra. Emptying the bladder after sexual intercourse helps flush any bacteria that entered the urethra. Seeking prompt treatment of bladder infections helps prevent the pathogens from traveling up the ureters to the kidneys themselves where they could directly attack kidney cells.

Controlling blood pressure within normal limits and keeping serum glucose levels normal helps slow the atherosclerotic process that affects the blood vessels. *Healthy blood vessels promote good kidney function.*

Carefully monitoring for adverse affects on the kidney of the drugs one takes and avoiding the use of chemicals known to be harmful to the kidney help preserve optimal kidney function (Table 23-1). When drugs that can be harmful to the kidney, such as sulfa

TABLE 23-1 ◆ *Substances That are Potentially Nephrotoxic*	
Antiinfectives/antibiotics	
◆ Amikacin	◆ Paramomycin
◆ Amphotericin B	◆ Polymyxin B
◆ Cephaloridine	◆ Rifampin
◆ Cephalothin	◆ Streptomycin
◆ Colistin	◆ Sulfonamides
◆ Gentamicin	◆ Tetracyclines
◆ Kanamycin	◆ Tobramycin
◆ Methicillin	◆ Vancomycin
◆ Neomycin	◆ Viomycin
Other drugs	
◆ Acetaminophen	◆ Indomethacin
◆ Captopril	◆ Mafenamic acid
◆ Cisplatin	◆ Methotrexate
◆ Cyclophasphamide	◆ Phenazopyridine hydrochloride
◆ Cyclosporine	
◆ D-Penicillamine	◆ Quinine
◆ Edetate disodium	◆ Salicylates
◆ Ethacrynic acid	◆ Many drugs when in combination with other drugs
◆ Furosemide	
◆ Halothane and fluorinated anesthetics	
Other substances	
◆ Carbon tetrachloride (cleaning solvent)	◆ Many pesticides
	◆ Many fungicides
◆ Ethylene glycol (antifreeze)	◆ Myoglobin from muscle tissue breakdown
◆ Heavy metals: arsenic, bismuth, copper sulfate, gold salts, lead, mercury compounds	◆ Xray contrast media dye

compounds, are prescribed, increasing the fluid intake to 3,000 to 3,500 mL per day can help reduce the problem. Avoiding routine use of over-the-counter drugs, such as acetaminophen, decreases exposure to potentially harmful chemicals.

Think about . . . What changes could you make in your dietary habits or lifestyle that might help you prevent urological problems?

DIAGNOSTIC TESTS AND PROCEDURES AND NURSING IMPLICATIONS

Patients experiencing problems with the urinary system undergo general systems tests, including a complete blood count (CBC) and chemistry panel and other diagnostic tests or procedures specific to the problem. Table 23-2 lists the diagnostic tests and procedures most commonly performed, along with their nursing implications. Other tests may also be ordered. A magnetic

TABLE 23-2 ♦ *Diagnostic Tests for Urological Problems*

Test	Purpose	Description	Nursing Implications
Urinalysis	Detects bacteria, blood, casts, and other abnormalities of the urine.	The urine is observed for color and clarity; the pH and specific gravity are determined; tests are performed to detect blood, protein, sugar, bilirubin and acetone; a microscopic exam is performed to detect the presence of red and white blood cells, casts, and crystals.	Obtain a urine specimen of at least 10 mL. A fresh morning specimen is preferred. Send specimen to lab immediately. Normal urine is clear, straw to dark amber in color, has a pH of 4.5 to 6.0, a specific gravity of 1.010 to 1.030, and is negative for protein, glucose, ketones, and bilirubin. It should have only a rare RBC, no more than 0 to 4 WBCs, and an occasional cast.
Fractional urine (two- to three-bottle routine)	Determines site and degree of bleeding after prostate surgery.	Patient voids into one urine container and then, without stopping the stream, continues to void into another container. The amount of blood in each container gives an indication of the degree and site of bleeding.	Provide two or three urine containers and instruct patient to switch containers midway through the voiding without stopping the stream.
Urine culture and sensitivity	Verifies urinary tract infection (UTI) and determines type of organism responsible. Usually done in conjunction with an anti-infective sensitivity screen.	A midstream clean catch or sterile catheterized specimen is obtained, and the urine is placed in a culture medium for growth of bacterial colonies. After incubation, the colonies are counted. If more than 100,000 organisms per milliliter are counted, there is a urinary tract infection. The organisms are then identified as to type. Gram-negative bacilli are the most common cause of UTIs. *Escherichia coli (E. coli)* found in the intestinal tract is a frequent cause of UTI. Sensitivity test involve exposing the bacteria to various antiinfectives to see which most effectively kills the organism.	Instruct patient in method for collection of a "clean catch" specimen. Instructions come with the specimen container. Allow time for questions after patient is familiar with directions. A sterile specimen can also be obtained via urinary catheterization. Send specimen to lab immediately to prevent change in pH, which can affect bacterial growth.
Urine osmolality	Determines whether the kidneys can concentrate urine normally.	The patient is either placed on fluid restriction or given a specific amount of fluid to drink before the test. Normal range for urine osmolality is 300 to 1,200 mOsm/kg.	Give a high-protein diet for 3 days prior to the urine collection. Restrict fluids for 8 to 12 hours before obtaining specimen. Collect a random urine specimen, preferably in the morning, label it (including the time), and send to lab.
Protein metabolites Blood urea nitrogen (BUN)	Determine ability of the kidneys to filter and excrete end products of metabolism.	Urea is the main protein metabolite excreted. Blood urea nitrogen (BUN) is measured to help evaluate kidney function; the extent of renal disease, and hydration status. High BUN levels can indicate poor kidney function, dehydration, or increased breakdown of body protein such as occurs with severe burns or excessive exercise. Lower BUN levels are found in severe liver damage, excessive hydration, and protein deficiency. Normal BUN levels average 8 to 20 mg/dL, depending on sex and age.	Usually done with patient NPO for 8 hours. Requires 5 mL of venous blood.

(Table 23-2 continued)

TABLE 23-2 ◆ *Diagnostic Tests for Urological Problems* (Continued)

Test	Purpose	Description	Nursing Implications
Serum creatinine	Evaluates kidney function.	Creatinine is produced in fairly constant amounts in the body in proportion to muscle mass. The measurement of the amount of creatinine in the blood makes it a good estimator of kidney function. Serum creatinine is measured first, and, if it is elevated, then urine creatinine is assessed. Urine creatinine helps assess glomerular filtration and goes up when renal perfusion is lessened or when the glomeruli cannot function properly. Normal serum creatinine is 0.4 to 1.2 mg/dL.	No food or drink restriction, but patient should not eat large amounts of meat beforehand. Requires 5 to 10 mL venous blood. List drugs patient is taking on lab slip, as certain drugs affect the test.
Creatinine clearance	Determines how well kidneys can excrete creatinine by examining both blood and urine.	A 12- to 24-hour urine specimen is obtained, and a blood specimen is drawn. Elevated serum creatinine with decreased urine creatinine indicates decreased kidney function. Normal creatinine clearance is 15 to 25 mg/kg body weight in 24 hours.	A 5-mL venous blood sample is collected before the test begins. Place a sign on the patient's door and over the toilet stating "24-hour urine test in progress" so that everyone will save the urine properly. Collect a 12- or 24-hour urine specimen: have patient void and discard the urine: note the time on the lab slip; put each successive voiding into the collection container. Check with lab as to whether the container must be kept on ice. At the time the test is to end, ask the patient to void and add this last urine to the collection bottle. Send the specimen to the lab.
Radiological studies KUB (kidneys, ureters, bladder)	Visualizes the structures of the urinary tract; locates stones or abnormalities.	X-ray of the lower abdomen done without contrast medium.	Explain purpose and procedure; have patient put on x-ray gown. Determine pregnancy status.
Intravenous pyelogram (IVP)	Visualizes the kidneys and ureters. Detects impairment of kidney function resulting from obstruction, stones, or tumor in the kidneys, ureters, or prostate.	After IV injection of an iodine-based dye, multiple x-rays are taken at 5 or more minutes apart, showing the flow of the dye through the renal system. A retrograde pyelogram is done during cystoscopy. Catheters are threaded into the ureters to inject the dye into the kidneys.	Explain purpose and procedure; check for allergy to iodine or shellfish and consult with physician if one exists. Patient may feel a hot flush when dye is injected; nausea sometimes occurs. Inform patient that the test takes 30 to 60 minutes.
Cystogram	Visualizes the contour of the bladder.	X-ray films are taken before and after sodium iodide is injected into the bladder through a urethral catheter.	Inform patient that the bladder may feel very full and he may feel like he needs to void after the dye is instilled. A Foley catheter is usually inserted prior to the procedure. The bladder is drained after the x-rays are taken.
Computed tomographic (CT) scan	Determines presence of a cyst or tumor in the kidney.	A combination of x-ray and computer techniques yields cross-sectional information and indicates the density of tissues.	Explain the purpose and procedure. Contrast medium may be given; check for allergy to iodine. Describe the CT scan machine and the sounds she might hear (clicking and whirring).

TABLE 23-2 ♦ *Diagnostic Tests for Urological Problems* *(Continued)*			
Test	**Purpose**	**Description**	**Nursing Implications**
Renal ultrasono-graphy	Determines size, shape, and location of each kidney, the ureters, and the bladder; indicates tumors and obstructions to urine flow.	Uses high-frequency sound waves and an oscilloscope screen. A probe is passed over the surface of the flank while the patient is positioned on a table.	Explain the purpose and procedure. Patient may be asked to drink fluid to fill bladder prior to sonogram. Test takes approximately 30 minutes.
Renal angiography	Assesses renal arterial system function and identifies areas of obstruction to blood flow.	Under local anesthesia, a catheter is threaded through the femoral artery, up the aorta to the renal artery, and a contrast agent is injected. Fluoroscopic examination is done while the agent enters and fills the blood vessels. Angiography is performed to detect complications in a transplanted kidney, to evaluate a kidney mass, or to determine the extent of kidney trauma.	Requires a signed permission form. Check for allergy to iodine-based dye. Pressure is applied to the entrance site for 20 minutes after procedure, a pressure dressing and a sandbag are applied, and the patient is kept flat in bed for 4 to 12 hours, assessed frequently for signs of bleeding, shock, or other complications, and kept on bedrest for 24 hours. Vital signs are taken q 15 to 30 min until stable, and popliteal and pedal pulses are checked at least q 4 h to evaluate peripheral circulation. The puncture site is watched for bleeding or hematoma formation.
Radionuclide renal scan	Studies renal blood flow or detects abnormal areas of kidney tissue (i.e., tumors or cysts).	A radioisotope is injected into the blood, and a scintillation scaner is passed over the area of the kidney. This yields a pattern of areas in which the isotope has been taken up. An interval of about 30 minutes is allowed before scanning if a tumor or cysts are suspected.	Explain that the isotope used is low-dose radiation and is quickly eliminated from the body. There usually is no danger to the patient or others from it. Describe the clicking sounds the scanner makes; test takes approximately 45 to 90 min.
Cystoscopy	Examines the interior of the bladder.	Under short-acting anesthesia, a cystoscope is passed up the urethra into the bladder. The scope can be guided into a ureter to extract a stone or to biopsy lesions in the bladder.	Requires a signed permission form, as it is a surgical procedure. Explain the purpose and procedure. Unless general anesthesia is to be used, a full liquid breakfast is given. A preoperative sedative/tranquilizer and analgesic is given 1 hour prior to the procedure. The patient will be placed in the lithotomy position on the operating table. Water may be instilled into the bladder to promote better visualization. The test takes about 1 hour. After the procedure, burning, frequency, and pink-tinged urine are normal. Warm sitz baths and mild analgesics are given for voiding discomfort. Urine is monitored for 24 hours for signs of frank bleeding.
Renal biopsy	Obtains tissue for pathological study.	With local anesthetic, the patient is placed in the prone position, and a biopsy needle is inserted into the lower lobe of the kidney. A tissue sample is extracted and sent to the lab.	The patient is placed in a prone position with a pillow wedged under the abdomen at the level of the kidney. The results of IVP or ultrasound are used to precisely locate the kidney, a local anesthetic is given, and a biopsy needle is inserted below the 12th rib. The patient must hold her breath while the needle is inserted and withdrawn.

(Table 23-2 continued)

TABLE 23-2 ◆ *Diagnostic Tests for Urological Problems* (*Continued*)

Test	Purpose	Description	Nursing Implications
			Afterward a pressure dressing is applied, and the patient is kept prone for 30 to 60 minutes. She is usually on bedrest for 24 hours. Vital signs are taken every 5 to 10 min for 1 h and then with decreasing frequency until stable. The patient is assessed for flank pain and for gross and microscopic hematuria (blood in the urine). She is not to lift heavy objects for 5 to 7 days. WBCs and temperature are monitored for signs of infection.
Cystometrography (CMG)	Determine the effectiveness and sensitivity of the detrusor muscle in the bladder wall.	The patient voids and the amount, rate of flow, and time of voiding are recorded. A urinary catheter is inserted and attached to a cystometer. Fluid is instilled into the bladder. The point at which a feeling of the need to void is felt is noted. Readings of bladder capacity and pressure are recorded graphically. When the instillation is complete, the patient is asked to void; the amount is recorded and urinary residual is noted. The catheter is removed.	Sterile technique must be used for catheter insertion and bladder fluid instillation. The patient is monitored for signs of infection postprocedure.
Urethral pressure study	Determine the nature of urinary retention and incontinence.	A catheter with pressure-sensing capabilities is inserted into the bladder. As the catheter is withdrawn, the varying pressures of the smooth muscle of the urethra are recorded.	Sterile technique must be used for catheter insertion. The patient is monitored for signs of infection postprocedure.
Electromyography of the perineal muscles	Evaluate the quality of the voluntary muscles used in voiding.	Electrodes are placed either in the rectum or the urethra to measure contraction and relaxation of the muscles involved in voiding.	Warn the patient that some short, mild discomfort may accompany the placement of the electrodes. Analgesics may be given after the procedure to relieve discomfort. The patient is monitored for signs of infection postprocedure.

resonance imaging (MRI) scan is sometimes done to detect a kidney tumor, but because it is very expensive, other methods of diagnosis are usually used first.

Elder Care Point . . . The aged kidney has less ability to concentrate the urine, and this phenomenon predisposes the patient to dehydration when fluid intake is restricted for diagnostic tests. The contrast agents used for x-ray tests, in conjunction with dehydration, can cause acute renal failure in the elderly patient. The nurse should pay particular attention to rehydrating the patient as soon as the test is finished to prevent this problem.

NURSING MANAGEMENT

◆ Assessment

Definition of Terms   The following terms are commonly used to describe various kinds of abnormal flow of urine:

- **Anuria:** absence of urine. This rarely occurs, but can be due to renal failure, usually acute.
- **Oliguria:** diminished or abnormally decreased flow of urine. It may be dehydration, renal failure, or obstruction to the flow of urine somewhere in the drainage system.

- **Polyuria:** abnormally high urinary output; the result of excessive solutes and increased excretion of water. Therefore, urine is very dilute. Possible causes include hypercalcemia, diabetes insipidus, uncontrolled diabetes mellitus, and increased fluid intake.
- **Urinary retention:** retaining or holding urine in the bladder. This can be due to anxiety; postoperative swelling; fear of pain on voiding, particularly following surgery; neurological disorders; and obstruction to flow of urine through the urethra, as in enlargement of the prostate gland. If a catheter is not passed to relieve urinary retention and bladder distention, the bladder will not rupture, but urine will begin to dribble out of the urethra. Retention of urine stretches the bladder walls, causing extreme discomfort. Nursing measures to induce voiding may be effective in some cases, thereby avoiding the danger of introducing infectious organisms by catheterization.
- **Residual urine:** that which is left in the bladder after voiding. Poor bladder tone or partial obstruction of the urethra can result in dribbling of urine or passing only the overflow, leaving the bladder partially full. Residual urine is measured by having the patient void as much urine as possible and then inserting a catheter immediately after. Fifteen milliliters is considered a normal amount of residual urine. Any amount over this can become more and more stagnant and concentrated over time, predisposing the patient to bladder infection and the formation of stones.
- **Suppression of urine:** inability of the kidney to produce urine. This is due to renal failure and results in oliguria or anuria.

History and Present Illness

At the time of admission the nurse will try to obtain background data related to urinary problems to establish a nursing data base for intervention. Because of the kidney's response to pathological conditions in virtually every other system of the body, a personal history of illness or injury to any system could be relevant to an assessment of kidney function. Previous disorders of the urinary tract, especially those that required surgery, are particularly relevant.

Family history of cardiovascular disease, diabetes, and kidney stone formation is pertinent to assessment of a patient's renal status. These diseases can adversely affect the kidney, and they tend to occur more often in family members than would be expected by chance.

Sexually transmitted diseases and other genital and reproductive disorders frequently have a negative impact on the urinary drainage system by interfering with normal urination. Examples include herpetic inflammation of the urethra and benign or malignant enlargement of the prostate gland. (See Chapters 27 and 28.)

Many drugs can be toxic to the kidney (i.e., nephrotoxic). Therefore the nursing history should include any drugs recently or currently being taken by the patient.

Information from the patient about his present illness should include observations of changes in urinary output, including amount and character of urine, pain or discomfort in either the bladder or the kidney region, and abnormal patterns of voiding. These kinds of data pertinent to assessment of urological status are discussed in detail in the following sections. Table 23-3 presents an assessment guide for the nurse.

Ongoing Assessment Nursing responsibilities in the daily assessment of urinary function include (1) measuring intake and output; (2) evaluating abnormal flow of urine; (3) noting the character of urine (color, odor, clouding); (4) noticing changes in the pattern of voiding; and (5) ascertaining pain and discomfort.

Characteristics of urine. The color of urine can give helpful information about the status of the patient

---

TABLE 23-3 ◆ *Assessment: Guide to Urological Assessment*

The following questions are asked when assessing the patient with a urological problem:

- Do you or any of your family have a history of hypertension, cardiovascular disease, diabetes, kidney stones, frequent urinary tract infections, or other kidney problems?
- Have you ever had a genital herpes infection?
- Do you have any pain when urinating? Any abdominal or flank pain?
- Do you have any difficulty in starting the stream of urine?
- Do you feel as though you empty the bladder completely when you urinate?
- Have you noticed any change in the appearance or smell of your urine?
- Have you needed to empty the bladder more frequently than usual?
- Have you been experiencing any urgency, where the desire to empty the bladder is so great that dribbling occurs before you reach the bathroom?
- How many times do you need to get up at night to empty the bladder? (Once a night is average.)
- Have you had any episodes of urinary incontinence?
- Have you ever noticed blood in your urine (other than when menstruating—for women)?
- Do you have any problem with sexual dysfunction?
- Are you experiencing excessive fatigue?
- Have you noticed any itching of the skin?
- How much fluid do you drink in a day?

Physical examination should include the following:

- Inspect the abdomen for any visible abnormalities.
- Palpate all four quadrants for areas of tenderness.
- Palpate above the pubic bone for evidence of bladder distention.
- Examine the urine for color, clarity, volume, and smell.

and the functioning of the kidney. Table 23-4 shows color variations in urine and the significance of abnormal coloration.

Another characteristic that should be noted is *odor*. Normal urine develops an ammonia-like odor after it has stood for a length of time, but this odor should not be present in freshly voided urine. A foul smell indicates infection. Acetone in the urine, which occurs during metabolic acidosis, causes it to have a sweet, fruity odor.

Hematuria means blood in the urine. Microscopic hematuria usually is not indicative of any abnormality in the urinary system. Gross hematuria, a common cause of abnormal changes in urine color, is a sign of continued bleeding from some point in the urinary tract. Red blood in the urine is not easily missed, but if the blood has been in the bladder or kidney for a long time, it could have deteriorated and will cause the urine to be a smoky gray or dark brown.

TABLE 23-4 ◆ *Common Causes of Variations in Color of Urine*

Color	Medication or Diet	Other Causes
Colorless or pale yellow	Diuretics Alcohol	Dilute urine due to diabetes insipidus, diabetes mellitus, overhydration, chronic renal disease, nervousness
Bright yellow	Riboflavin (multiple vitamins)	None
Dark amber to orange	Phenazopyridine HCl (Pyridium, Azo Gantanol, Azo Gantrisin) Nitrofurantoin (Macrodantin) Sulfasalazine (Azulfidine) Docusate calcium; phenolphthalein (Doxidan) (in alkaline urine) Thiamine (multiple vitamins) Excessive carotene (e.g., carrots)	Concentrated urine due to dehydration or increased metabolic state Urobilinogen Bilirubin
Pink to red	Phenothiazines Phenolphthalein (laxatives) (in alkaline urine) Phenytoin (Dilantin) Rifampin Phenolsulfonphthalein (PSP) dye (in alkaline urine) Cascara (in alkaline urine) Senna (X-Prep, Senokot) Beets Blackberries Rhubarb (in alkaline urine)	Hemoglobin Porphyrin Red blood cells Myoglobin Menstrual contamination
Brown	Cascara (in acid urine) Metronidazole (Flagyl) (if left standing)	Extremely concentrated urine due to dehydration or increased metabolic state Urobilinogen Porphyrin Bilirubin Red blood cells
Blue or green	Triamterene (Dyrenium) Amitriptyline (Elavil) Phenylsalicylate Methylene blue Indigo carmine Vitamin B complex	Bilirubin-biliverdin *Pseudomonas* infection

Dark brown to black	Nitrofurantoin (Macrodantin)
	Iron preparations (if left standing)
	  Levodopa (if left standing)
	  Methocarbamol (if left standing)
	Phenacetin
	Quinine
	Cascara (in acid urine)
	Senna (X-Prep, Senokot)
	Methyldopa (Aldomet)
		Melanin
		Porphyrin
		Red blood cells (old blood)
		Homegentisic acid in alkaptonuria

Source: Karlowicz, K. A. (1995). *Urologic Nursing Principles and Practice.* Philadelphia: Saunders, p. 41

When assessing a patient with hematuria, the nurse should try to find out at what point during the act of urinating the blood is noticed. This information can help locate the source of bleeding. If the blood is noticed as soon as voiding starts, it is likely that the bleeding is from somewhere in the urethra. If it is noticed at the end of urination, the site probably is near the neck of the bladder. Bleeding throughout voiding indicates that the blood is coming from a site above the neck of the bladder, because the blood has been well mixed with the urine in the bladder.

Changes in voiding pattern. These changes include the number of times during the day and night the patient has the urge to urinate (frequency). Other alterations could be in the size and force of the urinary stream, feeling of fullness even after voiding, and change in the amount urinated each time.

Increased frequency can be a manifestation of some abnormality in the urinary drainage system, particularly in the bladder and urethra. The frequency with which a person feels the urge to urinate can be related to psychological as well as physiological factors. Excitement, anxiety, and fear can produce increased frequency of urination. Caffeine and other diuretics found in foods and drinks and simply an increased intake of water can increase the number of times a person must urinate. Pathological conditions that can cause increased frequency include inflammation of the bladder (*cystitis*) or urethra (*urethritis*).

Urgency also is symptomatic of inflammation. Urgency refers to an almost uncontrollable desire to void. Sometimes it causes incontinence, because it is not possible to get to a bathroom soon enough when the urge to urinate is felt.

Pain and discomfort. In general, the locations in which the patient with a urinary problem is most likely to experience discomfort are either the bladder or suprapubic area, or the region over the kidney (flank pain). The third kind of discomfort may be painful urination, or **dysuria.**

Bladder pain can be due to an overfull bladder and stretching of its walls. Assessment of the size and location of the bladder is indicated when a patient reports pain in the bladder region. Normally the bladder cannot be felt. If a smooth, rounded mass is felt on palpation in the area above the pubic bone, the bladder is distended.

Bladder pain also can be caused by spasms of the bladder musculature as it attempts to empty itself of clots, bits of tissue, and other cellular debris. This can occur postoperatively or when there is moderate to severe inflammation and bleeding in the urinary tract. Relief sometimes can be obtained by irrigating the bladder and tubing to remove the clots and debris. Belladonna and opium (B&O) rectal suppositories often are ordered for bladder spasms.

Flank pain also can be due to obstruction and distention; in this case the affected organs are the ureters and kidney pelvis. **Spasmodic peristaltic contractions along the ureter can be caused by stones, clots, a tumor, inflammatory swelling, or any other condition that prevents the flow of urine from the kidney to the bladder.** In her evaluation of flank pain the nurse should ask the patient the location of the pain, to see if it tends to radiate from the kidney or ureter to the genitalia and thigh.

Dysuria usually is caused by inflammation in either the bladder or the urethra. It often is described as burning and can range from mild to moderate to severe. In addition to determining where the pain is and how it feels, the nurse also should ask the patient when the pain occurs and if it is related to and felt immediately before, during, or after voiding.

◆ Nursing Diagnosis

Nursing diagnoses frequently associated with urological problems and disturbances in urinary flow include the following:

- Altered pattern of urinary elimination related to inflammation or tissue damage.
- Fluid volume excess related to inability to form urine.
- Pain related to ureteral spasm, bladder spasm, or inflammation.
- Activity intolerance related to fatigue.
- Sleep pattern disturbance related to nocturia.
- Knowledge deficit related to management of disease and means of prevention.
- Fear related to cause of hematuria, possibility of malignancy, or treatment by dialysis.
- Body image disturbance related to maintenance of life by dialysis or urinary diversion.
- Risk of sexual dysfunction related to effects of kidney failure.

◆ Planning

General goals for patients with urologic disorders are:

- Absence of infection
- Absence of pain
- Restoration of normal urinary output
- Return to normal fluid balance
- Knowledge for appropriate self-care
- Resolution of body image disturbance
- Prevention of complications

Planning care of the patient with a disorder of the urological system involves considering the effect of the disorder on the other systems of the body. **Fatigue is** common when kidney function is impaired because of the effect of the buildup of waste products in the body and their effect on body cells. In the acute stages kidney failure patients often have self-care deficits. When wastes are circulating in the blood in greater than usual quantities, they can irritate the nervous system cells and make the patient irritable. The nurse must take these occurrences into account when working with these patients.

The patient undergoing hemodialysis undergoes considerable fluid volume shifts that affect homeostasis. The nurse will need to plan to assess this patient more frequently in the hours after dialysis treatment is completed.

◆ Implementation

Caring for patients with urological problems focuses on monitoring intake and output, weight, and signs of edema. Specific nursing interventions are presented in the nursing care plan, clinical pathway, and Table 23-5. The nurse must use strict aseptic technique when

TABLE 23-5 ◆ *Common Nursing Diagnoses, Expected Outcomes, and Nursing Interventions for Urological Disorders*		
Nursing Diagnosis	**Goals/Expected Outcomes**	**Nursing Interventions**
Fluid volume excess related to retention of sodium and water from inadequate kidney function.	Weight will return to previous level within 10 days. Lungs will be clear to auscultation. Foot and ankle edema decrease within 24 hours. No evidence of foot and ankle edema within 7 days.	Record objective assessment of foot and ankle edema. Administer diuretic as ordered. Restrict fluid intake to 1,200 mL/24 hours as ordered. Restrict sodium to 2 g/day as ordered. Obtain daily weight before breakfast and record. Auscultate lungs q shift. Assess for shortness of breath q shift. Assist to establish acceptable schedule for restricted fluids. Explain reason for fluid restriction. Provide hard candy and gum; give mouth care q 2 h. Carefully measure and record intake and output.
Activity intolerance related to decreased hemoglobin and hematocrit values.	Hemoglobin values will increase to 11 g/100 mL within 2 weeks. Hematocrit will increase to 28% within 2 weeks. Fatigue will be lessened as voiced by patient within 2 weeks.	Administer ferrous sulfate and folic acid as ordered. Instruct about foods with high iron and folic acid content. Administer Epogen as ordered; monitor hemoglobin and hematocrit. Transfuse with blood product if ordered; monitor for adverse effects. Monitor urine for blood. Alternate periods of activity with adequate rest.
Knowledge deficit related to scheduled diagnostic tests and side effects of drugs ordered.	Patient will be able to identify common side effects of drugs prescribed within 2 weeks. Patient will verbalize purpose of each diagnostic test and the preparation requirements before the test is performed.	Create teaching plan for side effects and purpose of each drug prescribed; perform teaching in short sessions; obtain feedback for evaluation of comprehension. Explain the purpose and preparation requirements for each diagnostic test ahead of time. Obtain feedback for evaluation of comprehension.
Fear of malignancy, renal failure, and death.	Patient will begin to talk about fear of renal failure and death within 7 days. Patient will verbalize specific fears about dialysis before it is instituted.	Establish trusting relationship. Encourage verbalization of feelings. Provide information on chronic renal failure and treatment options—peritoneal dialysis, hemodialysis, renal transplant. Emphasize that good quality of life can be attained with dialysis.
Body image disturbance related to maintenance of life by dialysis.	Patient will verbalize feelings related to loss of kidney function and reliance on artifical kidney within 3 weeks. Patient will demonstrate positive attitude toward the life-giving aspect of dialysis within 3 months.	Establish trusting relationship. Encourage verbalization of feelings and perceptions about how life has changed. Offer support from well-adjusted dialysis patient. Help patient to focus on positives of personality, capabilities, and life.
Risk of sexual dysfunction related to effects of kidney failure.	Patient will verbalize fears regarding sexual dysfunction within 3 weeks.	Encourage verbalization of fears. Counsel regarding the positive aspects of dialysis. Counsel in ways to obtain sexual satisfaction with mate or refer for counseling should sexual problems arise.

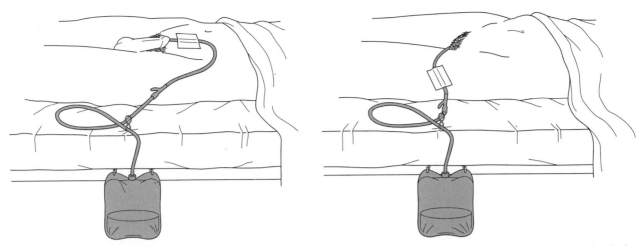

FIGURE 23-4   Catheter tubing attached to a collection bag with catheter secured to the abdomen for the male and the thigh for the female.

catheterizing patients, emptying drainage bags, handling drainage tubes and stents, and when performing peritoneal or hemodialysis. When cleaning patients incontinent of stool, or assisting with toileting, wipe the female perineum from front to back to avoid contaminating the urethral meatus.

If the patient has an indwelling catheter, the meatus and catheter should be gently cleansed with soap and water and rinsed thoroughly, just as the area would be cleansed if the patient were bathing normally. All indwelling catheter drainage bags should have a valve leading to the catheter that prevents backflow of urine from the bag. The catheter should be fastened to the upper leg with tape or a strap. Long-term catheter use in the male requires that the tube be secured to the abdomen (Figure 23-4). Connecting tubing should be positioned so that there is no pulling on the catheter when the patient turns, moves in bed, or arises to ambulate; this prevents pulling on the balloon that holds the catheter in place, which would cause tissue irritation and predispose to infection. When the drainage bag is emptied, care should be taken not to contaminate the drainage port and it should be cleansed before it is closed and replaced. Each patient should have a personal container into which the urine is drained for disposal. Such equipment should not be shared among patients. Table 23-6 presents the principles of urinary catheter and tube care. Bedpans should be thoroughly cleansed and rinsed after use and should *not* be stored on the floor.

When irrigation of a urinary catheter is needed, it should be done using a closed system technique whenever possible. Opening a urine drainage system invites the entrance of bacteria. Table 23-7 lists common urinary catheters and tubes used for urological disorders.

Measuring Intake and Output   The quantity of fluids entering the body, by whatever route, has a direct bearing on fluid balance. The importance of maintaining a normal fluid balance is covered in Chapter 5. Patients with urological disorders are very likely to suffer fluid imbalances, and therefore their intake and output should be measured and the totals recorded every 8 hours during hospitalization or acute illness. In critically ill patients the urinary output is often measured hourly.

For total output, amounts need to be measured for all urine excreted, drainage from all tubes, any vomitus, watery stools, and an estimate of the amount of fluid lost through perspiration. Any fluid used to irrigate urinary catheters and tubing must be measured and the amount added to the total intake.

A large part of nursing intervention is to assess for signs of infection and decreasing urinary function. Urine output should be at least 30 mL/hour. Monitoring the drug combinations patients are taking for potential nephrotoxicity and for possible urinary retention is very important.

◆ Evaluation

Evaluation requires reassessment to determine whether nursing actions are achieving the desired expected outcomes. If not, the actions need to be revised. The nurse compares intake and output data over a period of days to determine clinical improvement or the presence of problems. Urine output is evaluated and should be at least 30 mL/hour. Laboratory data, such as serum levels of blood urea nitrogen (BUN) and creatinine, potassium, and urinalysis reports, provide further information to evaluate the effectiveness of treatment. Decrease in symptoms that indicated a urinary problem indicates resolution of the problem.

The following principles should be followed when caring for a patient with a urinary catheter or drainage tube:

- Use aseptic technique and gentle handling when caring for any urinary drainage tube.
- Insert urethral catheters using sterile technique.
- Never open a urinary drainage system unless there is no other way to remedy a problem (i.e., the drainage bag must be changed for some reason).
- Remove collected urine from the bottom of the drainage bag by opening the drainage port; use aseptic technique and do not allow the drainage tube to touch the collection container. After reclamping the tube, wipe away residual urine from the tube with an antiseptic swab before securing it.
- Use each patient's own collection container for draining the urine storage bag.
- **Observe all tubes and level of drainage in the collection bag each time the patient is seen.**
- Keep the drainage bag below the level of the catheter or tube's entry into the body. If the bag must be raised above entry level, clamp off the tube briefly while repositioning the patient and bag to prevent backflow of urine unless bag has a one-way valve.
- Perform perineal care at least twice daily, cleaning the urinary meatus and catheter with soap and water; rinse well (see agency's policy).
- Keep an intake and output record to help monitor kidney function.
- Force fluids to 3,000 mL/day unless contraindicated; adequate fluid helps flush the bacteria and sediment from the urinary system.
- Prevent undue tension on the catheter by securing the tubing to the female's leg or the male's abdomen and securing the drainage tubing so it doesn't get caught in bed siderails or wheelchair parts.
- When irrigating, use the correct, ordered sterile solution in the correct amount. (Nephrostomy tube <5 mL; ureteral tube or stent <2 mL. **Amount of solution is by physician's order.**)
- Use a steady, gentle stream to irrigate. Avoid exerting pressure that may traumatize or cause discomfort.
- Do not pull back forcefully on an irrigating syringe attached to a urinary catheter or tube as this creates negative pressure that may damage delicate tissues.
- Allow for the backflow of solution as part of the irrigation.

INFLAMMATORY DISORDERS OF THE URINARY TRACT

♦ Cystitis

Cystitis is an inflammation of the urinary bladder. It is one of the most common urinary tract infections, especially in women, probably because the urethra is shorter in women and the urinary meatus is in close proximity to the vaginal and anal areas. The *Esche-*

richia coli bacterium, which normally resides in the intestinal tract as a nonpathogenic microorganism, accounts for about 80% of all urinary tract infections (UTI) in females.

Cystitis and urethritis are most often seen in women after they have become sexually active. This is because bacteria may enter the urethra due to friction during intercourse. They are more common in older women, its incidence increasing with age as the decreased muscle tone in the urinary tract prevents complete emptying of the bladder, causing stasis. Urine that sits in the bladder provides a good medium for bacterial growth.

Signs and Symptoms   **The most common symptoms of cystitis are painful urination, frequent and urgent urination, and lowback pain.** The urinary meatus may appear swollen and inflamed. Cystitis has a tendency to recur, producing less acute symptoms, such as fatigue, anorexia, and a constant feeling of pressure in the bladder region between flareups. The urine may appear cloudy or even bloody.

Elder Care Point . . .   One of the first signs of cystitis or UTI in the elderly may be confusion. If a patient who is normally alert becomes confused, assess the urine and check for signs of UTI.

Urinalysis and urine cultures are used to establish a definite diagnosis and to identify the specific causative organism in cystitis.

Treatment   Treatment of cystitis includes administering either urinary antiseptics or antibacterial drugs. Table 23-8 lists the most commonly used drugs and their implications for nursing. The patient is encouraged to

TABLE 23-7 ♦ *Common Catheters and Tubes Used for Urological Disorders*

Tube/Catheter	Purpose
Urethral catheter	Drain urine from the bladder.
Foley catheter	Indwelling catheter for continuous urine drainage from the bladder.
Suprapubic catheter	Continuous drainage of urine from the bladder; inserted in suprapubic area of abdomen through abdominal and bladder wall.
Ureteral catheter	Drain urine directly from the ureter or kidney.
Ureteral stent	Tube placed in ureter to hold it open during healing.
Nephrostomy tube	Placed into the pelvis of the kidney to provide drainage of urine directly from the kidney.

TABLE 23-8 ◆ Drugs Used for Urinary Tract Infections

Drug	Features and Action	Nursing Implications
Urinary antiseptics		
Methenamine (Cystamin, Cystogen, Urotropin, Mandelamine)	Bacteriostatic compounds of ammonia and formaldehyde.	Needs acid urine. Fluids encouraged.
Nalidixic acid (NegGram)	Effective against gram-negative organisms.	Give 1 hour before meals to maximize blood levels.
Nitrofurantoin (Macrodantin, Furadantin) Macrocystalline nitrofuradantin (Macrobid)	Wide range of antibacterial action against both gram-negative and gram-positive organisms.	Tints urine brown. Give with food.
Phenazopyridine (Pyridium)	Mildly antiseptic. Has analgesic effect on urinary mucosa.	Colors urine orange.
Antiinfectives: sulfonamides		Sulfonamides potentiate oral anticoagulants, methotrexate, and hypoglycemic agents that are sulfonylureas. Force fluids.
Sulfisoxazole (Gantrisin) Sulfamethoxazole (Gantanol) (Azo Gantanol)	Short-acting antiinfective. Intermediate-acting antiinfective. Sulfamethoxazole combined with phenazopyride provide analgesic action.	Protect preparations from light and moisture. Maitain fluid intake at minimum of 3,000 mL daily. Colors urine orange-red.
Sulfamethoxazole-trimethoprim (Bactrim, Septra)	Active against gram-negative and gram-positive organisms.	Maintain fluid intake at minimum of 3,000 mL daily. Stress need to take all of medication. Repeat urinalysis after course of medication.
Quinalones		
Norfloxacin (Noroxin) Ciprofloxacin (Cipro) Ofloxacin (Floxin)	Bactericidal.	Give 2 hours after a meal and with 2-hour spacing between it and antacids, H_2-receptor agonists, sulcrafate, or iron preparations. Notify doctor immediately of skin rash or other sensitivity reaction. Use with extreme caution in patients taking theophylline. Use cautiously in those patients with history of seizure disorder. Teach patient to increase fluids to prevent crystalluria. Instruct to avoid caffeine while taking this drug to prevent cumulative effects of caffeine. Warn the drug may cause dizziness or lightheadedness and to take precautions accordingly.
Penicillins		
Ampicillin (Omnipen, Polycillin) Carbenicillin (Geocillin)	Bacteriostatic and bactericidal.	Watch for signs of hypersensitivity. Do not give to patients with known allergy to penicillin.
Amoxicillin-clavulanate (Augmentin)	Bactericidal.	Give with food to decrease GI irritation. Observe for rash indicating sensitivity reaction. Tell patient to take all the medication as directed.
Tetracyclines		
Vibramycin Minocin Doxycycline	Long-acting antiinfective.	Avoid prolonged exposure to sunlight. Do not take with milk or milk products.
Cephalosporins		
Cephalexin monohydrate (Keflex)	Well absorbed from intestinal tract and excreted 90% unchanged in the urine in 8 hours.	Used to treat infections that do not respond to other, less expensive drugs. Candidal (yeast) vaginitis is common side effect of all drugs that destroy normal vaginal flora.

(Table 23-8 continued)

TABLE 23-8 ◆ *Drugs Used for Urinary Tract Infections* (Continued)		
Drug	**Features and Action**	**Nursing Implications**
Cefazolin (Ancef, Kefzol) Cephalothin (Keflin) Ceftazidrine (Fortaz) Ceftrialone (Rocephrin) Cefepime (Maxipime)	Bacteridical	Reconstitute for IV infusion strictly according to package directions. Monitor for sensitivity reactions. Check for possibility of drug interaction with other drugs patient is taking. May cause false-positive glucose urine test with Clinitest, Clinistix, or Tes-Tape. Use cautiously in those with allergy to penicillin. Doses may need to be reduced in the elderly.
Aminoglycosides (tobramycin, gentamicin)	Effective against resistant infections; used cautiously, as they are nephrotoxic.	Monitor BUN and creatinine levels. Monitor for signs of ototoxicity.

drink large amounts of fluids during treatment and to continue the habit once the acute symptoms subside. Vitamin C can help acidify the urine and decrease the frequency of cystitis. Drinking cranberry juice also has proven to be beneficial as it alters urine pH.

Nursing Intervention   Some measures that can be taken to reduce the possibility of bacterial growth and resultant cystitis are presented in Table 23-9. Measures to relieve the discomfort of cystitis include the application of heat in the form of sitz baths and hot water bottles on the back or directly over the bladder region.

TABLE 23-9 ◆ *Patient Education: Measures to Prevent Recurring Urinary Tract Infection*
The patient should be taught the following:

The patient should be taught the following:

- Always wipe the anus from front to back after a bowel movement.
- Avoid wearing nylon pantyhose, tight slacks, or any clothing that increases perineal mositure.
- Do not wash underclothing in strong soap powders or bleaches; rinse clothing repeatedly until water is clear.
- Do not sit around in a wet bathing suit for a long time.
- Wear cotton underwear.
- Do not use bubble bath, perfumed soap, feminine hygiene sprays, or products containing hexachlorophene.
- Prolonged bicycling, motorcycling, horseback riding, or traveling involving prolonged sitting can contribute to urethritis and cystitis.
- Get into the habit of drinking at least 8 full glasses of water each day.
- Do not ignore vaginal discharge or other signs of vaginal infection. *Candida* and *Trichomonas* infections should be treated promptly to prevent their spread to the bladder.
- Empty the bladder promptly after sexual intercourse and then drink two glasses of water to help flush out microorganisms that may have entered the urethra and bladder during intercourse.

Think about . . . If your patient who is prone to recurrent cystitis states that she just doesn't like water that much and has a hard time drinking more than a glass or two of it a day, what could you suggest?

◆ Urethritis

Urethritis is an inflammation of the urethra and can be caused by many different organisms. Urethritis is one of the most common symptoms of gonorrhea, however, and should be investigated as soon as it is first noticed. Nonspecific urethritis (NSU) is a sexually transmitted inflammation of the urethra caused by a variety of organisms other than gonococci. It is thought to be the most common sexually transmitted urethritis in males in the United States, but this cannot be validated because NSU is not a reportable disease. NSU usually responds to treatment with antibiotics.

Inflammatory involvement of the urethra from the herpes virus is found in males and females. In women, trauma during childbirth and the proximity of the urethra to external genitalia and the anus predispose the urethra to infection and inflammation. Chemical irritation secondary to use of spermicidal jellies, bath powders, feminine hygiene sprays, and bubble bath also may cause urethritis.

Signs and Symptoms   The chief symptoms of urethritis are burning, itching, frequency in voiding, and painful urination. There is a discharge, which becomes increasingly more purulent if gonorrhea is present. The urinary meatus is swollen and inflamed.

Treatment   Treatment of urethritis begins by determining the causative organism by smear and Gram stain, or culture of the discharge, and by administering specific drugs to combat the infection.

Nursing Assessment and Intervention   The nursing care is similar to that for the patient with cystitis. The nurse should be especially aware of the possibility of a gonorrheal infection until a definite diagnosis has been established and should carry out the necessary teaching to prevent spread of the infection to the eyes.

◆ Nephritis

Nephritis, sometimes called *Bright's disease,* refers to a general inflammation of the kidneys and the resultant degeneration of the cells. The inflammation is not the result of an invasion of bacteria, although it is often preceded by a bacterial infection and is therefore classified as a *noninfectious disease.*

◆ Acute Glomerulonephritis

Glomerulonephritis is an immunological problem caused by an antigen-antibody reaction and results from a variety of diseases. It most commonly occurs about 2 to 3 weeks after a group A beta-hemolytic streptococcal infection, such as "strep throat" or impetigo. It is primarily seen in children and young adults and affects males more than females. The glomerular basement membrane is damaged, causing altered permeability. It can occur in response to bacterial, viral, or parasitic infection elsewhere in the body.

Diagnosis   **The patient with acute glomerulonephritis usually becomes suddenly ill with fever, chills, flank pain, widespread edema, puffiness about the eyes, visual disturbances, and marked hypertension.** The urine may be smoky, contains red blood cells and protein, and has an increased specific gravity. Serum BUN and creatinine levels rise above normal. If treatment is not successful, the disease will rapidly progress to uremia and death.

Treatment   A sodium-restricted diet is indicated if edema is present, and fluids may be limited if there is oliguria or anuria. A low-protein, high-carbohydrate diet may be ordered.

Nursing Intervention   The nurse's first responsibility in treating acute glomerulonephritis is to decrease the work of the kidney. **Absolute bedrest usually is ordered until the clinical signs are gone.** If the patient responds quickly to treatment and wishes to be more active, the nurse must emphasize the need for continued rest.

The nurse should be sure the patient understands the importance of diet restrictions in the treatment of the disease and should do all she can to encourage his cooperation.

Edema that is obvious from external signs may very well be present in the internal organs. For this reason, blood pressure and pulse must be checked frequently for indications of cerebral edema with increased *intracranial* pressure. Cardiac failure or pulmonary edema also may develop, and the patient must be watched closely for extreme restlessness, increased respiratory difficulty, or cyanosis. Antihypertensives and diuretics are ordered to control hypertension and edema.

The prognosis for acute glomerulonephritis varies, depending on the extent of permanent damage done to the kidneys or other vital organs.

◆ Chronic Glomerulonephritis

Chronic glomerulonephritis may develop rapidly or progress slowly over several years.

Symptoms and Prognosis   Insidious edema, headache associated with hypertension, fatigue, and dyspnea accompany glomerulonephritis. The prognosis for this disease is ultimately poor. However, the speed with which it progresses to renal failure and uremia varies with the individual. The exact reason for this is not known. Some patients who develop chronic glomerulonephritis may have acute exacerbations (flareups) that subside. They may live for several years before damage to the glomeruli of the kidneys brings about the symptoms of renal failure.

Treatment   The treatment for chronic glomerulonephritis in the latent stage is primarily *symptomatic,* with emphasis on avoiding fatigue and infections, particularly of the upper respiratory tract. When renal failure develops, dialysis and possibly a kidney transplant are the only alternative modes of therapy. Chronic renal failure is discussed later in this chapter.

◆ Nephrotic Syndrome

Signs and Symptoms   Nephrotic syndrome sometimes occurs after the glomeruli have been damaged by glomerulonephritis or some other disease. It is characterized by extensive proteinuria, hyperlipidemia (elevated blood lipids), hypoalbuminemia (low blood albumin), and severe edema. The outcome is variable. Some patients recover without further incidence, and others experience repeated episodes and eventual kidney failure.

Treatment   Treatment consists of an adequate-protein, low-fat, low-sodium, ample-potassium diet; diuretics; supplemental multiple vitamins and minerals; and antibiotics if infection is present. Some patients are treated with cortisone and cyclophosphamide (Cytoxan), chlorambucil, or cyclosporine. Information about diuretic drugs is located in Chapter 19.

Nursing Intervention   Nursing care includes monitoring intake and output, recording daily weight, encouraging rest, and providing excellent skin care.

◆ Nephrosclerosis

The primary causes of nephrosclerosis are hypertension and atherosclerotic disease of the small arteries in the kidneys. As the blood supply decreases, the kidney cells degenerate and lose their ability to function, resulting in end-stage renal disease (ESRD, renal failure). Nephrosclerosis is classified as benign or malignant, depending on the severity of the disease and the speed with which hypertensive and atherosclerotic changes occur. The symptoms of nephrosclerosis are similar to those of chronic glomerulonephritis and renal failure. Treatment is the control of hypertension.

◆ Pyelonephritis

Acute pyelonephritis is an infection of the kidneys. It is thought to occur when bacteria from a bladder infection travel up the ureters to infect the kidneys. A frequent cause of pyelonephritis is an obstruction causing stasis of urine and stones that cause irritation of the tissue. Both situations provide an environment in which bacteria can grow.

Signs and Symptoms   **In the acute state of pyelonephritis, the symptoms include fever, chills, headache, malaise, nausea and vomiting, and pain in the flank radiating to the thigh and genitalia.** The chronic phase is more often insidious, with gradual scarring of the kidney tissues. This results in loss of weight, low-grade fever, and weakness. Eventually the urine becomes loaded with bacteria and pus.

Treatment   Prompt treatment of cystitis and prevention of recurrence can help prevent acute pyelonephritis. Correction of obstruction, removal of stones, and prevention of stone formation are essential to correct chronic pyelonephritis. Bedrest, analgesics, and antipyretics are prescribed.

Special diagnostic tests may be done to determine the location of the obstruction if one is suspected. Specific drugs to destroy the bacteria are usually chosen according to the sensitivity of the causative organism, so that the most effective antibiotic is given (see Table 23-9).

The prognosis of the patient depends on the success of the treatment of the active infection before destruction and scarring of the kidney cells can occur. With chronic pyelonephritis, the patient may live for years without significant symptoms before renal damage leads to hypertension or uremia.

Nursing Intervention   The nurse encourages high fluid intake, records intake and output, monitors the urine for changes, and keeps the patient comfortable. Intravenous fluids may be given to flush the kidneys, especially if the patient is nauseous and vomiting.

Think about . . . What characteristics of a fresh urine specimen might indicate an infection? Why should UTIs be treated promptly?

OBSTRUCTIONS OF THE URINARY TRACT

◆ Hydronephrosis

Whenever the normal flow of urine is obstructed, there follows a backward flow of fluid into the renal pelvis. If this condition is not relieved by removing the obstruction, the kidney will become dilated and continue to fill with fluid. Soon, the kidney cells will atrophy until all normal function ceases and the kidney becomes merely a thin, walled cyst. This condition is known as *hydronephrosis*. It can eventually result in complete destruction of the kidneys. Hydronephrosis may be *unilateral* or *bilateral* (one or both kidneys). If it occurs only on one side, the other kidney may enlarge and efficiently carry on the work of two kidneys. This is called *compensatory hypertrophy.*

Signs and Symptoms   Severe pain is present only if hydronephrosis develops rapidly. Otherwise, there are no outstanding symptoms, and the patient may develop signs of uremia only after serious damage has occurred. A definitive diagnosis is obtained by extensive urological examination and detailed x-ray studies of the kidney and ureters, which usually reveal the site and cause of obstruction and distention of the renal pelvis.

Treatment and Nursing Intervention   The primary goal of treatment for hydronephrosis is to remove the obstruction so the kidney may drain properly. The ideal remedy is to drain the kidney in the early stages with a nephrostomy tube. If the damage is irreparable, surgery is necessary to remove the damaged kidney (nephrectomy).

Nursing care of the patient with hydronephrosis is concerned with close observation and accurate reporting of urinary output and early signs of impending uremia. If nephrectomy is performed, the nursing care is the same as for any patient with kidney surgery.

◆ Renal Stones

A renal or kidney stone is a crystalline mass that forms in the urinary system. Stones can be as small as a grain of sand or quite large. Renal stones also vary in composition and in the environment in which they form. Some stones form more readily in an acid urine, whereas others occur in alkaline urine.

There are four major types of renal stones and one that is hereditary. Table 23-10 shows the cause and dietary interventions for each type. Identifying the type and cause of particular kinds of stones can be very effective in preventing further formation and deciding the appropriate method of treatment for each patient. However, in about half the cases the precise cause of stone formation cannot be identified. It is known, however, that certain conditions predispose a person to having renal calculi.

Causative Factors   Among the most common causative factors are: (1) supersaturation of the urine with crystalloids that do not readily dissolve (e.g., calcium, uric acid, and cystine); (2) urinary infections, which produce bacteria and other debris in the urine that form the core around which a stone can form; (3) inadequate fluid intake, which leaves the urine concentrated and does not allow for adequate flushing of the urinary tract; (4) sluggish flow of urine as may occur with bedrest; and (5) certain substances in the urine (for example, urate, which encourages the formation of crystals of calcium oxalate or calcium phosphate).

Prevention   **An essential factor in preventing stone formation is high fluid intake to prevent urinary stasis.** A continuous flow of dilute urine flushes the tract and removes substances that could form stones. To prevent stone formation by diluting the urine, the adult must put out at least 3,500 mL of urine every 24 hours.

Preventing urinary infections and maintaining adequate drainage when tubes and catheters are in place also can help prevent stone formation. In those cases in which the urine pH is crucial to stone formation, changing the pH to a less favorable level can prevent or reduce the incidence of renal calculi.

A very small percentage of patients with calcium stones have a tumor of the parathyroid. This gland produces a hormone that raises the level of serum calcium and thus calcium in the urine. Treatment of the parathyroid condition removes the cause of the stones. Treatment and prevention of the recurrence of renal stones must be based on identification of the specific type of stone being produced.

Signs and Symptoms   Some renal stones do not cause noticeable symptoms and can be passed without the person being aware of them. Others may lodge in the renal pelvis and cause symptoms only after they begin to destroy kidney cells. The stones that cause the severe pain typically associated with kidney stones are those that are small enough to be moved along the ureter with the urine. Moving stones can get trapped somewhere along the ureter, causing obstruction to the flow of urine and swelling of the ureter.

Many renal stones have sharp little spikes on their surface. As a stone rolls along the ureter, it can scrape the ureteral lining, causing excruciating pain and bleeding. **The pain is typically felt in the flank over the affected kidney and ureter, and radiates downward toward the**

TABLE 23-10 ◆ *Causes of and Treatments for Renal Stones*

Stone Type	Cause	Dietary Interventions	Rationale
Calcium oxalate	Supersaturation of urine with calcium and oxalate.	Avoid oxalate sources, such as spinach, chard, parsley, chocolate, peanuts, etc.	Reduction of urinary oxalate content may help prevent these stones from forming. Urinary pH is not a factor.
Calcium phosphate	Supersaturation of urine with calcium and phosphate.	Decrease intake of foods high in calcium, such as milk and other dairy products.	Reduction of urinary calcium content may help prevent these stones from forming.
Uric acid (urate)	Excess dietary purine. Gout (primary or secondary).	Decrease intake of purine sources, such as organ meats, gravies, red wines, and sardines.	Reduction of urinary purine content may help prevent these stones from forming.
Struvite (magnesium ammonium phosphate)	Urea splitting by bacteria.	Limit high-phosphate foods, such as dairy products, red and organ meats, and whole grains.	Reduction of urinary phosphate content may help prevent these stones from forming.
Cystine	Hereditary cystine crystal formation.	Encourage PO fluids, up to 3 L/day.	Increased fluid helps dilute the urine and prevent the cystine crystals from forming.

Source: Ignatavicius, D. D., Workman, M. L., Mishler, M. A. (1995). *Medical–Surgical Nursing: A Nursing Process Approach,* 2nd ed. Philadelphia: Saunders, p. 2067.

genitalia and inner thigh. Nausea and vomiting often occur because of the severity of the pain.

Diagnosis   Diagnostic tests include urinalysis and x-ray studies to locate stones that are radiopaque and an IV pyelogram (IVP) to find those that are not. The IVP will not show the stone itself, but there will be gap in the stream of dye being excreted in the urine. Once the stone has been found and dealt with, further studies of the blood and urine might be done to determine the levels of substances, such as calcium, uric acid, and cystine that can form stones.

Elder Care Point . . .   The possibility of a renal stone should be ruled out in any elderly patient who has sudden onset of severe abdominal pain. Obtain a urine specimen and test for presence of blood as well as assess for signs of infection.

Treatment   At first, the physician may try to flush the stone out by increasing the patient's fluid intake and managing pain by prescribing analgesics and antispasmodics such as propantheline bromide (Pro-Banthine) or oxybutynin chloride (Ditropan). Fluids may be administered IV to augment oral intake. If there is pus in the urine, an antibiotic is prescribed to deal with infection.

When the stone is not passed spontaneously, surgical intervention is necessary. Some stones can be broken up and dissolved by irrigation through a ureteral catheter or percutaneous nephrostomy tube or crushed by ultrasound. Extracorporeal shock wave lithotripsy (ESWL) has largely replaced surgery for renal stones. Newer refinements of this form of ultrasound are occurring frequently. The latest technique is percutaneous ultrasonic lithotripsy (PUL), which can pulverize larger stones than can ESWL. Others require cystoscopy and surgical removal of the stone. Extremely large stones in the renal pelvis require surgical excision from the kidney, *nephrolithotomy or pyelolithotomy*. Once stones have been removed, chemical analyses of the urine, blood, and the stone itself are necessary to plan effective preventive measures for the future.

Nursing Assessment and Intervention   The nurse should assess for kidney stone formation in all patients who are at risk such as:

◆ Males, who are much more at risk than women for development of calcium stones.

◆ Those who have a family history of renal stones.

◆ Those who have had intestinal bypass surgery for obesity. They absorb too much oxalate from foods; this oxalate is excreted in the urine and sets up conditions that favor the formation of calcium oxalate stones.

◆ Those who are immobilized for any reason and are in danger of developing urinary stasis.

◆ Those who have recurrent urinary infections. During initial assessment of a patient with kidney stones, the nurse will need to gather information about changes in urinary output, characteristics of the urine, and other assessment data presented earlier in this chapter.

While attempts are made to have the patient pass the stone spontaneously, all urine is strained to recover the stone or fragments of it for analysis. Fluids are forced during this time to encourage removal of the stone without surgery. Nursing interventions for selected problems in a patient with a renal stone are summarized in Nursing Care Plan 23-1.

CANCER

◆ Cancer of the Bladder

Approximately 52,900 new cases of bladder cancer were expected in the United States in 1996. The cancer occurs three times more often in men than in women. **Smokers have double the risk of developing this cancer.** People living in urban areas and those who are exposed to nitrates, dyes, rubber, or leather processing are at higher risk.

The main symptom of a bladder tumor is **hematuria**, blood in the urine. Frequency, urgency, or dysuria also may be present. Diagnosis is confirmed by IVP and by examining the bladder wall with a cystoscope and biopsy of the tumor.

Treatment is surgery, either alone or in combination with chemotherapy or radiation. Surgical treatment depends on the clinical stage of the tumor. Every effort is made to preserve the bladder if the tumor is confined to the mucosa or submucosa. In this case, a partial cystectomy or transurethral resection of the bladder tumor (TURB, TURBT) is performed.

A new therapy is the use of BCG live vaccine (Intravesical, TheraCys). This was originally used as a vaccine against tuberculosis. It has been found to help patients with bladder carcinoma in situ by reducing tumor recurrence and by eliminating residual malignant cells after surgery. It is instilled into the bladder via a urinary catheter beginning 1 to 2 weeks after surgery. Treatments are continued weekly for 6 weeks. Maintenance doses are given at 3-, 6-, 12-, 18-, and 24-month intervals.

Trials are currently under way for small bladder tumor treatment with photodynamic therapy. A drug is administered IV that makes the tumor tissue sensitive to light. The area in the bladder is then treated with a laser via a cystoscope.

Nursing Care Plan 23-1

Selected nursing diagnoses, goals/expected outcomes, nursing interventions, and evaluations for a patient with a renal stone

Situation: Herbert Simpson, 29 years old, has been admitted with severe flank pain radiating downward into the scrotum, a history of renal stone formation, and blood-tinged urine.

Nursing Diagnosis	Goals/Expected Outcomes	Nursing Intervention	Evaluation
Pain related to ureteral spasm. SUPPORTING DATA Severe flank pain.	Pain will be controlled with analgesia within 2 hours. No pain at time of discharge as verbalized by patient.	Administer analgesic as ordered; assess for effectiveness within 30 to 60 minutes; assess for side effects.	Obtaining good pain control with analgesic; Demerol 50 mg IM at 8 A.M., 11 A.M., and 2:20 P.M.; continue plan.
Risk of alteration in urinary elimination related to obstruction of flow. SUPPORTING DATA Flank pain indicative of ureteral stone; history of stone formation; blood-tinged urine.	Stone will be passed within 24 hours. No signs of hydronephrosis evident at time of discharge.	Force fluids to 3,000 to 4,000 mL in each 24 hours. Strain all urine. Send any stones to laboratory for analysis. Assess characteristics of urine; have patient stand to void.	Taking 8 oz fluids q h; straining urine; no sign of stone yet; urine dark amber; continue plan.
Risk of urinary tract infection related to disruption in urinary system. SUPPORTING DATA Blood-tinged urine; flank pain indicative of stone.	Urinalysis will show no abnormality at discharge. Temperature will be within normal limits at discharge.	Force fluids. Administer prophylactic antimicrobial agent as ordered. Monitor temperature; instruct to report chills or dysuria.	Forcing fluids; temperature normal; urine not cloudy; odor normal; continue plan.
Knowledge deficit related to prescribed regimen to prevent renal stone formation. SUPPORTING DATA Cannot verbalize need for increased fluids daily, foods to avoid in diet.	Patient will verbalize rationale for intake of 3,000 to 4,000 mL of fluid per day within 24 hours. Patient will verbalize foods to avoid in diet before discharge. Patient will not experience stone recurrence in next 5 years.	Explain rationale for high fluid intake. Reinforce dietitian's dietary instructions to alter urine pH and prevent stone formation. Explain rationale and action of medication ordered to alter urine pH.	Discussed need for continuous high fluid intake after discharge; dietitian to see patient; continue plan.

More invasive tumors require removal of the bladder, *cystectomy*, with urinary diversion. These surgeries are covered later in this chapter. If the disease is caught early, prognosis is quite good.

◆ Cancer of the Kidney

Cancer of the kidney is fairly uncommon, actually constituting less than 1% of all malignant tumors of the body. They are, however, nearly always cancerous and are extremely difficult to treat in the later stages. Except for Wilms' tumor, which occurs in infants and small children, neoplasms of the kidney occur mostly between 50 and 70 years of age. Males are affected twice as often as females.

Diagnosis   The principal symptom of malignant tumors of the kidney is **hematuria** (blood in the urine),
which usually is not accompanied by pain in the early stages. The affected kidney may be enlarged. Tests such as the renal angiogram, arteriogram, computed tomography (CT) and magnetic resonance imaging (MRI) scans and ultrasound are performed to determine whether the symptoms are being caused by a cyst (nonmalignant) or a tumor.

Treatment   The only treatment that has met with any degree of success is surgical removal of the affected kidney before *metastasis* has occurred. Unfortunately, this is difficult to achieve, because the patient usually does not have symptoms severe enough to send him to the doctor until metastases have occurred. Chemotherapy with a variety of drug regimens is utilized for metastatic cancer. Immunotherapy is sometimes attempted for recurrent tumors.

Nursing Intervention   Nursing care of the patient is the same as that for patients following nephrectomy, as discussed later in this chapter.

COMMON PROBLEMS OF UROLOGICAL DISORDERS

◆ Urinary Incontinence

Incontinence affects over 10 million residents in the United States, particularly the elderly. About 30% of the elderly who are not in long-term care facilities suffer from incontinence. In the nursing homes, over 50% of residents have incontinent episodes several times a day. In the over-65 group, women experience incontinence twice as frequently as men. The problem is more common among women who have experienced childbirth. Men do not experience the problem unless they have a prostate problem, have had prostate surgery, have a spinal cord injury, or a neurological disorder.

Diagnosis   Urine flow out of the bladder is controlled by two circular muscles called *sphincters*. The internal sphincter lies close to the lowermost part of the bladder, and the external sphincter surrounds the urethra. Many factors can cause loss of sphincter control. Unconsciousness, UTI, paralysis, interference with nerve transmission to and from the brain, and loss of muscle tone of the bladder and sphincters are some of the conditions that frequently cause patients to become incontinent. The Agency for Health Care Policy and Research (AHCPR) has published guidelines for managing acute and chronic urinary incontinence. Incontinence is identified as being of several types: urge, stress, mixed, overflow, functional, or incontinence due to neurological dysfunction. *Urge incontinence* occurs when there is involuntary loss of urine in response to a strong sensation of need to empty the bladder (urinary urgency). *Mixed incontinence* is a combination of different types such as stress and urge incontinence. *Stress incontinence* occurs when there is urethral sphincter failure and is usually associated with increased intraabdominal pressure, as occurs with sneezing, laughing, coughing, and aerobic exercise. *Overflow incontinence* occurs when there is poor contractility of the detrusor muscle, obstruction of the urethra as in prostate hypertrophy in the male, or genital prolapse or abnormality in the female. *Functional incontinence* is caused by cognitive inability to recognize the urge to urinate, extreme depression, or dementia. Inability to reach the bathroom due to restraints, siderails or an out-of-reach walker, can also result in *functional incontinence*. *Neurologic incontinence* is caused by disorders of the neurological system such as multiple sclerosis, spinal cord injury, etc.

Drugs such as alpha-adrenergic agents, beta-adrenergic agonists, and calcium-channel blockers may contribute to the problem of incontinence. Drugs most often contribute to urinary retention problems with overflow incontinence.

Nursing Assessment and Intervention   When incontinence is occurring, the first step is to identify factors that may be contributing to the patient's incontinence. Immobility, UTI, atrophic urethritis or vaginitis associated with menopause, stool impaction, prostate surgery, delirium or confusion, endocrine problems, and various types of medication may be contributing to the problem. Obesity also is a factor as it causes increased pressure on the bladder. The second step in the assessment is to take an incontinence history such as that presented in Table 23-11.

When incontinence is not remedied by correcting an underlying cause, the nurse attempts to help the patient by setting up a voiding schedule. The nurse first assesses when the patient is experiencing incontinence. By tracking the times when this occurs, toileting assistance can be offered at set times just prior to when incontinence usually occurs.

Spacing fluid intake, with the majority of fluids taken during the day, can assist in keeping the patient dry at night and make voidings more predictable. Getting the patient on to a voiding schedule takes a great deal of patience and persistence on the part of the nurse and the patient. However, the patient's joy at being dry is more than enough reward for the effort.

Patients often experience transient incontinence after removal of an indwelling catheter that has been in place for several days. Usually the catheter is clamped

---

TABLE 23-11 ◆ *Assessment: Incontinence History*

Questions such as those listed are useful in the initial identification and assessment of urinary incontinence.

- ◆ Can you tell me about the problems you are having with your bladder?

or

   Can you tell me about the trouble you are having holding your urine (water)?
- ◆ How often does urine escape when you don't want it to?
- ◆ When do you leak urine when you don't want to? What activities or situations are linked with leakage? Is it associated with laughing, coughing, sneezing, or getting to the bathroom?
- ◆ How often do you wear a pad for protection?
- ◆ Do you use other protective devices to collect leaked urine?
- ◆ How long have you been having a problem with urine leakage?

Source: U. S. Department of Health and Human Services, Public Health Service. (1996). *Managing Acute and Chronic Urinary Incontinence: Quick Reference Guide for Clinicians,* No 2, 1996 Update. Rockville, MD: Agency for Health Care Policy and Research, p. 5.

TABLE 23-12 ♦ *Patient Education: Exercises to Strengthen Pelvic Floor Muscles (Kegel Exercises)*

The best way to locate the correct muscle is to stop the flow of urine while urinating on the toilet. Tightening the anus as if preventing the evacuation of stool locates the correct muscle also. Practice this for several days each time you urinate. Then begin the exercise program.

♦ While lying down, slowly count 1-2-3 while tightening the pelvic muscles. Release slowly to count 1-2-3. Do this 15 times.

♦ While sitting, repeat the above sequence 15 times; tightening while counting 1-2-3, and then slowly releasing to the count 1-2-3.

♦ Stand and repeat the sequence 15 times; tighten to the count 1-2-3, and slowly release to the count 1-2-3.

♦ Do the exercises once a day. If you can do them twice each day, improvement in continence will occur more quickly.

♦ Improvement may be noted in 6 to 8 weeks, but may take as long as 3 months.

♦ **This method has been proven effective if the exercises are performed as instructed and done faithfully.**

for intervals and then opened to drainage before it is removed to help rebuild bladder muscle tone. After this has been done for 12 to 24 hours, the catheter is removed. The patient should then be instructed to void every hour to prevent incontinence. It takes time to retrain the bladder to hold greater capacity. Gradually the interval between voidings is lengthened to 2, 3, or 4 hours. Because it is not practical to continue a frequent voiding schedule at night, external drainage is used. A condom catheter is used for males, and absorbent pads and moisture-proof pants or incontinence pads can be used for women. Accidents will happen during the retraining period, and patients need to be assured that this is expected. They should be treated with kindness, not scolding.

Stress incontinence that occurs with exercise, such as aerobics or playing ball, laughing, coughing, may be corrected or improved by exercises to strengthen the pelvic floor muscles (Table 23-12). Women who have experienced childbirth, particularly those who have had several children, may have anatomical changes that make stress incontinence more likely. Maintaining normal weight and using estrogen therapy after menopause decreases the incidence of this disorder. Avoiding alcohol and caffeine also helps. Various medications, such as phenylpropanolamine, pseudoephedrine, propantheline (Pro-Banthine), oxybutinin (Ditropan), dicyclomine hydrochloride (Bentyl), imipramine (Tofranil), desipramine (Norpramin), nortriptyline (Pamelor), and other tricyclic antidepressants, have been found helpful. Estrogen replacement therapy may help postmenopausal women.

Vaginal weight training with a set of five small, cone-shaped weights that are used along with pelvic muscle exercise is another option. The lightest cone, which has a string attached, is inserted into the vagina and held in place by muscle tightening for 15 minutes twice a day. When there is no problem holding this cone in place, the next heaviest cone is used. This continues until the heaviest cone can be held in place for the 15-minute period. The cones are produced and sold by Dacomed Corporation located in Minneapolis. A prescription is not necessary.

When these measures do not improve continence, the physician may choose to evaluate the condition with a series of diagnostic tests, including urodynamic studies. Further treatment options include biofeedback therapy, electrical stimulation therapy, and surgery, such as bladder neck suspension, or implantation of an artificial urinary sphincter, to correct anatomical problems. Details of bladder training for the patient who has a neurological problem or urge incontinence are given in Chapter 14.

When these measures do not solve the problem, incontinence is managed by intermittent catheterization, indwelling urethral catheterization (Figure 23-5), suprapubic catheter, external collection system (such

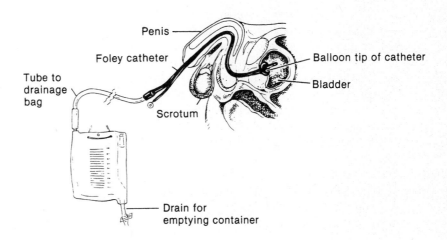

FIGURE 23-5 Foley (indwelling) catheter drainage system shown in male patient. (*Source:* deWit, S. C. [1994]. *Rambo's Nursing Skills for Clinical Practice,* 4th ed. Philadelphia: Saunders, p. 646.)

Penis —
Foley catheter —
Balloon tip of catheter
Tube to drainage bag
Bladder
Scrotum
Drain for emptying container

as condom catheters), protective pads and garments, pelvic organ support devices, or penile compression devices.

RENAL FAILURE

Renal failure is the inability of the kidneys to maintain normal function. Impairment of renal function affects most of the body's major systems because of the role the kidneys play in maintaining fluid balance, regulating the electrochemical composition of body fluids, providing protection against acid–base imbalance, and eliminating waste products. The kidneys also take part in red blood cell formation and regulation of calcium levels and, in conjunction with the endocrine system, control of blood pressure.

Renal failure is classified as acute or chronic. The final stage of chronic and irreversible renal failure is called *end-stage renal disease* (ESRD).

◆ Acute Renal Failure (ARF)

Acute renal failure occurs suddenly as a result of physical injury, infection, inflammation, or damage from toxic chemicals. Nephrotoxic agents are those that are poisonous to kidney cells and include many drugs, iodine substances used as x-ray contrast media, and heavy metals. These toxins may inflict damage on the renal tubules, causing acute tubular necrosis (ATN) and loss of function. They also can indirectly harm the tubules by causing severe constriction of blood vessels that serve the kidney, producing renal ischemia. Acute tubular necrosis is responsible for 90% of acute renal failure. Other causes of renal ischemia include circulatory collapse, severe dehydration, and prolonged hypotension in certain compromised surgical or trauma patients.

There are three types of acute renal failure, depending on the cause. *Prerenal ARF* is caused by circulatory problems, such as hypoperfusion, massive vasodilation, or decreased cardiac output (pump failure). Decreased blood flow to the kidney causes a decrease in the kidney's ability to function. *Intrarenal ARF* occurs from glomerular damage, vascular disease that affects the vessels in the kidney, renal ischemia or acute tubular necrosis, or nephrotoxicity causing ATN. *Postrenal ARF* is caused by obstruction in the ureters, bladder, or urethra that causes eventual backup of urine into the kidney that leads to tissue damage. Acute renal failure is potentially reversible, especially if identified early. Often the patient regains kidney function.

The course of acute tubular necrosis is divided into three phases: oliguric/nonoliguric, diuretic, and recovery phase. In the *oliguric/nonoliguric phase,* the patient either puts out a great deal of urine or very little urine.

Oliguria (diminished urine secretion in relation to intake) usually occurs with disorders producing ischemia. Urine output is 100 to 400 mL of urine in 24 hours and for an average of 8 to 15 days; BUN and creatinine levels rise. When this occurs there may be volume overload, which can precipitate heart failure, multiple electrolyte imbalances, metabolic acidosis, catabolism, and uremia. Dialysis is needed. Nonoliguric ATN is often due to nephrotoxic agents. Urine output is greater, but the kidneys cannot eliminate waste products efficiently and BUN and creatinine levels rise and electrolyte imbalances occur. Dialysis is needed less often and, if used, is necessary for a shorter time.

The *diuretic phase* only occurs if dialysis has not been started early and extracellular fluid volume has built up. This phase was more common before dialysis was started early. The diuretic phase represents excretion of the excess fluid retained in the oliguric phase.

The *recovery phase* begins as the patient's kidneys begin to concentrate urine normally and urine output and electrolytes return toward normal. This is followed by 1 to 2 weeks of rapid improvement and then a period of slower recovery. About one-third of ARF patients are left with residual renal insufficiency, and about 5% do not recover sufficiently to discontinue dialysis.

Think about . . . When caring for a patient at risk for ARF, what assessments would you make to determine whether ARF is occurring?

Treatment   Treatment of ARF is geared toward correcting the underlying cause and preventing or controlling complications. The goal of treatment is to restore and maintain a tolerable internal environment until the kidneys are able to recover and resume their normal functions.

Symptomatic treatment includes measures to maintain fluid and electrolyte balances, manage the accompanying anemia and hypertension, and cleanse the blood and tissues of uremic waste products with peritoneal dialysis or hemodialysis.

Volume overload is treated with diuretics and sometimes low-dose dopamine to promote better kidney perfusion. Dialysis may be necessary if the volume overload cannot be reduced with the drugs.

Electrolyte imbalances are monitored and treated; they include hyperkalemia, hypocalcemia, hyperphosphatemia, and mild hypermagnesemia. Metabolic acidosis, if severe, is treated with IV sodium bicarbonate and close monitoring. Dialysis with buffer in the dialysate may be utilized.

The catabolic state is treated with nutritional management via total parenteral nutrition (TPN). This is necessary to provide adequate nutrients. Potassium, phosphate, and magnesium are omitted from the solution while the patient is oliguric.

Uremia signs generally appear when BUN concentration passes the 100-mg/dL mark. The presence of uremic signs is the absolute indicator for initiating dialysis. The goal is to maintain BUN below 100 mg/dL and to keep creatinine below 8 mg/dL.

Anemia occurs because the kidney cannot produce normal amounts of erythropoietin. The lifespan of RBCs is shortened because of the toxic wastes circulating in the blood and because of hemodilution from fluid overload. Infection frequently occurs in people with ARF and is the leading cause of death in these patients. The nurse must be vigilant in monitoring for beginning signs of infection and must follow strict asepsis. Clinical Pathway 23-1 shows the nursing diagnoses and collaborative care needed for the patient with ARF.

◆ Chronic Renal Failure

Chronic renal failure is a progressive loss of kidney function that develops over the course of many months or years. In the early stages of the disease, renal function can remain adequate, but the waste products normally filtered out by the kidney and excreted in the urine begin to accumulate in the plasma. The patient does not experience symptoms until about 65% of the kidney tissue is damaged. As the disease progresses, nitrogenous waste products, such as urea nitrogen and creatinine, build up to higher levels in the blood. In the final or end stage of renal failure, 90% or more of kidney function is lost. Chronic renal failure indicates permanent renal damage. Figure 23-6 shows a schematic of the pathophysiology of renal failure.

Causes of Chronic Renal Failure (CRF)   Chronic renal failure is caused by destruction of the nephrons. All of the causes of acute renal failure may also cause chronic renal failure. Hypertension, diabetes mellitus, sickle cell disease, glomerulonephritis, nephrotic syndrome, lupus erythematosus, heart failure, and cirrhosis of the liver contribute to CRF. The most common causes of chronic renal failure are glomerulonephritis and nephrosclerosis. **Diabetic nephropathy (pathological condition of the kidney associated with diabetes mellitus) is the most common cause of death in patients with diabetes mellitus.**

Diagnosis   The physician uses a variety of diagnostic tests and procedures to establish a diagnosis of renal failure. A renal biopsy sometimes is done to identify the specific cause because in some patients the original cause cannot be identified in any other way.

Evaluation of kidney function is usually based on measurements of creatinine clearance. Clearance is the volume of plasma that can be cleared of a substance by the kidneys in a given period of time. It also is a reflection of the flow of plasma through the renal circulation, which can be severely impeded by narrowing of the renal arterioles. Effective clearance depends on the ability of the renal tubular cells to handle substances that have been filtered by the glomeruli. **Determining the blood urea nitrogen (BUN) level and the serum creatinine are the two tests most often used to screen for kidney problems.** Measurement of creatinine clearance involves collecting a 12-hour or 24-hour urine specimen.

There are three stages of CRF. In stage 1 there is diminished renal reserve, but no accumulation of metabolic wastes. The healthier kidney works harder. Urine concentration is decreased and polyuria and nocturia occur. Stage 2 is renal insufficiency and is heralded by a rise in circulating metabolic wastes; BUN and creatinine levels begin to rise. The glomerular filtration rate (GFR) falls and oliguria and edema occur. Stage 3 is end-stage renal disease. Circulating metabolic wastes accumulate in the blood, homeostasis cannot be maintained, electrolyte and fluid imbalances are serious, and dialysis or kidney transplant is necessary to maintain life.

Signs and Symptoms   The symptoms of chronic renal failure do not appear early in the disease. Renal insufficiency, which occurs before renal failure (end-stage renal disease), can produce occasional headaches and fatigue, but these symptoms usually either go unnoticed or are not reported by the patient. At this point in the process kidney function is about 20% to 40% of normal. When symptoms do become readily apparent, kidney function can be as little as 5% to 10% of normal.

One of the earliest signs of renal impairment is the inability of the kidneys to concentrate urine. This produces polyuria and a very dilute urine. The patient may complain of having to get up frequently during the night to urinate (**nocturia**). Later on, as renal insufficiency progresses, the kidneys may not be able to produce much urine at all. This causes oliguria and eventually anuria.

The symptoms of end-stage renal disease constitute a syndrome called **uremia**. Clinical signs and symptoms of uremia are related to pathological changes in the various body systems and depend on the extent of these changes and the degree of renal impairment. The skin is dry, scaly, and a pallid yellow-gray color. **Pruritus** (severe itching) occurs. Uremic frost appears on the skin. Hyperkalemia is present, and there is a sodium imbalance. Hypocalcemia and hyperphosphatemia occur. The patient is hypertensive from fluid overload and pulmonary edema and heart failure may occur. The patient's weight increases. Metabolic changes occur including triglyceride elevation and carbohydrate intolerance. Serum protein decreases as protein is lost

CLINICAL PATHWAY 23-1 ◆ Acute Renal Failure: Medical Management

Nursing Diagnosis/ Collaborative Problem	Expected Outcome (The Patient Is Expected to . . .)	Met/ Not Met	Reason	Date/ Initials
Altered renal tissue perfusion.	Have a return of usual renal function with stable renal function tests.			
Fluid volume deficit or excess.	Have adequate urinary output and no indications of dehydration or edema.			
Altered nutritional status.	Understand rationale for dietary restrictions and follow recommended diet.			
Fatigue.	Perform ADLs independently.			
High risk for infection.	Exhibit no signs or symptoms of infection.			

Aspect of Care	Date ___ Day 1	Date ___ Day 2	Date ___ Day 3	Date ___ Day 4	Date ___ Day 5
Assessment	Systems assessment q shift with particular attention to renal: decreased urine volume, frequency, change in color, odor. Vital signs and neurological signs q 4 h. Assess for underlying cause. Check for Chvostek's or Trousseau's sign, neck vein distention, cap refill. Monitor medication levels; assess need to adjust medication (e.g., those excreted or metabolized in kidney). Monitor for complications: acidosis, hyperkalemia; hypertension, overload; infection, uremia, ileus; pneumonia, gastrointestinal bleed. Psychosocial assessment.	Same as Day 1. Monitor closely for renal failure, progression, uremia. Assess need for dialysis (severe acidosis and/or hyperkalemia).	Same as Day 2.	Same as Day 3. Vital signs and neurological signs q 8 h.	Same as Day 4.

Education	Orient to hospital and unit. Prepare for diagnostic tests. Provide information about diagnosis. Involve family in care of patient as appropriate. Review plan of care/clinical pathway with patient and family.	Continue to provide information regarding diagnosis and diagnostic tests. Explain dialysis if needed.	Diet education and fluid restriction. Medication: action, side effects, time. Importance of rest and gradually increasing activity.	Same as Day 3. Instruct in signs and symptoms of renal failure, infection. Based on identified cause of renal failure, provide prevention or management information.	Review medications, diet, lab work, fluid and activity restriction. Instruct to do daily weight using same scale. Instruct in signs and symptoms of renal failure, infection.
Consults	Dietician Nephrologist Social worker	N/A	N/A	N/A	N/A
Lab tests	Electrolytes, blood urea nitrogen (BUN), creatinine Mg^{+2}, phosphorus, bicarbonate, calcium, protein, albumin, lipids. Complete blood count (CBC) with differential. INR (PT)/APTT Urine for: C & S, Cr, osmolality, lytes	Electrolytes, BUN, creatinine (Cr), hematocrit (Hct), and hemoglobin (Hgb).	Same as Day 2.	Lytes, BUN, Cr, Hgb, Hct, Mg^{+2}, phosphorus, albumin, protein.	Serum: BUN, Cr, electrolytes. Urine: urinalysis, electrolytes, osmolality.
Other tests	Chest and kidney, ureter, and bladder (KUB) x-ray. CT scan with contrast. Renal sonogram, ECG.	Aortorenal angiography. Possible cystoscopy or retrograde pyelography.	Possible renal biopsy.	N/A	
Medications	*Acidosis and/or hyperkalemia:* Kayexalate followed by sorbitol. If K^+ >6.5 mEq, give 50% glucose and regular insulin. Sodium bicarbonate citrate or calcium gluconate. *Antihypertensives:* Hydralazine. Methyldopa. Propranolol. Cardiotonic such as digoxin.	Antihypertensive. Cardiotonic. Diuretic. Vitamin and mineral supplement. Stool softener.	Same as Day 2.	Antihypertensive.	Same as Day 4.

Continued on following page

CLINICAL PATHWAY 23-1 ◆ *Acute Renal Failure: Medical Management* (*Continued*)

Aspect of Care	Date Day 1	Date Day 2	Date Day 3	Date Day 4	Date Day 5
Treatments/interventions	*Hyperphosphatemia:* Calcium carbonate or other phosphate binders. Vitamins and minerals (vitamin D, folic acid). Stool softener. Strict intake and output (I&O) measure of all body fluid output. Urine specific gravity each void. Daily weights. Frequent skin and oral care. O$_2$ per nasal canula if needed. Safety precautions. Incentive spirometer q 2 h while awake. Strict aseptic techniques for all procedures. Guaiac all stools.	Same as Day 1.	Same as Day 2.	Strict I&O. Daily weights. Skin and mouth care.	Same as Day 4.
Nutrition	High-fat and carbohydrate, low-protein diet with NA$^+$ and K$^+$ restriction. Fluid restriction based on electrolytes.	Same as Day 1.	Same as Day 2.	Same as Day 3.	Same as Day 4.
Lines/tubes/monitors	IV fluids (depends on phase)	Same as Day 1.	Convert IV to saline loc.	Saline loc.	D/C saline loc.
Mobility/self-care	Bedrest. ROM q 4 h while awake. Prevent complications of immobility.	Out of bed (OOB) as tolerated. ROM.	OOB as tolerated. Ambulate in room as tolerated.	OOB and ambulate as tolerated.	OOB and ambulate as tolerated.
Discharge planning	Social worker to assess need for social services, financial status, health insurance and coverage, home environment, need for placement and family support.	Same as Day 1.	Assess ability to perform ADLs, home environment, and need for assistive/adaptive devices.	Arrange for outpatient blood and urine tests. Ensure transportation available. Verify ability to pay for meds and lab work. Continue ADL assessment. Refer to home health.	Continue as Day 4. Arrange for follow-up visit with MD.

Source: Ignatavicius, D. D., Hausman, K. A. (1995). *Clinical Pathways for Collaborative Practice.* Philadelphia: Saunders, pp. 146–150.

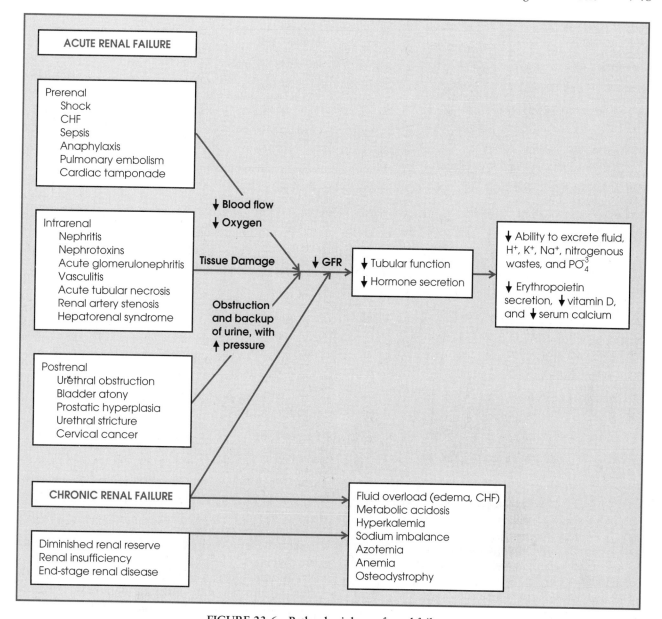

FIGURE 23-6 Pathophysiology of renal failure.

because of the dietary restriction on protein in an attempt to decrease the waste products that the kidney can no longer handle. Anemia is present. Anorexia, nausea, and vomiting occur because of gastrointestinal mucosa irritation from waste products circulating in the blood. Constipation often occurs from drug therapy and fluid restriction. Changes occur in just about every body system. These effects and some of their clinical signs and symptoms are shown in Figure 23-7.

Treatment Managing chronic renal failure is highly complex because of the impact kidney failure has on homeostasis and major body systems. Medical treatment and nursing intervention include measures to correct fluid and electrolyte imbalance and acid–base-imbalance whenever possible. A restricted protein diet

often is necessary, and it has been found that decreasing protein in the diet of patients with beginning renal insufficiency may help slow down the disease process. Dialysis and kidney transplant, which are discussed later in the Common Therapies section, are two major alternatives that offer hope to the patient with end-stage renal failure. A variety of drugs are used to counteract the fluid and electrolyte imbalances, treat metabolic acidosis, and control the complications (Table 23-13). Diuretic drug information is contained in Chapter 19.

Nursing Assessment and Intervention Appropriate medical and nursing intervention for the management of renal insufficiency and renal failure can help patients remain relatively free of symptoms until the final stages of renal failure. The accomplishment of this

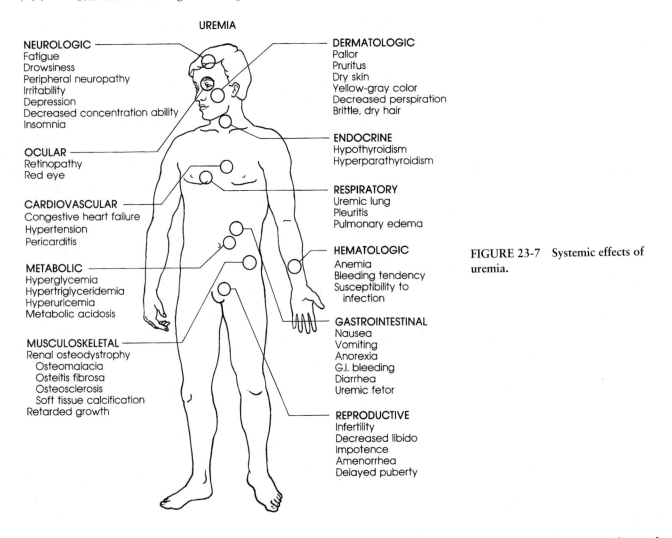

UREMIA

NEUROLOGIC
Fatigue
Drowsiness
Peripheral neuropathy
Irritability
Depression
Decreased concentration ability
Insomnia

OCULAR
Retinopathy
Red eye

CARDIOVASCULAR
Congestive heart failure
Hypertension
Pericarditis

METABOLIC
Hyperglycemia
Hypertriglyceridemia
Hyperuricemia
Metabolic acidosis

MUSCULOSKELETAL
Renal osteodystrophy
   Osteomalacia
   Osteitis fibrosa
   Osteosclerosis
   Soft tissue calcification
Retarded growth

DERMATOLOGIC
Pallor
Pruritus
Dry skin
Yellow-gray color
Decreased perspiration
Brittle, dry hair

ENDOCRINE
Hypothyroidism
Hyperparathyroidism

RESPIRATORY
Uremic lung
Pleuritis
Pulmonary edema

HEMATOLOGIC
Anemia
Bleeding tendency
Susceptibility to
   infection

GASTROINTESTINAL
Nausea
Vomiting
Anorexia
G.I. bleeding
Diarrhea
Uremic fetor

REPRODUCTIVE
Infertility
Decreased libido
Impotence
Amenorrhea
Delayed puberty

FIGURE 23-7   Systemic effects of uremia.

goal requires cooperative effort on the part of every person on the health care team, especially the patient and family.

A major role of the nurse is to assess the patient's health status and learning needs throughout the illness to help provide information to manage symptoms and prevent further damage whenever possible. A thorough and careful nursing assessment can lead to accurate identification of specific nursing diagnoses. Nursing diagnoses commonly used for patients with renal insufficiency and failure are listed in Table 23-5. Assessment and nursing intervention for many of these nursing diagnoses have already been covered earlier in this text. For example, anemia, bleeding tendency, and susceptibility to infection are discussed in Chapter 17; nausea, vomiting, anorexia, gastrointestinal bleeding, and other gastrointestinal problems are covered in Chapter 20. Congestive heart failure is covered in Chapter 19.

Because fluid and electrolyte balance are major concerns in the management of renal failure, the nurse must be especially aware of hydration status. **Daily weight, measurement of intake and output, determining the pattern of urination, and restricting fluid are** essential to the well-being of the patient with renal damage.

In addition to these rather basic procedures, the nursing care plan should include monitoring the serum levels of electrolytes, BUN, and creatinine. The presence of accumulations of these nitrogenous products is called **azotemia**. This condition requires frequent monitoring of the patient for nausea and vomiting and changes in mental awareness and levels of consciousness.

High levels of serum potassium (5 to 7 mEq/L) can adversely affect the heart, causing dysrhythmia and arrest. By watching for earlier signs of hyperkalemia and promptly reporting them, the nurse can help avoid serious cardiovascular problems.

The patient with end-stage renal disease does not absorb calcium from the intestinal tract. This causes a loss of calcium from the body and a corresponding drop in serum calcium. If the hypocalcemia is not corrected, the patient will eventually suffer from muscle cramps, twitching, and possibly seizures. Complaints about "restless leg syndrome" are frequent, and the leg discomfort may interfere with sleep.

TABLE 23-13 ◆ Drugs for the Patient with Renal Failure

Drug	Purpose/Rationale
Diuretics	Promote urine flow; rid body of excess fluid; used in early stages of acute and chronic renal failure.
Vitamins and minerals	Supplement during catabolic state and to treat anemia. If patient is on hemodialysis, these are given after treatments.
Epoetin alpha (Epogen)	Treat the anemia; promotes red blood cell formation.
Phosphate binders (Basalgel, Amphogel)	Prevent problems of calcium loss. Given with meals to bind phosphate. Constipation is a common side effect.
Cardiotonics (Digitalis preparations)	Treat cardiac failure; promotes increased strength of cardiac contractions.
Calcium supplements	Dietary supplement; given when phosphate levels are normal. Give after meals.
Stool softeners and laxatives	Treat constipation caused by drugs and fluid restrictions.

Think about ... How would you know whether the patient is suffering from hyperkalemia or hypocalcemia?

As kidney cells cease to function, they are less and less able to secrete phosphorus in the urine. This results in an elevated serum phosphate level (hyperphosphatemia), which only serves to exaggerate the problem of inadequate calcium absorption. That is because phosphate binds with the calcium, making its absorption from the intestinal tract even less likely to occur. Specific electrolyte imbalances, their symptoms, and nursing intervention for imbalances are discussed in Chapter 5.

Maintaining adequate nutrition for the patient with chronic renal failure is a very real challenge. Because of the buildup of nitrogenous wastes from protein metabolism, restriction of protein intake is necessary. The reduced intake of protein requires that only high-quality protein foods be used in the diet. These include meat, eggs, milk, and cheese, which provide all of the essential amino acids in relatively small servings.

Potassium restriction also is necessary because of the inability of the kidney to excrete it. Sodium intake often is restricted, especially if the patient is hypertensive (Table 23-14). Phosphate binders (basic aluminum carbonate [Basalgel]) are given with meals to prevent the absorption of phosphorus.

The complexity of diet restrictions and modifications makes understanding and compliance very difficult for the patient. The expertise of nutritionists and other professionals is needed to help accomplish the goals of (1) minimizing uremic toxicity; (2) maintaining acceptable electrolyte levels; (3) controlling hypertension; (4) providing sufficient calories; and (5) maintaining good nutritional status. The therapeutic communication that follows presents a scenario of how the nurse can reaffirm the importance of diet restrictions with the noncompliant patient.

Therapeutic Communication

Mr. John T. is a 48-year-old male who has end-stage renal disease and is on hemodialysis twice a week. He has not been compliant with his treatment regimen, diet, and fluid restrictions and has been increased to three dialysis treatments a week. He gained 5 lb over the weekend.

TABLE 23-14 ◆ Dietary Restrictions for the Patient with Renal Failure

Dietary Component	With Chronic Uremia	With Hemodialysis	With Peritoneal Dialysis
Protein	0.55–0.60 g/kg of body weight per day.	1–1.3 g/kg of body weight per day.	0.8–1.5 g/kg of body weight per day.
Fluid	Depends on urinary output, but may be as high as 1,500 to 3,000 mL/day.	500–700 mL/day plus amount of urinary output.	Restriction based on fluid weight gain and blood.
Potassium	60–70 mEq/day.	70 mEq/day.	Usually no restriction.
Sodium	1–3 g/day.	2–4 g/day.	Restriction based on fluid weight gain and blood pressure.
Phosphorus	700 mg/day.	700 mg/day.	800 mg/day.

Source: Ignatavicius, D. D., Workman, M. L., Mishler, M. A. (1995). *Medical–Surgical Nursing: A Nursing Process Approach,* 2nd ed. Philadelphia: Saunders, p. 2125.

"John, I see that you have gained 5 lb since Friday. Could you tell me a little about your weekend?"

"Yeah, but what's the difference? I just got tired of never having any fun or doing the things others around me are doing. I went fishing with some buddies and we drank a lot of beer. It was hot. We barbequed our fish and some sausage and had a real feast!"

"How are you feeling today?"

"I feel rotten. I don't have any energy, and my thinking is slow. My legs are really swollen, and I'm having trouble breathing."

"Do you think that might have something to do with the beer drinking and the eating binge?"

"I suppose it does, but can't a guy have a little fun?"

"John, it is your body and your life and you must make your own decisions. We have explained to you several times that each time you get so overloaded with fluid and wastes, your whole body gets out of balance and damage occurs in other organs. It's especially hard on the heart."

"Yeah, I know you've told me. It's just so hard to stay on the diet and the fluid restrictions. You don't understand what it is like."

"You are right, I don't have kidney disease, and I don't know what a battle it is to stay on the diet and fluid restrictions. I think it would be very difficult for me, too. I do know that with my family, I would want to live, though. Keeping that goal in mind might help me."

"Well, you know that my wife left me, and I don't see much of the kids. I sure do enjoy my granddaughter, though. She is the cutest little thing. We go to the zoo, and the park, and to McDonald's sometimes. I really enjoy my times with the guys at the Lodge, too."

"What can we do that would help you to stick to the diet and fluid restrictions? Do you have any friends who are in a similar situation that you can talk to when it begins to really get you down?"

"I don't know. I do pretty well, and then I just get fed up and feel like I have to do something "normal" for once. No, I don't have any friends with kidney disease."

"Would you like me to see if we can find you a "buddy" among our patients who could give you some encouragement and support? Perhaps you could do the same for him at times."

"I don't know; I don't make friends with strangers easily."

"There is a young man who comes here for dialysis treatments who is always talking about fishing. Maybe the two of you would hit it off."

"Well, maybe. . . ."

"I see on the schedule that he will be here on Wednesday. How about if we schedule your treatment for the same time. Perhaps you could get acquainted."

"O.K., that seems fine."

"Meantime, do you think you can stick to your diet, fluid restrictions, and medication schedule?"

"Yeah, well for you I will try. . . ."

Think about . . . What would be the first steps to take in trying to assist a patient who is to begin hemodialysis make dietary modifications necessary to treat end-stage renal disease?

◆ Trauma to the Kidneys and Ureters

Accidental injury to the kidneys, ureters, bladder, or urethra occurs frequently and should always be considered a possibility whenever there has been trauma to the abdominal cavity or thoracic cage.

Symptoms and Diagnosis　Signs and symptoms characteristic of trauma to the kidneys include massive hemorrhage, hematuria, abdominal or flank pain, and possibly an enlarged mass in the kidney area. Diagnostic tests include serial urinalyses, hemoglobin and hematocrit tests, and measurements of electrolytes. Rising BUN levels and creatinine indicate diminishing renal function. Radiological studies including films of the kidney, ureters, and bladder (KUB), and IVP can demonstrate the extent of damage to the urinary system. Hourly measurements of urinary output and observation of the characteristics of the urine can help determine the type and extent of injury.

Treatment　Bleeding in the kidney often is self-limiting. Lacerations and contusions without interruption of urinary function usually can be treated conservatively by bedrest. For this reason the urologist may advocate a period of watchful waiting to see whether the kidney can be saved.

Nursing Assessment and Intervention　During this time the patient is monitored closely for signs of hypovolemic shock, cardiovascular changes, urinary output, and size of the flank mass. Nursing intervention in the care of all patients with trauma to the kidney must not be focused only on renal function. Most patients with injuries of this kind also have had damage to the colon, spleen, or pancreas. A comprehensive plan for dealing with problems associated with multiple trauma is usually necessary.

◆ Trauma to the Bladder

Any violent blow or crushing injury to the lower abdomen may result in rupture or perforation of the bladder wall, with resulting leakage of the urine into the pelvic tissues or peritoneal cavity. This brings about a severe inflammation in these areas. Bladder trauma is more likely if the bladder is full at the time of an accident than when it is empty.

Signs and Symptoms Early symptoms of bladder injury are painful hematuria or inability to void, marked tenderness and spasm in the suprapubic area, or the development of a large mass in that area.

Treatment If the bladder has ruptured or is perforated, treatment consists of a suprapubic cystostomy to drain blood and urine. Care of the patient demands meticulous attention to drains and dressings to avoid infection and maintain good drainage. Cold applications to the surgical site both before and after surgery may be ordered.

Nursing Assessment and Intervention The nurse should observe the patient carefully for postoperative shock and massive hemorrhage. Any mass formation in the suprapubic area before or after surgery or any change in the vital signs should be reported immediately.

In addition to physical distress, the patient with bladder injuries is likely to have emotional difficulties in dealing with the problems arising from the sudden loss of control over the urinary flow and the intimate procedures and treatments necessary. The nurse must be prepared for this and show consideration for the patient's concerns.

COMMON THERAPIES FOR UROLOGICAL PROBLEMS

◆ Catheterization

When a patient cannot expel urine from the bladder (void) because of effects of anesthesia, paralysis, trauma, neurological causes, partial obstruction, or after surgical procedures, a urethral catheter may be inserted into the bladder to remove urine. An indwelling catheter may be inserted when urine flow must be monitored closely, as in many critically ill patients. Urethral catheters are available in several sizes. For the adult, a small 12 French up to a large 20 French catheter is used. Urinary catheters are of one of two types: straight or retention (indwelling). Straight catheters are the Robinson or the whistle-tip; retention catheters are the Foley, coude, Malecot, and Pezzer. The Foley, double-or triple-lumen catheter is the most

common one. The Malecot or Pezzer catheter often is used as a suprapubic, rather than urethral, catheter (Figure 23-8).

A straight catheter is used for a single "in-and-out" catheterization where the inability to empty the bladder is temporary or where the patient has permanent paralysis and must use intermittent catheterization to empty the bladder. Straight catheterization also is used to check for residual urine (urine left in the bladder after voiding) during bladder retraining. **To check for residual urine, catheterization must occur immediately after the patient has voided.**

Urinary catheters and tubes must be handled with strict aseptic technique. **Urinary catheters are the most common cause of hospital-acquired infection.** Techniques for insertion of urethral catheters are found in fundamentals of nursing textbooks. Table 23-6 reviews the principles of urinary catheter care.

A *retention catheter* in the urethra should always be kept open and draining freely unless there are specific orders to clamp it off. Clamping is sometimes done as part of a bladder training program or when a urine specimen is needed.

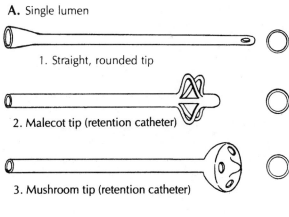

A. Single lumen

1. Straight, rounded tip

2. Malecot tip (retention catheter)

3. Mushroom tip (retention catheter)

B. Double lumen (Retention catheter with rounded tip)

Drainage
Sterile water for balloon inflation

C. Triple lumen (Retention catheter with coude tip)

Drainage
Irrigation
Sterile water for balloon inflation

FIGURE 23-8 Types of urinary catheters. (*Source:* Lammon, C. B. et al. [1995]. *Clinical Nursing Skills.* Philadelphia: Saunders, p. 482.)

When the physician orders removal of the retention catheter, the nurse accepts responsibility for removing the catheter and carefully observing the patient for signs of retention of urine and for signs of infection. The time of removal of the catheter is recorded, and the patient is observed for signs of difficulty in voiding. Any bleeding, dribbling, or incontinence of urine should be reported as these are possible signs of an excessive amount of residual urine or bleeding from the bladder or urethra.

Alternatives to indwelling urethral catheters should always be considered when there is evidence that the patient cannot remain continent of urine. Such alternatives can be used temporarily, as in a bladder control program, or permanently. They include condom (external) drainage for males, drainage by suprapubic catheter, and self-catheterization.

◆ Renal Dialysis

Hemodialysis and peritoneal dialysis are two procedures commonly used to remove waste products normally excreted by the kidneys. Both procedures rely on diffusion to remove elements normally excreted in the urine. The principle of diffusion states that *solute* molecules that are in constant motion tend to pass through a semipermeable membrane from the side of higher concentration to the side of lower concentration.

Hemodialysis Hemodialysis removes nitrogenous waste products from the blood by pumping the blood from the arterial circulation through a dialysate bath and back to the venous circulation. A dialysis membrane separates the blood from the dialyzing solution. The molecules of waste pass through this membrane out of the blood and into the dialyzing solution until the two solutions are equal in concentration (Figure 23-9).

A temporary access for hemodialysis can be achieved by inserting a subclavian, jugular, or femoral vein dialysis catheter. This access is used for ARF. The subclavian site is preferred if more than one or two treatments are probable. The catheter can be inserted by the physician at the bedside.

Two kinds of internal access are used to withdraw arterial blood, bathe it in dialyzing solution, and return it to the venous system for the patient with chronic renal failure who requires ongoing hemodialysis. An arteriovenous (AV) fistula is formed by joining an artery and a vein together (Figure 23-10A). In other words, the vein is "arterialized"; that is, it is made into a large superficial vein with an arterial supply that is easily accessible by venipuncture. Most often the radial or brachial artery is joined to the cephalic vein in the arm. A period of 6 to 8 weeks after surgery is needed for the vessel walls to become thickened and usable for the repeated insertion of the hemodialysis needles. When an AV fistula is no

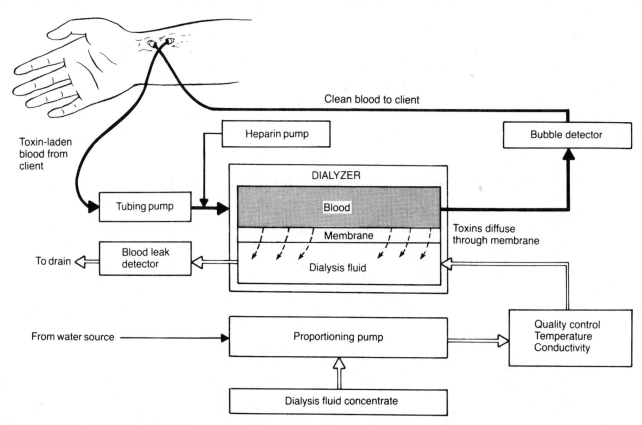

FIGURE 23-9   Typical hemodialysis system. (*Source:* Modified from Black, J. M. Matassarin-Jacobs, E, [1993]. *Luckmann and Sorensen's Medical Surgical Nursing: A Psychophysiologic Approach,* 4th ed. Philadelphia: Saunders, p. 1512.)

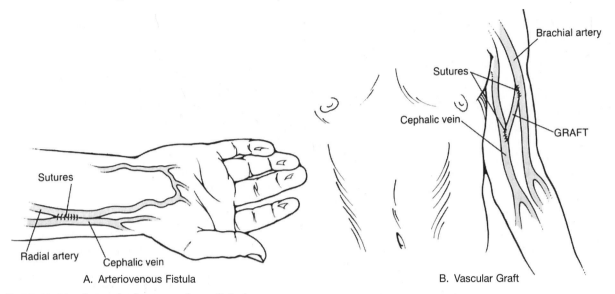

FIGURE 23-10   **Access for long-term hemodialysis.** (*Source:* Modified from Ignatavicius, D. D., Workman, M. L., Mishler, M. A. [1995]. *Medical–Surgical Nursing: A Nursing Process Approach,* 2nd ed. Philadelphia: Saunders, p. 2135.)

longer functional and another cannot be created, the second form of access is utilized.

The second kind of arteriovenous (AV) access is accomplished by connecting an artery and a vein with a graft of a piece of synthetic material (GoreTex). The hemodialysis needles are then placed directly into the graft (Figure 23-10B).

When caring for the hospitalized patient who has an arteriovenous graft or an AV fistula, it is important to protect the graft from injury and check its status. The site should be observed at least four times a day for signs indicating clotting or infection, and the fingers of the arm with the graft should be checked for adequate circulation. There should be a palpable thrill and a bruit should be clearly heard upon auscultation. The arm or leg in which the arteriovenous shunt has been created should never be used for checking blood pressure or performing venipuncture. When a graft has been inserted, the extremity is elevated postoperatively and kept at a level above the heart for 24 to 72 hours. Thereafter, the patient should sleep with that extremity free rather than on the side with it tucked underneath the body. **Care is taken never to compress the extremity containing the vascular access.**

The scheduling of hemodialysis sessions varies from patient to patient, but treatments usually are done two to three times a week, most often on an outpatient basis at a dialysis center. The problems that a patient on hemodialysis may experience include fluid overload (hypervolemia), electrolyte imbalance, alterations in blood components leading to anemia, and platelet abnormalities that produce a tendency to bleed abnor-

mally. Other major problems are infection in either the access site or the blood.

Medications frequently prescribed for the dialysis patient include multivitamins, antacids, iron supplements, antihypertensives, digitalis, vasodilators, H_2-receptor antagonists, and phosphate binders. Epoetin alpha (Epogen), a synthetic substance that stimulates red blood cell production, is given to combat the suppression of natural erythropoietin that occurs in renal failure. **Antihypertensive drugs are not given the morning of dialysis, as they can cause severe hypotension during the treatment. Nitroglycerin (NTG) patches, digitalis, and anticoagulants also are held.**

Patients who depend on hemodialysis for survival require extensive instruction in the care of their cannulas and access sites. They also must understand the rationale for various fluid and food restrictions and the medications prescribed. Patient compliance is a major challenge to nurses who care for patients on dialysis.

Hepatitis and acquired immunodeficiency syndrome (AIDS) are dangers because of occasionally needed transfusions and because of the exposure to multi-user dialysis machines, even though the machines are cleaned with acid and bleach. Patients who had multiple transfusions before reliable testing of blood for the human immunodeficiency virus (HIV) existed may have been exposed to the virus.

Perhaps an even greater challenge for the nurse is to help dialysis-dependent patients cope with the stress of prolonged intensive treatment and the frustrations of dealing with an incurable illness. Rigid dietary restrictions, fatigue, malaise, occasional limited mobility, and possibly sexual difficulties take their toll on the patient as well as significant others. Family members usually are profoundly affected by the patient's chronic illness and the demands long-term dialysis places on them. Their needs, as well as the patient's, are considered when planning nursing intervention. **The major goals of nursing care are to facilitate acceptance of the diagnosis of chronic renal failure and adaptation to dialysis treatment.**

Guidelines for facilitating positive adaptation to dialysis are as follows:

- Enhance nursing assessment and observation skills and detect complications.
- Genuinely care for the patient, accepting him as an individual and allowing him to realize his full human potential.
- Practice empathetic listening and provide opportunities for the patient to express feelings.
- Monitor verbal and nonverbal behavior that might indicate depression or suicidal behavior.
- Work closely with the family to assess the impact the patient's illness and treatment are having on them. Encourage them to achieve a balance between supporting the patient and allowing as much independence as possible. Encourage communication between patient and spouse to express feelings about changes in sexual activity, role reversal, and family responsibilities.

Postdialysis nursing care includes monitoring the access site for bleeding, assessing the patient for signs of confusion or disorientation, monitoring vital signs, and continuing assessment of the access site for patency and signs of infection. **Invasive procedures are postponed for 4 to 6 hours after dialysis because the clotting time is extended from the heparin used during dialysis and prolonged bleeding could occur.**

Peritoneal Dialysis   Peritoneal dialysis is an alternative procedure that can be used instead of hemodialysis to remove waste products or toxins that have accumulated as a result of renal failure. Peritoneal dialysis operates on the same principles as hemodialysis, the difference being that in this procedure the semipermeable membrane is in the peritoneum and the dialyzing solution is introduced into and withdrawn from the peritoneal cavity.

Peritoneal dialysis has the advantages of being initiated more quickly than hemodialysis because there is no need for a dialyzing apparatus, anticoagulants are not necessary, and maturation of the access and canalization of blood vessels is not required. And, because chemical and fluid exchanges occur more slowly in peritoneal dialysis, there is less stress on the cardiovascular system.

Acute and chronic renal failure can both be treated with peritoneal dialysis. Some patients with renal failure fare better on a gentler dialytic therapy. With available equipment, it is possible for a patient to have intermittent or continuous peritoneal ambulatory dialysis or continuous cycling peritoneal dialysis at night (Figure 23-11). The patient is taught to operate a portable, manual device and to perform her own dialysis as often as necessary to manage her disease and prevent symptoms.

For continuous ambulatory peritoneal dialysis (CAPD), where the process goes on 24 hours a day, 7 days a week, the bag of dialyzing solution is suspended above the level of the abdomen and the tubing is attached to the permanently implanted peritoneal di-

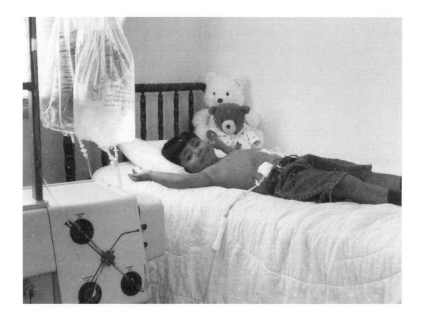

FIGURE 23-11   Peritoneal dialysis at home.
(Photo by Glen Derbyshire; courtesy of Santa Barbara Visiting Nurse Association, Santa Barbara, CA.)

alysis catheter. The clamp on the tubing is opened and the dialysate solution is allowed to run into the abdomen by gravity flow. When the bag is empty, the tubing is reclamped, the bag rolled up and secured, and the patient can move about during the dwell time (time the fluid remains in the peritoneal cavity) of 4 to 8 hours while dialysis occurs. At the end of the dwell time, the bag is unrolled and placed below the level of the abdomen (Figure 23-12). The dialysate solution containing waste products drains from the abdominal cavity.

Peritoneal dialysis cannot be done when there is severe trauma to the abdomen, after multiple abdominal surgeries, if there are adhesions in the abdominal cavity, or if the patient has a severe coagulation defect, paralytic ileus, or diffuse peritonitis.

During the procedure, warm fluid equal in osmolarity and similar in composition to normal body fluid is introduced into the peritoneal cavity via a catheter. The fluid infuses by gravity; its rate of flow can be controlled by lowering or raising the container of dialysate or by manipulating a clamp on the tubing.

The solution is left in the peritoneal cavity a specified time (dwell time) until the concentrations of the solutions on either side of the peritoneal membrane are equalized. After the solution has remained in the peritoneal cavity the correct time, the fluid is drained from the cavity. This either completes the dialysis or prepares the cavity for instillation of fresh dialysate.

Complications such as peritonitis, leakage, obstruction or other problems with the catheter, respiratory problems, and fluid overload can occur.

Specific nursing care for the patient undergoing peritoneal dialysis includes obtaining the patient's weight before and after the treatment; maintaining careful intake and output records; maintaining strict aseptic technique in handling the dialysate bags, peritoneal catheter, and all equipment; monitoring vital signs; observing for complications such as peritonitis; and keeping the patient as comfortable as possible. The solution should be at room temperature and must be instilled slowly. The patient and family are taught all the steps of the procedure before discharge.

Think about *...* What signs and symptoms might indicate that your peritoneal dialysis patient has peritonitis?

◆ Continuous Hemofiltration

Another method of treatment for acute renal failure is continuous venovenous hemofiltration (CVVH). A double-lumen catheter is inserted into the subclavian or femoral vein. A pump sends blood through a hemofilter, through an air and clot trap, past an air detector, and

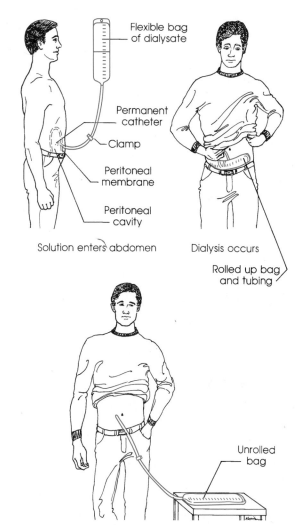

FIGURE 23-12   Continuous ambulatory peritoneal dialysis.

back into the patient. The blood passes through a special hollow-fiber filter and returns to the vein. A dialysis machine is not needed. This method filters out wastes much more slowly than hemodialysis, but does not cause such rapid fluid and electrolyte shifts. CVVH is used for critically ill patients who cannot tolerate hemodialysis and is continued for an average of 10 days. Other similar methods of dialysis are slow, continuous ultrafiltration (SCUF), continuous arteriovenous hemofiltration (CAVH), continuous venovenous hemodialysis (CVHD), and continuous arteriovenous hemodialysis (CAVHD).

◆ Kidney Transplantation

An alternative to dialysis for treatment of renal failure is to transplant a kidney from a blood relative of the patient, another tissue-compatible donor, or from a cadaver whose kidney tissue is compatible with that of the recipient.

Tissue typing to determine donor–recipient compatibility is performed, along with extensive psychological assessment and counseling for both the live donor and the recipient. The closer the tissue match, the greater the chance of successful retention of the kidney. Transplant candidates must be free from medical problems that might increase the risks of the procedure or jeopardize the success of the transplant. Malignancy, IV drug abuse, severe obesity, active vasculitis, and severe psychosocial problems eliminate some candidates.

Hypertension is brought under the best possible control, any infection is treated, and the patient is dialyzed immediately before transplantation. Immunosuppressive drugs are started and are continued postoperatively in decreasing dosages to prevent organ rejection. Previously cyclosporine was the drug of choice to prevent kidney transplant rejection. Now the drug tacrolimus (Prograf) has been found useful when cyclosporine fails to prevent signs of rejection. Long-term problems for transplant patients are increased susceptibility to infection and a 35% higher risk of malignancy, both directly related to the necessary immunosuppressive therapy.

Renal transplant patients are transferred to critical care or specialty units after surgery, where they are closely monitored for signs of rejection: fever, increased blood pressure, and pain over the iliac fossa where the new kidney was placed (Figure 23-13). **Ongoing assessment includes watching for the signs of renal failure, particularly oliguria, anuria, and rising BUN levels and serum creatinine. Protection from sources of infection is a top priority.** Once the new kidney is functioning properly, the primary physician may lift the previous dietary restrictions.

Renal failure and dialysis are very expensive for the patient and his family. However, lack of funds does not exclude anyone from needed care. Since July 1973 an amendment to the Social Security Act allows Medicare to pay 80% of the cost of treating end-stage renal disease, including dialysis and renal transplant. Medical expenses continue after transplant, as the drugs needed to prevent rejection are very expensive.

◆ Lithotripsy

When extracorporeal lithotripsy is performed to break up a renal stone, the patient is placed in a specially designed tub with the trunk of the body submerged in water. Straps are secured to help maintain correct position and immobility for the 30 to 40 minutes needed for the procedure. Sedation may be given. Shock waves are generated under water, bounce off of a reflector and strike the stone, breaking it up. The patient may experience cramping pain after the procedure and is given antispasmodics if this occurs. A fluid increase to 3,000 to 4,000 mL is necessary to help wash the stone fragments from the kidney. The fragments travel in the urine down the ureter and into the bladder for excretion. Early ambulation helps mobilize the fluid and the stone fragments so that they can be eliminated in the urine. For percutaneous ultrasonic lithotripsy, ultrasound waves are percutaneously delivered to the stone to break it up.

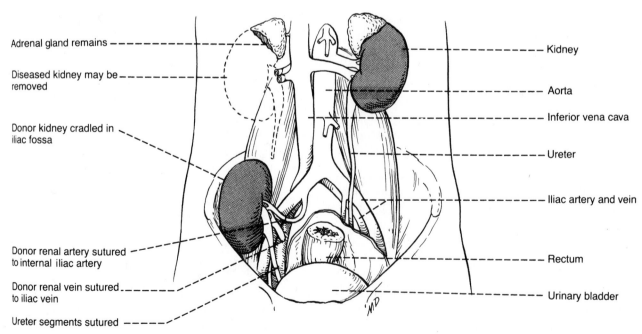

FIGURE 23-13   Placement of transplanted kidney. (*Source:* Modified from Black, J. M. Matassarin-Jacobs, E. [1993]. *Luckmann and Sorensen's Medical–Surgical Nursing: A Psychophysiologic Approach,* 4th ed. Philadelphia: Saunders, p. 1517.)

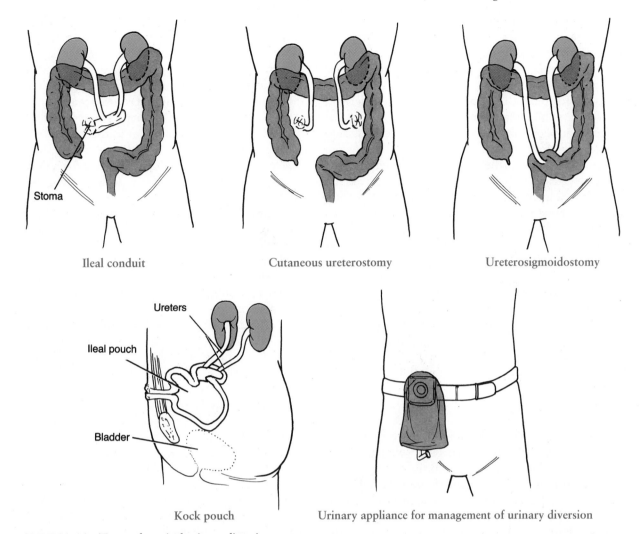

Ileal conduit   Cutaneous ureterostomy   Ureterosigmoidostomy

Kock pouch   Urinary appliance for management of urinary diversion

FIGURE 23-14   Types of surgical urinary diversion. (*Source:* Bollander, V. R. [1994]. *Sorensen and Luckmann's Basic Nursing: A Psychophysiologic Approach,* 3rd ed. Philadelphia: Saunders, p. 1164.)

◆ Surgery

Bladder surgery may be minor, such as removing polyps from the bladder interior using a cystoscope, or major such as a *cystectomy*, removal of the bladder. Cystectomy is performed for bladder cancer. A variety of procedures may be performed to correct the anatomical position of the bladder, such as bladder neck suspension. These surgeries are most often performed to correct urinary incontinence in women.

Nursing care following cystectomy is always difficult because of the danger of hemorrhage and infection. There also are problems involved in devising a satisfactory arrangement for urine collection.

When the bladder is surgically removed, a urinary diversion procedure is necessary to handle the excretion of urine. There are several ways in which urinary diversion can be accomplished (Figure 23-14), including *ileal conduit* or *ileal loop, cutaneous ureterostomy, ureterosigmoidostomy or sigmoid conduit, vesicostomy,* and *ileal reservoir (Kock or Indiana pouch).*

Ileal Conduit   This procedure also is called urinary *ileostomy* and *ileal loop or Bricker's procedure.* A portion of the ileum is used as a tube or conduit through which urine flows to the outside. It is important to realize that the section of ileum is removed from the intestinal tract. Urine does *not* flow through it to the intestines, as when the ureters are sutured to the sigmoid. The open ends of the intestines where the section of ileum was removed are rejoined by anastomosis.

The surgeon cuts out a portion of the ileum, leaving nerve and blood supply intact so that it remains a viable tissue. The two ends of the intestine from which the section of ileum is removed are rejoined. The "borrowed" section of ileum is sutured together at one end to form a pouch, while the other end is brought outside to form a stoma. The ureters are attached to the ileal conduit so that urine can flow through the conduit to the outside.

Cutaneous Ureterostomy and Vesicotomy   *Ureterostomy* is a surgical incision into the ureter that diverts the flow of urine. In a cutaneous ureterostomy, the surgeon detaches one or both ureters from the bladder and brings them to the surface of the body, usually in the region of the flank. The patient may have one or two stomas.

A vesicotomy is an incision into the bladder just above the pubic area. After incising the bladder, the surgeon moves it forward and sutures the cut edges to the skin, forming a stoma.

An obstruction to the flow of urine through a ureter causes a backflow of urine into the renal pelvis and eventually a hydronephrosis. If the patient has a cutaneous ureterostomy with two stomas (one from each ureter), the flow of urine from each stoma must be measured. Any tubing leading from the ureterostomy should be kept open so that urine can flow freely. The tube is checked frequently for signs of obstruction by mucus or blood clots.

Ureterosigmoidostomy or Sigmoid Conduit
A sigmoid, or colonic, conduit is similar to an ileal conduit, the difference being that a portion of the sigmoid colon is used to form the conduit. The ureters are implanted in the conduit.

Ileal Reservoir (Kock Pouch)
This procedure creates a continent ileal reservoir. The ureters are implanted into a segment of ileum that has been isolated. Special nipple valves connect the pouch to the exterior of the skin. The pouch can then be catheterized via the nipple valve by the patient, providing continence with no exterior collection device. The distal nipple valve is brought flush to the skin on the right side of the abdomen, forming a stoma. The patient is continent of urine, but needs to catheterize the pouch several times a day to empty the urine. An adhesive bandage or gauze pad over the stoma will absorb the mucus it secretes. One daily irrigation of the pouch is performed to empty it of the mucus that has collected there.

Threads of mucus in the urine are to be expected; these are secreted by the mucous membrane of the ileal or colonic segment of the conduit. Whitish crystals or encrustations in or near the stoma indicate an alkaline urine; this should be reported so that treatment can be prescribed to prevent stone formation.

Indiana Pouch
This type of pouch is constructed from portions of the ileum and cecum, and the ileocecal valve provides a means of continence. It is larger than the Kock pouch and spherical in shape with lower internal pressure that helps prevent incontinence. The ureters are tunneled into the pouch wall to help prevent reflux into the kidneys. The pouch is emptied via self-catheterization of the nipple valve in the same manner as for Kock's pouch.

Postoperative Nursing Care General postoperative care for a urinary ostomy is the same as for an intestinal ostomy (see Chapter 20). Additional workup for the patient with a stoma for urinary diversion includes assessing the amount and characteristics of the urine and mucus it is expelling and recording accurate output of urine every hour for the first 24 hours and then every 4 to 8 hours. After the Kock or Indiana pouch is formed there will be six drains, including two ureteral stents, a cecostomy tube, a red rubber catheter from the stoma, and two abdominal drains. To keep it open, the cecostomy tube is irrigated four times a day with 30 to 60 mL of normal saline. The tube will need to be irrigated by the patient four times a day after discharge. When catheterization of the stoma begins, the catheter is lubricated with a water-soluble lubricant. At night the cecostomy tube can be attached to a urinary drainage pouch so that catheterization is not needed during hours of sleep.

About 4 weeks after surgery, self-catheterization will begin on a schedule of every 3 hours during the day and every 4 hours at night. After about a week, if the pouch is continent, the schedule is altered to every 4 hours during the day and once at night. The Indiana pouch may take 6 to 12 months to begin to function ideally. The patient needs a lot of support and encouragement during this recovery period.

Skin irritation and breakdown can be a problem, and every effort is made to keep urine from touching the skin when the patient has an external stoma. A well-fitted and properly adhering collection appliance is essential. A thin gauze roll or tampon is placed into the stoma during appliance change and cleansing to prevent leakage of urine on to the skin. Most ostomy bags can be used for 3 to 5 days. To prevent infection, the bag must be changed at least weekly. The bag should be emptied when it becomes 1/3 to 1/2 full. This prevents the weight of the urine from pulling the bag loose. At night the bag can be connected to a larger urine container. The bag should be changed in the morning when urine flow is less. The area around the stoma is washed with a solution of 1/2 vinegar and 1/2 warm water to remove any crystals. If no crystals are present, warm, soapy water may be used. The area is thoroughly rinsed and patted dry with a towel before a new bag is attached. Any remaining moisture may interfere with the seal of the new appliance. A bath or shower may be taken with the bag on or off.

Odor may be a problem and result from poor hygiene, alkaline urine, normal breakdown of urine when it is exposed to air, and the ingestion of certain foods, such as asparagus. Acidifying the urine helps reduce odor. Dilute urine is less odorous as well and this is accomplished by increasing fluid intake. Reusable appliances must be washed with soap and water and soaked in dilute white vinegar solution or a commercial deodorizing product for 20 to 30 minutes. The pouch is then rinsed and allowed to dry. Deodorant tablets that may be placed in the appliance to decrease odor are available.

Retropubic Suspension (Marshall-Marchetti-Krantz Procedure)

This procedure is performed to correct a cystocele and urinary incontinence. A low abdominal incision is made and the urethral position is elevated in relation to the bladder. A urethral and suprapubic catheter are in place for several days postoperatively.

Needle Bladder Neck Suspension (Pereyra or Stamery Procedure)

A needle vaginal approach is combined with a small suprapubic skin incision to elevate the urethral position in relation to the bladder. Direct visualization of the operative area is not possible with this procedure, and it tends to result in more complications than the retropubic suspension. However, the success rate for preventing incontinence is higher.

Artificial Sphincter Implant

This is implanted more frequently in men than in women. A mechanical device is placed around the urethra to open and close it. Its purpose is to correct incontinence.

Nephrolithotomy and Pyelonephrolithotomy

These procedures for removing a kidney stone may be done percutaneously or with an open procedure. Fiberoptic equipment has made percutaneous procedures first choice. A special forceps is introduced through the nephroscope to retrieve the stone. A nephrostomy tube is inserted as the scope is removed and this remains in place for 1 to 5 days. A fluid intake of 3,000 to 4,000 mL per day is required to flush any residual stone fragments out of the kidney. The patient is monitored for infection, hemorrhage, and leakage of fluid into the retroperitoneal cavity. When a stone cannot be retrieved by percutaneous procedure, an open procedure is used. If a stone is lodged in a ureter and will not descend on its own with fluid increases, a *uretolithotomy* is performed.

Nephrectomy and Nephrostomy

The two main types of surgical procedures that may be performed on the kidney are *nephrectomy* and *nephrostomy*. *Nephrectomy* is the surgical removal of the kidney to eradicate a tumor or to remove a severely damaged kidney. Although this is always a serious operation, a person may live with only one kidney. The remaining kidney enlarges and is usually able to carry on the work formerly done by two kidneys.

Nephrostomy is a surgical incision into a kidney to drain the kidney artificially. This procedure may be done to treat obstructions from large stones or strictures of the ureter or to drain purulent material from an infected kidney.

Postoperative Nursing Care

Continual postoperative assessment is necessary to detect complications. Nursing interventions focus on promoting unimpeded urine flow by properly caring for catheters and tubes. Abdominal procedures require the same care as for any abdominal surgery. Vaginal procedures require monitoring for vaginal bleeding.

In both nephrectomy and nephrostomy, the surgical incision may be lumbar, transabdominal, or thoracic. When the patient returns from surgery, the nurse must check carefully for the location of the surgical wound and the presence of any drains or tubes that may have been inserted during the operation.

Dressings over the surgical wound may be reinforced. The drainage on these dressings will be blood-tinged at first, but it should gradually become clearer. If bright red blood appears or there is a sudden change in the amount of drainage, the doctor should be notified. Extreme care must be taken when changing dressings to ensure that the drains or tubes are not dislodged or pulled from the surgical incision.

Positioning of the patient depends on the wishes of the surgeon, who may prefer to have the patient lie only on the affected side. Turning the patient may be difficult at first because it is usually quite painful for her to move about. The nurse should explain the need for frequent turning and deep-breathing so that complications may be prevented.

Hemorrhage always is a danger after surgery of the kidney. It will be remembered that the kidneys have a very rich supply of blood directly from the aorta and vena cava. The vital signs are carefully checked and any indication of shock or hemorrhage reported immediately.

Adequate drainage from the opposite kidney after surgery is of great importance. Urinary output must be very carefully measured and recorded. Fluids are usually restricted immediately after surgery and then gradually increased as the remaining kidney compensates for the loss of its partner. If a nephrostomy has been done, fluids are restricted until the affected kidney can recover sufficiently and resume its functions.

Psychological care of the patient facing malignancy and an operation that will radically change his body image should be a primary nursing concern. The nurse must encourage the patient to talk about his fears and concerns. The spouse must also be encouraged to share feelings. There are always sexual concerns when cystectomy and urinary diversion are performed. Some of the more radical procedures will produce impotence in the male. The caring nurse should not leave the patient and family to sort out these concerns alone.

COMMUNITY CARE

A major function of nursing in the community is to assist hypertensive and diabetic patients to achieve good control of their disease. Adequate control of blood pressure and blood sugar helps prevent damage to the kidneys.

Nurses who work in dialysis centers often are the primary nurses for the patient in renal failure. They are the ones who constantly assess the patient for complications, watch for medication-related problems, continue with teaching regarding diet and lifestyle to promote compliance with the treatment program. Considerable psychosocial support and counseling may be necessary as dialysis patients often experience depression, hopelessness, sexual problems, role changes, and relationship problems.

Home care nurses are constantly on the alert for signs of acute or chronic renal failure among their patients. Many illnesses and the variety of drugs that patients have prescribed may cause kidney damage. Many home care patients have indwelling catheters and must be assessed for signs of infection and their catheters replaced with new ones periodically. Problems of incontinence also are treated in the home.

Nurses in long-term care facilities deal with a variety of urinary problems. Bladder training for incontinence is a prime consideration. Knowing that the elderly have diminished renal reserve makes monitoring for drug toxicities in this population imperative as drugs are not excreted as quickly as in the younger person. Keeping residents dry and odor free is very important. Monitoring for obstruction to the flow of urine is another priority in the elderly population and is particularly pertinent in those who are ill.

Nurses in outpatient clinics will be assisting with urological procedures such as cystoscopy and removal or destruction of renal stones. They will be teaching and monitoring the patient with bladder or kidney cancer. Clinic nurses also do a great deal of teaching to help with problems of incontinence.

Nurses working in long-term care or with families of home care patients who have patients who usually need to get up frequently at night to urinate might try ambulating the patient for at least 10 minutes an hour or two before bedtime. This tends to greatly decrease trips to the bathroom during the night because the muscular activity helps to mobilize fluid.

All nurses can help the people in the community to promote healthy kidney function by encouraging the intake of more water and by encouraging prompt recognition and treatment of urinary tract infections.

CRITICAL THINKING EXERCISES

Clinical Case Problems

Read each of the clinical situations and discuss the questions with your classmates.

1. A friend of yours tells you that she has been very uncomfortable during the past week because of frequency of urination and burning when she voids. Last night, she had a severe chill and some elevation of temperature. She has been told that she probably has a very common ailment in women and that if she drinks a lot of fluids, it will probably go away.

   a. What would be your advice to your friend?

   b. How would you explain the need for her to follow your advice?

2. Mrs. Simpson, age 54, has had hypertension since she was in her early twenties. She now has developed symptoms of chronic renal failure. She was referred to a nephrologist, who, after a series of diagnostic tests, recommended hemodialysis and kidney transplant when an organ is available.

   a. What diagnostic tests do you think the nephrologist would have ordered for Mrs. Simpson?

   b. Why might Mrs. Simpson's renal disease not have been diagnosed earlier?

   c. If Mrs. Simpson does not agree to hemodialysis, what symptoms is she likely to experience eventually? What other alternatives are available to her besides hemodialysis?

   d. What psychosocial problems would you expect Mrs. Simpson to have? Write specific nursing diagnoses for each and list nursing interventions that might be effective in helping her deal with them.

3. Mrs. Diaz is a 35-year-old patient who has had a nephrostomy for treatment of hydronephrosis resulting from obstruction by a renal stone in the pelvis of the kidney. She returns from surgery with a nephrostomy tube, a urethral catheter, and a rubber Penrose drain in place.

   a. How would you explain the purpose of the nephrostomy tube?

   b. What is the specific nursing care for these tubes and the drain?

   c. What is the likely treatment for the renal stone?

BIBLIOGRAPHY

American Journal of Nursing. (1995). Tacrolimus (Prograf): A new choice to prevent organ rejection. *American Journal of Nursing.* 95(4):55–56.

Applegate, E. J. (1995). *The Anatomy and Physiology Learning System: Textbook.* Philadelphia: Saunders.

Bennett, J. C., Plum, F., eds. (1996). *Cecil Textbook of Medicine,* 20th ed. Philadelphia: Saunders.

Black, J. M., Matassarin-Jacobs, E. (1997). *Medical–Surgical Nursing: Clinical Management for Continuity of Care,* 5th ed. Philadelphia: Saunders.

Brooks, M. J. (1995). Assessment and nursing management of homebound clients with urinary incontinence. *Home Healthcare Nurse.* 13(5):11–19.

Catanzaro, J. (1996). Managing incontinence: An update. *RN.* 59(10):39–44.

Connor, P. A., Kooker, B. M. (1996). Nurses' knowledge, attitudes, and practices in managing urinary incontinence in the acute care setting. *MEDSURG Nursing.* 5(2): 87–117.

Copstead, L. C. (1995). *Perspectives on Pathophysiology.* Philadelphia: Saunders.

Cotran, R. S., Kumar, V., Robbins, S. L., Schoen, F. J., eds. (1994). *Robbins Pathologic Basis of Disease,* 5th ed. Philadelphia: Saunders.

Czarapata, B. J. R. (1994). Clinical highlights: management of interstitial cystitis. *Urologic Nursing.* 14(3):145–148.

Dambro, M. R. (1996). *Griffith's 5 Minute Clinical Consult.* Baltimore: Williams & Wilkins.

Damjanov, I. (1996). *Pathology for the Health Related Professions.* Philadelphia: Saunders.

Davis, J., Sherer , K. (1994). *Applied Nutrition and Diet Therapy for Nurses,* 2nd ed. Philadelphia: Saunders.

DeGroot-Kosolcharoen, J. (1995). Combating infection: thirteen ways to protect your patient from bacteriuria: how to keep catheters from causing harm. *Nursing 95.* 25(4):30.

Deutsch, N. (1995). Keeping current. Laparoscopic bladder repair. *Canadian Nurse.* 91(7):21.

deWit, S. C. (1994). *Rambo's Nursing Skills for Clinical Practice,* 4th ed. Philadelphia: Saunders.

Dirkes, S. M. (1997). A dialysis alternative more nurses can run. *RN.* 60(5):20–25.

Dirkes, S. (1994). How to use the new CWH renal replacement systems. *American Journal of Nursing.* 94(5): 67–68, 69, 70, 72–73.

Duffield, P. (1996). Managing urinary tract infections: Part 2: Caring for children and the elderly. *American Journal of Nursing.* 96(10):16i–16j.

Fiers, S. (1994). Indwelling catheters and devices: avoiding the problems. *Urologic Nursing.* 14(3):141–144.

Fiers, S. (1995). Management of the long-term indwelling catheter in the home setting. *Journal of Wound.* 22(3): 140–144.

Giddens, J. F., Vigil, G. J., Sanchez, A. (1993). Risks and rewards of kidney transplant. *RN.* 56(6):56–61.

Goshorn, J. (1996). Kidney stones. *American Journal of Nursing.* 96(9):40–41.

Gurklis, J. A., Menke, E. M. (1995). Chronic hemodialysis patients' perceptions of stress, coping, and social support. *ANNA Journal.* 22(4):381–388.

Guyton, A. C., Hall, J. E. (1996). *Textbook of Medical Physiology,* 9th ed. Philadelphia: Saunders.

Higley, R. R. (1996). Continuous arteriovenous hemofiltration: A case study. *Critical Care Nurse.* 16(5):37–40.

Hoffart, N., Stein, P. (1995). Vascular access. *AORN Journal.* 61(5):801–802.

Ignatavicius, D. D., Hausman, K. A. (1995). *Clinical Pathways for Collaborative Practice.* Philadelphia: Saunders.

Ignatavicius, D. D., Workman, M. L., Mishler, M. A. (1995). *Medical–Surgical Nursing: A Nursing Process Approach,* 2nd ed. Philadelphia: Saunders.

Jarvis, C. (1996). *Physical Examination and Health Assessment,* 2nd ed. Philadelphia: Saunders.

Karlowicz, K. A., (1995). Urologic Nursing Principles and Practice. Philadelphia: Saunders.

Kee, J. L., Hayes, E. R. (1993). *Pharmacology: A Nursing Process Approach.* Philadelphia: Saunders.

Kelly, M. (1997). Acute renal failure. *American Journal of Nursing.* 97(3):32–33.

Kelly, M. (1996). Clinical snapshot: chronic renal failure. *American Journal of Nursing.* 96(1):36–37.

Kirton, C. A. (1997). Assessing for bladder distension. *Nursing 97.* 27(4):64.

Larsen, P. D., Martin, J. H. (1994). Renal system changes in the elderly. *AORN Journal.* 60(2):298–301.

Laycock, J. (1994). Pelvic muscle exercises: physiotherapy for the pelvic floor. *Urologic Nursing.* 14(3):136–140.

Lehne, R. A. (1994). *Pharmacology for Nursing Care,* 2nd ed. Philadelphia: Saunders.

Linton, A. D., Matteson, M. A., Maebius, N. K. (1995). *Introductory Nursing Care of Adults.* Philadelphia: Saunders.

Malarkey, L. M., McMorrow, M. E. (1996). *Nurse's Manual of Laboratory Tests and Diagnostic Procedures.* Philadelphia: Saunders.

Matteson, M. A., McConnell, E. S., Linton, A. D. (1997). *Gerontological Nursing.* Philadelphia: Saunders.

McConnell, E. A. (1994). Clinical do's & don'ts: how to apply a self-adhesive condom catheter. *Nursing 94.* 24(11):26.

McConnell, E. A. (1995). Clinical do's & don'ts: maintaining a peritoneal dialysis catheter. *Nursing 95.* 25(5):26.

McConnell, E. A. (1995). What's wrong with this patient? Assessing flank pain. *Nursing 95.* 25(11):74–75.

McCorkle, R., Grant, M., Frank-Stromborg, M., Baird, S. B. (1996). *Cancer Nursing: A Comprehensive Textbook.* Philadelphia: Saunders.

McEwen, D. R. (1994). Arteriovenous fistula: vascular access for long-term hemodialysis. *AORN Journal.* 59(1):223, 225–230, 232, 235–237, 239–240.

McKinney, B. C. (1995). Cut your patients' risk of nosocomial UTI. *RN.* 58(11):20–23.

Miller, C. A. (1995). Drug consult. Medications can cause or treat urinary incontinence. *Geriatric Nursing.* 16(5):253–254.

Monahan, F. D., Drake, T., Neighbors, M. (1994). *Nursing Care of Adults.* Philadelphia: Saunders.

Mondoux, L. C. (1994). Patients won't ask. *RN.* 57(2):35–40.

Moore, D. A., Edwards, K. (1997). Using a portable bladder scan to reduce the incidence of nosocomial urinary tract infections. *MEDSURG Nursing.* 6(1):39–43.

Moore, S., et al. (1993). Treating bladder cancer: new methods, new management. *American Journal of Nursing.* 93(5):32–39.

Mrazik, M. J. (1994). Drug hot line. Hemodialysis: when to give drugs. *Nursing 94.* 24(1):74.

Neskey, K. L., Loehner, D. (1994). Urinary diversion with an Indiana pouch. *Nursing 94.* 24(1):32C–32D, 32F, 32H.

Nursing 96. (1996). Peritoneal dialysis: Making a clean sweep. Adapted from *Nurses' Photo Library,* 1995. Springhouse Corp.:58–61.

Palumbo, M. V. (1995). Continence consultation for the rural homebound. *Home Healthcare Nurse.* 13(4):61–70.

Peterson, K. J., Solie, C. J. (1994). Interpreting lab values in chronic renal insufficiency. *American Journal of Nursing.* 94(5):56B, 56E, 56H, 56J.

Polaski, A. L., Tatro, S. E. (1996). *Luckmann's Core Principles and Practice of Medical–Surgical Nursing.* Philadelphia: Saunders.

Price, C. A. (1994). Acute renal failure: a sequela of sepsis. *Critical Care Nursing Clinics of North America.* 6(2): 359–372.

Ruth-Sahd, L. A. (1995). Renal calculi. *American Journal of Nursing.* 95(11):50.

Shellenbarger, T., Krouse, A. (1994). Treating and preventing kidney stones. *Medsurg Nursing.* 3(5):389–394.

Springhouse Corporation. (1996). *Nursing 96 Drug Handbook.* Springhouse: PA: Author.

Stark, J. (1997). Dialysis choices. *Nursing 97.* 27(2):41–46.

Stark, J. L. (1994). Interpreting B.U.N./creatinine levels: it's not as simple as you think. *Nursing 94.* 24(9):58–61.

Winslow, E. H. (1993). Myth of the clean catch. *American Journal of Nursing.* 93(8):20.

Wood, J. M., Bosley, C. L. (1995). Acute postrenal failure: Reversing the problem. *Nursing 95.* 25(3):48–50.

Wozniak-Petrofsky, J. (1994). Basic elements of urodynamic evaluation in urinary incontinence. *Urologic Nursing.* 14(3):125–129.

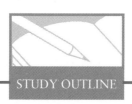

STUDY OUTLINE

I. Introduction

A. The urological system is responsible for maintaining proper balance of the fluids, minerals, and organic substances necessary for life.

B. Disease in other systems of the body may have a direct effect on the urological system.

C. Kidney failure can affect the heart, lungs, circulatory system, and other parts of the body.

II. Causes and Prevention of Disorders of the Urological System

A. Bacterial infections, immunological disorders, metabolic disorders such as diabetes mellitus, and circulatory disorders may all cause dysfunction.

B. Circulatory shock or heart failure may cause reduced blood flow to the kidney, decreasing its ability to filter wastes.

C. Stones may obstruct the flow of urine.

D. An enlarged prostate may obstruct urine flow.

E. Tubular necrosis from bacterial or chemical destruction of the nephron affects the functional ability of the kidney.

F. A lack of oxygen may cause tubular necrosis.

G. Disorders that systemically affect the blood vessels restricting blood flow also may affect the kidney vessels.

H. Tumors may destroy kidney tissue or cause obstruction to urine flow.

I. **The best way to prevent disorders of the urological system is to drink plenty of water.**

J. Emptying the bladder at regular intervals prevents stasis of urine that may predispose to renal stone formation or urinary tract infection.

K. Good hygiene practices help prevent urinary tract infections.

L. Seeking prompt treatment for signs of bladder infection helps prevent more serious kidney infection.

M. Controlling blood pressure to within normal limits and keeping serum glucose levels within normal helps slow the atherosclerotic process that affects the kidney vessels.

N. Monitoring for adverse effects on the kidney of the drugs one takes and avoiding the use of harmful chemicals help optimize kidney function.

O. Increasing fluid intake when taking drugs harmful to the kidney helps reduce potential damage.

III. Diagnostic Tests and Procedures and Nursing Implications (Table 23-2)

IV. **Nursing Assessment of Renal Function and the Urinary Drainage System**
  A. Definition of terms.
    1. Anuria: absence of urine.
    2. Oliguria: decreased flow of urine.
    3. Polyuria: increased flow of urine.
    4. Urinary retention: urine held in bladder.
    5. Residual urine: urine left in the bladder after voiding.
    6. Suppression of urine: inability of the kidney to produce urine.
  B. History and present illness.
    1. Previous illness affecting any of the major systems.
    2. Previous surgery involving the urinary system.
    3. Family history of cardiovascular disease, diabetes, and kidney stone formation.
    4. Sexually transmitted diseases.
    5. Drug history to identify nephrotoxic drugs.
  C. Ongoing assessment.
    1. Characteristics of urine: abnormal color, odor, clarity.
    2. Changes in voiding pattern: frequency, urgency.
    3. Pain and discomfort.

V. **Nursing Diagnosis**
  A. Fluid volume excess.
  B. Altered patterns of urinary elimination.
  C. Pain.
  D. Activity intolerance
  E. Sleep pattern disturbance.
  F. Knowledge deficit
  G. Fear.
  H. Body image disturbance.
  I. Risk of sexual dysfunction.

VI. **Planning**
  A. Consider effect on other systems of the body.
  B. Fatigue is common.
  C. Irritability may occur.
  D. Dialysis causes fluid volume shifts that affect homeostasis.

VII. **Implementation**
  A. Care focuses on monitoring intake and output, weight, and signs of edema.
  B. See Clinical Pathway 23-1 and Table 23-5.
  C. Use strict aseptic technique when catheterizing, emptying drainage bags, handling drainage tubes and stents, and performing peritoneal or hemodialysis.
  D. Provide regular catheter care.
  E. Stabilize the catheter and the tubing.
  F. See principles of catheter and tube care in Table 23-6.
  G. Maintain a closed urine drainage system.
  H. Assess for signs of complications.

VIII. **Evaluation**
  A. Reassess to determine whether actions are effective.
  B. Determine whether expected outcomes are being met.
  C. Evaluate whether urine output is at least 30 mL/hour.
  D. Evaluate drugs being taken for nephrotoxicity.
  E. Evaluate lab data: BUN, creatinine, uric acid, potassium, and urinalysis results to determine the effectiveness of treatment.

IX. **Inflammatory Disorders of the Urinary Tract**
  A. Cystitis: more common in females.
    1. Preventive measures aimed at reducing contamination of urinary meatus, especially by intestinal bacteria.
    2. Most common symptoms: painful urination, frequent and urgent urination, and low-back pain.
    3. Measures to prevent recurrent cystitis: see Table 23-9.
    4. Medical treatment includes urinary antiseptics and systemic antiinfectives.
  B. Urethritis: may be associated with sexually transmitted disease, especially gonorrhea. Nonspecific urethritis caused by a variety of organisms.
  C. Nephritis: general inflammation and resulting degeneration of the renal cells.
    1. Acute glomerulonephritis an immunological disorder most often associated with systemic streptococcal infections.
      a. Assessment: widespread edema, visual disturbances, marked hypertension.
      b. Medical treatment and nursing intervention: rest, low-sodium diet, and observation for signs of increased intracranial pressure, cardiac failure, or pulmonary edema.
    2. Chronic glomerulonephritis can develop rapidly or over a period of years.
      a. Assessment: observe for insidious edema, headache associated with hypertension, and dyspnea.
      b. Medical treatment and nursing intervention as for patient with chronic kidney failure.
    3. Nephrotic syndrome sometimes occurs after glomerulonephritis.

    a. Signs and symptoms: severe edema, proteinuria, hyperlipidemia, hypoalbuminemia.

    b. Treatment: diuretics, bedrest, ample-protein, low-sodium, low-fat diet; sometimes cortisone, chlorambucil, cyclosporine, or cyclophosphamide (Cytoxan).

    c. Excellent skin care required because of edema.

4. Nephrosclerosis: hardening and narrowing of renal arterioles, leading to degeneration of renal cells. Symptoms and treatment similar to those of chronic renal failure.

5. Pyelonephritis: infection of the kidney caused by bacterial invasion.

    a. Bacteria from bladder travel up ureters to kidneys.

    b. Increase in strength and number of bacteria in bloodstream.

    c. Back pressure of urine because of obstruction to drainage.

6. Assessment: fever, chills, nausea and vomiting, and pain in flank radiating to the thigh and genitalia. Later symptoms: weight loss, weakness, and bacteria and pus in the urine.

7. Medical treatment and nursing intervention: bedrest, fluids, careful observation of urine for amount, color, and odor; administer urinary antiseptics and antibiotics.

X. Obstructions of the Urinary Tract

A. Hydronephrosis: flow of urine from the kidney is obstructed; kidney dilates and fills with fluid.

  1. Symptoms and medical diagnosis.

    a. Severe pain occurs only if condition develops rapidly; otherwise, symptoms are mild and patient may not be aware of condition until uremia develops.

    b. Definitive diagnosis made by radiological studies.

  2. Surgical treatment and nursing intervention:

    a. Aimed at removal of obstruction.

    b. Patient observed for signs of impending uremia, urinary output noted and recorded; nephrectomy may be necessary if damage is extensive.

B. Renal stones: types: listed in Table 23-10.

  1. Causative factors.

    a. Supersaturation of urine with crystalloids that do not dissolve easily.

    b. Urinary infection.

    c. Inadequate fluid intake and concentrated urine.

    d. Urinary stasis.

    e. Urate and other substances in the urine.

  2. Prevention.

    a. High fluid intake.

    b. Prevention and prompt treatment of urinary infections.

    c. Removal of parathyroid tumor.

    d. Identification of specific kind of stone so as to change urinary pH to one less favorable to stone formation.

  3. Symptoms and medical diagnosis.

    a. Clinical manifestations include pain, blood in urine, and nausea and vomiting.

    b. Radiological studies include x-rays and IVP.

  4. Medical-surgical treatment.

    a. Force fluids to encourage spontaneous passing of stone.

    b. Analgesics and antispasmodics to manage pain.

    c. Break up stones with irrigation or ultrasound.

    d. Surgical removal.

  5. Nursing assessment and intervention.

    a. Identify patients most at risk.

    b. Gather data about changes in urinary output, etc.

    c. Strain all urine to recover stone.

    d. Encourage increased fluid intake.

    e. Education of patient to prevent further stone formation.

XI. Cancer of the Bladder

A. Symptoms and medical diagnosis: intermittent, gross hematuria. Diagnosis confirmed by cystoscopy and biopsy.

B. Treatment: surgical removal of all or part of the bladder; combined with chemotherapy or radiation.

C. Photodynamic therapy (PDT) for carcinoma in situ is undergoing trials.

XII. Cancer of the Kidney

A. Neoplasms fairly uncommon but nearly always malignant.

B. Symptoms and medical diagnosis.

  1. Hematuria and enlargement of affected kidney are major signs.

  2. Diagnosis confirmed by radiological studies, renal ultrasonography, and MRI.

C. Surgical treatment and nursing intervention.

  1. Surgical removal of affected kidney before metastasis has occurred.

  2. Nursing care as for patient having kidney surgery, malignancy, or radiation therapy.

XIII. Common Problems of Urological Disorders

A. Urinary incontinence affects over 10 million residents in the United States of America.

1. Various types of incontinence: stress, urge, overflow, mixed, functional, or neurologically induced.
2. Drugs may help or cause incontinence.
3. Nursing intervention.
   a. Assessment of type and contributing factors.
   b. Assistance with correction of underlying causes.
   c. Spacing fluid intake and using a voiding schedule.
   d. Bladder training program.
   e. Patient education for muscle strengthening.
4. Medical diagnosis if condition persists. Basic exam and laboratory workup plus urodynamic studies if needed.
5. Treatment.
   a. Bladder retraining.
   b. Muscle exercises.
   c. Surgery.
   d. Indwelling catheter or condom catheter, pelvic organ support devices, or penile compression devices.

B. Renal failure: failure of the kidneys to function normally.
1. Classified as acute or chronic renal failure.
2. Acute renal failure (ARF): results from infection, physical injury, inflammation, or damage from toxic chemicals.
   a. Prerenal, intrarenal, and postrenal failure classification depending on cause.
   b. May resolve or progress to chronic renal failure.
3. Acute tubular necrosis (ATN) is most common type of acute renal failure.
   a. Three phases: oliguric/nonoliguric, diuretic, and recovery.
   b. Nonoliguric ATN less commonly requires dialysis; has high urine output, but wastes are not efficiently excreted.
   c. Diuretic phase only seen when dialysis has not been started early in oliguric failure.
   d. About one-third of patients with ARF are left with residual renal insufficiency.
4. Medical treatment: correct underlying cause and control or prevent complications.
   a. Maintain fluid and electrolyte balance.
   b. Manage anemia.
   c. Control hypertension.
   d. Cleanse blood and tissues of uremic waste products with peritoneal dialysis or hemodialysis.
   e. Correct acid–base imbalances.

   f. Correct catabolic state with nutritional supplementation.
5. Chronic renal failure causes.
   a. Infection, inflammation, and upper urinary tract obstruction.
   b. Obstruction in lower urinary tract.
   c. Systemic diseases and toxic states, such as hypercalcemia, hypokalemia, hypertension, heart failure, cirrhosis of the liver and diabetes. Diabetic nephropathy is the third major cause of chronic renal failure and the most common cause of death in persons with diabetes.
   d. Medical diagnosis.
      (1) Renal biopsy.
      (2) Evaluation of BUN, serum creatinine, and creatinine clearance.
      (3) Clinical manifestations usually do not appear until large percentage of renal function is lost.
      (4) Symptoms of end-stage renal disease comprise the syndrome known as uremia.
      (5) Systemic effects of renal failure (see Figure 23-7).
   e. Medical treatment.
      (1) In acute renal failure, goal is to restore and maintain tolerable internal environment until kidneys resume normal function. Peritoneal dialysis used in some cases.
      (2) In chronic renal failure, management is highly complex. Patient has two major alternatives to sustain life: renal dialysis and kidney transplant.
   f. Nursing assessment and intervention.
      (1) Patient and family will need help in learning to manage the symptoms of renal failure.
      (2) Fluid and electrolyte balance and acid–base balance are of major concern.
      (3) Symptoms of azotemia require careful monitoring of patient for changes in level of consciousness, nausea and vomiting, fluid and electrolyte imbalance.
      (4) Relevant laboratory data to plan nursing care include serum levels of calcium, potassium, magnesium, and phosphorus.
      (5) Maintaining nutritional status is very difficult.

XIV. Trauma to the Kidney and Ureters
   A. Always a possibility when there has been injury to the abdominal cavity or thoracic cage.

B. Symptoms: gross hematuria, pain and tenderness in renal area, enlarged mass in flank.

C. Medical treatment and nursing intervention.

   1. Observe for signs of shock and hemorrhage.

   2. Strict bedrest.

   3. Surgical intervention, usually nephrectomy.

XV. Trauma to the Bladder

A. Caused by violent or crushing blow to lower abdomen.

B. Symptoms and medical diagnosis: painful hematuria, spasm or large mass in suprapubic area.

C. Surgical treatment and nursing intervention.

   1. Suprapubic cystostomy to provide drainage.

   2. Meticulous care of drains and dressings to avoid infection and maintain good drainage of urine.

XVI. Common Therapies for Urological Problems

A. Catheterization: performed when patient cannot expel urine from the bladder.

   1. Size 12 French to 20 French commonly used for adult.

   2. Urinary catheters of two types: straight or retention (see Figure 23-8 for types of catheters).

   3. Catheterization performed with sterile technique.

   4. Urinary catheters are the most common cause of hospital-acquired (nosocomial) infection.

   5. Catheterization may be performed to check for residual urine; this must be done immediately after voiding.

   6. When a catheter is removed, the patient is monitored for voiding and should void within 8 hours.

B. Renal dialysis: removal of waste products normally excreted in urine.

   1. Hemodialysis utilizes the principle of diffusion to remove from the blood those waste products normally excreted by the kidneys. It does this by pumping blood from arterial circulation through a dialysate bath and back to the venous circulation.

      a. Temporary access by catheter into subclavian, jugular, or femoral vein.

      b. Internal access: Arteriovenous fistula or arteriovenous graft.

         (1) Protect access from injury: no needle sticks or blood pressure readings on that extremity.

         (2) Assess for thrill and bruit qid.

      c. Dialysis carried out two to three times a week usually.

      d. Problems/complications include: fluid overload, electrolyte imbalance, alterations in blood components (anemia), platelet abnormalities, and infection.

      e. Medications for hemodialysis patients may include: multivitamins, antacids, iron supplements, antihypertensives, digitalis, vasodilators, H_2-receptor antagonists, and phosphate binders.

      f. Antihypertensives, digitalis, anticoagulants, and nitroglycerin patches are held the morning of dialysis and given afterward if needed.

      g. Hemodialysis patients are placed on dietary and fluid restrictions (see Table 23-14).

   2. Long-term hemodialysis creates many difficulties for patient and family. Goals of nursing are to facilitate acceptance of the diagnosis of chronic renal failure and adaptation to continued dialysis treatment.

C. Peritoneal dialysis uses the peritoneal lining as the semipermeable membrane. Dialyzing solution is instilled via a catheter into the peritoneal cavity, left in the cavity for some time, and then removed.

   1. Continuous ambulatory peritoneal dialysis is performed 24 hours a day.

   2. Intermittent peritoneal dialysis may occur only at night time using a peritoneal dialysis cycling machine.

   3. Advantages of peritoneal dialysis.

      a. Can be initiated more quickly than hemodialysis.

      b. Anticoagulants are not needed.

      c. Less stress on the cardiovascular system.

      d. Dietary restrictions are less strict.

   4. Disadvantages of peritoneal dialysis.

      a. Slower process of removal of excess water and wastes.

      b. Constant danger of infection (peritonitis) from indwelling catheter.

   5. Nursing care.

      a. Weigh patient before and after.

      b. Use strict aseptic technique.

      c. Warm dialysate solution.

      d. Measure intake and output accurately.

      e. Monitor for signs of infection.

      f. Monitor vital signs.

      g. Keep patient as comfortable as possible.

      h. Instill solution slowly.

D. Continuous hemofiltration used for critically ill patients who cannot undergo peritoneal or hemodialysis.

E. Kidney transplantation.
   1. Most successful of all organ transplants.
   2. Major problem is organ rejection by the recipient's immune response system.
      a. Immunosuppression can help avoid rejection of the kidney, but carries the risk of increased susceptibility to infection and the development of cancer.
      b. Renal transplant patients require close monitoring for signs of rejection: elevated blood pressure, fever, pain over transplant, fatigue, oliguria, increased BUN, creatinine.
      c. Dietary restrictions may no longer be necessary once donor kidney begins to function.
      d. Medicare or state assistance may pay for 80% of cost of treating end-stage renal disease.
F. Lithotripsy: performed to break up a renal stone.
   1. Patient is placed in special tank and trunk is submerged in water.
   2. Patient is subjected to underwater shock waves.
   3. Sedation may be given.
   4. Takes 30 to 40 minutes.
   5. Fluids are forced after the procedure to flush the fragments from the system.
G. Surgery.
   1. Cystectomy: partial or total. Usually performed for bladder cancer.
   2. Total cystectomy requires urinary diversion procedure.
      a. Ileal conduit: portion of ileum is formed into a tube into which ureters are implanted. A stoma is created on the abdomen to drain urine.
      b. Cutaneous ureterostomy and vesicostomy: May have one or two stomas where ureters are moved to exit sites on abdominal wall. Vesicostomy is an opening from the bladder to the abdominal wall, forming a stoma.
      c. Ureterosigmoidostomy or sigmoid conduit: sigmoid colon is used to form the conduit; ureters are implanted in the tube.
      d. Ileal reservoir (Kock pouch): reservoir created from a portion of the ileum, ureters are implanted, and a nipple valve is created at the abdominal opening to prevent the release of urine. A catheter is inserted to drain the urine periodically.
      e. Indiana pouch: larger than Kock pouch. Constructed from portions of the ileum and cecum; uses the ileocecal valve. Ure-

ters are implanted and a nipple valve is used. Self-catheterization is used to empty the reservoir.
   3. Postoperative nursing care.
      a. Same as for intestinal ostomy (see Chapter 20).
      b. Assess amount and characteristics of the urine.
      c. Expect mucous to be expelled in the urine.
      d. Care for all drains and stents using aseptic technique.
      e. Monitor for complications; watch intake and output closely.
      f. Teach self-catheterization technique.
      g. Protect stoma and skin from irritation and breakdown.
      h. Bag should be emptied when half full.
      i. Skin must be completely dry for a new appliance to adhere.
      j. Odor can be prevented by good hygiene, dilute urine (increase fluid intake), avoiding foods such as asparagus, and acidifying the urine. Deodorant tablets may be added to the bag.
   4. Other surgical procedures.
      a. Retropublic suspension (Marshall-Marchetti-Krantz procedure).
      b. Needle bladder neck suspension (Pereyra or Stamery procedure).
      c. Artificial sphincter implant.
      d. Nephrolithotomy and pyelonephrolithotomy to remove stone.
      e. Nephrectomy and nephrostomy.
         (1) Postoperative nursing care.
            (a) Monitor for unimpeded urine flow.
            (b) Monitor for bleeding.
            (c) Reinforce dressings PRN.
            (d) When changing dressings use extreme care not to dislodge drains and tubes.
            (e) Position according to physician's orders.
            (f) Carefully assess intake and output ratio.
            (g) Provide psychological support for changes in body image.
            (h) Encourage verbalization of fears.

XVII. Elder Care Points
   A. Sometimes the urethra in the elderly female is displaced into the vaginal outlet, predisposing to urinary tract infection.

B. Many elderly purposely restrict fluid intake to decrease the incidence of incontinence. Others are on fluid restrictions for heart failure, renal failure, or other disorders. Restricting fluid intake deceases urine flow and makes one more susceptible to urinary tract infection.

C. The aged kidney is less able to concentrate the urine, which predisposes to dehydration when fluid is restricted for diagnostic tests. The contrast media used for some x-rays in conjunction with dehydration may cause acute renal failure in these patients.

D. One of the first signs of urinary tract infection in the elderly may be confusion.

E. The possibility of a renal stone should be ruled out in any elderly patient who has sudden onset of severe abdominal pain; obtain a urine specimen and test for blood and assess for signs of infection.

XVIII. Community Care

A. Major nursing function is to assist hypertensive and diabetic patients in achieving good control of their disease.

B. Dialysis center nurses must constantly assess patients for complications, watch for medication-related problems, provide teaching regarding diet and lifestyle changes, and provide psychosocial support.

C. Home care nurses must be constantly on the alert for signs of acute or chronic renal failure in their patients.

D. Home care nurses insert and monitor indwelling catheters and assess and treat urinary incontinence.

E. Long-term care facility nurses deal with a variety of urological problems.

1. Bladder training for incontinence is a primary consideration.

2. Observing for signs of urinary tract infection is essential.

3. Monitoring for nephrotoxic drug problems is important; increase fluid intake when patient is taking such a drug.

F. Nurses in outpatient clinics will be assisting with diagnostic procedures; teaching patients about the procedures and instructing regarding postprocedure care.

G. All nurses can promote healthy urological function by encouraging an adequate intake of water and by teaching people to get prompt assistance for urinary tract infections.

CHAPTER 24

Care of Patients with Endocrine Disorders: Pituitary, Thyroid, Parathyroid, and Adrenal Glands

OBJECTIVES

Upon completing the chapter the student should be able to:
1. List four major problems associated with hyposecretion of pituitary hormones and give at least three nursing interventions appropriate for each of them.
2. Teach patients about the diagnostic tests performed for symptoms of endocrine disorders.
3. Identify specific areas of assessment needed for patients with a possible endocrine disorder.
4. From an appropriate list of nursing diagnoses, plan nursing care for patients with endocrine problems, such as hypothyroidism, hyperthyroidism, Addison's disease, or Cushing's syndrome.
5. Plan pre-and postoperative assessment and nursing care for a patient who has had a hypophysectomy.
6. Describe pre- and postoperative assessment and nursing care for a patient who has had a thyroidectomy.
7. List six signs and symptoms of adrenocortical insufficiency (Addison's disease).
8. List four major causes of Cushing's syndrome.
9. Identify nursing diagnoses and appropriate interventions for patients with diabetes insipidus.
10. Prepare a teaching plan for the patient taking a corticosteroid.

The endocrine system is made up of groups of cells whose primary function is to synthesize and release hormones directly into the bloodstream and body fluids. The endocrine hormones are transported by the blood to various parts of the body, where they act on cells to control their physiological functions. The cells and tissues that are affected by a specific hormone are called its *target cells* or *target tissues*.

Some of the endocrine hormones, such as the thyroid hormones, affect practically every cell in the body. Others, such as the sex hormones, exert their special effects on only one kind of organ. Moreover, hormones from one endocrine gland can affect another endocrine gland. The pituitary, for example, secretes several different kinds of hormones that affect other endocrine glands.

The endocrine, or hormonal, system and the nervous system are the two major control systems of the body, and their regulatory functions are interrelated.

However, the primary regulatory activities of the hormonal system are concerned with (1) altering chemical reactions and controlling the rates at which chemical activities take place within the cells; (2) changing the permeability of the cell membrane and thus selecting the substances that can be transported across the membrane; and (3) activating a particular mechanism in the cell (e.g., the system that controls cellular growth and reproduction).

The secretion of a particular hormone normally depends on the physiological need for it at any given moment. Thus if an endocrine gland receives a message that its particular hormone is in short supply, it will synthesize and release more of the hormone. If, on the other hand, the hormonal need of a target tissue is being satisfied, production or secretion of the hormone will be inhibited.

Some glands, such as the adrenal medulla and posterior pituitary, receive their information about hormone levels in the body directly and respond only to appropriate stimulation of nerve endings in the glands themselves. However, the posterior pituitary gland indirectly receives notice either to release or to inhibit hormones. Stimulation comes by way of the hypothalamus and the anterior lobe of the pituitary gland (the adenohypophysis). The hypothalamus contains special nerve endings that produce releasing and inhibiting hormones (factors) that are absorbed into capillaries of a portal system that transports them to the adenohypophysis. **Thus the hypothalamus controls the secretion of hormones from the pituitary, which in turn controls the release or inhibition of hormones from other glands.** Many of the hormones of the anterior pituitary are "tropic" hormones; that is, they tend to cause a change in the endocrine gland which is the target of the specific pituitary hormone. An example is corticotropin (adrenocorticotropic hormone, or ACTH), which acts on the adrenal cortex. The various tropic hormones and their target tissues are shown in Table 24-1.

The interrelationships between endocrine glands, the hormones they synthesize and release, and the systems and subsystems that affect and are affected by hormones are complex. There are many steps between a need for a particular hormone and its eventual release is recognized. Thus, endocrine disorders cannot be thought of in terms of simply overproduction or underproduction of hormones, even though many disorders (e.g., hypothyroidism) are named in this way.

In this chapter, as well as in Chapter 25, only those endocrine disturbances most frequently encountered in nursing practice will be covered. To understand better the content of these chapters, it is necessary to recall the structure and functions of the endocrine system.

OVERVIEW OF ANATOMY AND PHYSIOLOGY

What Are the Structures of the Endocrine System?

⅄ The major glands of the endocrine system are the pituitary, thyroid, parathyroids, adrenals, pancreas, ovaries, and testes. The minor glands are the pineal and thymus glands. (Figure 24-1).

⅄ The pituitary gland, 1 cm in diameter, is located in the cranial cavity at the base of the brain. It connects to the hypothalamus via the hypophyseal stalk. It is divided into the anterior pituitary and the posterior pituitary.

⅄ The thyroid gland has two lobes and lies below the larynx over the thyroid cartilage in front of and on either side of the trachea.

⅄ The parathyroids are four small glands that are located on the posterior surface of the thyroid gland.

⅄ The adrenal glands are located on the anterior upper surface of each kidney. Each adrenal gland is composed of the cortex and medulla.

⅄ The pancreas sits in the upper left aspect of the abdominal cavity. The pancreas is divided into the head and the tail. Islets of Langerhans, or beta cells, are located in the pancreas.

⅄ The ovaries are located in the pelvic cavity of the female.

⅄ The testes hang suspended in the scrotum of the male.

⅄ The pineal gland is in the midbrain in the cranial vault.

⅄ The thymus gland lies at the base of the neck in the front of the thoracic cavity.

What Are the Functions of the Endocrine System?

⅄ The endocrine system works in the body by:

⅄ Altering chemical reactions and controlling the rates at which chemical activities take place within the cells.

⅄ Changing the permeability of the cell membrane and thus selecting the substances that can be transported across the membrane at a particular time.

⅄ Activating a particular mechanism in the cell, such as the system that controls cellular growth and reproduction.

⅄ The hormones produced by the endocrine system, the target organs on which they act, and the principal action of each hormone are presented in Table 24-1.

What Are the Effects of Aging on the Endocrine System?

⅄ There is an increase in antidiuretic hormone in the elderly that may contribute to more rapid dehydration when illness strikes.

TABLE 24-1 ◆ *The Principal Endocrine Glands and Their Hormones*

Gland	Hormone	Target Tissue	Principal Actions
Hypothalamus	Releasing and inhibiting hormones	Anterior lobe of pituitary gland	Stimulates or inhibits secretion of specific hormones.
Anterior lobe of pituitary	Growth hormone (GH)	Most tissues in the body	Stimulates growth by promoting protein synthesis.
	Thyroid-stimulating hormone (TSH)	Thyroid gland	Increases secretion of thyroid hormone; increases the size of the thyroid gland.
	Adrenocorticotropic hormone (ACTH)	Adrenal cortex	Increases secretion of adrenocortical hormones, especially glucocorticoids such as cortisol.
	Follicle-stimulating hormone (FSH)	Ovarian follicles in the female; seminiferous tubules of testis in male	Follicle maturation and estrogen secretion in the female; spermatogenesis in the male.
	Luteinizing hormone (LH); also called interstitial cell-stimulating hormone (ICSH) in males	Ovary in females, testis in males	Ovulation; progesterone production in female; testosterone production in male.
	Prolactin	Mammary gland	Stimulates milk production.
Posterior lobe of pituitary	Antidiuretic hormone (ADH)	Kidney	Increases water reabsorption (decreases water lost in urine).
	Oxytocin	Uterus; mammary gland	Increases uterine contractions; stimulates ejection of milk from mammary gland.
Thyroid gland	Thyroxine and triiodothyronine	Most body cells	Increases metabolic rate; essential for normal growth and development.
	Calcitonin	Primarily bone	Decreases blood calcium by inhibiting bone breakdown and release of calcium; antagonistic to parathyroid hormone.
Parathyroid gland	Parathyroid hormone (PTH) or parathormone	Bone, kidney, digestive tract	Increases blood calcium by stimulating bone breakdown and release of calcium; increases calcium absorption in the digestive tract; decreases calcium lost in urine.
Adrenal cortex	Mineralocorticoids (aldosterone)	Kidney	Increases sodium reabsorption and potassium excretion in kidney tubules; secondarily increases water retention.
	Glucocorticoids (cortisol)	Most body tissues	Increases blood glucose levels; inhibits inflammation and immune response.
	Androgens and estrogens	Most body tissues	Secreted in small amounts so that effect is generally masked by the hormones from the ovaries and testes.
Adrenal medulla	Epinephrine, norepinephrine	Heart, blood vessels, liver, adipose	Helps cope with stress; increases heart rate and blood pressure; increases blood flow to skeletal muscle; increases blood glucose level.
Pancreas (islets of Langerhans)	Glucagon	Liver	Increases breakdown of glycogen to increase blood glucose levels.
	Insulin	General, but especially liver, skeletal muscle, adipose	Decreases blood glucose levels by facilitating uptake and utilization of glucose by cells; stimulates glucose storage as glycogen and production of adipose tissue.
Testes	Testosterone	Most body cells	Maturation and maintenance of male reproductive organs and secondary sex characteristics.
Ovaries	Estrogens	Most body cells	Maturation and maintenance of female reproductive organs and secondary sex characteristics; menstrual cycle.
	Progesterone	Uterus and breast	Prepares uterus for pregnancy; stimulates development of mammary gland; menstrual cycle.
Pineal gland	Melatonin	Hypothalamus	Inhibits gonadotropin-releasing hormone, which consequently inhibits reproductive functions; regulates daily rhythms, such as sleep and wakefulness.
Thymus	Thymosin	Tissues involved in immune response	Immune system development and function.

Source: Applegate, E. J. (1995). *The Anatomy and Physiology Learning System: Textbook.* Philadelphia: Saunders, pp. 209–210.

▲ Ovarian function declines with age, reducing estrogen production after menopause, and affects calcium levels in the body; gonadal function decreases causing deterioration of secondary sex characteristics.

▲ Decreased glucose tolerance may occur, predisposing to hyperglycemia and the onset of type II diabetes.

▲ Thyroid function decreases and hypothyroidism may occur, especially in older women.

▲ The amount of hormones secreted changes, decreasing the individual's ability to adapt to stress and respond to environmental changes as readily as someone younger.

▲ Because of decreasing liver and kidney function in the elderly, hormone replacement therapy must be done very cautiously to prevent overdosage.

CAUSES AND PREVENTION OF ENDOCRINE PROBLEMS

Endocrine disorders are caused by an imbalance in the production of hormone or by an alteration in the body's ability to use the hormones produced. Dysfunction can occur at any point in the production–secretion–feedback–regulation cycle.

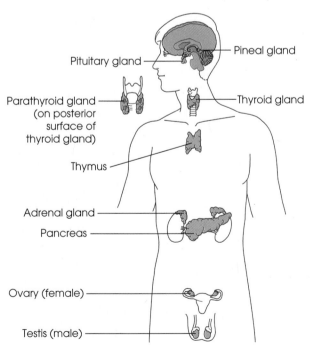

FIGURE 24-1   Major endocrine glands.

Pituitary gland

Pineal gland

Parathyroid gland (on posterior surface of thyroid gland)

Thyroid gland

Thymus

Adrenal gland

Pancreas

Ovary (female)

Testis (male)

Primary endocrine dysfunction means that an endocrine gland is either oversecreting or undersecreting hormone(s). Tumor or hyperplasia of the gland may lead to hypersecretion. Hyposecretion usually is caused by tumor or an inflammatory process that destroys glandular tissue or interferes with function. Infection, mechanical damage, or an autoimmune response may cause such an inflammatory response in a gland.

Secondary endocrine dysfunction occurs from factors outside of the gland itself. Medications (especially corticosteroids), trauma, hormone therapy, and other factors may cause secondary dysfunction. Such dysfunction may be temporary or permanent; often function will return to normal if the cause of dysfunction is corrected.

Preventing of most endocrine disorders is not possible by lifestyle changes, (although goiter, an overgrowth of the thyroid gland, may be prevented by sufficient intake of iodine. Iodine is available in foods grown near the ocean and seafood. Iodized salt is the major source for most people.

Secondary Cushing's syndrome produced by long-term cortisone therapy is often reversible if the medication is tapered off and stopped. However, most people taking cortisone are taking it for other health disorders and cannot manage without it. No one should take steroids for a condition other than the specific health disorder for which they are prescribed.

DIAGNOSTIC TESTS AND PROCEDURES

Tests of the endocrine system are performed on blood samples, urine samples, or by scans, sonograms, x-rays, or magnetic resonance imaging (MRI). Table 24-2

TABLE 24-2 ◆ *Diagnostic Tests and Procedures of the Endocrine System*

Test	Purpose	Description	Nursing Implications
Pituitary hormone levels: luteinizing hormone (LH), follicle-stimulating hormone (FSH), growth hormone (GH), adrenocoticotropic hormone (ACTH), thyroid-stimulating hormone (TSH), prolactin	Detect oversecretion or deficiency of pituitary hormones.	Sample of venous blood is drawn; requires at least 1 mL for immunoassay test; check lab procedure manual.	Monitor venipuncture site for bleeding; apply bandage or dressing.
Hypertonic saline test	Stimulates release of ADH to evaluate ADH secretion and to detect diabetes insipidus (DI).	The patient is loaded with water. An infusion of hypertonic saline is administered. Urine output and urine specific gravity are measured hourly.	Tell patient to produce a urine specimen in the marked container each hour.
Fluid deprivation test	Detect DI.	While patient is NPO for specified time, hourly urine output, specific gravity, osmolality are measured; body weight and vital signs are measured hourly. Dose of vasopressin is given SC and the hourly measurements are continued for several hours.	Explain the procedure to the patient. Provide urine collection containers. Remind patient to void hourly.
Serum T_4 (total thyroxine) Normal value: 4.5–11.5 µg/dL	Assess thyroxine in blood to evaluate thyroid function.	Requires a venous blood sample of at least 1 mL.	Aspirin, iodine-containing medications, contrast media, and other drugs may affect the result. Check with lab regarding these substances.
Serum T_3 (total triodothyronine) Normal value: 70–220 ng/dL	Used with T_4 to evaluate thyroid function.	Requires a venous blood sample of at least 1 mL.	Same as for serum T_4.
TSH (thyroid-stimulating hormone) Normal value: 1–10 µU/mL	To differentiate between pituitary dysfunction and primary thyroid dysfunction; assist with diagnosis of hypothyroidism.	Requires a venous blood sample of at least 1 mL.	Same as for serum T_4.
Antithyroid antibody titer Normal value: <1:100	Detect the presence of thyroid antibodies and differentiate between autoimmune thyroid disorders and toxic thyroid adenoma.	Requires a venous blood sample.	Radioactive iodine will interfere if given within 24 hours of withdrawal of blood sample.
Calcitonin Normal value: <100 pg/mL	Used for differential diagnosis of cancer of the thyroid.	Requires a venous blood sample.	If base level is within normal, pentagastrin may be administered by injection. Blood samples are then drawn 1½ and 5 minutes after injection.
Radioactive iodine uptake Normal values: <6% uptake in 2 h; 2%–25% in 6 h; 15%–45% in 24 h. 24-hour urine: 40%–80% RAI excreted in 24 h.	Assess function of thyroid gland. Measures the rate of iodine uptake by the thyroid.	Trace dose of radioactive iodine (RAI) is given orally. A gamma counter or scintillation counter is placed over the gland at intervals to measure the amount of RAI absorbed. Concurrent 24-hour urine specimen may be collected to assess iodine secretion.	Test must not be done during pregnancy or lactation. Explain that the amount of radioactive iodine used is small and that it will not make the patient "radioactive." Explain the procedure and the time it will take (check with nuclear medicine department). Instruct how to collect a 24-hour urine specimen if one is required.

(Table 24-2 continued)

TABLE 24-2 ◆ *Diagnostic Tests and Procedures of the Endocrine System* (*Continued*)

Test	Purpose	Description	Nursing Implications
Thyroid scan	Determine size, shape, and activity of the thyroid gland. Detects hyperactive "hot" spots and hypoactive "cold" spots.	After administering radioactive iodine, a scintillation camera moves back and forth across the gland to obtain an image of iodine concentration and distribution in the thyroid gland. A computer may be used to provide a three-dimensional image. Often done in conjunction with RAIU.	Same implications as for radioactive iodine uptake (RAIU). Patient must lie perfectly still without swallowing during the scanning procedure. Scan takes about 20 minutes. Rescanning is performed at intervals of 6 and 24 hours after RAI is administered.
Cortisol Normal value: 8 A.M., 6–23 μg/dL; 4 P.M., 3–15 μg/dL; 10 P.M., <50% of 8 A.M. value	Assess cortisol production by adrenal glands.	Requires sample of venous blood.	Explain that a specimen may be collected 2 to 3 times in 24 hours to evaluate circadian effects on cortisol secretion. Stress should be kept to a minimum during test period. Note time collected on laboratory slip.
ACTH Normal value: morning, 20–100 pg/mL; afternoon, 10–40 pg/mL	Assess ACTH production from pituitary gland.	Requires venous blood sample. Place specimen in ice water immediately after drawing.	Prepare ice bath before venipuncture. Note collection time on laboratory slip. Single specimen is best collected in morning.
ACTH stimulation test Normal value after ACTH; serum cortisol >20 μg/dL	Assess adrenal response to ACTH. Used to detect adrenal cortical insufficiency (Addison's disease).	Baseline venous sample taken for cortisol determination. ACTH is administered IV or IM. Blood sample is withdrawn at 30 and 60 minutes for further cortisol determinations.	Note time ACTH is administered; note time each specimen is drawn. Instruct patient to avoid strenuous activity on the day before the test. Check with laboratory regarding food restrictions.
Dexamethasone suppression test Normal value: after dexamethasone, serum cortisol <5 μg/dL	Help diagnose Cushing's syndrome. Assess response to dexamethasone.	Morning baseline serum cortisol levels are measured. Oral dexamethasone is administered at bedtime. Blood sample is collected the next morning to measure cortisol levels.	Explain the procedure to the patient. Check orders for drugs to be withheld. Both cortisol levels must be drawn at the same time on each day. Note time specimens were drawn on laboratory slips; note any medications patient is taking on laboratory slip. Instruct patient to avoid strenuous activity the day before the test.
Urine tests 17-Hydroxycorticosteroids (17-OHCS) Normal values: females, 3–13 mg/24 h; males, 3–15 mg/24 h	Determine levels of glucocorticoid metabolites.	Collect a 24-hour urine specimen in a container with appropriate preservative (check with laboratory). Many medications can interfere; consult with physician and laboratory about medications patient is taking.	Instruct patient in collection procedure. Note start and end time of collection on laboratory slip. Note medications patient is taking on laboratory slip.

TABLE 24-2 ◆ *Diagnostic Tests and Procedures of the Endocrine System (Continued)*			
Test	**Purpose**	**Description**	**Nursing Implications**
17-Ketosteroids (17-KS) Normal values: females, 5–15 mg/24 h; males, 8–15 mg/24 h, >65 yr, 4–8 mg/24 h	Determine amount of androgen metabolites in the urine.	College 24-hour urine specimen. Check with laboratory regarding need to keep specimen chilled.	Same as for 17-hydroxycorticosteroids test.
Aldosterone	Determine urinary aldosterone levels to assist in diagnosis of aldosteronism.	Requires 24-hour urine specimen with preservative; specimen must be kept chilled.	Instruct in dietary and medication restrictions (consult physician). Record diet and medications on laboratory slip.

presents the various tests and procedures with their nursing implications.

The nurse should be aware of factors that can distort test results. Thyroid test results are altered by iodine-based contrast media for radiological studies. Betadine used for skin preparation may also affect thyroid studies. Oral contraceptives, aspirin, and other drugs may render thyroid hormone assays useless, because they either increase or decrease the levels of various thyroid hormones.

Think about . . . How would you instruct a patient who needs to collect a 24-hour urine specimen for hormonal studies?

NURSING MANAGEMENT

◆ Assessment

A full physical assessment and history are needed to evaluate the patient who is possibly experiencing an endocrine disorder because the hormones produced by the glands of this system affect the body in so many different ways. History taking collects data about how the patient perceives function of the various body systems affected by the endocrine glands (Table 24-3). Data elicited by history and physical assessment are evaluated, and the nurse then selects appropriate nursing diagnoses for the patient.

◆ Nursing Diagnosis

Table 24-4 presents the most common nursing diagnoses, expected outcomes, and nursing interventions for patients with endocrine problems. Further nursing diagnoses may be found in the nursing care plans in this chapter. The vocational nurse assists with the construction of the plan of care.

◆ Planning

Planning care for a patient with an endocrine problem will depend on what type of problem the patient has. One thing is certain, stress has an effect on the problem. Therefore, measures to help the patient decrease stress

TABLE 24-3 ◆ *Assessment: Guide to History Taking for the Endocrine System*

The nurse asks the following questions when assessing a patient with a potential endocrine problem:

◆ Have you gained or lost weight over the past 6 months?
◆ Has your appetite increased or decreased?
◆ Have you noticed any changes in thinking? Any difficulty concentrating? Any difficulty with memory?
◆ Have you become more anxious or nervous? Do you cry a lot?
◆ Has your personality changed?
◆ Has your energy level changed?
◆ Have you experienced muscle cramping or numbness or tingling in your hands and legs?
◆ Have you been experiencing diarrhea or constipation?
◆ Have you had more gas or abdominal bloating?
◆ Have you noticed any facial or ankle swelling?
◆ Has your voice become huskier?
◆ Have you been thirstier than usual? Do you find you urinate more now?
◆ Have you noticed any heart palpitations? Do you know if your pulse rate has changed?
◆ Have your sleep patterns changed? Do you need more sleep? Are you finding it difficult to sleep?
◆ Have your menstrual periods altered? (for women)
◆ Is there any history in your family of thyroid, pituitary, adrenal disease, or diabetes?
◆ Have you ever had radiation treatments to the head or neck?
◆ Have you noticed a difference in the way you react to the environmental temperature? Are you cold or hot when others are comfortable?
◆ Have you noticed any changes in the texture or thickness of your hair or eyebrows? What about your fingernails? Are they brittle?
◆ Has your skin become dry and rough?

TABLE 24-4 ◆ *Nursing Diagnoses, Goals/Expected Outcomes, and Nursing Interventions Commonly Used for Patients with Endocrine Problems*

Nursing Diagnoses*	Goals/Expected Outcomes	Nursing Interventions
Fluid volume deficit related to increased urine output (DI, HyperT, AD)	Patient will display balance between intake and output.	Monitor for dehydration and signs of decreased cardiac output. Measure and record intake and output q 2 h; maintain ordered IV fluid rate; encourage oral fluid intake.
Constipation related to: loss of fluid from intestine, slowed intestinal peristalsis (DI, HypoT, AD)*	Patient will display normal bowel pattern within 6 weeks.	Provide high-bulk diet; encourage fluid intake; administer stool softener or laxatives as ordered. Encourage exercise to promote better bowel function.
Body image disturbance related to changes in physical appearance (PT, HyperT)	Patient will verbalize acceptance of alteration in body appearance within 6 months.	Allow time for verbalizing feelings. Assist to identify strengths and positive aspects of self and of life. Focus on strengths and positive aspects. Give sincere compliments.
Sexual dysfunction related to decreased libido, amenorrhea, or impotence (PT, HyperT)	Patient will acknowledge need for patience until therapy improves the symptoms.	Help patient understand how therapy might help the problem. Assist patient to recognize and maintain personal worth as an individual. Assist to maintain roles within family or living unit. Help significant others understand patient's illness.
Knowledge deficit related to illness and treatment (all endocrine disorders)	Patient will verbalize understanding of concepts taught at end of 6 weeks.	Teach patient and significant others about the disease and each aspect of treatment. Provide written instructions regarding medications, their side effects, and what should be reported to the physician. Provide instructions for "sick" days. Alert to signs and symtoms of too much or too little medication. Emphasize the importance of follow-up care. Stress the need for Medic-Alert tag or bracelet and wallet card.
Alteration in nutrition, less than body requirements related to anorexia, constipation, increased metabolic rate (PT, HyperT)	Patient will regain and maintain weight within normal limits within 6 months.	Weigh × 2 per week. Alter diet as needed to increase fiber and carbohydrate content; provide small, frequent, meals of preferred foods.
Fatigue related to weakness, somnolence, lethargy (PT, DI, HypoT, CS)	Weakness and fatigue will resolve with medical therapy; patient will show improved energy within 3 months.	Provide periods of rest. Assist with ADLs as needed. Set slower pace for activities. Give patient time to respond to verbal communications. Encourage physical activity to highest level of tolerance. Monitor electrolyte and fluid status; provide electrolyte replacement as needed.
Risk for injury related to potential increased intracranial pressure (PT), inability to think clearly (HyperT, HypoT), mental and physical sluggishness (HypoT)	Patient will not experience damage from increased intracranial pressure. Patient will exercise caution in making decisions, operating dangerous machinery, and moving about quickly until symptoms resolve.	Conduct regular checks of neurological status, monitoring for signs of increased intracranial pressure. Continue hormone replacement therapy as needed to decrease symptoms from tumor or hypofunction.
Sleep pattern disturbance related to insomnia, hypermetabolic state (HyperT, CS)	Patient will utilize relaxation methods to induce sleep.	Assist with rest periods during the day if fatigue is severe. Assure that therapy can resolve the problem. Instruct in relaxation methods to help induce sleep. Provide noise-free, sleep-inducing environment.
Ineffective individual coping related to emotional lability (HyperT, AD, CS)	Patient will devise plan to cope with mood swings until they resolve.	Encourage verbalization of feelings and concerns. Assure patient that, as disease is controlled, moods will be more stable. Help patient identify strengths and focus on them. Teach relaxation techniques to handle stressful times. Explain physiological causes of changes in mood.

TABLE 24-4 ◆ *Nursing Diagnoses, Expected Outcomes, and Nursing Interventions Commonly Used for Patients with Endocrine Problems* (Continued)

Nursing Diagnoses*	Expected Outcomes	Nursing Interventions
Decreased cardiac output related to fluid depletion (DI, AD), hypometabolic state (HypoT), hypermetabolic state (HyperT)	Patient will be free of signs of heart failure.	Explain to patient how disease process is affecting heart function. Monitor for signs of dysrhythmia and heart failure. Assure that treatment of underlying disease should alleviate heart symptoms.
Risk for infection related to surgical incision (PT, HyperT), antiinflammatory effect of excess cortisol (CS)	Patient will not develop infection as evidenced by normal temperature, WBC within normal range, and absence of visible signs of wound infection.	Maintain strict asepsis for invasive procedures and dressing changes. Monitor temperature, WBC, and subtle signs of infection as steroids can suppress usual signs. Advise to stay away from individuals who have colds or other infections.
Alteration in nutrition, more than body requirements, related to altered glucose metabolism (CS), hypometabolic state (HypoT)	Patient will regain and maintain weight within normal limits within 6–12 months of beginning therapy.	Teach signs and symptoms of hyperglycemia and how to administer ordered insulin; teach regarding correct diet for condition. Assist in designing diet according to food preferences. Teach to balance diet and exercise.

*Endocrine disorders to which these nursing diagnoses apply are in parentheses: PT, pituitary tumors and hypopituitary syndrome; DI, diabetes insipidus; HyperT, hyperthyroidism; HypoT, hypothyroidism, AD, Addison's disease; CS, Cushing's syndrome.

should be planned. Supplemental hormones such as corticosteroids are given in the early morning when such hormones will not interfere with the body's normal release and use of them.

General goals for the patient with an endocrine disorder are:

- ◆ Prevention of injury
- ◆ Fluid and electrolyte balance
- ◆ Hormone balance
- ◆ Reduction of stress
- ◆ Improved coping mechanisms
- ◆ Knowledge for self-care
- ◆ Activity tolerance
- ◆ Normal bowel function
- ◆ Improved mental-emotional status
- ◆ Integration of body image

Expected outcomes are written for each individual patient depending on the nursing diagnoses chosen.

◆ Implementation

Interventions vary depending on the type of endocrine problem present and are discussed with disorders in the following sections. Common specific nursing interventions are listed in Table 24-4 and in the nursing care plan in this chapter.

◆ Evaluation

Evaluation is assessed by determining whether symptoms are resolving and by laboratory testing to see whether treatment is effective. Many of the symptoms of endocrine disorders are subjective, and the nurse must collect reliable data from the patient about levels of fatigue, feeling cold or hot, parasthesias, and so on. **Each patient is questioned about the presenting symptoms and their improvement during the evaluation of care and treatment.**

PITUITARY DISORDERS

In view of the varied functions of the pituitary gland it is difficult to classify the many syndromes that can occur as a result of a pituitary disorder. Figure 24-2 shows the effects of hormones secreted by the pituitary gland. When the gland dysfunctions, one or more of these hormones is affected. In turn, the target organ for that hormone will be affected. Among the more common disorders are tumors of the pituitary, which account for about 10% of all intracranial tumors, and diabetes insipidus (DI).

◆ Pituitary Tumors

Tumors of the pituitary gland can produce local and systemic symptoms. Local symptoms are more likely to

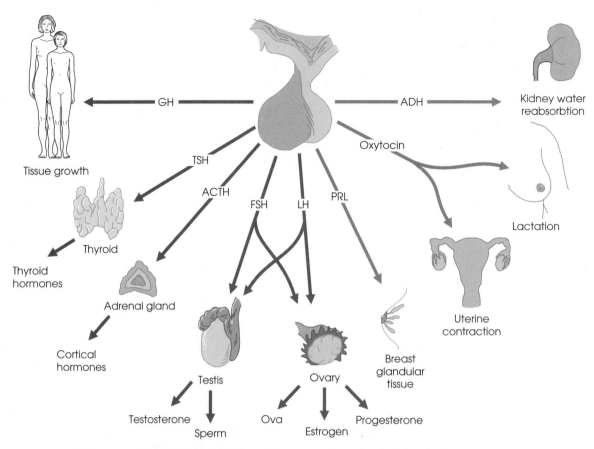

FIGURE 24-2   Effects of hormones from the pituitary gland.

occur when the tumor is large and creates pressure within the brain. Smaller tumors, as well as the larger ones, can cause various endocrine dysfunctions, depending on whether they stimulate or inhibit the secretion of particular hormones.

Signs and Symptoms   Local symptoms include headache and visual disturbances, the latter being due to pressure within the optic chiasm. **If the pressure is not released, continued pressure will destroy the optic nerve and produce blindness.** Systemic symptoms may be vague and, like the local symptoms, progress very slowly. Personality changes, weakness, fatigue, and vague abdominal pain can be present for years before the condition is diagnosed correctly.

Hyperplasia or tumor of the anterior pituitary may cause excessive secretion of growth hormone. In children this results in *gigantism.* In adults the resulting disorder is *acromegaly* (hyperpituitarism). The patient's facial features change with the lips thickening, the nose enlarging, and the forehead developing a bulge. The hands and feet become enlarged. Sometimes the first thing the patient notices is that shoes no longer fit. Muscle weakness may occur and osteoporosis and joint pain are common. Headaches and other symptoms from the pressure of the tumor occur.

Diagnosis is established by immunoassay tests for anterior and posterior pituitary hormones. Other diagnostic tests for pituitary dysfunction include a computed tomographic (CT) scan of the skull and an MRI.

Treatment   In some cases the physician may choose to treat the pituitary tumor conservatively with hormone replacement therapy and periodic monitoring of the patient's progress. If the tumor continues to grow or presents serious hormonal imbalances, it may be treated surgically or by irradiation. Some specialists prefer to remove the tumor surgically and then apply radiation to the site to be sure that all tumor cells have been destroyed. Hypophysectomy is the surgical procedure. It most often is done with microsurgical techniques. The approach may be transphenoidal via the nose.

Nursing Intervention   After the surgery, the patient is kept in a semi-Fowler's position and monitored for signs of increased intracranial pressure. A nasal drip pad is in place and is changed as needed. Table 24-4 presents the nursing diagnoses and interventions commonly used for patients with pituitary tumor or *hypopituitary* syndromes.

◆ Diabetes Insipidus

This condition is characterized by the production of copious amounts of dilute urine, often as much as 15 to 20 L in every 24-hour period. **Diabetes insipidus occurs as a result of decreased production of the antidiuretic hormone (ADH), which regulates reabsorption of water in the kidney tubules.** When ADH is not present in sufficient amounts, the water remains in the tubules and is excreted as urine. **Restriction of fluid intake does not control the excessive flow of urine.**

Diabetes insipidus is treated by vasopressin tannate (Pitressin tannate in oil) via nasal inhalation 4 to 6 times a day or by injection every 2 to 3 days. Nursing diagnoses and interventions for patients with pituitary diabetes insipidus are listed in Table 24-4.

◆ Syndrome of Inappropriate Antidiuretic Hormone (SIADH)

Syndrome of inappropriate antidiuretic hormone (SIADH) is the opposite of diabetes insipidus. Excessive amounts of ADH are produced, resulting in fluid excess. Many things can cause SIADH including malignancies and tumors pressing on the pituitary.

Signs and symptoms are confusion, seizures, and loss of consciousness accompanied by weight gain and edema. Serum sodium drops to less than 120 mEq/L and hyponatremia from fluid excess is present.

Treatment is to correct the underlying cause, restrict fluids, and administer sodium chloride, diuretics, and demeclocycline (a tetracycline) to increase free water clearance. Enemas may be prescribed to draw out excess water. Electrolytes and weight are monitored closely. Good cardiovascular assessment is essential to prevent serious complications of fluid shifts. Neurological status also is closely monitored.

THE THYROID

Recall that the thyroid gland secretes the hormones thyroxine (T_4), triiodothyronine (T_3), and thyrocalcitonin. The more potent form of thyroid hormone is T_3, but there is about 20 times more T_4 than T_3 in normal circulating blood. When T_3 is needed, it is converted from the abundant supply of T_4. Sufficient quantities of dietary protein and iodine are needed to synthesize both of these thyroid hormones.

Thyroid hormones influence many metabolic functions within the cell. They activate the cellular production of heat; stimulate the synthesis of protein and lipids and their mobilization and degradation; stimulate the manufacture of coenzymes from vitamins; regulate many aspects of carbohydrate metabolism; and affect tissue response to epinephrine and norepinephrine.

The secretion of thyroid hormones is regulated by the hypothalamic-pituitary-thyroid control system (Figure 24-3). In other words, all three organs are involved in the closed-loop negative feedback system. Internal conditions, such as low thyroid and norepinephrine (NE) serum levels, can activate the hypothalamus, as can external conditions such as cold. In response to feedback received by the hypothalamus, thyrotropin-releasing hormone (TRH) is secreted. The TRH acts on the pituitary gland, bringing about its release of thyroid-stimulating hormone (TSH). The TSH then acts on the thyroid cells, causing them to release thyroid hormones. When sufficient heat has been produced by increased metabolic activities (if cold was the stimulus), or when there are sufficient levels of thyroid hormone in the body fluids (if a deficit was the stimulus), feedback to the hypothalamus causes it to stop releasing TRH (Figure 24-3).

There are three major abnormalities of the thyroid gland: (1) enlargement of the gland (goiter); (2) overactivity of the gland (hyperthyroidism); and (3) underactivity of the gland (hypothyroidism).

Elder Care Point... Tissue changes of the thyroid gland do occur during aging, and thyroid nodules are not uncommon among the older age group. The only significant change seen in this age group is that T_3 levels are decreased.

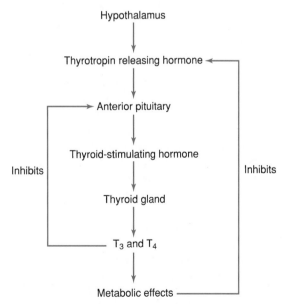

FIGURE 24-3   Regulation of thyroid hormone secretion by negative feedback control. (*Source:* Monahan, F. D., Drake, T., Neighbors, M. [1994]. *Nursing Care of Adults.* Philadelphia: Saunders, p. 1303.)

◆ Overactivity and Underactivity of the Thyroid

Abnormalities in the activity of the thyroid gland and resultant changes in the levels of thyroid hormones are some of the most common disorders affecting the endocrine system. More than one test is necessary to determine whether the thyroid gland is functioning properly. Usually a group of tests, called a *thyroid panel,* is performed.

Diagnostic Tests And Nursing Responsibilities
Tests currently used to evaluate thyroid function involve little more than a venipuncture and collection of blood samples. The nurse should be aware of factors that can distort test results. Contrast media for radiological tests, such as gallbladder studies and intravenous pyelogram, contain iodine, Betadine used for skin preparation contains iodine, and so do some drugs taken internally. **Moreover, oral contraceptives, aspirin, and other rather commonly used drugs can render thyroid hormone assays useless, because they either increase or decrease the levels of various thyroid hormones.** When assessing a patient prior to diagnostic tests for thyroid function that involve radioimmunoassay or competitive binding analysis, the nurse should be sure to ask about any drugs the patient is taking, any previous x-rays, and other possible sources of iodine.

Patients with primary hypothyroidism will have low levels of T_3 and T_4 and high levels of thyroid-stimulating hormone (TSH). The latter is the result of the body's attempt to compensate for low thyroid hormone levels by producing more TSH to stimulate the gland to produce more hormones.

◆ Goiter

The person with a goiter has a greatly enlarged thyroid gland. The serum levels of the thyroid hormones may or may not be within normal limits. One type of goiter is caused by a deficiency of iodine in the diet. It can be prevented by providing iodine intake, such as using iodized salt. Although the administration of iodine will not cure goiter, it will stop the continued enlargement of the gland. Another type of goiter occurs as a result of unknown causes.

Signs and Symptoms   Because there may be no systemic symptoms or changes in the metabolic rate of a person with simple goiter, the first sign that is usually noticed is an enlargement in the front of the neck. Later, if the gland continues to grow bigger, it presses against the esophagus and causes some difficulty in swallowing. The goiter also can press against the trachea and interfere with normal breathing.

Treatment   If goiter resulting from iodine deficiency is treated early, the growth of the gland can be arrested, and in some cases the enlargement will eventually disappear. Medications prescribed include preparations containing elemental iodine (the iodide ion).

A very large goiter that continues to grow and produce local symptoms of pressure or presents the possibility of developing into a malignant growth or a toxic goiter is surgically removed in a procedure similar to the one sometimes done for hyperthyroidism.

Nursing Intervention.   Iodine preparations should be given well diluted and administered through a straw, as they can stain the teeth a dark brown. Adverse effects of iodine preparations can include gastrointestinal upset, metallic taste, skin rashes, allergic reactions, and epigastric pain.

◆ Hyperthyroidism

Patients most at risk for hyperthyroidism are adult women between the ages of 30 and 50. Women over 50 years of age often do not show the typical signs of hyperthyroidism, but do exhibit the shortness of breath, palpitations, and chest pain typically thought of as indicative of angina pectoris and congestive heart failure. Hence hyperthyroidism might be overlooked, and they could be treated for a cardiovascular rather than an endocrine disorder. When assessing older women, the nurse should be alert for the possibility that an overactive thyroid gland is the cause of cardiovascular symptoms.

Primary hyperthyroidism is the result of an abnormality of function involving the thyroid gland itself and causes excessive circulation of thyroid T_4 and T_3 hormones. However, it is possible that only the T_3 level will be above normal if the patient has Graves' disease, toxic adenoma of the thyroid, or toxic nodular goiter. These conditions are discussed later.

High serum levels of T_4 can be caused by either overactivity of the thyroid gland or excessive doses of T_4 given in replacement therapy. Primary hyperthyroidism is more common in women 30 to 50 years of age. *Secondary* hyperthyroidism usually is the result of an abnormality in another gland, such as the pituitary gland, that could produce too much TSH and therefore overstimulate the thyroid gland.

Primary hyperthyroidism also is known as *Graves' disease, toxic goiter,* and *thyrotoxicosis.* Medications containing iodine, such as amiodarone, an antidysrhythmic heart medication, can predispose to thyrotoxicosis.

Signs and Symptoms   *The earliest symptoms of hyperthyroidism may be weight loss in spite of a good appetite and nervousness.* However, symptoms can vary from mild to severe and also include weakness, insomnia, tremulousness, agitation, tachycardia, palpitations, exertional dyspnea, ankle edema, difficulty concentrating, diarrhea, increased thirst and urination, decreased libido, scanty menstruation, and infertility. The condition sometimes is not diagnosed in its early stages because of the vagueness of the symptoms. In some cases hyperthyroidism is misdiagnosed as a cardiovascular disease because the symptoms are so similar. If hyperthyroidism is not diagnosed correctly and continues untreated for any length of time, the patient can develop true organic heart disease.

The symptoms manifested by a hyperthyroid patient are the result of an accelerated metabolic rate and a speeding up of all physiological processes. Emotional upheaval occurs as a result of the action of thyroid hormones on the nervous system. The patient often reports episodes of emotional extremes with uncontrollable crying and depression followed by intense physical activity and euphoria. **The patient with Graves' disease also exhibits an enlarged thyroid gland (toxic goiter) and abnormal protrusion of the eyeballs (*exophthalmia*).**

Medical diagnosis is based on clinical manifestations of hyperthyroidism and the results of laboratory tests for thyroid hormone levels. An excellent indicator of thyrotoxicosis is assessment of the heart rate while the patient is sleeping. A rate that is consistently above 80 could signify a toxic state resulting from excessive levels of thyroid hormone.

Treatment   Hyperthyroidism may be treated medically by administering radioactive iodine and antithyroid drugs, mild sedatives, and antiadrenergic drugs to control tremor, temperature elevation, restlessness, and tachycardia.

Radioactive iodine (131 I) is the drug of choice for middle-aged persons and nonpregnant women. Its main disadvantage is the possibility of hypothyroidism caused by "overeffective" treatment. The hypothyroidism can occur immediately after treatment or long after it is completed; hence the patient must have ongoing follow-up.

Dosage depends on the size of the gland and the thyroid's sensitivity to radiation. **Patients receiving small doses can be given the drug orally for several doses and on an outpatient basis. Larger doses require isolation of the patient for 8 days, which is the half-life of 131 I.** Because the iodine circulates in the blood and is excreted by the kidneys, precautions must be taken when handling needles, syringes, and other equipment likely to be contaminated with blood and bedpans, urinals, and specimen bottles likely to be contaminated by urine.

All patients receiving radioactive iodine must be observed for signs of thyroid crisis resulting from radiation-induced thyroiditis. (Thyroid crisis is discussed later.) If hyperthyroidism is not controlled within several months of therapy with radioactive iodine alone, the patient will require adjunctive therapy in the form of potassium iodide and antithyroid drugs.

Throughout therapy the patient is checked frequently to ensure that thyroid activity is being reduced to normal levels. This is not easily accomplished, as hypothyroidism may be induced by an overly aggressive treatment regimen and persistent hyperthyroidism may result if treatment is ineffective.

Antithyroid drugs are prescribed as the initial treatment of hyperthyroidism in children, young adults, and pregnant women. Iodine preparations such as propylthiouracil and potassium iodide (SSKI) have only a temporary effect. Methimazole (Tapazole) is the main drug utilized. **The patient must take the antithyroid drug at the prescribed time and strictly according to schedule. A dangerous side effect is agranulocytosis, which can develop rather quickly.**

Iodine preparations also may be given for a period of 10 to 14 days before surgery of the thyroid to reduce the vascularity of the gland, minimizing the danger of releasing large amounts of thyroid hormone into the bloodstream during surgery and to decrease the risk of hemorrhage during surgery.

Thyroidectomy. Patients who do not respond well to antithyroid drug therapy, are unable to take radioactive iodine, or have greatly enlarged thyroid glands, are candidates for a subtotal thyroidectomy. Patients with thyroid malignancy undergo a total thyroidectomy. In the subtotal procedure two thirds of the glandular mass is removed. The remaining portion of the gland is left intact so there can be continued production and release of thyroid hormones.

Nursing Intervention   Because of the effect hyperthyroidism has on physical and mental health status, caring for these patients presents a very real challenge to the nurse. Physical and mental rest are extremely important, because physical stress and emotional upset can stimulate the thyroid gland to become even more active. Adequate rest is essential to conserve the strength of the patient, but it is difficult for a person with hyperthyroidism to relax and get sufficient rest.

The diet of the patient should be sufficiently high in calories to meet metabolic needs. This will vary from person to person, but continued loss of weight is an indication that more high-calorie foods are needed in the diet. It may be necessary to refer the patient to a dietitian who can work out a satisfactory diet that helps maintain normal body weight.

Patients who are being treated medically for hyperthyroidism must understand that they have an illness that requires ongoing medication and frequent monitoring to assess the effectiveness of treatment. Sometimes it is difficult for the patient's family to accept and deal with the emotional outbursts and mood changes that are present when the disease is not under control. Once hormone levels return to the normal range, the mental and physical symptoms should subside.

Many patients will be rendered hypothyroidic because of surgery or radiation therapy that alters thyroid function. It is then necessary to manage their illness with long-term thyroid replacement therapy. Nursing interventions for selected problems of patients with hyperthyroidism are summarized in Nursing Care Plan 24-1.

Preoperative nursing care. The responsibility of the nurse for preparation of the patient who is to have a thyroidectomy is essentially the same as for other types of major surgery. If the patient does appear nervous, tense, and apprehensive, his condition should be reported to the physician. These symptoms may indicate improper control of the thyroid gland and may predispose the patient to the postoperative complication of "thyroid crisis" (see the following section).

Postoperative nursing care. The patient is placed in the *Fowler's* position to facilitate breathing and reduce swelling of the operative area. The head may be supported with sandbags on either side to relieve tension on the sutures.

Close observation of the patient is of dire importance. The vital signs are checked at frequent intervals, and the patient is watched closely for signs of bleeding and swelling at the operative area. **Any rise in temperature, pulse, or respiration rate should be reported when first noticed, because it may indicate a high level of thyroxine in the blood stream.** External swelling may cause constriction of the bandage around the neck.

> Difficulty in swallowing or breathing should also be reported immediately, as it may indicate internal edema and pressure on the esophagus and trachea.

In many hospitals, a tracheostomy set is kept at the bedside of the postoperative thyroidectomy patient in case severe respiratory embarrassment develops. Other symptoms to be reported are persistent hoarseness or loss of the voice, as they may indicate damage to the vocal cords. *Tetany* and *thyroid crisis* are other possible complications. These are rare, but when they do occur, the nurse must be alert for the beginning signs and report her observations immediately.

Tetany actually is a symptom and results from injury to, or accidental removal of, the parathyroid glands. These small glands are located on the posterior surface of the thyroid gland. *Parathormone*, or *parathyroid hormone*, is secreted by the parathyroid glands and is important in regulating the calcium and phosphorus levels in the body tissues. **A deficiency of parathyroid hormone produces muscle cramps, twitching of the muscles, and, in some cases, severe convulsions.**

These symptoms represent a medical emergency and must be reported to the physician at once.

This complication is treated by the IV administration of calcium gluconate during the emergency stage and subsequent maintenance doses of parathyroid hormone to maintain the proper calcium and phosphorus balance in the body.

Thyroid crisis, sometimes called *thyroid storm*, is another complication following a thyroidectomy. The condition is caused by a sudden increase in the output of thyroxine caused by manipulation of the thyroid as it is being removed. Another cause may be improper reduction of thyroid secretions before surgery.

The symptoms of thyroid crisis are produced by a sudden and extreme elevation of all body processes. The temperature may rise to 106°F (41.1°C.) or more, the pulse increases to as much as 200 beats per minute, respirations become rapid, and the patient exhibits marked apprehension and restlessness.

> Unless the condition is relieved, the patient quickly passes from delirium to coma to death from heart failure.

Treatment of thyroid crisis must begin immediately after the first symptoms are noticed. Measures are employed to reduce the temperature, cardiac drugs are given to slow the heart beat, and sedatives, such as a barbiturate, are given to reduce restlessness and anxiety.

Think about . . . Can you list the specific assessments you would make for the patient assigned to you who returned from having a thyroidectomy 4 hours ago?

◆ Hypothyroidism

Hypothyroidism can be caused by inflammation of the thyroid gland (thyroiditis) or by treatment of hyperthyroidism that results in destroying too many thyroid cells and a resultant deficit of thyroid hormone. Genetic defects can cause congenital hypothyroidism (cretinism). Cretinism is caused by a severe lack of thyroid hormone during fetal life and infancy and is characterized by growth failure. Underactivity of the thyroid gland can also be caused by a pituitary or hypothalamus dysfunction that causes inadequate stimulation of the thyroid, inducing secondary hypothyroidism.

Signs and Symptoms   The child with hypothyroidism will have retarded physical and mental growth and will become very sluggish within a few weeks after birth. Adults who have *myxedema* (very low thyroid production) have a decrease in appetite but an increase in weight because of a lower metabolic rate. Other typical signs are bagginess under the eyes and swelling of the face. In both children and adults there is a tendency to

Nursing Care Plan 24-1

Selected nursing diagnoses, goals/expected outcomes, nursing interventions, and evaluations for a patient with hyperthyroidism

Situation: Mrs. Jackson, age 35 years, has been having symptoms of hyperthyroidism. She complains of feeling "hot and soaked with perspiration all the time." She is 25 pounds underweight, even though she reports a "ravenous" appetite. Her vital signs are: pulse, 110, bounding; respirations, 30; and somewhat irregular; blood pressure, 170/90. Her serum calcium level was found to be 11.5 mg/dl when she had a physical examination at her physician's office. She has been admitted for control of hypercalcemia and for more diagnostic tests. Mrs. Jackson is very apprehensive, agitated, and irritable.

Nursing Diagnosis	Goals/Expected Outcomes	Nursing Interventions	Evaluation
Anxiety related to nervousness and agitation. SUPPORTING DATA "I don't understand what is happening to me. I feel so nervous all of the time." Wringing her hands, eyes darting around the room, fidgeting in bed.	Anxiety and agitation will be controlled with medication within 3 days.	Keep environmental stimuli at a minimum. No visitors other than family as requested by patient. Approach in a calm and unhurried manner. Provide 30-minute rest periods before lunch, in afternoon, and after supper. Change sweat-soaked linens and gown as needed. Keep room as cool as possible.	Linens changed × 2; rested after bath and lunch; door to room kept closed; encouraged to play quiet, low music; continue plan.
Knowledge deficit related to lack of information about disease and treatment. SUPPORTING DATA States she does not know anything about hyperthyroidism or its treatment.	Patient will verbalize basic understanding of disease and treatment before discharge.	Explain disease process; teach about diagnostic tests and what to expect for each one. Encourage questions and supply answers. Explain options for treatment.	Teaching for diagnostic tests done; questions answered.
Alteration in nutrition, less than body requirements, related to increased metabolic rate. SUPPORTING DATA Has lost 25 lb over last 6 months, although appetite has increased considerably.	Will gain 2 lb/week when thyroid production is under control.	Weigh daily; encourage high-calorie between-meal snacks. Increase caloric intake to 3,000 calories per day. Try to accommodate food preferences.	Eating entire meals; two between-meal snacks taken; weight up ½ lb; continue plan.
Risk for injury related to excess circulating thyroid hormone and excess serum calcium. SUPPORTING DATA Thyroid levels: T_3, 230 mg/dL; T_4, 16 μg/dL; calcium, 16 mg/dL	No permanent cardiac problems will develop; thyroid production will be controlled with medication within 2 weeks; serum calcium will be within normal levels before discharge.	Check vital signs q 4 h. Assess cardiac function each shift and watch for symptoms of thyrotoxicosis such as increased pulse, dyspnea, edema, and rising blood pressure; report such signs at once. Medicate with calcium-channel blocker as ordered; observe for side effects. Give medication to decrease calcium levels (diuretic) and monitor electrolyte levels.	Heart rate, 86; rhythm regular; BP, 132/86; electrolytes within normal limits except for calcium (11.2 mg/dL); continue plan.
Ineffective individual coping related to labile moods. SUPPORTING DATA States she has been very moody; family says that she keeps changing her mind about things.	Return to former emotional stability when thyroid production returns to normal.	Assure her that mood swings are manifestations of her thyroid disorder. Stress importance of complying with treatment regimen after discharge and keeping appointments with doctor. Give positive reinforcement for correct behavior; encourage verbalization of feelings. Establish trusting relationship; be accepting of behavior; spend uninterrupted time with her each shift; display acceptance of her and her behavior.	Expressing frustration with being "highly emotional"; discussed mood swings and how to cope; encouraged walking daily to reduce stress; continue plan.

be lethargic and to sleep for abnormally long periods during the day and night. The speech may be slurred, and the individual will appear sluggish in both mental and physical activities. Other signs and symptoms of hypothyroidism are cold intolerance, constipation and abdominal distention, flatulence, impaired memory, depression, husky voice, thinning eyebrows, hair loss, brittle nails, easy bruising, fatigue, muscle cramps, numbness and tingling, dry, scaly skin, and nonpitting edema. Gastrointestinal symptoms are the result of decreased peristaltic activity and can lead to paralytic ileus if the hypothyroidism continues untreated. Medical diagnosis is based on clinical signs and symptoms and laboratory testing of serum levels of thyroid hormones and TSH.

Elder Care Point . . . Elderly patients who are lethargic, slow in thinking, and unenthusiastic about whatever is going on around them could be showing signs of hypothyroidism rather than senility or some other convenient label. Hypothyroidism is particularly common in older women.

Treatment   Hypothyroidism can be treated effectively with replacement of thyroid hormones. The dosage is gradually increased until a proper level has been reached, and then a delicate balance must be maintained so that the patient does not suffer from either hypothyroidism or hyperthyroidism.

Nursing Intervention   The results of treatment of hypothyroidism are very striking, and most patients show a remarkable abatement of their symptoms. The nurse may not see many cases of hypothyroidism in the hospital because treatment usually does not require hospitalization. If the patient is admitted for some other condition or illness and is also being treated for hypothyroidism, some special considerations must be made. As stated, these patients have very rough and dry skin, and they will need massage with lotions and creams to prevent cracking and peeling of the skin. Provisions for extra warmth must also be made for those patients who have an increased sensitivity to cold as a result of their hypothyroidism. **It is important that the patient receive thyroid medication every day.**

The nurse must also bear in mind the psychological aspects of hypothyroidism. She must avoid rushing these patients or giving them the impression that she is annoyed and inconvenienced by their sluggishness. Forgetfulness, inability to express themselves verbally, and physical inertia are mannerisms that are a direct result of the thyroid deficiency, and the nurse must recognize them as unavoidable as long as the condition is uncontrolled. Nursing diagnoses, expected outcomes, and other nursing interventions are presented in Table 24-4.

◆ Myxedema Coma

Although rare, myxedema coma is life-threatening. It can be precipitated by abrupt withdrawal of thyroid therapy, acute illness, anesthesia, use of sedatives or narcotics, surgery, or hypothermia in the hypothyroid patient. Signs and symptoms are loss of consciousness along with hypotension, hypothermia, respiratory failure, hyponatremia, and hypoglycemia. Treatment is administration of levothyroxine sodium IV, fluid replacement, maintenance of an airway and respiration, IV glucose administration, corticosteroids, and provision of warmth.

THE PARATHYROIDS

Production and secretion of the hormone parathormone from the parathyroids is regulated by the plasma calcium level, which is part of the feedback mechanism that either stimulates or inhibits the release of parathormone. A low calcium level will stimulate the release of parathormone, which increases the level of calcium in the plasma. Conversely, a high calcium level will inhibit the release of parathormone.

Parathormone raises the calcium level in the plasma by acting on the renal tubules to increase the excretion of phosphorus in the urine and the reabsorption of calcium. It also acts on bone, causing the release of calcium from the bone into the bloodstream.

◆ Hypoparathyroidism

Hypoparathyroidism is caused by atrophy or traumatic injury to the parathyroid glands. This can occur as a result of accidental removal or destruction of parathyroid tissue during a thyroidectomy or irradiation of the thyroids or from idiopathic atrophy of the glands.

Signs and Symptoms   A deficiency of parathormone will result in a drop in serum calcium levels and an increase in phosphorus levels. **The chief symptom resulting from a lowered serum calcium level is *tetany*.** Muscular twitching and spasms occur because of extreme irritability of neuromuscular tissue. If the calcium level continues to fall, the patient will suffer from convulsions, cardiac arrhythmias, and spasms of the larynx. Other symptoms related to hypocalcemia are discussed in Chapter 5 and summarized in Table 5-3. Medical diagnosis is established by clinical signs and laboratory data.

Treatment   Acute hypoparathyroidism is treated by measures to raise serum calcium levels to normal range. Oral or parenteral administration of calcium salts is used in the acute phase. In chronic hypoparathyroidism, treatment is aimed at restoring and maintaining normal calcium levels in the blood. This can be accomplished by parathormone replacement therapy, administration of vitamin D in massive doses to enhance absorption of calcium from the small intestine, and oral administration of calcium salts.

♦Hyperparathyroidism (Von Recklinghausen's Disease)

Hyperparathyroidism is another common disorder of the endocrine system. In recent years a greater number of cases have been diagnosed because of improved radiological and laboratory screening procedures. The disorder occurs most often in postmenopausal women. Excessive synthesis and secretion of parathormone can occur as a result of benign enlargement of the parathyroid glands (adenoma) or hyperplasia of two or more glands.

Hypercalcemia (calcium level above 10.5 mg/dL) occurs with hyperactivity of the parathyroid glands. Signs and symptoms may be mild or severe and include dehydration, confusion, lethargy, anorexia, nausea, vomiting, weight loss, constipation, thirst, frequent urination, and hypertension. If serum calcium levels are high, indicating hypercalcemia, there may be skeletal changes, including thinning of the bone and bone cysts. A fracture often causes the patient to seek medical attention.

Signs and Symptoms   Many cases of hyperparathyroidism are now being diagnosed in the earliest stages of the disease before the clinical manifestations of hypercalcemia become apparent. Laboratory testing for serum calcium and phosphate levels helps confirm the diagnosis.

Excessively high levels of calcium in the blood (hypercalcemia) are manifested in virtually every major system in the body (Table 24-5).

Treatment   The treatment of hyperparathyroidism will depend on the severity of the symptoms produced by hypercalcemia and hypophosphatemia. Methods of therapy include the infusion of isotonic sodium chloride and administration of diuretic agents to promote excretion of excess calcium in the urine; phosphate therapy to correct the deficit; administration of mithramycin to inhibit skeletal resorption (release) of calcium; and administration of calcitonin to decrease the rate of skeletal resorption.

Surgical removal of a major portion of the parathyroids (subtotal parathyroidectomy) is recommended for patients who have severe systemic disorders associated with excessively high levels of parathormone. The remaining parathyroid tissue will continue to function and prevent the problem of hypoparathyroidism.

TABLE 24-5 ♦ *Characteristics of Hyperparathyroidism and Hypoparathyroidism*

Hyperparathyroidism	Hypoparathyroidism
Increased bone resorption	Decreased bone resorption
Elevated serum calcium levels	Depressed serum calcium levels
Depressed serum phosphate levels	Elevated serum phosphate levels
Hypercalciuria and hyperphosphaturia	Hypocalciuria and hypophosphaturia
Decreased neuromuscular irritability	Increased neuromuscular activity, which may progress to tetany

Source: Polaski, A. L., Tatro, S. E. (1996). *Luckmann's Core Principles and Practice of Medical–Surgical Nursing.* Philadelphia: Saunders, p. 1223.

Nursing Intervention   Nursing intervention for patients receiving diuretic therapy includes accurate measuring of intake and output, daily weight, monitoring of serum electrolytes, ongoing assessment of the patient for electrolyte imbalance, and appropriate nursing intervention (see Chapter 5).

THE ADRENAL GLANDS

The adrenal glands are composed of two distinct parts that have no direct functional relationship. The *adrenal medulla* (middle portion) secretes two hormones, *epinephrine* and *norepinephrine.* These substances are secreted in response to stimulation from the sympathetic nervous system, and **their effects are, in turn, almost the same as direct stimulation of the sympathetic nerves.** Epinephrine prepares the body to meet stress or emergency situations and prevents hypoglycemia (Figure 24-4). Norepinephrine functions as a pressor hormone to maintain blood pressure.

The hormones secreted by the *adrenal cortex* (outer covering) are called *adrenal corticosteroids.* The word *steroid* is sometimes used as an abbreviated form to designate an adrenal corticosteroid or a synthetic compound with similar properties. The two major types of hormones secreted by the adrenal cortex are the *mineralocorticoids* and the *glucocorticoids* (Figure 24-5). It also secretes small amounts of *androgenic hormones,* which have effects similar to those of the male and female sex hormones. Normally, the androgenic hormones have very little effect in comparison with the sex hormones secreted by the gonads, but in some abnormalities of the adrenal cortex, such large amounts of androgenic hormones are poured into the bloodstream that they can present symptoms of sexual changes in the patient.

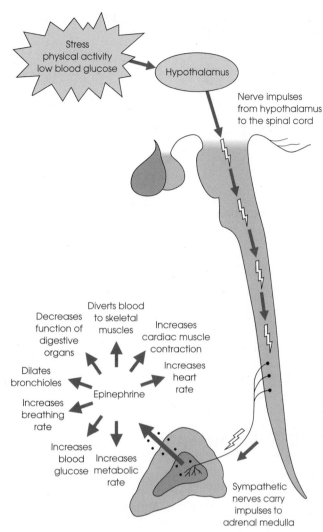

FIGURE 24-4   Epinephrine—its effects and control of its secretion. (*Source:* Applegate, E. J. [1995]. *The Anatomy and Physiology Learning System: Textbook.* Philadelphia: Saunders, p. 218.)

The mineralocorticoids and glucocorticoids are so named because of the effects they have on the body. The mineralocorticoids affect the electrolytes, particularly sodium, potassium, and chloride. **The principal mineralocorticoid is aldosterone, which works to conserve sodium and water in the body.** Without the mineralocorticoids, a person would die within 3 to 7 days, because these hormones directly control fluid balance, blood volume, cardiac output, exchange of nutrients and wastes in each cell, and, in effect, all chemical processes and glandular functions within the body. Little wonder that they are said to be "lifesaving hormones." The glucocorticoids are almost equally important because they are essential to the metabolic systems for proper utilization of carbohydrates, proteins, and fats. **The primary glucocorticoid is cortisol, or hydrocortisone.** Cortisol acts to increase glucose levels in the blood. It also helps counteract the inflammatory response. Both aldosterone and cortisol are

controlled by ACTH-releasing hormone from the hypothalamus and ACTH secreted by the anterior pituitary (Figure 24-5).

◆ Pheochromocytoma

Pheochromocytoma is a rare tumor of the adrenal medulla that secretes catecholamines. It often causes severe hypertension. Treatment is surgical removal (adrenalectomy). Prior to surgery, the patient may be in hypertensive crisis and needs vigilant nursing care.

◆ Adrenocortical Insufficiency (Addison's Disease)

In this condition, overall decreased function of the adrenal cortex leads to a deficit in all three hormones secreted by the adrenal cortex. The major problems presented by this disorder are, however, related to insufficiencies of the mineralocorticoids and the glucocorticoids. The insufficiency of the androgenic hormones can be compensated for by the ovaries and testes.

Insufficient production of the adrenocortical hormones can result from a disorder affecting the adrenal

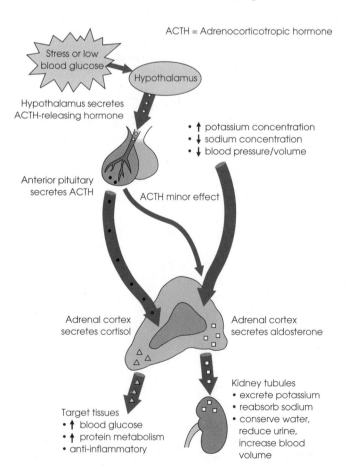

FIGURE 24-5   Regulation of aldosterone and cortisol secretion. (*Source:* Applegate, E. J. [1995]. *The Anatomy and Physiology Learning System: Textbook.* Philadelphia: Saunders, p. 217.)

cortex itself *(primary insufficiency)* or from a disorder affecting the pituitary gland that stimulates adrenal secretion *(secondary insufficiency)*. Disorders causing a primary insufficiency include idiopathic atrophy, inflammation, infection, and nonsecreting tumors of the adrenal cortex. Secondary insufficiency is the direct result of failure of the pituitary gland to secrete corticotropin (also known as adrenocorticotropic hormone, or ACTH). This can occur because the pituitary is underfunctioning or the gland was surgically removed, *(hypophysectomy)* or because of certain pituitary tumors **and abrupt withdrawal of steroid therapy.**

Think about . . . What signs and symptoms would you see in a patient who was developing Addison's disease after stopping steroid therapy?

Signs and Symptoms   In the early stages of Addison's disease the clinical manifestations may be so vague as to be annoying to the patient but not serious enough to consult a physician. Hence it is easily missed altogether or misdiagnosed. Later, as the hormone insufficiency becomes more pronounced, **the patient will begin to exhibit more severe symptoms associated with fluid and electrolyte imbalance and hypoglycemia.** Considering the functions of the mineralocorticoids, **a major problem is depletion of sodium (hyponatremia), which in turn causes depletion of extracellular fluid and potassium retention (hyperkalemia).** The patient experiences generalized malaise and muscle weakness, muscle pain, orthostatic hypotension, and vulnerability to cardiac dysrhythmias. The problems of hyponatremia, fluid volume deficit, and hyperkalemia are discussed in Chapter 5.

Insufficiency of the glucocorticoids affects blood glucose levels and causes symptoms of hypoglycemia. There is also decreased secretion of gastrointestinal enzymes, which results in anorexia, nausea and vomiting, flatulence, and diarrhea. These symptoms, as well as anxiety, depression, and loss of mental acuity, are thought to be related to absence of the peaks of cortisol output that normally occur every 24 hours. In fact, abnormal serum electrolyte levels, decreased glucose tolerance, and abnormally low levels of free cortisol are among the criteria used to diagnose Addison's disease.

Treatment   Replacement therapy to provide the missing adrenocorticoid hormones is the major component of treatment. **Replacement therapy usually brings about a rapid recovery, but the patient must continue taking the hormones for the rest of his life.**

Nursing Intervention   Nursing intervention is concerned with:

◆ Intensive care and support during *Addisonian crisis* when the patient is in a critical condition and in danger of death from fluid volume depletion, hypotension and shock, and impairment of cardiac function.
◆ Prevention of problems related to fatigue and orthostatic hypotension.
◆ Alleviation of gastrointestinal problems.
◆ Instruction of the patient in self-care.

Two important nursing measures are to provide both regular feedings throughout the day and adequate rest. The patient may feel well in the morning but becomes progressively weaker and more fatigued as the day goes on. If fasting is necessary for diagnostic studies or surgery, the patient with Addison's disease probably will need IV feedings of glucose to avoid developing profound hypoglycemia. Maintenance doses of exogenous (originating outside) glucocorticoids are especially important whenever fasting is required.

Gastrointestinal problems bring on the possibility of altered nutritional status related to anorexia, nausea and vomiting, and diarrhea. Specific fluid and electrolyte imbalances have already been discussed and are covered in more depth in Chapter 5.

Stress, even relatively mild physical or emotional stress, can quickly bring on an Addisonian crisis. The patient should be cautioned to avoid undue stress whenever possible and to learn effective coping mechanisms to deal with the emotional stresses everyone faces. Table 24-6 presents guidelines for instruction of the patient with Addison's disease and Nursing Care Plan 24-2 outlines the nursing care.

TABLE 24-6 ◆ *Patient Education: Managing Addison's Disease*

The nurse should teach the patient about the signs and symptoms of inadequate or excessive steroid levels, the importance of reporting either promptly, and the following points:

◆ The nature of the illness and what can be done to control it.
◆ The purpose of each medication and the side effects to be reported.
◆ The importance of taking the medication every day and of never stopping corticosteroids suddenly; they need to be tapered off slowly.
◆ Methods of adjusting medication dosage to combat the effects of stress.
◆ Signs and symptoms to report to the doctor immediately (worsening weakness, hypotension, confusion, infection).
◆ Diet adjustments to provide food throughout the day and a bedtime snack.
◆ The importance of following the prescribed diet to avoid gastrointestinal problems.
◆ Planned rest periods during the day and sufficient sleep at night as well as avoidance of physical stress.
◆ The need for a Medic-Alert tag or bracelet stating Addison's disease and that the patient is on steroid therapy.

Nursing Care Plan 24-2

Selected nursing diagnoses, goals/expected outcomes, nursing interventions, and evaluations for a patient with adrenocortical insufficiency (Addison's Disease)

Situation: Mr. Cox, age 49, is admitted with a tentative diagnosis of adrenocortical insufficiency (Addison's disease). He has recently experienced weight loss, weakness and poor coordination, vomiting, changes in skin coloration, and loss of body hair. During initial assessment, Mr. Cox is found to be very irritable and easily upset by the questions. His blood pressure is 90/50; pulse, 70 and slightly irregular; respirations, 16 and deep. He reports that he feels pretty good when he awakens in the morning but quickly becomes tired and his muscles begin to ache. He is concerned about his weight loss and change in appearance and also has noticed that he has been unable to "think straight." Admission laboratory data: blood glucose, 50 mg/dL; sodium, 90 mEq/L; and potassium, 5.6 mEq/L.

Nursing Diagnosis	Goals/Expected Outcomes	Nursing Interventions	Evaluation
Activity intolerance related to weakness and electrolyte imbalance. SUPPORTING DATA States that with the least little exertion, he tires and has muscle aching.	Serum sodium will return to normal within 24 hours.	Administer glucocorticoids and mineralocorticoids as prescribed; observe for side effects. Weigh daily; measure and compare intake and output. Monitor electrolyte levels. Force fluids until steroid therapy takes effect. Encourage him to eat to maintain adequate blood glucose and sodium levels.	Cortisone and fludrocortisone administered as ordered; weight unchanged; intake, 2,860; output, 2,320; continue plan.
Risk for injury related to possible severe drop in blood glucose. SUPPORTING DATA Blood glucose on admission, 50 mg/dL.	Blood glucose will be maintained within normal limits. Crisis will not develop.	Observe for signs of hypoglycemia and report promptly. Check to see that meals are served on time; provide snacks as needed. Teach signs of hypoglycemia and instruct him in what to do when this occurs.	Blood glucose, 95; no signs of hypoglycemia; continue plan.
Ineffective individual coping related to excess cortisol and mood swings. SUPPORTING DATA Very irritable and impatient; states he is unable to "think straight"; tentative diagnosis of Addison's disease; serum cortisol results pending.	Patient will develop effective coping mechanisms; relaxation techniques will be used before discharge. Patient will not be subjected to infection during hospitalization.	Protect him from exposure to infection. Monitor vital signs, WBC count, and lung fields each shift. Observe for signs of infection. Teach relaxation techniques and supervise practice; work with patient on other ways to decrease stress in daily life. Teach him how to handle anticipated stress by adjusting dosage of medications. Encourage verbalization of concerns and fears; answer questions. Discuss alterations in body image and changes that can be expected with therapy.	Lung fields clear; WBC count, 6,800; taught relaxation exercises and encouraged to practice; began survey of usual coping mechanisms and ways to decrease daily stress; continue plan.

Nursing Care Plan 24-2 *(Continued)*

Nursing Diagnosis	Goals/Expected Outcomes	Nursing Interventions	Evaluation
Knowledge deficit related to illness, medications, and necessary changes in lifestyle. SUPPORTING DATA States that he knows nothing about Addison's disease, its diagnosis, or treatment. Unfamiliar with corticosteroid therapy.	Patient will simply describe problems of Addison's disease. Patient will verbalize understanding of medications and dosage schedule before discharge. Patient will verbalize plans for obtaining adequate rest before discharge.	Help to identify stressors in his life and assist in determining ways to avoid them. Answer questions and discuss expected effect of continued therapy on his ability to resume pre-illness activities. Help him develop a schedule that allows for periods of rest, work, social interaction, and recreation. Stress importance of balancing rest and activity. Provide written instructions that give warning signs and symptoms of insufficient corticosteroid medication and those of excess medication (Cushing's syndrome). Instruct him to report either set of symptoms to the physician promptly so medication can be adjusted. Discuss how to adjust medication for periods of extra stress (minor illness, such as a cold, an emotional upset, or unusual physiological or psychological stress). Instruct him to wear a form of Medic-Alert identification with data concerning steroid therapy.	First teaching session complete; written guidelines regarding medications given; continue plan.

Think about . . . What interventions would you use to help a patient with Addison's disease learn to decrease and/or cope with stress?

Addisonian crisis. Physical stress from the flu or other minor infection can tip the scales for the patient with Addison's disease and send him into crisis. The stress of surgery also presents problems. The nurse must be especially watchful and closely monitor vital signs in these patients.

Addisonian crisis requires immediate fluid replacement therapy, or the patient will go into irreversible shock. Intravenous hydrocortisone is given along with sodium, fluids, and dextrose until blood pressure becomes stable. The hydrocortisone is then tapered off slowly.

◆ Excess Adrenocortical Hormone (Cushing's Syndrome)

Cushing's syndrome is a rare disorder. The group of symptoms typical of Cushing's syndrome are manifestations of excess levels of the hormones from the adrenal cortex. The condition can be caused by:

◆ Excessive secretion of corticotropin (ACTH) by the pituitary gland, which may actually result from faulty release of corticotropin-releasing factor (CRF) from the hypothalamus.

◆ A secreting tumor of the adrenal cortex.

◆ Ectopic production of corticotropin by tumors outside the pituitary, most commonly lung carcinoma, medullary thyroid carcinoma, and thymoma.

◆ *Iatrogenic* Cushing's syndrome due to overzealous use of exogenous steroid therapy.

Symptoms and Diagnosis   The symptoms and signs presented by the patient are the outcome of excessive levels of this hormone. They include painful fatty swellings in the intrascapular space (buffalo hump) and in the facial area (moon face), an enlarged abdomen with thin extremities, bruising following even minor traumas, impotence, amenorrhea, hypertension, and general weakness due to abnormal protein catabolism with loss of muscle mass. The diagnosis of Cushing's syndrome is established by laboratory findings indicating consistently high levels of free plasma cortisol rather than the usual 24-hour (diurnal) fluctuations.

Unusual growth of body hair (hirsutism) can occur in women, and streaked purple markings in the abdominal area can occur due to collections of body fat. Patients with Cushing's syndrome who have a familial predisposition to diabetes mellitus frequently develop insulin-dependent diabetes mellitus as a result of the antiinsulin, diabetogenic properties of cortisol.

Treatment   Pituitary Cushing's syndrome can be treated by microsurgical procedures on the pituitary gland. In some instances disorder can be prevented by using steroids cautiously and restricting their administration to patients who do not respond to other forms of therapy.

If Cushing's syndrome is arising from an adrenal tumor, adrenalectomy is indicated. In this instance replacement of glucocorticoids will be necessary (Table 24-7).

TABLE 24-7 ◆ *General Nursing Implications for the Administration of Corticosteroids*

When giving a corticosteroid drug, the nurse should:

- Question the patient about history of peptic ulcer, glaucoma, cataracts, diabetes, or psychiatric problems (these conditions may contraindicate the use of steroids).
- Take baseline vital signs and particularly note blood pressure before the start of therapy; steroids may elevate the blood pressure.
- Assess for signs of infection before starting the therapy as steroids may mask the signs and symptoms of infection.
- Check dosage very carefully and administer only the amount ordered. Spread topical ointment or cream very sparingly.
- Never stop steroid therapy abruptly; such abrupt withdrawal may cause death in the patient who has been on long-term therapy.
- Increased stress such as major infection or surgery may cause acute adrenal insufficiency.
- Give a daily dose in the morning.
- When not contraindicated, give a diet low in sodium and high in potassium.
- Give oral doses with food to decrease gastrointestinal irritation.

Regarding possible side/adverse effects of the drug, the nurse should:

- Assess for side effects when patient has been on glucocorticoid therapy for more than 10 days.
- Monitor the older adult for signs of osteoporosis. Give vitamin D and recommend exercise to prevent osteoporosis.
- Assess for changes in muscle strength.
- Instruct to report slow healing of wounds to the doctor.
- Watch for signs of depression in patients on high-dose steroid therapy.
- Monitor for signs of hypokalemia, such as nausea, muscle weakness, abdominal distention, and irregular heart rate.
- Monitor blood sugar of diabetic patients closely as glucocorticoids may cause hyperglycemia.
- Check blood pressure regularly during therapy to monitor for hypertension.
- Patients on long-term steroid therapy should have regular checkups for glaucoma and cataracts.

- Observe stool for signs of gastrointestinal bleeding.
- Monitor weight as steroids may cause increased appetite and weight gain.

The nurse should teach the patient taking a corticosteroid drug to:

- Take oral doses in the morning with food.
- Not to discontinue the drug abruptly but taper down the dosage before stopping it.
- Watch dietary intake as patient may be hungrier and this could cause weight gain.
- Watch for signs of hypokalemia, such as muscle weakness, fatigue, anorexia, irregular heart beat.
- Take the drug only as prescribed.
- Eat foods such as fresh and dried fruits, juices, potatoes, meats, and nuts that are high in potassium.
- Report signs of Cushing's syndrome, such as moon-shaped face, puffy eyelids, edema in the feet, increased bruising, dizziness, bleeding, and menstrual irregularity.
- Carry a Medic-Alert card and wear a bracelet stating patient is on steroid therapy when on long-term steroids.
- Avoid people with infections and stay away from crowds, especially during cold and flu season.
- Advise all other physicians and dentists seen that patient is on steroid therapy.
- Be aware that more insulin may be needed if patient is diabetic.
- Be aware that antibody response from immunization while taking steroids may be reduced; do not take a live-virus vaccine.
- Use aspirin and NSAIDs cautiously as they will increase the risk of gastrointestinal bleeding when taken during steroid therapy.
- Be aware that steroids decrease the effect of barbiturates, phenytoin, and rifampin and that the doses of these drugs may need to be increased.
- Have clotting time monitored closely when taking anticoagulant at the same time as the steroid.
- Taking steroids along with potassium-wasting diuretics may cause hypokalemia; increase potassium intake in diet.

Nursing Assessment and Intervention   The nursing care of patients with Cushing's syndrome is primarily concerned with helping each patient cope with the many systemic problems presented by the disorder. The more common problems and suggested nursing interventions are summarized in Table 24-4. The nurse must assist the patient with psychosocial concerns presented by emotional lability and depression when they occur. The patient needs assurance that the symptoms will improve with proper treatment.

COMMUNITY CARE

Many of the patients with endocrine disorders are cared for in outpatient settings. Often times home care nurses find that the patient with heart disease, neurological problems, diabetes, or respiratory problems also has a thyroid problem. Careful assessment by the clinic nurse may uncover a developing endocrine problem.

Nurses in long-term care facilities must be on the alert for signs of hypothyroidism and hyperparathyroidism among their elderly female patients. The nurse often is the one who picks up subtle changes in the patient that have occurred over many months.

Nurses can be instrumental in preventing secondary Cushing's syndrome by cautioning patients to seek other means of possible treatment than long-term steroid therapy for arthritis or allergy. Every nurse must teach the patient who receives a new prescription for steroid therapy that the drug must not be stopped abruptly, but must be tapered off slowly.

CRITICAL THINKING EXERCISES

Clinical Case Problems

Read the following clinical situation and discuss the questions with your classmates.

1. Mrs. Timms has a tentative diagnosis of hyperthyroidism. She is 45 years old, 5 feet 7 inches tall, and weighs 102 pounds.
   a. What subjective and objective signs and symptoms would you expect Mrs. Timms to present during nursing assessment?
   b. How would you go about preparing Mrs. Timms for laboratory diagnostic tests for thyroid function?
   c. If Mrs. Timms' physician decided to treat her condition with large doses of radioactive iodine, what special nursing care will she require?
   d. What other forms of therapy are used to treat hyperthyroidism?

2. Mr. Lau, age 37, is receiving adrenocorticoid hormones for Addison's disease as replacement therapy.
   a. What kinds of problems does insufficiency of the adrenal cortex hormones bring about?
   b. What should be included in your instructions to Mr. Lau to help him manage his illness?

3. Mrs. Josten, age 48, is hospitalized for a cholecystectomy. She has Cushing's syndrome as well as gallbladder disease. She is 35 pounds overweight and depressed.
   a. What kinds of problems is Mrs. Josten likely to have as a result of her Cushing's syndrome?
   b. What would be your concerns in the immediate postoperative period?
   c. What would you want to include in your discharge teaching plan?

BIBLIOGRAPHY

Applegate, E. J. (1995). *The Anatomy and Physiology Learning System: Textbook*. Philadelphia: Saunders.

Angelucci, P. A. (1995). Caring for patients with hypothyroidism. *Nursing 95*. 25(5):60–61.

Bennett, J. C., Plum, F., eds. (1996). *Cecil Textbook of Medicine*, 20th ed. Philadelphia: Saunders.

Bianco, C. M. (1996). Diabetes insipidus. *American Journal of Nursing*. 96(8):30–31.

Black, J. M., Matassarin-Jacobs, E. (1997). *Medical–Surgical Nursing: Clinical Management for Continuity of Care*, 5th ed. Philadelphia: Saunders.

Bryce, J. (1994). S.I.A.D.H.: Recognizing and treating syndrome of inappropriate antidiuretic hormone secretion. *Nursing 94*. 24(4):33.

Copstead, L. C. (1995). *Perspectives on Pathophysiology*. Philadelphia: Saunders.

Corsetti, A., Buhl, B. (1994). Managing thyroid storm. *American Journal of Nursing*. 94(11):39.

Cotran, R. S., Kumar, V., Robbins, S. L., Schoen, F. J., eds. (1994). *Robbins Pathologic Basis of Disease*, 5th ed. Philadelphia: Saunders.

Croce, J. (1986–1996). Parathyroid disorders: hyperparathyroidism, hypoparathyroidism, and other problems. In *Nurse Review Series*, ed. Goldberg, K. Springhouse, PA: Springhouse Corporation.

Dambro, M. R. (1996). *Griffith's 5 Minute Clinical Consult*. Baltimore: Williams & Wilkins.

Davies, P. (1996). Caring for patients with diabetes insipidus. *Nursing 96*. 26(5):62–63.

Gaedeke, M. K. (1993). Evaluating T.S.H. . . . thyroid-stimulating hormone. *Nursing 93*. 23(10):72.

Guyton, A. C., Hall, J. E. (1996). *Textbook of Medical Physiology*, 9th ed. Philadelphia: Saunders.

Howser, R. L. (1995). What you need to know about corticosteroid therapy. *American Journal of Nursing*. 95(8):44–48.

Ignatavicius, D. D., Workman, M. L., Mishler, M. A. (1995). *Medical–Surgical Nursing: A Nursing Process Approach*, 2nd ed. Philadelphia: Saunders.

Jankowski, C. B. (1996). Irradiating the thyroid: How to protect yourself and others. *American Journal of Nursing.* 96(10):51–54.

Jones, S. (1986). Thyroid disorders: hyperthyroidism, hypothyroidism, and other problems. In *Nurse Review Series,* ed. Goldberg, K. Springhouse, PA: Springhouse Corporation.

Kee, J. L., Hayes, E. R. (1993). *Pharmacology: A Nursing Process Approach.* Philadelphia: Saunders.

Kim, T. S. (1994). Primary hyperparathyroidism. *Orthopedic Nursing.* 13(3):17–25.

Lammon, C. A., Hart, G. (1993). Recognizing thyroid crisis. *Nursing 93.* 23(4):33.

Lee, L. M., Gumoski, J. (1992). Adrenocortical insufficiency: a medical emergency. *AACN Clinical Issues in Critical Care Nursing.* 3(2):319–330.

Lehne, R. A. (1994). *Pharmacology for Nursing Care,* 2nd ed. Philadelphia: Saunders.

Lindaman, C. (1992). S.I.A.D.H.: is your patient at risk? *Nursing 92.* 22(6):60–63.

Malarkey, L. M., McMorrow, M. E. (1996). *Nurse's Manual of Laboratory Tests and Diagnostic Procedures.* Philadelphia: Saunders.

Matteson, M. A., McConnell, E. S., Linton, A. D. (1997). *Gerontologic Nursing: Concepts and Practice,* 2nd ed. Philadelphia: Saunders.

McConnell, E. A. (1996). Myths & Facts . . . about thyroid disease. *Nursing 96,* 26(4):17.

McMorrow, M. E. (1996). Myxedema coma. *American Journal of Nursing.* 96(10):55.

Monahan, F. D., Drake, T., Neighbors, M. (1994). *Nursing Care of Adults.* Philadelphia: Saunders.

Peterson, A., Drass, J. (1993). How to keep adrenal insufficiency in check. *American Journal of Nursing.* 93(10): 36–39.

Polaski, A. L., Tatro, S. E. (1996). *Luckmann's Core Principles and Practice of Medical-Surgical Nursing.* Philadelphia: Saunders.

Spittle, L. (1992). Diagnosis in opposition: thyroid storm and myxedema coma. *AACN Clinical Issues in Critical Care Nursing.* 3(2):300–308.

Ulrich, S. P., Canale, S. W., Wendell, S. A. (1994). *Medical–Surgical Nursing Care Planning Guides,* 3rd ed. Philadelphia: Saunders.

Young, W. F. (1993). Pheochromocytoma: a brief management guide. *Hospital Medicine.* 29(10):67–72, 76–79, 98–101.

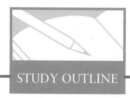

STUDY OUTLINE

I. Introduction

A. Endocrine glands secrete their hormones directly into bloodstream or body fluids.

B. Cells and tissues affected by a specific hormone are called its *target cells* or *tissues.*

C. Hormonal regulation concerned with changing chemical activities within the cells, altering cell membrane permeability, and activating a particular mechanism in the cell.

D. Endocrine glands, their hormones, and target cells are summarized in Table 24-1.

E. Regulation of secretion of hormones is a negative feedback system that acts in response to a biological need.

F. Many endocrine disorders are related to overactivity or underactivity of a gland.

II. Causes and Prevention of Endocrine Problems

A. Problems are caused by an imbalance in the production of hormone or by alteration in the body's ability to use the hormone.

B. When there is dysfunction in one endocrine gland, function of one or more of the other endocrine glands is affected.

C. Primary dysfunction is due to either oversecretion or undersecretion of a hormone.

D. Tumor or hyperplasia of a gland may lead to hypersecretion.

E. Hyposecretion usually is caused by inflammation or tumor.

F. Inflammation may be from infection, mechanical damage, or an autoimmune response.

G. Secondary dysfunction is due to factors outside the gland itself; medications may cause secondary dysfunction.

H. Prevention of most endocrine disorders is not preventable by lifestyle changes.

I. Goiter may be prevented by sufficient intake of iodine.

J. Secondary Cushing's syndrome may be resolved by tapering off and stopping steroid medication.

III. Diagnostic Tests and Procedures

A. Tests are performed on blood samples, urine samples, or by scans, sonograms, x-rays, or MRI.

B. See Table 24-2 for information and nursing implications regarding diagnostic tests.

IV. Nursing Management

A. Assessment.

1. A full physical assessment and a thorough history are needed for the patient with a possible endocrine disorder.

2. A guide for history taking is found in Table 24-3.

B. Nursing diagnosis.

1. Diagnoses are chosen based on assessment data; the nurse designates the diagnoses to be used for the patient.

2. Table 24-4 presents the most common nursing diagnoses for the patient with an endocrine disorder.

C. Planning.

1. Measures to decrease and cope with stress are part of the care for each patient with an endocrine disorder.

2. Supplemental hormones, such as thyroid and corticosteroids, are planned for early-morning administration so as not to interfere with the body's normal release of them and to prevent insomnia.

3. Expected outcomes are written for each individual patient for the nursing diagnoses chosen.

D. Implementation.

1. Common specific interventions are included in Table 24-4.

2. Nursing Care Plans 24-1 and 24-2 also show specific nursing interventions.

E. Evaluation.

1. Determination is made as to whether symptoms of the disorder are resolving or not.

2. Lab data are compared to determine improvement.

3. Subjective data are sought from the patient about the decrease in symptoms.

V. Pituitary Gland

A. The pituitary is a pea-sized gland located at the base of the brain and connected to the hypothalamus.

B. The anterior pituitary (adenohypophysis) and posterior pituitary lobe (neurohypophysis) secrete completely different hormones.

C. Among the more common disorders of the pituitary are tumors and diabetes insipidus.

D. Pituitary tumors.

1. Large tumors can create pressure within the brain, causing local symptoms of headache or visual disturbances.

2. Small tumors may present vague symptoms, such as personality change, weakness, fatigue, and abdominal discomfort.

3. Acromegaly is caused by hyperplasia or tumor of the anterior pituitary; it causes excessive secretion of growth hormone.

a. Signs and symptoms include change in facial features with nose enlargement, lip thickening, and a forehead bulge; the hands and feet enlarge. Headaches may occur. Patient may notice that shoes do not fit.

b. Treated by hypophysectomy to remove tumor.

4. Symptoms can be present years before diagnosis is made.

5. Medical diagnosis established by immunoassay for hormone levels, CAT scan of skull, and MRI.

6. Medical and surgical treatment and nursing intervention.

a. Conservative treatment: administration of pituitary hormones.

b. Surgical procedure involves removal of tumor, radiation, or both.

c. Common problems and nursing intervention for patients with hypopituitarism are summarized in Table 24-4.

E. Diabetes insipidus results from decreased production of ADH; characterized by production of copious amounts of dilute urine.

1. Treatment consists of injections of vasopressin every 2 to 3 days or nasal spray of vasopressin several times daily.

F. Syndrome of inappropriate antidiuretic hormone (SIADH).

1. Occurs from excessive production of ADH.

2. Results in fluid excess.

3. Caused by tumor, malignancy, and many other things.

4. Signs and symptoms: confusion, seizures, loss of consciousness, weight gain and edema.

5. Treatment of underlying cause, fluid restriction, administration of sodium chloride, diuretics, and demeclocycline.

VI. The Thyroid

A. Has two lobes and is highly vascular.

1. Principal hormones are thyroxine (T_4) and triiodothyronine. (T_3).

2. These hormones stimulate protein and lipid synthesis, regulate many aspects of carbohydrate metabolism, and stimulate the synthesis of coenzymes from vitamins.

B. Overactivity and underactivity of the thyroid.

1. Diagnostic tests and nursing responsibilities.

a. Involve little more than venipuncture to obtain blood sample.

b. Test results can be altered by presence of iodine in body from previous radiological studies using contrast media, certain drugs.

c. Patients with hyperthyroidism usually have high levels of both T_3 and T_4.

d. Patients with hypothyroidism have low levels of T_3 and T_4, and high levels of thyroid-stimulating hormone (TSH).

C. Goiter.

1. Marked enlargement of the thyroid gland; thyroid hormone levels may or may not remain within normal range.

2. May be prevented by adequate intake of iodine for one type.

3. Medical diagnosis based on enlargement of thyroid, local symptoms, absence of systemic changes.

4. Medical treatment and nursing intervention.

   a. Large goiters not responsive to medical treatment are removed surgically. Smaller ones may respond to administration of iodine.

      (1) Iodine preparations must be given diluted and through a straw to avoid staining the teeth.

D. Hyperthyroidism: systemic condition resulting from overactivity of thyroid and overproduction of thyroid hormones.

1. Patients most at risk: women between ages of 30 and 50.

2. Older women might be misdiagnosed and treated for cardiac disorders.

3. Primary hyperthyroidism also known as Graves' disease, toxic goiter, and thyrotoxicosis.

4. Symptoms and medical diagnosis.

   a. Clinical signs and symptoms indicative of increased metabolic rate; exophthalmos and nervousness.

   b. Sleeping pulse rate elevated.

   c. Serum levels of thyroid hormones elevated.

5. Medical treatment.

   a. Radioactive iodine. Small doses given P.O. to outpatients. Large doses require isolation and precautions in handling blood and urine.

   b. Antithyroid drugs include propylthiouracil, SSKI, and Tapazole. Frequently given in preparation for surgery of thyroid.

6. Nursing intervention.

   a. Provide physical and mental rest.

   b. Diet sufficiently high in calories to meet metabolic needs.

c. Administer medications and instruct patient about them.

d. Explain relationship between symptoms and pathology associated with disease.

e. Subtotal thyroidectomy.

   (1) For patients who do not respond well to drug or radiation therapy, have greatly enlarged thyroid glands, or have actual or potential malignancy of the thyroid.

   (2) Two thirds of gland is removed.

   (3) Preoperative care: observe patient for signs of overactivity or other indications that metabolic rate may be too high for safety during surgery.

   (4) Postoperative care.

      (a) Patient placed in high-Fowler's position.

      (b) Vital signs checked frequently and carefully.

      (c) Patient watched for signs of bleeding or swelling in operative area.

      (d) Two most dangerous complications are thyroid crisis and tetany (from damage to parathyroids).

E. Hypothyroidism: underactivity of the thyroid with insufficiency of thyroid hormones. Can be genetic or acquired.

1. Symptoms and medical diagnosis.

   a. In children, symptoms of cretinism are retarded physical and mental growth.

   b. In adults, condition (myxedema) is characterized by bagginess under the eyes, facial swelling, weight gain, abdominal distention and bloating, constipation, flatulence, diminished mental acuity, impaired memory, dry and scaly skin, and increased sensitivity to cold.

2. Diagnosis based on clinical manifestations and serum levels of T_3, T_4, and TSH.

3. Medical treatment and nursing intervention.

   a. Condition usually responds to replacement therapy.

   b. Meticulous skin care necessary.

   c. Provide warmth if patient is sensitive to cold.

   d. Avoid rushing patient.

   e. Educate patient of necessity for taking medication daily.

4. Myxedema coma: life-threatening, but rare.

   a. Precipitated by abrupt withdrawal of thyroid therapy, acute illness, anesthesia, use of sedatives or narcotics, surgery, or hypothermia in hypothyroid patient.

b. Signs and symptoms: loss of consciousness with hypotension, hypothermia, respiratory failure, hyponatremia, and hypoglycemia.

c. Treatment: administration of levothyroxine sodium IV, fluid replacement, maintenance of airway, IV glucose, corticosteroids, and provision of warmth.

VII. The Parathyroids

A. Parathyroids located on the posterior aspect of the thyroid.

B. Parathyroid hormone regulates calcium and phosphorus serum levels. Acts on renal tubules to increase excretion of phosphorus and reabsorption of calcium. Also acts on bone to release calcium into bloodstream.

C. Hypoparathyroidism.

1. Caused by atrophy or traumatic injury to parathyroids, as in thyroid surgery or radiation.

2. Medical diagnosis based on abnormal calcium and phosphorus serum levels, symptoms of hypocalcemia, tetany, cardiac arrhythmias.

3. Signs and symptoms: decreased serum calcium level with elevated phosphorus level, fatigue, muscular twitching, muscle spasm, possible tetany.

4. Medical treatment.

a. Measures to raise serum calcium levels.

b. Parathormone replacement therapy.

D. Hyperparathyroidism.

1. One of the most common endocrine disorders. Often diagnosed during routine physical examination and screening techniques.

2. Results from benign secreting tumors of parathyroid or hyperplasia of the gland.

3. Signs and symptoms: elevated serum calcium, gastrointestinal complaints, dehydration, confusion, weight loss, thirst, and hypertension.

4. Medical diagnosis based on clinical manifestations and laboratory tests.

5. Medical treatment and nursing intervention.

a. Saline infusions, diuretics to remove excess calcium.

b. Phosphate therapy, mithramycin, and calcitonin to correct skeletal release of calcium.

c. Nursing measures as for patients receiving diuretic therapy, monitoring serum electrolytes, measuring intake and output.

6. Surgical treatment: subtotal parathyroidectomy.

VIII. Adrenal Glands

A. Adrenal medulla secretes epinephrine and norepinephrine; adrenal cortex secretes mineralocorticoids, glucocorticoids, and androgenic hormones.

B. Dysfunctions of adrenal cortex are more likely to be related to abnormal levels of cortical hormones other than androgenic ones because testes or ovaries can compensate for insufficiency of sex hormones.

C. Pheochromocytoma: tumor of adrenal medulla that secretes catecholamines.

1. Causes severe hypertension.

2. Treatment is surgical removal of the affected adrenal gland.

D. Adrenocortical insufficiency (Addison's disease).

1. Primary insufficiency due to malfunction of adrenal gland; secondary related to disorders of pituitary.

2. Primary insufficiency can be caused by idiopathic atrophy of gland, inflammation, infection, and nonsecreting tumors of adrenals.

3. Symptoms and medical diagnosis.

a. In the early stages of Addison's disease clinical manifestations can be very vague.

b. Eventually patient will show signs of fluid and electrolyte imbalance: hyponatremia and fluid water deficit, hyperkalemia, low blood pressure, and hypoglycemia.

4. Medical treatment and nursing intervention.

a. Replacement therapy usually brings about rapid recovery.

b. Nursing intervention.

(1) Intensive care during Addisonian crisis.

(2) Problem of fatigue and orthostatic hypotension.

(3) Alleviation of anorexia, nausea and vomiting, diarrhea.

(4) Preventive and coping mechanisms for stress.

(5) Patient education.

(a) Medications.

(b) Signs and symptoms of insufficient or excess adrenocorticoid hormones.

(c) Prescribed diet.

(d) Need for extra rest.

(e) ID card and tag.

E. Excess adrenocortical hormone (Cushing's syndrome).

1. Can be caused by excess corticotropin, secreting tumor of adrenal cortex, overzealous administration of steroids.
2. Symptoms and medical diagnosis.
   a. Laboratory testing of 24-hour levels of cortisol. Constantly high level indicative of Cushing's syndrome.
   b. Clinical manifestations include painful fatty swellings, large body with thin extremities, bruising after mild trauma, impotence, amenorrhea, hypertension, and general weakness.
   c. Patients with family history of diabetes can develop IDDM.
3. Medical treatment and nursing intervention.
   a. Surgical removal and radiation or destruction of pituitary gland when pituitary disorder is primary cause.
   b. Nursing diagnoses common to patient with nursing interventions located in Table 24-4.

IX. **Elder Care Points**
   A. Thyroid tissue changes include formation of nodules in many patients in this age group.
   B. Elderly patients who are lethargic, slow in thinking, and unenthusiastic about whatever is going on may be hypothyroid.
   C. T_3 levels decrease with age.

X. **Community Care**
   A. Most patients with endocrine problems are outpatients.
   B. Home care nurses may find that many patients with other problems also have a thyroid problem.
   C. Nurses in long-term care facilities must be on the alert for signs of hypothyroidism and hyperparathyroidism among elderly females.
   D. Nurses can be instrumental in prevention of secondary Cushing's syndrome by cautioning patients to seek other means of treatment for arthritis and allergy than steroids whenever possible.

CHAPTER 25

Care of Patients with Endocrine Disorders: Diabetes Mellitus and Hypoglycemia

OBJECTIVES

Upon completing this chapter the student should be able to:

1. State significant differences in the two major types of diabetes mellitus.
2. Identify each of the four kinds of factors that influence the development of diabetes mellitus.
3. Describe laboratory tests used in the diagnosis of diabetes mellitus.
4. Describe nursing assessment and intervention for the management of type I and type II diabetes mellitus.
5. Prepare to teach a newly diagnosed diabetic patient about the disease, treatment, and self-care.
6. Describe the early signs and symptoms that might indicate that the diabetic patient is in early ketoacidosis.
7. List the signs and symptoms of an insulin reaction (hypoglycemia) and describe the appropriate nursing interventions.
8. Identify sources of support and information for diabetic patients and their families.
9. Describe the acute and long-term complications and results of poorly controlled diabetes mellitus.
10. Identify signs and symptoms of hypoglycemia and its treatment in nondiabetic patients.

Diabetes mellitus is a complex group of disorders that have in common a disturbance in metabolism and use of glucose that is secondary to a malfunction of the beta-cells of the pancreas. The beta cells are responsible for producing and secreting insulin and glucagon. Glucose cannot enter the cells when insulin is absent, and the cells enter a state of starvation even though there is an excess of glucose in the blood.

The pancreas is both an **endocrine** and **exocrine** gland. Its endocrine function is to produce the hormones *insulin* and *glucagon*. The exocrine function is to produce pancreatic enzymes that enter the duodenum to assist digestion. Figure 25-1 shows the effects of insulin and glucagon in the body. Because insulin is involved in the metabolism of carbohydrates, proteins, and fats, diabetes mellitus is not limited to a disturbance of glucose homeostasis. However, the one disorder that all diabetic persons share is an intolerance to glucose. Figure 25-2 shows the action of insulin on blood glucose.

Elder Care Point... Blood glucose levels rise with age, with fasting levels climbing about 1 mg/dL for each decade and postprandial levels increasing 6 to 13 mg/dL. The elderly experience hypoglycemia more quickly than a younger person, making tight control of diabetes difficult in the elderly person.

TYPES OF DIABETES MELLITUS

Of the approximately 16 million cases of diabetes mellitus in the United States, there are at least two major types and five subtypes. The categories of diabetes are not defined by hard-and-fast rules. Table 25-1 summarizes the major characteristics of various forms of diabetes mellitus. This section reviews primarily type I and type II.

Type I, or insulin-dependent, diabetes mellitus (IDDM) accounts for about 5% to 10% of all cases. It

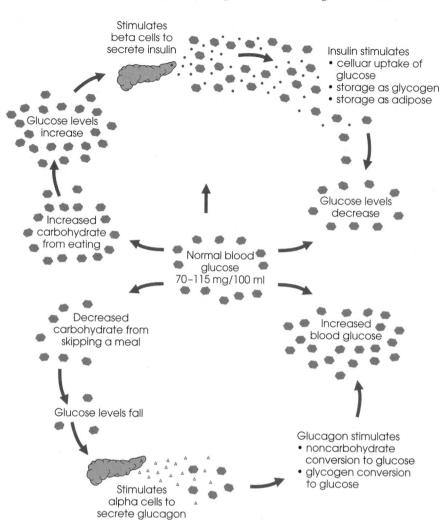

FIGURE 25-1   Effects of insulin and glucagon. (*Source:* Redrawn from Applegate, E. J. [1995]. *The Anatomy and Physiology Learning System: Textbook.* Philadelphia: Saunders, p. 220.)

occurs twice as frequently in women as in men. Black Americans are twice as likely to develop the disease as white Americans, and **Hispanic Americans have a five times greater incidence of diabetes mellitus than the rest of the population.** As the name implies, persons who have this type of diabetes require injections of **exogenous** (from outside the body) insulin to maintain life because they produce little or no endogenous insulin on their own. In general, persons with IDDM are more prone to a serious complication (ketosis) associated with an excess of ketone bodies, leading to metabolic acidosis (ketoacidosis). Moreover, IDDM is more likely to appear early in life. In fact, this type of diabetes was formerly called *juvenile diabetes* and *ketosis-prone diabetes* because of its typical early onset and potential for ketoacidosis.

Type II, or non-insulin-dependent diabetes mellitus (NIDDM), affects about 14.4 million Americans, 90% of the total diabetic population. **It is believed to be related to inappropriate insulin production, such as an insufficient amount or a delayed response to a glucose load (increased glucose in the blood). This type of**

diabetes also is related to an increased resistance to insulin at the cell level. A genetic defect has been found to cause a rare form of this disorder. Geneticists at the University of Texas at Houston are working on isolating a gene that they feel is responsible for up to 75% of type II diabetes in Mexican Americans.

In general NIDDM has a tendency to develop later in life than IDDM, and these patients rarely develop diabetic ketoacidosis. Table 25-2 compares the signs and symptoms of Type I and Type II diabetes.

Elder Care Point . . . Type II diabetes has its onset in adulthood and often is not discovered until the sixth or seventh decade. Many patients in these age groups have difficulty adjusting to the new diet, medication, and required exercise. Income is generally lower, and some patients have difficulty obtaining the necessary foods or medicine because of financial constraints.

Gestational diabetes may occur as a result of the stress of pregnancy. It is treated with insulin. After delivery, the condition must be reevaluated; the patient

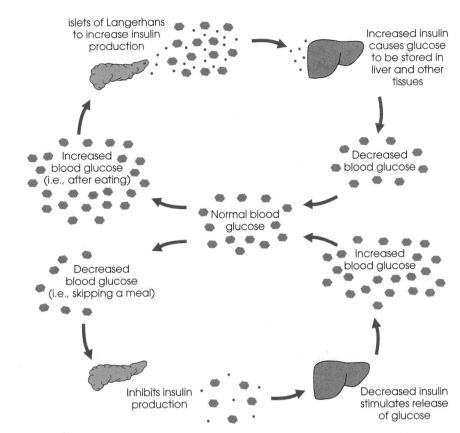

FIGURE 25-2   Interaction of blood glucose and insulin. (*Source:* Redrawn from: Applegate, E. J. [1995]. *The Anatomy and Physiology Learning System: Textbook.* Philadelphia: Saunders, p. 208.)

may revert to impaired glucose tolerance, or she may prove to have true IDDM or NIDDM, especially if she is overweight.

◆ Contributing Factors

At least four sets of factors influence the development of diabetes mellitus: genetic, metabolic, microbiological, and immunological.

Genetic factors are included in the etiology of diabetes because diabetes tends to run in families, even though research has not yet pinpointed the responsible genes. It is known that the risk of having some form of diabetes increases in proportion to the number of relatives who are affected, the genetic closeness of the relatives, and the severity of their disease.

Metabolic factors involved in the etiology of diabetes are many and complex. Emotional or physical stress can unmask an inherited predisposition to the disease, probably as a result of glucogenesis induced by increased production of hormones from the adrenal cortex, especially the glucocorticoids.

Perhaps even more significant than metabolic factors and the occurrence of diabetes is the association of NIDDM and obesity. About 80% of NIDDM patients are obese, and there is a higher incidence of NIDDM in persons who lead a sedentary life and eat a high-calorie diet. With weight reduction and increased physical activity, blood glucose can be restored to normal levels and maintained there—hence the importance of diet and exercise in the management of NIDDM. In this type of diabetes there also seems to be a relationship to aging and a reduction in the function of the pancreatic beta-cells and how they synthesize insulin.

Microbiologic factors have to do with the suspicion that some forms of IDDM are related to viral destruction of the beta-cells. The mumps or Coxsackie virus is thought to be the trigger. Evidence that supports viruses as causative factors include the following:

◆ Both IDDM and viral infections tend to have sudden onsets.

◆ Seasonal fluctuations in the onset of IDDM—late autumn and early spring—correspond with the times of the year when "flu" and other viral illnesses are most common.

◆ Viral infections can and often do attack the pancreas; many viral infections are characterized by inflammation of the pancreatic beta-cells.

There are known cases in which children developed IDDM after having had a recent viral infection.

Immunologic factors are considered because research studies have presented strong evidence that some types of IDDM are an autoimmune reaction associated with the HLA-DR3 gene. At the time IDDM is diag-

TABLE 25-1 ♦ *Clinical Categories of Diabetes Mellitus and the Characteristics of Each*	
Type and Former names	**Characteristics**

Type I (IDDM)
    Juvenile diabetes
    Juvenile-onset
    Ketosis-prone
    Brittle diabetes
	Little or no endogenous insulin produced. New patients can be any age but usually are young. Patient must receive exogenous insulin and follow prescribed diet and exercise program.
	Renal, cardiovascular, retinal, and neurological complications likely if disease is not kept under tight control.

Type II (NIDDM)
    Adult-onset diabetes
    Maturity-onset diabetes
    Ketosis-resistant
    Stable diabetes
	Rarely develop ketosis; may develop hyperglycemic, hyperosmolar nonketotic syndrome (HHNS). Patients vary in need for exogenous insulin. New patients usually over 30 and most are obese. Disorder often responds to diet and exercise.

Impaired glucose intolerance
    Asymptomatic diabetes
    Chemical diabetes
    Subclinical diabetes
    Borderline diabetes
	Glucose levels between those of normal people and those of diabetics. Are at high risk for atherosclerotic disease and cardiovascular problems. Do not seem to be particularly susceptible to renal and retinal complications

Gestational diabetes	Occurs only during pregnancy. Greater risk of developing diabetes after pregnancy.
Statistical risk of diabetes	Those who have had impaired glucose tolerance in the past but have normal glucose tolerance now; prediabetes; latent diabetes, subclinical diabetes. Those who are predisposed to diabetes because of family history, age, race, or obesity.

♦ Incidence and Prevalence

For reasons not yet fully understood, the incidence of diabetes mellitus is increasing at an alarming rate. The prevalence of diabetes mellitus in the United States is 6%, affecting an estimated 16 million people.

The rate of increase can be explained in part by improved methods of diagnosing and reporting and by more effective management of the disease, which has increased the life span of diabetic persons. **Successful management has saved the lives of many diabetic infants who formerly could not survive more than a few months.** Moreover, improved methods of control have allowed young diabetic adults to have children safely, and their offspring are more likely to develop diabetes.

DIAGNOSTIC TESTS

The most common diagnostic tests for diabetes mellitus are those that test for glucose in the blood and urine. Laboratory blood tests require the withdrawal of 5 to 7 mL of blood. Table 25-3 presents the tests most commonly used to diagnose and monitor diabetes mellitus.

Glucose normally is excreted by the kidneys in minute amounts, whereas uncontrolled diabetes causes a "spilling" of excess glucose in the blood over the renal threshold and into the urine. Before the invention of the glucometer for blood testing, urine testing was the mainstay of monitoring therapy. However, as a person grows older, urine tests for glucose are less reliable because of the kidneys' inability to rid the blood of excess sugar. Older persons' eyesight may not be able to detect the subtle color changes needed to correctly interpret a urine test. The presence of glucose in the urine (**glycosuria**) may be normal if the specimen is checked im-

TABLE 25-2 ♦ *Comparison of Symptoms of Type I and Type II Diabetes*	
Type I—Insulin Dependent (IDDM)	**Type II—Non-insulin-dependent (NIDDM)**
Very thirsty (polydipsia) Frequent urination (polyuria) Extremely hungry (polyphagia) Rapid loss of weight Irritability Weakness and fatigue Nausea and vomiting	May experience polydipsia, polyuria, and polyphagia. More commonly experience: excessive weight gain. Family history of DM. Poor healing of scratches, abrasions, and wounds. Blurred vision Itching Drowsiness Increased fatigue Tingling or numbness in the feet

nosed, about three fourths of the cases studied have islet cell antibodies circulating in the blood. Such antibodies are not found in normal individuals. Diabetics who continue to produce insulin will eventually stop producing normal amounts of the hormone if islet cell antibodies remain in the blood.

Think about . . . What is one way in which you or your family members might decrease the risk of NIDDM in later life?

TABLE 25-3 ◆ *Diagnostic Tests for Detecting and Monitoring Diabetes Mellitus*			
Test	**Purpose**	**Description**	**Nursing Implications**
Serum tests			
Fasting blood glucose Normal value: 70–115 mg/dL; elderly: rises 1 mg/dL per decade of age.	Determine level of circulating glucose; detect hyperglycemia or hypoglyemia.	Requires a fasting venous blood sample.	Explain importance of fasting state to the patient.
2-h postprandial blood glucose Normal value: <140 mg/dL; elderly: rises 5–10 mg/dL with age.	Determine need for glucose tolerance test; determine need for change in diabetes therapy.	Venous blood sample drawn 2 hours after a meal.	Explain the importance of presenting self for blood sampling exactly 2 hours after finishing a meal.
Glucose tolerance test Normal values: Fasting <140 mg/dL; 2 h <200 mg/dL.	Detect abnormal glucose metabolism; assist in diagnosis of diabetes mellitus.	A venous blood sample is drawn after a 10- to 12-hour fast; patient is given a glucose "load," usually a prepared liquid drink of 300 mL, that contains a specified amount of glucose. Venous blood samples are drawn at ½-hour intervals for 2 hours. Phenytoin (Dilantin), birth control pills, diuretics, and glucocorticoids will adversely affect results; consult physician regarding taking these medications.	Instruct patient to eat a balanced diet with at least 150 g of carbohydrate for a minimum of 3 days before the test as well as maintain a normal level of physical activity. Explain the need for a 10- to 12-hour fast prior to beginning the test. Explain the procedure. Advise that during the test the patient will not be able to smoke, drink liquids, or eat and must remain at rest for the 2 hours. During the test, request that the patient report feelings of severe weakness, dizziness, nervousness, and confusion, which indicate hypoglycemia.
Glycosolated hemoglobin (HbA1$_c$) Normal value: 2.2%–4.8%.	Determine degree of diabetic control of blood sugar over the preceding 6 to 8 weeks.	A sample of venous blood is required. Fasting is not necessary.	Explain to the patient the need for this test to be done several times a year to monitor effectiveness of diabetic therapy and determine degree of control over the disease process.
C-peptide Normal values: 0.78–1.89 ng/mL.	Evaluate endogenous secretion of insulin when the presence of insulin antibodies interferes with direct assay of insulin.	A fasting sample of 1 mL of venous blood is used.	Caution the patient to fast for 8 to 12 hours before the test. Water is permitted.
Urine test			
Ketone bodies	Determine presence of ketones in the urine, which indicates a state of ketoacidosis.	A fresh urine sample is tested with a dip stick or with acetest tablet. Follow instructions on bottle of test material.	Instruct diabetic patient that ketone testing should be done whenever illness has interfered with normal eating and activity for more than 24 hours and whenever signs of hyperglycemia are present, such as increased thirst, excessive urination, fatigue, nausea, irritability, and/or change in level of consciousness.

mediately after ingestion of a high-carbohydrate meal. Blood testing is much more accurate.

The following is used to establish a diagnosis of IDDM: a fasting glucose level over 200 mg/dL, along with the classic symptoms of diabetes; fasting glucose level of 140 mg/dL or more on least at two occasions; or a fasting glucose level less than 140 mg/dL plus two oral glucose tolerance tests with 2-hour values of over 200 mg/dL and one intervening level over 200 mg/dL.

The 2-hour postprandial test may be done to determine whether a full glucose tolerance test is necessary. A single blood specimen is taken 2 hours after a normal meal. A result above 140 mg/dL is considered abnormal.

The glucose tolerance test does not always give a definitive diagnosis of diabetes mellitus, and cannot be depended on to rule out the disease in every case either. It is, however, commonly used as one of the criteria for diagnosing diabetes mellitus. The glucose tolerance test is a challenge test, in which the patient is given a set amount of glucose to evaluate insulin secretion and the body's ability to metabolize glucose. A drink containing 75 g of glucose is an amount frequently administered. Additional hourly monitoring is sometimes done to aid in the diagnosis of hypoglycemia. **Normal plasma glucose levels reach their highest level of 160 to 180 mg per 100 mL within 30 minutes to 1 hour after the glucose preparation is ingested. The plasma glucose should return to fasting level or lower after 2 to 3 hours.**

The glycosylated hemoglobin test is used not to diagnose diabetes, but to monitor the progress of a person who is already known to be a diabetic. Commonly called *hemoglobin A₁c* (pronounced *A-one-see*), the test measures blood glucose control over a period of many weeks rather than at any one time. No preparation is necessary for the test. The test involves only a venipuncture to obtain a small sample of blood and can be done at any time of the day. Hemoglobin A₁c is hemoglobin with glucose attached to it. Hemoglobin A, the normal type of adult hemoglobin, is "sticky"; therefore glucose in the bloodstream attaches itself to the hemoglobin A molecules and remains there for the life span of the red blood cell. **Because red cells live about 120 days, a measurement of the amount of glucose attached to the hemoglobin can give an average blood glucose level for the past 3 to 4 months.** This test offers advantages for both the patient and the physician who is helping her gain and maintain control over her blood sugar. Patients who monitor their own blood glucose levels at home and follow the prescribed control regimen can determine whether the methods they are using for control are working. Physicians can use test results to change and improve prescribed programs to manage diabetes. **Knowing the test results every 3 to 4 months also can work as a motivator to patients who can see for themselves whether their compliance with the prescribed program is keeping their blood glucose at**

an acceptable level over time. A normal value for hemoglobin A₁c depends on the laboratory method used. Table 25-4 shows the ratings designating degree of control based on glycosylated hemoglobin A₁c levels.

In the future, fructosamine assays may be used more often to determine diabetic control over a shorter time (3 weeks). This test is less influenced by age, which would be an advantage.

SYMPTOMS AND MEDICAL DIAGNOSIS

In addition to the results of laboratory tests, the physician depends on clinical signs and symptoms of diabetes mellitus to establish a diagnosis. **The classic symptoms of the disorder, regardless of type, are related to an elevated blood glucose level.** The excess glucose in the bloodstream (**hyperglycemia**) increases the concentration of the intravascular fluid, raising its osmotic pressure and pulling water from the cells and interstitial fluid into the blood. This causes cellular dehydration and the loss of glucose, electrolytes, and water in the urine.

Cellular dehydration causes thirst and a resultant increased intake of water (**polydipsia**) and diuresis with increased urination (**polyuria**). Hunger (**polyphagia**) is the result of the body's effort to increase its supply of energy foods, even though the intake of more carbohydrates does not meet the energy needs of the cells.

Classic signs and symptoms of diabetes mellitus are polydipsia, polyuria, and polyphagia.

Fatigue and muscular weakness occur because the glucose needed for energy simply is not metabolized properly. **Weight loss in patients with IDDM occurs partly because of the loss of body fluid and partly because in the absence of sufficient insulin, the body begins to metabolize its own proteins and stored fat.** The oxidation of fats is incomplete, however, and so fatty acids are converted into ketone bodies: beta-hydroxybutyric acid, acetoacetic acid, and acetone. When the kidney is unable to handle all of the ketones accumulated in the blood, the patient has what is called *ketosis*. **The overwhelming presence of the strong organic acids in the blood lowers the pH and leads to a severe and potentially fatal acidosis.** The metabolism of

TABLE 25.4 ◆ *Degrees of Control of Blood Glucose Based on Glycosylated Hemoglobin (HgbA1c) Levels*

Glycosylated Hemoglobin Level	Rating
4.9%–6.7%	Excellent
7.6%–8.5%	Good
9.4%–10.0%	Fair
12.1%–13.0%	Poor

body protein when insulin is not available causes an elevated blood urea nitrogen (BUN) level because the nitrogen component of protein is discarded when the body metabolizes its own protein to obtain the glucose it needs.

Diabetic persons are prone to infection, delayed healing, and vascular diseases. **The ease with which poorly controlled diabetics develop an infection is thought to be partly a result of decreased normal function of leukocytes and abnormal phagocyte function.** Another contributing factor to infection and delayed healing probably is decreased blood supply to the tissues because of atherosclerotic changes in the blood vessels. An impaired blood supply means a deficit in the protective cells brought by the blood to a site of injury.

Moreover, it is believed that the neurological, vascular, and metabolic complications of diabetes predispose the diabetic person to infections by allowing organisms to enter tissues that are normally better defended and less accessible. For example, a neurogenic bladder predisposes the patient to stagnant urine and accumulations of bacteria, and a leg ulcer resulting from peripheral vascular disease is without the protection of the skin as a barrier to organisms. Chronic neurological and vascular complications of diabetes are discussed later in this chapter. *Weight gain* is common in persons with NIDDM because of high caloric intake and the availability of endogenous insulin fully to use the food that is eaten.

Think about . . . If a relative complains of fatigue, thirst, and frequent urination, what questions would you ask? What would you suggest this person do?

MANAGEMENT OF DIABETES

There is no cure for diabetes mellitus; the goal is to maintain blood glucose and lipid levels within normal limits and to control these factors as tightly as possible to prevent complications. Although there is some controversy over the need for rigid control of diabetes, the American Diabetes Association wholeheartedly supports the concept that many of the sequelae of diabetes can be minimized by optimal control.

The National Institute of Diabetes and Digestive and Kidney Diseases did a 10-year study that showed that tight control of type I diabetes mellitus (average blood sugar of 155 mg/dL) decreased the incidence of eye, nervous system, and kidney problems by 50%. Patients attempting tight control follow an intensive therapy plan of blood glucose testing at least four times daily and insulin injections three or more times a day or use an insulin pump.

There are some risks associated with perfect control of blood glucose levels. The most serious of these is hypoglycemia or insulin reaction. Weight gain is another problem with tight control and this can present other problems. Type II diabetics tend to be overweight in the first place and extra pounds make these diabetics more insulin resistant. For these reasons, such tight control is not indicated for every diabetic.

Elder Care Point . . . Elderly patients are more prone to hypoglycemia. Severe hypoglycemia in the elderly patient may precipitate myocardial infarction, angina, stroke, or seizures. For this reason, "tight" control may not be the best thing for an elderly patient.

In general, "good" or "tight" control is thought to be achieved when fasting blood glucose stays within normal limits, glycosylated hemoglobin tests show that blood glucose has stayed within normal limits from one testing period to the next, the patient's weight is normal, blood lipids remain within normal limits, and the patient has a sense of health and well-being.

The protocol for control of diabetes mellitus is highly individualized and depends on the type of diabetes a person has; her age, general state of health, ability to follow the prescribed regimen, and acceptance of responsibility for managing her illness; and a host of other factors. Both IDDM and NIDDM patients must follow their prescribed diets and carry out some form of regular exercise. These are the cornerstones of management, regardless of the specific problem with glucose intolerance.

Insulin therapy can be prescribed for NIDDM patients as well as IDDM patients. **In most cases, those who have NIDDM can control their blood glucose by reducing caloric intake and increasing physical exercise.** In addition, oral hypoglycemic or antidiabetic agents may be prescribed for NIDDM patients to help keep their blood glucose levels under control. If control is difficult to maintain, then insulin may be added to the treatment plan.

◆ Diet

Diet is the cornerstone of diabetic treatment. Weight loss is a goal for most patients with type II diabetes. The diet of each diabetic patient is calculated on an individual basis. There is no such thing as a "typical" diabetic, and because diabetes is an unstable and changing process, each patient's needs will change from time to time. In general, the diabetic diet is geared toward providing adequate nutrition with sufficient calories to maintain normal body weight and to adjust the intake of food so that blood glucose is kept within safe limits. **Since 1994, less emphasis has been placed on caloric intake and restriction of carbohydrates and more atten-**

tion paid to the regulation of body weight and control of cholesterol and blood glucose levels in each patient. Sweets have been added to one of the carbohydrate lists as new evidence has revealed that eating sugar as part of the meal plan need not interfere with blood glucose control. There is also a "very lean meat" list now and the fat group has been divided into monosaturated, polyunsaturated, and saturated fat. Fat-modified foods, such as fat-free cookies and fat-reduced waffles, have been added. Vegetarian foods also are included. The combination food lists now contain such things as fast food burritos, chicken nuggets, and a variety of sandwiches. These changes make the lists easier to use, and most diabetics now find it less difficult to stick with their designed diet.

The individual diet is based on the patient's type of diabetes, her height-to-weight ratio, usual dietary intake, cultural preferences, exercise level, and daily schedule. Meal plans are generally made up of 55% to 60% carbohydrate, 12% to 20% protein, and 30% fat. Concentrated sweets are limited, and meals should include an adequate amount of fiber. This is accomplished by taking in mostly complex carbohydrates from the carbohydrate group. Fats should be mainly polyunsaturated or monosaturated.

Elder Care Point . . . Weight-loss is seldom a goal for the elderly type II diabetic unless weight is more than one and a half times normal for height and frame. Elderly people are more susceptible to nutritional deficiencies from teeth problems, illness, and decreased appetite. Diet is frequently managed by reducing concentrated sugars and adhering to a meal schedule.

The American Diabetes Association and the American Dietetic Association have worked together to devise a simplified method of calculating a diabetic diet and planning a diabetic's meals. The booklet containing this information is entitled "The Exchange Lists for Meal Planning." The principal foods are divided into three clusters.

Each cluster contains foods that are similar in kind and have equal nutritional value in regard to carbohydrate, protein, and fat. For example, more than 30 fruits from which the diabetic can choose are listed, each providing 10 gm of carbohydrate, a negligible amount of protein and fat, and 40 calories per serving. Other lists contain similar information for a great variety of foods. The booklet also includes instructions for substitutions among the food groups, as well as a table for the conversion of weights and measures. With this simple method of choosing a menu from the exchange lists, a diabetic or a member of her family can calculate caloric and nutritional value with ease. Copies of the 32-page booklet may be purchased by calling 1-800-ADA-ORDER.

It is important that the diabetic patient not develop a defeatist or negative attitude toward her diet. Emphasis should be placed on the positive aspects of the diet, on the foods she is allowed rather than those that are forbidden. Cultural preferences must be considered when helping the patient devise meal plans. **A patient should not be made to feel guilty about experiencing difficulty with staying on the diet or the times when deliberate "cheating" occurs and foods that are not allowed are eaten.** We all have moments when we are likely to yield to the temptation to do what we know is not in our best interest.

One of the most effective means of helping the diabetic patient follow her diet is by teaching her about food values and how they affect diabetes so that she can understand how food elements affect her health and well-being. To help the diabetic and her family learn which foods she should eat and those she should avoid, the physician, the dietitian, and the nurse must all participate in the instruction. Fortunately, many well-written and clearly illustrated booklets and pamphlets are available and are very helpful to the diabetic and her family. Organizations such as the American Diabetes Association (National Service Center, 1660 Duke Street, Alexandria, VA 22314, 1-800-232-3472) and the Joslin Diabetes Center (One Joslin Place, Boston, MA 02215, 617-732-2415) will send instructive material on request. This material not only covers diets but also warns the diabetic against misleading or fraudulent information about quick "cures" or special diets that are supposed to cure diabetes.

Think about . . . How would you assess whether your diabetic home care patient is eating a "correct" diet to treat diabetes?

◆ Exercise

Physical exercise is an important part of managing diabetes. Muscular activity improves glucose utilization for energy and also improves circulation. In addition to lowering blood glucose levels by "burning up" the glucose, exercise makes the insulin receptors on cells more sensitive to the hormone and thus improves utilization of the available glucose. Because diabetic control also considers blood lipid levels, exercise contributes to that control by reducing triglyceride levels and increasing high-density lipoprotein (HDL) levels.

The exercise program should be designed for the individual patient.

The plan should consider the age and overall physical condition of the patient, ability to carry out the exercises regularly, and how well controlled the diabetes is. For some patients a brisk walk of 1 or 2 miles daily

TABLE 25.5 ◆ *Patient Education: Home Treatment for Hypoglycemia*

When signs of hypoglycemia are present and the patient is able to swallow, give one of the following:

- ½ cup of juice (apple or orange).
- ½ cup of 2% or skim milk.
- ½ cup of regular soda (not sugar free).
- 6 to 7 hard candies, such as Life-savers (not sugar free).
- 1 small box of raisins (2 tablespoons).
- 3 glucose tablets.
- 1 tablespoon of honey.
- 1 tablespoon of sugar.
- 5 small cubes of sugar.
- 1 small tube of cake icing (2 oz).
- 1 small tube of glucose gel.

If the patient is unable to swallow (groggy or unconscious):

- Turn the patient on the side.
- Administer 1 mg of Glucagon by injection after mixing the solution in the bottle until it is clear.
- Feed the patient as soon as he or she is awake and able to swallow.
- Give a fast-acting source of sugar (see above list) and a longer-acting source, such as crackers and cheese or a meat sandwich.
- If the patient does not awaken within 15 minutes, give another dose of Glucagon and inform a physician of the situation immediately.
- If a physician cannot be contacted, call 911 or the local emergency service.

is as much exercise as they can tolerate. Others may be able to perform more strenuous exercises, but they must be cautioned against extremes, especially if they are taking insulin. Exercise can rapidly lower blood glucose levels and cause serious hypoglycemia.

All exercise programs should begin with milder forms of exercise and gradually increase until the patient's level of tolerance or the desired therapeutic effect is reached. **A program should not be started until the blood glucose is under control.** The exercise program should be planned so that the exercises are performed at the same time every day, preferably after a meal when the blood glucose is highest. **Blood glucose should be checked before beginning to exercise.** The patient is encouraged to wear a Medic-Alert bracelet and to exercise with a friend who knows the signs and symptoms of hypoglycemia and how to treat it (Table 25-5). **Every diabetic should have emergency supplies for treatment for hypoglycemia available when exercising.**

Elder Care Point . . . Physical limitations may discourage older diabetic patients from exercising. The elder diabetic is at risk of developing hypoglycemia up to 24 hours after exercising if the exercise is too strenuous. Walking, swimming, or riding a stationary

bicycle are considered the safest activities for this group. Exercise should begin slowly and build up to 30 to 45 minutes three or four times a week. The gradual increase helps prevent hypoglycemia, stress fractures, and cardiovascular complications.

Increasing Food Intake during Exercise During moderate exercise, such as brisk walking, bowling, or vacuuming, 5 g of simple carbohydrate should be consumed at the end of 30 minutes and at 30-minute intervals during the continued activity. Jogging, swimming, or scrubbing floors should be preceded by consumption of 15 to 20 g of complex carbohydrate plus protein 15 to 30 minutes prior to beginning the exercise, and then, if the activity continues for more than 30 minutes, 10 g of simple carbohydrate should be taken every 30 minutes. Vigorous exercise, such as fast jogging, skiing, or playing tennis, requires intake of 30 to 40 g of complex carbohydrate plus protein 15 to 30 minutes ahead of time and then 10 to 20 g of simple carbohydrate intake every 30 minutes after the first half-hour.

Performing exercise when insulin or an oral antidiabetic agent is at its peak of action can bring on an acute hypoglycemic reaction. Another precaution for insulin-dependent patients is to avoid injecting insulin into an area that will soon receive extra exercise (for example, the leg). **The abdomen is a good site for insulin injection as absorption is steady, rapid, and not affected by exercise.** Eating a piece of fruit before even light exercise, if done between meals, also can help prevent hypoglycemia in insulin-dependent diabetics.

Once a patient begins to follow a regular exercise program, her insulin dosage and diet may need to be revised. In general, she may need to take less insulin and to increase her caloric intake if she exercises regularly. Keeping a daily record of her exercise, along with her weight, insulin dosage, and blood glucose levels can help motivate the patient to continue with her exercises.

◆Administration of Insulin

Insulin is a potent drug that must be treated with respect by the patient and any others involved in its administration. Many exogenous insulins are a liquid hormonal preparation obtained from the pancreas of animals. Since the advent of genetic engineering techniques, human insulin (sometimes called *humulin*) is the preferred form because it is less likely to cause allergies and other problems associated with insulin from an animal source. Human insulin is produced in the laboratory by splicing genetic material into the deoxyribonucleic acid (DNA) of a bacterium. The interjected genetic material contains information for the structure of the insulin protein. The bacteria use this information to produce the insulin over and over again in successive generations.

TABLE 25-6 ◆ *Common Types of Insulins and Their Onset, and Duration of Action*

Type	Source	Therapeutic Effects (Average Range)*		
		Onset (h_r)	Peak (h_r)	Duration (h_r)
Short-acting insulin				
Insulin injection (regular crystalline zinc insulin)				
Iletin I R	Beef or pork	½	2–4	6–8
Iletin II R	Pork (purified)	½–1	2–4	6–8
Regular	Pork	½	2½–5	8
Pork Regular	Pork (purified)	½	2½–5	8
Humulin R	DNA technology	½–1	2–4	6–8
Novolin R	DNA technology	½	2½–5	8
Novolin Penfill	DNA technology	½	2½–5	8
Velosulin R	DNA technology	½	1–3	8
Iletin II U-500	Pork (purified)	1–3	6–10	12–18
Prompt insulin zinc suspension (semilente insulin)				
Semilente	Beef	1–2	5–8	10–16
Intermediate-acting insulins				
Isophane insulin suspension (NPH insulin)				
Iletin I	Beef or pork	1–2	6–12	18–26
Iletin II	Pork (purified)	1–2	6–12	18–26
NPH	Beef	1½	4–12	24
NPH pork	Pork (purified)	1½	4–12	24
Insulatard	Pork	1½	4–12	24
Humulin N	DNA technology	1–2	6–12	18–24
Novolin N	DNA technology	1½	4–12	24
Novolin Penfill	DNA technology	1½	4–12	24
Insulatard	DNA technology	1½	4–12	24
Insulin zinc suspension (lente Insulin)				
Iletin I	Beef or pork	1–3	6–12	18–26
Iletin II	Pork (purified)	1–3	6–12	18–24
Lente	Beef	2½	7–15	24
Lente Pork	Pork (purified)	2½	7–15	22
Humulin L	DNA technology	1–3	6–12	18–24
Novolin L	DNA technology	2½	7–15	22
Fixed-combination insulins				
Mixtard 70/30	Pork	½	4–8	24
Humulin 70/30	DNA technology	½	2–12	24
Novolin 70/30	DNA technology	½	2–12	24
Mixtard 70/30	DNA technology	½	4–8	24
Long-acting insulins				
Extended insulin zinc suspensions (ultralente insulins)				
Ultralente	Beef	4	10–30	36
Humulin U	DNA technology	4–6	8–20	24–28
Buffered insulins for use in external pumps				
Velosulin BR	Pork (purified)	½		

*Peak action and length of action may vary, depending on the amount of insulin injected and the client's response. These times depend on the species of insulin.
Source: adapted from Ignatavicius, D. D., Workman, M. L., Mishler, M. A. (1995). *Medical–Surgical Nursing: A Nursing Process Approach,* 2nd ed. Philadelphia: WB Saunders, p. 1879.

Exogenous insulin was first developed in 1921 by Sir Frederick Banting and Dr. Charles Best. The plain insulin, known today as *regular insulin,* acts for no longer than 6 to 8 hours after injection. In 1936, Hagedorn, a Danish physician found that by adding a protein (protamine) to insulin, its action could be prolonged to a period of 12 hours. It was later discovered that by adding zinc to the insulin, blood glucose levels could be reduced for as long as 26 hours with a single injection. After continued research, scientists developed an intermediate-acting insulin that reaches its peak of action at some time between that of the fast-acting regular insulin and the long-acting zinc suspensions. The first to be used was globin insulin. Later, neutral protamine Hagedorn (NPH), lente, and semilente insulin were developed. Long-acting insulins using protamine and zinc were used for many years. However, it has been found that better control of blood glucose can be achieved with shorter- and intermediate-acting insulins and the production of the longer-acting insulins has almost been stopped. Today NPH insulin is one of the most popular types.

The variety of rapid-acting, slow-acting, and intermediate-acting insulins provides alternative types from which to choose to find the one best suited for the individual patient (Table 25-6). To achieve a level of insulin throughout the day that is as near as possible that of endogenous insulin, some patients may take both a regular and a longer-lasting insulin once or twice a day. Humulin 70/30 is a combination of NPH and regular insulin (70% NPH and 30% regular insulin) and is often prescribed so that patients do not have to mix insulins. Figure 25-3 shows various regimens in which regular (short-acting) and longer-acting insulins are used.

Lente insulin and NPH are cloudy and milky in appearance and must be thoroughly mixed before they are administered so that the patient will receive the prescribed dose. This is done by gently rolling the bottle between the palms of the hands. The bottle is not shaken, because this produces very fine air bubbles that are almost impossible to see but can alter the dosage given and may contribute to breakdown of the insulin.

The type of insulin prescribed for a patient should not be confused with its strength. Insulin labeled "U100" means that there are 100 units of insulin per milliliter of solution; that is, each milliliter contains 100 units. The syringe used for measuring and administering U100 insulin is calibrated to accommodate insulin of this strength. A "lo-dose" syringe will accommodate up to 50 units of insulin. If the dose is higher than this amount, the larger 100-unit syringe is needed. **If regular insulin and a longer-acting insulin are to**

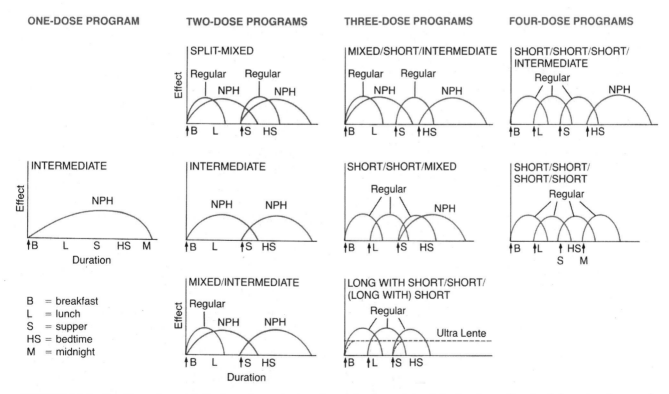

FIGURE 25-3   Insulin regimens. Split doses (two, three or four injections of the daily dose) or split mixed doses (a mixture of short-acting and longer-acting insulins) may give better control. (*Source:* Ignatavicius D. D., Workman, M. C. Mishler, M. A. [1995]. *Medical–Surgical Nursing: A Nursing Process Approach,* 2nd ed. Philadelphia: Saunders, p. 1880.)

be mixed in one syringe, the regular insulin is drawn up first to prevent any contamination of the regular bottle of insulin with the longer-acting variety. Nursing Procedure 25-1 shows how to mix two types of insulin in one syringe.

No matter what the type, insulin must be given by injection. It cannot be taken orally or given via a feeding tube, because it is destroyed by gastric juices. Oral hypoglycemic drugs, which are prescribed for some non-insulin-dependent diabetics, are not an oral form of insulin. Jet injectors are available for patients who are unable to self-inject with a needle.

Insulin injections are rotated within one body area to enhance absorption. Patients are given charts showing the places on the arms, legs, buttocks, and abdomen where insulin can be injected (Figure 25-4). They are then encouraged to keep a daily record of injection sites to help them remember which sites have been used and to avoid the problem of altered or erratic absorption. Pain at the injection site may be caused by injecting insulin that has been refrigerated. The current vial of insulin in use may be stored at room temperature for up to 1 month. If insulin is refrigerated, it should be warmed by gently rotating the filled syringe between the hands. Table 25-7 presents guidelines for teaching a patient how to give insulin subcutaneously.

Insulin requirements change as metabolic needs are altered by diet, exercise, age, and even changes in seasons. In the summer, for example, many people are outdoors and exercising more than during the winter months. Also, as a person grows older, her level of physical activity may decrease. **Insulin requirements also are altered when the patient has an infection or illness or is under added stress.**

If a patient is monitoring her own blood glucose at home and her physician has recommended adjustments of insulin dosage on the basis of daily blood glucose levels, she will need to be taught how to calculate the amount of insulin she should take to achieve the desired blood glucose level.

Nursing Procedure 25-1 Mixing Two Types of Insulin

Steps	Rationale
1. Check expiration dates on both bottles of insulin.	Outdated insulin is not reliable and should not be used.
2. Follow correct vial and syringe preparation technique, and pull back syringe plunger until tip reaches mark for correct number of units for the "cloudy" intermediate or long-acting insulin.	Swabbing the top of the vial with an alcohol swab removes bacteria or other particles; an insulin syringe must be used. This prepares the syringe to inject air into the vial.
3. Push needle into vial above fluid level and inject the air; withdraw the empty needle and syringe and set the "cloudy" vial aside.	Places air in the vial that helps to smoothly draw out the same amount of insulin.
4. Pull syringe plunger back until the mark for the correct number of fast-acting "clear" insulin units is reached.	Prepares to inject air into the "clear" vial.
5. Push the needle into the "clear" vial and push the plunger down, injecting the air. Leave the needle in the vial.	Placing air in the vial promotes smooth withdrawal of the correct number units of insulin as it prevents a vacuum from forming in the vial.
6. Turn vial and syringe upside down and hold together in one hand at eye level. Pull plunger back to any unit marker slightly beyond the desired dose of "clear" insulin.	This action pulls insulin into the syringe. Pulling in the clear insulin first prevents contaminating the fast-acting insulin with the longer-acting "cloudy" insulin.
7. Check the syringe for air bubbles. If any are present, flick the syringe firmly with a finger. Push the plunger up to the mark for the desired dose of "clear" insulin.	Flicking the syringe barrel causes bubbles to rise to the needle where they can be expelled when the plunger is pushed up. *Another nurse should verify that you are drawing up the correct amount of both insulins by watching you.*
8. Remove the needle from the "clear" vial and insert the needle into the "cloudy" vial, immediately turning the vial and syringe upside down while holding firmly onto the plunger.	Holding the plunger firmly prevents pushing some of the "clear" insulin dose into the "cloudy" insulin vial.
9. Pull back very slowly on the plunger to the exact mark for the number of units of "cloudy" longer-acting insulin desired. Remove the needle from the vial and recap it if the insulin is not to be injected at this time.	Pulling slowly on the plunger helps prevent air bubbles from being pulled into the insulin, changing the actual dose.
10. Verify that the amount of units contained in the syringe is equal to the amount of "clear" insulin units ordered, plus the amount of "cloudy" insulin units ordered. Ask the other nurse verifying the insulin dose whether the correct dose is in the syringe.	This acts as a third check that the correct amount of insulin ordered is prepared in the injection for the patient.

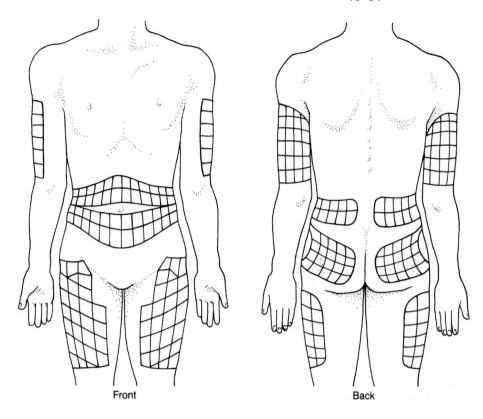

FIGURE 25-4 Rotation sites for injection of insulin.
(*Source:* Ignatavicius, D. D., Workman, M. L., Mishler, M. A. [1995]. *Medical–Surgical Nursing: A Nursing Process Approach,* 2nd ed. Philadelphia: Saunders, p. 1881.)

Front   Back

TABLE 25-7 ◆ *Patient Education: Guidelines for Subcutaneous Insulin Injection*

Instruct the patient to do the following:

◆ Wash hands thoroughly.
◆ Check type of insulin and expiration date on the bottle label.
◆ Check that syringe type is correct (e.g., U100 for U100 insulin).
◆ Roll the bottle of insulin between the palms of the hands to mix it gently.
◆ Cleanse the top of the rubber stopper with an alcohol swab.
◆ Remove the needle cover and pull the plunger back to a point equal to the desired amount of insulin you will draw up; place the needle into the bottle above the surface of the insulin and inject the air (this prevents bubbles).
◆ Turn the bottle and syringe upside down, holding them with one hand; with the bevel of the needle well into the insulin, slowly draw up the correct amount of insulin.
◆ Remove air bubbles in the syringe by tapping on the barrel of the syringe, reinjecting into the bottle, and then redrawing up the correct dosage of insulin without bubbles.
◆ Remove the needle from the bottle; select a site for injection that has not been used in the past month.
◆ Clean the site with an alcohol swab; pinch up the area of skin and insert the needle all the way at a 90-degree angle; inject the insulin.
◆ Pull the needle straight out quickly. Blot the site with the alcohol swab; do not rub the site.
◆ Do not recap the needle; dispose of the syringe and needle in a puncture-proof container.

Think about . . . How would a patient know that his or her insulin requirement has changed?

Research is in progress to determine whether it is possible effectively to deliver insulin dosages by eye drop or nasal inhalation. Someday insulin by injection may be obsolete.

Insulin Pump   An alternative to insulin therapy by daily injections is the *insulin pump.* These pumps can deliver a continuous infusion of insulin through an automated system composed of a battery-driven electronic "brain," an electric motor and drive mechanisms, and a syringe. The syringe is attached to plastic tubing and a subcutaneous needle, which is inserted into the abdomen or thigh. Insulin pumps are especially useful for "brittle" diabetics (those whose blood glucose levels swing widely each day).

The pump partially imitates the action of the beta-cells by delivering insulin continuously. Current models do not yet have a mechanism by which the pump can sense the body's ever-changing needs for insulin, as happens in a normal physiological closed-loop feedback system. In all of the commercially available models, the patient still must check the blood glucose to determine the amount of insulin needed on a day-to-day or moment-to-moment basis.

At the present time insulin pumps are recommended only for a select few patients who are able to discipline themselves to monitor their blood glucose frequently during the day, who can understand the principles of continuous insulin infusion, who are compliant with their diet and self-care, and who have no physiological and pathological contraindications.

Soon a programmable implantable medication system may be available to deliver continuous insulin directly into the peritoneal cavity. The device technically would have to be replaced only every 5 years. A small, handheld external radio transmitter is used by the patient to program insulin release from the pump. The patient will still have to do regular blood glucose monitoring. The advantage of the system is the decreased risk of infection compared with the external pump and needle system.

♦ Oral Hypoglycemic Agents

Oral hypoglycemic or antidiabetic agents are sometimes prescribed for patients with NIDDM to help control their blood glucose. Some of these drugs are sulfonylureas, which stimulate the beta-cells to release more insulin. They are related to the sulfonamide antibiotics. In addition to their ability to stimulate the beta-cells, they also appear to inhibit glucose produc-

tion and facilitate the transport of glucose into the muscle cells. Recent research indicates that the sulfonylureas also increase the number of receptor sites where insulin is bound and where it initiates the process of breaking down glucose. This action is particularly beneficial to diabetics who produce enough insulin but whose cells resist it.

Because the sulfonylureas are from the same family of drugs as the sulfonamide antibiotics, they must be given with caution to persons known to have an allergy to sulfa drugs.

There are four first-generation oral hypoglycemic agents in use: acetohexamide (Dymelor, Dimelor), chlorpropamide (Diabinese), tolazamide (Tolinase), and tolbutamide (Orinase) (Table 25-8). Side effects occur in less than 5% of patients. Those that do occur are common to all four agents, which belong to the sulfa family and have similar properties. **Side effects include hematological and gastrointestinal disorders, jaundice, skin rash, photosensitivity, and a reaction to alcohol similar to that associated with disulfiram (Antabuse).** The symptoms of alcohol intolerance include severe vomiting, throbbing headache, respiratory difficulty, blurred vision, and confusion.

TABLE 25-8 ♦ *Oral Hypoglycemic Agents*

Name	Dosage	Metabolism	Duration of Effect
First generation			
Tolbutamide (Orinase)	500–3,000 mg daily total, taken bid or tid. Available in 250- and 500-mg tablets.	Metabolized by liver. Excreted in urine.	6–12 hours.
Acetohexamide (Dymelor)	250–1,500 mg daily total, taken once a day or bid. Available in 250- and 500-mg tablets.	Metabolized by liver. Excreted in urine.	12–24 hours.
Chlorpropamide (Diabinese)	100–500 mg daily total, taken once daily. Available in 100- and 250-mg tablets.	Very little metabolized by liver. 99% excreted in urine.	Up to 60 hours.
Tolazamide (Tolinase)	100–1,000 mg daily total, taken once daily or bid. Available in 100-, 250-, and 500-mg tablets.	Metabolized by liver. Excreted in urine.	12–24 hours.
Second generation			
Glyburide (Diabeta, Micronase)	1.25–20 mg daily with breakfast or in two doses.	Metabolized by liver. Excreted in urine.	12–24 hours.
Glipizide (Glucotrol, Minidiab)	5–15 mg daily before breakfast or in two doses.	Metabolized by liver. Excreted in urine.	12–24 hours.
Newer drugs			
Metformin (Glucophage)	1000 mg–2,550 mg daily. Taken once or twice daily. Available in 500- or 850-mg tablets.	Excreted unchanged in the urine.	
Acarbose (Precose)	25 mg–300 mg daily. Taken three times a day with meals. Available in 50- and 100-mg tablets.	About ½ of dose is excreted in feces; 2% is metabolized in liver and excreted by the kidneys	Approximately 2 hours.

Elder Care Point . . . The elderly patient metabolizes and excretes drugs more slowly than the younger patient. Drugs stay active in the body longer. Some first-generation oral hypoglycemic agents (Diabinese) have a long half-life and remain active even longer in the elderly patient. These drugs may cause hypoglycemia in these patients and for that reason are not the first choice for treatment in the elderly patient.

Second-generation sulfonylurea hypoglycemics include glyburide (Micronase and Diabeta) and glipizide (Glucotrol). These hypoglycemics are more potent, meaning that lower dosages can be used to control blood glucose. Their primary side effects include gastrointestinal distress and skin reactions. When used in pregnant women, glyburide is discontinued 2 weeks before delivery to prevent severe hypoglycemia in the newborn. Glipizide has not been released for use during pregnancy.

A newer drug, metformin (Glucophage), helps body tissues take up and use insulin naturally available in the body more efficiently in the type II diabetic by reducing insulin resistance. It reduces the liver's production of glucose, lowering the demand for insulin. Unlike the sulfonylureas, this drug does not cause hypoglycemia or hyperinsulinemia, and it does not lead to weight gain. The drug also seems to decrease blood lipids. Metformin is recommended for use in type II diabetics in whom blood glucose cannot be managed by dietary measures alone. It can be used in combination with a sulfonylurea.

Another new drug, acarbose (Precose) works by reducing the demand for insulin. It slows the digestion of complex carbohydrates in the small intestine by inhibiting two enzymes that are responsible for conversion of glucose. This curtails the after-meal jump in blood glucose that occurs in type II diabetics. The drug is used with dietary modification for NIDDM patients when hyperglycemia isn't sufficiently controlled by diet alone. Troglitazone (Rezulin), a new drug used to treat insulin resistance, increases the action of insulin in skeletal muscle and decreases glucose production in the liver.

Among the drugs that enhance or increase the effect of the sulfonylureas are NSAIDs, sulfonamide antibiotics, ranitidine, and cimetidine. Drugs that can inhibit or decrease the action of the oral antidiabetic agents include calcium-channel blockers, combination oral contraceptives, glucocorticoids, phenothiazines, and thiazide diuretics. Beta-blockers interfere with the action of tolbutamide. **The nurse should always check for drug interactions for other drugs a diabetic patient is taking.**

Patients receiving hypoglycemic agents should know that the drug does not eliminate the need for following their prescribed diet and exercise program. Some may be under the mistaken notion that if they go off their diet and indulge themselves, they can just take more oral hypoglycemic pills to make up for this. Others who have been on a diet and exercise program for a while and then have an oral hypoglycemic agent prescribed for them think it is all right to stop planning their meals and exercising regularly.

All hypoglycemic agents are capable of producing gastric irritation, nausea, vomiting, and diarrhea. There also can be liver damage with resultant jaundice, bone marrow depression, and allergic skin reactions in some patients.

Research at the University of Pittsburgh Medical Center is under way on transplanting insulin-producing islet cells. The islet cells from the pancreas of a cadaver donor are injected into the patient's portal vein. The islet cells lodge in the liver and begin to produce insulin, functioning just as they did in the pancreas. Someday this treatment may eliminate the need for insulin injections.

◆ Pre- and Postoperative Insulin Management

The emotional and physical stress of surgery can increase the blood glucose level and alter the amounts of medication needed for good control. Patients with NIDDM may be taken off of oral hypoglycemic medication up to 48 hours prior to surgery and are started on insulin by injection to achieve adequate control of their diabetes during this stressful period. The patient should be reassured that this does not indicate that his diabetes is worse and that the insulin injections are only a temporary measure. IDDM patients will have sliding-scale insulin orders along with their usual insulin order. Blood sugar determinations are done more frequently.

For all diabetic patients, intravenous fluids are begun as soon as the patient is NPO and are continued until he is eating again after surgery. During surgery an insulin "drip" may be used; this is the IV administration of regular or short-acting insulin with a 5% to 10% glucose solution. Blood glucose is monitored closely during surgery and every 2 to 4 hours postoperatively, and urine is checked for signs of acetone when glucose levels are high. The nurse must be especially alert for signs of hypoglycemia in patients who are receiving insulin IV. Blood glucose should be monitored every hour. Insulin dosage often is ordered by injection according to a sliding scale in which increments of regular short-acting insulin are used to attempt to keep the blood glucose within a safe range.

NURSING MANAGEMENT

◆ Assessment

The nurse should always assess each patient, regardless of her complaint, for signs and symptoms of diabetes mellitus. Table 25-9 presents guidelines for history taking. The nurse should physically assess the skin for signs of poor wound healing or areas of infection. The feet should be inspected for signs of tight-fitting shoes and beginning sores. The nurse should weigh the patient and determine whether her weight is within normal limits.

For the newly diagnosed diabetic, the nurse must assess whether the patient is a good candidate for using a blood glucose–monitoring machine, a glucometer. The patient must have adequate peripheral circulation to obtain a drop of blood for the test easily. Manual dexterity is needed to perform the finger stick, to obtain a large enough drop of blood, and to place the drop on the right spot. Patients with arthritis may have difficulty with these steps. Vision must be good enough to perform the finger stick, correctly place the drop of blood, and to read the result on the meter. The patient must be able to time the test, remember the correct

---

TABLE 25-9 ◆ *Assessment: Guide for History Taking Related to Diabetes*

The following questions should be asked to establish a data base that either indicates that the patient may have diabetes, has poorly controlled diabetes, or has no signs of diabetes.

- Has anyone in your family ever been told he or she has diabetes? What about your parents and grandparents?
- Have you had any recent weight loss?
- Have you become increasingly hungry over the past few months?
- Has your thirst increased? Are you drinking more fluids than you used to?
- Do you have to urinate (go to the toilet) more than you used to?
- Have you noticed that you are more tired than you were 6 months ago?
- Do you have any trouble with scratches and wounds healing?
- Do small scratches or abrasions become easily infected?
- Have you noticed any numbness or tingling or "funny" sensations in your hands, legs, or feet?
- Is constipation becoming a problem?
- Are you having any sexual difficulties? Any impotence (men)? Any frequent vaginal infections (women)?

If the patient is a known diabetic ask these questions also:

- Do you feel that you can easily and correctly perform your blood glucose determinations? (Check the patient's performance using her own machine.)
- How do you calibrate your blood glucose monitor?
- Are you having any trouble sticking to your dietary plan?
- How are you planning your meals?
- Are you taking your insulin/oral medication regularly?
- Are you having any problems in relation to the medication?
- Are you keeping records of your blood glucose readings and your insulin injections? (Check the records kept.)
- Are you seeing your primary doctor at regular intervals?
- Are you having your eyes examined regularly?
- Are you visiting the dentist regularly?

---

sequence of the steps, and remember to do it at the designated times of day. Determining whether the patient can cope with the frustration of learning the procedure and whether there is willingness to fit it into the daily routine are other assessment factors. Periodic assessment of glucose monitoring techniques, medication administration, and compliance with treatment regimen is essential.

◆ Nursing Diagnoses

The following nursing diagnoses are common for patients with diabetes mellitus:

- Alteration in nutrition, less than (or more than) body requirements, related to food and energy needs.
- Knowledge deficit related to disease process, possible complications, and self-care.
- Risk for infection related to elevated blood glucose level.
- Ineffective individual coping related to denial of need for effective self-care.
- Sensory perceptual alteration related to effect of elevated blood glucose on nervous system.
- Sexual dysfunction related to effect of elevated blood glucose on nervous system.
- Risk for injury related to severe decrease in tissue perfusion in feet and possibility of gangrene requiring amputation.
- Self-esteem disturbance related to diagnosis of chronic disease requiring insulin injections for survival.

There are many other nursing diagnoses related to the various complications that the diabetic patient may develop over the years. Nursing care plans must be carefully individualized to the particular problems and needs of each patient.

◆ Planning

The nurse must plan his time carefully when caring for diabetic patients. Times for frequent glucose monitoring should be noted on the daily worksheet. Remembering to check calibration of the glucometer before beginning testing is essential. The nurse should know the times of dietary tray delivery to plan glucose testing and insulin injections at the appropriate times in the morning and throughout the day. Fingersticks for blood glucose testing should be performed 30 minutes before breakfast. **If an hour has elapsed without insulin being given after the reading was obtained, the test should be repeated before insulin is administered.**

When a patient is NPO for tests, the nurse must plan to monitor for signs of hypoglycemia and to obtain the patient's food tray immediately when the patient is back. The insulin dose should be adjusted according to physician order during the NPO period, not withheld. Assessment for hyperglycemia must be planned for various times during the shift when the patient is undergoing the added stress of illness or surgery.

Making certain that the patient's insulin, appropriate syringes, or oral medication are on the unit ahead of scheduled medication time prevents delays. **Every insulin dose should be verified by another nurse as it is drawn up for injection.** Asking another nurse to be present at an appointed time saves having to hunt for another nurse at the time of injection preparation. Sliding scale doses of regular insulin should be mixed in the same syringe as the standard daily dose for the patient. Being certain the patient is in the room before drawing up the insulin also saves time.

General goals for the diabetic are:

◆ Maintain blood glucose levels within set limits
◆ Maintain electrolyte and acid-base balance
◆ Maintain optimal weight
◆ Acquire knowledge for self-care
◆ Comply with treatment regimen
◆ Prevent complications

Individual expected outcomes are written for each nursing diagnosis to be included on the nursing care plan. Both long- and short-term goals are considered when writing expected outcomes.

◆ Implementation

Intervention is geared toward assisting the patient with self-care, performing blood glucose determinations, and administering medication when she is ill and cannot do so for herself, observing for signs and symptoms of complications, assessing learning needs, and carrying out a teaching plan as indicated.

The nurse should monitor the trend of blood glucose and glycosylated hemoglobin readings over time, rather than focus only on the current reading. The nurse assesses how well the patient is eating and her fluid intake. Intake and output recordings are appropriate if the patient is ill or having surgery. **Any type of stress can alter the control of her diabetes.** Electrolytes should also be monitored, with particular attention to potassium levels, which can shift suddenly when insulin is insufficient.

Every patient on insulin should be monitored for hypoglycemia after her insulin injections. The nurse must know how many hours after injection of each type of insulin this might occur and should then assess her patient at that time (refer to Table 25-6). Patients are taught to report signs of hypoglycemia promptly to avoid a crisis.

Monitoring for signs of ketoacidosis also is essential. Some of the earliest symptoms may be polyuria, fatigue, anorexia, abdominal pain, and a "fruity" smell to the breath. Look for beginning signs of dehydration with decreased tissue turgor, sunken eyeballs, and dry mucous membranes (Table 25-10). Report such findings to the physician promptly.

Patient Education   Successful management of diabetes requires that the patient be so well informed about the illness and the protocol for controlling it that responsibility can be assumed for changing former dietary habits, administering medication, and monitoring progress. In addition adjustments in lifestyle, recreational choices, and self-image will probably need to be made. The patient must be taught the correct steps for blood glucose monitoring or how to use dip sticks to monitor urine correctly (Figure 25-5).

The problem of noncompliance can be devastating to the welfare of the patient and can mean the difference between leading a nearly normal life or becoming an invalid; eventually it may mean the difference between life and death for the diabetic person. Many hospitals and clinics have developed standardized teaching programs for diabetes education because the task of teaching the diabetic patient is very challenging and complex. (Figure 25-6).

Major topics covered in a standardized program usually include the following:

◆ Pathophysiology of diabetes mellitus, including functions of the pancreas and potential contributing or precipitating factors in the development of diabetes.
◆ How to manage a diabetic diet program.
◆ Blood glucose monitoring at home using either a visually read test or a glucose monitoring meter. (Specific step-by-step instructions come with each individual device.)
◆ Foot care (Table 25-11).
◆ Urine testing when blood glucose level is over 240 mg/dL to check for acetone. (Dipstick instructions are included with each particular type of testing material.)
◆ Identification tag, ID card, and medical information (Figure 25-7).
◆ Information on what to do on "sick" days, especially when nauseous or vomiting and unable to maintain diet (Table 25-12).
◆ Community resources and help groups available to diabetic and family.
◆ Devices that make insulin administration easier (especially for the elderly, visually impaired, or arthritic patient).

TABLE 25-10 ◆ *Comparison of Hypoglycemia and Ketoacidosis*

	Hypoglycemia	Ketoacidosis
Causes	Overdosage of insulin Skipped or delayed meal Unplanned strenuous exercise	Failure to take insulin Illness or infection Overeating or too many carbohydrates Severe stress (surgery, trauma, emotional upset)
Symptoms	Headache Weakness Hunger Pallor Irritability Lack of muscle coordination Apprehension Shakiness Diaphoresis with cool, clammy skin Blurred vision Rapid heart beat Confusion Coma (late)	Increased thirst Increased urination (polyuria) Acetone breath odor ("fruity") Dry mucous membranes and sunken eyeballs (dehydration) Nausea and vomiting Deep respirations (Kussmaul's respiration) Abdominal pain and rigidity Parasthesias, weakness, paralysis Hypotension Oliguria or anuria (late sign) Stupor or coma (late sign)
Treatment	If patient can swallow, give 3 glucose tablets or equivalent glucose gel, 6 oz of orange juice, 6 oz regular cola, 6 oz of 2% or skim milk, or 6 to 8 Life-savers. If patient cannot swallow, administer glucagon by injection. If at the hospital: give D50W solution.	Insulin and correction of electrolyte imbalances Severe cases are hospitalized for stabilization
Prevention	Eat meals 4 to 5 hours apart, plus prescribed snacks. Take correct dose of insulin. Test blood glucose level regularly and more frequently during illness. Eat extra food when exercising more than usual.	Take correct dose of insulin. Consult physician when ill. Follow diet; don't overeat and don't overload with carbohydrates.

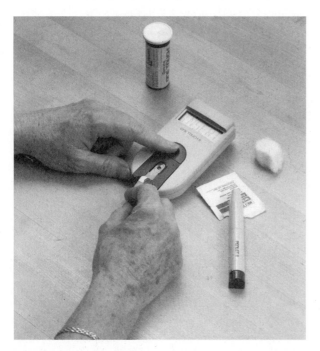

FIGURE 25-5   Blood glucose monitoring. (Photo by Glen Derbyshire; courtesy of Rehabilitation Institute of Santa Barbara, CA.)

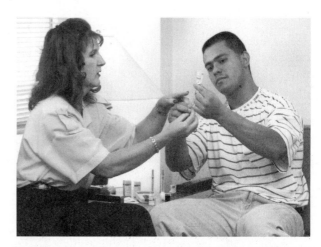

FIGURE 25-6   Nurse teaching diabetic patient. (Photo by Glen Derbyshire; courtesy of Rehabilitation Institute of Santa Barbara, Ca.)

Every diabetic should be taught the following points for proper care of the feet.

- Inspect each foot daily for cuts, cracks, blisters, abrasions, or discoloration of the toes; report any abnormality to your health care provider. Use a mirror if unable to bend to see the bottom of the foot. Be certain to check between the toes.
- Wash the feet in warm (not hot) water, using mild soap; do not soak the feet as this can cause cracking of the skin.
- Thoroughly dry the feet after washing, paying special attention to drying between the toes. Rub in a nonscented, nonmedicated cream if the skin is dry; do not put the cream between the toes.
- Cut the nails straight across; have corns, calluses and ingrown nails managed by a podiatrist. Smooth the nails with an emery board after cutting to prevent cuts on the legs from rough nails while sleeping.
- Wear a clean pair of cotton socks each day.
- Wear properly fitted shoes with a firm sole that do not pinch or bind the foot; never walk barefoot.
- Break in new shoes gradually.
- Never wear open sandals or sandals with straps between the toes.
- Use socks and blankets to warm the feet; do not use a heating pad or hot water bottle near them.
- Test the temperature of bath water before stepping into the tub or shower.
- Elevate the feet whenever possible to improve circulation.

Elder Care Point... Elderly patients have special learning needs. The nurse must be certain that the patient can hear adequately, that vision is enhanced as much as possible by aids and by lighting. Noise and distractions in the environment should be eliminated as much as possible so that the patient can concentrate more fully. Table 25-13 presents suggestions for assisting the elderly patient to learn about diabetes and self-care.

The health care team helping the diabetic manage her illness should include a diabetic specialist, nurse educator, dietitian, podiatrist, periodontist, and, of course, the patient and her significant others. Because of frequent updates and changes in diabetes management, all persons responsible for the care of diabetic patients should read and continue to study and learn about the current protocols. Table 25-14 provides traveling tips for diabetic patients. Common nursing diagnoses, expected outcomes, and nursing interventions for diabetic patients are listed in Table 25-15.

Sources of Information   There are at least two free publications that are published regularly and made available to diabetics, their families, and others interested in learning more and keeping current with new developments in diabetes management. *Diabetes in the News*, published by the Ames Education Corporation, can be obtained by sending your name and address to *Diabetes in the News*, Subscription Department, 1201 N. Clark Street, Suite 405, Chicago, IL 60610-2270. The second publication, a newsletter published bimonthly by the American Diabetes Association, can be obtained by writing to that organization at 1660 Duke Street, Alexandria, VA 22314.

A third publication, also published by the American Diabetes Association, is called *Diabetes Forecast*. It is written and edited by health care specialists and is aimed at providing information for diabetics so that they can manage their illness more effectively. There is a charge for this publication, which can be obtained by writing to the American Diabetes Association, National Service Center, at the address given above. Another helpful resource from the ADA is *101 Tips for Improving Your Blood Sugar* (approximately $12.50). Pharmaceutical companies, local chapters of the American Diabetes Association, and the American Dietetic Association also are excellent sources of information for continuing education in the diabetes management.

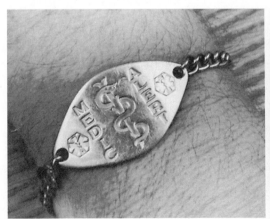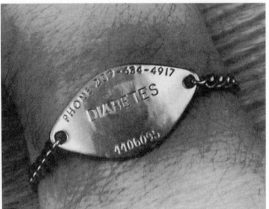

FIGURE 25-7   Medic-Alert emblem worn as bracelet (also may be worn as necklace). Reverse side denotes specific medical problem of the wearer. (Photos by Ken Kasper.)

TABLE 25-12 ◆ *Patient Education: What to Do on Sick Days*

The following instructions should be followed whenever you have a bad cold, flu, or minor gastrointestinal upset.

Medication

- Take your insulin as prescribed. Adjust the dosage as directed depending on your blood glucose readings.
- If taking an oral hypoglycemic, take your usual dose. Do not increase the dose unless ordered to do so by your physician. If you are vomiting and unable to take medication by mouth, the doctor may place you *temporarily* on insulin.

Diet

- Eat your normal diet on schedule.
- If you have nausea and vomiting, replace carbohydrate solid foods in your normal diet with liquids that contain sugar (fruit juice, regular soft drinks, or jello).
- Take at least 1 cup of water or calorie-free, caffeine-free liquid each hour. If you are nauseous, take small sips to help avoid vomiting.

Monitoring

- Test blood glucose at least every 4 hours and record result. If severely ill, check blood glucose every 2 hours.
- Test your urine for ketones if your blood sugar level is over 240 mg/dL.

Notifying the physician

- Call the physician right away if you are vomiting or have abdominal pain or a temperature above 100.2° F (38.8 C).
- Notify the physician if your blood glucose is above 200 mg/dL or your urine test shows ketones in the urine.
- Report to the physician if your blood glucose level that was above 200 mg/dL does not come down with an additional dose of insulin.
- If you cannot reach your physician, go to your hospital emergency room.

Further treatment

- Rest as much as possible.
- Treat vomiting, diarrhea, and fever with fluids and appropriate medication as recommended by your physician.

◆ Evaluation

Evaluation is based by determining whether the expected outcomes have been met. For a diabetic patient this usually means assessing whether learning has taken place and whether there is compliance with the treatment regimen. Monitoring glycosylated hemoglobin levels provides data about the degree of control of blood glucose. Questioning the patient about exercise and diet provides data about those areas. Observing demonstrations of learned skills for insulin injection, good foot care, dietary planning, and glucose monitoring tells how well these tasks have been integrated.

If the expected outcomes are not being met, then the nursing care plan must be revised. Collaboration with the physician and dietitian may be necessary to design a plan that is effective for the patient.

COMPLICATIONS

In general, diabetic patients are susceptible to two types of complications: short-term, or acute, problems and long-term problems.

◆ Short-Term Problems

Acute complications arise when the blood glucose suddenly becomes either too high (hyperglycemia) or too low (hypoglycemia; Table 25-5 and Table 25-10). Ketoacidosis is treated with fluids, insulin, and correction of electrolyte imbalances. Electrolytes and serum glucose are monitored closely. When a patient is admitted to the hospital with hyperglycemia, decisions about the proper modes of therapy are based on whether the patient has type I or type II diabetes and the objective and subjective symptoms presented. Type I diabetes is more likely to be complicated by ketoacidosis, whereas type II diabetics may suffer hyperglycemic hyperosmolar nonketotic syndrome (HHNS, HHNC, HNKC, and HHNK are common abbreviations).

Diabetic Ketoacidosis Diabetic ketoacidosis is a serious condition caused by incomplete metabolism of fats due to the absence or an insufficient supply of insulin. When insulin is not present in adequate amounts to meet metabolic needs, the body breaks down proteins

TABLE 25-13 ◆ *Patient Education: Working with Elderly Diabetic Patients*

The following guidelines are helpful when teaching elderly patients:

- Set a time for the teaching session that is agreeable to the patient.
- Arrange a quiet, nondistracting environment for the session.
- Be certain that the patient is comfortable before beginning.
- Keep the sessions short—no more than 15 to 20 minutes at a time.
- Limit information to a few major concepts per session.
- Go slowly and seek feedback that the patient has understood each point when finished presenting it.
- Allow time for the patient to jot down important points.
- Repeat key concepts frequently; if the patient does not understand, try rephrasing the concept.
- Use bold type printed materials with a white or yellow background.
- Leave printed materials that are illustrated with simple drawings and that are not crowded with text.
- Printed materials should be written at a 5th- to 10th-grade reading level depending on the patient.
- If the patient becomes frustrated or distracted, stop the session and reschedule it.
- Summarize what has been taught and what has been learned at the end of the session.

TABLE 25-14 ◆ *Patient Education: What to Do When Traveling*

Instruct the patient who will be away traveling to do the following:

♦ Carry extra medication or insulin in case a bottle gets lost or broken. Keep one set of pills or insulin with 48 hours of syringes in your purse, briefcase, or carry-on lugguage, along with your blood glucose–monitoring device.

♦ Wear a Medic-Alert bracelet or tag, and carry a medical information card in your purse or wallet.

♦ Carry an emergency supply of fast-acting sugar at all times in case of a hypoglycemic episode. Also carry longer-acting foods, such as peanut butter and crackers.

♦ Plan ahead at least 2 days for replenishing supplies for blood glucose monitoring, insulin, and syringes in case the correct items are hard to find in a foreign city. (It is best to take supplies with you for the entire time you will be gone.)

♦ If you become severely ill, seek medical attention immediately before you get into a dangerous condition.

♦ Stick to prescribed meal plans as well as possible, substituting available foods according to food group classification.

♦ Obtain sufficient rest and avoid stressful situations as much as possible to prevent stress-induced hyperglycemia.

♦ If you are a "brittle" diabetic, it is best to travel with someone who is familiar with your condition and treatment. It is best to advise the airline or ship personnel that you are diabetic when you embark.

♦ Obtain your usual amount of exercise or adjust food and medication intake accordingly.

♦ Drink a glass of water every 2 hours to prevent dehydration.

♦ Check your blood glucose level frequently.

♦ Obtain a letter from your physician stating that you have diabetes as well as extra prescriptions for your medications.

♦ Protect your insulin from temperature extremes.

♦ Eat something at least every 4 hours.

♦ Call airlines and ship companies ahead of departure to request diabetic meals.

♦ Research food substitutions for the type of food in the places you will be traveling before departure so that you will be able easily to accommodate your personal meal plan.

♦ Remember time zones: going westward lengthens your day; take more insulin. Going eastward shortens your day; take less insulin.

and fats for energy. This produces an abundance of the by-products of fat metabolism, which are potent organic acids called *ketones*. In an attempt to rid itself of the excess ketones, the body excretes some of them via the lungs. This produces a characteristic fruity odor to the breath. Acetone, a ketone body, is excreted in the urine, causing acetonuria or ketonuria. **As the kidney excretes excess glucose and ketones, it also eliminates large quantities of water and electrolytes. These pathological changes are responsible for metabolic acidosis, dehydration, and electrolyte imbalances.**

Signs and symptoms of diabetic ketoacidosis include hyperglycemia; thirst; abdominal pain; nausea and anorexia; vomiting; excessive urine output; alteration in level of consciousness; fruity odor to the breath; flushed face; rapid, thready pulse; hypotension; Kussmaul's respirations; and possibly coma.

Treatment of ketoacidosis is aimed at restoring normal pH of the blood and other body fluids, correcting the fluid and electrolyte imbalance, lowering the blood glucose level gradually, providing life-support measures as necessary if the patient is comatose, and eventually correcting the underlying cause of poor control of insulin-dependent diabetes.

Hyperglycemic Hyperosmolar Nonketotic Syndrome (HHNS)   Hyperglycemic hyperosmolar nonketotic syndrome, (HHNS) occurs in type II diabetics who are suffering an illness and experience high levels of blood glucose because of the illness or added stress. Glucose levels between 600 and 1,000 mg/dL are not unusual. **The extremely high levels of glucose in the blood precipitate severe dehydration** that results in circulating volume depletion. Blood osmolality is considerably elevated (>350 mOsm/kg). **Ketones and acidosis are absent.** Because ketosis and acidosis are absent, the gastrointestinal symptoms do not occur and the patient does not seek early medical care in the course of illness. The patient's mental state may progress from confusion to complete coma. In contrast to ketoacidosis, the patient may suffer generalized or focal seizures.

Elder Care Point...   Elderly patients are at greater risk for HHNS syndrome as they become dehydrated more quickly than the younger patient. HHNS may be the first indicator that the patient is diabetic. It most frequently occurs after a febrile illness or gastrointestinal flu in which the patient has stopped eating properly and possibly discontinued her oral hypoglycemic agent.

Things that may precipitate HHNS in a type II diabetic are (1) medications, such as steroids, thiazides, phenytoin, and beta-blockers; (2) acute illnesses, such as infection, myocardial infarction, and trauma; (3) chronic illnesses, such as cerebrovascular accident and psychiatric illnesses, such as dementia; (4) treatments, such as total parenteral nutrition and peritoneal dialysis.

Treatment focuses on fluid replacement and correction of electrolyte imbalances. Because fluid replacement will initially be quite rapid, the nurse must closely monitor cardiovascular status. Small amounts of insulin may be used until the patient is stabilized. Blood glucose and intake and output must be monitored closely. The underlying illness that triggered the HHNS is treated. HHNS can be fatal, and mortality is directly correlated with higher elevations of blood glucose.

Somogyi Phenomenon   Another condition sometimes encountered in patients with IDDM is the

TABLE 25-15 ◆ *Common Nursing Diagnoses, Expected Outcomes, and Nursing Interventions for Patients with Diabetes*

Nursing Diagnosis	Goals/Expected Outcomes	Nursing Interventions
Alteration in nutrition, less than (or more than) related to food and energy needs.	Patient will develop meal plan that will assist in maintaining normal weight and blood sugar within normal limits. Glycosylated hemoglobin levels will show compliance with dietary plan within 6 months.	Perform dietary assessment. Instruct in diabetic meal planning. Assist with construction of an acceptable meal plan for attaining desired weight and to normalize serum glucose levels.
Knowledge deficit related to disease process, possible complications, and self-care.	Patient will verbalize basic knowledge about disease process within 1 month. Patient will verbalize ways to prevent the complications of diabetes within 3 months. Patient will demonstrate proper foot care within 1 month. Patient will demonstrate knowledge of correct meal planning within 3 months.	Instruct patient about the disease process of diabetes. Instruct regarding the potential complications of diabetes and how to decrease the risk of complications. Instruct in proper foot care techniques. Instruct in meal planning. Instruct in insulin or oral medication administration. Seek feedback regarding material taught by verbalization and demonstration of skills.
Risk of infection related to elevated blood glucose level.	Patient will demonstrate blood glucose levels within acceptable limits within 1 month. Patient will demonstrate an absence of infection as evidenced by no signs of skin infection, absence of fever, and feeling of well-being.	Instruct in glucose monitoring technique appropriate to patient. Ask to chart blood glucose findings after testing. Instruct in signs of infection to report. Explain why diabetics are more prone to infection than the general public.
Risk for injury related to severe decrease in tissue perfusion in feet.	Patient will verbalize process of blood vessel deterioration that is caused by diabetes. Patient will demonstrate proper foot care technique. Patient will not experience amputation.	Explain how diabetes hastens arteriosclerosis and decreased circulation, especially in the feet. Verify that patient can perform correct foot care. Ascertain whether patient complies with need for daily foot assessment and proper self-care of feet. Praise for efforts at self-care. Encourage to report even minor injuries of the foot to the physician.
Ineffective individual coping related to denial of need for effective self-care.	Patient will express desire to prevent the complications of diabetes. Patient will express commitment to the self-care techniques that when regularly practiced can help decrease the risk of complications.	Assess usual coping methods for dealing with stress or adversity. Reinforce positive coping techniques. Refer to diabetes support group and/or diabetes educator. Monitor progress toward learning and using regular self-care techniques to prevent complications. When glycosylated hemoglobin levels indicate only fair or poor control of disease, explore problems patient may be having with diet, exercise, medication, or glucose testing. Reinforce teaching for self-care as needed. Offer praise and encouragement for all efforts at self-care and control of disease.

TABLE 25-15 ◆ *Common Nursing Diagnoses, Expected Outcomes, and Nursing Interventions for Patients with Diabetes* (Continued)		
Nursing Diagnosis	**Expected Outcomes**	**Nursing Interventions**
Sensory perceptual alteration related to effect of elevated blood glucose on nervous system.	Patient will use self-care techniques to prevent injury due to changes in sensation or vision.	Reinforce the importance of foot care if patient has reduced sensation in the feet. Encourage at least yearly opthalmological exams. Institute measures to prevent bladder infection if patient experiences neurogenic bladder. Increase fluid intake; encourage timed toileting. Institute measures to counteract constipation if neurological bowel problems occur. Increase fluid and fiber within meal plan.
Sexual dysfunction related to effect of elevated blood glucose on nervous system.	Patient will explore treatment for impotence. Female patient will seek treatment for frequent vaginal infections that interfere with pleasure of intercourse.	Explain that taking a concentrated glucose source such as 5 to 6 Life-savers before attempting intercourse may cure the problem of inability to maintain an erection in the earlier phases of diabetes. Advise of the availability of penile injections or use of a vacuum suction device to achieve and maintain an erection. Provide information on how to obtain information and prescriptions for these measures. Assess female for vaginal infection; advise to seek treatment. Instruct on ways to prevent further infections. Advise couple on means other than intercourse to satisfy sexual needs.
Self-esteem disturbance related to diagnosis of chronic disease requiring lifestyle changes or insulin injections for survival.	Patient will verbalize own strengths within 1 month. Patient will express that control over the disease and life is possible.	Encourage verbalization of feelings related to diagnosis of diabetes and need for lifestyle changes. Allow expression of frustrations. Encourage exploration of strengths and positive measures of self-worth; i.e., roles, accomplishments. Explain how control over disease and life is possible. Provide the knowledge and tools to achieve control. Praise efforts at learning and practice of self-care techniques.

Somogyi phenomenon, a rebound hyperglycemia resulting from overtreatment with insulin. This rebound follows a period of hypoglycemia. When hypoglycemia occurs, the body secretes glucagon, epinephrine, growth hormone and cortisol to counteract the effects of low blood sugar. This increase in circulating hormones with falling insulin levels and the rise in glucose production from the liver raises blood glucose excessively. Insulin resistance also may occur for 12 to 48 hours because of the action of the released hormones. Often the Somogyi phenomenon occurs when unrecognized hypoglycemia occurs during sleep. By morning, when the patient checks her blood glucose, the released hormones have caused elevated serum glucose. The insulin dose increases and this just worsens the problem. **The patient may report nightmares and night sweats along with morning elevated serum glucose and ketones in the urine.**

When this phenomenon occurs, the blood glucose should be measured between 2 A.M. and 4 A.M. and again at 7 A.M. If the blood glucose is low (i.e., 50 to 60 mg/dL) and then is more than 189 to 200 mg/dL at 7 A.M., the Somogyi phenomenon is occurring. Effective treatment usually is to lower the insulin dosage or to move the time of the intermediate-acting insulin to bedtime. Changing or increasing the bedtime snack also helps.

Whenever a diabetic person is subjected to additional stress, as in an unrelated medical illness or when surgery is necessary, her metabolic needs change, and thus the delicate balance between hyperglycemia and hypoglycemia is threatened.

Hypoglycemia   The word *hypoglycemia* means low blood glucose. Hypoglycemia is a rather common complication of type I diabetes mellitus. Most often it is a response to either too large a dose of insulin or too much exercise in relation to the amount of food eaten. **Signs and symptoms of hypoglycemia include tremulousness, hunger, headache, pallor, sweating, palpitations, blurred vision, and weakness; symptoms may progress to confusion and loss of consciousness.** Individual reactions vary considerably. Some patients are alert with a glucose level of 40 mg/dL, and others are comatose.

Treatment depends on the degree of hypoglycemia and level of consciousness. If the patient can take oral feedings, glucose levels of 40 to 60 mg/dL respond to ingestion of food such as milk, crackers, or 4 oz of orange juice. Glucose levels of 20 to 40 mg/dL respond best to concentrated sugars, such as honey, table sugar, or juice. In the hospital, if the person is experiencing seizures or is comatose as a result of severe hypoglycemia or has a very low blood sugar, a solution of 50% glucose is given IV. When an IV access cannot be established, 1 mg of glucagon is administered. The injection is repeated in 15 minutes if symptoms are not resolved.

When there is doubt as to whether the patient is suffering from hyperglycemia or hypoglycemia, treatment is begun for hypoglycemia until a blood glucose determination is obtained to prevent brain damage from extremely low cerebral glucose levels.

Diabetic patients must be taught to monitor themselves for beginning signs of hypoglycemia and always to carry a source of concentrated sugar with them to be taken if the symptoms occur. Glucose tablets or Lifesavers are easily portable sources of glucose.

◆ Long-Term Problems

The long-term consequences of diabetes mellitus are chiefly the result of damage to the large and small blood vessels. There is no doubt that elevated blood glucose levels over a period of years will seriously damage blood vessels and the organs they serve. Diabetes remains among the three leading causes of death in the United States, the other two being cardiovascular disease and cancer. In addition, cardiovascular disease and other causes of death often can be attributed to diabetes.

Patients who have had diabetes for more than 10 years are likely to develop one or more of the complications of the disease. The less closely the blood glucose has been controlled, the more likely the development of cardiovascular, eye, and renal complications. Although not every diabetic person will suffer from long-term

complications, many will be hospitalized for one reason or another in some later stage of the disease.

Cardiovascular Disease   Thickening of the vessels occurs when blood glucose is elevated over a long time. The basement membrane grows thicker. The vessels of the retina, renal glomeruli, peripheral nerves, muscles, and skin are affected. Larger vessels also are affected, which predisposes the patient to atherosclerosis and vascular occlusion. **A person with diabetes has a 50% higher chance of suffering from heart disease or stroke than does a nondiabetic person.** About half of all diabetics suffer premature death from myocardial infarction; the survival time for those diabetics whose first heart attack was not fatal is about 50% less than that of nondiabetic heart attack victims.

Nephropathy   Diabetic *nephropathy* (disease of the kidney) occurs directly from changes in the renal blood circulation. As damage from inadequate blood circulation is done, the patient experiences signs of renal failure. Researchers at Tel-Aviv University have discovered that Enalopril (Vasotec) 10 mg a day may be beneficial for those at risk of nephropathy. It seems to slow the blood vessel changes. Proteinuria (protein in the urine) and hypertension are early signs of renal failure.

Micro-Bumintest strips can alert patients to extremely small quantities of albumin in the urine. A reading greater than 2 μcg/minute may signal the onset of renal complications. This can provide the patient with an opportunity to become more aggressive about diabetes treatment and thereby slow the vascular deterioration. A large percentage of diabetics develop chronic renal failure and are on renal dialysis. Perhaps with albumin monitoring and more aggressive therapy, the need for dialysis can be averted.

Peripheral Vascular Disease   Gangrene, which often necessitates amputation, is 40 to 50 times more common in diabetic persons. Vascular changes frequently cause very poor circulation in the feet and lower extremities. Healing of wounds in these areas is difficult because of the poor blood supply and also because increased levels of glucose in the blood provide a good medium for bacterial growth, making it harder to eradicate infection. Learning and practicing excellent foot care are essential to prevent eventual amputation.

Retinopathy   Visual impairment and blindness are common sequelae of diabetes mellitus. **The three most common problems are diabetic retinopathy, cataracts, and glaucoma.** Retinal damage, which can cause visual impairment and blindness, occurs in most diabetics within 10 years of diagnosis. Changes in the retinal vessels lead to hemorrhages and also to retinal detachment. Recent surgical techniques using photocoagulation of destructive lesions of the retina with laser beams now offer hope for preserving sight by preventing further progress of diabetic retinopathy. Good glucose control, frequent eye examinations, and treatment can help preserve vision.

Neuropathy   Pathological changes in the nervous system cause deterioration, with symptoms such as paresthesia, numbness, and loss of function. Diabetic neuropathies primarily affect the peripheral nerves, causing sexual impotence in the male, constipation, neurogenic bladder, and pain or anesthesia (lack of feeling) in the lower extremities. It is for this reason that foot care and daily inspection of the feet are so important. Because the patient often cannot feel cuts, blisters, or abrasions on the foot, there is great danger that a neglected sore might become infected. The patient typically experiences an anesthesia beginning about 10 years after onset of diabetes. There eventually may be almost total anesthesia of the affected part, bringing with it the potential for serious injury to the patient without her being aware of it. In contrast, some patients experience debilitating pain and hyperesthesia; some lose deep-tendon reflexes. Other problems related to diabetic neuropathies are the result of autonomic nervous system involvement. These include orthostatic hypotension, delayed gastric emptying, diarrhea or constipation, and asymptomatic retention of urine in the bladder.

Impotence often can be helped by using a vacuum device such as Erec Aid. With this device most men can obtain and maintain an erection and achieve orgasm during intercourse. These devices have greatly improved the quality of life for diabetic men.

Prevention of the potentially devastating long-term consequences of diabetes is a major goal of management. Preventive measures related to heart disease, stroke, and peripheral vascular disease are discussed in Chapter 18. Tight control of blood glucose levels is especially beneficial in preventing pathological changes in the small blood vessels serving the kidneys, thereby preventing renal failure. Care of patients with urological disorders is discussed in Chapter 23.

Research is in progress at Colorado State University to determine whether a deficiency of insulin-like growth factor (IGF) may be the key in preventing diabetic neuropathy. Someday replacement therapy with IGF may prevent or relieve this common diabetic complication.

Elder Care Point . . . Diabetic patients in the sixth, seventh, or eighth decade are more likely to have developed complications of the disease. Hypertension and renal insufficiency or renal failure are common problems. Failing vision from retinopathy is very common and causes problems with insulin administration as well as self-care. Total blindness occurs in many patients.

Cardiovascular problems occur in the normal population in these age groups and are compounded for those with diabetes mellitus. There is a much higher incidence of stroke and myocardial infarction in those with diabetes. Peripheral vascular disease and infection lead to amputation of the toes or foot in approximately 50,000 diabetics per year. Neuropathy is yet another complication, leading to bladder and bowel problems as well as limb numbness and paralysis, especially of the legs.

HYPOGLYCEMIA

Diagnosis   A low blood glucose state can exist whenever the homeostatic mechanisms designed to maintain blood glucose within a rather narrow range fail to function as they should. The organs involved in meeting the challenge of carbohydrate ingestion include the intestines, liver, and pancreas (specifically, the beta-cells that produce insulin). Thus any condition affecting these organs and their systems can lead to hypoglycemia. Examples other than diabetes mellitus include gastrectomy and surgical bypass procedures. These types of surgery provide more rapid access of glucose to the absorptive sites in the small bowel. Tumors of the pancreas (insulinomas), liver disease, and disorders of the adrenal cortex and pituitary gland can produce abnormally low blood glucose levels. Alcoholics and drug addicts also are prone to hypoglycemia.

Functional hypoglycemia, for which there is no known cause, may be a very early indicator of diabetes mellitus. In fact, studies have shown that almost one-third of the people who have functional hypoglycemia may eventually develop diabetes if the hypoglycemia is not effectively controlled.

Reactive and spontaneous hypoglycemia. The pathophysiology of hypoglycemia and its attendant symptoms are quite different after eating from what they are in a fasting state. These differences are the basis for classifying the disorder into *hypoglycemia in the fed state* (also called *reactive hypoglycemia*) and *hypoglycemia in the fasting state (spontaneous hypoglycemia)*. Reactive hypoglycemia has been the subject of the most debate about its cause, effect, and treatment. The term *hypoglycemia* often is mistakenly used to explain symptoms that may or may not be indicative of reactive hypoglycemia. These symptoms include rapid heart beat, tremulousness, weakness, anxiety, nervousness, and hunger, and they occur rather suddenly several hours after carbohydrates are eaten. The diagnosis of reactive hypoglycemia is very difficult to confirm, as abnormally low blood glucose levels often cannot be demonstrated.

Treatment   Treatment of hypoglycemia is through modifying eating patterns. Smaller and more frequent meals that are relatively free of simple sugars are recommended. The diet should be high in proteins and low in carbohydrates, and carbohydrates should be complex ones such as those found in fruits, vegetables, and whole grains. Refined sugar and white flour are omitted. Cases in which gastric surgery and intestinal bypass are believed to be the cause of hypoglycemia may be treated with drugs that reduce intestinal motility.

Nursing Assessment and Intervention   One of the most unfortunate consequences of hypoglycemia from any cause is that the physiological symptoms may be mistaken for indications of a psychiatric illness. These symptoms include irritability, personality change, temper tantrums, and other psychoneurotic manifestations.

Nurses are in an excellent position to observe and help identify patients who might be hypoglycemic. In addition to information about her physical and mental symptoms, assessment should include a rather detailed history of the patient's eating habits. Does she eat regularly? How often during each day? What kinds of foods constitute a typical meal for her? Does she crave sweets? Has she had episodes of weakness, sweating, visual disturbances, and confusion or inability to concentrate? If these symptoms have occurred, when are they most noticeable (that is, in a fed or fasting state)?

Nursing interventions for patients with hypoglycemia include explaining the nature of the disorder and the need for diagnostic testing to confirm or rule out reactive hypoglycemia, objective and nonjudgmental observation and reporting of symptoms, and reinforcement of dietary instruction and restrictions.

COMMUNITY CARE

There is a great need for home care and monitoring of the diabetic elderly population. If nurses could follow the progress of these patients over the years with good assessments, the incidence of complications could probably be decreased. As the national trend shifts toward preventive medicine and health care, perhaps the funds for such a program will be forthcoming.

Long-term care nurses must be alert to the signs of diabetes in their residents. When a resident does not properly recover from a viral illness, in-depth assessment for signs of diabetes is wise.

Home care and clinic nurses must be persistent in assessing compliance with diabetic regimes and instrumental in teaching the public about the signs and symptoms of diabetes and the measures for self-care to prevent complications. Far too many diabetic patients do not understand the ramifications of poor control of their disease. Presently, diabetes is costing the United States over $1 billion a year in health care expenditures. This is one area in which nurses could be instrumental in cutting health care costs.

CRITICAL THINKING EXERCISES

Clinical Case Problems

Read each clinical situation and discuss the questions with your classmates.

1. Mrs. Lopez is 42 years old and has had non-insulin-dependent diabetes mellitus (NIDDM) for the past 10 years. She is admitted to the hospital for treatment of an infection of the great toe on her left foot, which is the result of improper care of an ingrown toenail. She is 45 pounds overweight and admits to frequent binges of eating foods not on her diet. She does not exercise regularly because she says the housework she does gives her enough exercise. When asked about the oral antidiabetic agent and diet that have been prescribed for her, she tells you that she only takes her medicine and follows her diet most of the time.

   a. Devise a specific teaching plan for Mrs. Lopez to help her manage her illness better.

   b. What could you suggest to Mrs. Lopez to help her lose weight?

   c. What do you think might motivate Mrs. Lopez to accept more responsibility for managing her illness?

   d. What laboratory testing would be recommended to track Mrs. Lopez' compliance with her treatment regimen?

2. Mr. Tobin is a 22-year-old construction worker who has recently experienced fatigue, excessive thirst and urination, and weight loss. A routine urinalysis revealed glycosuria and a trace of acetone. His physician has arranged for Mr. Tobin to have an oral glucose tolerance test to determine whether he has diabetes mellitus.

   a. What is the significance of the findings of the routine urinalysis?

   b. What is involved in an oral glucose tolerance test?

   c. If Mr. Tobin is found to have insulin-dependent diabetes mellitus, what kinds of information will he need to manage his illness?

   d. How would you explain the importance of good or tight control of his blood glucose levels to Mr. Tobin?

   e. What criteria could be used to determine whether his diabetes is under control?

3. Mr. Smith, a 76-year-old male, has recently been diagnosed with NIDDM. It has been difficult to control his blood sugar and his physician has added insulin to his treatment regimen. Mr. Smith was issued a glucometer by the hospital, but says that the test strips are too expensive for him to buy very

often. Mr. Smith lives alone, cooks for himself, and likes a glass of wine with dinner. Other than an occasional fishing trip, he does not exercise regularly.

a. How would you approach a teaching program for this patient?

b. What resources could you suggest that might assist him to purchase the test strips for the glucometer?

c. How can a glass of wine be incorporated into an acceptable diabetic meal plan?

d. What sort of exercise program could you recommend to this gentleman?

BIBLIOGRAPHY

American Diabetes Association. (1994). Nutrition recommendations and principles for people with diabetes mellitus. *Diabetes Care.* 17(5):519–522.

American Journal of Nursing. (1996). Newdrugs: acarbose (Precose): a new approach to diabetes control. *American Journal of Nursing.* 96 (4):57–58.

American Journal of Nursing. (1995). Newdrugs: Metformin (glucophage): a different kind of oral diabetes drug. *American Journal of Nursing.* 95 (9):57–58.

Anderson, L., Bruner, L. A., Satterfield, D. (1995). Diabetes control programs: New directions. *The Diabetes Educator.* 21(5):432–437.

Applegate, E. J. (1995). *The Anatomy and Physiology Learning System: Textbook.* Philadelphia: Saunders.

Arbour, R. (1994). Acute hypoglycemia: responding quickly to prevent hypoglycemic seizures. *Nursing 94.* 24(1):33.

Bak, L. B., Heard, K. A., Kearney, G. P. (1996). Tube feeding your diabetic patient safely. *American Journal of Nursing.* 96(12):47–49.

Bennett, J. C., Plum, F., eds. (1996). *Cecil Textbook of Medicine,* 20th ed. Philadelphia: Saunders.

Berry, R., Mohn, K.R., Holzmeister, L. A. (1995). Monioring diabetes therapy. *Home Healthcare Nurse.* 13(1): 39–42.

Bodzin, B. J. (1997). Type II (Noninsulin-Dependent) diabetes: new treatment options. *Home Healthcare Nurse.* 15(1):41–47.

Caffrey, R. M. (1996). Diabetes update and implications for care. *Home Healthcare Nurse.* 14(10):756–766.

Cirone, N. (1996). Diabetes in the elderly, Part I: Unmasking a hidden disorder. *Nursing 96.* 26(3):34–39.

Cirone, N., Schwartz, N. (1996). Diabetes in the Elderly Part II: Finding the balance for drug therapy. *Nursing 96.* 26(3):40–45.

Conti, S. F., Chaytor, E. R. (1995). Foot care for active patients who have diabetes. *The Physician and Sportsmedicine.* 23(6):53–54, 56, 61, 65, 68.

Conti, S. F., Chaytor, E. R. (1995). Steps to healthy feet for active people with diabetes. *The Physician and sportsmedicine.* 23(6):71–72.

Copstead, L. C. (1995). *Perspectives on Pathophysiology.* Philadelphia: Saunders.

Cotran, R. S., Kumar, V., Robbins, S. L., Schoen, F. J., eds. (1994). *Robbins Pathologic Basis of Disease,* 5th ed. Philadelphia: Saunders.

Davis, J., Sherer, K. (1994). *Applied Nutrition and Diet Therapy for Nurses,* 2nd ed. Philadelphia: Saunders.

Deakins, D. A. (1994). Teaching elderly patients about diabetes. *American Journal of Nursing.* 94(4):38–42.

deWit, S. C. (1994). *Rambo's Nursing Skills for Clinical Practice,* 4th ed. Philadelphia: Saunders.

Dorgan, M. B., et al. (1995). Performing foot screening for diabetic patients. *American Journal of Nursing.* 95(11): 32–36.

Dowdell, H. R. (1995). Diabetes and vascular disease: a common association. *AACN Clinical Issues: Advanced Practice in Acute and Critical Care.* 6(4):526–535.

Drass, J. A. (1996). Caring for patients with insulin-dependent diabetes mellitus. *Nursing 96.* 26(8):46–47.

Drass, J. A. (1996). Caring for patients with non-insulin dependent diabetes mellitus. *Nursing 96.* 26(9):48–49.

Drass, J. (1995). Insulin injections. *C. E. Test Handbook.* Vol 6:75–78.

Drass, J. A., Peterson, A. (1996). Type II diabetes: exploring treatment options. *American Journal of Nursing.* 96(11): 45–49.

Fishman, T. D., Freedline, A. D., and Kahn, D. (1996). Putting the best foot forward. *Nursing 96.* 26(1):58–60.

Gaedeke, M. K. (1995). Lab test tips. Evaluating glycosylated hemoglobin. *Nursing 95.* 25(2):31.

Goldharn, R. E. (1996). I'm a born again diabetic. *RN.* 59(12):33–35.

Guthrie, D. W., Guthrie, R. A. (1991). *Nursing Management of Diabetes Mellitus,* 3rd ed. New York: Springer.

Guyton, A. C., Hall, J. E. (1996). *Textbook of Medical Physiology,* 9th ed. Philadelphia: Saunders.

Harris, M. D. (1995). Medicare and the nurse. Current research findings related to individuals with diabetes mellitus. *Home Healthcare Nurse.* 13(1):79–81.

Hempy, A. (1995). Caring for the home-bound elderly client with diabetes mellitus. *Journal of Home Health Care Practice.* 7(2):56–61.

Hogue, J. K., Kinahan, J. J., Delcher, H. K. (1996). A hospital-based home health diabetes education model. *Home Healthcare Nurse.* 14(5):373–377.

Holzmeister, L. A. (1996). Diabetes: nutrition therapy in homecare. *Home Healthcare Nurse.* 14(3):179–184.

Hoyson, P. M. (1995). Diabetes 2000: oral medications. *RN.* 58(5):34–38.

Ignatavicius, D. D., Workman, M. L., Mishler, M. A. (1995). *Medical–Surgical Nursing: A Nursing Process Approach,* 2nd ed. Philadelphia: Saunders.

Jonaitis, M. A. (1995). Diabetes 2000: complications during pregnancy. *RN.* 58(10):40–44.

Kestel, F. (1994). Are you up to date on diabetes medications? *American Journal of Nursing.* 94(7):48–52

Lehne, R. A. (1994). *Pharmacology for Nursing Care,* 2nd ed. Philadelphia: Saunders.

LeMone, P. (1996). Differentiating and treating altered glycemic responses. (1996). 5(4):257–261.

Lilley, L. L., Guanci, R. (1997). Knowing your antidiaetic agents. *American Journal of Nursing.* 97(1): 12–14.

Matteson, M. A., McConnell, E. S., Linton, A. D. (1997). *Gerontological Nursing: Concepts and Practice,* 2nd ed. Philadelphia: W. B. Saunders.

McConnell, E. A. (1997). Monitoring blood glucose levels at the bedside. *Nursing 97.* 27(4):28.

Norton, R. A. (1995). Diabetes 2000: the right mix of diet and exercise. *RN.* 58(4):20–24.

O'Hanlon-Nichols, T. (1996). Clinical snapshot: hyperglycemic hyperosmolar nonketotic syndrome. *American Journal of Nursing.* 96(3):38–39.

Parker, C. (1994). Responding quickly to hypoglycemia. *American Journal of Nursing.* 94(6):46.

Peragallo-Dittko, V. (1995). Diabetes 2000: acute complications. *RN.* 58(8):36–40.

Polaski, A. L., and Tatro, S. E. (1996). *Luckmann's Core Principles and Practice of Medical–Surgical Nursing.* Philadelphia: Saunders.

Reising, D. L. (1995). Acute hypoglycemia: keeping the bottom from falling out. *Nursing 95.* 25(2):41–48, 50.

Reising, D. L. (1995). Acute hyperglycemia: putting a lid on the crisis. *Nursing 95.* 25(2):33–40, 49.

Robertson, C., (1995). Diabetes 2000: chronic complications. *RN.* 58(4):34–40.

Robertson, C., Cerrato, P. L. (1993). Managing diabetes: a major study injects good news. *RN.* 56(10):26–29. *RN.* 58(9):34–40.

Savinetti-Rose, B., Bolmer, L. (1997). Understanding continuous subcutaneous insulin infusion therapy. *American Journal of Nursing.* 97(3):42–48.

Shapiro, M., Stegall, M. D. (1995). Diabetes 2000: when insulin isn't enough. *RN.* 58(7):34–36.

Springhouse Corporation. (1996). *Nursing 96 Drug Handbook.* Springhouse, PA: author.

Steil, C. F., Deakins, D. E. (1995). Oral hypoglycemics. *C. E. Test Handbook,* Vol. 6:69–74.

Strowig, S. (1995). Diabetes 2000: insulin therapy. *RN.* 58(6):30–36.

Tomky, D. (1995). Diabetes 2000: advances in monitoring. *RN.* 58(3):37–44.

Wilson, J. P. (1995). New diabetes nutrition guidelines: do you know the score? *Nursing 95.* 25(7):65–66.

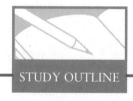

STUDY OUTLINE

I. Diabetes Mellitus

A. Diabetes is defined as a complex group of disorders that have in common a disturbance in metabolism and use of glucose that results from a malfunction of the beta-cells of the pancreas.

B. Beta-cells in the islets of Langerhans in the pancreas secrete insulin and glucagon.

C. The types of diabetes are summarized in Table 25-1.

   1. Type I diabetes, called insulin-dependent diabetes mellitus (IDDM) generally occurs at an earlier age than type II and causes more instances of serious complications.

   2. Type II diabetes, called non-insulin-dependent diabetes mellitus (NIDDM), usually occurs after age 30 and affects about 90% of the diabetic population.

D. Contributing factors.

   1. Genetic: tends to run in families (genetic predisposition); gene has not been identified yet.

   2. Metabolic: obesity, emotional and physical stress.

   3. Microbiological: some cases of IDDM related to viral infections.

   4. Immunological: IDDM thought to be an autoimmune disorder because of islet cell antibodies found in the blood of about 75% of diabetics.

E. Incidence and prevalence.

   1. Incidence increasing at an alarming rate; currently there are about 16 million diabetics in the United States.

   2. Increasing incidence can be explained in part by improved methods of case finding and reporting.

F. Symptoms and medical diagnosis: see Table 25-2.

   1. Classic symptoms: polydipsia, polyuria, polyphagia.

   2. Fatigue, muscle weakness, weight loss, ketoacidosis found in IDDM.

   3. Weight gain common in NIDDM.

   4. Frequent and slow-healing infections, proneness to vascular disease.

G. Diagnostic tests (Table 25-3).

1. Fasting blood glucose levels above normal are indications for further assessment and testing.

2. Fasting blood and urine samples taken, then patient given large amount of glucose. Samples taken after 30 minutes and then at hourly intervals for up to 4 hours. Point system used to avoid misinterpretation of blood and urine values.

3. 2-hour postprandial blood glucose test can indicate need for glucose tolerance test.

4. Glycosylated hemoglobin (hemoglobin A$_{1c}$) is not a diagnostic test. Gives information about average blood glucose levels over period of 2 to 3 months. Useful in determining effectiveness of prescribed protocol for diabetes management.

H. Management of diabetes.

1. Strict control decreases risk of nerve, vascular, and eye complications.

2. In general, good control indicated by:

a. Fasting blood sugars within normal limits.

b. Hemoglobin A$_{1c}$ indicating average blood glucose within normal range.

c. Weight staying within normal range.

d. Serum lipids within acceptable range.

e. Patient having sense of health and well-being.

3. Diet: prescribed for individual patient.

a. Intended to provide adequate nutrition from each of major food groups.

b. Patient must learn to use food exchange list or other dietary planning system.

c. Patient encouraged to avoid concentrated sweets, excess fats in diet.

4. Exercise: patient encouraged to follow a program of regular exercise daily.

a. Helps metabolize glucose.

b. Makes insulin receptors more sensitive to insulin.

c. Helps lower serum lipid levels.

d. Patient will need instruction in precautions to take during exercise, especially if she has IDDM.

5. Insulin: types shown in Table 25-6.

a. Type of insulin not to be confused with strength, which usually is 100 units of insulin per milliliter (U100).

b. Insulin must be given by injection.

c. Dosage varies according to patient need. Some may require two or more daily injections of two types.

d. Patient or family member will need instruction in how to administer insulin. Insulin

pump: a system for delivering continuous infusion of insulin. Recommended only for selected patients.

6. Synthetic hypoglycemic agents (oral antidiabetic drugs) sometimes prescribed for NIDDM patients.

a. Not an oral form of insulin.

b. Examples: Dymelor, Diabinase, Tolinase, Orinase, Diabeta, Micronase, and Glucotrol, Glugophage, Precose.

c. Sulfonylureas, akin to sulfa antibiotics.

(1) Lower blood glucose by stimulating beta-cells to produce insulin.

(2) Inhibit glucose production.

(3) Facilitate transport of glucose into cell.

(4) Increase number of receptor sites.

d. Certain drugs enhance the action of oral antidiabetic agents, whereas others inhibit their action.

e. Patient receiving oral antidiabetic drugs will require instruction in how to take the drug and how to avoid drug-to-drug interactions.

II. Nursing Management

A. Nursing assessment.

1. Every patient should be assessed for signs of diabetes mellitus.

2. General assessment should include questions about family history of diabetes, weight loss, increased hunger, thirst, or urination, poor wound healing, and fatigue (see Table 25-10).

3. Patients known to be diabetic should be assessed for signs of complications.

4. Assessment of performance on blood glucose monitoring and of technique for insulin injection should be done.

B. Common nursing diagnoses for diabetic patients.

1. Alteration in nutrition, less than (or more than) body requirements.

2. Knowledge deficit.

3. Risk for infection.

4. Ineffective individual coping.

5. Sensory perceptual alteration.

6. Sexual dysfunction.

7. Risk for injury related to severe decrease in tissue perfusion in feet.

8. Self-esteem disturbance.

9. Many other nursing diagnoses become appropriate as the patient experiences the many complications of the disease.

C. Planning.

1. Consideration of times for glucose monitoring should be incorporated into the daily work schedule.

2. Glucose monitoring and insulin injections should be scheduled in relation to the time meal trays are delivered in the hospital and extended care facility.

3. When a patient is NPO for diagnostic tests, monitoring for signs of hypoglycemia is necessary.

4. When the patient is undergoing added stress from illness or surgery, the nurse must monitor for hyperglycemia.

5. All insulin doses should be verified by another nurse for accuracy when drawn up.

6. Expected outcomes are written based on the chosen nursing diagnoses and the specific patient needs.

D. Nursing interventions are geared toward assisting the patient with self-care, monitoring blood glucose, administering medication, observing for signs and symptoms of complications, assessing learning needs, and carrying out a teaching plan (see Table 25-15).

1. The trend of blood glucose readings over time should be monitored.

2. Food and fluid intake should be checked.

3. Electrolytes, especially potassium, should be checked to see that they are within normal limits.

4. The patient should be monitored for hypoglycemia after insulin injections.

5. Monitoring for early signs of ketoacidosis also is essential: polyuria, fatigue, anorexia, abdominal pain, dehydration, irritability.

6. Patient education: an extremely important component of management.

   a. The patient must learn enough about her disease and treatment to take charge of her own care. Topics to be covered include:

      (1) Blood glucose monitoring.

      (2) Urine testing for acetone when blood glucose is 200 mg/dL.

      (3) Pathophysiology of diabetes mellitus.

      (4) Type of medication, side effects, and method of administration (insulin injections).

      (5) Signs and symptoms of hyperglycemia and hypoglycemia and treatment.

      (6) Skin and foot care.

      (7) Diet planning and adherence.

      (8) Balance of diet, exercise, and medication.

      (9) Need for ID tag.

      (10) What to do on sick days (Table 25-12).

      (11) Pointers for traveling (Table 25-14).

      (12) Community resources and help groups available.

      (13) Devices that make insulin preparation and administration easier.

      (14) Need for close medical follow-up.

7. American Diabetes Association and American Dietetic Association and their local chapters and pharmaceutical companies are excellent sources of information for patient education.

E. Evaluation.

1. Evaluation is performed to determine whether expected outcomes are being met.

2. Monitoring glycosylated hemoglobin values and blood glucose reading trends helps determine whether the patient is compliant with therapy.

3. Observing demonstrations of learned skills evaluates the effectiveness of teaching.

4. Plan may need revision if expected outcomes are not being met; revision is by collaboration with physician and dietitian.

III. Complications

1. Short-term problems.

   a. Hyperglycemia and hypoglycemia: symptoms, causes, prevention, and treatment summarized in Tables 25-5 and 25-10.

   b. Diabetic ketoacidosis: caused by incomplete oxidation of fats with resultant accumulation of organic acids (ketones) in the urine.

      (1) Symptoms include fruity odor to breath, acetonuria, and signs and symptoms of acidosis and fluid and electrolyte imbalances.

      (2) Treatment aimed at restoring normal blood pH, correcting fluid and electrolyte imbalances, and treating underlying cause.

   c. Somogyi phenomenon: a rebound hyperglycemia caused by administration of too much insulin.

   d. Hypoglycemia: response to too much insulin (insulin reaction) or too much exercise in relation to food intake.

      (1) Signs and symptoms: tremulousness, hunger, headache, pallor, sweating, palpitations, weakness, and blurred vision.

      (2) May progress to confusion and unconsciousness.

      (3) Treated with a form of glucose.

      (4) Glucagon is an alternative treatment.

   e. Hyperglycemic hyperosmolar nonketotic syndrome (HHNS).

      (1) Occurs in NIDDM, especially elderly patients.

      (2) Is life-threatening and is fatal about 30% of the time.

(3) Often brought on by illness, such as gastrointestinal flu or febrile illness that causes dehydration.

(4) Glucose levels between 600 mg/dL and 1,000 mg/dL are not unusual.

(5) Medications such as steroids, thiazides, phenytoin, and beta-blockers may cause the disorder in some patients.

(6) Treatment is with fluid replacement, small amounts of insulin, and electrolyte replacement as needed.

2. Long-term consequences are chiefly the result of atherosclerotic changes and damage to large and small blood vessels.

   a. Diabetes is among the three most common causes of death in the United States.

   b. Cardiovascular disease: a person with diabetes has a 50% higher chance of suffering from heart disease or stroke than does a nondiabetic person. About half of all diabetic persons die from heart attack, and those who survive live about half as long as others after heart attack.

   c. Nephropathy: large percentage of patients on renal dialysis are diabetic.

   d. Peripheral vascular disease: gangrene is 40 to 50 times more prevalent among diabetics.

   e. Neuropathy: can lead to impotence, neurogenic bladder, and pain or loss of feeling in the lower extremities.

   f. Retinopathy: can cause visual impairment and blindness.

3. Stages of diabetes mellitus vary in relation to complications.

   a. Stage I: no ketoacidosis or other complications, but blood glucose is above normal.

   b. Stage II: diabetes with infection, acetone in serum, retinopathy, and other complications.

   c. Stage III: diabetes with acidosis and coma, retinopathy and loss of vision, or azotemia.

IV. Hypoglycemia

A. Disturbance of glucose metabolism resulting in abnormally low blood glucose levels.

B. Failure to meet the challenge of carbohydrate ingestion can occur.

   1. Following intestinal surgery.

   2. In tumors of the pancreas.

   3. In liver disease.

   4. In disorders of the adrenal cortex and pituitary.

C. Alcoholics and drug addicts also prone to hypoglycemia.

D. Functional hypoglycemia: no known cause.

E. Fasting hypoglycemia: result of insufficient intake of glucose.

F. Reactive hypoglycemia (person in a fed state): the most controversial type.

   1. Diagnosed only when symptoms are correlated with abnormally low blood glucose levels as determined by extended glucose tolerance test.

   2. Treatment.

      a. Patient placed on diet of complex sugars, high-protein foods; refined sugar and starches restricted or omitted.

      b. Persons with abnormally rapid passage of food through the bowel may also be given medications to decrease motility.

   3. Nursing assessment and intervention.

      a. Recognize physiological, psychological, and emotional symptoms of hypoglycemia.

      b. Assess patient's eating habits thoroughly.

      c. Explain nature of illness and need for testing to confirm a diagnosis.

      d. Reinforce dietary instruction and restrictions.

V. Elder Care Points

A. Blood glucose levels rise with age.

B. Type II diabetes has its onset in adulthood and often is not discovered until the sixth or seventh decade.

C. Older patients have difficulty adjusting to the diet, medication, and exercise routine.

D. Financial constraints sometimes make it difficult to obtain needed food and medicine.

E. By the sixth, seventh, and eighth decades, many diabetics have developed the complications of the disease: kidney failure, visual impairment, neuropathy, and severe cardiovascular and peripheral vascular disease.

F. Elderly develop hypoglycemia more quickly than a younger person, making tight control of diabetes difficult and often undesirable.

G. Severe hypoglycemia in the elderly patient may precipitate myocardial infarction, angina, stroke, or seizures.

H. Older NIDDM patients are prone to develop hyperglycemic hyperosmolar nonketotic (HHNK) syndrome, which can be fatal.

I. Weight loss for elderly type II diabetics is not a goal unless the weight is more than one and a half times normal for height and frame.

J. Physical limitations may discourage older patients from exercising; walking, swimming, and riding a stationary bicycle are recommended; begin slowly and work up to a full schedule.

K. Hypoglycemia from exercise may occur in the elderly patient up to 24 hours past the time of exercise.

L. Second-generation oral hypoglycemics are a better choice than some of the first-generation drugs because they do not have as long a half-life and are eliminated from the body more quickly.

M. Elderly patients have special learning needs; be certain patient can hear and see adequately before beginning teaching and that the environment is free of noise and distractions (Table 25-13).

VI. **Community Care**

A. Closer monitoring of the diabetic population could assist in reducing the number of complications experienced.

B. Long-term care nurses must be constantly alert for the signs of diabetes in residents.

C. Home care and clinic nurses must be persistent in assessing and improving compliance in diabetic patients.

D. Reinforcement of teaching for control and self-care periodically is needed for most diabetic patients.

CHAPTER 26

Care of Patients with Disorders of the Female Reproductive System

OBJECTIVES

Upon completing this chapter the student should be able to:

1. Discuss the female reproductive organs and their role in the overall health of the individual.
2. Identify interventions that are helpful in relieving dysmenorrhea.
3. State interventions that may help alleviate the discomforts associated with menopause.
4. List nursing responsibilities for patients undergoing gynecological tests and examinations.
5. Describe the procedure for breast self-examination (BSE) and vulvar self-examination (VSE).
6. Utilize the nursing process to care for the gynecological patient.
7. State the signs and symptoms of common vaginal infections.
8. List the risk factors for cancer of the breast, cervix, endometrium, and ovary.
9. Discuss methods of treatment for endometriosis.
10. Describe the various types of surgical procedures for gynecological dysfunctions, including postoperative nursing care.

The female reproductive system is highly complex. It depends on hormones produced by the endocrine system for correct development and function. A variety of hormones released in a specific order at specific times triggers the formation of internal and external sexual organs in the developing fetus. Puberty and sexual maturation also are dependent on accurate release of hormones at the appropriate time. As the childbearing years draw to a close, hormone production slows until the reproductive cycle ceases altogether.

Reproductive health can be disrupted by a variety of disorders, such as infertility, premature labor, spontaneous abortion, infection, and the growth of abnormal tissue, including cancerous and noncancerous tumors. Nursing care of patients with diseases of the female reproductive system is further complicated by the emotional effects of such disorders. The reproductive organs represent the biological aspect of sexual identity, and women may feel their personal identity is threatened by disorders of this system. Hormone imbalances that occur as primary disorders or as a result of other reproductive diseases may affect how women view themselves and their interactions with others.

OVERVIEW OF ANATOMY AND PHYSIOLOGY

What Are the Primary External Structures of the Female Reproductive System?

⮦ The *vulva*, or *pudendum*, is the name given to the external female genitalia. It is made up of the following structures:

⮦ The *mons pubis* is a rounded mound of fatty tissue immediately below the abdomen. It is covered with pubic hair.

⮦ The *labia majora* are two elongated, raised folds of pigmented skin that enclose the vulvar cleft. The pubic hair extends along these folds.

⮦ The *labia minora* are soft folds of skin within the labia majora. They are soft, shiny, made up of erectile tissue, and have no hair follicles.

⮦ The *clitoris* is located at the top of the vulvar cleft, between the labia majora and immediately above the labia minora. It is made up primarily of erectile tissue and is highly sensitive to touch. It is a primary source of pleasurable sensation during sexual activity.

⮦ The *urethral meatus,* or external opening of the urethra of the urinary bladder, is located 1 to 2 finger breadths below the clitoris within the folds of the labia minora.

⮦ The *vaginal vestibule* is situated 1 to 2 finger breadths below the urethral meatus within the labia minora and is the entrance to the vagina.

⮦ The *perineum* is the flat muscular surface lying between the vagina and the anus.

What Are the Primary Internal Structures of the Female Reproductive System?

⮦ The *vagina* is a muscular tube lined with mucous membrane that connects the external and internal female sexual organs (Figure 26-1).

⮦ The *uterus* (womb) is a hollow, pear-shaped organ with a thick muscular wall. It lies at the upper end of the vagina. It is capable of expanding to many times its normal size to accommodate a growing fetus. The lower opening of the uterus is the *cervix,* which dilates during labor to allow for delivery of the infant.

⮦ There are two *fallopian tubes* (sometimes called *oviducts* or *uterine tubes*) that branch outward from the right and left side at the top of the uterus. They form the pathway for the *ovum* (egg) from the ovary to the uterus.

⮦ There are two *ovaries,* one located near the end of each fallopian tube. These almond-shaped glands excrete estrogen and progesterone into the bloodstream. At birth, the ovaries contain all the eggs (*oocytes*—primitive ova or eggs) the woman will ever produce, approximately 400,000 in each ovary, most of which will never mature for possible fertilization.

⮦ The *bony pelvis,* located at the base of the body between the hips, supports the pelvic organs, including the growing uterus during pregnancy. It is assisted by the *pelvic floor,* a collection of strong muscles and supportive tissues that brace the pelvis and provide both support and protection for the pelvic organs.

What Are the Accessory Organs of the Female Reproductive System?

⮦ The breasts or *mammary glands,* located on the upper chest, are the accessory organs. They are composed of fibrous, adipose, and glandular tissue, and are the organs of *lactation* (milk production), which provide nourishment for the infant.

What Are the Phases of the Female Reproductive Cycle During the Childbearing Years?

⮦ The *ovarian cycle* has two phases.
Follicular phase—this is the first 14 days of a 28 day cycle. *FSH (follicle stimulating hormone)* and *LH (luteinizing hormone)* cause the maturing of an immature ova in preparation for fertilization. Estrogen peaks at the end of the ovarian cycle and the ovum is released (ovulation) for possible fertilization about the 14th day. The period of time during which the ovum is capable of fertilization is believed to be 6 to 24 hours.
Luteal phase—15th to 28th day. LH and progesterone are the primary hormones in this phase. The blood supply to the uterus increases in preparation for possible implantation of a fertilized ovum. If fertilization and implantation do not occur, the lining of the uterus will degrade and be shed during menstruation, and the cycle begins again.

⮦ The *menstrual cycle* has four phases, depicted in Table 26-1.

When Does Sexual Development Occur in the Fetus?

⅄ During the first weeks of pregnancy the male and female sexual organs are undifferentiated. After the seventh week rapid changes occur, and by the twelfth week the external genitalia are formed and fully differentiated as male or female. The internal structures also are forming during this period.

What Changes Take Place as Girls Mature into Women and Become Capable of Reproduction?

⅄ The period of sexual maturation is called *puberty*. It usually occurs between ages 9 to 17 for girls, with the average onset being 12 years of age and lasts 1 to 5 years. First is a period of accelerated growth, then the hips begin to widen and the breasts begin to develop. Axillary and pubic hair appears. Puberty is completed by the onset of the menstrual cycle or **menses**. The beginning of menstruation is called **menarche**. Menstruation (shedding of the uterine lining) will continue at intervals of approximately 4 weeks throughout the childbearing years except when pregnancy occurs.

What Changes Take Place as a Woman Enters Menopause?

⅄ Toward the end of the childbearing period, women enter the period known as the **climacteric**. The menses become irregular in both pattern and flow and eventually cease altogether. **Menopause** has occurred when the menses have completely ceased.

What Changes Occur with Aging?

⅄ After menopause, some atrophy of the female organs, loss of elasticity, dryness of the vaginal membranes, and reduction of bone mass occur because of the decrease in estrogen levels. Loss of natural elasticity may allow internal organs to sag, or *prolapse*, into the vagina.

MENSTRUATION

During the first year following menarche, the menstrual cycle may be somewhat irregular, but by the second year a regular cycle of approximately 28 days is normally established.

Attitudes and ideas regarding menstruation are formed early. They are based on the thoughts and beliefs expressed by other women and on personal experience. Incorrect perceptions about this normal process may increase physical discomfort or cause the young woman unnecessary embarrassment or fear. Although there has been significant improvement in communication with preadolescent young women about the changes they will experience, many still have incorrect ideas and need further education whenever the opportunity arises. **It is important that the nurse understands her own attitudes about sexuality and the reproductive process before attempting to provide information for**

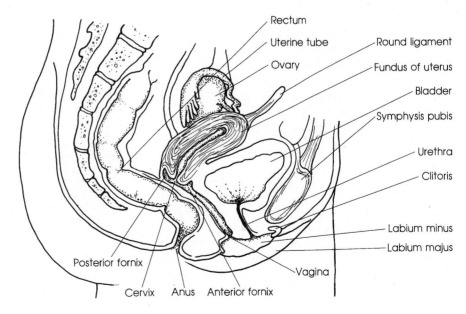

FIGURE 26-1   Female reproductive organs.

Rectum
Uterine tube
Ovary
Round ligament
Fundus of uterus
Bladder
Symphysis pubis
Urethra
Clitoris
Labium minus
Labium majus
Posterior fornix
Vagina
Cervix   Anus   Anterior fornix

TABLE 26-1 ◆ *Stages of the Menstrual Cycle*		
First to Fifth Day	**Sixth to Fourteenth Day**	**Fifteenth to Twenty-eighth Day**
*Menstrual stage (dismantling stage)**	*Stage of growth and repair (estrogen or proliferative stage)*	*Secretory stage (postovulatory or progesterone stage)*
1. Endometrium sloughs away as menstrual flow begins.	1. Follicle grows and egg matures.	1. Corpus luteum secretes progesterone.
2. Progesterone and estrogen are no longer secreted.	2. Endometrium returns to normal state and then begins to thicken in response to estrogen.	2. Endometrium continues to thicken in response to estrogen and progesterone. Prepares to receive fertilized ovum.
3. New follicle starts to mature.	3. Ovulation occurs 14 days before menses, regardless of length of menstrual cycle. Takes place when follicle ruptures and releases egg.	

*For menstruation to occur, two organs are essential: (1) the uterus because menstruation is the sloughing away of about three fourths of the lining of the uterus; and (2) at least part of one ovary, because the ovary secretes the hormones that cause the endometrium to thicken.

women on these sensitive issues. A healthy view of menarche as a natural physiological process marking reproductive maturity should be encouraged.

MENSTRUAL DYSFUNCTIONS

◆ Amenorrhea

Amenorrhea means absent menstruation. Primary amenorrhea refers to women who have not had a normal onset of menstrual periods. Secondary amenorrhea applies to women who began normal menses that later ceased. The causes are varied and complex. They include (1) anatomical defects, such as an imperforate (closed) *hymen* (the membrane which normally partially covers the vaginal opening until broken either by sexual intercourse or as a child during vigorous activity such as sports); (2) endocrine dysfunction affecting production of female hormones; (3) chronic disease and obesity; (4) emotional disturbances; (5) side effects of some drugs; (6) poor nutrition, including that caused by eating disorders such as bulimia and anorexia nervosa; (7) excessive vigorous exercise causing body fat to drop below 10%; and (8) abrupt discontinuation of oral contraceptives. Amenorrhea also occurs with pregnancy, but this is a normal occurrence.

◆ Dysmenorrhea

Dysmenorrhea is painful or difficult menstruation. Symptoms include cramping, aching in the lower back or pelvic region, nausea, vomiting, diarrhea, headache, dizziness, fatigue, and emotional instability. Primary dysmenorrhea is not accompanied by any specific pathology, although there is a known relationship to the presence of elevated amounts of prostaglandins, naturally occurring substances that have the ability to stim-

ulate contractions of the smooth muscles. Emotional and psychological stress also may increase primary dysmenorrhea. **Prostaglandin synthetase inhibitors, such as ibuprofen, naproxen sodium and mefenamic acid, seem to offer the greatest relief of symptoms.** Traditional self-treatment methods, including aspirin or acetaminophen, heat applied to the back and abdomen, mild exercise, rest, and relaxation techniques also may help alleviate symptoms. See Table 26-2 for medications commonly used to relieve dysmenorrhea.

Secondary dysmenorrhea is related to an infection or inflammation of the pelvic organs, endometriosis (discussed later in this chapter), or the presence of an intrauterine device (IUD). In such cases, treatment of the underlying cause usually provides relief.

◆ Premenstrual Syndrome

Premenstrual syndrome (PMS) is a group of symptoms that may be experienced in the several days preceding menstruation. They include accumulation of body fluid, acne-like skin eruptions, food cravings, crying spells, severe headaches, and depression, anger, and fatigue. **Helpful dietary interventions include lowering intake of refined sugar, red meats, caffeine, salt, and alcohol and increasing intake of carbohydrate-rich foods, particularly during the week before menstruation.** Regular exercise and relaxation techniques also may help. Progesterone therapy and antidepressants such as Prozac have been helpful for some women. PMS clinics and support groups provide opportunities for women with severe PMS to talk with each other. The sharing of ideas, experiences, and knowing that they are not alone in the experience has been very helpful.

◆ Dysfunctional Uterine Bleeding

Dysfunctional uterine bleeding is uterine bleeding that occurs at times other than the normal menstrual cycle.

It can be relatively insignificant, or it can be an early sign of a serious disorder such as a malignancy. **Metrorrhagia** refers to uterine bleeding or spotting that occurs outside the normal cycle, and **menorrhagia** refers to excessive blood loss during menses, either because the flow is excessively heavy or excessively prolonged.

In very young women dysfunctional bleeding can occur before hormones fully regulate the cycle. Decreasing hormones during the climacteric also can cause dysfunctional uterine bleeding. The presence of an IUD or the discontinuance of oral contraceptive pills can cause a heavier-than-normal menstrual flow. These situations usually regulate themselves over time, but women with excessive bleeding associated with IUDs may need to have the device removed.

Heavy bleeding caused by an infection of the *endometrium* (lining of the uterus) is usually accompanied by a foul-smelling vaginal discharge. The presence of the infection interferes with normal clotting and causes the heavy bleeding. Antibiotic treatment is required to resolve the infection.

In the childbearing years dysfunctional bleeding may be caused by spontaneous abortion, **ectopic pregnancy** (pregnancy which implants in the fallopian tube rather than the uterus), benign **fibroid** (thickened vascular masses in the uterus), and endometriosis (discussed later in the chapter). Malignancy of the cervix, adenocarcinoma of the vagina, and uterine cancer are other potential serious causes of such bleeding.

Elder Care Point... Vaginal bleeding in elderly women is a possible warning sign of cervical or uterine cancer. An immediate pelvic examination to determine and treat the cause of such bleeding is advised. The incidence of these cancers increases with age.

Think about... What is a very important aspect of a nurse's knowledge base when working with patients with female reproductive disorders?

CONTRACEPTION

The majority of sexually active women of childbearing age are concerned about regulating or preventing pregnancy. With the assistance of a gynecologist, trained nurse, or reproductive clinic they can select the birth control method best suited to their physical health, sexual activity, desire for children at a future date, and religious beliefs concerning family regulation. See Table 26-3 for information on the current methods of contraception.

TABLE 26-2 ◆ *Medications Used to Relieve Dysmenorrhea*

Medication	Side Effects	Nursing Implications
Aspirin	Gastrointestinal (GI) irritation, ringing in ears in high doses.	Contraindicated in bleeding disorders or anticoagulation therapy such as warfarin, GI ulcers. Do not combine with nonsteroidal antiinflammatory drugs (NSAIDs).
Fenoprofen	Diarrhea, abdominal distention, nausea and vomiting, and dyspepsia, constipation.	Contraindicated in hemophilia, bleeding ulcers, bleeding disorders. Avoid alcohol.
Ibuprofen	Nausea, dyspepsia, itching, rash.	Contraindicated in hemophilia, bleeding ulcers, bleeding disorders Do not take with aspirin. Take with meals. Avoid alcohol.
Indomethacin	Nausea, dyspepsia.	Contraindicated in hemophilia, bleeding ulcers, bleeding disorders. Side effects more likely.
Mefenamic acid (potent prosta-glandin synthesis inhibitor)	Diarrhea, nausea, abdominal distention.	Contraindicated in hemophilia, bleeding ulcers, bleeding disorders. Incidence of GI side effects increased.
Naproxen sodium	Nausea, abdominal distress, dyspepsia, rash, itching.	Contraindicated in hemophilia, bleeding ulcers, bleeding disorders. Do not take with aspirin. Take with meals. Avoid alcohol.

TABLE 26-3 ◆ *Methods of Contraception*

Contraceptive Method	How Method Works	Side Effects/Precautions	Degree of Effectiveness
Fertility awareness methods			
Basal body temperature (BBT)	Basal body temperature is measured and charted daily upon awakening. Coitus is avoided on the day of temperature rise and for 3 subsequent days.	Temperature must be taken before any activity, or it will rise above its basal level. Thermometer should be right at bedside.	80%–98% for all fertility awareness methods.
Calendar or rhythm method	Woman charts her monthly menstrual cycle on a calendar and avoids intercourse during fertile period.	Not effective for woman with irregular menstrual cycles. Several months of charting are necessary to establish clear pattern.	Fertility awareness methods that monitor multiple parameters (e.g., symptothermal method) may be more effective, but most important aspect of success is faithful adherence to the method. Also, the woman must feel comfortable enough with her body to make the necessary observations each month.
Ovulation or Billings method	Cervical mucus changes are assessed. During ovulation mucus is clear with high stretchability ("egg white" consistency). Degree of stretch is tested by pinching a small amount of cervical mucus between the thumb and forefinger and stretching it between them. During ovulation, mucus smeared on a glass slide will dry into a "fern" pattern.	Woman must feel very comfortable about her body and confident in her ability to detect and assess changes.	
Symptothermal method	Variety of parameters are recorded, including cervical mucus changes, basal temperature pattern, mittelschmerz (brief sharp abdominal pain that may occur with ovulation), increased libido (sexual drive).	More effective for women with regular menstrual cycles. Requires significant record keeping.	
Mechanical or barrier contraception			
IUD (Intrauterine Device)	A small, sterile, flexible plastic device which is inserted by a physician into the uterus. Presence in uterus is believed to prevent conception by interfering with normal sperm activity.	May increase menstrual flow or cause cramping or low-back pain. Increased incidence of pelvic inflammatory disease in women with multiple sex partners, women whose partners have multiple partners, and women with previous incidence of PID. Client must check placement by feeling for string once each month.	Up to 99% effective, can be left in place up to ten years. Must be removed by physician.
Male condom	A sheath commonly made of latex* that is placed over the erect penis prior to intercourse.	Inexpensive, readily available, easy to use correctly. Precautions: (1) leave space at tip for semen to collect rather than being forced upward out of the condom; (2) store in a cool place and not for excessively long to avoid breakage due to aging of the latex or heat damage; (3) handle carefully to avoid spilling semen and possibly introducing it into the vagina. Effectiveness enhanced with use of spermicide. Provides protection against sexually transmitted diseases (STDs).	88%–98%. Use of spermicide increases effectiveness to 98% to 99%.

TABLE 26-3 ◆ Methods of Contraception (Continued)

Contraceptive Method	How Method Works	Side Effects/Precautions	Degree of Effectiveness
Female condom	Sheath with retaining ring that is placed in the vagina prior to intercourse. Open end with large entrance ring extends outside the vagina.	The penis must remain inside the sheath, not between the sheath and the vaginal wall. Acceptance of the method has been slow as it is more expensive and more difficult and time-consuming to place properly than the male condom. Effectiveness enhanced with use of spermicide. Provides protection against STDs.	79%–90%. Most failures occur when the penis is withdrawn too far and reenters the vagina beside rather than within the condom.
Diaphragm	Spermicide is applied to the cervical side of the diaphragm and it is inserted into the vagina so the fitted ring holds it securely in place at the top of the vagina to wall off the cervix. The spermicide enhances effectiveness should there be a leak around the edge or tear in the diaphragm.	A diaphragm must be fitted professionally and should be refitted periodically, particularly after pregnancy.	82%–94%
Cervical cap	Cervical cap fits over the cervix. Filled with spermicidal jelly and applied over the cervix. See diaphragm.	See diaphragm.	82% to 94%
Spermicidal methods Gels, foams, creams	Work by killing sperm within the vagina. Some also provide a degree of barrier effect to contain sperm within the vagina.	Available without prescription. More effective used as an adjunct to condoms, diaphragms, and caps.	Foam alone 79%–90%; creams and gels alone 79%.
Hormonal methods Oral contraceptives	"The pill" contains synthetic female hormones that prevent ovulation and thicken cervical mucus, making it difficult for sperm to travel upward (also true for injectable and time-released hormonal methods).	Prescription required. Must be taken faithfully to be effective. Precautions: not recommended for women over 35 who smoke or women with a history of heart or liver disease, breast or uterine cancer, blood clots or venous inflammation, or unexplained vaginal bleeding.	97%–99.9%.
Injectable contraceptives	Synthetic time-released progesterone is injected every 12 weeks, preventing ovulation.	Injections given in clinic or office. Must be repeated every 12 weeks to remain effective. Precautions: see oral contraceptives.	99.7%.
Sustained-release implants	Thin, flexible capsules containing synthetic hormone are placed under the skin of the forearm in a minor surgical procedure. Work over a period of 5 years without renewal.	Small incision required to place and to remove. Less popular now that injection is available. Precautions: see oral contraceptives.	98.4%–99.4%.
Morning-after pill	Taken orally the day following unprotected intercourse, it induces menses and prevents implantation.	Not to be used as a routine form of contraception. Women receiving the "morning-after" pill should also get assistance in choosing an effective, ongoing method of contraception.	

(Table 26-3 continued)

TABLE 26-3 ◆ Methods of Contraception (Continued)

Contraceptive Method	How Method Works	Side Effects/Precautions	Degree of Effectiveness
Sterilization			
Female: tubal ligation	The fallopian tubes are cut or tied to prevent sperm from reaching the ovum.	Sterilization procedures should be considered permanent as surgical reversal is difficult and may not be effective. Vasectomy is an office procedure, tubal ligation usually an outpatient surgical procedure.	99.6%.
Male: vasectomy	The *vas deferens* (sperm ducts) are cut and tied to prevent sperm from entering the ejaculatory fluid.		

*Contraceptive devices made of latex should be avoided by individuals with a known allergic sensitivity to latex.

INFERTILITY

◆ Causes and Risk Factors

Primary infertility is the inability of a couple to conceive a child, and is usually diagnosed if conception does not occur after 1 year of regular, unprotected intercourse. *Secondary infertility* refers to the inability to maintain a pregnancy and deliver a viable infant. It is estimated that about 17% of U.S. couples experience infertility and that about 60% of these couples can be effectively treated.

Causes and risk factors for women include failure to ovulate, ovarian tumors, inappropriate consistency of cervical mucus, poor endometrial development, endometriosis, blockage of the fallopian tubes, and infections of the reproductive tract. Other causes include a vaginal/cervical environment inhospitable to sperm motility or viability and immunological reaction to the sperm. See Chapter 27 for a discussion of male infertility.

◆ Emotional Impact

The emotional impact of infertility can be very intense. Some infertile couples become almost desperate to conceive. The nurse must be alert to evidence that emotional or psychological intervention is needed to assist these couples in dealing with the stress of their situation. Indications would include inability to focus on anything other than the desire to have a child and tension in the relationship, including blaming of the other partner.

◆ Diagnostic Studies

Initial intervention often addresses the mechanics of conception. Couples are counseled on techniques to increase the possibility of pregnancy. These include having intercourse every other day during the ovulatory period of the woman's cycle; use of the male-dominant position, with the woman remaining supine with hips elevated for 1 hour after intercourse; avoidance of artificial lubricants and douches, which may create an inhospitable environment for sperm; and use of basal temperature recordings and assessment of cervical mucus to determine time of greatest fertility. Couples also need to be encouraged to maintain the romance of sexual encounters and not let the desire for pregnancy override the opportunity for loving intimacy.

A variety of diagnostic tests are available to determine the cause of infertility. Frequently, sperm counts and analyses are done first because these studies are relatively simple, inexpensive, and noninvasive. Testing of the woman may include hormone assays to evaluate the function of the fertility cycle; vaginal and cervical secretion studies and cultures; hysterosalpingogram to evaluate the patency of the fallopian tubes; endometrial biopsy to determine whether the uterus provides an appropriate environment for implantation of the fertile ovum; and examination of the reproductive organs via laparoscopy or culdoscopy.

◆ Medical and Surgical Intervention

Major centers in various parts of the world are working actively on infertility treatment. One common intervention is artificial insemination using sperm from the prospective father or a suitable donor. Donor sperm is necessary when a poor sperm count or motility is the cause of infertility. Artificial insemination with the male partner's sperm is possible when the cause of infertility is problems with cervical mucus or other factors that cause an inhospitable environment for sperm or when the sperm count is low but still within a range that makes conception possible. In such cases, the sperm is frequently introduced directly into the uterus via the cervix rather than being deposited at the cervical opening.

Chemical stimulation of the ovaries may be used to induce ovulation. Drugs used include clomiphene citrate, menotropins, gonadotropin-releasing hormone, bromocriptine mesylate, and thyroid-stimulating hormone, depending on the underlying cause of failure to ovulate. Ovarian stimulation may cause release of several ova, increasing the possibility of a multiple-fetus pregnancy.

In vitro fertilization (IVF) is being used with increasing frequency in cases of persistent infertility where the problem is conception rather than the ability to maintain pregnancy. Ova may be harvested via laparoscopy from the woman or from a donor. After fertilization, using the male partner's sperm if viable, the ovum is implanted in the uterus through the cervix. More than one fertile ovum may be implanted to increase the possibility of success, which may also cause multiple-fetus pregnancy.

Another technique is *gamete intrafallopian tube transfer (GIFT)*. In this procedure, sperm and oocytes are placed into the fallopian tube via laparoscopy, allowing normal fertilization to occur.

Sometimes specific surgical interventions are required to allow a woman to conceive. These include repair of uterine or tubal abnormalities and surgical treatment of blockages in the fallopian tubes that prevent fertilization.

The greatest percentage of success exists in those couples who respond to the more basic interventions, such as reproductive counseling or treatment of an underlying infection. Invasive procedures such as IVF and GIFT currently have moderate success rates, are very expensive and may not result in the desired pregnancy. Couples receiving this level of infertility treatment may need professional assistance in making decisions regarding continued treatment versus adoption versus coming to terms with not having children. They must be allowed to make their own decisions in a supportive and informative environment.

MENOPAUSE

Sometime between the ages of 45 and 50, the climacteric usually begins. Climacteric is taken from a Greek word meaning *a rung on a ladder* and represents another step on the path of life. **When the menstrual flow has been completely absent for 1 year, menopause is said to have taken place.** This marks the end of the woman's reproductive period. Prior to actual menopause, pregnancy is still possible, and women wishing to avoid this should continue to use contraception for 1 year after the menstrual flow has ceased.

The average age for menopause is 50. It may occur at any time between the ages of 35 and 58, with the average age being 48 to 55. Menopause prior to age 35 is called *premature menopause*, and after age 58 it is termed *delayed menopause*. Either of these may be a normal, often inherited characteristic. However, they also may be the result of a primary disorder affecting the endocrine glands or the reproductive organs, so medical evaluation should be obtained.

During the climacteric the hormonal changes may cause some physical and emotional disturbances which may be severe enough to interfere with daily activities. Only about 25% of women, however, experience enough discomfort to seek medical attention. It is interesting to note that women who experienced an early menarche usually experience menopause later than average.

Surgically induced menopause occurs when the ovaries are removed or irradiated. The symptoms are usually more severe because the cessation of hormonal secretion is abrupt rather than gradual. Removing the uterus while leaving the ovaries does result in cessation of menses but will not induce climacteric symptoms.

Symptoms   At least three groups of factors affect the symptoms experienced by women during the climacteric: (1) decreased ovarian function resulting in hormone deficiency; (2) social-cultural factors influencing a woman's attitudes about the end of childbearing and growing older; and (3) psychological factors related to inner resources, personal coping skills, and support from family and friends. The change of life can bring feelings of freedom and new opportunities for personal growth or fears regarding a loss of identity and purpose in life.

A common symptom of beginning menopause is menstrual irregularities that affect the frequency, duration, and intensity of flow. Periods may be close together at times, widespread at others. Flow may be scant or heavy. This often is accompanied by patchy flushing of the skin and a sudden uncomfortable rush of physical warmth, called *hot flashes* or *hot flushes*. Hot flashes may be accompanied by excessive perspiration, particularly night sweats during sleep. The frequency and degree of intensity varies greatly from woman to woman, but tend to be more severe when the decline in ovarian hormones, specifically estrogen, is rapid rather than gradual. **Relaxation exercises such as deep, slow breathing and mental imagery of feeling cool and calm may help reduce the intensity of hot flashes.**

Other symptoms include fatigue, insomnia, emotional instability, and depression. Some women also experience back pain, headache, irritability, and decreased libido. The cause of these symptoms is not as defined, but appears to be related in part to hormonal changes and in part to psychological factors and coping skills. **A woman engaged in work or projects that are of interest and value to her is less likely to suffer serious emotional upheaval during menopause than the woman who sees herself as useless or unattractive.** Contrary to popular belief, the postmenopausal woman remains sexually attractive and may even find sexual intercourse more enjoyable because of the freedom from fear of pregnancy.

Treatment Estrogen replacement remains a controversial treatment. Possible benefits include decreased loss of bone mass (*osteoporosis*) with decreased danger of fractures; control of estrogen deficiency symptoms such as hot flashes and night sweats; decrease in vaginal and urethral dryness, decrease in skin surface thinning, wrinkling, and bruising; increased libido and stabilization of hormone-related mood swings; and protection against cardiovascular disease. This last benefit is receiving considerable attention. Before menopause, women have a significantly lower rate of cardiovascular disease, but this begins to change after menopause, and by age 70 rates are the same as for men.

Possible adverse effects of estrogen replacement therapy include an increased risk of breast and endometrial cancer; weight gain, fluid retention, nausea, headache, breast discomfort, leg cramps, hypertension, hypotension, gallbladder disease, lethargy, and a worsening of glucose tolerance in diabetic women.

Elder Care Point... The significant reduction in estrogen after menopause (about 80% less than during the reproductive years) causes a decrease in natural vaginal lubrication. Women may be prescribed vaginal creams containing estrogen to restore moisture and elasticity to vaginal tissues. They should be cautioned not to use the estrogen cream as a lubricant for sexual intercourse as their partner may absorb the estrogen. Nonmedicated lubricants should be used for this purpose if needed.

Nursing Management and Intervention Despite improved education and communication, women frequently are misinformed about menopause. Many women still have a strong reluctance to discuss sexual matters and need a receptive, nonjudgmental attitude from the nurse if any effective teaching is to be done. In addition, the nurse can provide information regarding healthy lifestyle choices in diet and exercise to maintain proper weight and physical well-being.

Women should be instructed to report any spotting or bleeding occurring between menstrual periods during the climacteric or after menopause has occurred. Such bleeding can be an early sign of uterine or cervical cancer and should be evaluated. Table 26-4

TABLE 26-4 ◆ *Risk Factors for Common Female Reproductive Cancers*

Type of Cancer	Risk Factors	Age Most Common	Common Warning Signs	Screening
Cervix	Diethylstilbestrol exposure. Sexually active as teenager. History of human papilloma virus, genital warts, herpes. Multiparity. Smoking. Higher with oral contraceptives? Race: African Americans.	In situ, 30–40 Invasive, 40–60	Vaginal bleeding between periods. Bleeding after menopause.	Pelvic exam with Pap smear every 3 years before age 40 (yearly if high risk); yearly after age 40.
Endometrium	History of diabetes, hypertension, breast cancer. Family history. Nulliparity. Higher with prolonged estrogen use (>3.5 years)? Obesity. Race: Caucasian.	50–65	Vaginal bleeding between periods. Bleeding after menopause.	Endometrial biopsy annually if high risk or on unopposed estrogen therapy. Pelvic exam every 3 years, annually if high risk or after age 40. No practical screening available for asymptomatic women.
Ovary	History of breast, colon, or endometrial cancer. Family history, especially mother. Nulliparity. High-fat diet. Oral contraceptives may have preventative effects.	Over 50	Often no obvious signs. Abdomen enlarged. Digestive problems.	No practical screening for asymptomatic women. Pelvic and physical exam every 3 years, annually if high risk or after age 40.
Vulva	History of vulvar disease, possibly diabetes. Genital warts, genital herpes. Possibly obesity.	60–70	Sores that do not heal. Ulcers. Bumps under skin. Itching. Skin color changes.	Monthly vulvar self-exam. Pelvic exam every 3 years before age 40, yearly after age 40.

gives symptoms of common female reproductive cancers.

Think about . . . How does attitude affect a woman who is when going through menopause?

DIAGNOSTIC TESTS AND PROCEDURES AND NURSING RESPONSIBILITIES

When assisting with or preparing patients for diagnostic tests and procedures, the nurse must first provide appropriate education and support. **Tests that require viewing and manipulating the sexual organs, such as pelvic exams, or that may lead to treatments that will change the appearance or function of these organs can be extremely stressful for the patient.** The nurse must give clear, concise information and answer all questions or arrange for the patient to speak with the physician or other health care professional qualified to answer. This must take place in an atmosphere of warmth, safety, and respect for the patient and her needs and concerns. Be sure the patient has received all the necessary information and explanations before the procedure. It is particularly important to correct any misconceptions in a manner that does not make the patient feel stupid or silly for her ideas or lack of knowledge.

Many procedures require a signed consent. It is the nurse's responsibility to ensure that this is done prior to the procedure. Consents are usually obtained immediately following the preprocedure teaching.

When setting up for any type of invasive exam or procedure, it is important to observe both *Standard Precautions* and aseptic technique to prevent exposure to bloodborne pathogens and infection. **The nurse must carefully review the facility's written policy before assisting with any unfamiliar procedure.** See Table 26-5 for descriptions of common diagnostic tests and procedures, reasons for performing, and the nursing implications.

◆ Breast Self-Examination (BSE)

Breast self-examination (BSE) should be done monthly 1 week after menstruation begins, or on a specific date each month after menopause. The nurse can play a major role in teaching and encouraging women to perform the procedure to detect breast lumps and thickened areas early. Currently only about 20% of American women perform BSE. See Figure 26-2 for the steps in the procedure. In addition, the American Cancer Society has videotapes available that demonstrate BSE.

◆ Vulvar Self-Examination (VSE)

Many women are unaware of the importance of vulvar self-examination (VSE). Although serious lesions in this area are less common than in the breast, delay in detection can lead to severe surgical disfigurement and death. Early detection allows rapid, often minimally invasive treatment.

Just like BSE, VSE should be done monthly. It usually is done in a sitting position. One hand is used to hold a mirror, the other to separate the labia and expose the area surrounding the vagina. Using both touch (to palpate for lumps or thickening beneath the skin) and visualization, the self-exam begins at the top of the vulvar area and works downward, examining first the mons pubis, then the clitoris, the labia minora, labia majora, the perineum, and finally the area around the anus. The woman should note any changes and report them to her primary health care provider. These include new moles, warts, or growths; new areas of pigmentation, especially white, red, or dark skin areas; ulcers or sores, and areas of continuing pain, inflammation, or itching. Most of these will not be malignant and will require little, if any, treatment. Treatment of malignancies detected early often is relatively easy and can avoid deformative surgeries such as *vulvectomy* (excision of the vulva) and prevent *metastasis* (spread of a malignancy to other areas of the body).

Think about . . . What is a very important aspect of maintaining personal reproductive health?

NURSING MANAGEMENT

◆ Assessment

Assessing patients with gynecological diseases or concerns can be difficult for both the patient and the nurse, as it involves aspects of the body and personal life often considered private. Cultural ideas and attitudes regarding sexuality and sexual identity, reproduction, and body image all affect the assessment process. **The nurse needs to ask questions in a tactful, yet matter-of-fact, manner, as well as appreciate that the patient has the right to choose not to answer.** See Table 26-6 on taking a gynecological history.

◆ Nursing Diagnoses

Nursing diagnoses commonly associated with gynecological disorders include:

◆ Activity intolerance related to anemia from excessive blood loss, weakness, or disabling discomfort.

TABLE 26-5 ◆ *Common Gynecological Diagnostic Tests and Procedures*

Test	Purpose	Description	Nursing Implications
Pelvic examination	Visual inspection of the external genitalia, vagina, and cervix to obtain specimens such as a Pap smear.	*Equipment:* gloves, vaginal speculum, lubricant, light, table/stirrups. *Process:* inspection via the vaginal speculum; manual palpation through abdominal wall, vaginally, and rectally of internal organs.	Some discomfort during exam (decreased or eliminated if the patient remains fully relaxed). Nurse to assure that patient is appropriately draped and correctly positioned in the stirrups. Exam time is usually 5 to 10 minutes.
Smears and cultures	To obtain samples of cells and fluids for pathology/cytology studies.	*Equipment:* sterile specimen collection equipment. *Process:* exudate, mucus and cells obtained from surface with sterile swab or scraping tool and placed on lab slide for pathology evaluation.	Cultures and smears of the cervix (e.g., Pap smear) may cause mild bleeding and cramping.
Endometrial biopsy	Postmenopausal bleeding, menstrual difficulties, infertility workup.	*Equipment:* same as pelvic exam plus suction biopsy apparatus. *Process:* a suction biopsy of the endometrium is performed via the cervical opening.	Severe cramping may occur during procedure. Patient is usually premedicated. Normally some vaginal bleeding following, flow should not be heavy.
Colposcopy	Endoscopic exam of the vagina and cervix to evaluate abnormal cells and lesions, particularly after a positive Pap smear.	*Equipment:* same as pelvic exam plus colposcope. *Process:* area is visualized through the scope, with photos and possible biopsies of lesions requiring further study.	Patient is positioned as for pelvic exam. Procedure takes a few minutes. Biopsy may cause a small amount of bleeding and minor cramping. No tampons should be used until healing has occurred.
Laparoscopy	Endoscopic exam of the abdominal cavity that allows the physician directly to visualize possible problems and to perform procedures such as biopsy, release of adhesions, and tubal ligation without a major incision.	*Equipment:* done in operating room. *Process:* exam is done through small abdominal incision just below the navel through which the laparoscope is passed. Instruments for procedures may be passed directly through the scope or through a small secondary incision.	May experience cramps, shoulder, and neck pain from gas used to inflate the abdomen during the procedure; vaginal bleeding, incisional pain may be present for 1–2 days. Occasionally the bowel or other organ will be nicked or perforated by the laparoscope. Anesthesia is used and postoperative recovery is required.
Hysteroscopy	Endoscopic exam of the interior of the uterus; may also involve procedures such as biopsy or removal of fibroids, adhesions, and septums. Endometrial laser ablation (destruction of uterine lining in some cases of severe bleeding) may also be performed.	*Equipment:* done in operating room. *Process:* hysteroscope is inserted vaginally (may also be inserted through an abdominal incision and uterine incision) usually under local anesthesia. May also be done in combination with laparoscopy.	Essentially the same as laparoscopy. Occasional injury to cervix or uterine wall. If endometrial ablation is done, the woman will not be able to become pregnant as the lining destruction is permanent.
Dilatation and curettage (D&C)	Diagnosis of cause of excessive bleeding; removal of hypertrophied uterine lining, retained placenta, or tissue remaining from incomplete abortion.	*Equipment:* done in operating room. *Process:* The cervix is dilated and the interior of the uterus is cleansed by scraping, suction, or both.	Mild cramping and bleeding for up to 1 week. Next period may be either early or late. Complications include uterine perforation, excessive bleeding, infection. Instruct patient to report heavy bleeding, clotting, sharp/severe abdominal pain, abnormal or foul discharge.

TABLE 26-5 ◆ *Common Gynecological Diagnostic Tests and Procedures* (Continued)			
Test	**Purpose**	**Description**	**Nursing Implications**
Mammography	To screen the breasts for abnormal growths, particularly cancer.	Done in the radiology department with special x-ray equipment.	Breast discomfort from compression of the tissue during the test; occasional mild bruising. Instruct patient to wear no deodorant or lotion on the upper body and to wear clothing that allows top to be easily removed.
Ultrasound (sonogram)	Pregnancy: to determine gestation; screen for birth defects or placental abnormalities. Gynecology: determine presence, location and size of abdominal mass; determine whether a mass is cystic (fluid filled) or solid; locate intrauterine device; monitor ovulation in infertility.	*Equipment:* ultrasound machine *Process:* sound wave transducer emits inaudible sound waves which record interior structures on the ultrasound screen. A videotape is made so results can be restudied and evaluated.	Some tests require a full bladder, which may be uncomfortable during the test. There are no known complications of ultrasound examination. Skin should be clean, dry, and free of lotions or powder.
Therapeutic abortion	Termination of a pregnancy.	Similar to a D&C.	Same as D&C. Termination of a pregnancy is a sensitive and emotionally painful experience for most women and appropriate supportive care is necessary. Nurses with strong feelings against the procedure should probably not care for these patients.

◆ Ineffective individual coping related to unhealthy attitude about human sexuality or menstruation.

◆ Body image disturbance related to surgery, fear of mutilating surgery, loss of femininity.

◆ Fluid volume excess related to premenstrual fluid retention.

◆ Knowledge deficit about practices of personal feminine hygiene, normal anatomy and physiology of the female reproductive organs, or safe methods of contraception.

◆ Sexual dysfunction related to **dyspareunia** (painful intercourse) or emotional block.

◆ Disturbance in self-concept related to sterility, menopause, and surgery of a reproductive organ.

◆ Impairment of skin integrity related to pruritus, genital lesions, and vaginal discharge.

◆ Pain related to menstruation, decreased vaginal lubrication, or vaginal irritation.

◆ Planning

Planning the care of a patient with a gynecological problem depends on the specific disorder. However, prevention of infection, effective patient education, and emotional support are appropriate goals for all.

The needs of a patient facing gynecological surgery would include pain management, education regarding the procedure and follow-up care, infection prevention, and supportive care specific to the procedure. A woman who will lose the ability of bearing children because of an early hysterectomy has very different supportive needs from those of the postmenopausal woman undergoing the same procedure. Surgery for breast cancer brings fears of a major change in body image and the possibility of death if the disease is not controlled. These need to be addressed in the plan of care.

The plan for the patient with an infection would include an appropriate medication schedule, monitoring for effectiveness of treatment (e.g., fever, swelling, pain resolving), and monitoring for signs of allergic response to antibiotics.

In the clinic setting, patients may be coming for annual visits, reproductive or contraceptive counseling, treatment of infections or sexually transmitted diseases (STDs), pre- and postnatal care, and a variety of other reasons. **If standardized care plans are used, they must be adapted to express the needs of the individual client**

1 Positions

Visual Inspection: Standing

In each position, look for changes in contour and shape of the breasts, color and texture of the skin and nipple and evidence of discharge from the nipples.

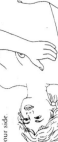

arms raised above head

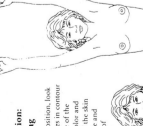

hands on hips

bending forward

arms relaxed at side

Axillary Examination:

Examine the breast tissue that extends into your armpit while your arm is relaxed at your side.

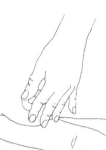

3 Palpation With Pads of Fingers

Use the pads of three or four fingers to examine every inch of your breast tissue. Move your fingers in circles about the size of a dime.

Do not lift your fingers from your breast between palpations. You can use powder or lotion to help your fingers glide from one spot to the next.

Palpation: Flat and Side-lying

Use your left hand to palpate the right breast, while holding your right arm at a right angle to the rib cage, with the elbow bent. Repeat the procedure on the other side. The side-lying position allows a woman, especially one with large breasts, to most effectively examine the outer half of the breast. A woman with small breasts may need only the flat position.

Side-lying Position: Lie on the opposite side of the breast to be examined. Rotate the shoulder (on the same side as the breast to be examined) back to the flat surface.

Flat Position: Lie flat on your back with a pillow or folded towel under the shoulder of the breast to be examined.

2 Perimeter

The exam area is bounded by the line which extends down from the middle of the armpit to just beneath the breast, continues across the underside of the breast, to the middle of the breast bone, then moves up to and along the collar bone and back to the middle of the armpit. Most breast cancers occur in the upper outer area of the breast (shaded area).

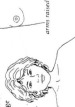

5 Pattern of Search

Vertical Strip:

Using the following search pattern to examine all of your breast tissue, palpate carefully beneath the nipple. Any incision should also be carefully examined from end to end. Women who have had any breast surgery should examine the entire area and the incision.

Start in the armpit, proceed downward to the lower boundary. Move a finger's width toward the middle and continuing palpating upward until you reach the collarbone. Repeat this until you have covered all the breast tissue. Make at least six strips before the nipple and four strips after the nipple. You may need between 10 and 16 strips.

Nipple Discharge:

Squeeze your nipples to check for discharge. Many women have a normal discharge.

4 Pressure

Use varying levels of pressure for each palpation, from light to deep, to examine the full thickness of your breast tissue. Using pressure will not injure the breast.

6 Practice With Feedback

It is important that you perform breast self-examination (BSE) while your instructor watches to be sure you are doing it correctly. Practice your skills until you feel comfortable and confident.

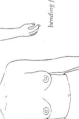
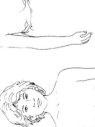
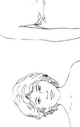

FIGURE 26-2 Patient education: recommended breast self-examination procedure.

TABLE 26-6 ◆ *Assessment: Guide to Gynecological History Taking*

Ask the following questions when assessing a patient with a gynecological problem:

- How old are you? (Gynecological disorders frequently are age related. Breast and endometrial cancers are more common in postmenopausal women, and STDs are more common among sexually active women in their teens and twenties.)
- How old were you when you began menstruating?
- Are your periods regular? How often do they occur? How long do they last?
- How heavy is your flow? Do you ever pass clots or pieces of tissue? (Particularly important when miscarriage is suspected.)
- Do you have cramps, headaches, abdominal or back pain before or during your period?
- Do you have cramps, headaches, abdominal or back pain at other times of the month?
- Do you have mood swings, depression, or periods of tearfulness associated with your menstrual cycle?
- Are you having any vaginal discharge or itching?
- Do you have bleeding or spotting between your periods?
- Do you have any pain, swelling, tender areas, lumps or dimpled skin areas on your breasts?
- Do you have any problems urinating, including burning, pain, or incontinence? (If "yes" to incontinence, ask if this is spontaneous or related to physical activity such as coughing, sneezing, or lifting.)
- How old were you when you became sexually active?
- Are you currently sexually active? Have you had, or do you currently have, more than one sexual partner? (Multiple partners increases the risk of STDs and some forms of female cancer.)
- Does your partner have other partners?
- Do you use a method such as condoms to prevent STDs?
- Do you experience pain during intercourse?
- Are you currently using any method of birth control, and if so, which method?
- Do you feel comfortable with your method or have a desire to change methods?

- How many times have you been pregnant?
- How many children do you have?
- Did you have any serious depression or "postpartum blues" after childbirth?
- Have you had any miscarriages?
- Have you had any therapeutic abortions?
- Have you ever had an STD or a pelvic infection?
- Do you perform breast and vulvar self-exam? If yes, how often? (Provide information on these techniques as needed.)
- When was your last Pap smear?
- Have you ever had an abnormal Pap smear?
- When was your last mammogram, and were there any problems?
- Are you taking any medications routinely?
- Have you ever been diagnosed with cancer?
- Has anyone in your family ever had cancer of the breast or reproductive organs?
- During her pregnancy with you, did your mother take diethylstilbestrol to prevent miscarriage? (Such women have a much greater risk for developing vaginal or cervical cancer.)
- Do you have diabetes mellitus, thryoid disease, sickle cell trait or disease? Does anyone in your family?
- Do you have any specific concerns or questions that we have not talked about?

The physical examination should include the following:

- Normal or abnormal secondary sex characteristics (distribution of body hair, breast development, pitch of voice, texture of the skin).
- Any signs of physical abuse, such as abnormal bruising, abrasions, or burns.
- Any indication of infection, such as copious discharge or foul odor.
- Any lumps, swelling, redness, surface discoloration, pain or tenderness, open or closed sores, moles, warts, rashes, orange peel appearance to skin surface.

or patient. Such plans are frequently used in hospitals, care facilities, and clinics.

The plan of care must address education, pain management needs, emotional and physical care, family impact, cultural influences, and financial constraints. Specific goals of care for any patient are based on nursing observation and assessment, physician orders, the patient's personal desires and goals, and input from other members of the health care team. The patient must agree to the goals, and they must be clearly communicated to other care providers through well-written care plans and documentation, as well as team conferences when appropriate. Nursing Care Plan 26-1 provides one example of an appropriate nursing care plan.

Cultural considerations can be particularly significant in the area of women's health care. **Cultural views regarding sexuality, reproduction, and the role of**

woman in society will have a direct bearing on the type of care sought and the amount and type of information the woman is willing and able to give. The nurse cannot pass judgement based on her own cultural bias, but must be open and supportive to the needs of women who continue to be under the influence of their own cultural experience.

The influence of culture is very strong. A few years ago, the author worked in a hospital that served an area with a large Spanish-speaking population. Among this cultural group it was not unusual for women to bottle-feed their newborns in the hospital then switch to breastfeeding at home, thus avoiding having strangers assist them in what they regarded as a personal process. Older women in their own community provided the support and counseling they needed once they were back in their own environment.

Nursing Care Plan 26-1

Selected nursing diagnoses, goals/expected outcomes, nursing interventions, and evaluations for a patient who has had an abdominal hysterectomy

Situation: Marilyn Blair, age 52, has just returned to the unit after abdominal hysterectomy for multiple fibroids, metrorrhagia, and greatly increased uterine size that caused abdominal pain. She has an IV of 1,000 mL normal saline in the left forearm, an indwelling urinary catheter, an abdominal dressing, and a patient-controlled analgesia (PCA) pump containing morphine. Her vital signs are blood pressure 138/82; pulse 86: respirations 16: temperature, 98.2°F.

Nursing Diagnosis	Goals/Expected Outcomes	Nursing Intervention	Evaluation
Pain related to surgical incision. SUPPORTING DATA Abdominal hysterectomy; moaning and grimacing.	Pain will be controlled by analgesia. Pain will be controlled by oral analgesia at time of discharge.	Instruct her in use of PCA pump. Give booster medication as ordered if needed. Assess location, type, and quality of pain q 3 to 4 h. Assist with repositioning and support with pillows to attain comfort. Provide quiet, darkened atmosphere for sleep and rest. Monitor for side effects of morphine, especially respiratory rate; administer antiemetic as ordered at first signs of nausea to prevent vomiting and further pain. Check catheter and tubing for patency frequently to prevent bladder distention and further pain.	Using PCA pump with good relief; sleeping long intervals on side with pillow behind back and between knees for comfort; respirations 14; no nausea or emesis; bladder not distended, Foley draining clear urine; continue plan.
Risk for fluid volume deficit related to possible hemorrhage from surgery. SUPPORTING DATA Abdominal hysterectomy	Vital signs will remain stable; no signs of shock. No hemorrhage as evidenced by lack of signs of excessive bleeding.	Monitor vital signs frequently per postoperative routine. Check abdominal dressing and beneath patient for signs of bleeding with each set of vital signs; assess for bleeding from vaginal cuff. Assess for signs of intra-abdominal bleeding; increasing abdominal girth, decreasing bowel sounds, increasing abdominal pain and rigidity.	Abdominal dressing clean and dry; no visible vaginal drainage; VS BP 118/68; P 84; R 16; abdomen soft; no bowel sounds, continue plan.
Risk for ineffective breathing pattern related to pain, anesthesia, and analgesia. SUPPORTING DATA Shallow respirations; groggy, sleeping for long periods; states "It hurts too much to cough."	Patient will perform deep-breathing and coughing exercises. No signs of atelectasis or pneumonia as evidenced by clear breath sounds in all areas and normal temperature.	Assist patient to sit up to deep-breathe and cough q 2 h; give small pillow to splint incision before coughing. Encourage her to take four deep breaths each time a commercial comes on the television while it is on. Enlist aid of family or significant others in reminding patient to deep-breathe. Auscultate lung sounds q shift, report diminished or absent breath sounds or crackles. Ambulate as soon as ordered.	Deep-breathing and coughing at 8, 10, 12, and 2 sitting on side of bed; lung sounds clear bilaterally; temperature, 98.8°F continue plan.

Nursing Care Plan 26-1 *(Continued)*

Nursing Diagnosis	Goals/Expected Outcomes	Nursing Intervention	Evaluation
Risk for infection related to surgery. SUPPORTING DATA Abdominal hysterectomy.	Patient will be without signs of infection at discharge.	Administer prophylactic antibiotics as ordered. Monitor incision for signs of redness, swelling, purulent drainage, hardness. Keep dressing clean and dry. Use careful aseptic technique when changing dressings. Monitor WBC count and temperature. Assess vaginal drainage for signs of odor or change in character. Assess abdomen for signs of abscess or peritonitis: increasing pain, localized tenderness, swelling, decreased bowel sounds.	Taking antibiotics; dressing clean and dry; white blood cell (WBC) not repeated, is afebrile; vaginal drainage moderate in amount, serosanguine in character; abdomen soft, no bowel sounds; no signs of infection; continue plan.
Risk for injury related to possibility of thrombophlebitis from bed rest and abdominopelvic surgery. SUPPORTING DATA Abdominal hysterectomy; reluctant to ambulate.	Patient will not exhibit signs of thrombophlebitis.	Encourage ambulation as soon as it is ordered; explain benefits. Encourage added fluid intake as soon as diet order allows. Assist with leg and ankle exercises q 2 h; encourage her to do them during commercials while watching television. Inspect lower legs q shift; check for positive Homans' sign beginning third postoperative day.	Leg and ankle exercises at 8, 10, 12, and 2; will ambulate this P.M.; continue plan.
Body image disturbance related to removal of uterus. SUPPORTING DATA States "I wonder if my sex life will be different now; it seems strange to be missing a part."	Patient will express her concerns over loss of uterus. Patient will accept new body image within 3 months as evidenced by lack of depression and reinvestment in usual activities.	Provide openings for conversation regarding patient concerns over loss of uterus and its meaning to her. Explore her feelings regarding sexuality after hysterectomy. Encourage expression of positive aspects of having the hysterectomy and how she as a person is unchanged.	Patient still groggy; begin discussion of concerns tomorrow; continue plan.

◆ Implementation

The patient's needs must always be addressed when implementing aspects of the plan of care. Education must be done in a manner appropriate to the woman's knowledge base and ability to assimilate new information and should be an aspect of each nursing contact. Always try to schedule routine care at times that are the easiest for the patient. For example, scheduling a daily procedure, such as a dressing change during the only time a patient's family can visit, may cause resentment and decrease her cooperativeness. Scheduling the procedure at a different time shows respect for her feelings and needs.

Aspects of the plan of care may prove unworkable, or the patient's needs may change over time. It is important to update the plan whenever these situations occur.

◆ Evaluation

Each aspect of care must be evaluated. How effective were pain control measures? How is the patient tolerating the change in diet or new therapy? Have there been any adverse reactions to medications or treatments? Any action toward the patient requires evaluation of its effects.

COMMON DISORDERS OF THE FEMALE REPRODUCTIVE TRACT

♦ Pelvic Inflammatory Disease (PID)

Pelvic inflammatory disease (PID) refers to any inflammation in the pelvis but outside the uterus. The organisms causing the infection are usually introduced from the outside, traveling through the uterus to infect pelvic organs. For this reason, **PID is much more common in sexually active women, particularly women with multiple sexual partners.** An IUD also increases the incidence of PID, particularly in women with multiple partners, or whose partner has other partners.

If the infection locates in the fallopian tubes, it is called **salpingitis.** Infection of the ovary is called **oophoritis;** involvement of the pelvic peritoneum is called pelvic peritonitis. In some cases of uterine infection after delivery, the inflammation may extend outward and involve adjoining connective tissues, causing a PID called *pelvic cellulitis.* The majority of these infections are caused by two sexually transmitted organisms, *Neisseria gonorrhoea* or *Chlamydia trichomatis,* and the most common side effect is sterility due to damage to the fallopian tubes.

Symptoms of acute PID include severe abdominal and pelvic pain and fever, frequently accompanied by a foul-smelling purulent vaginal discharge, and the patient appears acutely ill. Chronic PID usually causes backache, a feeling of pelvic heaviness, and disturbances in menstruation. However, mild cases may produce no symptoms but still cause significant reproductive damage. Acute PID usually is treated with IV antibiotics. If the women has an IUD, it is removed, usually 1 to 2 days after treatment begins, and she is encouraged to select another form of birth control.

♦ Vaginitis

Inflammation of the vagina and the accompanying itching and discharge are among the most common gynecological problems. However, not all vaginal infections cause inflammation. *Bacterial vaginosis* is a common vaginal infection that does not produce inflammation and may therefore go undetected. See Table 26-7 for a comparison of the most common types of vaginal infections.

DISORDERS OF THE CERVIX, UTERUS, AND ENDOMETRIUM

♦ Tumors of the Cervix

Benign cervical polyps are not uncommon and occur most frequently in women 40 to 60 years of age who have had more than one child. Slight bleeding between menstrual periods, after **coitus** (sexual intercourse), and after vaginal examination are the only symptoms of cervical polyps, and they closely parallel the symptoms of early cervical cancer. **Malignant tumors of the cervix are the second most common cancer in women.** Several recognized risk factors are associated with cervical cancer, including having multiple sex partners or one partner who has multiple sex partners, being sexually active as a teenager, multiple pregnancies (even if not carried to term), infection with human papilloma virus (HPV, genital warts), and smoking.

Regular pelvic examinations and Pap smears often disclose cervical cancer in the early stage, when treatment is both easier and less invasive. Table 26-8 lists the current diagnostic and staging criteria on cancer of the cervix, called the Bethesda System. This system allows the pathologist to give very complete information on any cellular changes, both malignant and benign, and is much more specific than previously used screening information.

♦ Tumors of the Uterus

Tumors of the uterus are not uncommon among women between the ages of 25 and 40. They are usually benign **uterine myomas** (fibroids), which are frequently asymptomatic. **The most common malignant tumor of the female reproductive organs is endometrial cancer,** which is slow growing and usually occurs after menopause. Bleeding is common with all uterine tumors, but endometrial cancer usually causes postmenopausal bleeding, whereas fibroids more commonly bleed between regular menstrual periods, and the problem frequently ceases after menopause with the reduction in female hormones. Benign fibroids often are treated conservatively or not at all if the bleeding is not severe, whereas endometrial cancer requires hysterectomy and perhaps radiation therapy. Fibroids that bleed excessively may be surgically excised. In older women a hysterectomy or endometrial **ablation** (laser destruction of the uterine lining) may be performed in cases of prolonged excessive bleeding.

Elder Care Point . . . A large number of older women are now on long-term estrogen replacement therapy to prevent osteoporosis. The increased risk in endometrial

TABLE 26-7 ◆ *Signs and Symptoms of Common Vaginal Infections*

	Bacterial Vaginosis (BV)	Chlamydia	Trichomonas	Yeast Infection
Primary causative organism(s)	*Gardnerella* (most common). *Haemophilus. Corynebacterium.* Certain anaerobes.	*Chlamydia trachomatis.*	*Trichomonas vaginalis.*	Candidiasis (formerly called *Monilia*).
Onset	May note odor after intercourse.	May have no symptoms, onset 1 to 5 weeks after exposure.	May appear or worsen immediately following menstruation.	Abrupt; preceding menstruation.
Odor	Fishy, most noticeable after intercourse.	None.	Fishy or foul with heavy discharge.	None.
Itching	Usually none (does not invade vaginal wall).	Itching and burning may occur, also burning on urination.	Occasionally, varies according to degree of inflammation.	Severe, most prominent symptom.
Discharge	Thin, milky white or grey, may be frothy.	May have thin or purulent discharge.	Yellow, green or grey, may be frothy.	Thick, white, "cottage cheese" when colonization is heavy.
Sexually transmitted	Yes.	Yes.	Yes.	Possibly.
Vulvar signs	Absent.	Absent.	May have redness or edema if discharge is profuse.	Redness; excoriation from scratching; may have edema of labia.
Vaginal signs	Little or no redness; discharge adherent to vaginal wall, normal cervix.	Nonspecific or absent. Often diagnosed because sexual partner has been diagnosed with nongonococcal urethritis.	Widespread redness, possible vaginal/cervical petechiae (red dots from tiny surface hemorrhages), cervix may bleed easily.	Discharge adherent to vaginal wall, normal cervix.
Treatment	Metronidazole orally, sometimes vaginally; sexual partner treated if problem recurrent.	Antibiotics such as tetracycline, doxycycline, erythromycin; treat sexual contacts concurrently. Avoid sex until both partners cured.	Metronidazole orally, betadine douche bid × 1 week; treat sexual contacts concurrently.	Miconazole or clotrimaxole vaginally as directed. Oral treatment Diflucon 150 mg in 1 dose.

cancer, as well as the possible relationship to breast cancer, makes it particularly important that these women have annual pelvic exams and perform BSE regularly.

ENDOMETRIOSIS

Endometriosis is a rather common disorder in which *endometrial tissue* (the inner lining of the uterus) is found outside the uterus, particularly in the ovaries, *rectovaginal septum* (wall separating rectum and vagina), pelvis, and abdomen. It usually undergoes the same changes as the normal endometrium during the menstrual cycle and may bleed at the time of menses, which can cause irritation, pain, and the formation of adhesions. Other symptoms may include excessive menstrual flow, bleeding between periods, painful bowel movements and painful coitus.

Treatment options from least to most invasive include watchful waiting if symptoms are mild or absent; birth control pills, which may cause the misplaced tissue to slough off; an androgen such as danazol, which may shrink the implanted tissue; laparoscopic treatment involving laser destruction of the implanted tissue; surgical excision or **fulguration** (destruction by electric cautery; and hysterectomy with *oophorectomy* removal of ovaries) to inhibit the formation of the hormones necessary to support endometrial tissue.

TABLE 26-8 ◆ *Diagnosis and Staging of Cervical Dysplasia—Bethesda System*

Adequacy of the specimen	General categorization
Satisfactory for evaluation Satisfactory for evaluation but limited by (specify) Unsatisfactory for evaluation	Within normal limits Benign cellular changes, see descriptive diagnosis Epithelial cell abnormality, see descriptive diagnosis

Descriptive Diagnosis				
Benign Cellular Changes	**Reactive Changes**	**Epithelial Cell Abnormalities**	**Glandular Cell**	**Other Malignant Neoplasms (Specify)**
Infection *Trichomonas vaginalis* Fungal organisms morphologically consistent with *Candida* spp. Predominance of cocco-bacilli consistent with *Actinomyces* spp. Cellular changes associated with herpes simplex virus. Other.	Reactive cellular changes associated with: Inflammation. Atrophy with inflammation. Radiation. Intrauterine device. Other.	Squamous cell Atypical squamous cells of undetermined significance: qualify. Low-grade squamous intraepithelial lesion encompassing: human papilloma virus (HPV) mild dysplasia/CIN 1*. High-grade squamous intraepithelial lesion encompassing: moderate and severe dysplasia, CIS/CIN 2 and CIN 3. Squamous cell carcinoma.	Endometrial cells, cytologically benign in a post menopausal woman. Atypical glandular cells of undetermined significance: qualify. Endocervical carcinoma. Endometrial adenocarcinoma. Extrauterine adenocarcinoma. Adenocarcinoma not otherwise specified.	Hormonal elevation (applies to vaginal smears only). Hormonal pattern compatible with age and history. Hormonal pattern incompatible with age and history: specify. Hormonal evaluation not possible due to: specify.

CIN 1, 2, 3 refers to previous common screening technique, where cells were differentiated as normal or CIN 1, 2 or 3 (types of abnormality).

OVARIAN TUMORS

Approximately 70% of ovarian tumors are benign. Some are *cystic* (sac-like), others are solid. *Dermoid cysts* are believed to be caused by the spontaneous growth of an unfertilized ovum. Benign ovarian tumors can grow very large and may cause problems by crowding other structures.

Ovarian cancer frequently has few, often rather nonspecific, symptoms. These may include a slightly swollen abdomen; digestive problems; chronic discomfort in the lower abdomen, low-back pain, dysuria, pelvic pressure, unusual vaginal bleeding (rare in ovarian cancer, but a definite sign of some abnormality which should be evaluated). Treatment includes *panhysterectomy* (removal of uterus, fallopian tubes, and ovaries) and chemotherapy, either IV or intraperitoneal. Radiation is more controversial, but may also be used. (See Chapter 9 for care of the cancer patient.)

UTERINE PROLAPSE, CYSTOCELE, RECTOCELE

When age or childbearing cause significant weakening of the muscles of the pelvic floor, they may no longer adequately support the uterus, bladder, and rectum. The uterus may *prolapse* (protrude downward into the vagina) and the bladder may bulge into the vagina (*cystocele*), as may the rectum (*rectocele*). The procedure to correct cystocele and rectocele as one surgical process is called an *anteroposterior repair* (frequently called an A&P repair) or *anterosposterior colporrhaphy*. Hysterectomy is commonly performed for uterine prolapse. However, if a woman is a poor surgical risk (usually because of advanced age), a **pessary** (hard rubber ring) may be inserted in the vagina to help keep the abdominal organs in place.

GYNECOLOGICAL SURGICAL PROCEDURES

Gynecological surgery may be classified into three major types: (1) sterilization procedures; (2) reconstructive procedures; and (3) removal of the female reproductive organs (*hysterectomy*). While standard abdominal incisions are still necessary for many procedures, there is a growing use of **endoscopy** (use of an optical instrument to visualize and access enclosed spaces within the body). An endoscopic tool such as a *laparoscope* is introduced via a small incision or a natural opening such as the cervix. The area can be fully visualized and surgical instruments can be introduced through the scope to perform various procedures.

◆ Sterilization Procedures

Sterilization procedures work by obstructing the pathway of the ovum to the uterus as well as preventing the sperm from traveling to the ovum via the fallopian tubes. **Sterilization should always be considered a permanent procedure.** Even procedures designed to be reversible, such as placing plugs within the fallopian tubes rather than **ligating** (tying) or cutting and **cauterizing** them (destroying cut ends with electrocautery) frequently leave adhesions or scar tissue that prevent reversal.

The procedure may be performed through a small abdominal incision (or concurrently with another abdominal surgery such as Cesarean section—the Pomeroy procedure is common), via a vaginal approach using a culdoscope that involves no external incision, or as an endoscopic procedure using the laparoscope.

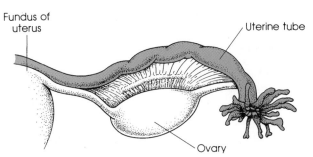

A. Intact tube and adjacent ovary.

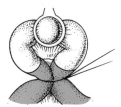 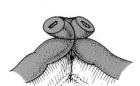

B. Portion of tube has been pulled through a ring to form a tight loop. Tube is severed.

C. Severed tube and destruction of its continuity so that ova can no longer pass through the uterus.

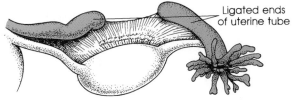

D. Severed tube.

FIGURE 26-3 Pomeroy procedure for sterilization.

Currently, most sterilization procedures are done with the laparoscope. The surgery and recovery times are both shorter than the abdominal approach, the incision is tiny and usually leaves minimal scaring, and the procedure has a much lower potential for infection than a vaginal approach. See Figures 26-3, 26-4, and 26-5 for diagrams of sterilization procedures.

◆ Vaginal and Abdominal Gynecological Surgery

Table 26-9 names and describes a variety of gynecological surgeries with teaching points and nursing care. General postoperative care for all patients includes monitoring during recovery from anesthesia or sedation, appropriate pain management, and monitoring for signs of infection. It should be noted that simple hysterectomy is now frequently done vaginally, with no abdominal incision. Recovery time is lessened, and in some areas these are now being done as an outpatient procedure. The surgeon often will specify a period of sexual abstinence following most of these procedures to allow for healing.

The patient undergoing these procedures frequently needs significant supportive care, as mentioned earlier. Fears of loss of femininity, loss of sexuality, loss of reproductive ability, and the potential of life-threatening illness are all possible reasons why such surgery may be extremely stressful.

BREAST DISORDERS

Although the breast is not a reproductive organ, it is affected by hormonal changes related to the menstrual cycle and pregnancy.

◆ Fibrocystic Breast Disease (FBD), or Fibrocystic Breast Change (FBC)

Fibrocystic changes affect more than 30% of the female population, causing experts to question whether it is actually a disease, thus the newer name *fibrocystic breast change*. The disorder is characterized by single or multiple benign tumors in the breast. These may be fluid-filled sacs (cysts) or solid fibrous growths containing connective tissue elements (*fibroadenomas*).

The phenomenon occurs most often during the reproductive years, beginning in the late teens or early twenties, and the symptoms seem to subside after menopause. The condition causes lumps in the breast with fullness and tenderness that is more noticeable during the premenstrual period. These lumps make breast self-exam more difficult and are a frequent source of anxiety.

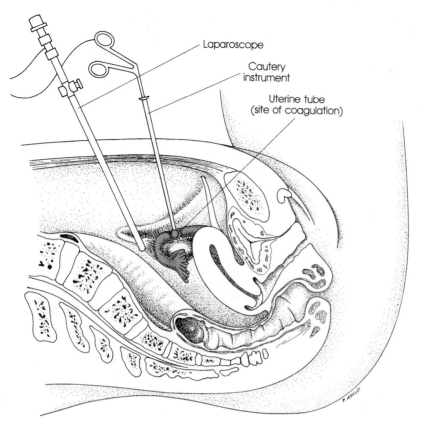

FIGURE 26-4   Laparoscopic procedure.

The laparoscope (visualizing instrument) has been inserted through one small incision in the lower abdomen after inflation of the peritoneal cavity. The cautery instrument has been inserted through a second small incision and is used to cauterize and thus destroy the continuity of the fallopian tube.

FIGURE 26-5   Culdoscopic procedure.

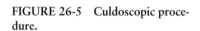

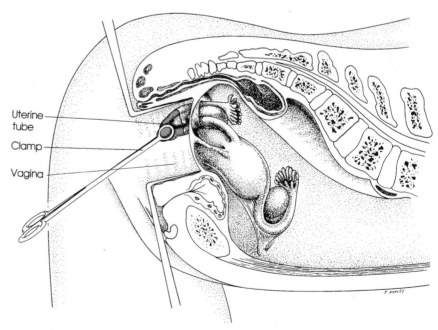

The culdoscope is introduced vaginally. The tubes are drawn into the vagina with a clamp, cut and tied, and then returned to their normal position.

TABLE 26-9 ◆ *Types of Gynecological Surgery*

Surgical Procedure	Reasons for Performing	Description	Nursing Care and Teaching Points
Dilatation and curettage (D&C)	Excessive vaginal bleeding; incomplete abortion; removal of placental fragments; therapeutic abortion.	Scraping away the inner lining of the uterus (endometrium) via the cervix.	Observe for excessive bleeding postoperatively.
Conization, or conical excision	Removal of abnormal or early cancerous tissue; biopsy.	Removal of cone of tissue with scalpel or electrical cutting wire.	Office procedure. May cause some bleeding.
Fistulectomy	Presence of rectovaginal fistula (channel between rectum and vagina) or urethrovaginal fistula (channel between bladder and vagina).	Surgical excision of the fistula and repair of the tissue to prevent passage of urine or feces into the vagina.	Observe for excessive bleeding or for vaginal fecal drainage postoperatively.
Hysterectomy	Prolapse of pelvic organs; pain associated with pelvic congestion; endometriosis; excessive/debilitating uterine bleeding; fibroids; noninvasive uterine or cervical cancer.	Removal of entire uterus, vaginally or abdominally.	Observe for excessive bleeding; paralytic ileus can occur. Ends childbearing if premenopausal, which may have profound emotional impact.
Panhysterectomy	Cancer; pain associated with pelvic inflammatory disease; recurrent ovarian cysts	Removal of entire uterus, fallopian tubes, and ovaries.	See hysterectomy. Removal of ovaries induces menopause in premenopausal women.
Radical hysterectomy	Invasive cancer.	Removal of uterus, tubes, ovaries, upper third of vagina and lymph nodes.	See hysterectomy and panhysterectomy. Vaginal alteration may affect ability to have sexual intercourse. Possible lymphedema due to removal of nodes.
Anterior and posterior colporrhaphy	Presence of prolapse of bladder and rectum into the vagina; may accompany a uterine prolapse.	Repair of the anterior and posterior wall of the vagina.	Observe for excessive bleeding.
Salpingectomy	Tubal pregnancy; tumor; traumatic injury.	Removal of a fallopian tube.	Will not cause infertility if other tube/ovary are intact.
Oophorectomy	Tumor; cystic disease; endometriosis; traumatic injury; severe hormonal disorder.	Removal of an ovary.	See salpingectomy. Only a portion of one ovary is necessary to provide normal hormonal balance prior to menopause.
Vulvectomy	Malignancy.	Radical vulvectomy: surgical excision of the labia, clitoris, perineal structures, femoral and inguinal lymphatic tissues.	Major disfigurement; extreme supportive measures, including professional counseling, often required.

Common treatment of FBC is vitamin or hormonal. A vitamin B complex is helpful, and vitamin E has shown dramatic improvement for some women. Hormonal therapy usually is given to women with significant FBC who do not get relief from more conservative therapies. Danazol, a synthetic androgen, gives good relief, but has possible side effects of menstrual irregularities, weight gain, edema, and acne. Bromocriptine, a prolactin antagonist, decreases cyclic breast pain. Possible side effects include nausea, vomiting, and dizziness.

Self-help measures include stress reduction and the use of stress-management techniques, and restriction of methylxanthines, particularly caffeine, which are found in foods such as coffee, tea, and chocolate. Many over-the-counter medications contain both caffeine and theobromine, both of which need to be avoided. Dietary treatment of FBC can be very difficult for some women

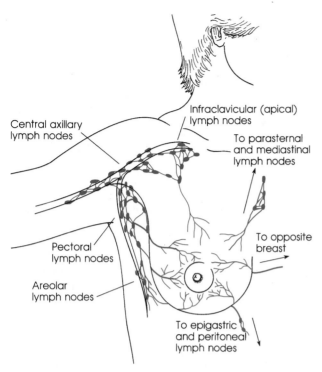

Infraclavicular (apical)
lymph nodes

Central axillary
lymph nodes

To parasternal
and mediastinal
lymph nodes

To opposite
breast

Pectoral
lymph nodes

Areolar
lymph nodes

To epigastric
and peritoneal
lymph nodes

FIGURE 26-6   Lymph drainage of the breast.

because the offending substances need to be totally eliminated and results usually take at least 2 months to become apparent. **Limiting sodium and taking a mild diuretic the week before menstruation may also help, as may warm compresses to the breast, wearing brassieres that give good support, and taking analgesic medications such as acetaminophen, aspirin, or ibuprofen.**

Breast self-examination should be performed 1 week after the beginning of menstruation as the swelling and tenderness are at a minimum at this point in the cycle. Women with FBC learn to recognize the size and shape of their normal lumps and should report any change in these findings, as well as change in breast contour, increased vein prominence, increased pain, and nipple changes. See Figure 26-6 for a diagram of the female breast.

Think about . . . Why is fibrocystic disorder no longer thought of as a disease by many practitioners?

◆ Breast Cancer

It is estimated that 184,300 new invasive cases of breast cancer will be diagnosed among women in the United States in 1996. The risk increases with age. Specific risk factors include (1) personal or family history of breast cancer, particularly mother or sister; (2) early onset of menstruation; (3) menopause later than age 50; (4) nulliparity or first child late in life; (5) higher education or socioeconomic level (involves lifestyle factors not yet determined); (6) high-fat diet; (7) fibrocystic disease with atypical cells. Absence of these risk factors does not make a woman immune to breast cancer. See Table 26-10 for the American Cancer Society recommendations for early detection.

A lump in the breast is the most common early symptom of breast cancer. These are usually painless, but there may be tenderness. All lumps and any tender or painful areas, including nipples, should be evaluated. Abnormal discharge from the nipple or retracting of the nipple, dimpling of the breast tissue, swelling or enlargement, increased firmness, and appearance of a reddened area or dry, flaky area are all symptoms that can mean cancer and need to be evaluated. Biopsy is required for a definitive diagnosis.

Elder Care Point . . . Women of advanced years may feel that they no longer need regular mammograms and Pap smears, particularly if they are not sexually active. They need to be aware that the incidence of breast and endometrial cancers increases with age and that annual screening becomes more, not less, important.

Treatment options are be based on the type of breast cancer, stage of the disease, patient's age, physical and menopausal status, and other health factors that may affect ability to undergo treatment. In general, the primary treatment is usually surgical removal of the tumor and varying amounts of surrounding tissue. The types of surgery are (1) lumpectomy (removal of tumor only); (2) partial or segmental mastectomy (removal of tumor and a portion of the surrounding breast tissue, axillary lymph nodes); (3) simple or total mastectomy (removal of entire breast, axillary lymph nodes); (4) modified radical mastectomy (breast, axillary lymph nodes, and lining over the chest wall muscles); (5) radical mastec-

TABLE 26-10 ◆ *Recommendations for Breast Cancer Screening*		
Age 20–40	**Age 40–49**	**Age 50 and older**
Monthly breast self-examination 1 week after menses begin.	Monthly breast self-examination 1 week after menses begin.	Monthly breast self-examination (do same day each month after menopause).
Mammography if M.D. feels that it is clinically indicated.	Mammography at age 40, then every 1–2 years.	Mammography every year.
Clinical breast examination every 3 years.	Clinical breast examination every year.	Clinical breast examination every year.

tomy (breast, axillary lymph nodes, and chest wall muscles under the breast). Radical mastectomy wasonce very common, but high success rates with a reduction in disfigurement are now made possible by using appropriate staging of the disease when making treatment decisions. Surgery may be delayed or deferred if the disease is widespread and the patient's overall condition is poor. Radiation often is done following lumpectomy or segmented mastectomy to further enhance cure. Chemotherapy also may be considered as part of treatment, in combination with surgery and radiation, or as the primary treatment in women who are poor candidates for surgical intervention.

Breast reconstruction following mastectomy is becoming increasingly common, and allows the return to a normal or near-normal appearance. It may be done as part of the mastectomy, or at a later date after treatment is completed. See Figure 26-7 for postmastectomy and post–breast reconstruction photos.

Body image and disfigurement issues, as well as the focus in our society on the breast as a marker of femininity or sexual attractiveness, make treatment for breast cancer a highly emotionally charged experience. Women require ongoing supportive care, and most will benefit greatly from participating in a support group and from visits by American Cancer Society's Reach to Recovery volunteers. These women have all undergone treatment for breast cancer and have been trained to do peer counseling. The local unit of the American Cancer Society can be contacted regarding Reach to Recovery visits.

◆ Pre- and Postoperative Care

Most women need extensive education prior to breast surgery. Many surgeons now provide educational programs for their patients, but it is important for the nurse to determine whether, in fact, the patient did receive adequate information and whether she has a good understanding of what was taught. Women often are particularly concerned about the change in their appearance following breast surgery. Talking with a Reach to Recovery volunteer or a nurse with extensive professional or personal knowledge prior to surgery can be very helpful. Teaching points will vary depending on the amount of tissue to be surgically removed and whether or not a prosthesis will be implanted either during the initial surgery or at a later date.

Postoperative care will include pain management, observation for signs of infection, and continued supportive and educational measures. Because breast tissue is very vascular, bleeding may be a problem. Surgical dressings should be observed frequently during the first 48 hours following the procedure. Some women will also benefit from professional counseling. The nurse should inform the physician if this appears to be an appropriate or needed intervention.

◆ Lymphedema

A common problem following invasive surgery for breast cancer is *lymphedema*. The removal of lymph tissue can cause lymph blockage that results in chronic swelling in the affected arm. **Use of lab tourniquets and blood pressure cuffs on the affected arm should be strenuously avoided to avoid aggravating the condition.** Information on a variety of ways of minimizing and controlling lymphedema can be obtained from the National Lymphedema Network, 2211 Post Street, Suite 404, San Francisco, CA 94115, phone 1-800-541-3259.

Following mastectomy, it is important that the woman exercise to regain normal arm movement on the

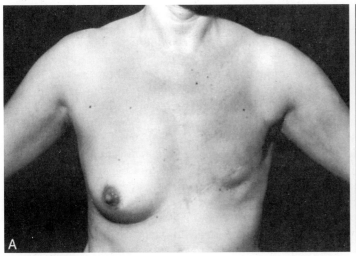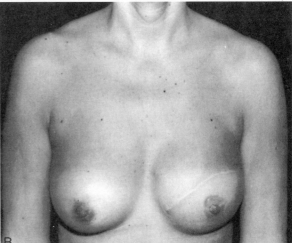

FIGURE 26-7 *(A)* Chest wall after modified radical mastectomy. *(B)* Appearance after reconstruction with a latissimus dorsi myocutaneous flap and an implant. *(Source:* Bland, K. I., Copeland, E. M. eds., (1991). *The Breast.* Philadelphia: Saunders.)

affected side. See Figure 26-8 for examples of postmastectomy exercises.

RECONSTRUCTIVE BREAST SURGERY

Plastic surgery of the breast may be done to enlarge the breasts, reduce their size, or to make the breasts equal in size and contour. As mentioned, reconstruction is becoming increasingly common among women who have been treated for breast cancer.

Plastic surgery of the breast includes the following procedures:

- **Reduction mammoplasty:** to reduce the size of the breasts when *hypertrophy* (excessive growth) of breast tissue causes physical and psychological problems. Problems related to excessively large breasts include back pain, shoulder pain and pressure on nerves from brassiere straps, inability to obtain appropriate clothing that fits, and psychological problems related to fear of ridicule and unwelcome sexual advances.
- **Augmentation mammoplasty:** to enlarge and possibly lift the breasts. This may be done for cosmetic reasons or to return the breast to normal size after a partial mastectomy.
- **Reconstructive mammoplasty:** to create a new breast when all the natural tissue has been removed during a mastectomy, either for cancer or traumatic injury.

COMMUNITY CARE

Community care can take many forms. In the area of general reproductive health, low-cost women's health care clinics and organizations such as Planned Parenthood offer pregnancy testing, counseling and instruction on contraception and sexually transmitted diseases, programs on breast and vulvar self-exam, and screening procedures such as pelvic exams and mammograms. Instruction and low-cost screening may also be made available by local chapters of organizations such as the American Cancer Society. These outreach programs seek to make information and services available to all women at a reasonable cost. Such programs assist in the prevention and early detection of disease, reducing the long-term effects of potentially serious illness and the cost of community health care.

Community care also takes the form of educational public service announcements on radio and television and in newspapers and magazines. These give the public valuable information on sexual health and disease prevention and treatment. The national AIDS Awareness program is an example of this type of community education.

School nurses can and should play a major role in reproductive education and health maintenance. Drugs, alcohol, and early sexual activity are major health care concerns for our adolescents. The rate of STDs, including HIV infection, is growing alarmingly among teenagers. The school nurse is in a position to become a trusted source of accurate, nonjudgmental information for young people who are confused and poorly educated in the realities of reproductive health.

In recent years, a variety of programs have been developed for women facing serious disease of the breast or reproductive organs. They may be sponsored by national organizations such as the American Cancer Society or by local groups or health care facilities and organizations. These programs provide both education and support groups for women undergoing treatment of serious health problems such as breast or uterine cancer, infertility, fetal loss, and other concerns of women. The nurse can be very helpful in referring women to these community programs or by volunteering as a group facilitator or resource person.

HOME CARE

Home health nursing is becoming a standard of care in the United States. Hospital stays are becoming progressively shorter, and women frequently go home very quickly after illness, surgery, or childbirth. Even IV antibiotic therapy is being done with increasing frequency in the home setting, with illnesses such as PID being treated outside the hospital setting.

Many women receiving reproductive home health care have undergone a surgical procedure. Nursing responsibilities would include pain management, observation of surgical site for signs of infection (redness, swelling, pain, presence of exudate, foul odor, fever), or reopening of the surgical wound because of trauma or a poor healing response. If the procedure involves the pelvic reproductive organs, the nurse must also assess the amount and duration of bleeding, any increase in the volume of flow, and any change (e.g., purulence or foul odor) that indicates the presence of infection.

Because hospital stays are frequently short, the majority of teaching often becomes the responsibility of the home health nurse. Even conscientious teaching by the hospital nurse frequently needs extensive follow-up because the patient's learning ability was impaired by immediate concerns such as acute pain, recovery from anesthesia, or emotional stresses associated with the diagnosis and the potential impact on daily living. The home health nurse must be prepared to give accurate, detailed information as part of home care. The nurse also should assess the client's need for more general

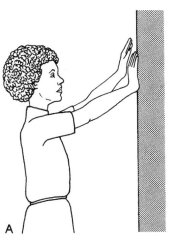

A

Front wall climbing

Patient stands facing the wall, elbows slightly bent. Palms are placed at shoulder level and fingers are flexed and unflexed as hands "walk" up the wall as high as possible. Hands are then walked back down to shoulder level. Patient moves toward wall as fingers climb higher and then away from wall as fingers move downward.

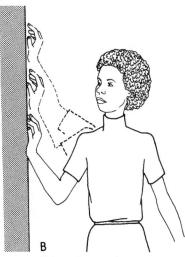

B

Side wall climbing

With operative side to wall, arm is extended until fingers touch wall. Patient moves toward the wall as fingers climb higher until body touches it. Maneuver is reversed as fingers climb back down wall.

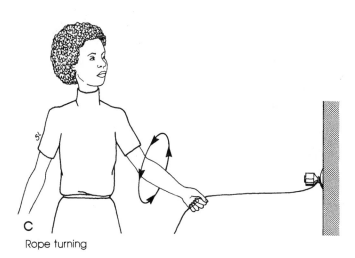

C

Rope turning

One end of rope is tied to door knob. Patient holds other end of rope and swings it in a circular motion, being sure entire arm and not the wrist is in motion.

Holding a yardstick or broom handle with both hands, the back is placed against a wall. Arms are extended straight downward and, with elbows straight, the stick is raised by the straightened arms until knuckles touch the wall over the head.

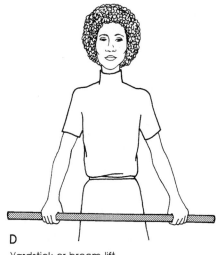

D

Yardstick or broom lift

FIGURE 26-8   Patient education: postmastectomy exercises.

education regarding reproductive health, such as regular BSE and VSE, Pap smears, and need for information regarding contraception or STDs.

The home health nurse must be able to function independently and needs actively to communicate with the other members of the care team by phone, written documentation, and group conferences. The nurse also is often the primary source of information about appropriate support groups and informational programs that would be of assistance to the client and family.

CRITICAL THINKING EXERCISES

Clinical Case Situations

1. Mrs. Long is a 45-year-old college instructor, married with two teenage children. She found a lump during breast self-examination that was diagnosed as malignant. Mrs. Long does not want to have the radical mastectomy recommended by her physician.

   a. What are some possible reasons for Mrs. Long's hesitation about having a radical mastectomy?

   b. What alternative surgical procedures are available to Mrs. Long?

   c. What types of resources are available to help Mrs. Long make this decision?

2. A neighbor, age 35, has fibrocystic disease that causes her considerable discomfort. She takes aspirin or acetaminophen if the pain becomes too intense. She has not tried any other approach to managing this problem.

   a. What might you suggest to this person to help her cope with the discomfort of this disease?

3. A favorite elderly maiden aunt confides to you that she is too embarrassed to go in for "female" exams and doesn't think she needs them anyway, since she has never been married or had children.

   a. What might you tell her about the importance of such exams?

   b. What might you suggest to make it easier for her to undergo a pelvic and breast exam?

BIBLIOGRAPHY

American Cancer Society. (1995). *Breast Cancer*. Document 004070.: Author.

American Cancer Society. (1996). *Breast Cancer Facts and Figures.*: Author.

American Cancer Society. (1995). *Cervical Cancer*. Document 10021.:Author.

American Cancer Society. (1995). *Ovarian Cancer*. Document 10025.: Author.

Appling, S. E. (1996). Hormone replacement therapy—helping your patient decide. *Medsurg Nursing*. 5(5):370–373.

Baron, R. H. (1995). Nine facts everyone should know about breast cancer. *American Journal of Nursing*. 95(7):29–33.

Dell, D. D. (1997). Common questions about ductal carcinoma in situ. *American Journal of Nursing*. 97(5):61–66.

Dest, V. M., Fisher, S. M. (1994). Breast cancer, dreaded diagnosis, complicated care. *RN*. 57(6):49–55.

Dillon, P. (1994). Ovarian cancer, confronting the "silent killer." *Nursing*. 24(5):66–67.

Garner, C. (1997). Endometriosis: what you need to know. *RN*. 60(1):27–31.

Harwood, K. (1996). Straight talk about breast cancer. *Nursing*. 26(10):39–44.

Hawkness, Dinches. (1996). *Medical Surgical Nursing: Total Patient Care*. 9th ed. St. Louis, MO: Mosby, pp. 831–834.

Holm, K., Penckofer, S., Chandler, P. J. (1995). Deciding on hormone replacement therapy. *American Journal of Nursing* 95(8):57–60.

Jeffries, E. (1997). One-day mastectomy. *Home Healthcare Nurse*. 15(1):31–37.

Johns Hopkins Medical Letter. (1995). Hormone therapy; is it the right choice for you? *Johns Hopkins Medical Letter*. 7(7):4.

Ivey, C., Gordon, S. I. (1994). Breast reconstruction: new image, new hope. *RN*. 57(7):48–53.

Ivey, C. (1994). When your patient has ovarian cancer. *RN*. 57(11):26–32.

Lewis, L. L. (1995) One year in the life of a woman with premenstrual syndrome: a case study. *Nursing Research*. 95(3):111.

Mogus, M. (1997). Pelvic floor surgery? *RN*. 60(4):36–41.

Scherer, Timby, D. (1995). *Introductory Medical–Surgical Nursing*, 6th ed. Philadelphia: Lippincott, pp. 822, 829–30.

Scura, K. W., Whipple, B. (1997). How to provide better care for the post-menopausal women. *American Journal of Nursing*. 97(4):36–43.

Sharts-Hopko, N. C. (1997). STDs in women: what you need to know. *American Journal of Nursing*. 97(4):46–53.

Shurpin, K. M. (1997). Ovarian cancer: when to suspect this silent killer is at work. *American Journal of Nursing*. 97(4):34–35.

Thompson, S. D., Szukiewicz-Nugent, S. M., Walczak, J. R. (1996). When ovarian cancer strikes. *Nursing*. 26(10):33–38.

Wasaha, S., Angelopoulos, F. M. (1996). What every woman should know about menopause. *American Journal of Nursing*. 96(1):24–32.

Whipple, B. (1995). Common questions about osteoporosis and menopause. *American Journal of Nursing*. 95(1):69.

Whitman, M., McDaniel, R. W. (1993) Preventing lymphedema, an unwelcome sequel to breast cancer. *Nursing*. 23(12):36–41.

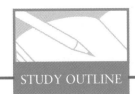

I. Introduction

A. The complex female reproductive system relies on hormones produced by the endocrine system for correct development and function.

B. Reproductive health can be disrupted by many physical disorders.

C. Emotional factors affect the care of women with reproductive disorders.

II. Reproductive Maturity

A. The period of sexual maturity is called puberty and usually occurs between the ages of 9 and 17.

B. Puberty begins with physical changes and is completed by the onset of menstruation.

C. Menses often are irregular for the first year or so.

D. Incorrect perceptions about menstruation are formed early and can increase physical and emotional discomfort.

III. Menstrual Dysfunction

A. *Amenorrhea* refers to absent menstruation, which may be related to anatomical defects, endocrine dysfunction, chronic disease, side effects of medications, poor nutrition, excessive physical exercise, or abrupt discontinuation of oral contraceptives.

B. *Dysmenorrhea* means painful or difficult menstruation, which may be increased by emotional or physiological distress.

C. A variety of medications to control pain associated with menstruation are listed in Table 26-2.

D. Infection or inflammation may be an underlying cause of menstrual dysfunction.

E. Premenstrual syndrome (PMS) symptoms include edema, acne-like eruptions, food cravings, crying spells, severe headaches, depression, anger, fatigue.

F. Dysfunctional uterine bleeding may be relatively insignificant or an early sign of a serious disorder.

　　1. *Metrorrhagia* is bleeding outside the normal cycle.

　　2. *Menorrhagia* is excessive bleeding during the cycle.

　　3. Common early in menses, during climacteric, with IUD use, and discontinuance of oral contraceptives.

　　4. May occur with infection of the endometrium.

　　5. May be caused by spontaneous abortion, ectopic pregnancy, benign fibroids, and malignancy of the cervix, vagina, and uterus.

IV. Contraception

A. Fertility awareness methods.

　　1. Basal body temperature method (BBT).

　　2. Calendar and rhythm methods.

　　3. Ovulation or Billings method.

　　4. Symptothermal method.

B. Mechanical contraception.

　　1. Male condom.

　　2. Female condom.

　　3. Diaphragm.

　　4. Spermicides.

　　5. Cervical cap.

　　6. Contraceptive sponge.

　　7. Intrauterine device (IUD).

C. Oral contraceptives.

D. Injectable contraceptives.

E. Sustained-release implants.

F. Sterilization.

　　1. Tubal ligation (female).

　　2. Vasectomy (male).

V. Menopause

A. Menopause marks the end of reproduction.

B. The average age is 50. Premature menopause occurs before 35, and delayed menopause occurs after age 58.

C. Hormonal changes during the climacteric may cause physical and emotional disturbances, which in about 25% of women are severe enough that they seek medical attention.

D. Menopausal symptoms are caused by hormone deficiency, social-cultural attitudes, and personal psychological factors.

E. Common symptoms include irregular menstruation, hot flashes or hot flushes, fatigue, insomnia, emotional swings, depression, back pain, headache, irritability, decreased libido.

F. Estrogen replacement therapy is controversial.

　　1. Possible benefits include decreased osteoporosis, control of hot flashes, decreased membrane dryness, decreased thinning of surface skin, decreased wrinkling and bruis-

ing, increased libido, decreased mood swings, and protection against cardiovascular disease.

2. Possible adverse affects include increased risk of breast and endometrial cancer, weight gain, fluid retention, nausea, headache, breast discomfort, leg cramps, hypertension, gallbladder disease, lethargy, worsening glucose tolerance in diabetic women.

G. Patient education can help women to overcome misconceptions, make healthy lifestyle choices, and realize the importance of reporting abnormal bleeding during or after menopause.

VI. Diagnostic Tests and Procedures and Nursing Responsibilities

A. The nurse must give clear, concise information and answers to questions, and provide an atmosphere that is warm, safe, and respectful of the woman's feelings, needs, and concerns.

B. A variety of common tests and procedures are listed in Table 26-5.

VII. Breast Self-Examination (BSE)

A. BSE should be done monthly 1 week after menstruation begins or on a specific date each month after menopause.

B. A specific pattern should be used. See Figure 26-2.

VIII. Vulvar Self-Examination (VSE)

A. Many women are unaware that VSE is just as important as BSE.

B. The exam is done by visualization with a mirror and palpation with the fingertips, and with the vulva held open to expose all externally visible structures.

C. Changes including new moles, warts, growths, new areas of pigmentation, ulcers, sores, pain, inflammation, itching should be reported to the patient's health care provider.

IX. Nursing Management—Assessment

A. The personal aspect of reproductive problems can make history taking difficult.

B. Necessary information includes current age; age at menarche; menstrual history, including problems; breast problems; whether sexually active and age became sexually active; number of pregnancies and outcome; history of STDs; whether BSE and VSE performed; date and outcome of last mammogram; history of PMS, postpartum depression, mood swings, menopausal depression; routine medications; family history of cancer of the breast or reproductive organs; use of diethylstilbestrol by her mother; history of diabetes mellitus, thyroid disease, sickle cell trait or disease.

C. Appropriate NANDA nursing diagnosis is based on assessment information.

X. Planning

A. Planning may include a wide variety of things, including pain management, education, and supportive care.

B. Specific goals are based on nursing observation, physician orders, information gathered during the assessment process, the patient's personal desires and goals, and input from other members of the health care team.

C. Planning must be communicated through written care plans and chart documentation.

D. Cultural considerations must be addressed in the planning process.

XI. Implementation

A. Education must be done in a manner appropriate to the woman's knowledge base and ability to assimilate new information.

B. The patient's needs must be addressed when implementing the plan of care.

C. Changes or aspects of the plan that prove unworkable must be addressed by changes in the plan of care.

XII. Evaluation

A. Each aspect of care must be evaluated for effectiveness.

B. Any action toward the patient requires evaluation of its effects.

XIII. Common Disorders of the Female Reproductive Tract

A. Pelvic inflammatory disease (PID) refers to any inflammation in the pelvis but outside the uterus, and is more common in sexually active women as infection is usually introduced from the outside.

1. Multiple partners and IUDs both increase the incidence of PID.

2. Specific types of infection include salpingitis, oophoritis, pelvic peritonitis, and pelvic cellulitis.

3. The most common organisms are *Neisseria gonorrhoea* and *Chlamydia trichomatis,* and the most common side effect is sterility.

4. Symptoms include pain, fever, foul-smelling vaginal discharge, acute illness.

B. Vaginitis is one of the most common gynecological problems (Table 26-7).

XIV. Disorders of the Cervix, Uterus, and Endometrium

A. Risk factors for cancer of the cervix include multiple sex partners, early sexual activity, multiple pregnancies, infection with HPV, and smoking.

B. Benign myomas (fibroids) of the uterus are common among women between 25 and 40 and may cause vaginal bleeding between menstrual periods.

C. Cancer of the endometrium usually occurs after menopause and is a frequent cause of dysfunctional bleeding. Risk is higher for women who are on long-term estrogen.

XV. Endometriosis

A. A somewhat common disorder where endometrial tissue is found outside the uterus and may bleed during menses, causing pain, irritation, and adhesions.

B. Treatment is based on severity; options include watchful waiting, birth control pills, hormone therapy, laser therapy, fulguration, and hysterectomy with oophorectomy.

XVI. Ovarian Tumors

A. Approximately 70% are benign and may be cystic or solid.

B. Ovarian cancer often has few symptoms, which makes early detection difficult.

C. Common treatment is panhysterectomy, chemotherapy, and possibly radiation.

XVII. Uterine Prolapse, Cystocele, Rectocele

A. Weakening of the pelvic floor can allow prolapse of the organs of the lower abdomen, requiring surgical repair.

B. Elderly women may be poor surgical risks, and a pessary may be used to help support these organs.

XVIII. Gynecological Surgical Procedures

A. Major types include sterilization, reconstructive procedures, and removal of the organs.

1. Sterilization should always be regarded as permanent. See Figures 26-3, 26-4, and 26-5 for examples of sterilization procedures.

2. Table 26-9 reviews common gynecological surgical procedures.

3. Women undergoing gynecological surgery frequently need significant emotional support.

XIX. Disorders of the Breast

A. Fibrocystic breast change (FBC) is characterized by benign tumors and may not be a disease, as it affects more than 30% of the female population.

1. It occurs most often in the reproductive years and makes BSE difficult.

2. Common treatments include vitamins such as B and E, and hormones, such as danazol.

3. Caffeine may aggravate the symptoms.

B. Breast cancer risk factors include personal or family history, early onset of menstruation, menopause later than age 50, nulliparity or first child late in life, higher education or socioeconomic level, high-fat diet, fibrocystic disease with atypical cells.

1. Symptoms include lumps, tender areas, redness, nipple discharge or retracting, dimpling, swelling, increased firmness.

2. Risk increases with age, making mammograms and exams particularly important for elderly women.

3. Surgical treatment includes lumpectomy, segmental mastectomy, simple mastectomy, modified radical mastectomy, and radical mastectomy.

4. Chemotherapy and radiation may be performed.

5. Breast reconstruction is becoming more common following mastectomy.

6. Supportive care is very important because of body image issues.

C. The primary aspects of preoperative care are education and establishing a support network.

D. Postoperative care includes pain management, observation for signs of infection and signs of excessive bleeding, and continued educational and supportive measures.

E. Lymphedema is a common problem following invasive breast surgery involving chronic swelling due to removal of lymph tissue.

F. Exercise to restore arm function is very important following mastectomy (Figure 26-8).

XX. Reconstructive Breast Surgery

A. Reconstructive surgery includes reduction mammoplasty, augmentation mammoplasty, and reconstructive mammoplasty following trauma or mastectomy.

XXI. Community Care

A. Community organizations may provide low-cost pregnancy testing, counseling, instruction on contraception and sexually transmitted diseases, programs on BSE and VSE, and screening procedures.

B. Public service health announcements are another form of community care.

C. School nurses can and should be a valuable resource to young women regarding issues of sexuality, reproduction, and disease.

D. A variety of programs are available for women facing serious disease of the breast or female reproductive organs.

E. The nurse should provide information to patients on these programs and assist her in making contact.

XXII. Home Care

A. Women frequently go home soon after major treatment or childbirth.

B. In the home, as in the clinic or hospital, the nurse must provide care as outlined by physician order and provide emotional support and education for the patient.

C. Nursing responsibilities include pain management, observation for signs of infection or poor healing, and amount of bleeding.

D. Patient teaching is an important aspect of home health nursing.

E. Communication between home health care team members is critical for the well-being of the patient.

CHAPTER 27

Care of Patients with Disorders of the Male Reproductive System

---

OBJECTIVES

Upon completing this chapter the student should be able to:
1. List the most common diagnostic tests and examinations of the male reproductive system and significant nursing responsibilities in the care of the patients undergoing each of them.
2. Describe systems and points included during assessment of the male reproductive system.
3. Choose nursing interventions for patients experiencing infection or inflammation of the reproductive organs.
4. Identify the patient teaching involved for early detection of testicular and prostate tumors.
5. Explain the nursing care for the patient who has a three-way catheter and continuous bladder irrigation system in the postoperative period.
6. Compare the nursing care plan for the patient who has had a perineal prostatic resection with that of a patient who has had a transurethral prostatic resection (TURP).
7. Discuss differences in treatment for cancer of the prostate based on the stage of the disease and the age of the man.
8. Identify causes of impotence and the methods used to treat it.

Many people are more open and comfortable talking about reproductive problems or concerns than they used to be. Frequently the nurse is the first person to discover a male reproductive concern. Many diseases and disorders, as well as medications, can affect the male reproductive system. The urinary system and reproductive system are so closely linked in the male that a disorder in one system often affects the other. The nurse needs to be comfortable with his or her own sexuality and knowledgeable about the male reproductive system to be helpful to the patient.

OVERVIEW OF ANATOMY AND PHYSIOLOGY

What Are the Structures of the Male Reproductive System?

⚴ The male gonads are the testes; they are oval shaped and are encased in the scrotum along with the epididymis, seminal vesicles, and vas deferens (Figure 27-1).

⚴ The scrotum is covered with wrinkled skin, *rugae*, and is very sensitive to temperature, pressure, touch, and pain.

⚴ The penis is a cylindrical, erectile organ that hangs in front of the scrotum. It contains three columns of erectile tissue that can cause it to extend and enlarge in circumference, becoming stiff. The penis is covered with skin and includes a foreskin unless circumcision has been performed (Figure 27-2). The scrotum and penis make up the external genitalia of the male.

⅄ The prostate gland is shaped like a walnut, encircles the urethra, and is located below and to the rear of the bladder.

⅄ The bulbourethral (Cowper's) glands are small pea-sized glands located in the urethral sphincter posterior to the urethra.

What Are the Functions of the Organs of the Male Reproductive System?

⅄ The seminiferous tubules within the testes produce sperm. Testosterone also is produced in the testes (Figure 27-3).

⅄ The scrotum, a thin-walled, muscular sac, holds the testes, the epididymis, and the vas deferens. The scrotum, which hangs from the pubic bone, suspends the testes outside of the body where they remain several degrees cooler than the body; the cooler temperature is needed for the production of viable sperm.

⅄ The spermatic cord attaches the testes to the body. It contains the blood vessels and nerves that supply the testes.

⅄ The epididymis is a long tube (almost 6 m) that conducts sperm from the testes to the vas deferens. Immature sperm mature as they travel through this tube. Mature sperm are stored in the lower portion of the epididymis.

⅄ The vas deferens is a muscular tube that connects to the epididymis. It stores sperm and then carries it to the ejaculatory duct by peristaltic movements.

⅄ The prostatic section of the urethra receives the sperm and carries it to the penile portion of the urethra for ejaculation. Secretions from the seminal vesicles and ducts of the prostate gland are mixed with the sperm.

⅄ The seminal vesicles produce a fluid that is thick and contains fructose to nourish the sperm and provide energy. The fluid also contains prostaglandins, which contribute to the motility of the sperm. This fluid mixes with the sperm to form seminal fluid, or **semen.** The average volume of semen ejaculated is 2.5 to 4 mL, but may vary from 1 to 10 mL.

⅄ The prostate gland produces thin, milky, and alkaline secretions that contribute to the seminal fluid and enhance the motility of the sperm.

⅄ The bulbourethral glands secrete an alkaline mucus-like fluid in response to sexual stimulation. These secretions neutralize the acid of residual urine in the urethra and provide some lubrication at the tip of the penis for intercourse.

⅄ The penis is flaccid until sexual arousal causes the arterioles to the erectile tissue to dilate and the veins to constrict, engorging the penis with blood until it is enlarged and rigid. This is an **erection.** Erections are stimulated by anticipation, memory, visual sensations, or by touch on the glans penis and skin of the genital area. If stimulation continues, **ejaculation** will occur. This is the forceful expulsion of semen from the urethra. Thoughts and emotions can sometimes inhibit erection.

⅄ The penis transfers semen to the vagina of the female. It also carries urine through the urethra to be excreted.

How Is Sperm Production Controlled?

⅄ The hypothalamus, the anterior pituitary, and the testes secrete hormones that control male reproduction.

⅄ The hypothalamus secretes gonadotropin-releasing hormone (Gn-RH) in response to an unknown stimulus.

⅄ Gn-RH stimulates the anterior pituitary to release lutenizing hormone (LH) and follicle-stimulating hormone (FSH). LH stimulates the testes to produce testosterone. FSH binds with cells in the seminiferous tubules, making them respond to testosterone. Testosterone and FSH stimulate the formation of sperm (spermatogenesis).

⅄ The male sex hormones are called **androgens.**

⅄ At puberty, testosterone levels rise and cause maturation of the male reproductive organs.

⅄ Sperm take 70 days to mature and are constantly being produced once puberty has occurred.

⅄ Normal sperm count is 100 million per milliliter. Sterility occurs when the sperm count, for one reason or other, drops to less than 20 million per milliliter.

What Changes Occur with Aging?

⅄ The scrotum becomes more pendulous and there is less rugae.

⅄ Prostate enlargement may occur with risk of urethral obstruction.

⅄ The penis becomes slightly smaller with increasing years.

▲ There is decreased sperm production, but fertility is intact. Ejaculate volume decreases.

▲ After age 60 the cycle of sexual response lengthens. Testosterone levels decrease slightly. Arousal takes longer and more direct penile stimulation is needed; the firmness of the erection may be decreased.

▲ Once an erection occurs, it can be sustained longer before ejaculation occurs.

▲ The time needed before another erection can occur is increased, often to between 12 and 24 hours or more.

▲ Transient inability to achieve an erection may occur. In the absence of disease, or side effects of medication, this will pass if the man has been consistently sexually active.

▲ Diabetes or hypertension, particularly if not well controlled, may cause **impotence** (inability to attain or maintain an erection).

CAUSES AND PREVENTION OF MALE REPRODUCTIVE DISORDERS

Disorders of the male reproductive system may be caused by infection, inflammation, trauma, metabolic disorders, endocrine disorders, or tumor. Cancer of the testicle is linked to history of undescended testicle and to prebirth exposure to DES. There is no known cause of cancer of the prostate, but there is a link to a genetic defect that makes some men more susceptible to the disease. Some physicians have questioned whether or not vasectomy predisposes a man to prostate cancer, but there is no research presently that verifies that vasectomy is a direct cause. Sexual activity may contribute to disorders of the male reproductive system if the man contracts a sexually transmitted disease.

Because the urinary system is so closely related to the male reproductive system, disorders in one affect the other system as well. Urethritis (inflammation of the urethra) certainly affects the male by making intercourse uncomfortable, if not impossible.

Good hygiene practices, careful choice of sexual partner, use of condoms for intercourse, and prompt attention to minor problems all can help prevent disorders of the male reproductive organs. Men between ages 15 and 40 should practice testicular self-exam and get immediate medical attention for any lump discovered. Obtaining a digital rectal exam and PSA test every year after age 50 helps detect cancers early enough to cure them.

Think about... Can you think of three ways you could educate people you know about prevention of disorders of the male reproductive system?

DIAGNOSTIC TESTS AND PROCEDURES AND NURSING IMPLICATIONS

◆ Digital Rectal Exam

To palpate the prostate and seminal vesicles a lubricated, gloved finger is inserted into the rectum. The examiner evaluates the consistency and size of the prostate and determines whether there are any nodules or tenderness.

During the examination the patient stands with his upper body bent over the examining table or lies on his left side with his hips and knees slightly flexed. Each step of the procedure is explained, and privacy is provided.

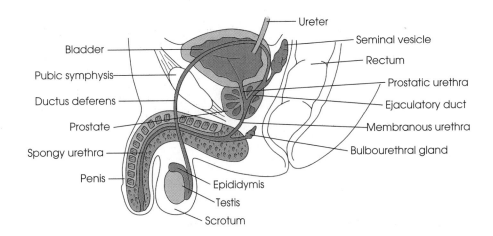

FIGURE 27-1 Structures of the male reproductive system.

Labels: Ureter, Seminal vesicle, Rectum, Prostatic urethra, Ejaculatory duct, Membranous urethra, Bulbourethral gland, Bladder, Pubic symphysis, Ductus deferens, Prostate, Spongy urethra, Penis, Epididymis, Testis, Scrotum

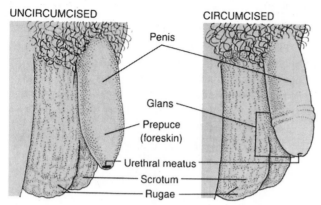

FIGURE 27-2 The external male genitalia. (*Source:* Ignatavicius, D. D., Workman, M. L., Mishler, M. A. [1995]. *Medical–Surgical Nursing: A Nursing Process Approach,* 2nd ed. Philadelphia: Saunders, p. 2166.)

◆ Semen Analysis

This test is most often done as part of a total evaluation for fertility. The specimen is analyzed for total volume of seminal fluid, and motility and number of sperm. A microscopic examination of the sperm and fluid also is done to identify infectious organisms. Semen analysis may be done for medicolegal purposes, for example, to verify the blood type in a case of alleged rape or to verify sterility as a defense in a paternity suit.

◆ Testicular Self-Examination

Testicular cancer is the third leading cause of death in young men between the ages of 20 and 35. In its concern for early detection and treatment of cancer of the testis the American Cancer Society encourages monthly self-examination of the testes by men, just as it encourages women to perform breast self-examination. If testicular cancer is treated in the early stages, it is one of the most curable forms of cancer.

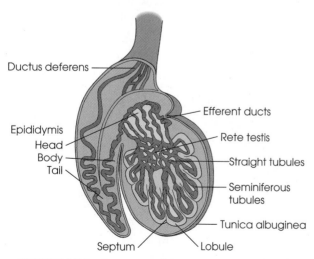

FIGURE 27-3 Structures of the testis and epididymis.

There are several sources of information for teaching testicular self-examination (TSE). The American Cancer Society publishes a pamphlet written for laypersons that is titled *For Men Only.* It also will provide a free film on TSE. Both give some basic facts about testicular cancer and explains the "how to's" of TSE.

It is recommended that TSE be done immediately after a warm shower or bath when the examiner's hands are warm and the scrotal sac is relaxed and the testicles are readily accessible. Each testicle is rolled between the thumb and fingers of both hands to detect any nodules in the testis or abnormalities in the epididymis and spermatic cord (Figure 27-4). The patient is instructed to contact his physician right away if any abnormality is found.

◆ Prostatic Specific Antigen (PSA)

The prostatic specific antigen (PSA) test is based on a glycoprotein produced only by the prostate. The test is performed on a sample of blood and costs about $50. Levels become elevated only when there is disease in the

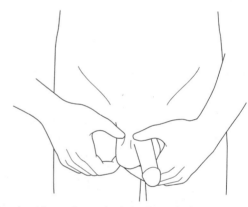

Your best hope for early detection of testicular cancer is a simple three-minute monthly self-examination. The best time is after a warm bath or shower, when the scrotal skin is most relaxed.

Roll each testicle gently between the thumb and fingers of both hands. If you find any hard lumps or nodules, you should see your doctor promptly. They may not be malignant, but only your doctor can make the diagnosis.

Following a thorough physical examination, your doctor may perform certain x-ray studies to make the most accurate diagnosis possible.

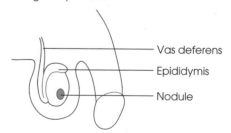

FIGURE 27-4 Testicular self-examination. (*Source:* redrawn from American Cancer Society. *For Men Only.* New York: Author.)

prostate. Normal values in males over age 15 are 0.81 to 0.89 ng/mL. Benign prostatic hypertrophy will cause PSA levels to rise, but they rarely exceed 10 ng/mL. PSA levels over 10 ng/mL are suspicious for prostatic cancer. The test is not totally diagnostic of cancer, however, as men without malignancy sometimes have a PSA elevation this high. More important, men with malignancy sometimes have a PSA within normal range. **The PSA test should be combined with digital rectal examination to detect prostate cancer.**

In patients who do have prostate malignancy, the degree of elevation may be predictive of metastases. In a group of patients who had PSA levels of 50 ng/mL or more, two thirds were found to have metastases. PSA testing is recommended annually for men over age 50. For men who have a family history of prostate cancer, testing should begin annually at age 40.

A new blood test, RT-PCR, for prostate cancer is under study. It has been 90% accurate in identifying the telltale antigen produced in response to prostate cancer cells. It is completely different from the PSA test and is more specific for prostate cancer.

◆ Transrectal Ultrasonography of the Prostate

Cancer of the prostate is the most common malignancy in men over 55 and is the second leading cause of cancer deaths in men. It is very difficult to detect in the early stages. A new tool using a transrectal probe with an ultrasound transducer at its tip can detect differences in tissue densities in the prostate gland, thereby picturing tumor location and size. This test usually is performed when PSA levels are elevated, but no mass can be felt in the prostate. The procedure takes 15 to 20 minutes to perform and can be done on an outpatient basis without anesthesia.

◆ Biopsy of the Prostate

The purpose of this test is to determine the cause of prostatic enlargement and rule out or confirm a diagnosis of malignancy. The prostate gland can be approached through the perineum, the rectum, or the urethra. A biopsy needle is inserted into several locations of the suspicious area in the prostate, and cells are aspirated and sent for histological examination.

During the procedure the patient may feel some discomfort, even though a local anesthetic is used. After the needle is withdrawn, slight pressure is applied to the insertion site to control bleeding and prevent hematoma. There are few, if any, complications expected from the procedure. Bleeding into the urethra can produce a small amount of blood in the urine.

The biopsy often is done on an outpatient basis, and the patient should be instructed to watch for signs of infection and hematoma and to report these promptly if they occur. The patient also should watch for gross hematuria and a change in urinary flow, such as frequency or inability to empty the bladder. If the patient is in the hospital at the time of the biopsy, the nurse monitors him for these signs of complications.

Think about... What sort of psychological care would the patient undergoing a prostatic biopsy need from the nurse? What might be some of the patient's concerns?

◆ Other Tests

Tests for general state of health, such as complete blood cell (CBC) count, urinalysis, chemistry profile, and thyroid tests are done initially for problems of the male reproductive tract. Serum acid phosphatase is usually elevated in the patient with prostate cancer. Serum alkaline phosphatase is elevated if malignancy of the prostate has metastasized to the bone. Kidney, ureters, bladder (KUB) x-ray; an IV pyelogram (IVP); and cystoscopy with urodynamic studies also may be done (Chapter 23).

Smears of urethral discharge and serum tests are done to detect sexually transmitted diseases (STDs). Tumor protein marker studies are performed for patients with testicular cancer for follow-up to determine the success of treatment or recurrence of the disease. The primary tumor markers are alpha-fetoprotein (AFP) and the beta-subunit of human chorionic gonadotropin (beta-hCG).

NURSING MANAGEMENT

◆ Assessment

Because of the predominance of certain kinds of reproductive disorders in males in certain age groups, the age of the patient is relevant to nursing assessment. In males over the age of 50, the assessment is directed more toward detecting prostate problems, whereas younger males are assessed for STDs and testicular cancer.

History Taking   It may be awkward for the new nurse to obtain a sexual and reproductive history, but with experience in interviewing male patients of all ages, she will soon become more comfortable and adept at obtaining necessary data. Because questions about urinary problems are usually less sensitive than those dealing with sexual dysfunction, it is best to begin with questions of this kind and then lead into more sensitive ones.

Open-ended questions that start out with "Tell me about . . ." or "When did you first notice . . ." give the

TABLE 27-1 ◆ *Guide to Assessment of the Male Reproductive System*

Ask the following questions:

◆ Have you noticed any changes in patterns of urination; any differences in the stream of urine?
◆ Do you ever have any discharge coming from the penis?
◆ Have you felt any masses or bumps in the scrotum or groin?
◆ Do you have any tenderness or pain in the scrotum or penis?
◆ Do you have any rectal or perineal pain?
◆ Do you perform regular testicular exam (if under 40 years of age)?
◆ How would you describe your sex life? Do you have any problems?
◆ Have you ever had a sexually transmitted disease?
◆ Have you had past infections of the reproductive system?
◆ What drugs do you take regularly?
◆ Do you use any recreational drugs? What about alcohol? How much do you drink? How often?
◆ Do you have diabetes? Is there a family history of diabetes?
◆ Do you have hypertension or heart disease? Have you had heart surgery?
◆ Do you have prostate problems? Have you had prostate surgery?
◆ Have you had a vasectomy?

---

patient room to discuss only those things he is comfortable talking about. It also is helpful to relate his problem to the inconvenience it has caused in his daily life. For example, tenderness and discomfort in the scrotal area could make sitting at a desk or walking very difficult and interfere with getting assigned work done. Frequent urination can cause distracting and sometimes embarrassing interruptions in his work schedule or recreational activities.

Good communication depends on the sender and receiver of messages using mutually understood language. Many people do not know the medical names of their sex organs. If the nurse suspects that the patient does not understand what particular part of the body she is talking about or if the nurse herself is not familiar with the term the patient is using, it is important to phrase questions differently or ask for clarification from the patient. Table 27-1 provides a list of questions helpful in eliciting needed information.

Physical Examination   Because most of the structures that comprise the male reproductive system are located outside the body, they are more easily inspected and palpated than the female reproductive organs.

The nurse can perform some of the physical inspection while assisting the male patient to bathe or dress or when performing catheterization. If the patient has complained of a problem with the penis or scrotum, the nurse could certainly ask to see the area involved. Providing privacy and using draping appropriately can reduce any embarrassment. With the concern for sexual harassment issues and legalities, perhaps it would be best to have a family member or another nurse in the room during such an examination. It usually is the physician, nurse practitioner, or physician's assistant who performs the routine physical examination of the male reproductive organs.

The penis and foreskin are inspected for signs of macules and papules, vesicles and pustules, erosions and ulcers, and abnormal growths. The foreskin, if present, is retracted (pulled back) to examine the surface of the penis under it. **Always replace the foreskin after examination. If left retracted, the foreskin can cause constriction of the penis.** The skin enclosing the scrotal sac is similarly examined for abnormalities. The glans is compressed slightly to see whether any discharge is emitted.

Each testis and scrotal sac is palpated for abnormal masses, localized and generalized swelling, and tenderness. The perineum is inspected for discoloration, lesions, swelling, growths, and masses.

◆ Nursing Diagnosis

Nursing diagnoses commonly used for problems of the male reproductive system may be:

◆ Urinary retention related to urinary obstruction.
◆ Anxiety related to inability to empty bladder completely or dribbling.
◆ Pain related to pressure of pelvic mass or of distended bladder; surgical incisions or bladder spasms.
◆ Sexual dysfunction.
◆ Altered sexuality pattern.
◆ Body image disturbance related to changes in sexual function.
◆ Risk for infection related to stasis of urine.

Additional nursing diagnoses may be appropriate for the patient undergoing surgery or who has cancer. See Chapters 4 and 9.

◆ Planning

General goals for the patient with problems of the male reproductive system are:

◆ Normal urinary elimination
◆ Prevention of infection
◆ Promotion of comfort
◆ Fluid volume balance
◆ Resolution or acceptance of sexual dysfunction
◆ Prevention of complications
◆ Intact self-esteem

Expected outcomes are written for individual patients based on the nursing diagnoses chosen. Interventions are planned to help the patient meet the expected outcomes. The nurse plans her interaction with the patient based on his age, educational level, degree of comfort in discussing reproductive problems, and culture.

◆ Implementation

Nursing actions for problems of the male reproductive system are found in the Table 27-2 and Clinical Pathway 27-1. Other interventions are included with the discussion of the various disorders. Privacy should always be provided when assessing the genitals, performing catheter care, or doing dressing changes. There are wide variances in the degree of modesty in men. The female nurse must be especially cautious and display a matter-of-fact, respectful manner when providing care. Sensitivity to embarrassment is necessary. Rather than stating "Don't worry; I'm used to this," it might be better to state, "I understand that this may be embarrassing for you; I will try to be as quick about it as I can."

If a male patient who is experiencing sexual dysfunction or is about to undergo surgery that may affect his sexuality makes sexual comments or advances to a female nurse, she should be tactful and matter of fact in setting limits on such behavior without taking it personally. Some patients make such remarks when they feel that their sexuality is threatened.

Think about . . . How would you begin your assessment interview with a 52-year-old male patient? Would you have any difficulty asking the questions necessary to obtain a good reproductive organ history and information about present problems?

◆ Evaluation

Evaluation is carried out by assessing the effectiveness of the nursing actions and treatments in helping the patient achieve the expected outcomes. If the actions and treatments are not achieving the desired effect, a revision in the plan of care is necessary.

INFLAMMATIONS AND INFECTIONS OF THE MALE REPRODUCTIVE ORGANS

Many of the inflammations and infections affecting the male reproductive system are similar to those of the female reproductive system in cause and effect. For example, urethritis in the male and female can be caused by common pyrogenic and colonic bacteria and by *Neisseria gonorrhoeae*. The male also can be infected with *Trichomonas vaginalis* or *Chlamydia*, which is transmitted by sexual contact. There always is the possibility that the sexual partners will reinfect one another until both are treated simultaneously.

Nonspecific genitourinary infections in the male, including nongonococcal urethritis (NGU), are not caused by any particular organism, but they present substantially the same clinical picture. Among the symptoms of nonspecific urethritis are mucopurulent discharge from the urethra, painful urination of varying degrees of severity, and occasionally the appearance of blood in the urine. A microscopic examination of a smear from urethral secretions usually does not show any specific organisms, but there may be an excessive number of white cells.

◆ Epididymitis

Epididymitis is an inflammation of the epididymis and may result from an infection of the prostate. The patient with epididymitis complains of groin pain plus swelling and pain in the scrotum. In men below the age of 35, the major cause of epididymitis is *Chlamydia trachomatis*, a sexually transmitted organism. Sometimes an inflammatory epididymitis occurs after vigorous exercise. Symptoms are scrotal pain, swelling, induration of the epididymis, and eventual edema of the scrotal wall. The adjacent testicle may become involved.

◆ Orchitis

Orchitis is inflammation of the testicle and may affect one or both testes. It may be caused by local or systemic infection or by trauma. *Mumps orchitis* occurs in about 20% of adult males who contract mumps. Serum immune globulin usually is given to lessen the severity of the orchitis. Bilateral orchitis is serious and very often causes sterility. The symptoms and treatment parallel those of epididymitis.

◆ Prostatitis

Prostatitis is inflammation that occurs from virus, bacteria, or congestion in the prostate gland. It can occur from a sudden decrease in sexual activity. *Acute prostatitis* is characterized by fever, chills, burning on urination, and urethral discharge containing many white blood cells (WBCs). Patients with chronic prostatitis complain of backache, perineal pain, urinary frequency and burning, and possibly blood in the urine.

Treatment   Treatment of nonspecific or nongonorrheal urethritis usually consists of oral administration of

TABLE 27-2 ◆ *Common Nursing Diagnoses, Expected Outcomes, and Interventions for Problems of the Male Reproductive System*

Nursing Diagnosis	Goals/Expected Outcomes	Nursing Interventions
Urinary retention related to obstruction of urine flow from urethra.	Patient will not experience cessation of urine flow. Patient will not experience hydronephrosis from urinary obstruction.	Determine usual urinary elimination pattern. Insert catheter as ordered for excessive urinary retention. Maintain patent drainage system for urine. Provide aseptic catheter care q shift. Monitor for signs and symptoms of urinary tract infection.
Risk of alteration in tissue perfusion related to possible hemorrhage at surgical site.	Vital signs will be within normal limits. Blood loss will be minimal as evidenced by lightened color of urine.	Assess color and characteristics of urine drainage q 15 minutes for first 2 h, then q 2 h for 24 h, then q 4 h. Maintain continuous bladder irrigation after TURP. Check for catheter patency, tube kinks, and distended abdomen at time of each patient assessment. Report change to dark red, viscous drainage with clots or drainage that is considerably darker in color for an extended time. Assess vital signs q 2 h for 24 h. Maintain traction on catheter for 8 h. Give stool softener daily and instruct not to strain at stool. Caution not to cough vigorously. Monitor dressings for signs of bleeding.
Risk of fluid volume excess related to continuous bladder irrigation.	Fluid balance maintained as evidenced by balanced intake and output. Absence of signs and symptoms of fluid overload: pulmonary crackles, increased blood pressure, confusion, weight gain, hyponatremia.	Accurately record intake and output (I&O). Auscultate lungs q shift, assess level of consciousness, check lab values for hyponatremia. Monitor blood pressure and assess for increase. Weigh daily and compare with previous weight.
Pain related to presence of catheter, surgical incisions, bladder spasms, and possible obstruction of catheter; or related to inflammation and swelling.	Pain will be controlled by medication as evidenced by patient's statements.	Check catheter and tubing for patency frequently to prevent obstruction and bladder spasm. Keep continuous bladder irrigation flowing to flush the bladder and prevent clot formation. Remind patient not to try to void around catheter as this can cause spasm. Teach to use patient-controlled analgesia (PCA) pump and monitor use. Assess for pain relief. Administer analgesics and antispasmodics as ordered; assess for side effects and effectiveness. Provide comfort measures and quiet environment. Apply ice packs and scrotal support for scrotal edema.
Risk for infection related to stasis of urine or possible invasion of infectious organisms at surgical site.	Patient will remain free of infection as evidenced by normal urinalysis, white blood cell (WBC) count, and temperature.	Maintain strict aseptic technique when handling catheter and drainage system. To flush bladder encourage drinking 10 to 12 glasses of water during the day after catheter is removed. Monitor temperature, WBC count, and urine for signs of infection. Provide catheter care q shift. Use aseptic technique for dressing changes. Administer prophylactic or treatment antibiotics as ordered. Encourage increased fluid intake to flush the urinary tract.

an antibiotic such as tetracycline, possibly followed by a sulfonamide. Because the infection typically is spread by sexual intercourse, it is possible that both partners have the disease and should be treated concurrently.

Untreated urethritis in the male can lead to acute infection of the epididymis.

Appropriate antibacterial drugs are prescribed to control other urogenital infections once the disorder has

TABLE 27-2 ◆ *Common Nursing Diagnoses, Expected Outcomes, and Interventions for Problems of the Male Reproductive System* (Continued)

Nursing Diagnosis	Goals/Expected Outcomes	Nursing Interventions
Knowledge deficit related to lack of knowledge regarding self-care after discharge.	Patient will list signs of infection, explain need for increased fluid intake, demonstrate care of wounds, dressings, and catheter and follow medication regimen.	Instruct to report signs of infection: fever, chills, malaise, increased pain, purulent drainage, excessive swelling. Instruct to avoid heavy lifting, driving, and sexual activity until permitted by urologist. Instruct to report new onset of burning on urination or cloudy urine. Explain what each medication is for and when and how to take it. Provide written information about signs and symptoms of urethral stricture or infection and instruct to report these symptoms to the urologist.
Sexual dysfunction related to outcome of surgical procedure or hormonal treatment for cancer.	Patient will verbalize problems and concerns within 1 month.	Encourage verbalization of problems and concerns. Provide information on alternative ways to achieve erection. Counsel in other ways to achieve intimacy. Include spouse or significant other in discussions. Assist to make plan to meet sexual needs.
Body image disturbance related to loss of testicles or loss of potency from hormone therapy.	Patient will accept new body image within 1 year.	Allow verbalization of grief over loss of testicles or potency. Encourage to focus on positives of therapy undergone on prolonging life. Ask to list the positives in present life. Help to visualize personal strengths and capabilities. Discuss success in roles that are continuing.

been diagnosed. When discharge is present, culture and antibiotic sensitivity studies determine the drug of choice for treatment. In some cases surgical intervention may be necessary to correct structural defects that help harbor infectious organisms.

Epididymitis is treated by bedrest for 1 to 2 days, ice packs, scrotal support and elevation by placing the scrotum on top of a folded towel. Specific antibiotics are administered to combat infection, and antiinflammatories or analgesics are given for pain. If epididymitis is from a sexually transmitted disease, the patient's sexual partner also must be treated. The nurse instructs the patient to avoid lifting, straining, or engaging in sexual activity until the infection is under control (which can take up to 4 weeks). A scrotal support should be worn when the patient is out of bed.

Treatment of prostatitis is vigorous to prevent abscess of the prostate and to eliminate urinary tract infection. Antimicrobials such as carbenicillin indanyl sodium (Geocillin) or fluoroquinolones (e.g., norfloxacin) are the drugs of choice for acute infection. Long-term therapy (30 days) with trimethoprim and sulfamethoxazole (Bactrim, Septra) is preferred for the patient with chronic prostatitis because the drug diffuses into the prostatic fluid. Frequent prostatic massage may be performed regularly to "milk" the prostate for clients who have recurrent episodes of prostatitis.

◆ Hydrocele

There is normally a small quantity of fluid in the space between the testis and tunica vaginalis within the scrotum. A larger-than-normal amount of fluid accumulating in this space is known as *hydrocele*. The fluid accumulation may be caused by infection, such as epididymitis or orchitis, or it may occur after trauma. Many times the cause is unknown. Hydrocele causes enlargement of the scrotum and usually is painless, but the weight and added bulk can cause discomfort.

Treatment, when indicated, is surgical incision of the sac. A pressure dressing and a drain are in place postoperatively. The patient will need to wear an athletic support for several weeks.

◆ Varicocele

Dilation and clumping of the tributary vessels of the spermatic vein cause this somewhat painful swelling. It usually occurs on the left side of the scrotum. The discomfort is rarely enough to warrant surgery. If infertility has been a problem, surgical correction will sometimes improve the sperm count.

Nursing measures to help the patient cope with fatigue, weakness, and fever are appropriate, because these problems often are associated with urogenital infections. **Fluid intake should be increased to helpprevent fluid deficit, reduce fever, increase urinary flow, and remove debris and bacteria.**

CLINICAL PATHWAY 27-1 ◆ *Transurethral Resection of the Prostate (TURP)*

Nursing Diagnosis/ Collaborative Problem	Expected Outcome (The Patient is Expected to ...)	Met/ Not Met	Reason	Date/ Initials
Potential for altered pattern of urinary elimination: retention. High risk for hemorrhage.	Have normal flow of clear urine. Have hemoglobin (Hgb) and hematocrit (Hct) within normal limits and void clear, yellow urine			
Pain.	State that pain is relieved and bladder spasms are managed with medication			

Aspect of Care	Date_____ Preadmission/Preop	Date_____ Day 1 (DOS)	Date_____ Day 2 (POD #1)	Date_____ Day 3 (POD #2)
Assessment	Systems assessment. Preop checklist. Psychological assessment.	*PACU* Vital signs (VS) q 15 min × 4, then q 30 min × 4. Systems and pain assessment. Check Foley for drainage and hematuria. *Postoperatively* Systems and pain assessment. Check Foley for drainage, hematuria, obstruction. Check Foley position (taped to abdomen or thigh). Monitor for complications Hemorrhage Hyponatremia Bladder perforation	Systems assessment q shift. VS q 4 h. Monitor for signs of catheter obstruction, complications. Assess for pain, bladder spasm. Assess for spontaneous voiding.	VS q 8 h. Continue to monitor for complications and pain.
Teaching	Orient to hospital and unit. Teach regarding Foley catheter, leg exercises, type of anesthesia, methods of pain relief. Review plan of care/ clinical pathway with patient and family.	Involve family in care of patient as appropriate. Leg exercises to prevent deep vein thrombosis.	Teach patient how to do Kegel exercises. Teach signs and symptoms of UTI. Instruct patient to avoid strenuous exercises for 2–3 weeks q surgery. Explain that slight hematuria may occur for up to 2 weeks.	Instruct patient to call MD if pain becomes severe, gross hematuria occurs, or if unable to void.
Consults	Medical clearance for surgery.	N/A	N/^	N/A
Lab tests	Complete blood count (CBC), lytes. Acid phosphatase. Type and screen urinalysis. INR(PT)/APTT.	N/A	Hgb and Hct.	N/A
Other tests	Chest x-ray. ECG.	N/A	N/A	N/A

CLINICAL PATHWAY 27-1 ◆ *Transurethral Resection of the Prostate (TURP)* (Continued)				
Aspect of Care	Date_____ Preadmission/Preop	Date_____ Day 1 (DOS)	Date_____ day 2 (POD #1)	Date_____ Day 3 (POD #2)
Medication	Prophylactic antibiotics before operation.	Analgesics (meperidine, acetaminophen) q 4 h. Antispasmodic (dicyclomine hydrochloride or oxybutynin).	PO analgesic. Continue antispasmodics if needed.	Continue as Day 2.
Treatments/ interventions	Thigh-high antiembolism stockings. Emotional support. Encourage to ventilate feelings about surgical procedure.	*PACU* Irrigate Foley catheter if needed. *Postoperatively* Thigh-high antiembolism stocking and sequential compression device. Irrigate Foley if needed. Strict I&O.	Thigh-high antiembolism stockings. I&O. Remove Foley. Progressive urine collection.	Thigh-high antiembolism stockings. I&O.
Nutrition	NPO after 12 midnight.	NPO until fully awake, then clear liquids.	Diet as tolerated. Encourage fluids to 2 L/day. Caffeine and spicy food in moderation.	Same as Day 2.
Lines/tubes/ monitors	N/A	Continuous IV fluids. Foley catheter to straight drainage. Continuous bladder irrigation with normal saline or other MD-specified fluid to keep urine clear.	D/C IV. D/C Foley catheter and continuous bladder irrigation.	N/A
Mobility/ self-care	N/A	*Epidural anesthesia* Flat in bed × 8 h, then increase head of bed. *General anesthesia* Out of bed to chair as tolerated. Bed rest if continuous bladder irrigation has been ordered.	Out of bed and ambulate as tolerated.	Same as Day 2.
Discharge planning	N/A	Determine if supplies are needed at home. Assess family support at home to assist with ADLs and other care needs after discharge.	Same as Day 1.	Refer to home health as needed. Arrange for follow-up visit with MD.

Source: Ignatavicius, D. D., Hausman K. A. (1995). *Clinical Pathways for Collaborative Practice.* Philadelphia: Saunders, pp. 162–165.

TESTICULAR CANCER

Testicular cancer most commonly occurs in men age 15 to 40 and is the leading cause of death in men 25 to 35 years of age. It is most frequently found in whites and is quite rare in blacks.

Men most at risk for testicular cancer are those who have had an undescended or partially descended testicle. This condition, called *cryptorchidism,* occurs during fetal development. As the unborn male child matures, the testes first appear in the abdomen at about the level of the kidneys. They develop at this site until approximately the seventh month of fetal life, when they start to move downward to the upper part of the groin. From there they move into the inguinal canal and then into the scrotum. If the descent of a testis is halted in its progress, it remains at that site as an undescended testis. Sometimes the undescended testicle will drop into the scrotum when the boy starts walking. If it remains undescended, surgical correction is done at 12 to 18 months of age. Treatment of cryptorchidism consists of surgical correction in a procedure called *orchiopexy.*

Men who were exposed to DES in utero also are at higher risk for testicular cancer. All males between the ages of 15 and 40 should practice testicular self-examination regularly on a monthly basis.

Think about . . . If you have a brother, son, nephew, or grandson, between the ages of 15 and 40 how would you go about talking to him about the importance of performing regular testicular exam?

Diagnosis   Assessment for testicular cancer includes questioning about any history of an undescended testicle, exposure to DES in utero, and the incidence of the disease in relatives. Testicular examination is performed by the physician, physician's assistant, or nurse practitioner. **Any testicular mass that will not transilluminate (allow light to shine through it) is assumed to be malignant until proved otherwise.** If a mass is found and thought to be malignant, diagnostic tests for tumor marker proteins are obtained to determine the likelihood of metastases. CT scans and/or MRIs are performed to detect any sites of metastases.

When testicular cancer is suspected, orchiectomy (unilateral removal of the testicle) is performed. Biopsy of a testicular mass is never done, as it can spread malignant cells. There are three stages for classifying the malignancy. In Stage I, the tumor is confined to the affected testis. In Stage II, malignant cells have spread to the regional lymph nodes, usually on the same side as the affected testis. In Stage III, there is metastasis to other organs, such as the lungs and liver. Figure 27-5 shows lymphatic drainage of the penis, testis, and scrotal wall.

Treatment   If the testicular tumor is limited to the scrotal sac and there is no metastasis, surgical removal of the testis *(orchiectomy)* may be all that is necessary to cure the patient of his disease. At the time of the orchiectomy a prosthesis is inserted into the scrotal sac cosmetically to simulate the removed testis. Removal of only one testis will not affect the patient's ability to produce the male hormone testosterone or render him impotent, as there remains another testis to carry on normal testicular function.

Further treatment for metastatic testicular cancer includes radical dissection of the lymph nodes and possibly radiation or chemotherapy. This extensive surgery can damage nerves necessary for normal intercourse and ejaculation. The patient could remain potent (that is, capable of having sexual intercourse), but there will be no ejaculation of seminal fluid, and so he will be sterile. A young man who is looking forward to fathering children might consider banking his sperm before surgery so that he could father children by artificially inseminating his partner.

The major chemotherapy protocol used is cisplatin in combination with vinblastine and bleomycin. When these three drugs are used, the patient may experience nephrotoxicity, pneumonitis, and peripheral neuropathy. Chapter 9 contains more information about chemotherapy and cancer treatment.

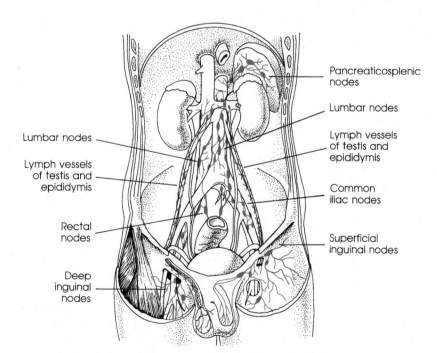

Pancreaticosplenic nodes

Lumbar nodes

Lymph vessels of testis and epididymis

Common iliac nodes

Superficial inguinal nodes

Lumbar nodes

Lymph vessels of testis and epididymis

Rectal nodes

Deep inguinal nodes

FIGURE 27-5   **Lymph drainage of the penis, testes, and scrotal wall.**

The lymphatics of the external genitals provide pathways by which gonorrheal and other infections of the urethra and epididymis, as well as malignancies of the testis, can spread.

Nursing Intervention   In addition to routine preoperative and postoperative nursing care and attention to the special needs of a cancer patient, the nurse helps the patient with testicular cancer deal with problems related to his masculinity and sexual activity. He will need time to think about and discuss the effects of surgery that have been explained to him by the surgeon.

Some men refuse to undergo orchiectomy because they view it as a loss of manhood. The nurse can be instrumental in assisting the patient to accept the procedure. Repeated explanation that removal of one testicle will not cause sterility and assurance that a prosthesis is implanted for normal appearance can overcome the patient's reluctance. Time for questions and discussion of concerns should be provided for the patient and his sexual partner.

TUMORS OF THE PROSTATE

Tumorous growth in the prostate can be either benign prostatic hypertrophy (BPH—growth of excessive tissue) or malignant growth. As the male ages, the glandular cells in the prostate undergo an abnormal increase in number (tissue hyperplasia), resulting in benign enlargement, or hypertrophy, of the gland. Benign prostatic hypertrophy occurs in all men over 40 to some degree. After age 50, 50% of men experience symptoms of this disorder. **As the prostate gland continues to enlarge, it extends inward, narrowing the urethral channel, and upward, narrowing the bladder opening and obstructing the outflow of urine.** These problems usually occur after age 60. Urinary retention and stasis can result in urinary tract infection. Obstruction to urine outflow can cause backup of urine into the ureters and kidney, causing hydronephrosis and eventual kidney damage. When these problems occur, surgery is recommended. After age 70, 80% of men have BPH.

Cancer of the prostate rarely occurs in men under 50 years of age and increases in incidence with each decade of life. It is the most common cancer in American men and occurs twice as frequently in blacks as in whites. Recent research has revealed that there is a genetic defect linked to prostate cancer that blocks the production of an enzyme that protects against environmental carcinogens. Some researchers believe that protective enzymes can be stimulated by consuming cruciferous vegetables such as Brussels sprouts and broccoli. However, this has not yet been proven. Tumor growth is associated with the presence of androgens and may act in combination with growth factors.

◆ Benign Prostatic Hypertrophy (BPH)

Signs and Symptoms   Benign prostatic hypertrophy (BPH) produces no symptoms until the growth becomes large enough to press against the urethra. Then the patient begins to **experience difficulty in urinating evidenced by a decrease in the caliber of the stream of urine, hesitancy, and dribbling after voiding.** There may be frequency, nocturia, and urgency due to irritation of the distended bladder wall. In the later stages there is complete obstruction of the urinary flow.

Treatment   When the patient is a poor surgical risk or there are no strong indications for surgery, BPH may be treated with alpha-adrenergic antagonists, such as prazosin (Minipress), terazosin, or doxazosin, and antiandrogen agents, such as flutamide, leuprolide, or finasteride (Proscar).

Not all men with BPH need surgery, but those who are experiencing recurrent urinary tract infection or hydronephrosis from bladder neck obstruction or are unable to obtain sufficient sleep because of frequency and nocturia are candidates for prostatic surgery. The type of surgical procedure depends on the size of the gland, the age and physical condition of the patient, and the preference of the patient and surgeon. All the common surgical procedures for BPH remove the hyperplastic tissue and leave the prostate capsule. Radical procedures performed for malignancy remove the capsule as well.

Think about... A patient has been experiencing increasing difficulty in emptying his bladder; he has BPH. Tests indicate that he has hydronephrosis. His physician has recommended prostate surgery. He is reluctant to have surgery. How would you interact with him to help him see the potential consequences of not having surgery? What other options are available to this patient that might prevent further organ damage?

Surgery. Surgical removal of all or part of the prostate gland (prostatectomy) is the treatment of choice for BPH. Transurethral resection of the prostate (TURP) is the most common procedure for removing an enlarged prostate gland. The location of the incision and the amount of tissue to be removed during surgical removal depend on the individual patient, his general physical condition, and the size of the gland or type of tumor present. A suprapubic, retropubic, or perineal approach may be used (Figure 27-6).

A transurethral incision of the prostate (TUIP) may relieve obstruction without more extensive surgery. With the patient under anesthesia, an instrument is passed through the urethra, and one or two small cuts are made in the prostate to reduce pressure on the urethra.

The newest treatment is transurethral laser incision prostatectomy. A laser is used for the incision, resulting in minimal blood loss. Irrigation of the bladder is not

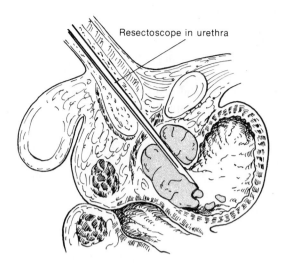

A. TRANSURETHRAL

Transurethral resection prostatectomy (TURP) is a closed method of treatment, i.e., no incision is made and the hyperplastic prostate tissue is removed through a resectoscope (like a cystoscope) inserted through the penis.

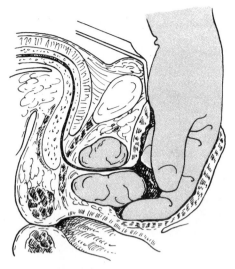

B. SUPRAPUBIC

Suprapubic (transvesical) prostatectomy is an open method of treatment in which the hyperplastic prostatic tissue is enucleated through the anterior walls of the abdomen and bladder.

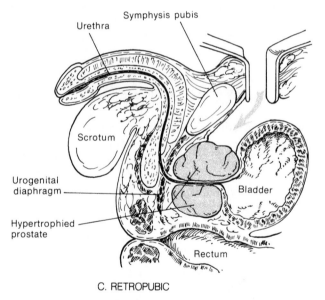

C. RETROPUBIC

Retropubic (extravesical) prostatectomy is an open method in which a low abdominal incision is made between the pubic arch and the bladder.

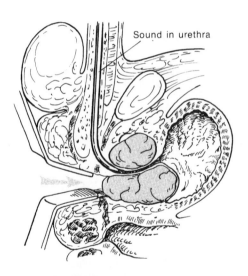

D. PERINEAL

Perineal prostatectomy is an open method involving an incision between the anus and the scrotum.

FIGURE 27-6   Four surgical methods of prostate removal. (*Source:* Black, J. M., Matassarin-Jacobs, E. [1993]. *Luckmann and Sorensen's Medical–Surgical Nursing: A Psychophysiologic Approach,* 4th ed. Philadelphia: Saunders.)

necessary postoperatively and the patient does not need a catheter.

Cryosurgical ablation is undergoing trials for prostate cancer. The procedure uses liquid nitrogen inserted into the prostate through thin metallic probes. Ultrasound is used to guide the probes to the correct location. The prostate cells are frozen by the liquid nitrogen. Upon thawing, the cancer cells burst. Although there is

less hospitalization time with this procedure, two-thirds of men become impotent, and one-third experience continuing incontinence. The procedure is more technically demanding than standard surgery.

Other procedures used to treat BPH are transurethral balloon dilation of the prostate and microwave hyperthermia. Transurethral balloon dilation, although not surgical, is invasive. A catheter is inserted into the urethra and the balloon is positioned in the section of prostatic urethra. The balloon is inflated for 15 minutes to apply pressure to the gland, causing it to dilate. Care must be taken not to damage the sphincter. The balloon is deflated and a urethral catheter is left to drain urine overnight. The procedure requires only local anesthesia and causes no blood loss. It is not known how long the procedure will last before growth and obstruction occur again.

Microwave hyperthermia is performed as an outpatient procedure without anesthesia. The treatment is delivered via a rectal probe and is repeated in a series of 4 to 10 sessions. Each treatment lasts about 60 minutes.

For very poor surgical risk patients, a prostatic stent may be inserted. This is done via an endoscope that can place the stent in the prostatic urethra. The stent mechanically holds the urethra open and does not seem to predispose to infection. However, the stent can be left in place for only 4 to 6 weeks, as after that epithelial cells will grow over it.

Preoperative nursing care. The preoperative care is the same as for any patient having abdominal surgery. An enema is given the night or morning before to prevent postoperative straining at stool, which can cause bleeding.

The patient with BPH who is admitted for a prostatectomy will inevitably have some difficulty in voiding. An indwelling catheter may be necessary to drain the bladder. An accurate record of intake and output is essential.

The average age for prostatectomy is about 73. Nursing care for this age group requires close attention to assistance with ambulation if a sedative has been given and appropriate use of siderails.

Elder Care Point... The elderly patient who has been suffering from urinary retention may have fluid and electrolyte imbalances that cause confusion. If the patient is confused pre- or postoperatively, the nurse should consider this possibility. Confusion usually clears in 24 to 72 hours. Extra safety measures are necessary in the meantime.

Preoperative teaching includes deep-breathing exercises, leg exercises, the preoperative and postoperative routine, and explanation of the care of the incision, catheters, irrigation system, and drains.

Postoperative nursing care. The postoperative nursing care of the patient varies according to the type of prostate surgery performed. The general principles of postoperative nursing care that apply to all patients having major surgery are necessary for the patient undergoing a prostatectomy. Potential postoperative complications are bleeding, urethral stricture, fistula, urinary incontinence, bladder neck constriction, and epididymitis.

Because hemorrhage always is a danger, vital signs are taken every 2 hours initially, then every 4 hours. The patient is monitored for pallor and rising pulse, which, along with blood pressure changes, may indicate excessive bleeding and shock.

Pharmacological therapy. Finasteride (Proscar) has recently been approved for pharmacological treatment of BPH. It acts on an enzyme responsible for the formation of a very potent androgen and in this manner suppresses testosterone production. It is taken orally on a once-a-day basis. Potential side effects are decreased libido, decreased volume of ejaculate, and impotence. The drug may decrease the effectiveness of theophylline.

Stool softeners may be given to prevent straining, which might cause further bleeding. Clinical Pathway 27-1 presents the collaborative care for the patient who has undergone a TURP.

Suprapubic prostatectomy and TURP patients will return from surgery with a three-way urethral catheter connected to continuous bladder irrigation (CBI) with sterile normal saline (Figure 27-7). **Bloody urine is usual for the first few days following the surgery.** To decrease clot formation, the flow rate is adjusted to keep the urine diluted to a reddish-pink, clearing to a pink tinge within 48 hours. Some pieces of tissue and small clots will be seen in the drainage. Additional intermittent irrigation with 20 to 30 mL of normal saline may be needed to clear the catheter of obstruction. **Hemorrhage is a possible complication and occurs most frequently in the first 24 hours.**

Persistent bleeding turning the urine darker than cherry red or bright red or viscous drainage with many clots should be reported to the surgeon. Traction may be applied to the catheter to supply pressure to prevent excessive bleeding. The surgeon does this by pulling against the balloon and then taping the catheter to the thigh or abdomen. The nurse checks frequently to see that the catheter and tubing are not kinked and that outflow is appropriate. Irrigation is continued for 2 to 3 days. **The patient may have some frequency and burning after catheter use is discontinued. Some blood in the urine is not unusual for several more days.**

The patient who has had a suprapubic prostatectomy will have a suprapubic catheter in addition to a urethral catheter. Each catheter is attached to a separate sterile drainage system. After the urethral catheter is removed (sometime after the third day), the suprapubic catheter is clamped, and the patient attempts to void. Residual urine is measured afterward by unclamping the suprapubic catheter. When there is no more than 75 mL of residual urine after voiding, the suprapubic catheter is removed. **Dribbling of urine often occurs after prostatectomy, but usually stops within about 6 months.**

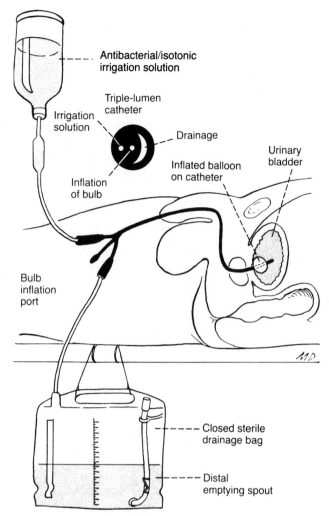

FIGURE 27-7   Closed bladder irrigation system (CBI).
(*Source:* Black, J. M., Matassarin-Jacobs, E. [1993]. *Luckmann and Sorensen's Medical–Surgical Nursing: A Psychophysiologic Approach,* 4th ed. Philadelphia: Saunders, p. 2100.)

When the urethral or suprapubic catheter is removed, the patient must be carefully monitored for ability to void. Intake and output are tracked closely. Any difficulty in voiding must be reported to the surgeon promptly as a distended bladder may cause bleeding.

The nurse monitors the incisional dressings and changes them as often as necessary to keep the patient dry and comfortable. Urine is very irritating to the skin, and any area that is exposed to drainage is thoroughly cleansed before a new dressing is applied.

Prophylactic antimicrobials and analgesics are administered in the early postoperative period. Bladder spasms often are a problem for the post–TURP and post–suprapubic prostatectomy patient. Before giving medication, the nurse checks to see that the tubing is not kinked and the catheter is draining well, as obstruction can cause bladder spasm. Abdominal distention may be a sign of catheter obstruction as well. Belladonna and

opium (B and O) rectal suppositories are effective if they are given when the spasms first begin. An anticholinergic, such as oxybutynin (Ditropan), may be used to help relieve bladder spasms. The patient who had a radical procedure may have a patient-controlled analgesia (PCA) pump to control pain.

Patients who experience incontinence are taught perineal muscle strengthening exercises for this problem and given instruction in bladder training. Teaching begins 24 to 48 hours after surgery (Chapter 23).

The patient who has had a radical prostatectomy needs good psychological care in addition to attention for his physical needs. If he is faced with orchiectomy as part of his treatment, he may become very depressed and angry. Fear of what awaits him in both treatment and the progression of the disease is a major concern. The nurse provides emotional support, acceptance of his moods, and a sympathetic ear.

Patients and their wives often worry about sexual activity after prostatectomy. Interference with sexual function depends on the type of surgical procedure performed and the general health and mental outlook of the patient. The nurse encourages questions and exploration of these concerns and suggests resources for information on issues of sexual function. Table 27-3 presents discharge teaching guidelines for the prostatectomy patient.

TABLE 27-3 ◆ *Patient Education: Postoperative Instructions for Prostatectomy*

The patient is instructed regarding the following points:

- Drink 12 to 14 glasses of water during the day to keep the urine flowing freely.
- Do not lift any object weighing more than 8 lb.
- For the next 2 to 3 weeks, depending on doctor's instructions, avoid strenuous activities: do not walk more than a few blocks, do not drive, play sports, or have sexual intercourse; avoid riding in the car for more than 25 minutes without a break.
- If blood is noticed in the urine, lie down and rest; drink more fluids and call the surgeon if the bleeding continues.
- Depending on the type of employment, it may be possible to return to work within 2 to 4 weeks. Consult the surgeon.
- Keep the catheter clean; cleanse catheter and around the meatus daily with soap and water and rinse thoroughly.
- Report any cloudiness or foul smell in urine.
- Report signs of infection such as fever, chills, or purulent wound drainage.
- After catheter removal, dribbling of urine may occur for up to 6 months. The problem usually will resolve. Perineal strengthening exercises help.
- After healing is complete, report changes in the force or size of the urine stream to the surgeon.
- Report for annual checkups to detect recurrence of tissue growth or the development of prostate cancer.

Think about . . . Can you identify the tubes, catheters, and dressings that a patient undergoing each type of prostate surgery might have postoperatively? Can you list the specific care needed for each one of them?

◆ Prostate Cancer

Diagnosis   Carcinoma of the prostate usually is not discovered until the later stages of development. This type of carcinoma is usually the slowest growing of all cancers. When palpated, a malignant nodule feels hard and immovable. Needle biopsy and tests to determine whether metastatic spread has occurred are performed to determine the best treatment. Whenever a biopsy shows a prostate tumor to be malignant, the entire prostate and its capsule may be removed. Table 27-4 presents the stages and the recommended treatment.

Surgery.   See the preceding section on BPH.

Radiation.   Radiation therapy may be added to surgical treatment for malignancy. Either interstitial radiation (brachytherapy), external beam radiation, or a combination of both are used. Interstitial radiation may involve placing radiation implants, such as iodine seeds, into the prostate with needles after a surgical pelvic lymphadenectomy. Or gold may be implanted in the prostate and external beam radiation treatments begun. Internal implants are left in place for life. An advantage of interstitial radiation treatment is that the ability for erection is saved. Cystitis often occurs 2 to 3 weeks after implantation. The patient is placed on radiation precautions for the first 2 weeks after implantation until the radiation danger to others passes.

External beam radiation is given in megavoltage doses to reach the prostate and is given over a period of 6 to 7 weeks. One side effect of such treatment is cystitis occurring about 1 week after treatment.

Other side effects of radiation therapy include fatigue, diarrhea, hematuria, skin reactions, urethral and rectal strictures, rectal inflammation or proctitis, and rectal bleeding. See Chapter 9 for particulars of care for the patient undergoing radiation therapy.

Pharmacological therapy.   For metastatic disease, hormonal therapy with progestational agents and androgen inhibitors is used. This therapy is based on the knowledge that prostate cells atrophy if they are deprived of androgens. Hormonal therapy removes the source of androgen and suppresses pituitary gonadotropin. These drugs can be used instead of bilateral orchiectomy to suppress testosterone production.

Treatment management is based on the stage of the disease and the age and physical condition of the patient. Flutamide (Eulexin) is an androgen blocker. Leuprolide (Lupron) and goserelin acetate (Zoladex) are gonadotropin-releasing hormone analogs. Finesteride (Proscar), another androgen inhibitor, also is used. Administration of DES, an estrogen compound, suppresses the release of pituitary gonadotropin and thereby reduces serum testosterone. However, the drug has many side effects, including gynecomastia and cardiovascular problems. Pretreatment external radiation to the breast area helps prevent the gynecomastia. Table 27-5 presents the nursing implications for hormonal therapy.

Chemotherapy may be added to the treatment, but only about 10% of patients respond. The chemotherapy drugs used are methotrexate (Rheumatrex), cyclophosphamide (Cytoxan), doxorubicin hydrochloride (Adriamycin), and mitomycin-C (Mutamycin) (Chapter 9). Bicalutamide (Casodex) is an antineoplastic agent used with a leutenizing hormone releasing hormone analog to treat advanced prostatic cancer.

Bone metastases are very common in the vertebra, pelvis, femur, or ribs. Pain is managed with radiation therapy and analgesics. Strontium-89 (Metastron) has proven helpful to control metastatic bone pain. It is a calcium analog that is taken up by the bone, particularly in areas of tumor. The drug locally irradiates tissue with beta-radiation. It is given by IV injection. Pain relief

---

TABLE 27-4 ◆ *Staging and Treatment Options for Prostatic Cancer*

Stage A
   Detected in about 10% of men with prostatic cancer. Tumor not palpable but detected by pathological exam of biopsy or surgically removed prostate tissue.
   In Stage *A1* in men over 70 who are not good candidates for surgical removal, watchful waiting is suggested. Monitor with physical examination and PSA tests every 3 to 6 months. *Watchful waiting is recommended only for men with a life expectancy of less than 10 years.*
   Stage *A2* or for patients younger than age 70, radical prostatectomy is recommended. If the patient declines this option, radiation may be performed.

Stage B
   Detected in about 15% to 20% of cases diagnosed. Palpable tumor is confined to the prostatic capsule and involves no more than one lobe of the prostate. Radical prostatectomy or radiation therapy are the options.

Stage C
   Detected in about 40% of cases diagnosed. Local extension of tumor beyond the prostate, but no evidence of distant metastases. Radical prostatectomy, radiation therapy, or both are options. Hormonal therapy may also be used.

Stage D
   Detected in 30% to 35% of new cases. The cancer is no longer localized and has spread to regional lymph nodes or beyond the pelvis to the bone or other organs. Prostatectomy is not an option as disease has spread beyond the prostate. Hormonal therapy is the treatment of choice. Radiation or chemotherapy may be combined with the hormonal therapy.

TABLE 27-5 ◆ *Major Nursing Implications for Hormone Management of Prostatic Cancer*

When giving a hormone to manage prostatic cancer, the nurse should:

◆ Follow the "five rights" of medication administration to prevent errors and injury to the patient (right patient, drug, dosage, time, route); pay special attention to dosage amount as it may vary for individual patients.

◆ Check other medications the patient is taking for interactions.

◆ Not handle crushed tablets of leuprolide if of childbearing age as it can affect a male fetus.

Regarding possible side/adverse effects of the drug, the nurse should:

◆ For flutamide, monitor for hot flashes, drowsiness, confusion, numbness or tingling of feet or hands, diarrhea, nausea, vomiting, loss of libido, and impotence.

◆ Monitor liver functions tests for patients taking flutamide or leuprolide, as they may cause hepatitis or liver enzyme elevations.

◆ Realize leuprolide takes 2 to 4 weeks to become effective.

◆ Watch for signs of myocardial infarction in the patient taking leuprolide.

◆ Monitor for congestive heart failure, arrhythmia, and myocardial infarction in patients taking goserelin.

◆ Monitor patients taking DES for signs of thrombophlebitis, cerebrovascular accident, pulmonary embolus, and myocardial infarction. Monitor for gynecomastia and impotence.

The nurse should teach the patient taking hormone therapy that:

◆ Flutamide must be taken in combination with leuprolide (Lupron) or goserelin acetate (Zoladex) to suppress testosterone production.

◆ Leuprolide and goserelin may cause an initial increase in symptoms of urinary obstruction and/or bone pain. Such effects are transient and disappear within about 1 week of therapy.

◆ Leuprolide or goserelin in combination with flutamide cause a chemical "castration" with less side effects than estrogen therapy.

◆ Leuprolide is given by subcutaneous injection daily or by an intramuscular "depot" injection once a month (for up to 6 months).

◆ Instruct patient giving SC injections of leuprolide to use only the syringes supplied by the manufacturer. A lo-dose insulin syringe is the only alternative syringe available. The drug must be stored at room temperature and protected from light and heat.

◆ Goserelin acetate is administered by implant injection into the abdominal wall. A local anesthetic is used prior to injection. Implantation must be repeated every 28 days.

◆ DES therapy may cause an increase in appetite and weight gain.

occurs 7 to 20 days after injection. During the first few days after injection, caution patients to flush the toilet twice, wipe up any spilled urine with a tissue and flush it down the toilet, and immediately launder any linens soiled with blood or urine.

VASECTOMY

Sterilization of the male by vasectomy is a popular method of permanent contraception. The term *vasectomy* refers to a surgical procedure performed on the vas deferens for the purpose of interrupting the continuity of this duct, which conveys the sperm at the time of ejaculation. This is considered a permanent procedure, but occasionally a vasectomy can be successfully reversed by vasovasotomy at a later time if a man's life circumstances change.

The procedure is done on an outpatient basis in a clinic or physician's office with a local anesthetic. An incision is made into the scrotal sac on each side, and the vas is lifted out. A segment of the vas is cut out, the ends are bound, and the incision is closed (Figure 27-8).

The nurse instructs the patient to use ice applications and aspirin, acetaminophen, or ibuprofen for scrotal pain and swelling the first 12 to 24 hours postoperatively. It is recommended that the patient wear jockey shorts or a scrotal support for comfort. Sexual intercourse may be resumed in about 1 week or whenever the patient finds it comfortable. The patient is told to use another method of birth control until sperm counts are negative, because active sperm are still present in the vas. A second sperm count should be done 1 year later to verify that the vas deferens is not intact.

IMPOTENCE

Impotence is the inability to achieve or maintain an erection that is firm enough for sexual intercourse more than 25% of the time. Although it was once thought that most cases of impotence were psychological in origin, it is now known that at least 50% of cases are related to physical disorders. Diabetes mellitus is one of the most common causes of impotence and occurs in about 55% of diabetic men. Certain drugs may cause problems with erectile function, and a thorough drug history is essential when assessing the patient experiencing impotence.

Elder Care Point... The elderly patient who has been consistently participating in intercourse through the years has the best chance of maintaining this capability. When abstinence has occurred over a con-

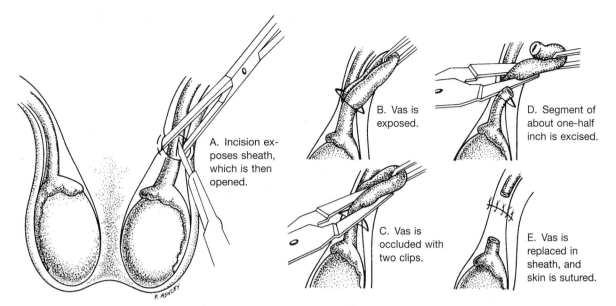

FIGURE 27-8   Vasectomy.

A. Incision exposes sheath, which is then opened.

B. Vas is exposed.

C. Vas is occluded with two clips.

D. Segment of about one-half inch is excised.

E. Vas is replaced in sheath, and skin is sutured.

siderable time, impotence may become a problem. With patience and treatment, this problem may be overcome. The male can reproduce as long as he can participate in intercourse.

One method of treatment is the use of self-intracavernosal injections into the penis using papaverine or prostin to achieve or maintain an erection. Vacuum erection devices have come into common use in the past few years, and many men are very successful with them (Figure 27-9). Such a device is available by physician's prescription.

If, after extensive testing, the problem is determined to be physiological, a penile prosthesis may be implanted surgically. There are various types of implants, including a semirigid type, a self-contained type acti-

vated by a pump device, and an inflatable prosthesis (Figure 27-10). A valve allows the device to be deflated. The semi-rigid type is the most common implant. It can be implanted under local anesthesia and is successful about 95% of the time.

Preoperative care is the same as for other types of general surgery. Postoperatively the patient is monitored for urinary retention, infection, atelectasis, deep vein thrombosis, and other complications of anesthesia and general surgery.

INFERTILITY

Approximately 30% of cases of infertility among couples can be attributed to the male. When the sperm

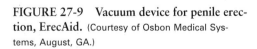

FIGURE 27-9   Vacuum device for penile erection, ErecAid. (Courtesy of Osbon Medical Systems, August, GA.)

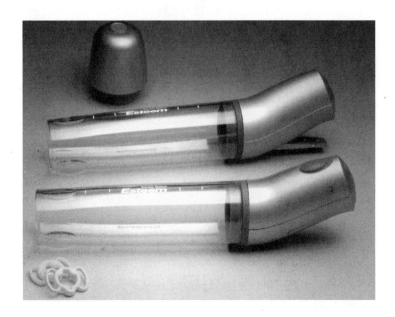

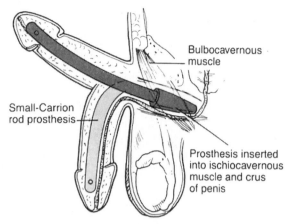

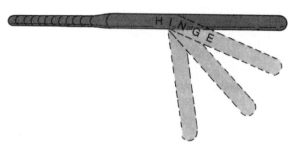

B. A Flexrod semirigid penile implant.

A. A Small-Carrion prosthesis consisting of plastic rods.

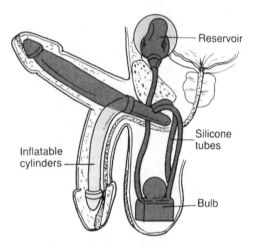

C. An inflatable penile prosthesis.

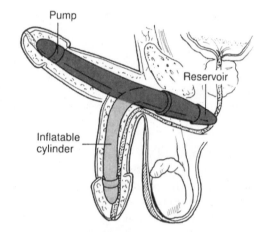

D. A self-contained penile prosthesis.

FIGURE 27-10   Penile prostheses. (*Source:* Black, J. M., Matassarin-Jacobs, E. [1993]. *Luckmann and Sorensen's Medical–Surgical Nursing: A Psychophysiologic Approach,* 4th ed. Philadelphia: Saunders.)

count is very low, or there is obstruction to the proper flow of sperm, infertility often results. Impotence prevents delivery of the sperm into the vagina. Viral diseases, such as mumps, tuberculosis, and pneumonia that cause orchitis or epididymitis, may induce infertility. All male children should receive mumps immunization to help avoid later infertility. Sexually transmitted diseases, such as syphilis, *Chlamydia trachomatis,* and *Neisseria gonorrhoeae,* if severe, or repetitive, may result in infertility due to scar tissue formation that interferes with normal function of the male reproductive organs. Undescended testicle (cryptorchidism) that is not remedied before 18 months of age may affect sperm production, thereby contributing to infertility. Varicocele may affect the testis, decreasing the formation of sperm. An episode of testicular torsion where the blood supply to the testis is cut off also will lower the sperm count.

Endocrine problems must be ruled out with hormonal studies, such as radioimmunoassay for follicle-stimulating hormone (FSH), luteinizing hormone (LH),

and testosterone. Semen analysis is necessary to determine whether a male is having fertility problems. The specimen is obtained by masturbation, and some men find this difficult or embarrassing.

A variety of other agents can reduce sperm counts. Pesticides such as ethylene dibromide and chlordeone (Kepone), inorganic lead or mercury exposure, neurotoxins from the manufacture of polyurethane foam, exposure to certain chemicals, and excessive exposure to ionizing radiation from x-rays and gamma-emitting radioisotopes all may affect spermatogenesis or sperm motility.

Medications, such as antipsychotics, antihypertensives, tricyclic antidepressants, monamine oxidase inhibitor antidepressants, tranquilizers, hormones, opiates, sedative-hypnotics, stimulants, chemotherapy drugs, and recreational drugs, may cause fertility problems by decreasing libido, erectile ability (impotence), ejaculatory ability, or by affecting sperm quality or motility. A thorough drug history should be obtained when a man is having infertility problems.

Treatment for infertility is based on the cause. Testosterone may be administered to correct low levels. Obstructions are treated surgically if possible. The man who is experiencing infertility is instructed to:

- Keep the scrotum cool by avoiding excessive heat, hot baths, jockey shorts, and tight clothing.
- Avoid excessive use of alcohol, tobacco, marijuana, and other recreational drugs.
- Develop effective stress-reduction techniques.
- Obtain sufficient sleep and exercise.
- Eat a well-balanced, nutritious diet.
- Avoid further exposure to harmful substances and radiation.

Artificial insemination is a possible option if viable sperm are being produced. Infertility brings considerable stress to a couple trying to conceive a child. When the problem is with the male, it can greatly affect his self-image. The nurse must be caring and considerate when interacting with these patients.

PENILE TRAUMA

Blunt or sharp trauma involving the penis may occur. Such trauma results in edema, bruising, or laceration. Ice packs are used to control bleeding and edema until consultation with a urologist is possible. If a penis is amputated, it may be possible to reattach it with microsurgical techniques. The amputated penis should be kept chilled and damp with sterile saline solution during transport, along with the patient, to the hospital.

COMMUNITY CARE

Nurses in the community can be instrumental in teaching and promoting the use of testicular self-exam in men between the ages of 15 and 40. Teaching the benefits of and encouraging all men over 50 to have an annual digital rectal exam and PSA test may help reduce the death rate from prostate cancer by promoting earlier treatment.

Each nurse should be knowledgeable enough about BPH and prostate cancer to direct patients who are trying to make a decision about treatment options to reliable information. The U.S.D.H.H.S. Agency for Health Care Policy and Research has available a publication detailing outcomes of BPH treatments.

Think about... Can you think of five relatives or friends you could provide with information on testicular self-exam? How would you approach them on this subject?

Nurses in long-term care facilities must be watchful for urinary obstruction in elderly male residents. Alert men should be questioned regularly about problems with urination; men with cognitive impairment who do not have a normal urinary stream should be placed on intake and output recording to detect any problems with urinary obstruction. Palpation just above the symphysis pubis may reveal a distended bladder.

All nurses can be instrumental in teaching perineal muscle exercises to decrease the incidence of incontinence. Incontinence is one of the greatest robbers of self-esteem in the elderly and can be corrected in many cases. Correcting incontinence also greatly decreases the nursing care time that needs to be spent with the patient, thereby cutting health care costs.

Home care nurses supervise or assist with dressing changes for the patient who has radical surgery; monitor side effects and complications in patients undergoing radiation; teach self-care; and provide psychosocial support for patients with prostate cancer and sexual dysfunction. Collaboration with the physician, social worker, and community agencies can provide avenues of help for the patient.

Nurses in the community can assist patients who are suffering from impotence by including assessment for this problem when working with male patients. Knowledge about treatment options, a matter-of-fact optimistic attitude, and a comfortable manner when speaking about this topic can provide hope and guidance. Sometimes this problem is brought to light when speaking with the spouse of the older patient. Many times a satisfying sexual life can be reinstituted for these couples, providing added fulfillment and joy in the autumn years.

CRITICAL THINKING EXERCISES

Clinical Case Problems

Read each clinical situation and discuss the questions with your classmates.

1. Your brother, who is 20 years old, tells you of a friend who has just learned that he has testicular cancer and is scheduled for surgery tomorrow. Your brother is concerned about the effect the surgery will have on his friend's "manhood." He also says that if ever he has that kind of cancer, he doesn't want to know about it, and he certainly wouldn't allow surgery.
   a. What information could you give your brother about testicular cancer and self-examination of the testes?
   b. How could you explain that removal of a testis does not render a man less masculine?
2. Mr. Watts, age 67, has been admitted to the hospital to undergo a transurethral resection of the pros-

tate. He is assigned to your care on his second postoperative day. Mr. Watts seems disoriented and restless, and when you begin to give him his bath, he tells you that his bladder is full and he needs to urinate. You check the catheter and find that it apparently is not draining as it should.

a. What would you tell Mr. Watts about his need to void?

b. What would you do about the catheter, which seems obstructed?

c. What observations should you make while caring for this patient?

d. What special precautions should be taken for his safety?

BIBLIOGRAPHY

American Cancer Society: Cancer Facts and Figures—1996. Atlanta: Author.

Andreoli, T. E., et al. (1993). *Cecil's Essentials of Medicine,* 3rd ed. Philadelphia: Saunders.

Anonymous. (1993). Drug news. Terazosin: easing prostate pain. *Nursing 93.* 23(5):108.

Applegate, E. J. (1995). *The Anatomy and Physiology Learning System: Textbook.* Philadelphia: Saunders.

Bennett, J. C., Plum, F., eds. (1996). *Cecil Textbook of Medicine,* 20th ed. Philadelphia: Saunders.

Black, J. M., Matassarin-Jacobs, E. (1997). *Medical–Surgical Nursing: Clinical Management for Continuity of Care,* 5th ed. Philadelphia: Saunders.

Brakey, M. R. (1994). Myths & facts about testicular cancer. *Nursing 94,* 24(9), 24.

Branch, W. T. (1994). *Office Practice of Medicine,* 3rd ed. Philadelphia: Saunders.

Brenner, Z. R., Krenzer, M. E. (1995). Update on cryosurgical ablation for prostate cancer. *American Journal of Nursing.* 95(4):44–48.

Cali-Ascani, M. A. (1994). Caring for patients with prostate cancer. *Nursing 94.* 24(6):32C–32D.

Carapella, J. S. (1994). Radical prostatectomy: a case study. *Journal of Post Anesthesia Nursing.* 9(6):344–349.

Copstead, L. C. (1995). *Perspectives on Pathophysiology.* Philadelphia: Saunders.

Cotran, R. S., Kumar, V., Robbins, S. L., Schoen, F. J., eds. (1994). *Robbins Pathologic Basis of Disease,* 5th ed. Philadelphia: Saunders.

Dambro, M. R. (1996). *Griffith's 5 Minute Clinical Consult.* Baltimore: Williams & Wilkins.

Davison, B. J., Degner, L. F., Morgan, T. R. (1995). Information and decision-making preferences of men with prostate cancer. *Oncology Nursing Forum.* 22(9):1401–1408.

Frank-Stromborg, M., Baird, S. B. (1996). *Cancer Nursing: A Comprehensive Textbook.* Philadelphia: Saunders.

Gregoire, I. (1995). Pharmacologic erection program: an alternative solution for the man with erectile dysfunction. *Urologic Nursing.* 15(1):10–13.

Greifzu, S., Tiedemann, D. (1995). Prostate cancer: the pros and cons of treatment. *RN.* 58(6):22–26.

Guyton, A. C., Hall, J. E. (1996). *Textbook of Medical Physiology,* 9th ed. Philadelphia: Saunders.

Ignatavicius, D. D., Hausman, K. A. (1995). *Clinical Pathways for Collaborative Practice.* Philadelphia: Saunders.

Ignatavicius, D. D., Workman, M. L., Mishler, M. A. (1995). *Medical–Surgical Nursing: A Nursing Process Approach,* 2nd ed. Philadelphia: Saunders.

Healy, S. A. (1995). Special focus: Prostate cancer. *Today's OR Nurse.* 17(3):3–36, 50–51.

Held, J. L., et al. (1994). Cancer of the prostate: treatment and nursing implications. *Oncology Nursing Forum.* 21(9):1517–1529.

Lassen, P. M., Thompson, I. M. (1994). Treatment options for prostate cancer. *Urologic Nursing.* 14(1):12–17.

Lehne, R. A. (1994). *Pharmacology for Nursing Care,* 2nd ed. Philadelphia: Saunders.

Matteson, M. A., McConnell, E. S., Linton, A. D. (1997). Gerontological Nursing Concepts and Practice, edition 2. Philadelphia: W. B. Saunders.

Meadus, R. J. (1995). Testicular self-examination (TSE). *Canadian Nurse.* 91(8):41–44.

Monahan, F. D., Drake, T., Neighbors, M. (1994). *Nursing Care of Adults.* Philadelphia: Saunders.

Newton, M., Moore, S., Gaehle, K. E. (1994). Prostate cancer: staging through laparoscopic lymphadenectomy. *AORN Journal.* 59(4):821, 823–829, 831, 833, 836–840.

Pobursky, J. (1995). Prostate cancer: detection and treatment options. *Today's OR Nurse.* 17(3):5–9.

Polaski, A. L., Tatro, S. E. (1996). *Luckmann's Core Principles and Practice of Medical–Surgical Nursing.* Philadelphia: Saunders.

Razanauzskas, M., Hoebler, L. (1994). Cold comfort: treating prostate cancer with cryosurgery. *Nursing 94.* 24(11):66, 68.

Springhouse Corporation. (1996). *Nursing 96 Drug Handbook.* Springhouse, PA: Author.

Swenson, K. K., Ferguson, J. (1995). Development of a prostate cancer support group. *Oncology Nursing Forum.* 22(2):379.

Ulrich, S. P., Canale, S. W., Wendell, S. A. (1994). *Medical–Surgical Nursing Care Planning Guides,* 3rd ed. Philadelphia: Saunders.

U.S. Department of Health and Human Services. (1994). *Treating Your Enlarged Prostate.* Rockville, MD: Agency for Health Care Policy and Research.

Walbrecker, J. (1995). Start talking about testicular cancer. *RN.* 58(1):34–35.

Walsh, P. C., et al. (1995). *Campbell's Urology,* 6th ed. Philadelphia: Saunders.

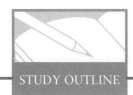

I. Introduction
   A. The nurse may be the first person to discover a male reproductive problem.
   B. The urinary and reproductive systems in the male are closely linked, and a disorder in one system often affects the other.

II. Causes and Prevention of Male Reproductive Disorders
   A. Infection, inflammation, trauma, metabolic disorders, endocrine disorders, or tumor may cause reproductive disorders.
   B. Cancer of the testicle is linked to history of undescended testicle or to exposure in utero to DES.
   C. Sexually transmitted diseases contribute to disorders of the male reproductive system.
   D. Good hygiene practices, careful choice of sexual partner, use of condoms, and prompt attention to minor problems can all help prevent disorders of the reproductive system.
   E. Practicing testicular self-exam between ages 15 and 40 and obtaining a digital rectal exam and PSA test annually after age 50 help detect cancer early.

III. Diagnostic Tests and Procedures and Nursing Implications
   A. Digital rectal exam: examiner inserts finger into rectum to palpate the prostate, checking for tenderness or nodules.
   B. Semen analysis: to determine volume of fluid and motility and number of sperm. Also to detect organisms causing infection and for medicolegal reasons.
   C. Testicular self-examination (TSE): to be done monthly to detect testicular tumors early.
   D. Prostatic specific antigen (PSA).
      1. Performed on a sample of blood.
      2. Levels become elevated when prostate disease is present.
      3. Normal values in males over age 15 are 0.81 to 0.89 ng/mL.
      4. Benign prostatic hypertrophy (BPH) causes a rise that rarely goes above 10 ng/mL.
      5. Levels over 50 ng/mL with history of prostate cancer often indicates metastases.
   E. Transrectal ultrasonography of the prostate performed when a nodule is found or when PSA levels rise and no nodule is palpable. Performed

as an outpatient procedure without anesthesia and takes about 20 minutes.
   F. Biopsy of the prostate: to rule out or confirm malignancy, determine cause of enlarged prostate.
      1. May experience pain or discomfort during procedure.
      2. After biopsy, pressure applied to needle insertion site to prevent hematoma.
      3. Instruct patient to watch for signs of hematoma, infection, and gross bleeding or urinary retention.
   G. Other tests are KUB, IVP, cystoscopy with urodynamic studies (Chapter 23), urethral discharge smears, and tumor marker studies if cancer is present.

IV. Nursing Assessment
   A. Age is relevant.
   B. History taking: do not assume male patient is reluctant to discuss problems related to reproductive organs and sexual activity.
      1. Begin with less sensitive questions about urinary function; then progress to questions about reproductive organs and sexual activity.
      2. Ask open-ended questions; relate symptoms to activities of daily living.
      3. Be sure you and patient are talking about the same things. Patient may not use terms understood by the nurse and vice versa.
      4. Gather information about patterns of urination, penile discharge, tumors or masses noted by patient or someone else, tenderness or pain, impotence, sterility.
      5. Personal and family history of endocrine disorders and prostate and testicular cancer (Table 27-1).
   C. Physical assessment.
      1. Examination of genitalia: by inspection and palpation.
      2. Provide privacy during examination; explain steps and purposes of examination.

V. Nursing Diagnosis
   A. Chosen based on findings from data collection.
   B. Diagnoses commonly chosen.
      1. Urinary retention.
      2. Anxiety.
      3. Pain.
      4. Sexual dysfunction.

5. Altered sexuality pattern.

6. Body image disturbance.

7. Risk for infection.

C. Additional diagnoses needed for the patient undergoing surgery or who has cancer.

VI. Planning

A. Expected outcomes written for individual patients based on nursing diagnoses chosen.

B. Interventions are planned to help patient meet expected outcomes.

C. Care planned based on patient's age, educational level, degree of comfort in discussing reproductive problems, and culture.

VII. Implementation

A. Nursing actions for problems found in Table 27-2 and Clinical Pathway 27-1.

B. Privacy when providing genital care is of great importance.

C. Matter-of-fact attitude and sensitivity to patient's feelings are essential.

VIII. Evaluation

A. Effectiveness of nursing actions and treatments is assessed.

B. Determination as to whether expected outcomes are being met is made.

C. Plan is revised as need indicates.

IX. Inflammations and Infections of the Male Reproductive Organs

A. Causative organisms include common pyogenic and colonic organisms and *Neisseria gonorrhoeae*, also organisms that cause vaginitis in women.

B. Nonspecific urethritis (also called nongonococcal urethritis [NGU]) not caused by any specific organism.

1. Symptoms include mucopurulent urethral discharge, dysuria, occasionally hematuria.

2. Treatment: oral antibiotics and sulfonamides.

C. Epididymitis: inflammation caused by strenuous exercise or infection; often caused by *Chlamydia trachomatis* in men under 35.

D. Orchitis: inflammation of the testis, usually caused by infection.

E. Prostatitis: inflammation of the prostate. Can be acute or chronic; can be difficult to eradicate.

F. Medical treatment and nursing intervention.

1. Antibacterials.

2. Surgical correction of existing structural defect.

3. Active and passive immunity to prevent effects of mumps.

4. Instruction of patient in personal hygiene and avoidance of factors that predispose to infections.

5. Encourage both sexual partners to be treated simultaneously to avoid reinfecting one another.

6. Warm sitz baths. Extreme heat to be avoided because of possibility of destroying spermatozoa.

7. Elevation of scrotum and application of ice bag. Athletic scrotal support when patient is ambulatory.

8. Other measures to deal with fatigue, weakness, and fever.

G. Hydrocele: larger-than-normal amount of fluid accumulates in the space between the testis and tunica vaginalis within the scrotum.

1. May be caused by infection, or trauma; cause is often unknown.

2. Usually is painless, but added weight and bulk may cause discomfort.

3. Treatment is surgical incision of the sac and pressure dressing.

H. Varicocele: dilation and clumping of the tributary vessels of the spermatic vein; usually occurs on left side; may be painful.

X. Testicular Cancer

A. One of the most common cancers in men between ages 15 and 40 years.

B. Cryptorchidism and exposure in utero to DES places person at greater risk.

C. Biopsy never performed, as it tends to spread malignant cells.

D. Surgical treatment: surgical removal of testis; more extensive surgery and radiation if metastasis has occurred. Effects of surgery and radiation on potence and ability to have children depends on type and amount of tissue damage.

E. Nursing intervention must include helping patient deal with perceived effects on his masculinity.

XI. Tumors of the Prostate

A. Prostate encircles urethra; enlargement of gland can cause urinary retention.

B. Benign prostatic hypertrophy (BPH) more common in older males.

C. Symptoms of BPH: usually none until growth obstructs urinary flow through urethra. Enlargement can be felt on rectal examination.

D. Cancer of the prostate treated by surgery and possibly radiation, hormonal therapy, and sometimes chemotherapy. If the man is over age 70, a watch-and-wait approach may be used for localized disease as prostate cancer is very slow growing. This is done only with men whose life expectancy is less than 10 years.

E. Surgical treatment: surgical removal of all or part of prostate (Figure 27-6).

1. Transurethral prostatic resection (TURP): part or all of the gland removed by way of the urethra, using an endoscope.

2. Suprapubic prostatectomy: gland removed by incision into bladder.

3. Retropubic prostatectomy: gland removed by low abdominal incision.

4. Perineal prostatectomy: U-shaped incision in perineum, through which gland is removed.

5. Radical prostatectomy: done by any of the above methods except TURP, but gland, capsule, neck of the bladder, and the regional lymph nodes are removed; performed for malignancy.

F. Other treatments: Transurethral balloon dilation, microwave hyperthermia, cryosurgical ablation.

G. Radiation: interstitial (brachytherapy) or external beam.

   1. Radiation implants may be placed directly into the prostate; left in place for life.

   2. Radiation precautions needed for first 2 weeks or until half-life point of isotope is passed.

   3. External beam radiation given in megavoltage doses. Course of treatment is usually 6 to 7 weeks.

   4. Side effects of radiation: cystitis, fatigue, diarrhea, hematuria, skin reactions, urethral and rectal strictures, rectal inflammation or proctitis, and rectal bleeding (Chapter 9).

H. Hormonal therapy.

   1. Androgen inhibitors are used to decrease testosterone production and thereby discourage growth of prostate tissue.

   2. Flutamide (Eulexin), leuprolide (Lupron, goserelin (Zoladex) and DES are androgen inhibitors.

   3. Finesteride (Proscar) is another androgen inhibitor that may be used to decrease growth for either BPH or prostate malignancy.

I. Strontium-89 (Metstron) is given IV to control metastatic bone pain.

J. Preoperative nursing care: maintain urinary flow, protect patient from injury from falls, explain all procedures.

K. Postoperative nursing care: guard against hemorrhage, but realize that bleeding is expected, maintain urinary flow, change dressing (if any) to keep patient dry and comfortable.

   1. Watch for signs of hemorrhage and shock: increasing cherry red urine, change in BP, rising pulse, rising respirations, decreased mental alertness.

   2. Maintain all drains, tubes, and catheters using aseptic technique; keep urine flowing.

   3. Have patient turn, cough, deep-breath, and do leg exercises; ambulate as soon as possible.

4. Watch for thrombophlebitis in patients having radical procedures.

5. Monitor for voiding after catheter removal; do not allow bladder distention to occur as it may cause further bleeding.

6. Monitor PCA analgesia; provide B&O suppository or antispasmodic for bladder spasms.

7. Teach perineal strengthening exercises for problems of incontinence or dribbling.

8. Patient education should include information about sexual activity.

XII. Vasectomy

   A. Removal of a section from each vas deferens to prevent impregnation (Figure 27-8).

   B. Performed as an outpatient procedure.

XIII. Impotence

   A. May be due to metabolic or endocrine disease (diabetes mellitus).

   B. May occur after prostatectomy.

   C. May be caused by medications.

   D. Perform thorough assessment to determine cause.

   E. Treatments include penile injection, vacuum pump device, medication, or penile implant.

XIV. Infertility

   A. 30% of infertility attributed to the male.

      1. Low sperm count caused by viral disease, sexually transmitted disease, cryptorchidism, varicocele, or torsion.

      2. May be an endocrine problem affecting testosterone levels.

      3. Some pesticides, heavy metal exposure, other chemicals, and ionizing radiation may affect sperm count.

      4. Obstruction of the vas deferens may be the problem.

   B. Some medications cause infertility by contributing to impotence; obtain a thorough drug history.

   C. Treatment is based on the cause.

      1. Testosterone is administered to treat low levels.

      2. Avoid harmful substances and radiation.

      3. Keep scrotum cool and avoid tight clothing.

      4. Surgery to correct obstruction.

   D. Artificial insemination is an option if viable sperm are being produced.

XV. Penile Trauma

   A. Blunt or sharp trauma may occur.

   B. Control bleeding with pressure and apply ice pack.

   C. Amputated penis should be kept chilled and damp with sterile saline solution and transported with patient to ER.

XVI. Elder Care Points

    A. Elderly patients suffering from urinary retention may have fluid and electrolyte imbalances that cause confusion.

    B. Elderly patients often become confused after prostatectomy because of fluid shifts; attention to safety is essential.

    C. May have slower and less intense response to sexual stimulation.

    D. Elderly patient who has consistently participated in intercourse through the years has the best chance of maintaining this capability into old age.

    E. Generally capable of reproduction into old age.

XVII. Community Care

    A. Nurses can be instrumental in teaching and promoting use of testicular self-exam and monitoring for prostate cancer by digital rectal exam and PSA testing.

    B. Nurses can educate regarding BPH and potential complications.

    C. Nurses in long-term care facilities must watch for signs of urinary obstruction in elderly men.

    D. Teaching and encouragement, along with bladder training, can help decrease the incidence of incontinence, thereby cutting health care costs.

    E. Home care nurses will be supervising or assisting with care of catheters, dressings, performing wound assessments, and providing teaching for self-care to post-prostatectomy patients.

    F. The home care nurse can provide assessment and counseling for patients experiencing sexual dysfunction; collaboration with physician, social worker, and community agencies can provide avenues of help.

CHAPTER 28

Care of Patients with Sexually Transmitted Diseases

OBJECTIVES

Upon completing this chapter the student should be able to:

1. Identity the signs and symptoms of the following sexual diseases: syphilis, gonorrhea, genital herpes, chlamydia, venereal warts (condylomata, HPV), hepatitis B, and AIDS.
2. Compare the symptoms of gonorrhea in the male and female.
3. Describe the treatment of gonorrhea and the potential consequences of failure to treat this disease.
4. Identify the three stages of syphilis and discuss treatment and the importance of early detection and intervention.
5. Describe the characteristics of genital herpes, its treatment, and the resources available to those who need information about it.
6. List the ways in which the AIDS virus and the hepatitis B virus are transmitted.
7. Identify specific things people can do that help prevent contracting sexually transmitted diseases.

Sexually transmitted diseases (STDs) refers to those particular diseases spread by intimate physical contact. Modes of transmission include sexual intercourse and contact with the *genitals* (sexual organs), rectum, or mouth. Some may be transmitted via blood contact, and several STDs also can be transmitted to the fetus via the placenta or to the newborn during the birth process.

The incidence of STDs continues to rise throughout the world. All sexually active people must be considered potentially at risk, and people with multiple sexual partners are at very high risk for contracting an STD.

Because a number of these disorders can lie dormant for many years, previous sexual encounters can result in disease being passed even within currently monogamous relationships.

Public attention tends to focus on acquired immunodeficiency syndrome (AIDS) because it is a progressive and fatal disorder. However, other STDs are more widely spread and have a major impact on reproduction and general health. Chapters 26 and 27 give detailed information and illustrations on female and male anatomy and physiology.

OVERVIEW OF SEXUALLY TRANSMITTED DISEASES, CAUSES, AND PREVENTION

STDs are primarily passed through some type of intimate contact, either genital to genital, mouth to genital, or genital to rectum. They occur in both heterosexual and homosexual relationships. Some, such as AIDS or hepatitis B, also may be passed through blood contact, including transfusion with contaminated blood. Accidental transmission may occur via needle injuries to medical personnel or by direct exposure to open wounds or body fluids.

The sharing of needles among IV drug users also promotes the transmission of AIDS or hepatitis B. Such bloodborne diseases may be transmitted to the fetus prior to birth. The newborn is at risk for contracting any STD that may reside in the vagina at the time of birth. Depending on the organism, such exposure can lead to a variety of serious problems for the infant, including pneumonia and blindness.

Think about... What are the four major modes of transmission for STDs?

In many states screening for some STDs, particularly syphilis, is required for a marriage license. However, it is impossible to screen for all possible STDs. **The greatest hope for controlling STDs is public awareness and willingness to take responsibility for prevention and for treatment should transmission occur.**

NURSING MANAGEMENT

◆ Assessment

Screening for potential STDs or risk for acquiring such an infection should be part of any patient history interview. However, it often is difficult to get accurate information. **Despite an outward appearance of extreme sexual freedom in society, people are frequently reluctant to discuss their sexual attitudes and practices.** They may hide symptoms such as inflammation, a rash, or discharge if they fear it is related to an STD. This is particularly true for adolescents, who may fear parental disapproval, rejection, or disciplinary action if they admit to being sexually active. Fear of finding a serious disorder such as AIDS also may make the patient reluctant to cooperate with information gathering.

When someone is diagnosed with an STD it is important to know the names of their sexual partners so that these people can be reached and treated. Many people do not wish to give out this information. The nurse must have a personal level of comfort with such discussions before attempting to take a sexual history. Professionals who deal with these issues regularly, such as public health nurses, often have special training in taking an appropriate history.

History Taking　**Obtaining a history on a client seeking treatment for an STD requires tact and sensitivity.** Such a history involves very intimate questions and may touch on a variety of cultural and personal issues. The nurse must maintain an open and nonjudgmental attitude. See Table 28-1 for specific information on taking the history.

Physical Examination　Physical examination involves exposure of the most private parts of the anatomy. Such an exam is usually performed by both a physician and a nurse, particularly when there are gender differences between the medical personnel and the patient. It is the nurse's responsibility to provide appropriate draping and to give the client privacy when he or she is undressing for the exam.

TABLE 28-1　◆ *Assessment: Guide to Sexual History Taking*
The following questions are asked when assessing the patient with or at risk for a sexually transmitted disease: ◆ Are you currently sexually active? ◆ At what age did you become sexually active? ◆ Do you currently have more than one sexual partner? ◆ Have you had other partners in the past? ◆ If yes to either of the last two questions, do you understand the risks associated with having multiple sexual partners? (Teaching opportunity: safer sex practices.) ◆ If sexually active female, are you having regular gynecological exams with Pap smears? If yes, when was your last exam? (Teaching opportunity: importance of such exams.) ◆ If sexually active female, are you currently pregnant or trying to become pregnant? (Important for potential affects of both disease and treatment on the fetus or newborn.) ◆ If currently in a nonmonogamous relationship, are you using comdoms to help prevent sexually transmitted diseases? (Teaching opportunity: proper use of condoms with appropriate spermicide for disease protection.) ◆ Have you ever had a sexually transmitted disease? If yes, ask for specific information (what, when, how treated, was follow-up done?) ◆ Do you have symptoms or reasons to believe you might have one now? If yes, ask for specific information (symptoms, duration, partner(s) symptomatic?)

Patients may request that a family member or significant other be allowed to remain with them, and they have this right. The nurse should escort such individuals into the room and have them sit or stand by the patient in a manner that allows them to provide support without interfering with the examination process. The nurse also should make sure that any required equipment, supplies, specimen containers, and lab slips are ready in the examination room.

◆ Nursing Diagnosis

Nursing diagnoses for the patient who has an STD may include:

◆ Knowledge deficit related to modes of transmission, signs and symptoms, and treatment.

◆ Pain related to inflammation.

◆ Anxiety related to need to contact partners.

◆ Fear of becoming *HIV* (human immunovirus, causative organism for AIDS) positive.

◆ Noncompliance related to repeated infection with STDs and refusal to use condoms.

◆ Planning

General goals for the patient with a sexually transmitted disease are:

- ◆ Compliance with treatment of the disease
- ◆ Control or elimination of pain
- ◆ Tissue integrity
- ◆ Knowledge of self-care to prevent recurrence or other STD
- ◆ Knowledge of safe-sex practices
- ◆ Effective coping
- ◆ Improved self-esteem
- ◆ Effective coping

In addition to managing the treatment protocol and any pain related to an STD, patient education and emotional support are primary aspects of planning for patients with or at risk for STDs.

Education in this area often is hampered by the client's reluctance to discuss sexual issues. This may result from cultural views or more personal feelings. Adolescents, for instance, may fear that parents or peers will find out about their sexual activity or the resultant disease. Clients of all ages may wish to protect themselves or their partners from possible condemnation or embarrassment through disclosure of sensitive information. The nurse must maintain a nonjudgmental attitude and give assurance that information will be kept confidential.

Think about . . . What factors make it difficult to take an accurate history or provide education for a patient with an STD?

When planning education, allow for the client's existing knowledge base and ability to understand. Select appropriate teaching aids, such as pictures, pamphlets, and three-dimensional models.

Emotional support is another important aspect of care of the patient with an STD. Allow time in your teaching plan for listening to the client's concerns and answering questions. Be prepared with information on support groups, counseling services, and informational programs that may be of assistance. In the case of serious disease, such as HIV infection, support programs and professional counseling are of particular importance.

◆ Implementation

Symptom Relief   STDs carry a variety of symptoms, some of which may cause mild discomfort or significant pain. Review Chapter 10 on pain-management techniques. Table 28-2 lists suggestions for specific pain-management techniques under Nursing Intervention.

Prevention of Spread   The spread of STDs is a major health concern in the United States and world today. People often become sexually active at a young age, and it is not uncommon for individuals to have had a variety of sexual partners over the years.

Although the only absolute prevention is abstinence, certain behaviors significantly reduce the risk of contracting an STD. These include the use of condoms with a spermicide containing nonoxynol-9, which both acts as a barrier and has viricidal and bacteriocidal action; limiting sexual contacts, preferably to one partner; and avoiding sexual contact if one of the partners is known to be infected or if lesions are observed in the genital, perianal, or oral regions. If the client or a client's sexual partner is an IV drug user, education regarding nonsharing of needles is important. HIV and hepatitis B in particular can be spread in this manner.

◆ Evaluation

Initially, each contact with the client should be evaluated for effectiveness by reviewing information discussed to determine whether learning has taken place. Over time it is necessary to evaluate whether the client is indeed following the recommendations. Negative follow-up cultures are a good indicator that medications were taken as ordered. During the follow-up interview the nurse can inquire about use of safer sex practices and evaluate retention of information previously taught.

DIAGNOSTIC TESTS FOR SEXUALLY TRANSMITTED DISEASES

Table 26-2 lists the more common STDs and contains information about modes of transmission, diagnosis, symptoms, treatment, and nursing responsibilities.

Think about . . . What safer sex practices can help prevent the spread of STDs?

A variety of types of tests are used for detecting STDs. *Smears and cultures* may be taken directly from the site (e.g., vaginal, cervical, or urethral swabs). In some instances, organisms also can be cultured from the blood. *Biopsies* are microscopic tissue exams performed on a sample taken from the affected area and are usually done to differentiate between benign and malignant tissues, but can also provide a differential diagnosis in

Text continued on page 891

TABLE 28-2 ♦ *Common Sexually Transmitted Diseases*

Disease	Modes of Transmission	Symptoms	Medical Diagnosis	Medical Treatment	Nursing Intervention
Chlamydia Trachomatis	Direct sexual contact. May be transmitted to the newborn during vaginal delivery. Most common STD in the United States.	*Male* Dysuria, frequency of urination, watery, mucus-like discharge. Causes about half the cases of epididymitis and nongonococcal urethritis. *Female* Approximately 75% have no symptoms. Vaginal discharge, urinary frequency, soreness, itching, pulling in vaginal area. May have unusual odor, "fishy" after intercourse. Causes up to 50% of cases of pelvic inflammatory disease (PID). *Neonate* Eye infections and pneumonia. Possible complications: Cervical dysplasia; carcinoma of cervix, penis, rectum; male urethral obstruction.	Usually by smear and Gram stain to identify polymorphonuclear leukocytes (WBCs) and rule out the presence of the gram-negative organism of gonorrhea. Fluorscein-labeled monoclonal antibody test gives results in 30 minutes. Cultures can also be done, but are expensive and take more time. Usually screened for gonorrhea as coinfection is not uncommon.	Doxycycline (a tetracy-cline) 100 mg PO bid × 7 days. Azithromycin 1 g single dose. Highly effective because of good compliance (only one dose), but expensive. Pregnant women: erythromycin base 250 mg PO qid × 14 days. PID: various regimens depending on organisms involved, as often a combination of organisms is present.	Education Encourage clients to seek attention for any unusual vaginal or penile discharge. Partner(s) must be treated concurrently to prevent "ping-ponging" the infection. Condom use for prevention of future infection, with abstinence until course of treatment completed. Must complete antibiotics to ensure effective treatment. Tetracyclines can cause photosensitivity, sunscreen recommended.
Condylomata acuminata (venereal warts)	Caused by human papilloma viruses (HPV) spread during sexual contact. Highly contagious. Can be transmitted to newborn during vaginal delivery.	Warts are flat or raised, rough, cauliflower-like growths on the vulva, penis, perianal area, vaginal or rectal walls, or cervix. The flat variety are more likely to lead to tissue changes that contribute to cervical or penile cancer. *Newborn* Laryngeal papillomas.	Biopsy, colposcopy, androscopy, anoscopy, Pap smear.	Freezing, laser therapy, surgical removal, topical chemotherapy. Podophyllin and podofilox are alternative treatments for external warts. No known cure, lesions may recur any time.	Education Teach about mode of infection and use of condoms to prevent spread. Regular Pap smears due to increased risk of cervical cancer. Risk factors include cigarette smoking and early age of onset of sexual activity.

| Genital herpes | Caused by herpes simplex virus (HSV) types 1 and 2. Highly contagious, spread by direct contact; not limited to sexual contact. Selfinoculation also possible, e.g., from lip ulcer (fever blister) to genitals. Invades nerve cells located near the site of infection. Lies dormant, flareups erratic and unpredictable. Some patients have frequent recurrence, others rarely or none. Neonate may be infected during delivery if mother has active disease (more common if initial episode occurs during pregnancy.) | *Primary* Fever, headache, malaise, myalgia, burning genital pain, dysuria (female), painful intercourse, possible aseptic meningitis, vesicles which ulcerate, crust over, and resolve spontaneously in about 2 weeks. *Secondary* Burning genital pain, possible numbness and tingling 24 hours before lesions appear, vesicles. *Male* Lesions may appear on glans penis, shaft of penis, prepuce, scrotal sac, inner thighs. *Female* Vulva, vaginal surface, buttocks, cervix. Cervical lesions may be small and superficial with diffuse inflammation, or a single, large, necrotic ulcer. Increased risk of cervical cancer. Primary infection during pregnancy associated with high risk of premature labor and spontaneous abortion. *Neonate* Severity ranges from clinically inapparent to local infections of eyes, skin, or mucous membranes to severe disseminated infection. The latter may be neurological and can cause severe damage or death. | Lesions usually easily identified by experienced clinician. Can be confirmed by viral cultures. Serological tests can help determine whether it is an initial or *recurrent* episode (return of symptoms from previous exposure, not a new infection). | No known cure. Treatment with acyclovir or valacyclovir HCL may reduce symptoms and accelerate healing. For individuals with frequent recurrence, continuous treatment may reduce frequency. Topical acyclovir is not as effective as systemic. | Lesions must be kept clean and dry to prevent secondary infection. Sitz baths, Burow's soaks, ice packs may decrease discomfort. Increased fluids will dilute urine for greater comfort during voiding, as will voiding in the shower or sitting in water. Application of topical steroids may hasten healing; topical anesthetics and oral analgesics may help manage pain. Strict gloving and observation of *Standard Precautions* are necessary.

Education
Use of condoms with spermicide to help prevent spread, avoidance of sex if lesions present; scrupulous handwashing; importance of informing physician if patient becomes pregnant that she has been infected with genital herpes (if disease is active, infant will be delivered by C-section to protect it from exposure); relationship to cervical cancer and need for annual Pap smears. Recurrence may be triggered by genital trauma, menses, other infections, emotional stress, exposure to sunlight. Information about education and support programs can be obtained by writing the Herpes Resource Center ASHA/HRC, P.O. Box 13827, Research Triangle Park, NC 27709-9940. Hotline: 919-361-8488. |

(Table 28-2 continued)

TABLE 28-2 ◆ *Common Sexually Transmitted Diseases (Continued)*

Disease	Modes of Transmission	Symptoms	Medical Diagnosis	Medical Treatment	Nursing Intervention
Gonorrhea	Easily transmitted by direct sexual contact. Transmitted to the newborn during vaginal delivery if mother has active disease. Autoinoculation via fingers to eye possible. Occasionally becomes bloodborne.	*Male* Dysuria with frequency; scant to copious purulent discharge from penis. If untreated, discharge increases and may continue for months; may develop urethral stricture, epididymitis. Can advance to inflammation of prostate and testes; can cause sterility. *Female* Vaginal discharge, burning urination, Bartholin's gland abscess; untreated spreads upward to fallopian tubes and ovaries (PID), with symptoms of abdominal pain and tenderness, abnormal menses, fever, cervical tenderness, chronic pelvic pain. PID is a leading cause of female sterility. *Homosexual males* Purulent or bloody rectal discharge, rectal burning or itching, asymptomatic rectal infection. *Male and female* May involve kidneys, bladder, rectum, eyes, oropharynx. May disseminate, causing septicemia, arthritis, dermatitis, meningitis, cardiac valve disease. *Neonate* At risk for ophthalmia neonatorum, which can cause blindness; scalp abscess at site of fetal monitor; rhinitis; meningitis; disseminated infection; anorectal infection. Note: As high as 40% of males and 90% of females with gonorrhea are asymptomatic.	Confirmed by presence of the causative organism, *Neisseria gonorrhoeae,* in vaginal or urethral smear. Additional confirmative tests, such as sugar fermentation, coagglutination, or fluorescent antibody may be required. Commonly also screened for syphilis and chlamydia.	Antibiotics. CDC recommends ceftriaxone (Rocephin) IM plus doxycycline 100 mg PO bid × 1 week. Penicillin, ampicillin, erythromycin, tetracycline in combination also may be used. All sexual partners must be treated simultaneously and no sexual contact should occur until treatment is completed. Resistant strains exist, so a patient is not considered cured until follow-up cultures are negative.	Observation of *Standard Precautions* and frequent handwashing if any contact with body fluids/vaginal or penile discharge. Education Teach about prevention and treatment, specifically importance of completing treatment, naming all contacts so everyone can be treated, and having follow-up cultures to assure that treatment has been effective. Encourage safer sex practices (use of condoms, limiting sexual contacts) to prevent reinfection. Be sure patient understands how to take ordered medication.

Hepatitis B	Caused by hepatitis B virus (HBV). Transmission via sexual contact, blood contact, and to the fetus via the placenta in an infected mother. Hepatitis C (non A non B), and delta hepatitis (seen only in persons with active HBV infection) also can be sexually transmitted. Hepatitis A is transmitted by the fecal-oral route and may be transmitted to a sexual partner.	May have anorexia, malaise, nausea, vomiting, abdominal pain, dark urine, jaundice, skin rashes, arthralgias, arthritis. Acute infection may be asymptomatic, and may resolve, resulting in permanent immunity. However, infection may be persistent and result in a chronic carrier state. Long-term patients may develop chronic persistent or chronic active hepatitis, cirrhosis, hepatocellular carcinoma, hepatic failure, and death. Infants born infected are at high risk for chronic hepatitis B infection.	Serological testing for HBV infection gives definitive diagnosis.	No specific therapy is available. Hepatitis B immune globulin (HBIG) is given prophylactically following known exposure. Hepatitis B vaccine is recommended for people at risk for exposure, including health care workers and intimate partners or immediate family members of persons who have hepatitis B. Hepatitis B vaccine is currently given as part of normal childhood immunizations. HBIG and hepatitis B vaccine are given to newborns of infected mothers at birth, with additional doses of vaccine at age 1 month and 6 months.	Appropriate handling of all blood or body fluids to prevent transmission of infection. Men in homosexual relationships are at increased risk for both Hepatitis B and HIV infection. Education Teach about vaccine, use of condoms, and screening of all pregnant women to provide optimal protection for the newborn. Importance of follow-up appointments for monitoring liver function studies.
Human immunodeficiency virus (HIV), AIDS, ARC (AIDS-Related Complex) (see Chapter 8 for detailed information on AIDS).	Sexual or blood contact. Presence of genital ulcers has shown increased risk of acquiring or transmitting the HIV virus.	May have mild viral illness at time of initial infection, then may remain asymptomatic except for HIV seropositivity for many years. HIV seropositivity may take several months to manifest. Symptoms may include fatigue, poor appetite, unexplained weight loss, generalized lymphadenopathy, persistent diarrhea, fever, night sweats, Kaposi's sarcoma, *Pneumocystis carinii* pneumonia, oral and esophageal candidiasis.	Diagnosis of HIV infection based on reactive enzyme immunoassay (EIA) confirmed by a more specific assay (e.g., Western blot or immunofluorescent assay). AIDS and ARC may be diagnosed based on lab results and/or specific diagnostic criteria (see Chapter 8).	Eight antiretroviral agents are currently available with active research in progress on others: Didanosine, lamiduvine, stavudine, zalcitabine, ritonair, saquinavir, indinavir, zidovudine (ZDV, formerly called AZT). Use may delay development of ARC and full-blown AIDS in HIV positive individuals. See Chapter 8 for more specific	People who have tested HIV positive or been diagnosed with AIDS or ARC should receive specific professionally trained counseling on lifestyle practices, treatment protocols, and follow-up procedures. AIDS is regarded as a terminal illness as currently no cure exists, and individuals with AIDS or the potential of developing AIDS need a significant support system. See Chapter 8 for more specific information.

(Table 28-2 continued)

TABLE 28-2 ◆ Common Sexually Transmitted Diseases (Continued)

Disease	Modes of Transmission	Symptoms	Medical Diagnosis	Medical Treatment	Nursing Intervention
				information on treatment for HIV, AIDS, and ARC.	Information sources National AIDS Hotline, 1-800-342-2437; Spanish, 1-800-342-7432. National Institute of Health AIDS Clinical Trials Group, 1-800-874-2572. American Foundation for AIDS Research, 1-212-719-0033.
Syphilis	Direct body contact; organism (*Treponema pallidum*, a spirochete) requires warm, wet environment to survive, can be destroyed with plain soap. Placental transmission to fetus in about 50% of women with active disease during pregnancy.	Syphilis has three stages *Primary* Chance (hard, painless sore) on the mucous membrane of the mouth or genitals, often unnoticed in women. Chance teeming with spirochetes, very contagious at this stage. Spirochetes enter blood stream 3 to 7 days after infection and begin to multiply rapidly. May have headache and lymph node enlargement near chancre; symptoms are often minor and disappear within 3 to 8 weeks. *Secondary* Symptoms vary. May have mild malaise, headache, skin rash, sore throat, patchy hair loss from scalp, arthritis, neuritis, retinitis. Symptoms may wax and wane, then disappear as the disease enters latent period. *Tertiary (late)* One to 20 years after infection. Spirochetes have had access to all body tissues, damage can cause a variety of symptoms. Nervous system, blood vessels, and eyes most often affected. *Congenital* Stillbirth, intrauterine growth retardation, multiple system damage, including central nervous system.	*Screening* VDRL (venereal disease research laboratory) and RPR (rapid plasma reagin) tests, performed on blood or spinal fluid if neurosyphilis is suspected. False-positive may be triggered by other infection, chronic systemic illness, nonsyphilitic treponemal disease, alcohol. May be negative in primary, but always positive in secondary cases. *Confirmation* Fluorescent treponemal antibody absorption (FTA-ABS) blood test.	*Antibiotics* (Benzathine penicillin) 2.4 million units IM for primary or secondary (less than 1-year duration). 2.4 million units IM weekly × 3 weeks for disease of undetermined length or duration greater than 1 year. Neurosyphilis: aqueous crystalline penicillin G, 2-4 million units IV q 4 h × 10-14 days. Other antibiotics, particularly tetracycline and erythromycin, may be used in cases of penicillin sensitivity.	Education Caution patients not to ingest alcohol for 24 hours prior to VDRL or RPR (may cause false-positive). Remember that chancre is highly infectious (gloved contact only). Encourage naming of contacts so everyone can be treated. Encourage condom use to prevent reinfection. Explain importance of follow-up (usually 3- and 6-month VDRL) to ensure treatment has been effective. Follow-up usually at 1, 2, 3, 6, 9, and 12 months for HIV-positive individuals.

diseases that have specific unusual cellular changes or organisms present.

Numerous types of blood tests can help detect STDs. They look for the presence of specific *antibodies* formed by the presence of certain microorganisms or for the effects of the presence of *antigens* (substances in the bloodstream that induce the production of antibodies). Such effects include the tendency for cells to *agglutinate* (clump together) in a variety of characteristic patterns.

Staining procedures differentiate organisms by using dyes that have been found to stain some bacteria in specific ways. An example of this would be a Gram stain, in which bacteria are first stained with crystal violet, then treated with a strong iodine solution, decolorized with ethanol or ethanol acetone, and then counterstained with contrasting dye. Those retaining the initial stain are considered Gram positive, those losing the stain but accepting the counterstain are considered Gram negative. Those neither retaining the initial stain nor accepting the counterstain are non-Gram positive or negative.

Identifying microorganisms is a complex procedure. **When collecting or assisting in the collection of specimens, the nurse has several specific responsibilities to ensure that the samples will allow appropriate studies to be performed.** These are as follows:

◆ Ensure that appropriate lab request slips have been prepared according to the physician's specific orders. If antibiotics have been started, note this on the lab slip.

◆ Check the lab manual for any specific restrictions or preparations for the tests ordered. Examples:

Urethral swabs should not be done within 1 hour of the last void as organisms will have been flushed away.

Female patients should not douche or tub-bathe for 24 hours before vaginal cultures or smears.

Some tests will give a false-positive reading if the patient is on specific medications, eats certain foods, or has other types of infection present.

Antibiotics may cause cultures to be negative even though the drug or the dose may not be sufficient to cure the infection.

Stool present in the rectum can prevent good rectal swabs from being obtained.

Cultures and smears usually are obtained with a sterile swab and sent to the lab for further handling. If slides or cultures are to be made as the physician collects the specimens, the nurse must obtain the appropriate supplies from the lab.

◆ Prepare the patient.

Explain what tests have been ordered and any dietary or activity restrictions. Answer all questions.

For smears, cultures, and biopsies provide appropriate draping and remain with patient during the procedure.

◆ Provide emotional support as needed.

◆ Make sure that specimens are appropriately labeled and delivered to the lab with the corresponding lab slips. Table 28-2 lists specific tests done for the STDs listed.

COMMUNITY CARE

Most communities have clinics, often through the public health system, that provide screening and treatment for STDs. These may be low cost or no cost, and they provide a valuable service by assisting the community to control the spread of STDs.

Some sexually transmitted diseases must be reported to public health authorities. The CDC and local health authorities establish these regulations and provide regular updates and reporting forms for monitored diseases.

Patient education is an important service provided by community clinics. The Health Department and Planned Parenthood are just two of the organizations that routinely provide pamphlets, posters, and classes on preventing and treating STDs. Confidential screening and education on safer sexual practices are important services provided by these clinics. Public service announcements, such as the TV spots on AIDS awareness, are another source of public education. In many areas, information and education are made available through the schools and colleges and are directed both at students and families and at the general community.

CRITICAL THINKING EXERCISES

Clinical Case Problems

Read each clinical situation and discuss the questions with your classmates.

1. A friend confides that she has a rash in her genital area that occurred since she began having sex with her latest boyfriend. She is afraid she may have syphilis or genital herpes and doesn't know what to do.

   a. What would you say to convince her that she needs to see an experienced clinician for diagnosis and treatment?

   b. Where can she go if she does not want to see her regular physician?

   c. What would you tell her about the differences between syphilis and genital herpes?

2. A patient confides in you that he has three girlfriends, all of whom are taking oral contraceptives, so he sees no reason to use condoms.

a. What could you tell him about the risks of multiple sexual partners and the importance of using condoms to prevent sexually transmitted diseases?

BIBLIOGRAPHY

Andreoli, T. E., et al. (1990). *Cecil Essentials of Medicine,* 2nd ed. Philadelphia: Saunders.

Barbier, S. (1995). Genital herpes, reducing outbreaks; a vaccine that shows promise. *Nursing.* 25(1):53.

Cibley, Laurence J., Leonard J. (1993). Detecting and treating HPV infection. *Clinical Advances in the Treatment of Infections.* 7(5):1–3, 11–12.

Cook, L. S., Kroutsky, L. A., Holmes, K. K. (1994). Circumcision and sexually transmitted diseases. *American Journal of Public Health.* 94(2):197.

Dambro, M. R. (1996). *Griffith's 5 Minute Clinical Consult.* Baltimore: Williams & Wilkins.

Ebel, C. (1995). *Managing Herpes; How to Live and Love with a Chronic STD.* American Social Health Association.

Genc, N., Mardh, P. (1996). A cost-effectiveness analysis of screening and treatment for *Chlamydia trachomatis* infection in asymptomatic women. *Annals of Internal Medicine.* 124(1):1.

Gurevich, I. (1990). Counseling the patient with herpes. *RN.* 47(2):22–28.

Pagana, K. D., T. J. (1995). *Mosby's Diagnostic and Laboratory Reference,* 2nd ed. St. Louis, MO: Mosby.

Rodgers, K. (1995). CDC recommends aggressive treatment of chlamydia. *Drug Topics.* 139(23):51.

Sargent, S. J. (1992). The "other" sexually transmitted diseases. *Post Graduate Medicine.* 91(4):359–362, 371–377.

Touchstone, D. M., Davis, D. D. (1992). Consider chlamydia. *RN.* 49(2):31–36.

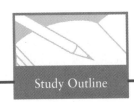

Study Outline

I. Sexually Transmitted Diseases: Causes and Prevention

　A. STDs are primarily passed though some type of intimate contact—genital to genital, mouth to genital, genital to rectum.

　B. Some, such as AIDS or hepatitis B, may also be passed by blood contact.

　　1. Transfusion.

　　2. Needle injuries.

　　3. Needle sharing.

　　4. Exposure to open wounds or body fluids.

　　5. Via placenta to the fetus.

　C. The greatest hope for controlling STDs lies in public awareness and willingness to take responsibility for prevention and for treatment should transmission occur.

II. Nursing Management

　A. Assessment.

　　1. People often are reluctant to discuss their sexual attitudes and practices.

　　　a. Fear of family rejection.

　　　b. Fear of a serious disorder such as AIDS.

　　2. It is important to get names of sexual contacts so everyone can be located and treated.

　　3. Taking the sexual history involves intimate questions and requires maintaining an open and nonjudgmental attitude.

　　4. The physical exam involves intimate exposure and is usually done with both physician and nurse present, particularly if there is a gender difference between the patient and the health professionals.

　　5. A patient has the right to have a support person in the room during the exam if requested.

　　6. The nurse is responsible for having required equipment and supplies ready in examination room.

　B. Nursing diagnosis

　C. Planning

　　1. Planning needs to include management of the treatment protocol and any pain related to the disease.

　　2. Education and emotional support are among the most important aspects.

　　　a. Education often is hampered by client's reluctance to talk about sexual issues.

　　　b. When planning education, allow for the client's existing knowledge base and ability to understand what is being taught.

　　　c. Allow adequate time for questions, answers, and just listening.

　D. Implementation

　　1. Pain-management techniques include oral analgesics, sitz baths, cold packs, and topical anesthetics.

　　2. The spread of STDs is a major health concern in the United States and world today.

3. Certain behaviors significantly reduce the risk of contracting an STD.
   a. Condoms.
   b. Spermicides containing nonoxynol-9.
   c. Limiting sexual contacts, monogamous relationships.
   d. Avoiding sexual contact during active disease or when lesions are present.
   e. Not sharing needles if IV drug user.

E. Evaluation
   1. Review information discussed to determine whether learning has taken place.
   2. Determine whether the client is indeed following recommendations.
      a. Medications completed.
      b. Safer sex practices.
      c. Follow-up testing.

III. **Tests for Sexually Transmitted Diseases**
   A. There are a variety of tests for STDs.
      1. Smears and cultures.
         2. Biopsy.
         3. Blood tests.
            a. Antibodies.
            b. Antigens.
            c. Agglutination.
            d. Staining.
   B. When collecting or helping collect specimens, the nurse has several specific responsibilities to ensure that the samples will allow appropriate studies to be performed.
      1. Correct lab slips.
      2. Specific guidelines from lab manual.
      3. Patient preparation.
      4. Specimens labeled and delivered to lab.

IV. **Community Care**
   A. Community clinics provide valuable screening and treatment programs, often at low or no cost.
   B. Some STDs must be reported to public health authorities.
   C. Community clinics also provide patient education.

CHAPTER 29

Care of Patients with Skin Disorders

The skin is an organ that is essential for the maintenance of life and good health. It functions very much like a built-in suit of armor; it is the first line of defense against invasion by pathogenic bacteria living in the environment.

Disorders that primarily affect the skin are numerous, but the skin also reflects systemic diseases. In this chapter the focus is on diseases that are primary skin disorders; however, a knowledge of the patient's health history greatly improves the chances of accurately diagnosing any skin abnormality.

When an area of the skin is destroyed by disease or trauma, its protective functions are immediately impaired, and the body is susceptible to infection. If very large areas of skin are destroyed, as in an extensive burn, fluid and electrolyte balance is disturbed, and body heat is lost.

Skin diseases are very common in humans. They also are extremely exasperating, because they often are difficult to diagnose and cure and they tend to recur. Although the physical effects of skin diseases usually are not extremely serious, it is difficult to measure the psychological impact of a disorder that renders the patient unattractive, threatens self-image, and damages self-esteem.

The word *dermatology* refers to the study of diseases of the skin. A *dermatologist* is one who specializes in the treatment of skin disorders. Many dermatologists have some standing orders or written instructions they wish followed when their patients are hospitalized. The nurse must check standing orders and agency protocols when caring for patients with skin disorders. To understand the discussion of the skin disorders better, a review of the anatomy and functions of the skin is necessary.

Pressure ulcers are discussed in Chapter 11, Care of the Immobile Patient. Pediatric disorders such as impetigo, eczema, and ringworm are discussed in pediatric nursing texts.

OVERVIEW OF ANATOMY AND PHYSIOLOGY

What Is the Structure of the Skin?

⊿ The skin consists of two layers of tissue, the epidermis and the dermis (Figure 29-1).

⊿ The skin is attached to underlying structures by subcutaneous tissue.

⊿ The epidermis consists of squamous epithelium and contains no blood vessels; cells receive nutrients by diffusion from vessels in the underlying tissue.

⊿ Cell growth occurs from the bottom of the epidermis and pushes cells above to the surface where they eventually die and slough off. This layer is called the stratum corneum.

⊿ The bottom layer of the epidermis contains melanocytes that contribute color to the skin.

⊿ The dermis, also called stratum corium, is thicker than the epidermis and consists of dense connective tissue.

⊿ The dermis contains both elastic and collagenous fibers that give it strength and elasticity.

⊿ The dermis contains blood vessels and nerves as well as the base of hair follicles, glands, and nails that are derived from the epidermis.

⊿ Fibroblasts that produce new cells to heal the skin are contained in the dermis.

⊿ Glands contained in the skin are sebaceous, sweat, or ceruminous (wax producing).

⊿ Nails are dead stratum corneum with a very hard type of keratin. They cover the distal ends of the fingers and toes.

What Are the Functions of the Skin and Its Structures?

⊿ The skin acts as a protective covering over the entire surface of the body.

⊿ The skin is waterproof, preventing water loss from the underlying tissues and too much water absorption during swimming and bathing.

⊿ Skin provides a barrier to bacteria and other invading organisms.

⊿ Skin protects underlying tissues from thermal, chemical, and mechanical injury.

⊿ The skin helps regulate body temperature by dilating and constricting blood vessels and by activating or inactivating sweat glands.

⊿ When the skin is exposed to ultraviolet light, molecules in the cells convert the rays to vitamin D.

⊿ Melanin pigment absorbs light and acts to protect tissue from ultraviolet light.

⊿ The nerve receptors in the dermis transmit feelings of heat, cold, pain, touch, and pressure.

⊿ Hair follicles contained in the skin produce hair.

⊿ Sebaceous glands secrete sebum that functions to keep hair and skin soft and pliable. Sebum also inhibits bacterial growth on the surface of the skin and, because of its oily nature, helps prevent water loss from the skin.

⊿ Sweat glands act to excrete water and salt when the body temperature increases; sweat evaporates, producing a cooling effect.

⊿ Sweat glands in the axillae and external genitalia secrete fatty acids and proteins as well as water and salts. They become active at puberty and are stimulated by the nervous system in response to sexual arousal, emotional stress, and pain.

What Changes Occur in the Skin and Its Structures with Aging?

⊿ The number of elastic fibers decreases and adipose tissue diminishes in the dermis and subcutaneous layers, causing skin to wrinkle and sag.

⊿ Loss of collagen fibers in the dermis makes the skin increasingly fragile and slower to heal.

⊿ The skin becomes thinner and more transparent.

⊿ Reduced sebaceous gland activity causes dry skin that may itch.

⊿ The thinned skin and decreased sebaceous gland activity reduces temperature control and leads to an intolerance of cold and a susceptibility to heat exhaustion.

⊿ A reduction in melanocyte activity increases risk of sunburn and skin cancer.

⊿ The number of hair follicles decreases and the growth rate of hair declines; the hair thins.

⊿ Decreased numbers of melanocytes at the hair follicle causes gradual loss of hair color.

⊿ Nail growth decreases, longitudinal ridges appear, and the nails thicken; nails become more susceptible to fungal infections.

⊿ Some areas of melanocytes increase in production producing brown age spots, senile lentigines (Color Figure 6).

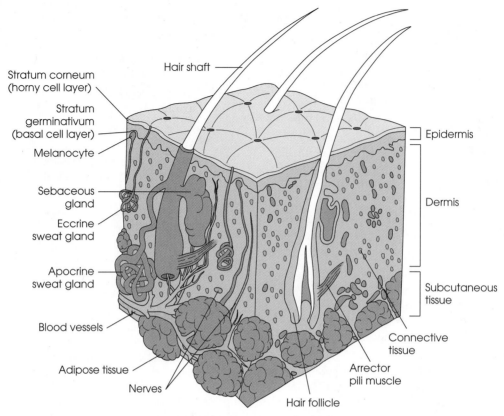

FIGURE 29-1   Structure of the skin.

CAUSES OF SKIN DISORDERS

Over 3,000 disorders of the skin have been officially named, and many more are not included in any official nomenclature. The majority of the recognized and named skin disorders arise from some pathology in the skin itself; the remainder are manifestations of some systemic disease. Skin disorders may occur from immunological and inflammatory disorders, proliferative and neoplastic disorders, metabolic and endocrine disorders, and nutritional problems. Physical, chemical, and microbiological factors also can damage the skin.

Many patients with dermatological disease are not hospitalized and are seen only in physicians' offices and outpatient clinics. Others do not seek medical attention but treat their skin disorder themselves with home remedies and over-the-counter drugs. In some cases self-care measures are successful, but they also have the potential for aggravating the condition or only temporarily relieving its more severe symptoms. This can lead to delay in treatment and allows the disease to progress to a chronic and sometimes untreatable state.

Caring for those who have a skin disorder can be particularly challenging to the nurse because of the recurrent nature of many skin disorders, the potential these disorders have for disfigurement, and the added burden they can place on the patient if the skin disease can be spread to others.

PREVENTION OF SKIN DISEASE

◆ Cleanliness

The ritual of the daily bath almost is an obsession with the average American, and nurses are perhaps guiltier than most in their insistence on using good, strong soap and plenty of hot water. No one will quarrel with the value of cleanliness, but it can be overdone, and the method of cleansing the skin deserves some consideration.

First, we must recognize that there are various skin types. Blondes and redheads usually have very delicate skin that requires special care to prevent drying and irritation. On the other hand, people with dark hair usually have skin that is more oily and less susceptible to excessive drying and irritation.

If the skin appears dry and scaly, frequent bathing with strong soaps and hot water only aggravates the condition. Oils and creams are available that cleanse the skin quite effectively and help replace the natural oils at the same time. The person with oily skin will need to clean the skin frequently, use a liberal amount of soap and water, and avoid applying additional oils to the skin.

◆ Diet

Adequate intake of vitamins and minerals is essential to the maintenance of healthy skin. Even borderline deficiencies in these nutrients will cause the skin to take on a sallow and dull appearance. Severe nutritional deficiencies lead to skin breakdown and the development of sores and ulcers. Many teenagers who are so concerned with their physical appearance that they refuse to eat properly for fear of gaining weight fail to realize that they are robbing themselves of one of the sources of real beauty—a healthy and radiant complexion.

◆ Age

Young people are not the only ones who should be concerned with the care of their skin. As we grow older, our skin undergoes certain changes that easily lead to irritation and breakdown if proper care is not given. The oil and sweat glands become less active, and the skin has a tendency to become dry and scaly. It also loses some of its tone, becoming less elastic and more fragile. Frequent cleansing of the skin becomes unnecessary as the skin ages, and alcohol and other drying agents must be used sparingly, if at all. As we grow older, we should establish a regular routine of massaging oils, creams, or oily lotions into the skin, if not for the sake of vanity, at least for the sake of preserving a very important organ.

Elder Care Point . . . The elderly patient who has dry skin does not need a full bath every day; cleansing of the axillae and genital-rectal area between bathing days should be sufficient. Elderly patients should use a mild lotion-based soap, such as Dove, for bathing. After showering or the bath, a lotion that helps seal in moisture should be applied while the skin is still damp.

◆ Environment

Several environmental factors can have a direct effect on the health of the skin. These include prolonged exposure to chemicals, excessive drying from repeated immersions in water, very cold temperatures, and prolonged exposure to sunlight. Some of these are occupational hazards and may necessitate a change of jobs to eliminate contact with a factor that is causing a skin disorder. See the discussion of contact dermatitis in allergic reactions in Chapter 7.

Overexposure to the ultraviolet rays of the sun can seriously and permanently damage the superficial and deeper layers of the skin, causing severe wrinkling and furrowing, loss of elasticity, and the skin to assume a tissue-paper transparency. In addition to the potential for premature aging and degenerative changes, solar damage also can result in malignant changes. Ultraviolet rays from the sun have long been known to be carcinogenic, especially in fair-skinned persons who have subjected their skin to prolonged exposure to sunshine. Although sunburns are especially harmful, it is the normal daily exposure of unprotected fair skin to sun that causes long-term damage.

Health teaching to inform the public about the dangers of solar ultraviolet radiation should include the following information:

- Although fair-skinned people who freckle easily are more likely to suffer sun-damaged skin, persons of all complexions and races can and do burn if exposed to sufficient sunlight.
- Although a good tan might be considered by many to be desirable, not everyone can acquire such a tan without serious damage to the skin. If one insists on lying out in the sun, the initial exposure should be slow and gradual, and an adequate sunscreen with a skin protection factor (SPF) of at least 15 should always be used. Too much sun too soon only leads to blistering and peeling.
- Select a sunscreen preparation on the basis of skin type and ability to tan, as well as its active ingredients and the amount of time to be spent in the sun. Remember that the sunscreen can be washed off by water or perspiration or rubbed off on sand and towels and must be periodically reapplied.
- Avoid exposure to the sun during the time its rays are most hazardous; that is, between 11 A.M. and 3 P.M. Local radio and television stations often give information about current weather conditions and the chances for being burned by the sun at particular times during each day.
- You can be sunburned on a cloudy or overcast day.
- Light, loosely worn clothing will not give adequate protection from the sun's rays.
- Remember that snow, water, and sand can reflect the sun's rays and increase the intensity of exposure.
- Do not try to gauge how much you are being burned while in the sun. It may be 6 to 8 hours before a painful burn becomes obvious.
- Wear a hat when you go out in the sun, and, when possible, wear protective clothing.

DIAGNOSTIC TESTS AND PROCEDURES AND NURSING RESPONSIBILITIES

◆ Skin Biopsy

Removing a sample of tissue (biopsy) from a skin lesion usually is performed with a local anesthetic. It can be done by shaving a top layer off a lesion that rises above the skin line *(shave biopsy)*, by removing a core from the center of the lesion *(punch biopsy)*, or by excising the entire lesion *(excisional biopsy)*.

Skin biopsy is used to differentiate benign from malignant lesions and to help identify the causative organism in bacterial and fungal infections.

No special patient preparation is necessary beyond a simple explanation of the procedure and its purpose. If a local anesthetic is to be used, the patient is asked about any personal or family history of allergies.

◆ Culture and Sensitivity Tests

When a bacterial, viral, or fungal infection of the skin is suspected, the dermatologist may wish to know the causative organism and the drug most appropriate for treating a specific kind of infection. A sampling of exudate is taken from the lesion and sent to the laboratory for culturing. Once the organism has been cultured, colonies can be tested for sensitivity to certain antiinfective agents. These tests take the guesswork out of treating infectious skin disease and very quickly determine which drug will be most effective in treating it.

As with the collection of any specimen for culture, care must be taken when handling the specimen and its container to avoid contaminating the person collecting and handling the specimen and the outside and inside of the container.

◆ Inspection under Special Light

Inspection of the skin is one of the principal means by which skin lesions are diagnosed. To facilitate the diagnosis of certain kinds of skin disorders, special lights may be used by the examiner.

A *cold light* is one in which the light is transmitted through a quartz or plastic structure to dissipate the heat. Because there is no danger of burning the skin, the cold light can be applied directly to the skin to illuminate its layers for visualization of malignant changes.

Wood's light is a specially designed ultraviolet light. The nickel-oxide filter holds back all but a few violet rays of the visible spectrum. This special light is especially useful to diagnose fungal infections of the scalp and chronic bacterial infection of the major folds of the skin (**erythrasma**). Under Wood's light, fungal lesions and erythrasma are fluorescent. Erythrasma usually is seen on the inner thighs, the scrotum, the axilla, and the area between the toes.

◆ Diascopy

Diascopy uses a glass slide or lens pressed down over the area to be examined, blanching the skin and thereby reducing the erythema caused by increasing blood flow to the area. The shape of the underlying lesion is then revealed.

◆ Patch Testing

When you suspect a rash to be of an allergic nature, patch testing is used to identify the responsible allergen. Test chemicals or substances are introduced to unaffected skin, usually on the forearm or back, by superficial scratches or pricks. If a localized reaction producing a **wheal** (smooth, slightly elevated area that is pale or reddened) occurs, the test is positive.

NURSING MANAGEMENT

◆ Assessment

History Taking   Diagnosing skin disorders often requires diligent detective work to identify factors that predispose a patient to or actually cause some type of skin disease. Data gathering on the potential etiological factors mentioned is necessary. Table 29-1 presents a guide for history taking.

Scabies, lice, and other parasites can be transmitted through close personal contact with infected persons at work, recreation, home, or school. If the patient has recently been exposed to severe cold, his skin may be drier than usual and he may complain of severe itching *(winter itch)*.

TABLE 29-1 ◆ *Assessment: A Guide to History Taking for Skin Disorders*

The following questions should be asked when seeking data on a skin disorder:

- ◆ When did the rash or lesion first appear?
- ◆ Can you think of any event or different food you ate or substance you were using just before it appeared?
- ◆ Have you noticed if anything makes it worse?
- ◆ What seems to make it better?
- ◆ Have you been using any chemicals lately for household cleaning or in pursuit of your hobbies?
- ◆ Have you been out in the country or the woods lately?
- ◆ Have you been traveling? Did you visit a tropical area?
- ◆ What drugs are you taking? Do you take any over-the-counter medications?
- ◆ Have you ever had a drug reaction?
- ◆ Do you have a history of any skin disorders in your family?
- ◆ Do you have any allergies?
- ◆ Are you experiencing itching? Pain?
- ◆ Have you had any gastrointestinal problems that began about the same time that the rash or lesion appeared? What about a runny or stuffed-up nose? Cough?

Almost all drugs can produce skin eruptions in certain individuals. Drug allergy or reaction can produce lesions and rashes that imitate any found in a long list of diseases including measles, chickenpox, fungus infections, skin cancers, and psoriasis.

Itching and pain are the most common complaints. If the disorder is due to an allergy, the patient also may complain of shortness of breath or cough or of some gastrointestinal symptoms. The patient also may be able to tell the nurse what other factors, such as stress or excitement, could be related to the appearance of his skin lesions.

Physical Assessment   Significant objective data include the following:

◆ Type of lesion (Table 29-2) and distribution, size, and appearance.
◆ Appearance of skin adjacent to lesions, noting whether reddened areas blanch when mild pressure is applied.
◆ Localized or generalized skin edema.
◆ Characteristics of secretions; that is, color, viscosity, amount.
◆ Odor: description of odor; strong or faint; source—local or generalized.
◆ General appearance of skin surface: texture, elasticity, thickness. Check the back and the soles of the feet.
◆ Observation of patient scratching, rubbing, or picking at lesions.
◆ Observation of scratching of the scalp or pubic areas.
◆ Temperature changes: location of hot spots or cold areas of the skin.

Seborrheic keratoses are common in the elderly. They appear as wart-like, greasy lesions on the trunk, arms, scalp, and sometimes the face. They are not cause for concern.

Darkly pigmented people will have areas that are darker than other parts of the skin. This is due to hormonal influences. The darker areas are the nipples, areola, scrotum, and labia minora. This is true among both blacks and Asians. Pallor in the dark-skinned person presents as an ashen-gray tone to the skin. In the brown-skinned person, pallor gives the skin a yellow-brown color.

The hair of blacks differs in texture. It varies from being long and straight to short, thick, tightly curled. It is very dry and fragile and requires daily grooming with oil. If a black child suffers from malnutrition, sometimes the hair will turn a coppery red. Asians tend to have straight, fine hair. When the skin of a darkly pigmented person is damaged, scar tissue may hypertrophy forming a **keloid** (a thick ridge of scar tissue that stands up from the surrounding skin) (Color Figure 7).

The skin should be lightly palpated to detect changes in texture and surface elevations. Palpation also is used to detect pain, areas of increased warmth, and tenderness. When checking the temperature of the skin, the back of the hand should be used. Skin turgor is assessed by lifting a fold of skin on the forearm between two fingers and seeing how fast it falls back into place.

Elder Care Point... When checking skin turgor on an elderly patient, it is best to test on the upper chest as the skin of the arms of the elderly has often lost elasticity and is not a reliable index.

Elderly patients bruise more easily as the skin becomes thinner and collagen is lost. Patches of senile purpura, deep red areas, may occur even from minor injuries. Women are more prone to this problem than men.

Teaching Self-Examination   All persons who have warts, moles, scars, or birthmarks should be taught how to do monthly evaluations of the lesions to detect malignant changes in their earliest stages. Examination can be done by the patient or by someone in the family if the patient cannot see well or has difficulty inspecting the area of the body where the lesions are located. Table 29-3 presents the information to be taught.

Think about... Can you describe how you specifically assess a patient who indicates that a rash has appeared on the legs?

◆Nursing Diagnoses

Nursing diagnoses are chosen based on the analysis of the data gathered from assessment. Diagnoses commonly associated with skin disorders include the following:

◆ Impaired skin integrity related to tissue destruction, autoimmune dysfunction, or infection.
◆ Pain related to itching, soreness, or tenderness of lesions; exposure of denuded skin to air; or involvement of nerve tissue.
◆ Self-esteem disturbance related to disfiguring skin lesions, scarring.
◆ Anxiety related to chronic, recurring nature of skin disorder and slow healing or potential for malignancy.
◆ Risk for infection related to loss of intact skin barrier.
◆ Knowledge deficit related to causative factors of skin lesions, appropriate therapy, and self-care.

TABLE 29-2 ◆ *Types of Skin Lesions, Example, and Description of Each*

Name of Lesion	Example	Description
Bulla	Second-degree burn	A blister; a circumscribed, fluid-filled, elevated lesion of the skin, usually more than 5 mm in diameter.
Burrow	Scabies	A linear or zigzag, slightly raised lesion, caused by parasite burrowing under the skin.
Comedo	Blackhead or whitehead	Plugged duct, formed from sebum and keratin.
Excoriation	Friction or chemical burn	Injury caused by scraping, scratching, or rubbing away layers of skin.
Macule	Freckle, purpura	A discolored spot or patch on the skin. Usually is not elevated nor depressed, and cannot be palpated.
Nodule	Intradermal nevus	Firm, raised lesion; deeper than a papule.
Papule	Measles rash	A solid elevation of skin. Can vary from the size of a pinhead to that of a pea. Usually red, resembling a pimple without pus.
Plaque	Psoriasis	Circumscribed, solid, elevated lesion greater than 1 cm in diameter.
Pustule	Acne, smallpox	A small elevation of the skin or pimple filled with pus.

TABLE 29-2 ◆ *Types of Skin Lesions, Example, and Description of Each* (Continued)		
Name of Lesion	**Example**	**Description**
Vesicle	Blister	A small sac containing serous fluid.
Wheal	Insect sting, hives, nettle rash	An area of local swelling, usually accompanied by itching.

- Sleep pattern disturbance related to itching or pain of skin disorder.
- Social isolation related to withdrawal from others because of unsightly appearance of skin.

◆ Planning

The goals for patient with skin disorders are to:

- Restore the skin to normal
- Decrease pain and itching
- Protect the skin from further damage
- Prevent infection
- Prevent scarring as much as possible

Goals may be long- or short-term. Specific expected outcomes are written for the individual nursing diagnoses chosen for the patient.

TABLE 29-3 ◆ *Patient Education: Self-Assessment of the Skin*

The skin should be examined every few months. If you are unable to see your back or other areas, have a family member or close friend examine the skin of that area for you. If you have any warts, moles, or discolorations of the skin, check them each month for:

- A darkening or spreading of color or increasing unevenness of color.
- An increase in size or diameter.
- A change in shape; that is, has the lesion become elevated, or its formerly regular edges become irregular?
- Redness or swelling of surrounding skin, or any other noticeable change around the lesion.
- Itching, tenderness, or other change in sensation.
- Crusting, scaling, oozing, ulceration, or other change in the surface of the lesion.

If any changes have occurred, consult your physician right away.

Planning of the daily work schedule should include consideration of time necessary for dressing changes, soaks, special baths, and other skin treatments.

◆ Implementation

The nurse must use *Standard Precautions* when caring for patients with a rash or skin lesion. Some general rules when caring for patients with a skin disease may be helpful as a guide until specific orders are obtained:

- Bathing with soap is usually contraindicated in all inflammatory conditions of the skin.
- Dressings covering the skin lesions that have been applied by a physician should not be removed when the patient is admitted unless there are specific orders to do so.
- Do not attempt to remove scales, crusts, or other exudates on the skin lesions until the physician has had an opportunity to examine the patient.
- Observe the skin very carefully at the time of the patient's admission, and record observations on the chart or report them to the nurse in charge.
- Avoid excessive handling or rubbing of the skin against the sheets and bedclothes when changing the bed.
- Lotions or other skin products should not be used on the skin unless the physician has approved their use.

Once the physician has determined the type of lesions present, specific treatments will be ordered to relieve the patient's symptoms and promote healing. The two most commonly used treatments are special dermatological baths and wet compresses or dressings. In addition, lotions, salves, or ointments may be applied locally at frequent intervals.

Although the vast majority of skin diseases are *not* contagious, nurses should be careful to observe rules of cleanliness and self-protection and *Standard Precautions* when caring for any patient with a skin eruption. **Special care is needed to avoid spreading infection from the fluid in all pustules and in the vesicles of fever blisters and cold sores.**

Giving Medicated Baths

Among the agents that may be added to the bath water are sodium bicarbonate, sodium chloride, cornstarch, oatmeal, medicated tars, oils, potassium permanganate, and special bath preparations.

During the bath, the patient must be protected from chilling, because the bath usually lasts from 30 minutes to an hour, and most patients with skin diseases have a lowered resistance to cold. When the patient is removed from the tub, the skin is dried by patting rather than by rubbing. If medication is to be applied locally, it should be put on as soon as the bath is completed in order to keep **pruritus** (itching) at a minimum. **Medication is applied in a thin layer unless otherwise ordered.**

The medicated bath has a very soothing and relaxing effect on the patient and also helps relieve the itching and burning commonly associated with skin diseases. The nurse should encourage the patient to rest in bed and perhaps to take a short nap after each bath.

Laundry Requirements

The bed linens and gowns used for patients with severe skin diseases may need special laundering to eliminate all traces of soap. If the patient is to be cared for at home, vinegar may be added to the rinse water to neutralize the soap. One tablespoon of vinegar is used for each quart of water.

Application of Wet Compresses or Dressings

Wet dressings may be applied to the skin in various ways. The two general types used are *open dressings* and *closed dressings*. Open compresses must be changed constantly and are never allowed to dry. They are used when the dermatologist wishes to have air circulating to the skin lesions. Closed dressings are thoroughly soaked with the prescribed solution and wrapped with an airtight, waterproof material. It is recommended that the nurse obtain specific instructions from the dermatologist before applying wet dressings to any skin lesions.

Application of Topical Therapy

Many skin lesions are treated by directly applying medications to the surface of the affected area. This method is called *topical therapy*. Lotion, cream, ointment, powder, or gel may be used. The physician prescribes the kind of medication to be used and the way in which the drug is to be applied. There are times, however, when a physician is not consulted and the nurse is asked for advice on using nonprescription medications. Patients with skin conditions do not always consult a physician and sometimes choose to treat themselves at home. **All patients should be instructed in the proper application of topical medications (Table 29-4).** Other nursing interventions are included with the discussion of the various disorders and in Nursing Care Plan 29-1.

***Think about* . . .** If a patient has a topical cream ordered to be applied to an area of rash on the right upper thigh, how would you apply this cream? (Describe every step you would take in detail.)

◆ Evaluation

Evaluation of treatment and nursing intervention for skin disorders is based on improved appearance of the skin, absence of signs of infection, relief from

---

> **TABLE 29-4 ◆ *Guidelines for Applying Topical Medications* ***
>
> ◆ **Powders.** Dry the area thoroughly before applying powder to prevent caking. Do not apply to raw and denuded areas. Some powders, such as cornstarch, can actually serve as glucose-rich culture media for the growth of bacteria.
>
> ◆ **Ointment.** Use only a small amount and gently massage into the skin until a thin film covers the area. Exception is when ointment is used as an occlusive dressing, as for a burn. Ointments tend to leave a greasy feeling to the skin. They are best for chronic lesions, because they help the skin retain moisture and natural oils. Avoid putting ointment on areas where the skin is creased and overlaps itself.
>
> ◆ **Gels.** A gel is a semisolid mixture that tends to liquefy when applied to the skin. It is absorbed into the skin and dries quickly, leaving a thin nonocclusive film. If applied to abraded or sensitive areas, alcohol in the base can cause a burning or stinging sensation.
>
> ◆ **Lotions.** These are actually powders suspended in water; they will leave a residue once the liquid evaporates from the skin. This residue should be washed off before a fresh dose is applied. Be sure powder is uniformly dispersed in solution before applying, then use a firm stroke to distribute the medication evenly. Do not "dab" on lotions, as this can be irritating to the skin.
>
> ◆ **All types.** Always apply topical medications sparingly and in a thin film that extends beyond the affected area about ¼ inch. Thick layers of topicals are wasteful, and some of these drugs, such as corticosteroids, are very expensive. Too much of some topicals (for example, antifungal agents) can chemically irritate the skin and delay healing. Thick layers also tend to soften the skin too much.
>
> If the skin condition appears to be getting worse after a topical agent is applied, or if the patient develops eczema, suspect an allergic contact dermatitis caused by the drug.
>
> *Allergies must be assessed before applying a topical medication.

Nursing Care Plan 29-1

Selected nursing diagnoses, goals/expected outcomes, nursing interventions, and evaluations for a burned patient

Situation: Mr. Young, age 33, sustained second- and third-degree burns over both arms when a container of gasoline he was carrying ignited. He also suffered first-degree burns on his hands and face. In the emergency department his wounds were cleaned, and a topical agent was applied; no dressings were applied. An IV line was established, and fluids were administered to avoid potential fluid and electrolyte imbalance. He received morphine for pain and on admission to his room was fairly comfortable, conscious, and oriented.

Nursing Diagnosis	Goals/Expected Outcomes	Nursing Intervention	Evaluation
Fluid volume deficit related to loss of fluids via open wounds. SUPPORTING DATA Second- and third-degree burns over both arms; weeping.	Adequate circulating blood volume as evidenced by blood pressure (BP), pulse (P), and urine output.	Monitor vital signs (VS) q 2 h. Monitor urine output, report drop below 50 mL/h. Monitor lab values for electrolyte imbalances. Maintain IV fluids on schedule. Encourage fluid intake of 3,000 mL q 24 h when bowel sounds are present.	BP maintaining 108/62; P, 92; urine output, 45 mL/h; continue plan.
Risk for infection related to damage to skin. SUPPORTING DATA Skin on both arms damaged by burns.	Burn wound will be free of infection as evidenced by normal vital signs and negative wound cultures.	Assess for sulfa allergy. Use strict aseptic technique when working with patient. Apply silver sulfadiazadine as ordered to wounds tid. Monitor WBC count for signs of infection; observe wounds tid. Encourage good nutrition.	Sulfadiazine applied q 8 h; WBC count, 7,800; temperature, 99.6° F.; wounds moist and clean; no purulent material evident; continue plan.
Pain related to open burn wounds. SUPPORTING DATA Is constantly asking for pain medication; grimacing and holding body rigid.	Patient will verbalize that pain control is adequate.	Administer pain medication as ordered before débridement procedures and PRN. Teach relaxation and imagery techniques to assist with pain control. Utilize diversionary activities such as television, card games, board games, to help diminish awareness of pain.	Demerol, 100 mg, 9, 12, and 3; relaxation and imagery techniques taught; encouraged to practice; states pain only controlled for 2½ hours; encourage diversional activities; continue plan.
Self-care deficit—bathing, feeding, toileting, grooming—related to inability to use arms and hands. SUPPORTING DATA Unable to perform self-care because of burns on arms and hands.	Patient will resume own self-care activities within 3 months.	Assist with toileting, bathing, grooming, and feeding. Allow him to make decisions as much as possible to lessen feelings of helplessness. Allow him to do as much as he is able to do.	Not ready to resume self-care activities; making decisions about time for bath, diversional activity, etc.; continue plan.

Continued on following page

Nursing Care Plan 29-1 *(Continued)*

Nursing Diagnosis	Goals/Expected Outcomes	Nursing Intervention	Evaluation
Self-esteem disturbance related to helplessness and fear of losing ability to work as a mechanic. SUPPORTING DATA "With my hands burned, I won't be able to work any-more."	Patient will verbalize improved sense of self-worth within 3 months; able to return to work as mechanic or to begin job retraining.	Establish trusting relationship; actively listen to concerns and frustrations. Help him establish his active role in recovery of use of hands and arms. Allow him to do whatever ADLs are possible for him. Praise him for his efforts with physical therapy exercises. Help him establish small, accomplishable goals on a weekly basis. Offer emotional support and encouragement that is realistic. Refer for job retraining if needed.	Verbalizing fears about the future and employment; working with physical therapist; established two small goals for the week; continue plan.

itching and pain, and signs of healing. Many skin disorders are slow to respond to treatment and patience is required on the part of the patient and the nurse. Even a minor fungal skin infection may take from 7 to 14 days to clear with topical medication. A major part of evaluation is to determine that treatment is not aggravating the condition. On occasion this happens when the patient who has sensitive skin may react badly to medication, heat, or light treatments. Further interventions are listed in Table 29-5 and Nursing Care Plan 29-1.

DISORDERS OF THE SKIN

◆ Infectious and Parasitic Skin Diseases

Many skin diseases result from infection by bacteria, viruses, or fungi or by infestation with parasites. Diseases of this kind require special precautions to avoid spreading the infectious organism or the parasite. The Center for Infectious Diseases, Centers for Disease Control and Prevention, recommends that *contact isolation,* as well as *Standard Precautions,* be implemented for a number of these diseases. Specifications for *contact isolation* are as follows:

- A private room is indicated. In general, patients infected with the same type organism may share a room.
- Gloves are worn when entering the room. Change gloves after contact with infective material, such as wound drainage or feces, and before treating a different location on the body. Wash hands before donning clean gloves.

- Remove gloves when leaving the room, and wash hands with an antimicrobial agent.
- Gowns are indicated if soiling is likely; particularly if there is drainage from an uncovered wound or the patient is incontinent.
- Articles contaminated with infective material should be discarded in a hazardous waste receptacle or bagged and labeled before being sent for decontamination and reprocessing.
- Patient care equipment should be used only for the one patient and should be left in the room until no longer needed.

Skin disorders that require contact isolation include:

- Diphtheria, cutaneous.
- Furunculosis, group A *Streptococcus.*
- Herpes simplex, disseminated, severe primary, or neonatal.
- Herpes zoster (varicella-zoster).
- Varicella (chickenpox)
- Impetigo.
- Infection or colonization by bacteria with multiple drug resistance (any site).
- Pediculosis.
- Scabies.
- Skin wound or burn infection, major (draining and not covered by dressing, or dressing does not adequately contain purulent material), including those infected with *Staphylococcus aureus.*
- Vaccinia (generalized and progressive eczema vaccinatum).

A variety of topical and systemic medications are used to treat infectious and parasitic skin diseases. A culture and sensitivity or biopsy are used to determine the causative organism and appropriate drug therapy.

Herpesvirus Infections   The herpesviruses are an extensive family of viruses, many of which are capable of infecting and causing disease in humans. Their nomenclature is complex and does not follow a consistent pattern. For example, some are named for the disease they cause (e.g., herpes simplex and herpes zoster [varicella]), and some for the persons who discovered them.

Herpes simplex.   Herpes simplex virus type 2 (HSV 2) is most often associated with genital herpes, whereas herpes simplex virus type 1 (HSV 1) lesions are

TABLE 29-5 ◆ *Common Nursing Diagnoses, Expected Outcomes, and Nursing Interventions for Patients with Skin Disorders*

Nursing Diagnosis	Goals/Expected Outcomes	Nursing Interventions
Impaired skin integrity related to injury and treatment; excoriation or scaling; infectious process.	Patient's skin will be intact within 2 weeks; 4 months for burns. Number of lesions will decrease within 2 months. Patient will exhibit no signs of infection within 3 months.	Cleanse skin and apply topical medications as prescribed. Monitor for signs of adverse reaction to topical medication. Preserve integrity of grafted areas with aseptic dressing technique and splinting. Apply light treatments as prescribed. Provide medicated baths as prescribed.
Anxiety related to chronic, recurring nature of skin disorder; reaction to diagnosis of cancer; slow healing.	Patient will verbalize feelings within 3 weeks. Patient will explore options for treatment of cancer. Patient will acknowledge that although healing is slow, disorder is self-limiting and will resolve.	Provide atmosphere of acceptance. Allow patient time to verbalize feelings. Assist to recognize positive coping techniques by looking at ways patient has coped with anxiety in the past. Provide information on treatment and prognosis for skin malignancy. Provide information on the skin disorder, treatment options, and prognosis.
Knowledge deficit related to cause and treatment of skin disorder.	Patient will verbalize knowledge of factors related to appearance of skin disorder. Patient will verbalize knowledge of treatment for disorder. Patient will demonstrate self-care techniques.	Explain the etiology of the skin disorder and measures to prevent recurrence, if possible. Instruct in various methods of treatment. Teach signs of side effects of medications. Instruct in self-care techniques for medication application, dressing changes, and so on. Obtain feedback of information and skills taught.
Sleep pattern disturbance related to itching or pain.	Patient will obtain at least 7 hours of rest per day.	Administer medication to relieve itching. Keep environment cool to decrease itching sensation. Caution patient to take cool or tepid baths or showers to decrease itching. Caution not to scratch lesions as this often makes itching worse. Advise in ways to use distraction to decrease focus on itching; i.e., card or game playing; intense concentration on learning something; or reading an absorbing book. Administer hypnotic as ordered. Administer analgesics as ordered. Encourage use of meditation, relaxation, or imagery techniques to decrease pain. Provide restful, quiet, environment. Use massage as appropriate to promote relaxation and sleep. Allow usual bedtime rituals that help patient induce sleep.
Social isolation related to long treatment process; disfigurement.	Patient will maintain social contact with family and friends. Patient will reintegrate into community within 24 months.	Encourage family and friends to send cards, call, and visit. Encourage patient to continue dialog with family and friends. Refer to psychologist or social worker for grief work and reintegration of new body image. Refer to support group for expression of feelings and realization they are not alone with such problems. Encourage return to employment or job retraining. Encourage return to church or community activities.

primarily nongenital (Color Figure 8). **It should be understood, however, that either type can cause lesions in the genital area as well as other regions of the body.** Autoinoculation of the virus is possible by direct contact; for example, lips to fingers to genitals or lips to fingers to eyes.

Signs and Symptoms   An infection with HSV 1 appears as lesions on the lips and nares that are commonly called cold sores or fever blisters. As with other types of herpesvirus infections, no drug will completely cure the infection.

Treatment and Intervention   The symptoms of itching and burning that accompany oral herpes infection sometimes can be minimized by warm compresses to the sores, followed by local application of tincture of benzoin or spirits of camphor to aid drying and facilitate healing. Sometimes topical and oral acyclovir (Zovirax) or valacyclovir (Valtrex) hastens healing. The disease usually is self-limiting, which means that it does not progress and will subside on its own, but it can recur.

Patients should be cautioned to use good personal hygiene to avoid spreading the virus to the eyes and genital area and other body parts. Handwashing is a very simple, but essential, part of preventing autoinoculation. Canker sores, which are shallow white ulcerations of the tongue and gums, often are mistaken for herpes simplex infection; however, they are not the same and are not known to be caused by any infectious organism.

Herpes zoster.   The causative organism for this skin disorder is herpes varicella–zoster. The virus causes chickenpox (varicella), mostly in young children, and shingles (herpes zoster). In herpes zoster the herpesviruses replicate in the peripheral nerve ganglia, where they lie dormant until reactivated by trauma, malignancy, or local radiation (Color Figure 9).

Signs and Symptoms   Herpes zoster begins with vague symptoms of chills and low-grade fever and possibly some gastrointestinal disturbance. About 3 to 5 days after onset, small groups of vesicles appear on the skin. They usually are found on the trunk and spread around the body, following the nerve pathways leading from the spinal nerve to the skin.

The vesicles eventually change from small blisters to scaly lesions and are accompanied by pain and itching. The lesions usually affect only one side of the body or face. The pain of shingles often is quite severe and can persist for several days or weeks after the skin lesions are completely healed.

Treatment   There is no cure for herpes zoster. **The condition can persist for months, especially in older and debilitated patients. Herpes infections may be recurrent**

as immunity does not occur. The earlier the condition is diagnosed and treatment begins, the better chance to decrease the amount and duration of the associated pain.

Symptomatic treatment usually involves administering an analgesic to relieve pain. Zostrix, an over-the-counter analgesic that is applied topically, decreases pain for some patients. Antibiotics may be prescribed prophylactically against secondary bacterial infection of the lesions. Most physicians prescribe oral acyclovir (Zovirax), famcyclovir (Famvir), or valacyclovir (Valtrex) to diminish the extent or duration of the lesions. Valacyclovir is used only in otherwise healthy patients. Famciclovir (Famvir), if given within the first two to three days of the outbreak, seems to shorten the duration of the chronic pain that frequently follows shingles.

Narcotic analgesics are avoided if possible, because they can lead to addiction when used for an extended time. If the pain persists and is intractable, the physician prescribes a corticosteroid to reduce inflammation. Vidarabine, administered IV, is sometimes given to patients who have an immune deficiency. It is usually effective in reducing, if not completely relieving, the pain.

Fortunately, even though shingles may be difficult to live with while it is running its course, there rarely are any serious complications from the disease. However, the prognosis is obviously less favorable in patients who have an underlying malignancy of the skin or who are immunocompromised.

Nursing Intervention   Nursing intervention is aimed at providing emotional support and symptomatic relief from the pain and itching and preventing a secondary bacterial infection. Cold compresses, calamine lotion, and diversional activities are sometimes helpful. Rest and adequate nutrition can promote healing and shorten the acute phase of shingles.

Fungal Infections   Fungal infections are called *mycoses;* systemic fungal infections involving the lungs and other internal organs are called *systemic mycoses.* There are actually two groups of fungi: (1) fungi that are truly pathogenic to humans; and (2) opportunistic infections (that can cause an infection when the host has an altered immune system).

True pathogenic fungi can cause infection in an otherwise healthy person, but relatively few fungi are able to do this. Fungal infections are rarely fatal if they involve only the superficial tissues of the body. Nevertheless, mycotic skin infections can be exasperating, because they progress slowly, are difficult to diagnose, and are often resistant to treatment.

The most common types of fungal infections involving the skin are *tinea pedis* (athlete's foot or dermophytosis), *tinea of the scalp* (commonly known as ringworm), and *tinea barbae* (barber's itch). *Moniliasis* (thrush) is a fungal infection that can attack the mucous membranes of the mouth, rectum, and vagina (*candidiasis*) (this condition is discussed more fully in Chapter 26).

All surface fungal infections produce itching, some swelling, and a breakdown of tissue. Because fungi thrive in warm, moist places, a tropical climate or other environmental factors that produce prolonged heat and moisture can encourage the development of fungal infections.

Elder Care Point . . . The elderly are prone to develop fungal infections of the finger or toe nails (onychomycosis), Color Figure 10. In the toenails, the condition may become quite painful. Treatment requires oral antifungal medication daily for several months. Itraconazole (Sporanox) is the newest medication for this disorder.

Diagnosis of fungal infections is confirmed by microscopic examination of skin scrapings that have been treated with potassium hydroxide solution (KOH). Fungal specimens generally show the typical filaments of fungal organisms. Instructions to patients for prevention of recurrent fungal infections are provided in Table 29-6.

Tinea Pedis (Athlete's Foot)   Tinea pedis affects the feet, particularly between the toes. The infection may spread to the entire foot and cause blistering, peeling, cracking, and itching. If it continues unchecked, it can spread to other parts of the body. The condition can be complicated by a severe bacterial infection.

TABLE 29-6 ◆ *Patient Education: Prevention of Recurrent Fungal Infections*

Instruct the patient to do the following:

- ◆ Wear shoes that provide ventilation for the feet. Wear cotton socks when rubber-soled shoes or sneakers must be worn.
- ◆ Wash and dry the feet at least daily, being careful to dry completely the skin between the toes.
- ◆ Spinkle an antifungal powder on the feet and between the toes if there is a tendency to have athlete's foot.
- ◆ Change hose or socks daily; do not wear them more than one day without washing.
- ◆ Change underpants or shorts daily; do not wear them more than one day without washing.
- ◆ Use only clean towels, changing them at least every other day.
- ◆ Change bed linens at least once a week.
- ◆ Do not use the toilet articles of others, and do not allow them to use yours.
- ◆ Inspect pets regularly for ringworm. Have veterinarian check the animal if an infection is suspected.

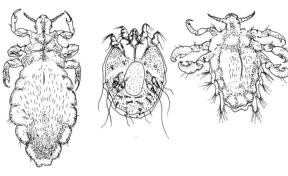

| Head louse, dorsal view (2–3 mm long) | Scab mite, ventral surface (0.4 mm long) | Pubic louse, dorsal view (1 mm long) |

FIGURE 29-2   Types of lice that infest human beings.

Treatment of tinea pedis consists of keeping the area dry, clean, and exposed to the air and sunlight as much as possible. Clean cotton socks should be worn every day, and the affected areas between the toes should be separated by gauze or cotton. Various topical antifungals can be prescribed, including ciclopirox (Loprox), miconazole, clotrimazole (Mycelex), econazole (Spectazole), ketoconazole (Nizoral), and naftifine (Naftin). Some medicated powders, such as undecylenic acid–zinc undecylate (Desenex), work to keep the feet dry and also help control fungi growth.

Because most cases are contracted and spread in swimming pools, showers, and other public facilities of this type, one should be careful to wash one's feet and dry them thoroughly after using such facilities. It is difficult to rid public facilities of fungi.

Parasitic Infestations: Pediculosis and Scabies
The parasites that cause pediculosis and scabies are found throughout the world in all types of climates, and they can infest anyone. The parasites are particularly troublesome, however, wherever people live under crowded conditions and are negligent in their personal hygiene. The occurrence of pediculosis and scabies in the United States has recently increased significantly because of communal living and other more natural lifestyles chosen by some people. It is often found in upper and middle class school children also.

Three basic types of lice that infest human beings are (1) the head louse, *Pediculus capitis* (Figure 29-2A); (2) the body louse, *Pediculus corporis;* and (3) the pubic or crab louse, *Phthirus pubis* (Figure 29-2C). In addition, human beings also may be infested by the *Sarcoptes scabiei*, the mange mite that produces scabies (Figure 29-2B). All types are acquired by contact with infested people or their clothing, bed linen, and bedding. Dogs have also been known to carry lice and the scabies mite.

Signs and Symptoms   The most prevalent symptom of louse infestation is severe itching. The resultant scratching can lead to excoriation of the skin and secondary infection causing impetigo, furunculosis, and cellulitis. Systemic infections are not commonly associated with louse infestation, but they can and do occur in the forms of glomerulonephritis, septicemia, pneumonia, and cystic abscesses. If the lice infest the eyelids and eyelashes, the eyelids become red and swollen. Swelling may also occur in the lymph glands of the neck of a person heavily infested with head lice. The body louse can transmit typhus fever, trench fever, and some other diseases. Other types of lice are not known to be transmitters of disease.

The scabies mites burrow under the top layers of the skin and live their entire life there. They are more likely to be found in the skin between the fingers and toes, in the groin, and in other areas where there may be folds of skin. Excretions from the mites produce irritation with intense itching and blistering. Secondary infection is not uncommon with scabies, and some deaths have occurred when the scabies infestation has led to pneumonia or septicemia.

Treatment The prescription drugs most commonly used and considered most effective against lice and scabies are 1% lindane (Kwell, Gamene) and 10% crotamiton (Eurax). They are available as creams, lotions, and shampoos. A-200 Pyrinate and Cuprex are nonprescription drugs used to treat louse infestations. The medication is left on the affected areas for 12 to 24 hours and then removed completely with soap and water. If needed, the treatment may be repeated once more 24 hours later.

Lindane also is available as a shampoo for head lice. The shampoo lather is rubbed on the hair and scalp for at least 4 minutes and then removed by thorough rinsing with water. A fine-toothed comb is then used to remove the nits (eggs) that may have remained on the hair.

Nursing Intervention Contact isolation is recommended. In addition, clothing, bedding, and other infested articles must be decontaminated to prevent reinfection. Laundering and dry cleaning can be effective for decontaminating clothing and bed covering. Mattresses, upholstered furniture, and other articles should be sprayed with a specific disinfectant.

Think about... How would you approach and instruct the parents of an 8-year-old who has scabies?

◆ Acne

Signs and Symptoms Acne is a disorder of the skin characterized by papules and pustules over the face, back, and shoulders. There are many kinds of acne, but the two major types are *acne vulgaris* and *acne rosacea*.

Of the two, acne vulgaris is the most common. It typically begins in early puberty, continues through the teens, and then begins to subside. Occasionally it persists, or it can recur several years later.

Some types of acne are related to cosmetics *(acne cosmetica)* or to chemicals in the environment; for example, occupational acne due to prolonged contact with oils and tars.

Acne occurs when the ducts leading from the sebaceous glands become plugged with sebum, the oily secretion of the glands.

The onset of acne vulgaris in adolescents is related to increased release of sex hormones, which stimulate activity of the sebaceous glands, causing increased production of sebum. It is not known why in some persons the ducts from these glands become plugged, but the increased production of sebum triggers the formation of blackheads and whiteheads. These lesions are not a sign of uncleanliness. The color of blackheads is due to the result of particles of melanin, the skin's own pigment.

Accumulations of sebum, skin particles, and dead skin cells can cause an inflammatory reaction. Bacterial infection leads to the formation of pustules. An extensive inflammation can lead to the formation of cysts, with swelling above and below the surface of the skin.

Treatment Mild, noninflammatory cases of acne respond well to efforts to remove blackheads and whiteheads by promoting dryness and peeling of the top layer of skin. The medication is applied directly on the skin. Nonprescription drugs, such as lotions, creams, and gels that contain sulfur, benzoyl peroxide, and sulfur combined with resorcinol usually are effective for noninflammatory acne.

Among the topical medications, retinoic acid (tretinoin, Retin-A) is the best agent for papular and pustular acne problems. It should be used once or twice a day. **Benzoyl peroxide is the most frequently used topical agent for acne and is available both by prescription and over the counter.** A new drug, azelaic acid (Azelex) is available and is applied topically twice a day.

Antibiotics such as tetracycline and erythromycin also are sometimes prescribed topically and orally for inflammatory acne to inhibit the growth of bacteria in the plugged ducts. The antibiotic can be given safely in low doses for months. Tetracycline should not be used for women who are pregnant.

Another drug given to treat cystic acne has been especially effective in controlling cases that are resistant to other forms of treatment. The drug is 13-*cis*retinoic acid and is marketed under the trade name Accutane. Almost all patients experience some adverse reaction to this drug, and it is not recommended for pregnant women. Accutane is taken by mouth daily for 2 to 4 months and inhibits activity of the sebaceous glands. Its effects are sustained for months to years after it has been discontinued. **Accutane is used only for severe cystic acne that is resistant to all other treatment.**

The appearance of the patient with deep scarring and pitting as a result of cystic acne can be improved by *dermabrasion.* This dermatological procedure involves mechanically scraping away the outer layers of skin and smoothing out its surface by applying motor-driven wire brushes or diamond wheels. Chemical dermabrasion is done by applying phenol or trichloroacetic acid to remove the scars.

Nursing Intervention   Nursing intervention is primarily concerned with teaching the patient about the nature of his particular skin disease and giving support while he is trying to cope with its physiological and psychosocial effects. He should feel that his problems are being taken seriously, even though they are certainly not life-threatening. Acne can be particularly distressing to adolescents, who are often deeply concerned about their appearance and acceptance by their peers.

There are many misconceptions about acne and its treatment. It is not a contagious disease. It is not due to uncleanliness or poor personal hygiene. It is not caused or made worse by lack of sleep, constipation, masturbation, venereal disease, or anger and hostility. Diet can contribute to the formation of lesions, but this is true of relatively few people who usually can find a relationship between the intake of certain foods and the appearance of the lesions of acne. In general, however, chocolate, colas, and the fried foods of which most adolescents are so fond need not be restricted or eliminated from the diet in an effort to prevent or cure acne. A well-balanced diet is all that is recommended in the management of acne.

The face should be washed gently and with a mild soap. Scrubbing the skin and using a harsh soap is damaging to the skin and contributes to inflammation. Special medicated soaps do not seem to be any better than a mild face soap. If the hair is oily, it should be shampooed frequently and kept off the face.

It is not a good idea to squeeze pimples and pustules. This can press the sebum and accumulated material more firmly in the clogged duct, increase the chance of inflammation, and spread an infection to other parts of the skin and body. Blackheads and whiteheads are best removed by applying a prescription medication that causes peeling of the skin.

Because the management of acne can go on for years and requires periodic evaluation by a dermatologist, patients and their families will need continued support and encouragement to follow the prescribed regimen. They will need to know the expected results of prescribed medications, any adverse reactions that might occur, and symptoms that should be reported immediately.

Think about . . . What skin care measures would you recommend to a young teenager who is just beginning to experience face blemishes such as blackheads or whiteheads?

◆ Psoriasis

Signs and Symptoms   Psoriasis is a chronic and recurring skin disorder that typically appears as patches or plaques covered with adherent silvery scales (Color Figure 11). These scales are the result of an abnormally rapid rate of proliferation of skin cells. The skin under the plaques is reddened, and when the scales are removed there is pinpoint bleeding. The plaques most often appear on the skin of the elbows, knees, and base of the spine. It also may affect the scalp, in which case it can be confused with seborrheic dermatitis. When the fingernails are involved there can be pitting of the surface of the nails. The palms and soles also can be affected, making it difficult for the patient to carry out activities of daily living. In some cases the skin eruptions are accompanied by inflammation of the joints, especially those of the fingers and toes. This is called psoriatic arthritis (Figure 29-3).

The cause of psoriasis is considered genetic, although the precise pattern of inheritance has not been defined. It is not contagious. A parent with psoriasis has a 50% chance of passing the presumed gene along to each child. However, as any individual with the gene has only a 50% chance of developing psoriasis, the offspring of a person with the disease only has a 25% chance of developing it.

Treatment   Each case of psoriasis is treated individually. The disease is unpredictable, tends to go into remission spontaneously, and sometimes will clear up temporarily with or without treatment.

Mild cases usually respond to steroid creams, but there is a possibility that eventually the disease will become resistant to steroids. Sunlight in moderate doses can help, because the ultraviolet rays slow down the rate at which epithelial cells are produced. Extremes of ultraviolet radiation can have the opposite effect, resulting in an aggravation of the condition. Calcipotriene (Dovonex), a new vitamin D analog cream helps to regulate skin cell production, decreasing the incidence of psoriasis plaques.

Tar preparations also act to impede the proliferation of skin cells and have long been used to heal psoriasis lesions. They may be administered in the form of baths, topical applications, or shampoos. Combinations of artificial ultraviolet radiation and a coal tar

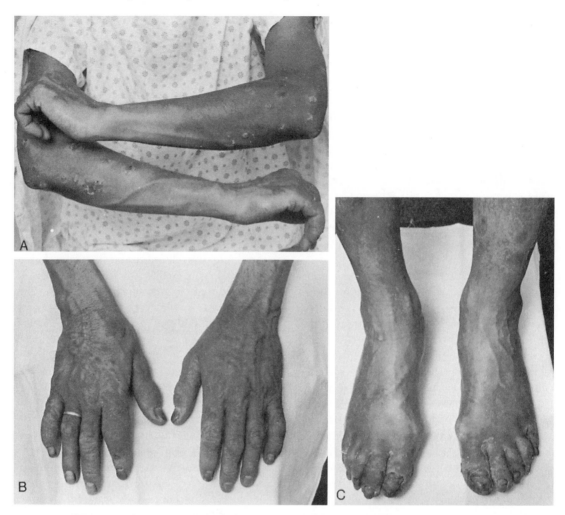

FIGURE 29-3   Classic lesions in psoriasis. Note arthritic changes in joints. (Photos by Ken Kasper.)

product often are prescribed for severe cases. This usually requires hospitalization so that the dosage of each component of therapy can be measured precisely. A form of therapy called PUVA combines application of the drug anthralin, which penetrates the skin, and exposure to ultraviolet light type A (UVA). Oral retinoids can also be added to this therapy.

The Goeckerman technique, named after the physician who developed it, combines ultraviolet light B (UVB) and a crude coal tar ointment for the treatment of psoriasis. This is often an inpatient treatment. Etretinate is used for severe psoriasis not responsive to other treatments.

Antimetabolites have more recently been used to treat severe psoriasis, helping to control the disorder by their antiproliferative action. Methotrexate is the most commonly used antimetabolite for this purpose. Hydrea is sometimes used.

Nursing Intervention   Patients with psoriasis will need instruction about the nature of their disease, the purpose of the prescribed treatment, and information about ways to avoid aggravating it. **The skin should be kept as moist and pliable as possible. Humidifiers to increase moisture in the environment are sometimes helpful.** Lubricating lotions and creams should be approved by the dermatologist before they are applied, but they usually can be used to maintain the integrity of the skin areas not affected by psoriasis.

Minor scratches and abrasions and bacterial infections can trigger the formation of lesions at a new site. **Because any irritation or break in the skin seems to stimulate the growth of psoriatic plaques in a person susceptible to psoriasis, the patient should be cautioned to avoid injury of any kind.** This includes hangnails, damaged cuticles, blisters from poorly fitting shoes, and potentially harmful agents in the environment such as radiation and chemicals.

◆ Skin Cancer

Skin cancer is often neglected because there is no pain associated with it and patients fear that treatment will involve extensive or mutilating surgery. Over 800,000 cases a year of basal cell or squamous cell cancers occur. These are highly curable cancers. It is expected that in 1996 38,300 persons will be diagnosed with melanoma, the most serious type of skin cancer and 7,300 deaths from melanoma will occur. There has been about a 4% a year increase in melanoma since 1973. Almost all these deaths could have been averted through early diagnosis and treatment.

Causes and Susceptibility   Several factors predispose an individual to developing skin cancer. Among these are internal changes in the cells that may be due to hereditary factors and external influences such as chronic exposure to ultraviolet radiation, chemicals such as coal tar, pitch, creosote, or arsenic compounds, or other irritants in the environment. Because children tend to inherit their skin characteristics from their parents, susceptibility to skin cancer tends to run in families. Blue-eyed blondes seem to be most susceptible, probably because they lack sufficient pigment to protect the skin cells from outside irritants. The incidence of skin cancer in blacks is very low.

A major cause of skin cancer today is the alteration in the ozone layer of the earth's atmosphere that causes more UV radiation to reach the earth's surface. This type of radiation is inflicting much quicker damage to skin with much less sun exposure than in years past. Another problem is that the quickly proliferating skin cells of the younger generation are even more susceptible to this type of damage and it is mostly the young who spend large amounts of time in the sun. Nurses should instruct all people about the dangers of sunning without an appropriate protective sunscreen.

Another danger is the tanning salon. Many use tanning beds that deliver dangerous UV radiation to the skin. **Dermatologists adamantly state that no one should use artificial tanning equipment.**

Types of Skin Cancer   The three main types of skin malignancy are basal cell carcinoma, squamous cell carcinoma, and melanoma. *Basal cell carcinoma* usually appears first as a small, scaly area and tends to become larger as the disease progresses (Color Figure 12). It occurs most often on the face and trunk. As the scales shed, there is a small amount of bleeding and a scab will form. When the scab is shed, the affected area becomes wider, and it is bordered by a waxy, translucent, raised area. **If such a sore has not healed within a month, it may be a basal cell carcinoma.** This spreading may continue very gradually during several months or years. Even though these malignancies do not metastasize, they can invade underlying tissues and death can result from complications such as infection, hemorrhage, or exhaustion. Small lesions can be removed under local anesthesia in a doctor's office. Larger lesions respond well to x-ray or radiation therapy.

Squamous cell carcinoma usually begins on the mucous membranes and can metastasize to other areas of the body. The tumor begins as a small nodule, which rapidly becomes ulcerated (Color Figure 13). Treatment must begin early if the condition is to be relieved before the skin cells sustain extensive damage. Surgical procedures involve total removal or destruction of the lesions and the surrounding tissues that have been invaded. Radiation therapy is advised for patients who are poor surgical risks or who are fearful of surgery.

Elder Care Point... Actinic keratoses occur very frequently on the skin of the elderly. They appear on fair-skinned people as a small, scaly, red or grayish papule particularly on areas of skin that are often exposed to the sun. These lesions should be removed as they can evolve into a squamous cell carcinoma that can grow rapidly and metastasize.

Malignant melanoma is the least common form of skin cancer. It arises from pigment-producing cells and varies in its course and prognosis according to its type (Color Figure 14). There are three kinds of malignant melanoma: superficial spreading, nodular, and lentigo malignant melanoma. In general, the superficial lesions can be cured, but the deeper lesions tend to metastasize more readily through the lymphatic and circulatory systems. Characteristics of the three types of melanoma are shown in Table 29-7.

Malignant melanoma always requires surgical removal of the tumor and excision of adjacent tissues and possibly nearby lymphatic structures. Chemotherapy may be employed to destroy tumor cells believed to have migrated beyond the tumor site. Radiation therapy usually is not indicated unless there is extensive metastasis. The radiation does not eliminate the disease, but it can relieve symptoms by reducing tumor size. Interferon alfa-2B has been found to prolong life in patients who have undergone malignant melanoma surgery and are at high risk for systemic recurrence. The medication is given for 1 year after the surgery.

Treatment and Nursing Intervention   Removal of cancerous skin tissue will depend on the type of malignant growth present. **In all but the most extensive growths, treatment is relatively simple and completely successful if started early.** Although benign precancerous lesions do not inevitably develop into malignant lesions, the most advisable course of action is to remove them when they are first diagnosed. Removal is performed by surgery, electrodessication (tissue destruction by heat), cryosurgery (tissue destruction by freezing), and laser therapy. Radiation therapy is sometimes used to destroy the cancer. The nurse often is in a position to notice these lesions in their early stages and should do her best to persuade the person with such a

TABLE 29-7 ♦ *Three Major Types of Skin Cancer*	
Type	**Characteristics**
Basal cell carcinoma	Slowly enlarging, firm, scaly papule. Crusted or ulcerated center that may be depressed; has pearly (semitranslucent) raised border. Dilated capillaries around lesion. Accounts for 70% of all skin cancers. Rarely spreads and is easily treated.
Squamous cell carcinoma	Appearance variable. Frequently seen as well-defined, irregularly shaped nodule or plaque. May be elevated, nodular mass, or fungated mass. Varying amounts of scale and crusting. May have ulcerated center. Predominantly on sun-exposed areas: head, neck, hands; 75% occur on the head. Spreads rapidly.
Malignant melanoma Superficial spreading melanoma (SSM)	Appears in a variety of colors: white, red, gray, black, blue over a brown or black background. Has irregular surface and notched border. Small tumor nodules may ulcerate and bleed. Horizontal growth can continue for years. Vertical growth worsens prognosis.
Nodular malignant melanoma (NMM)	Nodule with uniformly grayish-black color, resembles a blackberry. May be flesh-colored with specks of pigment around base of nodule. Itching, oozing, and bleeding may occur. Prognosis less favorable than superficial type.
Lentigo maligna melanoma (LMM)	Relatively rare. Arises from a lesion that resembles a large flat freckle that is of variable color from tan to black. Has irregularly spaced black nodules on the surface. Often located on the back of the hand, on the face, and under fingernails. Develops very slowly; may ulcerate. Tends to metastasize; prognosis poor.

lesion to seek prompt medical attention. Because victims of skin cancer run a high risk of eventually developing another malignancy, either at the former site or elsewhere in the body, they should visit a physician at least once a year after the skin cancer has been cured. Although most skin cancers are easily curable, they should not be considered harmless and something to forget about after treatment. See Chapter 9 for further information on care of the cancer patient.

Think about ... If you noticed a skin lesion on a person in line with you at the grocery store that looked like a skin cancer, how would you alert the person to the danger of such a lesion and the need for medical attention?

♦ Burns

Burns are injuries to the skin caused by exposure to extreme heat, hot liquids, electrical agents, strong chemicals, or radiation. Inhaling smoke or fumes also causes injury.

Classification of Burns   The classification of burns is based on the amount of the body surface that has been burned and the depth of the burn. The extent of a burn is roughly calculated outside of the hospital according to the **"rule of nines"** and is expressed as a percentage of total body surface (Figure 29-4). The figures used in this method are fairly accurate for gross assessment in adults; however, the rule of nines does not make allowances for the proportionate differences in children at various ages. The Lund and Browder or Berkow system computes the depth of the burn as well as the extent of the injury according to relative age, and the total burn estimate is used as the basis for treatment.

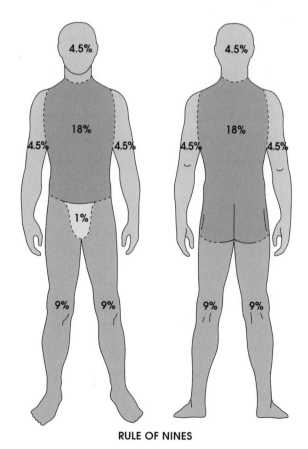

RULE OF NINES

FIGURE 29-4   Chart used for burn area estimate ("rule of nines").

The depth of a burn is more difficult to determine, because various graduations of injury are sustained in a major burn. Some small patches may be more deeply burned than the areas adjacent to them. Burn depth originally was classified according to degrees, a first-degree burn being the most superficial and a fourth-degree burn being the deepest.

A more current method to evaluate the depth of burns is based on the layers of skin that have been damaged (Figure 29-5). *Partial-thickness wounds* are those in which the epidermal appendages (sweat and oil glands and hair follicles) are not destroyed and the wound will heal by itself if no further injury occurs from either infection or inappropriate treatment. Partial-thickness burns are comparable to either first- or second-degree burns; grafting may or may not be necessary (Color Figure 15). A *deep-dermal* wound is a deep partial-thickness wound that can heal itself if infection does not destroy the epidermal appendages. *Full-thickness wounds* involve all layers of skin and the destruction of the epidermal appendages (Color Figures 16 and 17). Wounds of this type will require grafting for the wound to heal and for optimal function to be restored. Table 29-8 provides a guide for estimating the depth of a burn.

Electrical burns damage tissue deep within the body; the extent of damage is not visible. There is an entrance site and an exit site, but the course of the injury is difficult to know. An electrical injury may result in the loss of one or more limbs.

The *crust* is the dry, scab-like covering that forms over a superficial burn. **Eschar** is a hard, leathery layer of dead tissue that results when there has been a full-thickness injury. The eschar can act as a protective covering over the wound, serving as a barrier against infectious agents; however, removal of eschar and skin grafting are usually done within 1 week after the burn. Table 29-8 presents criteria for determining whether a burn is minor, moderate, or major.

Emergency Treatment   All burns should be considered potentially dangerous until they are thoroughly assessed. **The recommended treatment for minor burns is submersion in cool water or applications of cool compresses as soon as possible after the injury.** This helps relieve pain and edema and reduces the chances for a deeper burn.

Under no circumstances should burned clothing be removed in the field nor should salves or ointments or any greasy substance be applied to a burned area.

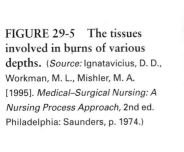

FIGURE 29-5   **The tissues involved in burns of various depths.** (*Source:* Ignatavicius, D. D., Workman, M. L., Mishler, M. A. [1995]. *Medical–Surgical Nursing: A Nursing Process Approach*, 2nd ed. Philadelphia: Saunders, p. 1974.)

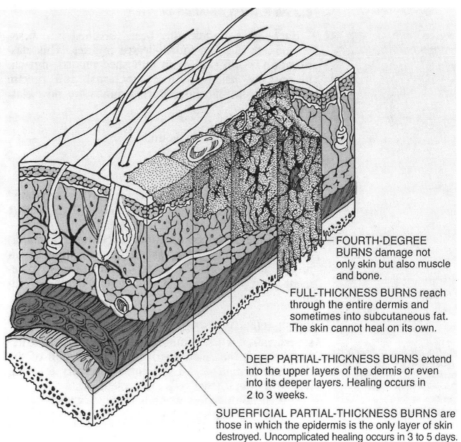

FOURTH-DEGREE BURNS damage not only skin but also muscle and bone.

FULL-THICKNESS BURNS reach through the entire dermis and sometimes into subcutaneous fat. The skin cannot heal on its own.

DEEP PARTIAL-THICKNESS BURNS extend into the upper layers of the dermis or even into its deeper layers. Healing occurs in 2 to 3 weeks.

SUPERFICIAL PARTIAL-THICKNESS BURNS are those in which the epidermis is the only layer of skin destroyed. Uncomplicated healing occurs in 3 to 5 days.

TABLE 29-8 ♦ Comparison of Burn Depth Classification Systems

Characteristic	Classification by Burn Degree				Classification by Burn Thickness			
	First-Degree	Second-Degree	Third-Degree	Fourth-Degree	Superficial	Partial-Thickness Superficial	Partial-Thickness Deep	Full-Thickness
Color	Pink to red	Red	Red, white, brown, yellow, black	Black	Pink to red	Pink to red	Red to white	Black, brown, yellow, white, red
Edema	Mild	Moderate	Severe	Absent	Mild	Mild to moderate	Moderate	Severe
Pain	Yes	Yes	Usually absent	Absent	Yes	Yes	Yes	Always absent
Blisters	No	Yes	No	No	No	Yes	Rare	No
Eschar	No	No	Yes; hard and inelastic	Yes; hard and inelastic	No	No	Yes, soft and dry	Yes; hard and inelastic
Healing time	3–5 days	2–6 weeks	Weeks to months	Weeks to months	3–5 days	~2 weeks	2–6 weeks	Weeks to months
Grafts required	No	Can be used if healing is prolonged	Yes	Yes	No	No	Can be used if healing is prolonged	Yes
Example	Sunburn, flash burns	Scalds, flames, brief contact with hot objects	Scalds; flames; prolonged contact with hot objects, tar, grease, chemicals	Scalds; flames; prolonged contact with hot objects, tar, grease, chemicals, electricity	Sunburn, flash burns	Scalds, flames, brief contact with hot objects	Scalds; flames; prolonged contact with hot objects, tar, grease, chemicals	Scalds; flames; prolonged contact with hot objects, tar, grease, chemicals, electricity

Source: Ignatavicius, D. D., Workman, M. L., Mishler, M. A. (1995). *Medical–Surgical Nursing: A Nursing Process Approach*, 2nd ed. Philadelphia: Saunders, p. 1973.

Because the removal of greasy substances is very painful, inappropriate treatment can cause unnecessary suffering and increase the possibility of infection. Blisters should not be disturbed as they serve as a protective covering over the wound.

If the burn is extensive, the area should be covered with a clean, dry dressing to protect it from bacteria. This can be a sheet, towel, or other freshly laundered piece of material. The patient is transported to a hospital as soon as possible.

Under ordinary circumstances the burned victim is given nothing by mouth until arrival at a medical facility. However, if there is an unavoidable delay of several hours before transport is possible, and the patient is conscious and able to swallow, fluids to drink are given. A solution of 1/2 teaspoon each of salt and baking soda in 1 quart of water is ideal. The patient is encouraged to drink small amounts of the solution at 10- to 15-minute intervals unless nausea develops and vomiting seems likely. Intravenous fluid therapy and more extensive medical treatment are started as soon as possible. Rings, bracelets, and watches should be removed from injured extremities to avoid a tourniquet effect when swelling occurs.

Immediate Care   Most major burn cases are transferred to a major burn unit for specialized care. However, many burn victims are initially treated and stabilized at the community hospital nearest the scene of the accident before being moved to a burn unit. The first hour of treatment after burning can be crucial to the eventual outcome of a serious burn.

If possible, details of the nature of the accident should be obtained so that a more thorough assessment can be made. The cause of the burn and whether there is any possibility of thermal damage to the respiratory tract can help identify more closely the specific needs of the patient. Once the depth and extent of the burn have been estimated, efforts are made to establish an IV line and infuse an isotonic balanced solution such as Ringer's lactate to maintain fluid balance. Oxygen is administered if blood gases indicate a problem with respiratory function or if inhalation injury is suspected. **Suspect inhalation injury if there are burns of the face or neck, singed nasal hairs, soot in nose or oral pharynx, or if sooty sputum is coughed up.**

Moist, cool towels are sometimes applied to help relieve pain. Analgesics may be withheld until the patient's vital signs are stable or fluid treatment is under way.

Preventing shock and infection.   **A major concern in the care of a burn victim is to prevent shock due to circulatory collapse.** The two most important measures used to relieve profound shock in a burn patient are (1) replacement of lost fluids and electrolytes (fluid resuscitation); and (2) relief of pain and anxiety. The loss of fluids and electrolytes results from the sudden shifting of the blood plasma and tissue fluids from their normal site to the area of the burn. This shift occurs in the first 24 to 48 hours postburn. The fluids are then lost by movement from the vascular space to the interstitial spaces. A foley catheter is inserted to monitor urine output and provides data to determine whether fluid resuscitation is adequate.

Unless these fluids are replaced immediately, the blood vessels will collapse and the resultant profound shock may be fatal to the patient. Plasma, fluids, and electrolytes are given IV through multiple lines and sometimes through an incision into a vein (a cutdown), for continuous replacement of fluids until normal fluid and electrolyte balance is established. In a severely burned patient, IV therapy may be necessary for several days or longer. The patient may receive additional nourishment by feeding tube. If tube feedings are not tolerated, total parenteral nutrition via a central line may be used as a last resort. Tetanus prophylaxis is given.

Managing pain.   Measures to relieve pain include the administration of morphine, hydromorphone hydrochloride (Dilaudid), or meperidine (Demerol) IV as soon as possible after the burn has been sustained. The massive fluid shifts that occur after a burn injury make absorption from an intramuscular site unpredictable in the first 24 hours postburn. An antianxiety drug also may be given.

The nurse must use gentleness and care in handling the patient as she turns him or administers treatments. Not only does this reduce the amount of pain the patient must suffer, but also the less the patient is handled, the less danger there is of contaminating the wounds.

Even though there usually is not much pain associated with full-thickness burns during the first few days, most burn patients sustain burns in varying depths and therefore suffer a great deal of pain. Also, burn victims do not lose consciousness. **Added to the physical discomfort is the patient's realization that he has been badly injured.** He no doubt thinks of all the horrifying sights and smells associated with burned flesh, and he can suffer much emotional shock from such a traumatic experience.

Nonpharmacological measures to reduce pain, such as relaxation techniques, meditation, guided imagery, and music therapy are used along with pain medication. Therapeutic touch may prove helpful.

Preventing other complications.   In addition to the dangers of shock and infection, there is a potential for respiratory failure if upper airway passages have been burned. Dyspnea may or may not be present at first, but if the burn victim inhaled smoke or superheated air at the time of injury, an inflammatory response could obstruct the air passages completely within 24 hours.

Patients who should be watched closely for signs of developing respiratory problems include those who have (1) burns of the face and neck; (2) singed nasal hair; (3) darkened membranes in the nose and mouth; and (4) a history of having been burned in an enclosed space.

Hemorrhage does not occur with burns. If a burned patient shows signs of bleeding, he must be checked for some other type of injury, such as a penetrating wound, fracture, or laceration that occurred at the same time that he was burned.

Although the physician chooses the type of medication to be applied topically or administered systemically, the nursing staff is responsible for continued assessment of the burn wounds to determine the effectiveness of the prescribed treatments.

The patient's vital signs must be checked at regular intervals and recorded accurately. The condition of the wounds also should be checked systematically to determine whether healing is taking place as it should and infection is being avoided.

> Three common conditions that the nurse should guard against and report immediately if signs appear are decreased urine output (indicating dehydration that can lead to shock), infection, and cellulitis.

It should be noted that a blood pressure reading taken by cuff from an extremity may not be reliable; an arterial line may be inserted for more accurate monitoring of blood pressure changes.

Dehydration may be indicated by thirst, increased heart rate, an elevated body temperature, decreasing urine output, and a dryness in the wound, with loss of skin turgor in the unaffected areas. **A very wet wound that has a foul odor indicates infection.** A greenish-blue exudate from the wound is a sign of *Pseudomonas* infection. A bluish-black discoloration at the edges of the wound and other signs of a generalized infection may indicate that the patient is developing septicemia. Signs of inflammation, such as redness and swelling of the tissues adjacent to the wound, may indicate **cellulitis** (acute inflammation of the subcutaneous tissues).

Every effort to maintain joint function is employed. Range of motion (ROM) exercises are instituted as soon as the patient is stable. Splints are applied to joints on injured extremities to prevent contractures and to hold them in a functional position.

Healthy granulation tissue does not emit exudate. **During the granulation stage of repair, the wound should look slightly pink and somewhat shiny. If there are any deviations from this description, such as those mentioned, the nurse should notify the physician.**

Treatment of the Wound   In general, two methods may be used to treat a burn wound: the *open technique*, which leaves the wound undressed; or the *closed technique* in which the wound is covered with a dressing. When the wound is left undressed, it usually is covered with a topical ointment to prevent infection and promote healing. The wound is cleansed at least once daily and the topical agent is reapplied, usually every 8 hours. If dressings are used, which is the more common method, they are composed of a few layers of sterile gauze saturated with one of the topical medications (Figure 29-6). The wound is then wrapped with a stretch gauze, such as Kling, or with an elastic bandage. Table 29-9 lists the most common topical medications and their nursing implications. The wound may be cleansed at the bedside, on a shower table in the burn unit treatment room, or in a whirlpool bath in the physical therapy department. Cleansing is done at least once a

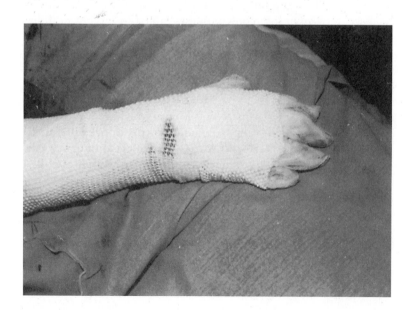

FIGURE 29-6   Occlusive dressing applied to a burned hand. (Courtesy of the Burn Center at Saint Agnes Medical Center, Philadelphia, PA.)

TABLE 29-9 ◆ *Topical Medications Commonly Used for Burns*		
Medication	**Action**	**Nursing Implications**
Silver sulfadiazine (Silvadene, Flamazine)	Interferes with DNA synthesis by binding to bacterial cell membrane.	Assess for allergy to sulfonamides. Observe for rash, itching, or burning, which may indicate allergic reaction. Observe for leukopenia, which may indicate an adverse reaction. Is not well absorbed into eschar. Not effective against *Pseudomonas* infections. Observe for suprainfection of wound evidenced by "soupy" appearance.
Mafenide acetate (Sulfamylon)	Bacteriostatic agent; effective against both gram-positive and gram-negative organisms.	Assess for allergy to sulfonamides. Observe for signs of allergic reaction. May cause metabolic acidosis; monitor blood gases and electrolyte levels. Application may cause pain for 30 to 40 minutes; medicate before applying. Penetrates eschar and is effective against *Pseudomonas*. Very effective for electrical burns.
Silver nitrate	Antimicrobial action.	Dressings must be kept continually wet with 0.5% solution. Stings upon application; stains fabric. Monitor electrolyte levels as may cause imbalances. Penetrates wound only 1 to 2 mm.
Sodium hypochlorite solution (Dakin's)	Bactericidal action; inhibits blood clotting and may dissolve clots.	Observe for signs of irritation. Keep dressings moist with the solution at all times. Helps dry wounds and assists debridement.
Nitrodurazone (Furacin)	Broad-spectrum antibacterial action.	Observe for allergic reaction. May cause contact dermatitis. Monitor renal function closely as can be toxic if used in large quantities.
Providone iodine (Betadine)	Bactericidal for gram-positive and gram-negative organisms.	May cause metabolic acidosis and elevated serum iodine levels; monitor electrolytes, serum iodine, and blood gases closely. May cause rash and burning sensation. Stains fabric.

*Other antibiotic solutions or creams may be used for infected wounds.

day and may be done as many as three times daily when the open technique is used.

There is no one best way to treat burns. Each patient must be evaluated according to his age, physical makeup, and type of burn and then treated on an individual basis. When the wound is exposed to the air, the nurse must guard constantly against infection. Usually, the serous fluid that exudes from the burns will harden and cover most of the burned area, but bacteria may enter through the cracks in the dried exudate.

Standard Precautions are used for all burn care. Protective isolation techniques are used in the burn unit. Those in attendance usually wear sterile caps, gowns, shoe covers, and gloves while caring for the patient. Contact isolation measures are used for infected wounds. Gloves are worn for all contact with open wounds and are changed when handling wounds on different areas of the patient's body and between handling soiled and sterile dressings. **Patient care items are not shared, and great attention is paid to maintaining asepsis for all patient care.** Bed linen is changed daily and whenever soiled, and a bed cradle or some other device is used to support the weight of the top covers to keep them off the burned areas.

Aside from preventing infection, the nurse also must provide additional warmth when the open method of treatment is used. Much body heat is lost through the parts of the body where the skin has been destroyed, and the patient is chilled easily. Heat lamps or radiant heat shields will usually provide the extra warmth needed and may be used in place of covers.

Wet compresses or soaks to cleanse the burned area and remove excess exudate and drainage must be used with extreme care and under sterile conditions to minimize the danger of infecting the wound.

Covering the wound protects it from infection. When the burned areas are covered, the patient does not have a constant visual reminder of his injuries. It also is true that patients who have pressure dressings are freer to move about and do things for themselves than those who do not have their wounds covered. An advantage of covering wounds is that when dressings are changed, dead tissue that is stuck to the bandage is debrided. The main disadvantages of the closed method are the need for frequent dressing changes and the trauma to the regenerating tissue. Other disadvantages of bulky dressings are that they (1) provide a culture medium for the growth of bacteria; (2) are difficult to apply properly to areas such as the face and perineum; (3) may increase fluid loss and heat retention; and (4) can mask bleeding. It is also much more difficult to assess the status of the wound when it is covered.

Debridement and grafting. Debridement involves removing the eschar and necrotic material from underlying tissues. This must be done with great care so that bleeding is kept at a minimum and healthy tissues are disturbed as little as possible. Some physicians prefer the method of soaking off eschar by placing the patient in a tub containing a temperature-controlled solution. Hibiclens, which is nonirritating, may be added to combat bacteria. The bath water is gently agitated to facilitate the debridement process. Patients do not object to the bath as they do to other methods of debridement, because the bath is soothing, relaxing, and less painful, and they can exercise more freely in the water. Debridement also can be done with a handheld shower instrument followed by the use of tweezers and scissors to remove loosened dead tissue.

Enzyme compounds, such as sutilains (Travase), containing proteolytic agents may be applied topically to digest necrotic tissue. They are used in conjunction with an antibiotic to prevent bacteria from entering the bloodstream from the wound.

Surgical removal of eschar and applications of biological dressings are done within the first week after the burn injury. *Biological* dressings are materials obtained from the patient's intact skin, cadavers, or animals. It is most desirable to graft the patient's own skin (**autograft**), but, when this is not possible, the skin of another person (homograft, **allograft**) obtained from a cadaver, heterograft (**xenograft**), usually obtained from a pig, or artificial skin (*Biosynthetic*) can be used as a temporary measure. Synthetic dressings consist of silicone, plastics, or alginate (brown seaweed) combined with other substances and remain in place for 1 to 14 days. **The patient's own skin is the only permanent graft material.** Some success has been achieved in growing skin cells harvested from the patient in cultures. The epithelial sheets grown are then used for grafting. However, these sheets are very fragile and take 3 to 4 weeks to grow.

Surgical debridement and grafting may require IV anesthetic agents, nitrous oxide, or narcotic analgesia.

Escharotomy. When tissue perfusion or quality of respiration are compromised because of eschar constriction, an escharotomy is performed. **An incision into the burn eschar with a scalpel or electrocautery relieves pressure caused by burns that encircle an extremity or that constrict movement of the chest.** The incisions extend into the subcutaneous tissue. If the pressure is not relieved, arterial blood flow in the extremity will be compromised, possibly causing necrosis; nerve damage from the pressure also may occur. An escharotomy on the chest improves lung expansion and oxygenation. The procedure does not cause discomfort as the nerve endings have been destroyed by the burn. No anesthesia is required.

Control of infection. Wound infection remains the major cause of death in burn victims. The necrotic tissue serves as an excellent breeding ground for microorganisms, which multiply rapidly in the burn wound. In the early 1960s, most patients with full-thickness burns over 50% of the body did not survive. Today, because of improved care to prevent infection and promote healing, many patients survive such extensive burns.

Some major reasons for the improved prognosis for extensive burns are (1) quicker, more aggressive fluid and electrolyte replacement; (2) better monitoring techniques for physiological parameters; (3) more adequate nutritional support with total parenteral nutrition or high-calorie, high-protein supplements and other measures to bolster the patient's defense system and meet metabolic needs; (4) contained burn units that can provide a truly aseptic environment; (5) specially trained nurses who understand and are competent in all aspects of burn care; and (6) better skin grafting techniques, both temporary and permanent.

Nursing Intervention   Care of the burn patient is interdisciplinary and includes the services of the physician, surgeon, nurses, dietitian, respiratory therapist, physical therapist, occupational therapist, psychologist or psychiatrist, and social worker. Other health professionals are added to the team as needed. Collaborative planning meetings are scheduled at least once a week initially. Input for the plan of care is contributed by all members of the team.

Goals of care include maintaining a patent airway; preventing or correcting hypovolemic shock; correcting metabolic acidosis, hyperkalemia, and hyponatremia; preventing infection; restoring skin integrity; preventing contractures and other complications; and restoring function to the individual as much as possible.

Humidified oxygen is given if the patient is experiencing respiratory distress; a tracheostomy and mechanical ventilation may be required. The nurse sees to it that the necessary equipment is at hand and constantly assesses the patient's respiratory effort. Measures such as use of an incentive spirometer, coughing, turning, and ambulation are used to maintain good respiratory function.

Preventing shock through fluid resuscitation is a primary objective. Various formulas are used to calculate the amount of fluid needed to maintain circulatory and kidney function. A large amount of fluid is given over a short time. One formula requires that half of the calculated fluid be given in the first 8 hours after the burn. The remainder of the fluid is given over the next 16 hours. After that fluids are based on specific volume and electrolyte imbalances and response to treatment. **Fluid replacement is calculated from the time of injury, not from the time of arrival at the medical facility.** An important nursing function is to keep IV access sites patent, monitor them constantly, and see that the fluids are administered at the ordered rates. Pressure from developing edema may cut off the fluid flow into a vessel. Urine output provides one measure of adequacy of fluid resuscitation. Urine flow should be equal to 1 mL/kg/percentage of burn up to 30 mL/hour. State of sensorium or level of consciousness is another measure. The nurse constantly assesses the patient's level of alertness and clarity of thinking.

Prevention of infection in the wound is important throughout the healing process. Applications of topical medications should be done under aseptic conditions, even if the burn is a minor one. When the patient is ready to accept some responsibility for self-care, and in preparation for release from the hospital, the nurse begins teaching how to apply topicals without contaminating the wound and how to change dressings if these are used.

Blood flow is shifted to the brain, heart, and liver because of the fluid shifts that occur. The gastrointestinal tract receives decreased blood and gastric motility is impaired. The nurse monitors peristalsis and is alert to signs of paralytic ileus. Severe abdominal distention may occur. Curling's ulcer may develop, inducing gastrointestinal bleeding. Stools are monitored for signs of occult blood. An H_2-receptor antagonist, such as cimetidine (Tagamet), ranitidine (Zantac), famotidine (Pepcid), or nizatidine (Axid), may be administered IV to prevent this complication.

She also will systematically assess scar tissue formation and help the patient adjust to the fact that burn scars may take as long as 12 to 24 months to mature completely. Maturing scars usually appear red, hard, and raised before they eventually begin to fade and soften. Pressure garments and masks help prevent thick and disfiguring scars but are uncomfortable. The patient may resist wearing them unless he understands their intended purpose.

Pain and itching often continue beyond the point at which the wound appears to have healed completely. Exercises to prevent contractures can cause pain, because they stretch the skin at a time when it is very tender. Splints to prevent musculoskeletal complications also can be uncomfortable for the burn patient. Analgesics will allow the patient to get sufficient rest, but they should be administered judiciously. If a patient begins to depend too much on one kind of analgesic, alternative drugs can be given. Itching can be controlled by giving regular doses of medication to prevent the problems, rather than waiting until the itching becomes intense and interferes with rest.

Contractures always are a threat to a patient with major burns and sometimes to one with minor burns. Proper positioning and regular exercise are essential to prevent musculoskeletal deformities following a burn. Painful as the motion of physical therapy exercises may be, the muscles and skin must be exercised and stretched every day if normal motion is to be maintained. Sometimes it is necessary for the patient to continue visiting the physical therapist for several months after discharge from the hospital. Ambulation two or three times a day is begun as soon as the fluid shift has stabilized for patients who have no fractures or serious injuries to the feet or legs.

Fluid intake and output are measured as long as there is a threat to fluid and electrolyte balance. Laboratory data are checked frequently for evidence of either a deficit or surplus of specific electrolytes.

The diet of the burn patient is an essential component of his therapy. Protein and calorie content is increased to several times that of a regular diet to help the body heal itself and rebuild lost tissue. Dietary supplements include vitamins, especially vitamin C; minerals such as iron and calcium; and electrolytes. Enteral feedings are started early in treatment if the patient cannot take in sufficient nutrients orally.

The odor of the burn and the patient's despondency over his predicament may initially affect his appetite. Perseverance and ingenuity in making meals and supplemental foods appealing are needed to help the patient meet his metabolic needs and promote healing and repair.

Pressure dressings are worn as soon as grafts heal to prevent the formation of contractures and decrease scarring that can inhibit mobility. The pressure dressing may be an elastic wrap or a custom-fitted, elasticized piece of clothing that provides uniform pressure over the burned area. These pressure dressings must be worn 23 hours a day, every day, until the scar tissue is mature. Scar maturity takes 12 to 24 months.

The emotional shock of a burn can be quite serious and long-lasting, especially if there is some loss of mobility and independence, or disfigurement involving the face or other parts of the body usually visible to others. Many burn patients experience posttraumatic shock syndrome. **The nurse should strive to develop an attitude of acceptance of the patient, a calm approach to dressing changes and discussions of scar formation, and an optimistic emphasis on what the patient can do and will be able to do in the future.** As is true in most long-term and slowly progressing disorders, the severely burned patient can become bored and apathetic and might even lose the will to live. Diversional and occupational therapy and a coordinated effort on the part of all members of the health team are needed to help the burn patient recover and adjust to the effects of his injury.

Psychological care is very important for the burn patient. When a patient has difficulty coping with the physical and psychosocial effects of a severe burn, effective nursing intervention can help him deal with his fears, anxieties, and sense of loss. The nurse assists the patient through the grief process. To be most helpful, the nurse should encourage the patient to relate what is experienced and feelings about what has happened or is happening. Questions about how the nurse and others who care for him can be most helpful and what changes in the environment might help are appropriate. It may be possible to change some elements of the environment. For example, noise, lights, or certain people—visitors or staff—may be very irritating to the patient; these factors usually can be adjusted. If the patient is unhappy about being isolated, bringing in a radio or magazines and books may help to stay in touch with the outside world. Regardless of whether every change desired by the patient can be made, at the very least assurance is given that there is someone who will listen and empathize.

The patient's self-esteem can be reinforced by emphasizing the strengths the nurse has noticed when he is coping with pain, inconvenience, or some other unpleasant situation. Involving the patient in performing self-care as much as possible and giving some sense of control over the situation are helpful. Words and actions can communicate the nurse's concern and caring.

The patient's body image may have been severely disrupted. This will require considerable adjustment. The nurse can assist the patient to grieve over the loss and integrate the present body image. Referrals to the psychologist, psychiatrist, social worker, or religious leader are made to help the patient address this issue. Nursing interventions for selected problems in a burned patient are summarized in Nursing Care Plan 29-1.

Rehabilitation   The patient who has experienced a major burn is referred for rehabilitation. Continued physical therapy and psychological care are essential to help the patient achieve his optimal level of function. Scar tissue maturation continues for many months and exercises must be religiously performed. Measures to prevent contractures must be continued. Some patients must learn to use adaptive devices or alter the way they formerly accomplished tasks.

Participation in a support group of burn victims is sometimes helpful. In this way the patient and family realize that they are not alone in their struggles with the many problems that the injury has brought.

Reintegration into roles, community activities, and employment take considerable time. Referral for job retraining may be required if the patient will be unable to return to a former occupation because of residual physical deficits. The nurse and health care team members can be very instrumental in helping the patient with these tasks. Rehabilitation goals and principles are covered in Chapter 12.

COMMUNITY CARE

Nurses in the community can do much to educate the public about the dangers of unprotected sun exposure and the signs of skin cancer. Skin self-screening is taught at every opportunity. Teaching fire safety to school children helps decrease fire injury. Home care nurses must continually assess patient homes for fire dangers and reinforce teaching to prevent home fires. School nurses perform assessments for signs of lice and scabies. They teach families how to deal with these problems and how to prevent their spread.

Long-term care nurses seek to promote good skin integrity in all residents, handling the elderly with special care so as not to tear the skin. Patients who are immobile are turned diligently to prevent pressure ulcers and skin is inspected regularly. Elderly patients are encouraged to use skin emollients to moisten and protect the skin surface. Nurses vigilantly assess changes in skin lesions that may indicate a cancer.

CRITICAL THINKING EXERCISES

Clinical Case Problems

Read each clinical situation and discuss the questions with your classmates.

1. You have been asked to give a presentation to your younger sister's ninth-grade class on skin care and prevention of skin disease.
   a. What specific information would you include on the subject of general skin care?
   b. Which skin disorders would you choose to talk about?
   c. What information would you plan to include about each of these disorders?

2. Mrs. Nash, age 32, has been assigned as your patient on the evening shift. She has severe dermatitis, probably allergic. Her physician has ordered a topical lotion, dermatological baths twice a day, and an antihistamine to relieve itching.
   a. What kinds of data would you include in your ongoing assessment of Mrs. Nash's skin disorder?
   b. What nursing care problems is Mrs. Nash likely to present?

c. What objectives and the nursing measures to meet them would you include in Mrs. Nash's nursing care plan?

d. What would you teach Mrs. Nash about the application of topicals when she returns home?

3. Ms. Moore, age 22, was badly burned when her clothing caught fire while she was grilling hamburgers on her patio. She has partial-thickness and full-thickness burns over her abdomen and down the front of both upper legs.

a. What is the priority of care after assessment when Ms. Moore reaches the emergency room?

b. What *nursing* measure should be taken to prevent infection of her burns?

c. What nursing measures would be included in the patient's nursing care plan to ensure that she did not suffer from an undetected fluid and electrolyte imbalance?

d. How is Ms. Moore's pain treated? Why?

e. List some specific things you and the other nurses could do to help her handle her sense of loss and altered self-image as a result of the appearance of the burns and scars.

4. Mrs. Hess, an 83-year-old resident of a long-term care facility has very dry skin. She asks you to look at a spot on her hand that is raised, scaly, and has a white flaky appearance.

a. What could this lesion on Mrs. Hess's hand be?

b. Why should such lesions be treated?

c. Mrs. Hess asks you why she bruises so easily. She says she hates these reddish-purple areas she gets on her arms and legs. What would you answer?

d. What nursing measures should be instituted for skin care for Mrs. Hess' dry skin?

BIBLIOGRAPHY

Allwood, J. S. (1995). The primary care management of burns. *Nurse Practitioner.* 20(8):74, 77–79, 83, 87.

Atwater, E. (1995). Acne assaults self-esteem and confidence of America's teens. (1995). *Dermatology Nursing.* 7(1): 61–62.

Bennett, J. C., Plum, F., eds. (1996). *Cecil Textbook of Medicine,* 20th ed. Philadelphia: Saunders.

Black, J. M., Matassarin-Jacobs, E. (1997). *Medical-Surgical Nursing: Clinical Management for Continuity of Care,* 5th ed. Philadelphia: Saunders.

Bolinger, B. (1995). Burn care in the home. *Journal of Wound, Ostomy and Continence Nursing.* 22(3):122–127.

Byers, J. F., Flynn, M. B. (1996). Acute burn injury: a trauma case report. *Critical Care Nurse.* 16(4):55–65.

Camisa, C. (1995). Treatment of severe psoriasis with systemic drugs. *Dermatology Nursing.* 7(2):107–120.

Cardona, V. D. (1994). *Trauma Nursing,* 2nd ed. Philadelphia: Saunders.

Dambro, M. R. (1996). *Griffith's 5 Minute Clinical Consult.* Baltimore: Williams & Wilkins.

Deutsch, N. (1994). New drug combats fungal infections. *Canadian Nurse.* 90(1):15–16.

Frankel, E. (1995). Psoriasis. *Journal of the American Academy of Nurse Practitioners.* 7(5):237–243.

Guyton, A. C., Hall, J. E. (1996). *Textbook of Medical Physiology,* 9th ed. Philadelphia: Saunders.

Halpern, J. S. (1994). Clinical notebook: recognition and treatment of pediculosis (head lice) in the emergency department. *Journal of Emergency Nursing.* 20(2): 130–133.

Hicks, L. E. M., Lewis, D. J. (1995). Management of chronic, resistive scabies: a case study. *Geriatric Nursing.* 16 (5):197.

Hill, M. J. (1995). Skin Cancer—the need for continuing education. *Dermatology Nursing.* 7(4):220, 222.

Holdcroft, C. (1995). Drug news: new topical psoriasis treatment. *Nurse Practitioner.* 20(3):15–16.

Ignatavicius, D. D., Workman, M. L., Mishler, M. A. (1995). *Medical–Surgical Nursing: A Nursing Process Approach,* 2nd ed. Philadelphia: Saunders.

Jarvis, C. (1996). *Physical Examination and Health Assessment,* 2nd ed. Philadelphia: Saunders.

Jeter, K., Lutz, J. (1996). Skin care in the frail, elderly, dependent, incontinent patient. *Advances in Wound Care.* 9(1):29–34.

Kravitz, M. (1993). Burn care. *ACCN Clinical Issues in Critical Care Nursing.* 4(2):349–442.

Lehne, R. A. (1994). *Pharmacology for Nursing Care,* 2nd ed. Philadelphia: Saunders.

Maguire-Eisen, M., Frost, C. (1994). Knowledge of malignant melanoma and how it relates to clinical practice among nurse practitioners and dermatology and oncology nurses. *Cancer Nursing.* 17(6):457–463.

Matteson, M. A., McConnell, E. S., Linton, A. D. (1997). *Gerontological Nursing Concepts and Practice Edition 2.* Philadelphia: Saunders.

McCorkle, R., Grant, M., Frank-Stromborg, M., Baird, S. B. (1996). *Cancer Nursing: A Comprehensive Textbook.* Philadelphia: Saunders.

McMahon, M. A. (1994). Clinical outlook: herpes zoster and the aging. *Journal of Gerontological Nursing.* 20(12): 42–46.

Monahan, F. D., Drake, T., Neighbors, M. (1994). *Nursing Care of Adults.* Philadelphia: Saunders.

Newland, J. A. (1995). Primary care protocol: pediculosis. *American Journal of Nursing.* 95(9):16A.

Nichols, P. H. (1994). When your resident has scabies. *Geriatric Nursing.* 15(5):271–273.

Quillen, T. (1996)... About psoriasis. *Nursing 96.* 26(10):25.

Sabatini, M. M. (1995). Skin cancer: the silent pandemic. *Dermatology Nursing.* 7(1):45–50.

Skewes, S. M. (1996). Skin care rituals that do more harm than good. *American Journal of Nursing.* 97(10): 33-35.

Sokoloff, F. (1994). Identification and management of pediculosis. *Nurse Practitioner.* 19(8):62–64.

Springhouse Corporation. (1996). *Nursing96 Drug Handbook.* Springhouse, PA: Author.

Talbot, L., Curtis, L. (1996). The challenges of assessing skin indicators in people of color. *Home Healthcare Nurse.* 14(3):167–171.

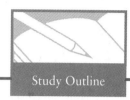

Study Outline

I. Introduction
A. Intact skin is essential to life and good health.
B. Skin is the first line of defense against bacteria in the environment.
C. There are many primary skin disorders, but systemic diseases also can affect the skin.
D. Skin diseases are among the most common afflictions in humans.
E. Dermatology is the study of diseases of the skin.
F. Diseases of the skin often are difficult to heal and have a tendency to recur.
G. People often try to treat skin diseases themselves.

II. Causes of Skin Disorders
A. Caused by immunological and inflammatory disorders, proliferative and neoplastic disorders, metabolic and endocrine disorders, and nutritional problems.
B. Damage from physical, chemical, and microbiological agents.

III. Prevention of Skin Disorders
A. Cleanliness; gentle cleaning with mild soap and water; lotions to combat dryness.
B. Well-balanced, nutritious diet.
C. Age: older persons experience dryness, loss of elasticity, and sometimes poor circulation to the skin.
D. Environment: avoiding irritants such as chemicals and ultraviolet radiation from the sun. Health teaching should warn general public of the hazards of overexposure to the sun.

IV. Diagnostic Tests and Procedures and Nursing Responsibilities
A. Skin biopsy: shave, punch, or excision. Done to differentiate benign from malignant lesions and to identify infectious organisms.
B. Culture and sensitivity tests.
C. Inspection under special lights.
　1. Cold light to illuminate layers of skin.
　2. Wood's light to diagnose fungal infections.
D. Diascopy uses a glass slide or lens to press down over the area, allowing the shape of the underlying lesion to be revealed.
E. Patch testing checks for allergy.

V. Nursing Management of Skin Disorders
A. Assessment.
　1. History taking: guide in Table 29-1.
　2. Teaching self-examination of the skin to recognize changes in warts, moles, birthmarks, and other lesions (Table 29-3).
　3. Physical assessment by inspection and palpation.
　　a. Appearance of adjacent skin.
　　b. Edema.
　　c. Characteristics of secretions.
　　d. Odor.
　　e. General appearance of skin surface; raised areas.
　　f. Observations: scratching, rubbing, picking at lesions or scalp.
　　g. Local changes in skin temperature.
B. Nursing diagnoses.
　1. Impaired skin integrity.
　2. Risk of impaired skin integrity.
　3. Pain.
　4. Disturbance of self-esteem.
　5. Anxiety.
　6. Risk for infection.
　7. Knowledge deficit.
　8. Sleep pattern disturbance.
　9. Social isolation.
C. Planning.
　1. Goals of care include
　　a. Restore skin to normal.
　　b. Decrease pain and itching.
　　c. Protect skin from further damage.
　　d. Prevent infection.
　　e. Prevent scarring as much as possible.

2. Short- and long-term goals are written as specific expected outcomes.

3. Planning of nursing time should consider time needed for therapeutic baths, dressing soaks and changes, and other skin treatments.

D. Implementation.

  1. *Standard Precautions* are used at all times.

  2. Careful handling of the skin; avoidance of alcohol, lotions, and other skin applications not specifically ordered by the dermatologist.

  3. Dermatological baths.

    a. Prepared by adding soothing agents or disinfectants to bath water.

    b. Avoid chilling patient.

    c. Pat, do not rub, the skin dry after bath.

  4. Laundering: bed linens and clothing may require special laundering to remove all traces of soap.

  5. Wet compresses and dressings often used.

  6. Topical therapy: administration of medication directly to surface of skin (Table 29-4).

E. Evaluation.

  1. Based on improved appearance of skin, absence of signs of infection, relief from itching and pain, and signs of healing.

  2. Skin disorders are slow to respond to treatment; patience is required.

VI. Skin Disorders

A. Infectious and parasitic skin diseases: Contact isolation measures recommended for certain skin disorders that can be transmitted to others by personal contact or contact with infective material.

  1. Private room, masks, gowns if soiling is likely, gloves upon entering room, handwashing, and decontamination of articles.

  2. Gloves to be changed between handling wounds or treating different areas on the body; wash hands when gloves are removed.

B. Herpesvirus infections: those caused by an extensive family of viruses.

  1. Herpes simplex: acute viral disease:

    a. Symptoms: lesions (blisters, ulcers) on lips and nares, also called cold sores and fever blisters.

    b. Treatment and nursing intervention.

      (1) Disease usually self-limiting. Treatment is symptomatic (no cure).

      (2) Oral acyclovir may be beneficial.

  2. Herpes zoster (shingles): caused by herpes varicella–zoster, which causes chickenpox (varicella) in children and shingles in older adults.

    a. Viruses replicate in the peripheral nerve ganglia, where they lie dormant until activated by trauma, malignancy, or local radiation.

    b. Symptoms begin with low-grade fever and possibly gastrointestinal upset. Lesions appear 3 to 5 days later, along the course of affected nerve. Pain and itching are chief complaints.

    c. Medical treatment and nursing intervention.

      (1) Non-narcotic analgesics.

      (2) Corticosteroids to reduce inflammation and pain.

      (3) Vidarabine IV for immune-deficient patients.

      (4) Acyclovir, valacyclovir, or famciclovir may diminish severity; corticosteroids used to relieve severe pain.

      (5) Emotional support and measures to relieve symptoms and prevent secondary bacterial infection.

C. Fungal infections.

  1. May be local or systemwide.

  2. Difficult to treat.

  3. Examples: tinea pedis (athlete's foot), tinea of the scalp (ringworm), and moniliasis (thrush).

  4. Symptoms: itching and some breakdown of skin.

  5. Treatment: fungistatic medicines.

  6. Patient teaching to avoid recurrent fungal infections (Table 29-6).

D. Parasitic infestations: pediculosis and scabies. Three kinds of lice: head, body, and pubic or crab lice.

    a. The most prevalent symptom of lice is severe itching. Scratching causes lesions and entry points for bacterial infection.

    b. Scabies mites burrow under skin and produce irritation with intense itching and blistering. Secondary infection is not uncommon.

    c. Lice and scabies treated with lindane (Kwell and Gamene) and 10% crotamiton (Eurax). A-200 Pyrinate and Cuprex do not require prescription.

E. Acne: characterized by papules and pustules over the face, back, and shoulders.

  1. Begins when ducts from sebaceous glands become plugged with sebum and cellular debris. Can cause inflammation and formation of cysts.

  2. Acne vulgaris most common type. Typically begins in early puberty.

  3. Medical treatment.

a. Mild noninflammatory type usually responds well to topicals that peel top layer of skin and remove blackheads and whiteheads.

b. Retin-A best for papular and pustular acne.

c. Benzoyl peroxide most used topical for acne.

d. Antibiotics, especially tetracycline, prescribed to inhibit bacterial infection.

e. 13-*cis*-retinoic acid (Accutane) effective in controlling most cases of treatment-resistant acne. Its effects are sustained for months or years after the drug is discontinued.

f. Scarring and pitting treated by dermabrasion.

4. Nursing intervention: health education and patient teaching.

a. Cleanliness, healthy diet, exercise recommended. No special diet needed unless patient notes relationship between certain foods and appearance of lesions.

b. Patient needs support and encouragement to continue treatment, which can last for months or years.

F. Psoriasis: chronic, recurring skin disorder. Patches of skin covered with adherent silvery scales (plaques).

1. Tends to run in families; cause unknown.

2. Comes and goes, often with or without treatment.

3. Medical treatment and nursing intervention:

a. Mild cases respond to steroid creams, moderate doses of sunlight.

b. Resistant cases treated with ultraviolet radiation and tar preparations.

c. Antimetabolites used in severe cases.

d. Patient education includes information about nature of disease, purpose of prescribed treatment, avoidance of factors that aggravate the condition or cause a flareup.

e. Skin should be kept moist and pliable; scratches and abrasions should be avoided because they can trigger the appearance of plaques at new sites.

G. Skin cancer.

1. Almost all cases can be treated successfully if caught early.

2. Cause unknown, but skin type, heredity, and exposure to environmental carcinogens, including sunlight, can increase susceptibility.

3. For types and characteristics, see Table 29-7.

4. Treatment: surgical removal, occasionally chemotherapy and radiation therapy once metastasis has occurred.

H. Burns.

1. Caused by exposure to heat, electrical agents, strong chemicals, and radiation.

2. Classified according to extent and depth of injury (Tables 29-8).

3. Emergency treatment: All burns should be considered potentially dangerous until they are thoroughly assessed.

a. Minor burns are treated by submersion in cool water, applications of cool compresses. Do not apply any ointment or greasy substance.

b. Cover major burns with a clean, dry, dressing.

c. Do not disturb blisters.

4. Immediate care (major burns).

a. First hour can be crucial to successful outcome; fluid replacement essential.

b. Obtain details of nature of accident; cause of burn, possibility of internal burns.

c. Determine depth and extent; establish IV lines.

d. Administer oxygen as needed.

e. Cover wound with clean sheet to protect from air.

f. Prevent or relieve profound shock.

(1) Replace fluids and electrolytes.

(2) Relieve pain.

(3) Manage pain.

(a) Administer morphine or meperidine IV as ordered.

(b) Handle gently.

(c) Consider emotional impact of burn.

g. Other immediate complications.

(1) Damage to respiratory tract; keep tracheostomy set handy.

(2) Hemorrhage not typical of burn. Check for other types of injuries.

(3) Insert Foley catheter to monitor for decreasing urine output.

(4) Insert nasogastric tube to decompress gastrointestinal tract; paralytic ileus may occur.

5. Nursing assessment.

a. Monitor vital signs frequently and regularly.

b. Check condition of wound for signs of infection, cellulitis. Note color, dryness, appearance of wound, swelling, and other signs of inflammation in adjacent tissues.

c. Monitor patient for fluid imbalance: urine output, vital signs.

6. Treatment of the wound.

a. Two general methods: open and closed.

(1) In open there is no dressing. Wound is left open to the air.

(a) Protective isolation.

(b) Provide additional warmth.

(c) Compresses and soaks done under sterile conditions.

(2) In closed method, wound is covered with dressing.

(a) Advantages are that the wound is not so obvious to the patient, infection is less likely, and the patient is able to move more freely.

(b) Disadvantages are pain involved in frequent dressing changes, potential bacterial growth on dressings, difficulty applying on certain body parts, potential increased fluid loss, and masking bleeding from healing wound.

b. Debridement and grafting to promote healing and cover wound; enzyme debridement may be used as well as biological dressings applied.

c. Escharotomy is performed to relieve constriction of chest or extremity.

d. Control of infection.

(1) Wound infection is the major cause of death from burns.

(2) Major reasons for improved prognosis are aggressive fluid replacement, more sophisticated physiological monitoring, better nutritional support, use of specialized burn units with highly skilled nurses, and better skin grafting techniques.

(3) Topical medications are used to prevent wound infection (Table 29-9).

7. Nursing intervention.

a. Use aseptic technique to avoid infecting patient while administering care.

b. Systematically assess scar tissue formation. Help patient adjust to possibility that scars will get worse before they begin to fade.

c. Measures to relieve pain and itching.

d. Exercises to prevent contractures.

e. Measure intake and output; check laboratory data for electrolyte imbalance.

f. Encourage adequate dietary intake of high-protein foods.

g. Help patient cope with emotional shock and sense of loss, altered self-image.

8. Rehabilitation

a. Long process; psychological and social service care is needed.

b. Physical therapy continues for months past injury.

c. Referral to support group or psychotherapy may be necessary for patients with major burns.

VII. Elder Care Points

A. Epidermis thins with advancing age, giving a translucent appearance to the skin.

B. Collagen decreases through the years, causing a decrease in skin strength and elasticity.

C. Elderly skin is more easily damaged and slower to repair as a result of the decreased vascularity of dermal layer.

D. Skin loses some of its ability to maintain body temperature.

E. Sebaceous gland secretion decreases, leading to dry, coarser skin.

F. Hair becomes thinner and more sparse, although baldness is related to genetic factors, rather than to aging alone.

G. Nails become dull, brittle, hard, and thick with aging.

H. Sun exposure over the years causes formation of actinic keratoses, which are premalignant lesions.

I. Age spots, skin tags, senile purpura are common among the elderly.

J. Skin cancers and fungal infections also are common problems among the elderly.

VIII. Community Care

A. Nurses must educate the public about the dangers of sun exposure.

B. Nurses in the community teach skin self-examination and the danger signs of skin cancer.

C. Teaching fire safety and monitoring patient homes for potential fire dangers are nursing functions.

D. Long-term care nurses must continually assess the skin of residents and provide care appropriate for aging skin.

E. School nurses and community clinic nurses are alert to the signs and symptoms of infestation with pediculosis or scabies.

CHAPTER 30

Care of Patients with Eye or Ear Disorders

OBJECTIVES

Upon completing this chapter the student should be able to:
1. Identify ways in which nurses can help patients preserve their sight and hearing.
2. Discuss tests and examinations used to diagnose eye and ear disorders.
3. State nursing activities associated with assessing the eye and ear.
4. Utilize the use of the nursing process for patients with disorders of the eye or ear.
5. Describe the signs and symptoms of selected disorders of the eye and appropriate medical treatment and nursing interventions for each.
6. Discuss nursing interventions to care for the visually impaired patient.
7. Explore the impact of hearing or vision loss on an individual and his or her family.
8. Identify aids and resources for persons with vision loss, impaired hearing, tinnitus, and dizziness or vertigo.
9. List the signs and symptoms of selected disorders of the ear, appropriate medical or surgical treatment, and nursing interventions for each.
10. State nursing interventions to care for the hearing-impaired patient.

Sensory losses such as the loss of vision or hearing may greatly affect the quality of life of an individual. This chapter discusses the eye first and then the ear.

Vision loss is one of the most profound and dreaded of physical disabilities. When a sighted person is no longer able to see, his world changes, and he is required to make many adjustments. There are two general kinds of patients with impaired vision: those who were born blind, and those who develop some degree of visual impairment later in life. This chapter focuses on the latter type of visually handicapped patient.

The nursing care of patients with severe visual handicaps demands a special awareness of the unique problems encountered by someone who has either a partial or a total loss of vision. The nurse must be sensitive to these patients' special needs. Patient education is especially important to these patients' acceptance of their visual disorder, their participation in diagnostic and therapeutic measures, and their adjustment to their new surroundings when they are hospitalized or admitted to a long-term care facility.

Within the past two decades, there have been many new developments in the treatment of a number of potentially blinding diseases. These new surgical techniques and medical treatments offer hope for eyesight preservation to increasing numbers of people. Efforts also have been made to educate the public about eye care, prevention of eye disease, and periodic examinations to detect eye disorders in their earliest and treatable stages.

Since 1986 another disease has begun to cause blindness, AIDS. Eye problems and resultant blindness are a result of opportunistic infections that the AIDS patient contracts. Ocular problems of the AIDS patient are discussed in Chapter 8.

Approximately 15 million people in the United States have some kind of hearing loss. The National Advisory of Neurologic Diseases and Stroke Council estimates that about 8.5 million Americans have either bilateral or unilateral hearing impairment sufficient to impose a serious handicap. In persons between 30 and 39 years of age, about 1.5% have a problem clearly understanding the spoken word. The figure rises to 4% in persons 50 to 59 years of age.

A loss of hearing, like a loss of sight, burdens its victims with physical, emotional, psychosocial, and financial problems. Hearing allows for communication with others in everyday conversations, in the classroom, and in business transactions. Without the ability to hear, one can be deprived of many of the joys and pleasures of life: music, drama, exchange of ideas, and the thousands of sounds in one's environment. Because hearing warns one of danger, an inability to hear can cause anxiety and fear. The adult who has a hearing deficiency might lose his job and alienate friends because of his communication handicap. Nurses must learn ways to help prevent hearing loss and to assist patients who already have such a loss.

Part I: Eye Disorders

To understand the causes of eye problems, and their effects, it is necessary to recall the anatomy and functions of the structures of the eye.

OVERVIEW OF ANATOMY AND PHYSIOLOGY

What Are the Structures of the Eye?

⅄ The eyeball is spherical in shape and 2 to 3 cm in diameter (Figure 30-1).

⅄ The sclera, which is part of the wall of the eyeball, is opaque white and covers the posterior ⅚ of the eyeball.

⅄ The transparent cornea is part of the wall of the eyeball and covers the anterior ⅙ of the eyeball.

⅄ The choroid is part of the middle layer of the eyeball. It is a highly vascular layer containing brown pigment located between the sclera and the retina.

⅄ The ciliary body is part of the middle layer of the eyeball and contains finger-like ciliary processes.

⅄ The iris is the third part of the middle layer of the eyeball; it is the colored portion of the eye and is a doughnut-shaped diaphragm with the pupil as the central opening. The iris contains two groups of smooth muscles that constrict and dilate the pupil.

⅄ The biconvex, transparent lens, together with the suspensory ligaments and the ciliary body, forms a partition that divides the interior of the eyeball into two chambers. The anterior chamber between the lens and the cornea is filled with aqueous humor. The posterior chamber, between the lens and the retina, contains vitreous humor.

⅄ The suspensory ligaments connect the ciliary body to the lens.

⅄ The retina is the inner coat of the eyeball and is found in the posterior portion of it. The retina contains several layers. The layer with rods and cones acts as the receptor for light images.

⅄ The optic nerve carries messages from the nerve cells in the retina to the brain.

⅄ The optic disk is formed by the axons of the ganglion cells of the retina.

⅄ The macula lutea is a yellow spot just lateral to the optic disk.

⅄ The fovea centralis is the area of the retina that produces the sharpest image.

⅄ The eyelids are composed of skin, connective tissue, and conjunctiva. The conjunctiva is a thin mucous membrane that lines the eyelid and covers the anterior portion of the eyeball except for the cornea.

⅄ Eyelashes line the edge of the eyelid.

⅄ Sebaceous glands are situated with the eyelashes.

⅄ The lacrimal glands are located in the upper outer area above the eyes. The lacrimal ducts and canals carry tears from the eye to the nose.

⅄ Six muscles attach to the eyeball and allow for movement. The muscles come from the bones of the orbit and insert on the outer layer of the eyeball.

What Are the Functions of the Eye Structures?

⅄ The bony orbit protects the eyeball.

⅄ The eyelashes help trap foreign particles, keeping them from landing on the eyeball.

⅄ The eyelids protect the eyes from foreign matter and help distribute moisture on the eye surface.

⅄ The sebaceous glands secrete an oily fluid that lubricates the lids.

⅄ Blinking of the eyelid 6 to 30 times a minute stimulates the lacrimal glands to produce tears.

⅄ The lacrimal gland secretes tears that moisten, lubricate, and cleanse the surface of the eye. Tears contain an enzyme that helps destroy bacteria and prevent infections.

⅄ The transparent cornea allows light to hit the lens. It assists with the bending of light rays, **refraction,** so that the rays will hit the retina in the right location for images to be transmitted to the brain.

⅄ The choroid's brown pigment absorbs excess light rays that could interfere with vision.

⊿ The ciliary processes secrete aqueous humor that helps maintain the shape of the anterior chamber; it also nourishes the structures in this part of the eye. The aqueous humor assists with refraction of light onto the retina. **The amount of aqueous humor present determines the internal pressure of the eye.** The aqueous humor is reabsorbed by the blood vessels located at the junction of the sclera and the cornea.

⊿ Muscles in the iris control dilation and constriction of the pupil.

⊿ The suspensory ligaments connected to the ciliary body and lens allow light to focus on the lens and retina, which is necessary for close vision.

⊿ The retina's rods and cones are photoreceptors for light and color. The nerves of the retina transmit the images perceived to the brain.

⊿ The optic nerve conducts nerve impulses from the retina to the brain.

⊿ Visualization of the optic disk provides information about the pressure within the eye and within the skull. When intracranial pressure gets higher, the optic disk appears "swollen" or "choked."

⊿ Visual impulses travel along the optic nerve to the optic chiasma just anterior to the pituitary gland; at this point some of the axons cross over to the other side. Images from the medial portion of the left eye and the lateral portion of the right eye are carried by the right optic tract. Images from the medial portion of the right eye and the lateral portion of the left eye are carried by the left optic tract (Figure 30-2). Images are conducted to the visual cortex in the occipital lobe of the brain.

⊿ Six muscles control movement of the eyeball. Table 30-1 lists the nerves that control these muscles.

What Alterations Occur in the Eye with Aging?

⊿ Subcutaneous fat and tissue elasticity decrease and the eyes appear to be sunken.

⊿ *Arcus senilis,* an opaque ring outlining the cornea, sometimes results from the deposition of fatty globules (Color Figure 18).

⊿ The cornea flattens and develops an irregular curvature after age 65, causing an astigmatism or making an existing astigmatism worse; vision becomes blurred. Cornea transparency also decreases.

⊿ The sclera develops a yellowish tinge due to fatty deposits; thinning of the sclera may cause a bluish tinge.

⊿ The ability of the iris to dilate decreases, causing difficulty for the older person in going from a bright area into a darkened area.

⊿ The lens of the eye changes after age 40, gradually losing water and becoming harder.

⊿ The ciliary muscle has less ability to allow the eye to accommodate, a process responsible for the gradual extension of distance from the eyes at which an item to be read is held *(presbyopia)*.

⊿ The farthest point at which an object can be identified decreases and the older person has a narrower visual field.

⊿ Color discrimination decreases with advancing age.

⊿ Moisture secretion decreases during the senior years, placing the eyes at greater risk for irritation and infection. This is especially common after age 70. Repeated episodes of keratitis may seriously compromise vision and can lead to loss of independence for an elderly person.

⊿ Eversion of the lower lid (ectropion) occurs because of loss of muscle tone and elasticity (Color Figure 19).

⊿ Decreased muscle tone and decreased elasticity may cause drooping of the upper lid to a point where it interferes with vision (Color Figure 20).

PREVENTION OF EYE DISORDERS

As health care providers, nurses share responsibility for maintaining good eyesight and for preserving vision throughout the patient's life span. Two major goals to promote good vision are (1) health education to inform the general public about basic eye care and (2) prevention of accidental injury to the eye.

◆ Basic Eye Care

The term *eyestrain* has often been used as a catchall to explain various visual defects and diseases of the eye. It is actually very difficult to strain the eye. Inadequate lighting or prolonged use of the eyes for close work can overwork the eye muscles, but this will not damage the eyes any more than straining to hear a distant sound can damage the ears. One should rest the eye muscles

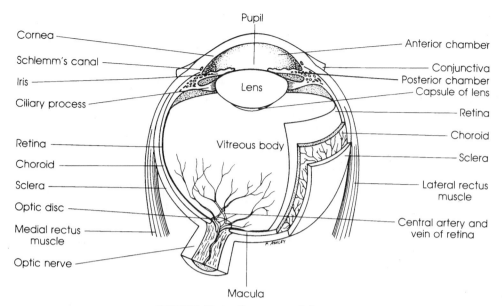

FIGURE 30-1   Structures of the eye.

periodically when watching television, doing needle-work, or performing any activity that demands intensive visual effort. If the eyes tire easily or if there is headache or burning, itching, or redness of the eyes, this is not eyestrain. These are symptoms of a visual problem and are an indication that the person's eyes should be examined.

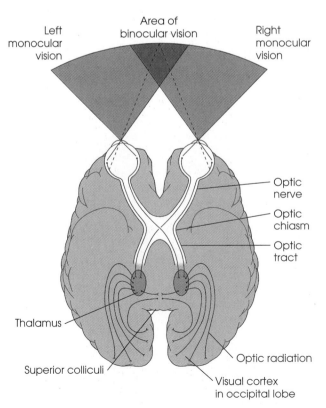

FIGURE 30-2   Visual pathway.

Adequate diet and good nutrition are important to conserve sight, but eating large amounts of carrots and other yellow vegetables will not improve eyesight. A vitamin A deficiency results in inflammation of the lids and conjunctiva and increased sensitivity to light. A serious deficiency of vitamin B can cause irreparable damage to the retina and permanent visual defects.

Normal eyes do not require irrigations or periodic "washing out" with over-the-counter eye solutions. Normal secretions of the conjunctiva and tear glands should be sufficient to lubricate the eye and wash away small particles of dust that may collect in the eye. **Accumulations of purulent material or excessive tearing usually indicates the need for an eye examination.** Dry eye syndrome that occurs in persons younger than 60 years of age could be symptomatic of an underlying disease.

Elder Care Point . . . Older persons sometimes suffer from "dry eyes." This is due to decreased production of tears and is treated by instilling "replacement tears," which are commercial preparations of solutions similar in composition to real tears.

Children do not outgrow crossed eyes (strabismus). Until a baby reaches the age of 6 to 9 months, he may have some difficulty focusing his eyes, but this problem should not persist. Neglect of strabismus can result in serious loss of vision. It is generally agreed by ophthalmologists that the sooner treatment is begun, the better the chance of correcting the condition and preserving the child's eyesight.

Every person over the age of 40 should have eye examinations every 2 to 3 years. It is particularly

TABLE 30-1 ◆ *Muscles of the Eye*

Muscle	Controlling Nerve	Function
Extrinsic (skeletal) muscles		
Superior rectus	Oculomotor (III)	Elevates eye or rolls it superiorly and toward the midline.
Inferior rectus	Oculomotor (III)	Depresses eye or rolls it inferiorly and toward the midline.
Medial rectus	Oculomotor (III)	Moves eye medially, toward the midline.
Lateral rectus	Abducens (VI)	Moves eye laterally, away from the midline.
Superior oblique	Trochlear (IV)	Depresses eye and turns it laterally, away from the midline.
Inferior oblique	Oculomotor (III)	Elevates eye and turns it laterally, away from the midline.
Intrinsic (smooth) muscles		
Ciliary	Oculomotor (III) Parasympathetic fibers	Causes suspensory ligament to relax, lens becomes more convex for close vision.
Iris, circular muscles	Oculomotor (III) Parasympathetic fibers	Decreases the size of the pupil to allow less light to enter the eye.
Iris, radial muscles	Sympathetic fibers from spinal nerves	Increases the size of the pupil to allow more light to enter the eye.

Source: Applegate, E. J. (1995). *The Anatomy and Physiology Learning System: Textbook.* Philadelphia: Saunders, p. 191.

important that a test for glaucoma be made at the time of the examination, because this disease usually is asymptomatic until damage to vision has occurred. Persons with a family history of glaucoma should be especially careful to have their eyes tested frequently for increased pressure within the eyeball, as this is the basic pathology of glaucoma and the disorder tends to be familial.

Accidental injury to the eye is a major cause of diminished or total loss of vision, especially in young children. Parents and teachers should be encouraged to teach children the danger of sharp pencils, paper wads, small stones, lawn darts, fireworks, and other small objects children may be tempted to hurl at one another while playing. Older children and adults should be cautioned to wear protective eyewear when engaging in sports such as raquetball and squash where small balls travel at high speeds. Protective eyewear should be worn when using machinery that might cause debris to fly into the eye, such as lawn mowers, sanders, or power saws.

The rate of occupational accidents has gone down since the establishment and enforcement of rules on wearing goggles and other protective devices for people working in a hazardous environment. The National Institute of Occupational Safety and Health (NIOSH) in Rockville, Maryland, provides information about eye safety and hazards in the workplace.

Cosmetics for the eyelids, eyelashes, and eyebrows can be a source of infection and allergy. Most dyes used for hair on the scalp are not intended for use on the eyelashes and eyebrows. Sometimes it is not the cosmetic but the way in which it is applied that causes eye disease. Saliva should not be used to moisten eye pencils, eye shadow, or mascara, as it may contain organisms that can cause eye infection. When eye cosmetics are being applied, it is important to have a steady hand to avoid accidentally scratching the cornea and eyelids. Cosmetics should never be shared, as this can transmit organisms. To promote prompt treatment of eye disease in its earliest stages, the National Society for the Prevention of Blindness has a list of danger signals (Table 30-2).

◆ Prevention of Visual Loss

Diabetes mellitus and hypertension are chronic diseases that, when uncontrolled, may cause visual loss. Patients

TABLE 30-2 ◆ *Patient Education: Danger Signals of Eye Disease*

- *Persistent redness of the eye.* Infections and inflammations of the structures of the eye that are not treated may leave scars that can produce loss of vision.
- *Continuing pain or discomfort about the eye,* especially following injury.
- *Disturbance of vision.* Although these symptoms may simply indicate a need for eyeglasses, blurred vision, loss of side vision, double vision, and sudden development of many floating spots in the field of vision may be symptomatic of more serious systemic diseases.
- *Crossing of the eyes,* especially in children.
- *Growths on the eye or eyelids* or opacities visible in the normally transparent portion of the eye.
- *Continuing discharge, crusting, or tearing of the eyes.*
- *Pupil irregularities,* either unequal size of the two pupils or distorted shape.

with these disorders are more susceptible to retinopathy. Helping patients gain good control over these disorders can prevent or control visual loss.

Encouraging people who experience an accident causing a corneal abrasion to seek medical attention quickly helps prevent infections that might cause corneal scarring and loss of vision. Promptly seeking medical attention when the eye is inflamed, secreting purulent discharge, or sore, assists in treatment of infection that may cause a residual visual loss.

Think about . . . Can you identify four specific ways in which you might help prevent eye disorders among your relatives and patients?

Assessing patients for the presence of cataracts and recommending regular periodic eye examinations should be a part of every nurse's practice. Cataract removal can greatly improve vision. Screening for glaucoma reduces the incidence of blindness from that disorder. Free screening clinics often are available in most communities. Nurses can inform patients of when and where such screenings are available.

Nurses must be aware that there are many types of visual loss. Some may affect only one area of the field of vision in one eye, others affect parts of the field of vision in both eyes. The degree of visual impairment varies greatly.

DIAGNOSTIC TESTS AND EXAMINATIONS

Diagnostic tests are performed to test visual acuity, to prescribe prescription lenses, inspect the interior of the eye, check intraocular pressure (IOP) and assess the health of the retinal blood vessels. Computed tomography (CT) and magnetic resonance imaging (MRI) may also be used to diagnose eye disorders. Table 30-3

TABLE 30-3 ◆ *Diagnostic Tests for Eye Problems*

Test	Purpose	Description	Nursing Inplications
Opthalmoscopy	Inspect the fundus (back portion) of the eyeball to detect abnormalities of the retina, macula, optic disk, and retinal vessels.	The examiner uses an opthalmascope (Figure 30-3) to focus light through the pupil on to the fundus.	The room is darkened before the examiner approaches the patient with the opthalmascope. Drops may be placed in the eye before this exam to dilate the eye and offer a wider area through which to view the fundus.
Visual acuity	Determine status of vision.	The Snellen chart is used. It is placed 20 feet from the patient, and first one eye is occluded and then the other eye is occluded. The person begins reading lines of letters that decrease in size. Visual acuity is expressed as a fraction for each eye. The numerator (top) figure indicates the distance between the patient and the chart. The denominator (bottom) figure expresses the distance at which the person could read at least half of the letters in the line correctly. Visual acuity of 20/20 in each eye is normal; vision of 20/200 is legally defined as blindness.	Explain the procedure to the patient. Have the patient hold the occluding card close to the nose so that the entire eye is covered. Start with the third line. If the patient cannot read that, progress upward; if the line is correctly read, go to the next line down; etc. Test the other eye. Record the findings.
Near vision test	Determine status of near vision.	The patient is a Jaeger's Test Type card with different sizes of type on it. One eye is occluded while the patient reads the lines of type. Determination of vision status is made on the basis of what a person with normal vision can read.	Explain that this is a simple test of vision to determine whether there are any problems that might require further testing.

(Table 30-3 continued)

TABLE 30-3 ◆ *Diagnostic Tests for Eye Problems* (Continued)			
Test	**Purpose**	**Description**	**Nursing Inplications**
Refraction	Determine amount of lens correction necessary to restore person's vision to as near normal as possible with glasses.	A series of glass lenses are placed in front of the patient's eyes to determine which lens provides the best vision correction. Each eye is tested separately.	A prescription for glasses will be written depending on the findings of the refraction test. The test may be performed for both near and far vision.
Intraocular pressure test	Determine the amount of pressure within the eye; aid in diagnosis of glaucoma.	A tonometer is used to measure the pressure. This may be a handheld instrument, but it usually is a device that measures pressure by taking a reading while air is directed at the eye by a pneumotonometer. Another type of tonometer is the applanation tonometer (Figure 30-4). Normal intraocular pressure is 15–21 mm Hg.	Explain that this is a test to determine whether a patient might have glaucoma. More than one reading on different days is necessary to confirm a diagnosis of glaucoma. If a diagnosis of glaucoma is made, medication can be prescribed to help control the intraocular pressure and preserve vision.
Slit lamp/ biomicroscopic examination	Examine the surface of the eye.	A beam of light is reduced to a narrow slit that illuminates only a small section of the eye, allowing examination of a thin section of the eye structures at a time.	Explain that this device helps detect "floaters" in the vitreous humor, abnormalities of the cornea and other structures of the eye. The eyes may be dilated with mydriatic drops for this test.
Topical dye	To detect abrasions of the cornea or the presence of a foreign body on the cornea.	Fluorescein dye drops are administered to the affected eye. The dye remains on the injured tissue or surrounds a foreign body. Such areas usually appear as green spots.	Explain the procedure and the rationale for the test. Warn that the drops may sting slightly for a few minutes. Give the patient a tissue to absorb the excess drops as they may stain clothing.
Fluorescein angiography	To detect tumors of the interior of the eye and to help diagnose and measure the extent of retinopathy.	An IV injection of sodium fluorescein is given. A short time later photographs of the fundus are taken with a special camera.	An IV injection is necessary. A signed permit is required to perform the procedure.

provides further information about diagnostic tests. See also Figures 30-3 and 30-4.

NURSING MANAGEMENT

◆Assessment

All nurses should be able to perform a basic eye examination. Only nurses who have had special training in ophthalmic nursing are qualified to conduct a complete eye assessment. Significant data can be obtained by nurses without such specialized education by taking an adequate history.

History Taking   Many systemic diseases, including acquired immunodeficiency syndrome (AIDS), hypertension, and diabetes mellitus, secondarily affect the eye and its functions. In the general assessment of any patient the nurse should be aware of the more obvious indications of an ophthalmic pathology, whether it be primary or secondary.

Normal vision depends in part on (1) adequately functioning nerve cells, including those in the retina as well as the optic nerve; (2) adequate circulation of blood to the retinal cells; and (3) intact and functioning structures of the eyeball itself.

A history of neurological disorders should be noted. Neuromuscular diseases are especially likely to cause diplopia, blurred vision, or inability to move the eyes. Endocrine disorders that secondarily affect the eyes include thyroid disease and diabetes mellitus. Acute hyperglycemia can alter the shape of the lens and temporarily cause blurred vision. **Prolonged hyperglycemia can adversely affect the blood vessels of the retina, causing bleeding and leading to loss of vision.** Liver and kidney failure can produce pathological changes in both neural and vascular structures within the eye. Retinal changes also can be caused by hypertension and atherosclerosis.

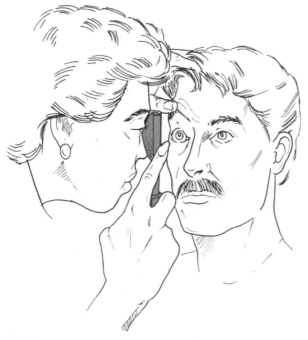

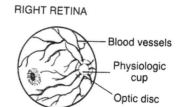

RIGHT RETINA

- Blood vessels
- Physiologic cup
- Optic disc

View of interior of eye and retina.

FIGURE 30-3 **Examination of the eye with an opthalmoscope.** (*Source:* Modified from Black, J. M., Matassarin-Jacobs, E. [1993]. *Luckmann and Sorensen's Medical–Surgical Nursing: A Psychophysiologic Approach,* 4th ed. Philadelphia: Saunders, p. 841.)

Some drugs are capable of producing either transient or permanent ocular changes that lead to disturbances in color vision and visual acuity and the formation of cataracts, retinopathy, and glaucoma. Among

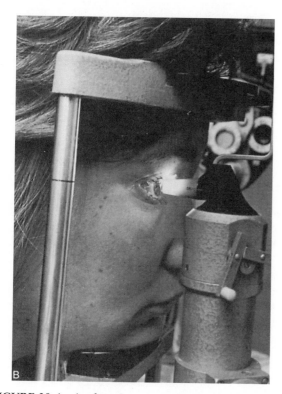

FIGURE 30-4 **Applanation tonometer.** (Photo by Ken Kasper; courtesy of Wills Eye Hospital, Philadelphia, PA.)

common drugs that have possible ocular side effects are digitalis leaf, corticosteroids, indomethacin (Indocin), and sulfisoxazole (Gantrisin).

A family history of eye disorders can be significant because disorders such as strabismus, retinitis pigmentosa, glaucoma, and cataracts tend to run in families or follow a pattern of inheritance.

Sometimes patients are not aware of gradual changes in vision, but have noticed that they have had more minor accidents lately, seem to be more easily fatigued, or are less interested in doing things that once gave them pleasure, such as sewing or some other hobby. Table 30-4 presents guidelines for history taking.

Physical Examination Observe for redness of the conjunctiva, swelling of the eyelids or in the periorbital space, excessive tearing, change in visual acuity, secretions and encrustations on the eyelids, abnormal position of the eyelid, and **exophthalmia** (protrusion of the eyeball) (Color Figure 21). Abnormalities of lid position are depicted in Table 30-5. *Xanthelasma,* soft, raised, yellow areas sometimes appear on the eyelid after age 50 (Color Figure 22). Signs and symptoms of selected eye diseases are listed in Table 30-6.

In addition to the more obvious signs of eye disease, visual impairment also can be assessed by noting the patient's head, hand, and eye movements. Tilting the head to one side to improve vision could mean that the patient has double vision or that one eye is much stronger than the other. Squinting could mean poor

The following questions should be asked when gathering history regarding an eye disorder:

- Have you noticed a change in your vision?
- Do you have any pain or discomfort in the eyes? Itching? Burning? Stinging? Excessive tearing or watering?
- Have you had any episodes of blurred vision? Double vision? or a loss in the field of vision? Blind spots? Floating spots?
- Do you have difficulty with vision at night?
- Is there any pain in the eyes when you are in bright light?
- Do you ever have headaches in the brow area?
- Do you see halos around lights?
- Have you ever injured an eye in any way?
- Do you experience frequent reddening of the eye (conjunctivitis)?
- Do you ever experience discharge or sticky matter in the eye?
- Do you find that your lids are crusty when you awaken?
- Do your eyes feel dry? Do you frequently use eye drops?
- Do you wear contact lenses? Use glasses?
- What medications do you take regularly?
- Is there any history of glaucoma in your family?
- Have you ever been told you have diabetes? Hypertension?
- When did you have your last eye examination?
- For those patients who have a previous visual loss: How do you cope with your loss of vision?

vision. Shading the eyes with the hands may indicate an increased sensitivity to light (**photophobia**).

Observation of the patient's ability to move his eyebrows and eyes can be helpful in diagnosing nerve damage. Inability to raise the eyebrows indicates damage to the facial nerve. Movement of the eyeball to direct the gaze is controlled by no less than six muscles, which are themselves under the control of three cranial nerves: the oculomotor nerve (third cranial), the trochlear nerve (fourth cranial), and the abducens nerve (sixth cranial).

◆ Nursing Diagnosis

Nursing diagnoses are based on the data obtained from assessment. The licensed practical nurse (LPN) collaborates with the RN in formulating the nursing care plan and selecting the nursing diagnoses. Some of the nursing diagnoses most frequently encountered in the care of patients with eye disease include:

- Visual sensory perceptual alteration related to decreased visual acuity.
- Risk for injury related to decreased visual field.
- Fear of blindness related to consequences of diabetic retinopathy.
- Impaired home maintenance management related to impaired vision.

TABLE 30-5 ◆ *Abnormalities of Lid Position*

Abnormality	Causes	Symptoms	Treatment
Entropion: inversion of lid margin; eyelids are turned inward toward eyeball so that lashes rub against it.	Scarring and contraction of skin near eyelid (*cicatricial entropion*); or aging of skin with laxness of tissues supporting the lid and contraction of obicularis muscle (*spastic entropion*).	Pain, tearing, redness, and corneal ulceration due to margin and eyelashes rubbing against cornea.	Splinting the lid, using a pressure patch, or taping lid into everted position. Surgical correction by tightening musculature and everting lid margin.
Ectropion: eversion or outward turning of the lower lid (Color Plate 30-2).	Aging and laxness of skin and muscle tissues, facial paralysis, edema of conjunctiva lining the lid, or contraction of scar tissue.	Irritation of palpebral conjunctiva, spilling of tears down the cheeks due to blocked outlet, irritation of skin of cheeks, symptoms of conjunctivitis.	Usually responds to patching of the eye. Surgical correction necessary if paralysis of orbicularis muscle is permanent or if there is severe scarring and contraction of skin near the lid.
Ptosis: drooping of the eyelid so that it partially or completely covers the cornea.	Congenital weakness of the levator superioris muscle or long-term presence of foreign body. One of first signs of myasthenia gravis.	Obvious drooping of eyelid. If not corrected in infants, can lead to blindness because light rays cannot enter and stimulate development of the eye. Patient may be observed tilting head back or raising eyebrows in an effort to see from under eyelids.	Surgical correction. Removal of foreign body, if that is the cause.

TABLE 30-6 ◆ *Clinical Signs and Symptoms of Selected Eye Diseases and Medical Treatment and Nursing Intervention*

Disease	Signs and Symptoms	Medical Treatment and Nursing Interventions
Blepharitis: Infection of glands and lash follicles along lid margin.	Itching, burning, sensitivity to light. Mucus discharge and scaling; eyelids crusted, glued shut, especially on awakening. Loss of eyelashes.	Warm compresses to soften secretions. Scrub eyelids with baby shampoo. Stroke sideways to remove exudate and scales. Antibiotic eyedrops. Systemic and topical antibiotics if skin is infected.
Chalazion: internal style; infection of meibomian gland.	Astigmatism or distorted vision, depending on size and location of chalazion. Small, hard tumor on eyelid.	Chalazion may require surgical excision and antibiotics to avoid chronic state and cyst formation.
Hordeolum: external style. Infected swelling near the lid margin on inside.	Sharp pain that becomes dull and throbbing. Rupture and drainage of pus bring relief. Localized redness and swelling of lid.	Hordeolum usually resolves spontaneously. Warm compresses qid for 10 to 15 min to bring stye to a head and hasten rupture. Caution patient never to squeeze swelling, as this could spread infection. Poor health status can predispose a person to recurrence of styes.
Conjunctivitis: inflammation of the conjunctiva. "Pink eye" is a specific type caused by chemical irritants, bacteria, or virus.	Varying degrees of pain and discomfort. Increased tearing and mucus production. Itching; sensation of a foreign body in the eye.	Depends on type of infecting organism. Antibiotic eyedrops and ointments. Special care when handling infective material.
Keratitis: inflammation of the cornea.	Varying degrees of pain and discomfort. Photophobia; blurred vision if center of cornea is affected.	Depends on specific causes. Could be allergy microbes, ischemia, or decreased lacrimation. Most superficial lesions are self-healing. Antibiotic eyedrops or ointment used for bacterial infections. Steroids can reduce inflammation and discomfort; however, herpes infection can rapidly worsen keratitis unless an antiviral agent is given simultaneously. Patient is encouraged to use good personal hygiene, frequent handwashing.
Corneal abrasion or ulceration	Moderate to severe pain and discomfort aggravated by blinking. History of trauma, contact lens wear.	Change or discontinue use of contact lens. Teach patient proper way to insert, remove, and care for contact lens. Caution not to moisten lens with saliva.

◆ Diversional activity deficit related to visual limitation.

◆ Knowledge deficit related to proper method and schedule of instillation of eye drops.

◆ Impaired home maintenance management related to visual loss.

◆ Planning

General goals for the patient experiencing a problem with the eye are:

◆ Promote optimal vision
◆ Prevent infection
◆ Prevent injury
◆ Promote coping with visual loss

◆ Knowledge for self-care to prevent deterioration of vision

Expected outcomes are individualized for each patient and are written for each nursing diagnosis. When a patient is visually impaired, the nurse must plan extra time to assist with personal care to allow the patient to perform as much self-care as possible. The instillation of preoperative eye drops is a very time-consuming nursing task. The nurse must plan for this when creating the work plan for the shift. Hands must be washed before and after instilling eye drops. Often an eye patch must be removed, and then a new one replaced after instilling eye medication. Planning also must be done to incorporate patient teaching on the administration of medication, self-care instructions for the patient with glaucoma, and postoperative instructions.

◆ Implementation

Nursing Interventions for the Visually Impaired
Considerable adjustments must be made by those who are deprived of optimum sight. A sense of hopelessness and despair may be experienced by those who have lost their eyesight. The patient goes through stages of grief in much the same way the dying person does. A different lifestyle must be learned, but it is not necessarily less meaningful.

Guidelines for Helping a Blind Person   *Remember that the person is blind, not deaf.* Speak normally.

Speak to the blind person as you enter the room, and do not touch him until after you have spoken to him. This prevents startling or frightening him when he may not have heard you enter the room.

Prevention of accidents is an important part of the care of the blind. Aside from the physical effects of bumping into objects or falling over them, the blind person also suffers from a loss of self-confidence and security if movement is not safe and independent. **Doors should be kept closed or completely open. They must never be left ajar.** If it is necessary to move any object in the patient's room, ask for consent and state its new location. *When you leave the room, tell the blind person that you are going.* This will prevent him from becoming frustrated by resuming a conversation only to find that no one is there.

Pity is neither expected nor appreciated by the blind. They only want to be treated as normal people and would prefer to ask for your help when they need it rather than have you do everything for them. If you are assigned to the care of a blind person, determine the amount of assistance the patient needs and wants. Do not assume that the person is helpless, but avoid neglect when help is needed.

When a blind or visually handicapped patient is admitted, *he will require special orientation to the room and surroundings.* If there is total blindness, describe the size of his room and the placement of furniture, using the bed as the focal point. An ambulatory patient can be walked around the room and to the bathroom to develop familiarity with the location of the commode, bath, and sink. As with any patient, show how to locate and use the call system, the radio, and the telephone if there is one at the bedside.

Most patients prefer to feed themselves if at all possible. However, it usually is necessary for the nurse to set up the meal tray of the visually handicapped patient, using the "clock" method for placement of food on the plate (Figure 30-5). The patient is told what food is in which area (i.e., "The potatoes are at 2 o'clock"). Setting up the meal tray includes opening containers of milk and juice, pouring coffee or tea, and cutting meat

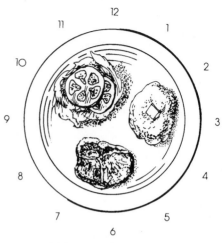

FIGURE 30-5   Clock system for food placement. (Telling the patient that the meat is at 6 o'clock, potato at 2 o'clock, and vegetable at 10 o'clock helps with location of items on the plate.)

into bite sizes, unless the patient is accustomed to doing these things.

Do not give a blind person a straw or drinking tube unless you are asked to, because it may be awkward to use. If you must feed the patient all of a meal, work slowly and calmly. Indicate about hot and cold foods on his tray, and alternate dishes rather than feeding all of one thing before offering another. Avoid talking too much, thus forcing the patient to either stop eating or answer you with a mouth full of food. Whenever possible, help the patient select finger foods such as sandwiches and raw fruit or vegetables from the menu. *Your goal is to help the patient maintain dignity and self-respect while meeting his personal needs.*

Think about . . . Can you think of three specific ways in which you can assist a blind patient who is admitted to the hospital maintain as much independence in this setting as possible?

Nursing Care of the Patient Having Eye Surgery
   Preoperative care.   Most eye surgery procedures are done on an outpatient basis unless the patient has other serious disorders such as cardiac arrhythmias, severe diabetes, or a chronic disability. Therefore a large part of nursing care is directed at discharge teaching for home care. One surgery that is performed as an inpatient procedure is a scleral buckle for retinal detachment. (See the section on retinal detachment.)

Stool softeners may be started a day or two before surgery to prevent constipation and the Valsalva maneuver postoperatively. Some physicians direct the patient to wash his face with surgical soap several times the evening and morning before surgery. The patient may be given instructions on the administration of eye drops the night before and the morning of surgery.

After admission, the patient is fully oriented to the outpatient surgery unit and given instructions about the layout of the room and area and the ways in which the nurse can be summoned. Siderails are usually necessary to prevent falls, and the patient should be cautioned against getting up without assistance. Preoperative eye drops and medications are instilled by the nurses in the outpatient surgery center the morning of surgery. Drugs must be given with extreme care and accuracy, especially if only one eye is affected.

> When the abbreviations "OD" (right eye) and "OS" (left eye) are used to designate the right eye and the left eye, the nurse must be sure that the medication is applied to the correct eye. The term "OU" means both eyes.

One way to remember this is to remember that in alphabetical order "OD" (right) comes before "OS" (left). Preoperative dilating (mydriatic) eye drops often are administered every 5 minutes for six doses. Other eye drops may be administered in between these doses. An IV infusion is started shortly before surgery.

Elder Care Point . . . Because the great majority of patients undergoing eye operations are elderly and therefore are most likely to be suffering from some additional chronic disease, the nurse must remember to apply the principles of geriatric nursing in administering care. Fear, anxiety over surgery, and confusion about the expected results of the surgery are all factors to be considered when preparing the patient for the operation. Instructions and information should be given both verbally and in writing. Measures to ensure patient safety are very important both pre- and postoperatively since vision is impaired.

Postoperative care. In caring for a patient undergoing any type of eye surgery, the key word is *gentleness*. The patient's head should not be jarred when transferring from the operating table or stretcher to the bed. Remember to speak before touching a patient who is blind or wearing bandages over the eyes.

Patients are usually kept in the recovery area of the Outpatient Surgery department for 2 to 3 hours postoperatively.

Nausea and subsequent vomiting can wreak havoc with delicate suture lines in the eye. **If the patient becomes nauseated, antiemetic medication should be administered immediately and all food and liquids withheld.**

> A sudden pain in the eye or change in vision may indicate hemorrhage and should be brought to the attention of the physician immediately.

An eye patch is usually placed over the eye that was operated on (Figure 30-6). If it is necessary to restrict movement of the eyes, then both eyes are patched. When placing a patch on the eye, the hands are washed, the skin of the forehead and cheek is cleansed with a skin prep solution or pad, and nonallergenic paper or other tape is prepared to secure the patch. Ask the patient to close both eyes and position the pad over the lid of the eye to be patched. Secure the patch by placing strips of tape diagonally over the patch from the cheek to the forehead. Use several strips of tape to ensure adhesiveness. If a pressure patch is needed (as in some retinal surgeries), two eye patches are used and the first one is folded in half, placed over the closed lid, and then the other patch is secured on top of the folded one. For further protection, or for sleeping, a plastic or metal eye shield may be placed over the patch; as healing occurs, the shield may be used over the eye without the underlying patch for sleeping. This is necessary for 2 to 6 weeks depending on the surgeon's instructions.

Instructions regarding postoperative medications and the times they are to be instilled are given before discharge. The patient or significant other is taught to wash the hands thoroughly, pull the lower lid of the eye downward while the patient is looking up (with the head tilted slightly upward), and squeeze the correct number of drops into the conjunctival sac without

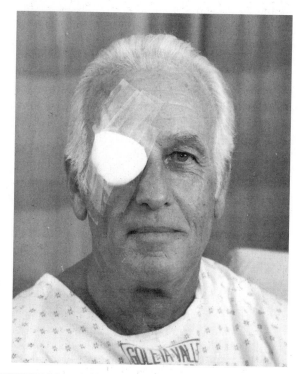

FIGURE 30-6   The eye is patched after surgery. (Photo by Glen Derbyshire; courtesy of Goleta Valley Cottage Hospital, Goleta, CA.)

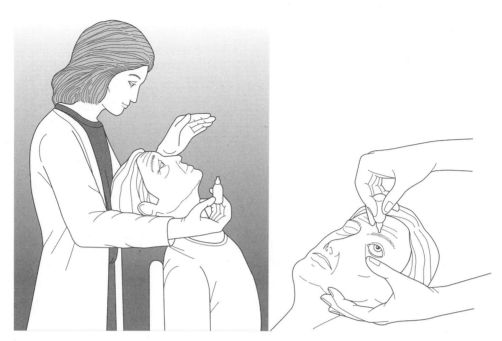

FIGURE 30-7   Placing eyedrops in the eye.

touching the tip of the medication container on the eye or lashes (Figure 30-7). The eye is to be closed gently so as not to squeeze all the medication out of it. Different types of eyedrop medications come with color-coded tops for easy identification. Eye drop bottles can be "labeled" by wrapping one, two, or three rubber bands around them so that the vision-impaired patient can differentiate one type of drop from another.

Should the patient need to stay in the hospital because of other problems, the nurse must be thoroughly familiar with his individual care needs. It should be known whether the patient can be turned on one or both sides or must remain flat on the back, can only be supine, whether pillows are allowed under the head, and how high the head of the bed may be raised. For certain types of retinal surgery, the head may need to be raised and positioned toward a particular side. If a gas bubble has been injected intraocularly, the patient is positioned supine toward one side or the other according to orders. If the patient is allowed out of bed, care must be taken not to jar the head or move too suddenly.

Sexual activity can usually be resumed in 1 to 8 weeks postoperatively, depending on the procedure performed. The surgeon will explain this to the patient. The nurse makes certain that the patient understands the time of the next appointment with the ophthalmologist. The patient and family should be encouraged to follow the physician's directions faithfully during the healing period at home so that nothing will jeopardize the success of the surgery.

Discharge planning for the patient having surgery from the outpatient department or the hospital is of utmost importance. Table 30-7 presents teaching points for home care.

TABLE 30-7 ◆ *Patient Education: Home Care After Eye Surgery*

Instructions for the patient and/or family caregiver:

◆ Always wash the hands before instilling medication. Be careful to check the label of the container of the medication to be certain it is the right medication. Do not contaminate the applicator tip of the medication.

◆ Instill only the number of drops ordered; apply pressure at the inner canthus to prevent systemic absorption; close the eye gently (do not squeeze the eye shut).

◆ Change the eye patch dressing at least once a day; change as needed to keep the area clean.

◆ Follow the medication schedule prescribed by the physician exactly. (Send home a written schedule.)

◆ Maintain designated head position and activity restrictions.

◆ Report signs of complications: sudden, increasing pain in the eye, which can indicate hemorrhage; purulent drainage; decreasing vision; signs of increased intraocular pressure, such as brow headache.

◆ Keep the follow-up appointment with the surgeon.

◆ Use caution to prevent water in the eye when showering or washing hair.

◆ Protect the eye during the day with glasses; use sunglasses for outside wear; wear a protective eye shield at night.

Care of an Artificial Eye   The procedure for cleansing and caring for an artificial eye is similar in many ways to care of dentures. Both require basic principles of cleanliness, careful handling, and proper storage. An artificial eye is very expensive and must be handled very carefully.

The artificial eye is cleansed with gentle soap and water, unless the patient, his family, or the physician directs otherwise. When the eye is to be reinserted, it should be cleansed again with soap and water. The patient's upper lid is lifted, and the eye is inserted with the notched end toward the nose. After the prosthesis is placed as far as possible under the upper lid, the lower lid is depressed allowing the eye to slip into place.

◆ Evaluation

Evaluation is based on reassessing data and determining whether expected outcomes have been met. This is an ongoing process. Some questions to be asked when gathering data for evaluation include: Is the patient compliant with the use of eye medications? Is an infection resolving? Is vision improving? If interventions have not been effective in helping the patient achieve expected outcomes, the plan of care should be altered.

COMMON DISORDERS OF THE EYE

The most common visual defects are those of refraction. This means that light rays entering the eye are not "refracted," or bent, at the correct angle and therefore do not focus on the retina. Errors of refraction may be caused by a number of structural defects within the eyeball itself. For example, if the eyeball is constructed so that the distance between the lens and retina is too short, the light rays focus behind the retina. This causes difficulty in seeing objects close at hand and is called farsightedness (**hyperopia**) (Figure 30-8).

If the opposite is true, and the eyeball is too elongated, the light rays will converge and focus in front of the retina. The individual then has difficulty seeing objects at a distance and is referred to as being nearsighted. Nearsightedness is called **myopia** (Figure 30-8).

Light rays from distant objects do not enter the eye at the same angle as light rays from near objects. When looking off into the distance and then quickly looking down at a book, the eyes must make an adjustment to the difference in the light rays entering the eye. This adjustment, which is called **accommodation**, is accomplished by ciliary muscles and ligaments that change the shape of the lens, making it more rounded or flatter, thereby allowing light rays to fall on the retina (Figure 30-9).

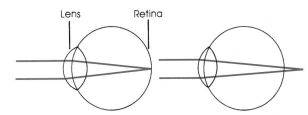

A The lens bends light rays so that they focus directly on the retina.

B Hyperopia. The lens is too close to the retina; light rays converge at a point beyond the retina.

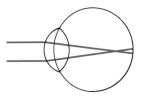

C Myopia. The lens is too far away from the retina; light rays converge before they reach the retina.

FIGURE 30-8   (A). Normal vision. (B). Hyperopia. (C). Myopia.

With age the ciliary muscles become less elastic and cannot readily accommodate the needs of distant and near vision. Hardening of the ciliary muscles occurs in many people over 40 years of age and is known as **presbyopia**. Bifocal glasses are usually prescribed for this condition because they allow for two sets of lenses

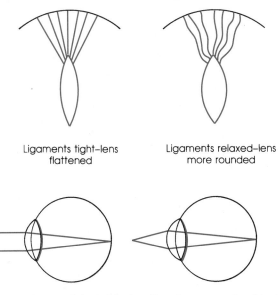

Ligaments tight–lens flattened

Ligaments relaxed–lens more rounded

Rays from a *distant* object are focused on the retina by a flattened lens

Rays from a *nearby* object are focused on the retina by a more rounded lens

FIGURE 30-9   Flattening and rounding of the lens during accommodation.

in one pair of glasses, one for viewing distant objects and one for seeing close objects.

Astigmatism is a visual defect resulting from a warped lens or an irregular curvature of the cornea, either of which will prevent the horizontal and vertical rays from focusing at the same point on the retina. Actually, very few people have perfectly shaped eyeballs, and thus there are very few who do not have some degree of astigmatism. If the astigmatism is very slight, the eye can accommodate for its imperfection by changing the shape of the lens. If there is a serious error of refraction, the eyes will tire very easily or the person will have defective vision because the eyes cannot change the shape of the lens enough to compensate for the abnormality.

Serious errors of refraction are treated with prescription artificial lenses and either eyeglasses or contact lenses that are fitted so that the light rays are brought into proper focus on the retina. In recent years, advances have been made in refractive surgery that permit correction of refraction problems for some people. Those who are nearsighted (myopic) can undergo *photorefractive keratectomy (PRK)*. An excimer laser is used to remove a thin layer of tissue from the cornea. This corrects the excessive curvature of the cornea that is interfering with the proper focus of light rays through the lens. The procedure takes less than a minute to perform; visual improvement is apparent within 3 to 5 days.

◆ Cataract

The word *cataract* literally means waterfall. It is used to designate an opacity of the lens that produces an effect similar to one a person would get when looking through a sheet of falling water (Color Figure 23). **A cataract causes a blurring of vision, because the lens, which is normally transparent, becomes cloudy and opaque.** Cataracts are sometimes present at birth *(congenital cataracts)*, but they most often occur as a result of aging and are found in people over the age of 50 *(adult-onset cataracts)*.

Traumatic cataracts may occur from a physical blow or exposure to sunlight, heat, or chemical toxins. **Cigarette smoking increases the risk developing cataract. Heavy drinking also is implicated.** Sometimes cataracts occur again after surgery if the lens capsule is left intact during original cataract surgery.

Symptoms and Diagnosis. In addition to the blurred vision that is typical of opacity of the lens, there may be distortion of vision when looking at distant objects. Vision may be better in low light when the pupil is dilated because there is more light transmitted around the opacity. Uncomplicated cataracts are usually painless, but the patient may have **photophobia** (intolerance of light). Assessment may reveal the following symptoms:

- Hazy, blurred, or double vision.
- Increasing complaints about glare.
- Increasing nearsightedness.
- Complaints that colors are faded or appear yellowish or brownish.
- Desire for increased light by which to read.
- Difficulty with night vision.
- Frequent need for eyeglass prescription change.

The loss of vision associated with cataracts is progressive and sometimes is partially due to secondary glaucoma. As an untreated cataract progresses, the lens of the eye becomes cloudy or milky white, then may turn yellow, and eventually become brown or black (Color Plate 30-3). The patient may have difficulty discriminating colors.

Diagnosis of a cataract is confirmed by examining the dilated pupil with a slit lamp, which enables the examiner to see opacities more clearly. Glaucoma should first be ruled out as a possible cause of the symptoms.

Treatment. **Cataract surgery is performed when the loss of vision greatly affects the quality of the person's life.** The only effective method of treating cataracts is surgical removal of the affected lens; cataract surgery is the most commonly performed surgical procedure in the United States. Surgical techniques are (1) *extracapsular extraction,* in which the lens capsule is excised and the lens removed along with the anterior portion of the lens capsule; and (2) *intracapsular extraction,* in which both the capsule and the lens are removed. Extracapsular extraction is most frequently performed because it allows an intraocular lens to be inserted inside the remaining capsule. A choice of lens for near vision or far vision is made by the patient. After surgery further correction of vision needed is by regular eyeglasses or contact lenses. Vision is usually fully recovered within 3 months of surgery. See Nursing Care Plan 30-1.

One technique for intracapsular cataract extraction (ICCE) utilizes *cryosurgery,* in which the lens is frozen by a super-cooled probe and then removed. *Phacoemulsification,* in which the tissue is pulverized and the debris is removed by suction, is often used for extracapsular cataract extraction (ECCE). These outpatient surgical procedures are performed under conscious sedation and local anesthesia. An intraocular lens implant is placed after extracapsular extraction. With the rising costs of medical care in the United States, there is talk of Medicare restricting payment for cataract surgery to only one eye.

When no intraocular lens is implanted, absence of the lens is corrected with the use of contact lenses or cataract eyeglasses. Cataract eyeglasses are used only by

Nursing Care Plan 30-1

Selected nursing diagnoses, goals/expected outcomes, nursing interventions and evaluations for a patient having a cataract extraction

Situation: Mrs. Fort, age 79, is admitted to the outpatient surgery unit for extraction of a senile cataract of the left eye with lens implant. The vision in her right eye also is affected by a cataract, but the visual loss is not as severe in that eye. Mrs. Fort suffers from a crippling osteoarthritis of the hands, but her general health is good. She is well-oriented, outgoing, and physically active. She lives alone in an apartment building for retired senior citizens. Her daughter and son-in-law live nearby and are in daily contact with her. Mrs. Fort has only been in the hospital once in her life for pneumonia and is concerned about what to expect pre- and postoperatively.

Nursing Diagnosis	Goals/Expected Outcomes	Nursing Interventions	Evaluation
Knowledge deficit regarding pre- and postoperative procedures and care. SUPPORTING DATA "I have never had surgery before."	Patient will verbalize preoperative routine activities and postoperative procedures and expectations.	Teach patient and daughter about eye medications to be used at home and how to instill them; how to dress and shield eye properly, how to remove bandage without contaminating eye.	Patient and daughter demonstrate proper way to instill eyedrops and apply eye patch and shield; patient states she understands pre- and postop routine and activities.
Risk for injury related to postoperative complications such as hemorrhage and increased intraocular pressure. SUPPORTING DATA Undergoing cataract extraction; hemorrhage and increased intraocular pressure are potential complications.	Intraocular hemorrhage will not occur, and there will not be an increase in intraocular pressure.	Teach signs and symptoms of complications that are to be reported to physician immediately: increasing eye pain, purulent discharge, decreasing vision, fever or chills, increasing brow headache. Instruct to refrain from straining at stool; encourage to use milk of magnesia or stool softener to prevent this as needed. Wash hands thoroughly before instilling eye medications or changing dressing; teach patient and daughter to wash hands before approaching eye area. Demonstrate how to put on eye shield for sleep. Instruct her to avoid rapid or sudden movements and bending from the waist. Instruct to take medication immediately for nausea and vomiting. Remind patient not to lie on affected side. Encourage her to seek assistance with ambulation while vision is blurred.	No complaints of increased eye pain; dressing dry and intact; no sign of complication; continue plan.
Self-care deficit related to disabilities imposed by osteoarthritis. SUPPORTING DATA Has severe osteoarthritis of the hands with limited dexterity.	Assistance with administration of postoperative eye medications and eye care will be given by daughter.	Explain pre- and postoperative routine to patient. Include daughter in all teaching regarding postoperative care; send home dosage chart and schedule for all postoperative medications. Teach patient and daughter about eye medications to be used at home and how to instill them; how to dress and shield eye properly; how to remove bandage without pressing on eye; importance of hand washing and not rubbing the eye and the importance of follow-up with physician.	Daughter verbalizes correct schedule for medications; lists signs of complications to report to doctor; states she understands postop and home care.

athose patients who cannot manage to insert and care for contact lenses.

Nursing intervention.   The patient must be told that there is a period of visual adjustment after cataract surgery. Postoperative care of the patient following implantation of an intraocular lens does not differ greatly from that of a patient with simple cataract extraction. The surgeon may prescribe miotic eyedrops after surgery to constrict the pupil and lessen the danger of lens dislocation. Teaching points for home care after cataract extraction are presented in Table 30-7.

Think about... Can you identify patients who should be carefully assessed for signs and symptoms of cataract?

◆ Glaucoma

The term *glaucoma* comprises a complex group of disorders that involve many different pathological changes and symptoms, but have in common an increased intraocular pressure (IOP) that damages the optic disc, causing atrophy and loss of peripheral vision. Glaucoma may come on slowly and cause irreversible visual loss without presenting any other noticeable symptoms, or it may appear abruptly and produce blindness in a matter of hours. The amount of increased pressure that causes damage differs from one person's eye to another. Blindness is preventable if the disorder is treated early.

The IOP is determined by the rate of *aqueous humor* production and the outflow of the aqueous from the eye. Aqueous humor is produced in the ciliary body

and flows out of the eye through the canal of Schlemm into the venous system. An imbalance may occur from overproduction by the ciliary body or by obstruction of outflow (Figure 30-10). Increased IOP greater than 23 mm Hg requires thorough evaluation. Increased IOP restricts the blood flow to the optic nerve and the retina. Ischemia causes these structures to lose their function gradually. **The vision impairment from damage to the optic nerve or retina is irreversible; it is permanent.** The terms *wide* and *narrow* (closed) *angle* refer to the angle width between the cornea and the iris. *Acute* and *chronic* refer to either the onset or duration of the problem.

Glaucoma can be present at birth or can develop at any age. It can result from genetic predisposition, trauma, or from another disorder of the eye. Glaucoma frequently is a manifestation of diseases and pathologies in other body systems. There are two major types of glaucoma: closed-angle (acute) glaucoma, and open-angle glaucoma. These two major types differ in their clinical signs and symptoms, treatment, and effects on vision.

Closed-Angle Glaucoma

Signs and Symptoms.   Closed-angle, or acute, glaucoma is a medical emergency in which there is severe pain in the eye accompanied by the appearance of colored halos around lights, blurred vision, and pain in and around the eye. Nausea and vomiting may occur. The cause of closed-angle glaucoma is the position of the iris, which lies too close to the drainage canal and bulges forward against the cornea, blocking the drainage of aqueous humor. The IOP rises suddenly, some-

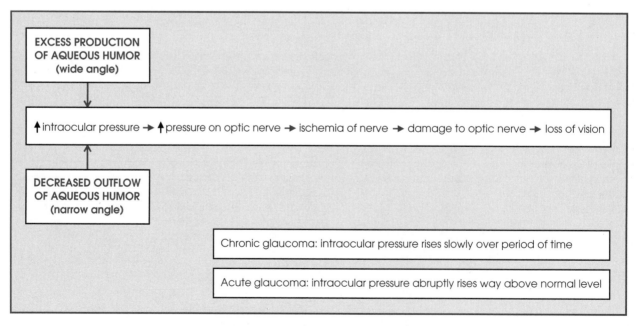

FIGURE 30-10   Pathophysiology of glaucoma.

times reaching a pressure of 50 to 70 mm Hg. Relief of the situation must be prompt, or damage to the optic nerve will cause blindness in the affected eye.

Treatment. Emergency treatment in closed-angle glaucoma consists of measures to reduce IOP as quickly as possible. During the attack, drugs such as pilocarpine, topical epinephrine, and acetazolamide are used IV. Surgery is performed as soon as inflammation subsides to relieve pressure against the optic nerve endings. *Trabeculectomy, laser trabeculoplasty,* or other procedures that allow filtering of the aqueous humor from the anterior chamber into the subconjunctival space are performed. If these procedures fail, sometimes *cyclocryotherapy* (the application of a freezing tip) may be used on the ciliary body to decrease the aqueous production.

Open-Angle Glaucoma Open-angle, or chronic, glaucoma, in which there is no angle closure, is much more insidious and more common, occurring in about 90% of the people with glaucoma. It often is an inherited disorder that causes degenerative changes in the aqueous humor outflow tracts. It usually is bilateral and can progress to complete blindness without ever producing an acute attack. Its symptoms are relatively mild, and many patients are not aware that anything is wrong until vision has been seriously impaired (Table 30-8).

Diagnosis. People at high risk for glaucoma are (1) diabetics; (2) blacks (at least five times as many blacks as nonblacks have glaucoma-related blindness); and (3) individuals with a family history of glaucoma.

A commonly used screening technique for early detection of glaucoma is to measure IOP with an air tonometer. A puff of air is directed at the cornea, which causes a momentary indentation while a pressure reading is taken. The test is painless, and nothing but the air touches the eye. Verification of the diagnosis of glaucoma may require the use of a more complex instrument called an *applanation tonometer* (Figure 30-4). The cornea is flattened and pressure is measured with a slit lamp biomicroscope.

TABLE 30-8 ◆ *Patient Education: Danger Signals of Glaucoma*

The National Society for the Prevention of Blindness lists the following symptoms as danger signals of open-angle glaucoma:

- Glasses, even new ones, don't seem to clarify vision.
- Blurred or hazy vision that clears up after a while.
- Trouble in getting used to darkened rooms, such as in movie theaters.
- Seeing rainbow-colored rings around lights.
- Narrowing of vision at the sides of one or both eyes.

Treatment. The initial treatment of choice for chronic (open-angle) glaucoma is medication rather than surgery (Table 30-9). If drugs are not effective or if they produce worrisome side effects, surgery is performed.

Drugs prescribed are intended to enhance aqueous humor outflow, decrease its production, or both. They do this by constricting the pupil (miotics) or by inhibiting the formation of aqueous humor. Commonly used miotics are pilocarpine hydrochloride (Isopto Carpine, Pilocar, Spersacarpine). Miotics cause blurred vision for 1 to 2 hours after use. Adjustment to dark rooms is difficult because of pupil constriction. Pilocarpine is available in an eye medication disk that resembles a contact lens. The disk is inserted into the conjunctival sac in a patient's lower eyelid, where it can remain for up to 7 days. The medication is slowly released. Use of the disk does not prevent the wearing of contact lenses. Drugs that decrease the formation of aqueous humor are beta-adrenergic–blocking agents, such as latanoprost (Xalatan), timolol (Timoptic) and levobunolol (Betagan). Carbonic anhydrase inhibitors also reduce aqueous humor production and include acetazolamide (Acetazolam, Diamox), dorzolamide (TruSopt) and methazolamide (Neptazane). Epinephrine (0.5%–2.0%) and dipivefrin hydrochloride (Propine) also decrease aqueous humor production. Diuretics may be prescribed to reduce the production of aqueous humor fluid. Not all diuretics reduce IOP, and a substitute should not be used for the specific drug prescribed.

Whenever glaucoma is being managed by medication, the patient must continue the eyedrops and oral medications on an uninterrupted basis. Patients admitted to the hospital for disorders other than glaucoma often are allowed to keep their glaucoma medication at the bedside if they are able to administer it themselves.

When drugs do not control glaucoma and increased intraocular pressure persists, surgery is an alternative. The goal is to create openings so that excess fluid can escape. A laser is used to create evenly spaced openings in the collecting meshwork (trabeculoplasty) to facilitate aqueous humor drainage in open-angle or chronic glaucoma (Figure 30-11). Filtering procedures such as *trephination, sclerectomy,* or *sclerostomy* create outflow channels from the anterior chamber to the subconjunctival space. Because scarring closes the openings in about 25% of the patients, an antimetabolite such as 5-fluorouracil may be injected subconjunctivally to inhibit fibroblast growth and decrease scarring. If all other surgical procedures fail, the ciliary body may be treated by applying a freezing tip *(cyclocryotherapy).* This permanently damages cells in the ciliary body and decreases the production of aqueous.

Laser surgery is performed with conscious sedation. The patient may experience a mild headache and blurring of vision during the first 24 hours. There is a

TABLE 30-9 ◆ *Pharmacological Management of Eye Disorders*		
Classification	**Examples**	**Action/Nursing Implications**
Glaucoma		
Miotics	Cholinergics: pilocarpine hydrochloride (Isopto-Carpine), pilocarpine nitrate (Ocusert Pilo-20, Pilo-40), carbachol (Miostat)	Constrict the pupil, promoting outflow of aqueous humor and reducing intraocular pressure. Reduces visual acuity in dim light; advise to avoid driving at night. Ocusert is placed in conjunctival sac and replaced weekly.
	Cholinesterase inhibitors: physostigmine salicylate (Isopto-Eserine), demecarium bromide (Humorsol), isofluorphate (Floropryl)	Produce miosis, increase aqueous humor outflow, and decrease intraocular pressure; avoid touching tip of bottle to eye; moisture may interfere with drug potency.
	Beta-adrenergic blockers: timolol maleate (Timoptic), betaxolol (Betoptic), levobunolol (Betagan), metipranolol (OptiPranolol), carteolol (Ocupress)	Reduce production of aqueous humor, thereby reducing intraocular pressure. Betoptic reduces intraocular hypertension. Monitor pulse and blood pressure during initiation of therapy. Blurred vision decreases with continued use. Use beta-blockers cautiously in patients with a history of asthma.
Carbonic anhydrase inhibitors	Action unknown: latanaprost (Xalatan), acetazolaminde (Diamox), dichlorphenamide (Daranide), methazolamide (Neptazane), dorzolamide (TruSopt)	Interfere with carbonic acid production, thereby decreasing aqueous humor formation and decreasing intraocular pressure. Taken orally or as eyedrops (TruSopt). When taken orally, these drugs have a diuretic action; observe for dehydration and postural hypotension. Monitor electrolytes. Confusion may occur in the elderly. Check interaction with other drugs patient is receiving.
Sympathomimetics	Epinephrine (Epitrate), dipivefrin (Propine)	Reduces intraocular pressure by increasing aqueous outflow. May cause brow ache, headache, eye irritation, and blurred vision. Used for open-angle glaucoma only. May cause tachycardia and rise in blood pressure.
Drugs used to facilitate diagnosis and surgery of the eye		
Cycloplegics and mydriatics anticholinergic agents	Atropine (Atropisol), cyclopentolate (Cyclogyl), homatropine (Isopto Homatropine), scopolamine (Isopto Hyoscine), tropicamide (Mydriacyl)	Dilate the pupils and paralyze the muscles of accommodation causing *mydriasis* and *cycloplegia.* Mydriasis facilitates observation of the eye's interior during an examination. Cycloplegia prevents movement of the lens during assessment of the eye.
Adrenergic agonists	Phenylephrine (Iospto Frin)	Induces mydriasis by action on the muscle of the iris. Causes blurred vision. Photophobia may be eased by using dark glasses.
Staining solution	Fluorescein sodium	Turns corneal scratches bright green; a green ring surrounds foreign bodies. Dye will filter through the lacrimal duct into the nasal secretions.
Anti-infective optic medications		
Antibiotics	Gentamicin sulfate (Garamycin Ophthalmic), erythromycin (Ilotycin), polymyxin B sulfate (Neomycin sulfate, Bacitracin), sulfonamides (Sodium sulamyd, gantrisin)	Used to treat infection or for prophylaxis. Caution patient to use a clean washcloth and towel on the face each time to prevent reinfection.
Antifungal	Natamycin (Natacyn Opthalmic)	To treat Fusarium. Caution as above.
Antivirals	Idoxuridine (IDV, Stoxil)	Store in refrigerator. Do not use with boric acid. If no improvement, discontinue after 1 week.
	Vidarabine (Vira-A Opthalmic)	Effective against DNA viruses; used for keratoconjunctivitis.

General guidelines for administering eye drops
- Wash hands before administering eye drops, and explain the procedure.
- Position the patient supine or with head tilted back, looking up at the ceiling.
- Provide a tissue for the patient to hold to blot gently excess fluid and keep if from running down the face.
- Verify the medication against the order one last time, and *consciously review which eye the drops are intended for.* Verify correct identification of the patient.
- Put on gloves.
- Remove the eye patch, if one is in place, and gently cleanse the closed eye with cotton and gauze moistened with irrigating solution or water if exudate is present.
- Remove gloves and rewash the hands.
- Remove the cap of the container, and place it so that the inside of the cap does not become contaminated.
- Pull the lower lid of the eye downward to expose the conjunctival sac.

TABLE 30-9 ✦ *Pharmacological Management of Eye Disorders* (Continued)		
Classification	**Examples**	**Action/Nursing Implications**

General guidelines for administering eye drops *(Continued)*

- Place pressure with another finger over the lacrimal duct at the inner canthus of the eye if you do not wish the medication to be absorbed systemically.
- Carefully drop the correct number of eye drops into the conjunctival sac without allowing the top of the dropper to touch the eye or surrounding tissue.
- Release the eye lid and ask the patient to close the eye gently without squeezing it shut (squeezing forces the medication out of the eye area). Direct the patient to rotate the eyeball while the lid is shut to distribute the medication over the eye surface.
- Instruct to blot the eye gently with the tissue to absorb expelled fluid.
- Repatch the eye if needed.

possibility that IOP may increase because of an inflammatory response. **Increasing pain in the eye should be reported to the ophthalmologist immediately.** The patient should be instructed to prevent increasing the venous pressure in the head, neck, and eyes by avoiding the Valsalva maneuver, not bending over, keeping the head up, and not making any sudden movements. A stool softener is given to prevent constipation. Strenuous exercise is to be avoided for 3 weeks. The head of the bed should be elevated 15 to 20 degrees to decrease pressure within the eyes during sleep. Elevated IOP will persist for a week or so in some patients. Glaucoma

medications are continued to meet the patient's individual needs. The patient must understand the importance of frequent checkups and the necessity of consistently following instructions. In other words, the surgical procedure may relieve the immediate problem of greatly increased IOP, but does not always eliminate the need for medication.

Nursing intervention. Education of the patient and his family is a major aspect of care, because 90% of all cases of glaucoma are chronic conditions for which there usually is no permanent cure. Failure to follow the prescribed treatment regimen to control of glaucoma

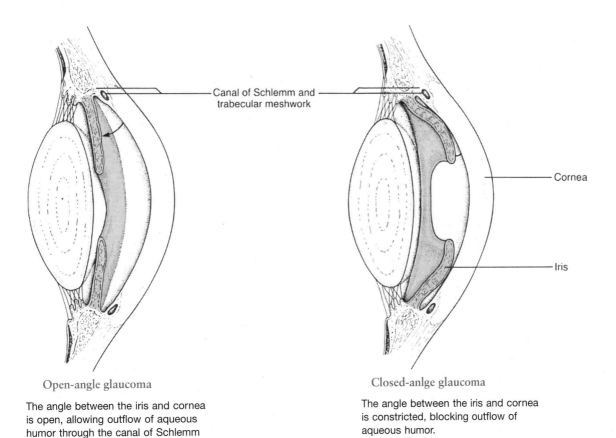

Open-angle glaucoma

The angle between the iris and cornea is open, allowing outflow of aqueous humor through the canal of Schlemm and the trabecular meshwork.

Closed-anlge glaucoma

The angle between the iris and cornea is constricted, blocking outflow of aqueous humor.

FIGURE 30-11 Comparison of open-angle (wide, chronic) and closed-angle (narrow, acute) glaucoma. (*Source:* Lehne, R. A. [1994]. *Pharmacology for Nursing Care,* 2nd ed. Philadelphia: Saunders, p. 877.)

and neglecting to maintain regular contact with the physician can result in progressive loss of vision and eventual blindness.

The patient who has glaucoma needs to be fully informed about the nature of this disorder, how it can affect vision, the treatments available, and the expected result of those treatments. An analogy that can be used to explain the nature of the disorder is to compare the eye to a sink with an open faucet (the ciliary processes), a drain (angle), and pipes (trabecular structures). As long as water flows into and out of the sink at the same rate, there is no problem. If something blocks the drain or the pipes, the water will fill the sink beyond its holding capacity. Treatment with miotics helps keep the pipes open so that drainage is possible; beta-blockers and diuretics can slow down the rate at which water flows from the tap. If the medications do not work or the sink suddenly is blocked by a clogged pipe, it may be necessary for the surgeon to clear the drainage system so that the water can drain from the sink.

In addition to learning about the nature of glaucoma and the expected results of prescribed treatments, the patient also must be made aware of the possibility of vision loss if the condition is not managed. **Teaching should emphasize that glaucoma medications prevent further vision loss but cannot restore vision.** This must be done with tact and sensitivity for the patient's feelings. The information should never be presented in such a way that the patient feels threatened or becomes so fearful that he is unable to participate in the management of his disorder. Table 30-10 summarizes a teaching plan for patients with glaucoma.

◆ Retinal Detachment

Retinal detachment is actually not a detachment of the whole retina but a separation of the sensory layers of the

---

TABLE 30-10 ◆ *Patient Education: The Patient with Glaucoma*

- ◆ Signs of IOP: pain in eye, redness, tearing, blurred vision, halos around lights, frequent need for change in eyeglasses.
- ◆ Measures to prevent increase in IOP: low-sodium diet, little caffeine, prevent constipation and Valsalva maneuver, decrease stress.
- ◆ Need to take prescribed medications and refrain from taking over-the-counter or other medications without physician's knowledge. Glaucoma medication must be take regularly for life.
- ◆ Use good aseptic technique when instilling eye medication.
- ◆ Wear ID tag or bracelet stating "Glaucoma" and carry card in wallet that states what medications are being taken.
- ◆ Keep extra bottle of eye medication on hand. Carry eyedrops.
- ◆ Maintain close medical follow-up with physician.
- ◆ Practice safety habits; avoid night driving if possible.

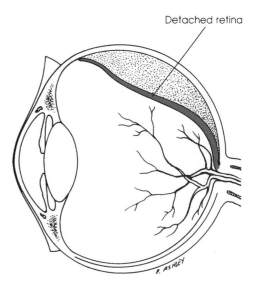

FIGURE 30-12   Retinal detachment.

retina from the pigmented epithelial layer, the choroid. Retinal detachment can cause vitreous fluid to leak under the retina, separating a portion of it from the vascular wall and thereby depriving it of its blood supply (Figure 30-12).

Retinal detachments often are classified as either primary or secondary. Primary retinal detachment is the result of spontaneous or degenerative changes in the retina or the vitreous. Secondary retinal detachment is associated with mechanical trauma, inflammation within the eye, or some other ophthalmic disorder, such as diabetic or hypertensive retinopathy. Retinal detachments frequently occur in persons with myopia. The incidence of retinal detachment increases dramatically after 40 years of age and is most common in persons between 50 and 60 years of age.

Symptoms and Diagnosis.   Onset can be either gradual or sudden, depending on the cause and extent of the detachment and location of the area involved. The patient may see flashes of colored light and then, days or weeks later, notice cloudy vision or loss of central vision. Another common symptom is the sensation of spots or moving particles (floaters) in the field of vision. In severe cases, there may be complete loss of vision.

Diagnosis of detached retina can be made with a direct ophthalmoscope, but it is greatly simplified by a stereoscopic indirect ophthalmoscope. This instrument permits visualization of the entire retina and produces an image of the retina with less magnification and distortion than the direct ophthalmoscope. Ultrasound can be used to detect retinal detachment when the eye is clouded by opacity from cataract or hemorrhage.

Treatment.   Retinal holes and tears sometimes can be repaired on an outpatient basis with laser therapy that creates an inflammatory reaction, causing the layers to adhere during healing. Those located in the posterior fundus can be coagulated and sealed with a laser beam or photocoagulator. Peripheral retinal holes through which no fluid has leaked can be closed by applying a freezing probe (cryotherapy). The frozen area scars over in a few days, and the hole is thus sealed.

A third procedure, called *scleral buckling*, requires more extensive surgery. In effect, it places the retinal breaks in contact with the pigmented epithelial layer. Adhesions are formed that bind the sensory, epithelial layers and choroid together. Prior to the procedure, air or gas is injected into the eye to apply pressure on the retina from the interior of the eye. This helps hold the layers together during healing.

In some instances when hemorrhage into the vitreous obstructs vision, the surgeon may perform a closed vitrectomy during retinal repair. The purpose of this procedure is to remove the cloudy vitreous humor and stabilize the retina against the choroid. Inert gas or air are used to fill the space until aqueous humor eventually refills the area.

Nursing intervention. Positioning of the patient and the level of activity allowed after surgery are prescribed by the surgeon. The head is positioned so that the area repaired is dependent, preventing the pull of gravity from disrupting the surgical site. The designated position for the head also is calculated to position the air or gas bubble, if one was used, in the best place to apply pressure to the retina. This requires a supine/lateral position for at least 16 out of 24 hours a day. Intraocular pressure is monitored closely for at least 24 hours. Vision does not return immediately because of postoperative swelling and the effects of the dilating drops. Vision improves on a gradual basis over several weeks to months. The eyes may both be patched, or pinhole occluders may be worn for 5 or 6 days. Eye patches are changed at least once a day. Several types of eye drops may be ordered for postoperative use as well as an antibiotic ointment. Strict asepsis is observed when instilling eye drops and ointment.

There usually is some degree of pain after all types of retinal surgery. Acetaminophen with codeine often is prescribed for this. If the patient is allergic to codeine, extra-strength Tylenol is usually sufficient to control the pain.

Flashing lights are common after retinal surgery for the first few weeks. These decrease over 2 to 6 months; if they worsen within several weeks of surgery, the doctor should be notified. Light sensitivity is common in both eyes after surgery and may cause tearing. This gradually lessens over a period of 4 to 6 weeks. Dark sunglasses when out of doors helps eliminate this problem. A moderate amount of discharge from the eye is not unusual; it should be yellowish or pink-tinged. If the amount of discharge increases markedly or is accompanied by severe pain, or if it has a foul smell or a greenish tinge, infection may be present; notify the surgeon. Cleanse the eyelid with a gauze pad or cotton ball moistened with irrigating solution or tap water. Wipe from the inner to the outer area of the eye.

The patient is allowed to sponge-bathe, brush teeth, shave, and comb hair as long as care is taken not to get water in the affected eye. At discharge the patient is cautioned to avoid heavy lifting and vigorous activity for several weeks. Eye glasses are worn during the day for protection, and the eye shield is worn at night after an eye patch is no longer necessary. Instructions for home care are listed in Table 30-11.

Think about . . . How do the signs and symptoms of glaucoma and cataract differ?

Retinopathy   The two major causes of retinopathy are diabetes mellitus and hypertension. Years of elevated blood pressure cause retinal vasospasm, which damages and narrows the retinal arterioles, thereby decreasing the blood supply to the retina.

Diabetic patients experience two different forms of retinopathy: proliferative and nonproliferative retinopathy. In the nonproliferative type of retinopathy, microaneurysms develop on the retinal blood vessels. These eventually swell and rupture, causing hemorrhage into the vitreous, which interferes with vision. The proliferative form of retinopathy occurs later in the course of diabetes. New blood vessels grow from the existing retinal vessels in a process called *neovascularization*. The new vessels are thinner and rupture more easily, causing hemorrhage. The blood from the hemorrhage causes scarring, which also interferes with vision.

Control of blood glucose levels is very important to prevent excessive diabetic retinopathy. There is no other known way to halt the process. The microaneurysms and the neovascularized vessels are treated with laser photocoagulation therapy to prevent hemorrhage and the consequent scarring and loss of vision. Vitrectomy also can be done if hemorrhage has caused serious impairment of vision.

Research is under way to determine whether a deficiency of insulin-like growth factor (IGF), a hormone that helps maintain nerve function, rather than uncontrolled glucose levels is the cause of diabetic retinopathy. If so, IGF injections may prevent the problem.

◆ Common Corneal Disorders

Keratitis   Keratitis is an inflammation of the cornea caused by irritation or infection. Patients who have had a stroke may develop irritation of the cornea because the eyelid does not close normally. Keratitis may occur in a comatose patient who is not receiving proper eye care. Some people with exophthalmos develop this disorder. Infection caused by bacteria, fungi, or protozoa also is a frequent cause of keratitis. Such an

TABLE 30-11 ◆ *Patient Education: Home Care Instructions for Retinal Surgery or Vitrectomy*

Instructions will vary if the patient has a gas bubble that was injected intraocularly. Positioning and activity are more restricted in this instance.

Activity

Restrict activity according to physician's instructions. Bedrest with bathroom privileges for the first few days is usual. The head may need to be positioned to the left or right most of the time. A head down or semi-prone position to the right or left will be required for the majority of the time if a gas bubble was injected into the eye.

The following activities are allowed immediately after discharge:
- Watching television from a distance of at least 10 feet.
- Tub bath or shower, using extreme care not to get soap or water into the eyes. Take care not to fall.
- Walking outdoors with the guidance of a companion.
- Reading for brief periods.
- Gentle shampooing of hair with head tilted backward and care not to get soap or water into the eyes *unless a gas bubble is present in the eye.*
- Riding in a car as a passenger, *except if a gas bubble is present in the eye.*

Eye Care

The operated eye is to be patched at all times and protected by an eye shield or glasses until you are told you may leave the eye uncovered. A patch or shield may still be recommended for use while sleeping. The eye patch is removed only to administer eye drops or ointment. The eyelid may be cleansed with cotton or gauze moistened with irrigating solution. Each time the patch is changed, check the movement of the eyeballs under the lids. Gently retract the upper lid, and look down as far as possible. Next, look up while retracting the lower lid. This helps break adhesions of the eyeball to the lids.

The following are expected and should not cause alarm: tearing, a small amount of blood on the eye patch, a scratchy sensation, blurred vision, unusual visual images, a few light flashes and floaters. Do call the doctor if these symptoms *significantly* increase after discharge.

Have someone else administer the eye medications. Assume a reclining position for eye drop or eye ointment placement. Pull down the lower lid, and with the patient looking up place the correct number of drops into the center of the conjunctival sac. Let the lid gently close. The patient should try not to squeeze the eye shut or blink excessively. Wait 3 to 5 minutes between types of eye drops so that they do not wash each other out and dilute the intended effect. Patch the eye after each set of drops or ointment is administered. If a shield is to be used, it is placed on top of the taped-down eye pad.

Comfort

Take prescribed analgesic or extra-strength acetaminophen to relieve pain. A cool washcloth or ice pack to the forehead may provide comfort. **Report pain that markedly grows worse or is accompanied by nausea and vomiting.**

Precautions

In case of cough, take cough syrup. Do not try to hold back sneezes. Do not strain at stool; take a stool softener or milk of magnesia if needed to prevent this.

Restrictions
- Avoid driving a car until visual acuity is 20/40 or better; your physician will tell you when you may resume driving.
- Avoid lifting heavy objects (those over 20 lb) for at least 4 months.
- Refrain from work for 2 to 6 weeks (depending on type of work); physician will tell you when you may return to work. Light housework that does not require bending over or vigorous scrubbing may be resumed within 1 to 2 weeks depending on the type of surgery performed.
- Avoid vigorous or strenuous activity for 4 months.
- Do not bend with your head down; keep the head upright, and bend at the knees.
- Avoid sports for 3 to 4 months.

---

infection is not uncommon in those who wear contact lenses. The infecting agent may be in home-prepared saline solution used for cleaning the lenses. The eye becomes reddened and there may be tearing along with a feeling of grittiness or pain. Discharge may occur. Treatment of irritation is instillation of artificial tears. Infection is treated by a medication to kill the organism. Drugs may be given topically, subconjunctivally, or by IV infusion.

Corneal Ulcer
A corneal ulcer may occur from irritation, infection, or injury. The ulcer is cultured to determine whether there is a causative organism. If so, appropriate medication is supplied. Scarring from corneal ulcers or severe infection is treated by keratoplasty.

Corneal Transplant (Keratoplasty)
Corneal transplants replace corneas that have been damaged by genetic disorders, trauma, ulcers, or disease, such as keratitis (inflammation of the cornea), and help restore corneal clarity. Two types of procedures are done: a full-thickness keratoplasty (corneal transplant), or a lamellar keratoplasty, which replaces only a superficial layer of corneal tissue. The full-thickness keratoplasty restores vision in about 95% of patients (Color Figure 24). Corneas for transplantation are harvested from cadavers soon after death. The procedure is performed with conscious sedation.

The patient must be "on call" to come for the transplant, as it is unpredictable as to when a matching donor cornea will become available. The patient must realize beforehand that it takes 1 week or 2 before any improvement in vision is noticeable and that improvement will continue for several months. Because the cornea does not have an abundant blood supply, healing is very slow and is not complete for about 1 year. **Prevention of infection is extremely important.** Preoperative care is much the same as for other eye surgeries.

The patient may remain in the hospital overnight postoperatively. A pressure dressing and eye shield are applied in the surgical suite after the procedure and should be removed only by the physician. The pressure dressing helps keep the donor tissue in contact with the eyeball. Nursing actions focus on caring for a patient with sensory/perceptual alteration (visual). Instructions regarding safety are provided before discharge. **The patient may lie only on his back and inoperative side postoperatively.** Should the first transplant fail, the procedure can be redone.

A new eye excimer laser has been approved to polish the cornea, restoring vision. A scleral lens has been developed, and is seeking U.S.FDA approval. It is like an oversized contact lens. It arches over the cornea. The space between the lens and the cornea is filled with artificial tears providing lubrication, and thus fulfills the optical functions of the damaged cornea. These innovations may eventually make corneal transplants unnecessary for many people.

◆ Macular Degeneration

The macular region of the retina gives us color vision, acute vision, and central vision. Macular degeneration (also called age-related macular degeneration, ARMD or AMD) occurs with aging and is the most common cause of visual loss in the elderly. Research is in progress to determine factors that seem to predispose to this disorder. There is a genetic tendency for the disease. Cigarette smokers seem to have two to three times the incidence of macular degeneration than nonsmokers. Wearing sunglasses regularly when outdoors may help protect against AMD. It also seems that people who take large doses of vitamin E are less likely to develop AMD.

There are two types of macular degeneration: dry (atrophic) and wet (exudative). In the dry form the problem lies with photoreceptors in the macula of the retina that fail to function and are not replaced because of advancing age. This form accounts for 85% to 90% of cases. In the wet form, degenerating retinal tissue allows fluid to leak into the subretinal space. A fragile vessel network grows into the subretinal space and may bleed into the macular region, causing central visual impairment. Fluorescein angiography may be performed to evaluate blood vessel abnormalities in the eye.

The problem usually is bilateral and progressive. Early symptoms may be an inability to see the vividness of colors or to see details. Objects may appear to be the wrong size or shape, or straight lines may appear crooked or wavy. As central vision deteriorates, there may be a large dark spot or empty place over the center of what is viewed. The patient retains peripheral vision and can walk, dress, cook, and even drive, but cannot read when the disorder becomes severe. Prompt laser treatment to destroy the fragile blood vessels can sometimes be done to prevent further bleeding and visual deterioration. For this reason, patients at risk for macular degeneration are taught to use an Amsler grid (a small card with lines in a grid formation) at home to assess for progression of the disorder (Figure 30-13). If macular degeneration is occurring, the lines appear wavy.

A technique under investigation is transplantation of healthy cells of retinal pigment epithelium (RPE) to replace or enhance degenerating RPE. It is hoped that transplantation of RPE before vision has greatly deteriorated will slow or eliminate the progression of AMD.

The nurse helps patients with permanent vision loss learn to use low-vision aids. A referral to a low-vision specialist and low-vision support groups often is needed. Devices are available to light and magnify reading material. Books with large print are easier to read. Learning to turn the head and move the eyeballs to work around the central scotoma may help. A closed-circuit TV system that magnifies a printed page on screen can be used for reading or doing cross-word puzzles. Telescopic lenses can help for watching movies, attending the theater, reading street signs, and seeing traffic lights. A head-mounted low-vision enhancement system (LVES) provides both distance and close-up enhancement. Easy-to-read watches with large numerals, TV-screen magnifiers, and guides that fit over checks to assist with writing on them are some of the less expensive low-vision aids that are available.

◆ Eye Trauma

Eye trauma occurs from accidents and from debris in the air. Not using safety goggles or glasses when sanding or operating weed-whackers and various types of power equipment accounts for most incidents of foreign bodies landing in the eyes.

Removal of Foreign Bodies in the Eye   If the foreign body is not deeply embedded in the tissues of the eye, it can easily be removed by irrigation. Irrigation with clear, lukewarm water or sterile water or saline is used to remove a foreign body sticking to the cornea. Continuous irrigation can be done with small tubing, and a bottle of solution or an irrigating syringe or bottle can be used. The nurse must be very careful not to touch the eye with the tip of the irrigating device used. Sometimes a speck of foreign matter on the cornea can be removed with a moistened, sterile cotton swab. Have the patient tilt the head back and move the eyes away from the site of the particle. Hold the eyelids open to prevent blinking.

If a foreign body is sticking out of the eye, no attempt to remove it should be made. Both eyes should

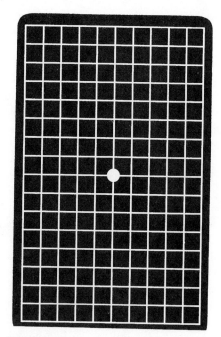

FIGURE 30-13   Amsler grid for assessing macular degeneration. The Yanuzzi card. (*Source:* Amsler grid; copyright © 1981 BMI. Courtesy of the Macula Foundation, Inc., NY.)

be patched to prevent further eye movement, and the patient should be transported to the emergency department or to an ophthalmologist.

If the patient continues to complain of a sensation that a foreign body is still in the eye after it appears to have been removed by irrigation or complains of continuing pain, refer to a physician immediately, as there may be a corneal abrasion.

The physician will apply a stain to the eye to assess whether the cornea is abraded. If there is an abrasion, medicated ointment will be prescribed, and the eye will be patched. The patient must be given instructions on how to instill the ointment. A thin line of eye ointment is applied from the inner canthus to the outer canthus along the lower eyelid inside the conjunctival sac (Figure 30-14). The patient closes the eye and moves the eyeball around in the socket to distribute the ointment. Excess medication is gently wiped away with a tissue from the inner to the outer canthus. If an eye patch is not applied, the patient is warned that the ointment may blur vision for a while. A corneal abrasion is painful; an NSAID may be used for discomfort.

Chemical Burns   Chemical burns should be treated by lengthy continuous irrigation. An IV bag of normal saline is the preferred solution; otherwise, tap water will do. Place the patient supine with his head turned to the affected side. With gloves on, direct the stream of fluid to the inner canthus so that the stream flows across the cornea to the outer canthus, holding the lids apart with your thumb and index finger. At intervals, stop and have the patient close his eyes to move secretions and particles from the upper eye to the lower conjunctival sac; then begin again. The patient should be seen by a physician as soon as possible.

Part 2: Ear Disorders

The inability to hear causes difficulty with communication. Approximately 1 in 1,000 babies born in the United States have some form of congenital hearing

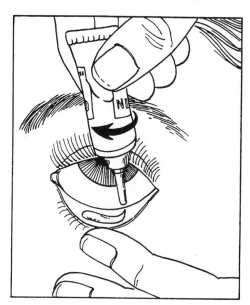

Twist tube to release ointment

FIGURE 30-14   Administering eye ointment. (*Source:* Lammon, C. B., et al. [1995]. *Clinical Nursing Skills.* Philadelphia: Saunders, p. 578.)

problem. After age 75, about one-half of the population has some degree of hearing loss. It is thought that the trend of playing very loud music, causing damage to the acoustic nerve, will result in considerably more hearing loss in the coming decades.

Inner ear disorders can cause problems with balance. Dizziness, vertigo, and ataxia can greatly interfere with an individual's ability to work or to perform usual activities of daily living (ADLs). Accidental injury and fractures from falls may occur. To understand the problems affecting the ear, it is necessary to recall its normal structure and functions.

OVERVIEW OF ANATOMY AND PHYSIOLOGY

What Are the Structures of the Ear?

- The external ear consists of the pinna (auricle) and the canal (auditory meatus). The pinna is the fleshy part of the ear situated on the side of the head (Figure 30-15).
- The auditory meatus is a tube about 2.5 cm long extending from the pinna to the tympanic membrane.
- The meatus is lined with numerous hairs and glands that secrete a waxy substance called cerumen.
- The middle ear contains the auditory bones (ossicles) and opens into the eustachian tube.
- The auditory ossicles are three small bones: the malleus (hammer), the incus (anvil), and the stapes (stirrup).
- The malleus attaches to the tympanic membrane.
- The stapes attaches to the oval window.
- The incus links the malleus and the stapes.
- The tympanic membrane (eardrum) separates the middle ear from the external ear.
- The eustachian tube connects the middle ear with the throat.
- The oval window and the round window connect the middle ear to the inner ear.
- The inner ear is divided into the vestibule, semicircular canals, and the cochlea.
- The inner ear contains a bony labyrinth with a membranous labyrinth lining and is located in the temporal bone of the skull.
- A clear fluid, endolymph, fills the membranous labyrinth.
- The cochlea contains the organ of Corti, which is comprised of sound receptors.

What Are the Functions of the Ear Structures?

- The pinna collects sound waves and channels them into the auditory meatus.
- The hairs and cerumen in the canal help prevent foreign objects from reaching the tympanic membrane.
- The tympanic membrane vibrates when sound waves hit it; the sound vibrations are conducted to the malleus.
- The bones of the middle ear transmit the sound vibrations to the inner ear. The malleus transmits them to the incus and the incus transmits them to the stapes. The stapes transmits the sound vibrations to the oval window, which transfers the motion to the fluid in the inner ear.
- Fluid motion in the inner ear stimulates the sound receptors in the cochlea and the organ of Corti.
- The organ of Corti transmits impulses to the cochlear branch of the vestibulocochlear nerve (cranial nerve VIII). This nerve carries the impulses to the medulla oblongata, the thalamus, and then to the temporal lobe of the brain that contains the auditory cortex.
- The eustachian tube helps equalize pressure in the middle ear.
- Receptors responsible for equilibrium (balance) are located in the inner ear within the bony vestibule and at the base of the semicircular canals.
- Impulses from the equilibrium receptors are transmitted to the brain via the vestibular branch of the vestibulocochlear nerve (cranial nerve VIII). The cerebellum is important in mediating the sense of equilibrium and balance.

What Changes Occur in the Ear with Aging?

- Cerumen becomes harder, containing less moisture, and its buildup within the ear may contribute to a hearing loss in the low-frequency range.
- The joints between the auditory bones become stiffer, which interferes with the transmission of sound waves, but this is not clinically significant by itself.
- There is a gradual loss of the receptor cells in the organ of Corti after age 40.
- With increasing age, the number of nerve fibers in the vestibulocochlear nerve decrease, contributing to hearing loss and sometimes affecting balance and equilibrium.

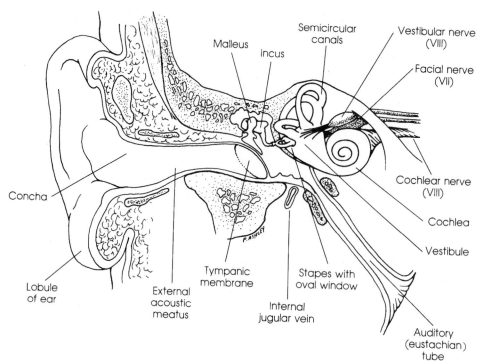

FIGURE 30-15   Outer, middle, and inner ear.

CAUSES AND PREVENTION OF HEARING LOSS

A glance at the causes of hearing loss listed in Table 30-12 will help identify some of the ways the nurse can help prevent hearing loss. Not all cases of hearing disability can be prevented, but education of the general public about causes of hearing loss can reduce its incidence. **Early and adequate treatment of ear infections helps preserve hearing.**

Hair pins, the ends of pencils, and other assorted objects should never be used to relieve tickling or itching in the ear, or to remove cerumen (earwax). Earwax normally moves on its own out of the ear canal to the outer ear, where it can be removed without danger of damaging the delicate lining of the ear canal or the tympanic membrane (eardrum). Obstructing cerumen should be removed by using drops that dissolve it or by a physician or nurse skilled in removing impacted cerumen. Foreign objects, such as beans, peas, and other vegetative substances, also should be removed by someone who is experienced and aware of the potential for ear damage.

Continued exposure to excessively high levels of sound can produce sensorineural loss called *noise-induced hearing impairment*. This condition is particularly likely to occur in industrial settings where machinery operation creates loud noise. The Occupational Safety and Hazard Administration's (OSHA) standards require the wearing of ear protectors in such settings.

A rather recent phenomenon is the potential damage to the inner ear caused by amplified music. **Authorities recommend that continual exposure to music amplified to more than 104 to 111 decibels be avoided.**

Many drugs can be toxic to the inner ear. This is especially true if a very high dose of the drug is given or if it is given incorrectly. Among the drugs that can be ototoxic are many of the antibiotics and potent diuretics, such as furosemide (Lasix). Aspirin and other salicylates can produce loss of hearing of high frequencies and ringing in the ears (tinnitus). Several chemotherapeutic agents used to treat malignancies are ototoxic.

Nurses should be aware of the potential for damage to the ear by potent drugs. Patients should be monitored

TABLE 30-12 ◆ *Common Causes of Sensorineural and Conductive Hearing Loss*	
Sensorineural Loss	**Conductive Loss**
◆ Congenital malformation of the middle or outer ear	◆ Heredity
◆ Degenerative changes of age (presbycusis)	◆ Infectious diseases such as measles, mumps, and meningitis
◆ Eardrum perforation	◆ Menière's syndrome
◆ Exposure to loud noise	◆ Otosclerosis
◆ Foreign object blocking the ear canal or wax plug (cerumen)	◆ Ototoxic drugs
	◆ Recurrent otitis media
◆ Head or ear trauma	◆ Rubella in utero
	◆ Tumor (acoustic neuroma)

carefully while receiving a potentially harmful drug. Any signs of ototoxicity, such as ringing in the ears, subtle changes in hearing ability, and difficulty in hearing should be reported immediately.

DIAGNOSTIC TESTS AND EXAMINATIONS

◆ Visual Examination of the Ear

The two instruments most commonly used to examine the ear canal and tympanic membrane are the otoscope and the aural speculum. The otoscope is fitted with a light and a magnifying lens to facilitate inspection (Figure 30-16). The aural speculum is used with a special circular, slightly concave head mirror that has a hole in its middle. The head mirror is positioned so that the central hole lies in front of one eye of the examiner. A source of light, such as a lamp, is placed behind the examiner so that it shines on the head mirror and is reflected into the ear.

The simple speculum can be modified by attaching a special tube and inflatable bag (pneumatic otoscope), thereby creating an airtight system. This allows the examiner to determine whether the tympanic membrane responds to positive and negative pressure. The normal eardrum moves in response to pressure. Healed perforations and scars on the eardrum can be seen when the tympanic membrane is moved.

A simple hearing test is the *whisper* test. The examiner stands behind the back of the patient and whispers a question to the patient. If the patient hears the question, an answer is forthcoming. The examiner backs up a step and whispers another question, and so on.

◆ Test for Nystagmus

To test for **nystagmus** (involuntary rhythmic jerking of the eyes), the nurse holds a finger directly in front of the patient at eye level. The patient is asked to follow the finger without moving the head. The nurse moves the finger slowly from the midline toward the right ear about 30 degrees. Then the finger is moved back to the midline and then slowly toward the left ear about 30 degrees. The patient's eyes are watched for any jerking movements.

◆ The Rhomberg Test

This is a test of equilibrium. The patient stands with his feet together, his arms out in front, and his eyes open.

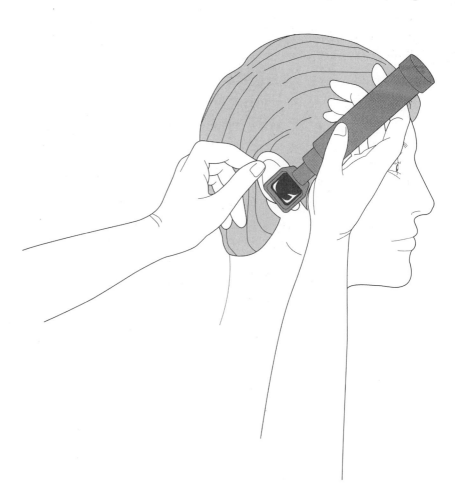

FIGURE 30-16   Examination of the ear with an otoscope.

The nurse notes ability to maintain an upright posture without swaying. The patient is then asked to close the eyes and posture is observed again. If the patient loses balance, it may indicate a problem with the inner ear or the cerebellum. Table 30-13 lists other diagnostic tests for the ear.

NURSING MANAGEMENT

◆ Assessment

Patients over the age of 60 should always be assessed for hearing loss. If a patient has a known hearing impair-

TABLE 30-13 ◆ *Diagnostic Tests for Ear Problems*

Test	Purpose	Description	Nursing Implications
Weber test	Determines loss of hearing in one ear or both.	Tuning fork is struck, and then the handle is placed on the patient's forehead. Normal hearing or equal loss in both ears is demonstrated by hearing the sound in the middle of the head.	Explain purpose and procedure to patient.
Rinne test	Determines whether hearing loss is sensorineural or conductive.	Tuning fork is struck, and then the handle is placed on the mastoid bone; the fork is removed and struck again and held beside the ear. The patient is asked in which position he heard the sound better or longer.	Explain procedure to patient.
Audiometry	Determines degree of hearing loss in each ear.	Earphones are placed on the patient's ears and with the use of an audiometry machine, the audiologist channels sounds of different decibels and pitch into one ear and then the other of the patient. The patient signals when he hears the tone.	Explain procedure to patient.
Caloric test	Checks for alteration in vestibular function in each ear.	With patient in a seated or supine position, each ear is separately irrigated with a cold and then a warm solution to determine vestibular response. Normal response is nystagmus, vertigo, nausea, vomiting, falling; decreased response indicates abnormality.	Explain procedure to patient; tell him he may experience nystagmus, vertigo, nausea and vomiting, but these will indicate a normal response.
Electronystagmography (ENG)	Assesses for disease of vestibular system.	Electrodes are placed near the patient's eyes. Caloric test is performed; movement of the eyes is recorded on a graph. Decreased response is abnormal.	Explain procedure and equipment to patient. Tell him that nausea, vertigo, etc., indicate a normal response.
Evoked response; auditory and brain stem response (ErA and ABR)	Determines abnormality of nerve pathways between eighth cranial nerve and brainstem.	Electrodes are attached to the client's head in a darkened room; similar to EEG. Auditory stimuli are directed to the patient, and a computer is used to track and separate the auditory electrical activity of the brain from other brain waves.	Explain procedure and equipment to patient. Tell him the room will be darkened.
Magnetic resonance imaging	Detects tumor of the eighth cranial nerve, acoustic neuroma.	Huge electromagnet is used to detect radio frequency pulses from the alignment of hydrogen protons in the magnetic field. A computer translates the pulses into cross-sectional images. Provides high-contrast views of soft tissue.	Explain that his head will be placed in a machine that looks like a huge doughnut. He will need to lie very still during the test; all metal must be removed before the test.
FTA-ABS blood test	Blood test for syphilis.	Blood is drawn and sent to the lab for determination of presence of syphilis. Syphilis can cause problems with nerve transmission from the ear.	Explain that a blood sample is needed.

ment, the nurse should assess how the patient is coping with it. Hearing and balance are subjective problems and require a good history from the patient. Table 30-14 presents guidelines for history taking. Diagnosis of infection requires an otoscopic exam. Table 30-15 shows a format for systematic examination of the ear by the nurse. It should be noted that the color, texture, and amount of cerumen varies among individuals. In Caucasians and African American it tends to be moist and rust-brown colored. Native Americans and Asians have cerumen that is lighter in color and drier. Normally, the top of each pinna is aligned with the corner of the eye on each side of the head. Lesions on the pinna may indicate skin cancer, particularly in the elderly patient. There should be no secretions other than cerumen from the ear. Ear pain may be referred from other parts of the head and neck and may occur from sinusitis, dental problems, or temporomandibular joint (TMJ) syndrome.

Elder Care Point . . . The ears of elderly in long-term care facilities should be checked with an otoscope at regular intervals for cerumen. Many long-term care residents have a correctable hearing loss related to impacted cerumen.

TABLE 30-14 ◆ *Assessment: Guide to History Taking for the Ear*

Ask the following questions:

◆ Have you had any pain in the ear?
◆ Have you had a recent temperature elevation?
◆ Do you suffer from allergies?
◆ Do you have frequent upper respiratory infections?
◆ Have you ever been exposed to very loud noise? Do you work in an area that is noisy? Do you listen to loud music?
◆ Have you ever had a head injury?
◆ Do you scuba dive, hunt or shoot skeet, or fly in small airplanes?
◆ Do you ever have ringing, buzzing, or odd sounds in the ears?
◆ Do you feel your hearing ability has decreased? Do people you live with think that you do not hear as well as you used to hear? Do you frequently have to ask people to repeat things that have been said to you?
◆ Is there a history of hearing loss in your family?
◆ Have you ever had a really high fever?
◆ What medications are you taking regularly? Are there other medications that you have taken for an extended period in the past? Do you take aspirin?
◆ How do you clean your ears?
◆ Do you ever suffer with dizziness, vertigo, loss of balance?

TABLE 30-15 ◆ *Assessment: Guide to Physical Examination of the Ear*

◆ Compare the pinna from one side to the other for symmetry and placement.
◆ Palpate the pinna for the presence of nodules.
◆ Observe for the presence of lesions on the pinna.
◆ Check for drainage (**otorrhea**) from the ear; color, and odor.
◆ Observe to see whether the patient can hear when across the room with the back turned toward the speaker.
◆ Observe the gait to detect any problem with balance.
◆ Observe for wavering when arising from a supine or seated position that might indicate dizziness or equilibrium problems.
◆ Observe for signs of bruising on the body from falls that may indicate problems with balance.
◆ Observe to see whether the person speaks in a voice louder than necessary.
◆ Observe to see whether facial expression indicates difficulty in understanding what is being said.
◆ Determine whether responses to statements are inappropriate.

Note: Someone qualified and experienced in using an otoscope should inspect the auditory meatus and the tympanic membrane.

◆Nursing Diagnosis

Nursing diagnoses are chosen based on the data provided during the assessment. Categories of nursing diagnoses associated with ear disorders and varying levels of hearing loss are as follows:

◆ Pain related to inflammation in the ear.
◆ Impaired verbal communication related to inability to receive messages or to decode and interpret them.
◆ Risk for injury related to inability to hear and follow directions or to loss of equilibrium and falls.
◆ Knowledge deficit related to nature of disability, self-care, availability of community resources for the hearing impaired.
◆ Social isolation related to difficulty in communicating.
◆ Activity intolerance related to dizziness, nausea, and vomiting associated with motion. (This condition often occurs when the inner ear is affected, as in Ménière's syndrome and labyrinthitis.)

Other nursing diagnoses may be appropriate depending on the individual's response to the disorder. Table 30-16 presents the most commonly encountered nursing diagnoses for patients with ear problems, along with the expected outcomes and nursing interventions.

◆Planning

General goals for the patient with problems of the ear or hearing are:

◆ Promote knowledge to protect hearing
◆ Prevent infection and injury

TABLE 30-16 ♦ *Nursing Diagnoses, Expected Outcomes, and Nursing Interventions for Patients with Ear Disorders*		
Nursing Diagnosis	**Goals/Expected Outcomes**	**Nursing Interventions**
Auditory sensory/perceptual alteration related to damage from infection or obstruction.	Patient will verbalize ways to prevent further hearing loss. Patient will be free of ear infection within 10 days.	If cerumen is obstructing the auditory canal, irrigate as ordered; warm the irrigation solution to body temperature. If infection is present, instruct regarding antibiotic medication and encourage to take entire prescription. Instruct in use of hearing aid if one is prescribed. Advise of ways to prevent further hearing loss: avoid loud noise or wear ear protectors; seek treatment immediately for signs of ear infection.
Pain related to inflammation in the ear.	Pain will be controlled with analgesia within 8 hours. Pain will be resolved within 7 days.	Administer analgesics as ordered PRN. Warm analgesic ear drops to room temperature before administration. Have patient rest head on heating pad turned on "low" setting if this seems to decrease pain.
Impaired verbal communication related to inability to receive messages or to decode and interpret them.	Patient will assist in choice of methods to improve ability to communicate. Patient will try hearing aid for 2 weeks if there is an indication that this device would help hearing.	Plan with patient the best way to communicate so that instructions and information are comprehended; explore tone of voice, level of volume, distance from patient when speaking, writing out communication, etc. Refer for evaluation by audiologist. Encourage daily use of hearing aid if one is prescribed. Explain that time and adjustments are necessary to obtain the optimum result. Give praise at efforts to use hearing aid.
Anxiety related to inability to hear warnings, perform at work, or communicate in social settings.	Patient will explore methods of maintaining safety within 2 weeks. Patient will verbalize ways in which assisted hearing devices might assist in performance in the work environment.	Encourage verbalization of fears. Utilize means to enhance communication (Table 30-17). Advise of assisted hearing devices, hearing aids, and of availability of "hearing" dogs. Introduce means of learning alternative communication methods, such as sign language and speech-reading. Explore methods of enhancing attention to visual cues of dangers in the environment, i.e., close attention to signal lights, or observing others at street crossings. Discuss problems of communication in social settings and explore possible solutions, i.e., masking devices for use in crowds, having interaction with only one or two people at a time, avoiding noisy restaurants, or using hearing aid.
Risk of injury related to impaired equilibrium.	Patient will verbalize methods to ensure safety within 3 days. Patient will not experience a fall or injury.	Adminsiter medication for vertigo as ordered. Encourage a low-sodium diet. Instruct to change positions very slowly. Encourage to hold on to something solid or someone when arising from a sitting to a standing position. If vertigo is present, do not ambulate without assistance. Teach or reinforce vestibular/balance exercises as prescribed. Assist to identify any aura (presence of symptoms that precede an attack). Instruct to lie down and keep the eyes open and focused straight ahead when experiencing vertigo.
Knowledge deficit related to the nature of disability, self-care, and availability of community resources for the hearing impaired.	Patient will verbalize ways to enhance safe self-care within 2 weeks.	Explain nature of hearing loss or vertigo and possible causes. Describe measures to assist the hard-of-hearing person to adapt; refer to support groups and sources for information. Refer to community agencies and resources for the hearing impaired.

◆ Promote effective communication

◆ Promote coping with hearing loss

Expected outcomes are written for each individual nursing diagnosis chosen for the patient's care plan. Writing the outcomes should be done in collaboration with the patient and other health team members. In addition to the nurse and physician, an audiologist, hearing aid specialist, and speech therapist may be involved in the patient's care. Both long- and short-term goals for the patient should be considered.

When a patient is severely hearing impaired, communication with the patient for treatments and activities of daily living may take longer than with normally hearing patients. The nurse should take this into consideration when creating the daily work plan. If the patient does not have adequate aids for hearing, the nurse must devise an acceptable method of two-way communication with the patient.

◆ Implementation

Interventions for the patient with a hearing or balance problem are geared toward patient education, treatment of infection, pre- and postoperative care and instructions, measures for communication, and referral to resources.

Instillation of Ear Medication   Ear drops may be ordered to dissolve cerumen, relieve pain, or combat infection in the auditory meatus. The patient should be positioned in a supine lateral position so that the affected ear is uppermost. The medication should be at room temperature. Cold ear drops may cause discomfort or dizziness. For the adult, the ear canal is straightened by drawing the pinna upward and toward the back of the head (Figure 30-17). For a child under age 3 the pinna is pulled down and back. Following the

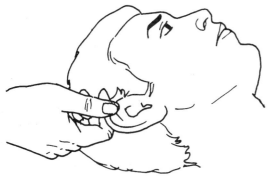

FIGURE 30-17 Straightening the ear canal to instill ear drops. (From deWit, S.C. [1994]. *Rambo's Nursing Skills for Clinical Practice,* 4th Ed. Philadelphia: Saunders, p. 912.)

"five rights" of medication administration, draw up the correct amount of medication. Insert the tip of the dropper into the external ear canal and instill the medication. Place cotton in the external meatus to prevent the medication from escaping. Have the patient remain in the lateral position for 2 to 5 minutes.

Interventions for Communication with the Hearing Impaired   The patient who is hearing impaired has unique problems of communication when in the hospital or long-term care facility. If he cannot hear well and misunderstands or misinterprets the voices and sounds in the unfamiliar surroundings, he is likely to be frustrated, fearful, and anxious. Unless a special effort is made to have frequent contact with the patient, social isolation may occur.

When trying to communicate with a person who is hearing impaired, bear in mind that attempts to answer questions without fully understanding what is asked may occur. Past experience has taught many hearing-impaired persons that to ask for repetition of questions irritates people and causes them to think the person is stupid. **For this reason, many people who cannot hear well frequently smile and say "Yes," when such an answer is either incorrect or inappropriate.** Another problem is that the individual may fill in parts of sentences with similarly sounding words. For example the words "Knott's Berry Farm" may be interpreted as "not very far." Some guidelines to help the hearing-impaired patient and improve the nurse's ability to communicate are given in Table 30-17.

TABLE 30-17 ◆ Communicating with the Hearing-Impaired Person

◆ Be certain you have the person's attention before beginning speaking.

◆ Speak slowly and very distinctly. Do not shout because this distorts speech and doesn't make the message any clearer. Keep the voice pitch at midrange, neither low nor high.

◆ The best distance for speaking to a hearing-impaired person is 2½ to 4 feet. Place yourself on eye level with the person. Do not speak directly into the person's ear as this prevents the person from obtaining visual cues while you are speaking.

◆ Do not smile, chew gum, or cover the mouth while speaking.

◆ Be aware of nonverbal communication. Facial expressions, gestures, and lip and body movements all give cues to the meaning of the message.

◆ Use short, simple sentences. If the patient does not appear to understand or responds inappropriately, rephrase the statement. Try to limit each sentence to one subject and one verb.

◆ Give the person time to respond to questions.

◆ Encourage the use of a hearing aide if the person has one, and allow time for the person to insert and adjust it before speaking.

◆ Avoid using the intercom system as it may distort sound.

Think about . . . What three techniques of communication with a hearing-impaired patient do you feel would be the most helpful?

A piece of tape or sign of some kind should be placed over the terminal on the "intercom" system that designates the room of a hearing-impaired patient. This serves to remind the person answering the light to go to the patient's room rather than try to talk over the intercom system.

Nursing Care of the Patient Having Ear Surgery

Most ear surgeries are performed as an outpatient procedure. Nursing care is focused on the immediate preoperative and recovery periods and on instructions for home care.

Preoperative care. Nursing care of the patient during the preoperative period usually is rather routine except for the administration of eardrops or other special medications. Physical preparation for ear surgery may or may not involve removing some of the hair from the scalp. Male patients should be clean shaven the morning of surgery. The external ear and surrounding skin should be thoroughly cleansed, preferably with a surgical soap. Female patients with long hair should have it braided or pinned back securely so that it will not become soiled by drainage from the ear or serve as a source of infection at the operative site.

Postoperative care. The patient will often return from major ear surgery with an ear dressing (Figure 30-18). Positioning of the patient after ear surgery depends on specific instructions from the physician. Usually the patient is placed flat in bed, and his head is supported so that he does not turn it from side to side. In addition to noting the vital signs, the nurse should watch for signs of injury to the facial nerve, including inability of the patient to close his eyes, wrinkle his forehead, or pucker his lips. The patient and family are advised to report such symptoms to the surgeon. If they appear later than 12 hours after surgery, they may be due to edema, and the physician may order a loosening of the dressings.

Safety precautions, such as raising siderails, should be taken to avoid injury due to dizziness and loss of balance during the recovery period. Balance is temporarily affected as a result of disturbance to the mechanism that maintains equilibrium. When the patient is allowed to get up and move about, assistance should be provided to prevent falls. The patient should arise slowly to a sitting position and sit for a few minutes. Then the patient stands while holding on or being supported. Dizziness must pass before the patient attempts walking.

Because the ear is so near the brain, a special effort must be made to avoid contamination of the surgical site. Dressings may be reinforced to keep them dry, but excessive drainage must be reported to the surgeon.

The patient should be instructed beforehand about what is to be expected from the surgery. Hearing is usually only slightly impaired immediately after surgery because of edema or bandages, but is expected to improve in time. Instructions for home care are in Table 30-18.

Myringotomy (incision of the ear drum) with placement of tubes is a lesser procedure and the only dressing may be a cotton ball in the ear. There is less occurrence of dizziness or nausea with this surgery.

◆ Evaluation

Evaluation involves reassessment to determine whether the expected outcomes are being met. Determining whether hearing has improved is the criterion by which effectiveness of treatment is evaluated. Improvement is verified by audiometry. Fading or resolution of dizziness and vertigo indicate that actions and treatments for these problems have been effective. Resolution of infection is determined by the appearance of the ear drum, absence of pain, and normal temperature.

COMMON DISORDERS OF THE EAR

◆ Hearing Impairment

Hearing impairment ranges from difficulty in hearing certain ranges of tones or in understanding certain words to total deafness. There are two types of hearing loss related to problems in the ear, *sensorineural* and

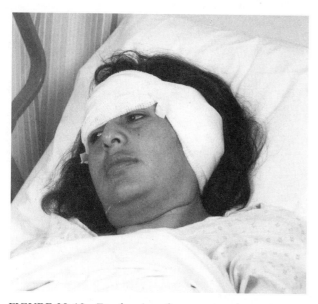

FIGURE 30-18   Ear dressing after tympanoplasty. (Photo by Glen Derbyshire; courtesy of Goleta Valley Cottage Hospital, Santa Barbara, CA.)

TABLE 30-18 ♦ *Patient Education: Home Care Instructions after Ear Surgery*

The following instructions are given to the patient after surgery at the time of discharge:

- Sneezing, coughing, and nose blowing are all ways in which the operative site may be disturbed. If necessary, blow the nose gently one side at a time. Cough or sneeze with the mouth open. Continue this for 1 week after surgery.
- Do not drink through a straw for 2 to 3 weeks.
- Limit physical activity for 1 week after surgery. Refrain from exercising and sports for 3 weeks or until the surgeon discharges you.
- Avoid heavy lifting for 3 weeks; Avoid bending over from the waist or moving the head rapidly for 3 weeks.
- Keep the ear dry for 4 to 6 weeks after surgery by placing a cotton ball covered with petroleum jelly (such as Vaseline) in the ear canal; refrain from shampooing hair with water for 1 week after surgery.
- After the initial dressing is removed, keep a cotton ball in the ear to protect it; change the cotton ball daily.
- Avoid people with colds.
- Do not fly until the surgeon allows it.
- Wear ear protectors when exposed to a loud environment.
- A return to work is usual after 3 to 7 days; strenuous work may not be resumed for 3 weeks.

Note: The surgeon will explain the specific time limitations for each activity based on the type of surgery performed.

conductive. About 80% of hearing loss is due to a disorder of the hearing nerve (sensorineural). Conductive hearing loss is caused by a problem of sound impulse transmission through the auditory canal, the tympanic membrane, or via the bones of the middle ear. Hearing impairment is the nation's number-one disability, affecting one in every 15 people. Causes of sensorineural and conductive hearing impairment are listed in Table 30-12.

Elder Care Point... Arteriosclerosis can cause decreased blood flow to the otic nerve (8th cranial nerve), resulting in sensorineural hearing loss. This often contributes to hearing loss in the elderly.

Persons with sensorineural hearing loss typically have more difficulty hearing high-pitched tones than low-pitched ones; thus they frequently can understand the speech of men better than that of women. Another characteristic of sensorineural hearing loss is difficulty hearing softly spoken and poorly enunciated words. Speaking slightly louder to the person with sensorineural hearing loss may help, but it is especially important to speak slowly and clearly and to face the person when communicating with him. Because persons with sensorineural hearing loss do not hear their own voices as well as a person with normal hearing, they tend to speak louder than necessary.

Hearing aids help some people with sensorineural hearing loss. Aids designed to amplify some pitches and block out others that do not need amplification are most helpful. Hearing aids are not always the answer to a problem of hearing loss, and for some persons the most effective therapy is focused on rehabilitation to facilitate acceptance of the loss and learning of new ways to communicate in spite of some degree of deafness.

Elder Care Point... The loss or decrease of hearing common to those over 75 years of age makes it important for the nurse to pay closer attention to communication with senior adults. Be certain you have the person's attention, face him or her, and speak distinctly. Validate communication by asking for feedback to know that what was said was correctly perceived.

Central hearing loss occurs in the brain as a result of some pathological condition above the junction of the eighth cranial nerve and the brain stem. Central hearing loss can be due to a problem of transmission of stimuli in the brain, an inability to decode and sort signals received from one or both ears, or a failure in the transmission of sounds from one hemisphere of the brain to the other. Causes include brain tumors, vascular changes that suddenly deprive the middle ear of its blood supply, and cerebrovascular accident.

Many people have a combination of two or more types of hearing impairment. Often there is a combination of sensorineural and conductive loss.

It should be noted that, when a person is fitted with a hearing aid, it takes considerable time of working with the audiologist on adjustments to the device to obtain the best result. Too many people give up on a hearing aid because they have not taken the time to work through the adjustment process.

♦ Otitis Media

This condition is an inflammation of the middle ear caused by various types of bacteria. Although it is mostly seen in infants and young children, it does occur in adults. It results in the accumulation of fluid behind the eardrum and some temporary impairment of hearing. Otitis media usually follows an upper respiratory tract infection or trauma to the ear. When the infection is sudden in onset and of short duration, it is termed *acute otitis media.* The eardrum is retracted inward because of negative pressure due to a closed eustachian tube. The pain can be very severe. When the infection is repeated, often causing perforation of the eardrum and drainage, it is called *chronic otitis media.*

Otitis media sometimes is accompanied by an allergy and may be aggravated by enlarged adenoids. Fluid may build up in the middle ear. This disorder is called *serous otitis media.* Symptoms are mild and may consist only of a feeling of fullness in the ear and evidence of impaired hearing. If the fluid remains over an extended time, it causes tympanic membrane contraction and can permanently impair its movement. Initially, the condition is treated conservatively with antihistamines and decongestants. If this approach is not successful, a *myringotomy* (incision into the eardrum) is done, and a ventilating tube is inserted to drain the excess fluid in the middle ear and to equalize pressure while the eustachian tube is blocked. The tympanic membrane is anesthetized locally. The procedure is painless and takes about 15 minutes. The incision heals within 24 to 72 hours unless a tube is placed in the opening. Tubes remain in place for 6 to 18 months before they are naturally expelled. The hole then heals.

Suppurative otitis media occurs when pus-producing bacteria infect the middle ear. It usually is associated with an upper respiratory tract infection, most often when organisms from the nasopharynx find their way into the middle ear. Treatment consists of systemic therapy with antibiotics, topical therapy with eardrops, *tympanoplasty* to repair a ruptured eardrum and damaged ossicles, and, sometimes, mastoidectomy to eliminate all sources of infection and prevent further degeneration of bone. See Nursing Care 30-2.

Infections in the middle ear always have the potential for spreading to the meninges and causing meningitis or to the mastoid bone and causing mastoiditis. With the advent of antibiotics, surgery to scrape and clean infected mastoid bone is performed far less frequently than it was previously. Although otitis media is a fairly common occurrence, it should always be treated immediately.

◆ Otosclerosis

Symptoms and Diagnosis. Otosclerosis is a hereditary degeneration of bone in the inner ear. It occurs twice as often in females and begins in the late teens or early twenties. It may become worse during pregnancy. The sense of hearing depends in part on the vibration of very small bones of the inner ear. The *stapes,* or stirrup, is particularly important, because it conducts sound waves to the fluid in the semicircular canals in the inner ear. Otosclerosis is a disease process that causes the formation of excess bone. This causes the footplate of the stapes to be fixed so that it no longer vibrates to transmit sound waves.

The patient often complains of difficulty hearing the voices of others, yet his own voice sounds unusually loud. In response to this, he may lower his voice to the point that he can scarcely be heard by others.

Treatment. The hearing loss of otosclerosis can sometimes be corrected by using a hearing aid. Micro-

surgical intervention can restore air-conductive hearing by providing a new moveable pathway for the sound waves.

During the operation, called a *stapedectomy,* the stapes is removed and is replaced with a prosthetic device. This device may be a steel wire and fat implant, a wire and a segment of vein, or a vein graft with polyethylene tubing. In any case, the prosthesis is attached to one end of the incus (anvil of the middle ear) so that sound can be transmitted to the inner ear.

The surgical procedure is extremely delicate and would not be possible without the dissecting binocular microscope and other modern surgical instruments that allow visualization and manipulation of the very small structures of the middle ear.

Nursing assessments and interventions. Postoperative care involves keeping the patient quiet and flat in bed for several hours. The head is turned so that the affected ear is uppermost. When the patient is allowed to move about, he must be warned that dizziness is likely to occur, especially if he turns his head suddenly. Position changes should be accomplished slowly. Tympanoplasty is now the more common procedure.

Tympanoplasty involves the surgical reconstruction of the tympanic membrane and ossicles to restore middle-ear function. There are five different types of procedures ranging from simple closing of a tympanic membrane perforation to extensive repair of the middle-ear structures. The procedure is performed with an operating microscope via the external auditory canal or through a postauricular incision. Although performed as an outpatient procedure, tympanoplasty requires general anesthesia.

◆ Labyrinthitis

Labyrinthitis is an inflammation involving the inner ear. It most commonly occurs as a complication of bacterial meningitis, chronic otitis media, or from a viral infection such as influenza, mumps, or measles. The symptoms include loss of hearing in the affected ear, severe dizziness with nausea and vomiting, and **nystagmus** (abnormal jerking movements of the eyes).

Treatment is aimed at removing the source of infection and controlling symptoms. Antibiotics may be given in massive doses to control a bacterial infection. Meclizine (Antivert, Bonine) or another antihistamine that assists in decreasing vertigo and its associated nausea and vomiting also is used. Scopalamine patches behind the ear can be used after the acute phase to control vertigo.

Initially the patient is kept on bedrest to prevent falls and injury. The family is cautioned not to let the patient get out of bed without assistance. If the source of the problem is chronic mastoiditis that won't re-

Nursing Care Plan 30-2

Selected nursing diagnoses, goals/expected outcomes, nursing interventions and evaluations for a patient having a tympanoplasty

Situation: Miss Cook, age 38, is a high school teacher who has had progressive hearing impairment as a result of recurrent otitis media of the right ear. She is admitted to outpatient surgery for tympanoplasty. During her initial assessment, the nurse found Miss Cook to be well informed about the nature of her disorder but somewhat anxious about the outcome of surgery. Her physical health status is good; her only previous hospitalization was for an appendectomy when she was 19 years old.

Nursing Diagnosis	Goals/Expected Outcomes	Nursing Intervention	Evaluation
Postoperative period			
Risk for injury related to graft displacement. SUPPORTING DATA Tympanoplasty.	Graft will be successful as evidenced by restored hearing in affected ear.	Position patient so that operative ear is uppermost. Reinforce preoperative instructions to remain in bed for 4 hours, avoid sudden movements, blowing nose, sneezing. Check vital signs, especially temperature, for evidence of infection bid. Take analgesic/sedative as ordered to promote rest. Provide quiet environment.	Temperature 99.2° F; maintaining bedrest; operative ear up; continue plan.
Risk for activity intolerance related to vertigo and instability. SUPPORTING DATA After tympanoplasty, states is very dizzy and nauseous.	Falls and trauma to head will be avoided.	Up only with assistance. Repeat explanation for safety precautions. Caution patient to change positions and turn her head very slowly. Provide well-lighted room when ambulating. Adminsiter medication prescribed for vertigo.	Cautioned to turn head slowly. Took dramamine for dizziness and nausea. Nausea relieved.
Knowledge deficit related to self-care after surgery. SUPPORTING DATA Asks about restrictions and self-care.	Patient will verbalize knowledge of home self-care before discharge. Patient will demonstrate dressing change correctly before discharge.	Instruct patient to avoid loud noises and pressure changes for 6 months, especially flying and diving. Stress importance of not blowing her nose for at least 1 week, avoiding an upper respiratory infection if at all possible, protecting her ear against cold, and refraining from any activity that might provoke dizziness or disturb the graft (e.g., straining, bending, and heavy lifting). Teach patient how to change dressing on the external ear. Reiterate importance of taking full course of prescribed antibiotic and reporting to surgeon at scheduled times. Reassure patient that because of swelling of tissues and presence of surgical pack, it may be several weeks before she can fully evaluate effectiveness of the surgery.	Discharge teaching done; obtain feedback by phone tomorrow and demonstration of changing ear dressing before discharge; continue plan.

spond to medical treatment, a mastoidectomy may be done.

♦ Menière's Syndrome

Symptoms and Diagnosis. Menière's syndrome is a group of symptoms in which there is an increase of fluid within the spaces of the labyrinths, with swelling and congestion of the mucous membranes of the cochlea. The symptoms include attacks of dizziness, ringing in the ear (tinnitus), poor coordination that makes walking difficult or impossible, and loss of hearing. **Any sudden movement of the head or eyes during an attack usually produces severe nausea and vomiting.** The exact cause is unknown, but the condition occurs most often in people who have had chronic ear disorders and allergic symptoms involving the upper respiratory tract.

Diagnosing Menière's syndrome usually is not difficult, but because these symptoms could indicate a tumor of the auditory mechanism, a *caloric test* may be performed, which involves instilling very warm or cold fluid into the auditory canal. A patient with Menière's syndrome will experience a severe attack; a normal person will complain of only slight dizziness. A person with a tumor of the auditory mechanism will have no reaction at all. Tympanometry and audiometry is ordered, and a brain stem evoked response (BSER) test is performed to rule out an acoustic neuroma or problem in the brain.

Treatment. Treatment of Menière's syndrome focuses on relieving symptoms; there is no cure for this condition, although it does disappear spontaneously in some cases. For an acute attack with disabling vertigo, atropine may be given subcutaneously, followed by diazepam (Valium), dimenhydrinate (Dramamine), meclizine (Antivert), or other drugs for motion sickness. To control edema and reduce pressure in the inner ear, the patient may be placed on a low-sodium diet, his fluid intake may be restricted, and diuretics may be ordered. Anticholinergic drugs, such as propantheline (Pro-banthine) or glycopyrrolate (Robinul), may be given to help control the vertigo and nausea. To improve circulation in the ear, papaverine (Vasospan) or niacin may be prescribed. Some patients find that Ginkgo biloba, which acts as a vasodilator, helps. The patient is kept quiet and in bed to avoid aggravating his symptoms. He may be very irritable and withdrawn and may refuse to eat or drink because of fear of vomiting. Care should be taken to avoid increasing his irritation by jarring his bed, turning on bright overhead lights, or making loud noises.

If attacks continue and are very severe despite medical treatment, the endolymph sac from the inner ear can be removed with microsurgical techniques. When hearing loss is total on the affected side, surgical destruction of the eighth cranial nerve may be done to resolve the symptoms. Although this produces permanent deafness in the affected ear, the severe attacks are eliminated. In most persistent cases of Menière's syndrome, the patient will eventually suffer a serious or even total loss of hearing regardless of the treatment used.

♦ Dizziness and Vertigo

The sense of balance and equilibrium is governed by the vestibular system in the inner ear. Increases in fluid pressure in the inner ear, inflammations, and vascular disorders that interrupt blood supply to the cochlea can produce dizziness, loss of balance, and nausea and vomiting. These symptoms can range from mildly annoying to completely incapacitating and should always be assessed whenever a person has an ear disorder and loss of hearing.

The patient who experiences dizziness and positional vertigo should be cautioned to avoid suddenly turning his head and other movements that aggravate the vertigo. He should be told to call for assistance whenever he needs to move from his bed or chair. When helping the patient to his feet, move slowly and give him time to stand for a moment before beginning to walk. **Typically, patients with this kind of vertigo feel that the room is spinning around during an attack, and any motion makes the sensation even worse.** While the patient is having an attack of vertigo, he should lie in bed and remain as motionless as possible. Stabilizing his head with a pillow on either side may encourage immobility. Attacks can last from a few minutes to hours.

Medications to reduce motion sickness and nausea should be given precisely as ordered. These are usually given every 3 to 4 hours or on a preventive basis *before* the patient's symptoms become severe.

When increased fluid pressure in the inner ear is suspected as the cause of dizziness, the physician may order a low-salt diet and limit fluid intake. Although there is some question about the effectiveness of this form of treatment, it does seem to be helpful in some cases.

Patients with recurrent attacks of vertigo are encouraged to stop smoking if they are habitual tobacco smokers. **Stress also is thought to affect the frequency of attacks of vertigo in patients with inner ear disorders.** Teaching the patient effective coping mechanisms to handle stress or adding rest periods into the work schedule may be helpful.

♦ Tinnitus

Signs and Symptoms. Ringing, buzzing, or other continuous noise in the ear *(tinnitus)* can be mildly annoying or so severe that it interferes with activities of daily living and prevents the patient from getting sufficient sleep and rest. Common causes of tinnitus include presbycusis, constant exposure to loud environmental noise, inflammation and infection in the ear, otosclerosis, Ménière's syndrome, and labyrinthitis. Systemic disorders, such as hypertension and other cardiovascular disorders, neurological disease including head injury, and hyper- and hypothyroidism also can cause ringing in the ears. Tinnitus frequently may be one of the first symptoms produced by an ototoxic drug.

Treatment. Medical treatment begins with efforts to determine the underlying cause and treat it. When the cause cannot be found, symptomatic relief is tried. However, some cases of intractable tinnitus resist all modes of conventional therapy. Less traditional measures that have varying degrees of success include biofeedback training and "masking."

Biofeedback training is especially helpful in those cases in which emotional stress and anxiety or hysteria are thought to be the underlying causes of tinnitus. Through visual or auditory signals the person learns to relax and exert some degree of control over his autonomic nervous system. This can lower blood pressure and pulse rate and relax muscles that are very tense.

Nursing intervention. *Masking* simply provides a low-level noise to block out, or "mask," the head noise heard by the person complaining of tinnitus. Some examples include playing soft music or a tape of sounds of nature such as a waterfall while the person is resting or sleeping, providing "white sound" in the working environment, using a hearing aid to amplify sound from the outside and overcome head noise, and wearing a special tinnitus instrument that is a combination hearing aid and tinnitus masker for persons who have both hearing loss and tinnitus. The therapeutic effect of masking is highly individualized. Some persons find instant relief, some partial abatement of the head noise, and some do not benefit from any attempts to mask the sounds of tinnitus. Earplugs or ear protection should be worn when noise exposure cannot be avoided.

REHABILITATION FOR HEARING LOSS

Specific measures to rehabilitate a patient with hearing loss depends on the age and aptitude of the patient. Adults who have acquired the skills of speech and language before their loss of hearing occurred are better able than children to pick up language cues and understand what is being said to them and therefore should have fewer problems with communication of language.

◆ Speech Reading

Instruction in reading lips is one mode of therapy for the hearing impaired, but it is not a panacea. Only about 60% of the sounds in the English language can be identified by watching the lips. Most experienced lipreaders do not catch more than half of the words spoken to them. Communication by lipreading is enhanced by other nonverbal clues, such as facial expressions and hand gestures.

Learning to lipread is difficult. It requires at least average intelligence, exceptional language skills, excellent eyesight, and much persistence and patience.

◆ Hearing Aids

An evaluation by a reputable audiologist should be completed before purchasing a hearing aid. In this way a prescription for a hearing aid designed to provide the best possible improvement of hearing is possible.

The hearing aids produced today can improve hearing for a variety of types of hearing loss. For the person who does not have a defect in the middle ear, a hearing aid can transmit amplified sound from the receiver through the eardrum to the inner ear. This is accomplished by amplifying sound waves transmitted by air conduction and bone conduction.

The design of a hearing aid varies. Some are worn in the ear, others behind the ear, and still others are built into the frame of eyeglasses (Figure 30-19). Persons with binaural hearing loss (both ears are affected) must wear a hearing aid in each ear. Regardless of the type of

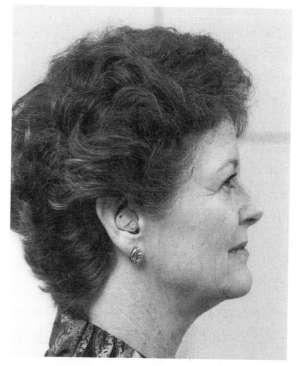

FIGURE 30-19   An in-the-ear hearing aid. (Photo by Glen Derbyshire; courtesy of Interpersonal Communications Hearing Aid Center, Santa Barbara, CA.)

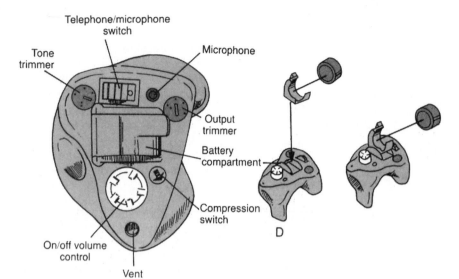

Tone trimmer

Telephone/microphone switch

Microphone

Output trimmer

Battery compartment

Compression switch

On/off volume control

Vent

D

FIGURE 30-20   Parts of a typical in-the-ear hearing aid. (*Source:* Black, J. M., Matassarin-Jacobs, E. [1997]. *Medical-Surgical Nursing:* Clinical Management for Collaborative Care, 5th ed. Philadelphia: Saunders, p. 997.)

hearing aid, it will have a microphone, an amplifier, a receiver, and a battery (Figure 30-20).

The hearing aid should not be handled roughly or dropped. The ear mold can be cleaned with soap and water, but the other parts of the aid should not get wet. Hair spray can damage the microphone of a hearing aid. Regular servicing by a dealer can keep the aid in good working order (Table 30-19).

There are many types of hearing aids on the market. Newer types can amplify the tones needed while masking other levels of noise. It takes time to become adjusted to a hearing aid and the audiologist must make repeated adjustments to the device to achieve optimum function.

◆ Cochlear Implant

Cochlear implants are now available for the patient who has no hearing at all. The device is a small computer that changes spoken words into electrical impulses that are transmitted via an implanted coil to the nerve endings in the cochlea. Success with the implant varies considerably from one person to the next. Bone hearing devices and semi-implanted devices are under development.

◆ Hearing Assistive Devices

Many devices on the market use hearing aid technology. These devices assist people to hear telephone conversations, television, and sound systems, such as those in church or the theater.

COMMUNITY CARE

Nurses in all settings should be conscious of eye safety for themselves and those around them. Public education about using sunhats, visors, and dark glasses when out of doors to protect the eyes from UVA and UVB rays is another function of all nurses. School nurses also should institute "case finding" methods with the teachers or faculty to identify students who may have vision problems that have not been identified.

Nurses working in home care often find patients who have not had eye care in many years; prescriptions have not been changed, and their quality of vision has decreased. Arranging for referral to an appropriate agency to arrange for eye examination should be done

---

TABLE 30-19 ◆ *Care Points for a Hearing Aid*

When a hearing aid doesn't work

- Check that the switch is "on."
- Examine the earmold for attached wax or dirt; clean the sound hole.
- Check the battery to see that it is inserted correctly.
- Check the connection between the ear mold and the receiver.
- Replace the battery. Batteries last an average of 2 to 14 days depending on type of aid.
- Check placement of the earmold in the ear; it should fit snugly.
- Adjust the volume.
- If all else fails, take the hearing aid to an authorized service center for repair.

To clean the hearing aid

- Turn the hearing aid off.
- Wash the earmold with mild soap and warm water; do not submerge in water.
- Use a pipe cleaner or toothpick to gently cleanse the opening or short tube that fits into the ear.
- Dry the mold completely before turning on the aid or before reattaching it to the hearing aid (if it is separate).

when the patient cannot afford an eye exam from a provider in the community. Glaucoma testing should be encouraged every 2 to 3 years for all adults over the age of 40.

A new innovation in providing vision care for low-income individuals is taking place in Long Beach, California. Residents of a public housing development have access to eye examinations via high-tech equipment that allows physicians 20 miles away to perform eye examinations by two-way interactive video and audio equipment. Residents at the housing project also have an opportunity to be trained as technicians at the eye clinic.

Both home care nurses and those working in long-term care should be alert to signs of progressing macular degeneration. The Amsler grid can assist in identifying this problem. Patients with known eye disorders should be periodically assessed to see how much vision has deteriorated and how much the patient's ability to perform ADLs and partake in usual hobbies is affected. Nurses should be instrumental in helping patients obtain low-vision aids.

All nurses should encourage the donation of corneas at death. Signing a donor card for organ harvest should be a consideration for all. The nurse may be the person to approach the terminal patient or the family about the possibility of donating corneas after death . . . the gift of sight to another.

Public education about the dangers of loud noise and music could do much to prevent thousands of people from becoming hearing impaired. Teaching people to seek medical attention for symptoms of otitis media quickly prevents damage to the tympanic membrane and preserves hearing ability.

Encouraging those with hearing impairment to have a thorough evaluation and to try a hearing aid could do much to improve the quality of their lives. Hearing aids from a reputable dealer usually have a money-back guarantee trial period. Most people do not know this. There is little economic reason for refusing to try a hearing aid. Nurses in home care and in long-term care settings should frequently assess the function of the patient's hearing aid.

Elder Care Point . . . The elderly person with arthritis or poor vision may have difficulty properly inserting the battery into a hearing aid. If the aid is not working, it may be that the battery simply is not inserted correctly.

◆ Resources for the Vision and Hearing Impaired

Loss of vision need not be devastating for a person if he is given support and encouragement for coping with his handicap. There are resources to help the visually handicapped person learn to care for himself, find employment, and enjoy educational and recreational activities. Many colleges provide special funds to enable blind students to hire readers and tape recorders to help them with their studies.

Resources for the Blind   The Library of Congress in Washington, DC, lends records and recording machines without charge to the blind and maintains a wide selection of recordings. Recordings of required textbooks may be obtained free of charge from Recording for the Blind and Dyslexic. Other resources include:

- American Printing House for the Blind, 1839 Frankfort Avenue, Louisville, KY 40206.
- Helen Keller International, 90 Washington Street, 15th Floor, New York, NY 10006; (212) 943-0890.
- Guiding Eyes for the Blind, 611 Granite Springs Road, Yorktown Heights, NY 10598; (800) 942-0149.
- Recording for the Blind and Dyslexic, 20 Roszel Road, Princeton, NJ 08540; (609) 452-0606.
- American Foundation for the Blind, 11 Penn Plaza, Suite 300, New York, NY 10001; (800) 232-5463.
- The Center for the Partially Sighted, 720 Wilshire Boulevard, Suite 200, Santa Monica, CA 90401-1713; (800) 481-3937.
- National Association for Visually Handicapped, 22 W. 21st Street, New York, NY 10010; (212) 889-3141.
- National Eye Institute, National Institutes of Health, 2020 Vision Place, Bethesda, MD 20892-3655.

Resources for the Hearing Impaired

- Self-help for Hard of Hearing People, Inc., 7910 Woodmont Avenue, Suite 1200, Bethesda, MD 20814.
- American Tinnitus Association, P.O. Box 5, Portland, OR 97207.
- Better Hearing Institute, Box 1840, Washington, DC 20013; (800) HEAR-WELL.

CRITICAL THINKING EXERCISES

Clinical Case Problems

Read each clinical situation and discuss the questions with your classmates.

1. Mr. Wilson, age 78, is scheduled for a right cataract extraction and intraocular lens implant. He has bilateral cataracts that have made him legally blind for years. He did not consult a doctor until recently, because he had always heard that cataracts had to

be "ripe" before they could be treated, and he felt he could not afford frequent trips to a doctor when nothing could be done for his condition. Mr. Wilson enters the outpatient surgery area, and you are assigned as his nurse.

- How would you approach and orient Mr. Wilson to his surroundings?
- What would you tell Mr. Wilson about the preoperative routine and medications at this time?
- What nursing diagnoses would be appropriate for Mr. Wilson at this time?
- What are the advantages of intraocular lens implants over cataract glasses and/or contact lenses?
- What discharge instructions will need to be given to Mr. Wilson?

2. Mr. Lavant, age 52, and his wife, who has diabetes, have heard about a glaucoma screening clinic being held in their community. They are interested in attending the clinic but are very apprehensive about the kind of tests that will be done. They ask you about the tests and whether you think they should go to the screening clinic when they have no symptoms of glaucoma or any other eye disease.

- How would you explain a test with a tonometer?
- How would you explain glaucoma in terms Mr. and Mrs. Lavant could understand?
- Who are among the people at high risk for glaucoma?
- What is the usual treatment for chronic, open-angle glaucoma?

3. Mrs. Como is admitted to the hospital for management of her hypertension. She has had sensorineural deafness for several years, and it is much worse in her left ear than in her right. Her inability to hear well causes additional stress for Mrs. Como, and she is especially anxious about being in the hospital among strangers. Mrs. Como also suffers from tinnitus, which adds to her stress and inability to relax and rest. This and the stress of not being able to hear adversely affect Mrs. Como's hypertension.

- What evidence would you expect to find that would indicate that Mrs. Como has a hearing impairment?
- What can the nurses do to improve communication with Mrs. Como and help allay her anxiety about being in the hospital?
- What measures might help Mrs. Como cope with her tinnitus?

4. Mr. Thompson is suffering from a severe attack of Menière's syndrome and vertigo. He is severely nauseated, and his vertigo prevents him from getting out of bed.

- What nursing actions would be appropriate for him?
- How would you explain this disorder to Mr. Thompson?
- The physician wants to rule out the possibility of tumor as a cause of Mr. Thompson's vertigo, and so he is scheduled for an electronystagmogram (ENG) with a caloric test and a magnetic resonance imaging (MRI) scan. How would you explain these tests to him?

BIBLIOGRAPHY

American Journal of Nursing. (1993). Clinical guidelines: cataract surgery and its alternatives. *American Journal of Nursing.* 93(7):59–61.

Applegate, E. J. (1995). *The Anatomy and Physiology Learning System: Textbook.* Philadelphia: Saunders.

Bennett, J. C., Plum, F., eds. (1996). *Cecil Textbook of Medicine,* 20th ed. Philadelphia: Saunders.

Black, J. M., Matassarin-Jacobs, E. (1997). *Medical-Surgical Nursing: Clinical Management for Collaborative Care,* 5th ed. Philadelphia: Saunders.

Brady, B. A. (1995). Macular degeneration: helping your patient cope. *Nursing 95.* 25(6):62–64.

Cleveland, P. J., Morris, J. (1990). Menière's disease: the inner ear out of balance. *RN.* 53(8):28–32.

Copstead, L. C. (1995). *Perspectives on Pathophysiology.* Philadelphia: Saunders.

Deutsch, N. (1995). Keeping current: diet behind ear trouble. *Canadian Nurse.* 91(2):19–20.

deWit, S. C. (1994). *Rambo's Nursing Skills for Clinical Practice,* 4th ed. Philadelphia: Saunders.

Erber, N. P. (1994). Communicating with elders: effects of amplification. *Journal of Gerontological Nursing.* 20(10):6–10.

Hunt, L. (1994). Eye safety tips: nutrients and the eye. *Insight.* 19(1):25–27.

Ignatavicius, D. D., Workman, M. L., Mishler, M. A. (1995). *Medical–Surgical Nursing: A Nursing Process Approach,* 2nd ed. Philadelphia: Saunders.

Jarvis, C. (1996). *Physical Examination and Health Assessment,* 2nd ed. Philadelphia: Saunders.

Kee, J. L., Hayes, E. R. (1993). *Pharmacology: A Nursing Process Approach.* Philadelphia: Saunders.

Kowalski, C. K. (1994). Cataracts: at any age. *Home Healthcare Nurse.* 12(2):43–46.

Lammon, C. B. et al. (1995). *Clinical Nursing Skills.* Philadelphia: Saunders.

Langseth, F. G. (1993). The use of 5-fluorouracil in glaucoma filtration surgery. *Insight.* 18(2):11–13.

Lehne, R. A. (1994). *Pharmacology for Nursing Care,* 2nd ed. Philadelphia: Saunders.

Lindblade, D. D., McDonald, M. (1995). Removing communication barriers for the hearing-impaired elderly. *Medsurg Nursing.* 4(5):379–385.

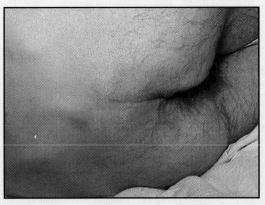

COLOR FIGURE 1 A stage I pressure ulcer.
(From Ignatavicius, D.D., Workman, M.L., Mishler, M.A. [1995].
Medical-Surgical Nursing: A Nursing Process Approach, 2nd ed.
Philadelphia: W.B. Saunders, Color Figure 67-2.)

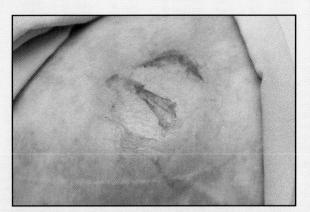

COLOR FIGURE 2 A stage II pressure ulcer.
(From Ignatavicius, D.D., Workman, M.L., Mishler, M.A. [1995].
Medical-Surgical Nursing: A Nursing Process Approach, 2nd ed.
Philadelphia: W.B. Saunders, Color Figure 67-3.)

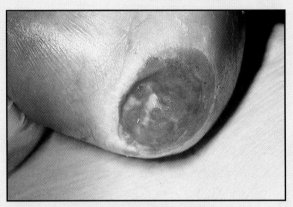

COLOR FIGURE 3 A stage III pressure ulcer.
(From Ignatavicius, D.D., Workman, M.L., Mishler, M.A. [1995].
Medical-Surgical Nursing: A Nursing Process Approach, 2nd ed.
Philadelphia: W.B. Saunders, Color Figure 67-4.)

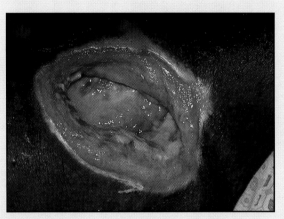

COLOR FIGURE 4 A stage IV pressure ulcer.
(From Ignatavicius, D.D., Workman, M.L., Mishler, M.A. [1995].
Medical-Surgical Nursing: A Nursing Process Approach, 2nd ed.
Philadelphia: W.B. Saunders, Color Figure 67-5.)

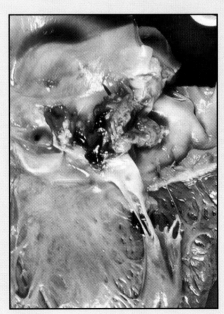

COLOR FIGURE 5
Bacterial endocarditis.
The valves are covered with extensive
vegetations. (From Damjanov, I. [1996].
Pathology for the Health-Related Professions.
Philadelphia: W.B. Saunders, p.177.)

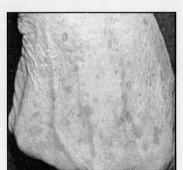

COLOR FIGURE 6
Senile litignes.
(From Lookingbill, D.P., Marks, J.G.
[1993]. *Principles of Dermatology*,
2nd ed. Philadelphia: W.B.
Saunders.)

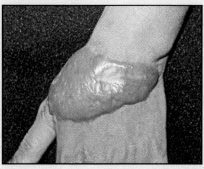

COLOR FIGURE 7 Keloid.
(From Lookingbill, D.P., Marks, J.G. [1993]. *Principles of Dermatology*, 2nd ed. Philadelphia: W.B. Saunders.)

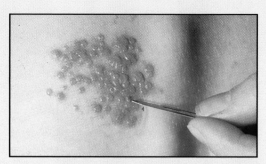

COLOR FIGURE 8 Herpes simplex.
(From Ignatavicius, D.D., Workman, M.L., Mishler, M.A. [1995]. *Medical-Surgical Nursing: A Nursing Process Approach*, 2nd ed. Philadelphia: W.B. Saunders, Color Figure 67-8.)

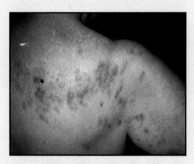

COLOR FIGURE 9 Herpes zoster.
(From Ignatavicius, D.D., Workman, M.L., Mishler, M.A. [1995]. *Medical-Surgical Nursing: A Nursing Process Approach*, 2nd ed. Philadelphia: W.B. Saunders, Color Figure 67-9.)

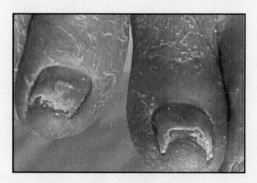

COLOR FIGURE 10 Onychomycoses.
(From Moschella, S.L., Hurley, H.J. [1992]. *Dermatology*, 3rd ed. Philadelphia: W.B. Saunders, p. 229.)

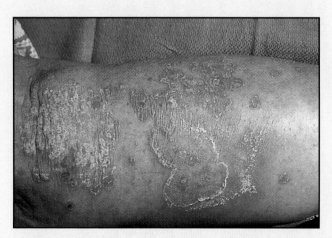

COLOR FIGURE 11 Psoriasis.
(From Black, J.M., Matassarin-Jacobs, E. [1997]. *Medical-Surgical Nursing: Clinical Management for Continuity of Care*, 5th ed. Philadelphia: W.B. Saunders, p. 2211.)

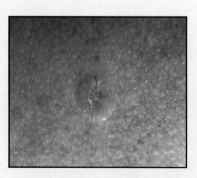

COLOR FIGURE 12 Basal cell carcinoma.
(From Ignatavicius, D.D., Workman, M.L., Mishler, M.A. [1995]. *Medical-Surgical Nursing: A Nursing Process Approach*, 2nd ed. Philadelphia: W.B. Saunders, Color Figure 67-16.)

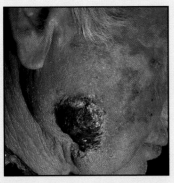

COLOR FIGURE 13 Squamous cell carcinoma.
(From Ignatavicius, D.D., Workman, M.L., Mishler, M.A. [1995].
Medical-Surgical Nursing: A Nursing Process Approach, 2nd ed.
Philadelphia: W.B. Saunders, Color Figure 67-15.)

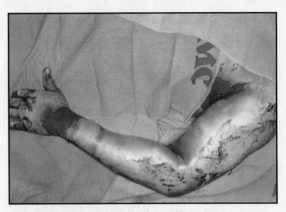

COLOR FIGURE 14 Melanoma.
(From Ignatavicius, D.D., Workman, M.L., Mishler, M.A. [1995].
Medical-Surgical Nursing: A Nursing Process Approach, 2nd ed.
Philadelphia: W.B. Saunders, Color Figure 67-17.)

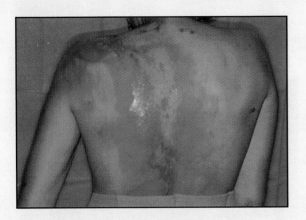

**COLOR FIGURE 15 Partial-thickness burn injury
(second-degree burn).**
(From Black, J.M., Matassarin-Jacobs, E. [1997]. *Medical-Surgical
Nursing: Clinical Management for Continuity of Care*, 5th ed.
Philadelphia: W.B. Saunders, p. 2238.)

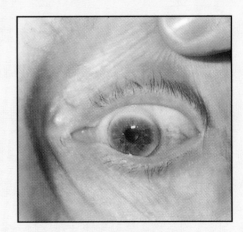

**COLOR FIGURE 16 Full-thickness burn injury
(third-degree burn).**
(From Black, J.M., Matassarin-Jacobs, E. [1997]. *Medical-Surgical
Nursing: Clinical Management for Continuity of Care*, 5th ed.
Philadelphia: W.B. Saunders, p. 2238.)

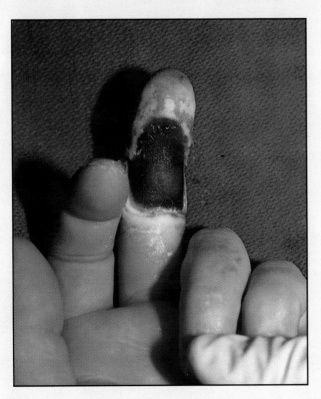

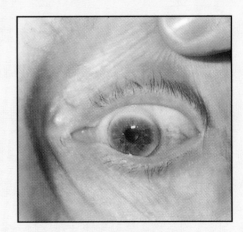

COLOR FIGURE 18 Arcus senilis.
(From Jarvis, C. [1996]. *Physical Examination and Health
Assessment,* 2nd ed. Philadelphia: W.B. Saunders, p. 334.)

**COLOR FIGURE 17 Full-thickness burn injury
(fourth-degree burn).**
(From Black, J.M., Matassarin-Jacobs, E. [1997]. *Medical-Surgical
Nursing: Clinical Management for Continuity of Care*, 5th ed. Philadelphia:
W.B. Saunders, p. 2238.)

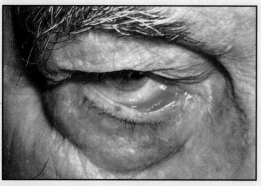

COLOR FIGURE 19 Ectropion.
(From Jarvis, C. [1996]. *Physical Examination and Health Assessment,* 2nd ed. Philadelphia: W.B. Saunders, p. 342.)

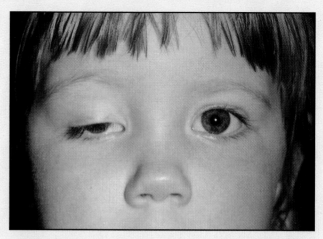

COLOR FIGURE 20 Ptosis.
(From Borodic, G.E., Townsend, D.J. [1994]. *Atlas of Eyelid Surgery.* Philadelphia: W.B. Saunders, p. 104.)

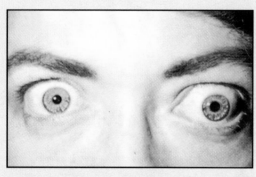

COLOR FIGURE 21 Exophthalmos.
(From Jarvis, C. [1996]. *Physical Examination and Health Assessment,* 2nd ed. Philadelphia: W.B. Saunders, p. 342.)

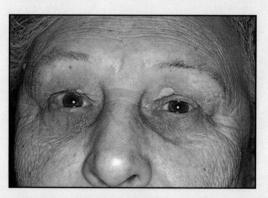

COLOR FIGURE 22 Xanthelasma.
(From Jarvis, C. [1996]. *Physical Examination and Health Assessment,* 2nd ed. Philadelphia: W.B. Saunders, p. 334.)

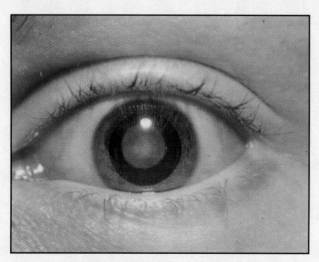

COLOR FIGURE 23 Cloudy appearance of an eye with cataract.
(From Polaski, A.L., Tatro, S.E. [1996]. *Luckmann's Core Principles and Practice of Medical-Surgical Nursing,* 4th ed. Philadelphia: W.B. Saunders, p. 441.)

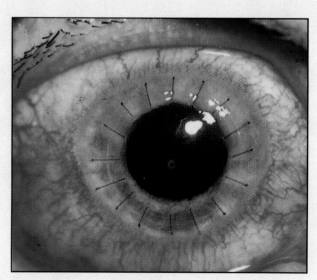

COLOR FIGURE 24 Keratoplasty.
(From Polaski, A.L., Tatro, S.E. [1996]. *Luckmann's Core Principles and Practice of Medical-Surgical Nursing.* 4th ed. Philadelphia: W.B. Saunders, p. 447.)

Long, K., Long, R. (1994). Pharmacology update: treating open-angle glaucoma. *Nurse Practitioner Forum.* 5(4):205–206.

Matteson M. A., McConnell, E. S., Linton A. D. (1997). *Gerontological Nursing: Concepts and Practice, Edition 2.* Philadelphia: W. B. Saunders.

McAllen, P. (1996). Managing Ménière's disease. *American Journal of Nursing.* 96(6):16E–16H.

McConnell, E. A. (1996). Caring for a patient who has a vision impairment. *Nursing 96.* 26(5):28.

McConnell, E. A. (1996). Handling your patient's hearing aid. *Nursing 96.* 26(7):22.

Meissner, J. E. (1995). Disease review: caring for patients with glaucoma. *Nursing 95.* 25(1):56–57.

Neatherlin, J. S., Egan, J. (1994). Benign paroxysmal positional vertigo. *Journal of Neuroscience Nursing.* 26(6):330–335.

Newland, J. A. (1994). Primary care protocol: adult otitis media. *American Journal of Nursing.* 94(9):16F.

Nursing 94. (1994). Opening your eyes to intraocular drug administration. *Nursing 94.* 24(6):44–45.

Olson, R. J. (1995). Now hear this! *RN.* 58(8):43–44.

Peralta, L. A. W., Adame, H. L. (1995). Corneal transplant: a new lease on life. *Seminars in Perioperative Nursing.* 4(4):227–233.

Polaski, A. L., Tatro, S. E. (1996). *Luckmann's Core Principles and Practice of Medical–Surgical Nursing.* Philadelphia: Saunders.

Pollock, K. J. (1995). Ménière's disease: a review of the problem. *ORL Head and Neck Nursing.* 13(2):10–13.

Sandler, R. L. (1995). Clinical snapshot: glaucoma. *American Journal of Nursing.* 95(3):34–35.

Smeltzer, C. D. (1993). Primary care screening and evaluation of hearing loss. *Nurse Practitioner.* 18(8):50–55.

Smeltzer, S., Bare, B. (1996). *Brunner & Suddarth's Textbook of Medical–Surgical Nursing,* 8th ed. Philadelphia: Lippincott.

Society of Otorhinolaryngology and Head Neck Nurses. (1994). Practice guidelines: stapedectomy. *ORL Head and Neck Nursing.* 12(4):22–23.

Spires, R. (1996). The ophthalmic ambulatory surgery patient. *Journal of Post Anesthesia Nursing.* 11(2):78–89.

Springhouse Corporation. (1996). *Nursing 96 Drug Handbook.* Springhouse, PA: Author.

Thobaben, M., Langlois, A. (1996). Patients with hearing impairments: implications for home healthcare professionals. *Home Healthcare Nurse.* 14(4):290–291.

Whitaker, V. B. (1995). Eye surgery. *Seminars in Perioperative Nursing.* 4(4):193–238.

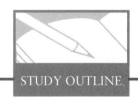

STUDY OUTLINE

I. Introduction
   A. Loss of vision or hearing may greatly affect quality of life.

   B. Nursing care of the visually impaired demands sensitivity to patient's unique needs, gentleness, and creativity in devising ways to help the patient accept and cope with his handicap.

   C. Newer surgical techniques and medical treatments have improved the chances for preserving sight and preventing blindness.

   D. Hearing loss is the most common handicap in the United States.

   E. Loss of hearing can create social, emotional, and financial burdens for the patient and family.

   F. Hearing loss may be gradual and therefore often is ignored.

II. Prevention of Eye Disorders
   A. Nurses share responsibility with other health care providers for preventing eye disease and loss of sight.

   B. Two major goals are to teach people how to take care of their eyes and to prevent eye injury.

   C. Basic eye care and prevention of injury.

      1. It is not possible to strain the eye. Headache, burning, itching, and redness of the eyes are symptomatic of eye disease, not eyestrain.

      2. Adequate nutrition conserves, but does not improve, eyesight.

      3. Normal eyes do not require irrigation. Persons with "dry eye syndrome" require replacement tears.

      4. Children do not outgrow crossed eyes. Amblyopia ("lazy eye") requires prompt treatment to avoid permanent loss of vision in the affected eye.

      5. Every person over the age of 40 should have periodic eye examinations.

      6. Teaching children and adults to practice eye safety could prevent many accidental injuries to the eyes.

7. Cosmetics for the eyelids, eyelashes, and eyebrows can be sources of infection and allergy.

8. Danger signals of eye disorders (Table 30-2).

III. **Diagnostic Tests and Examinations (Table 30-3)**

IV. **Nursing Management of Eye Disorders**

A. Assessment.

1. History taking (Table 30-4).

2. Physical examination: check for redness, swelling of eyelids or periorbital space, excessive tearing, exudate on eyelids, abnormal position of eyelids (Table 30-5), exophthalmia.

   a. Inflammation or infection (Table 30-6).

   b. Also note patient's posture and general behavior (e.g., tilting the head, squinting, shading the eyes, and matching clothes and colors).

   c. Ability to move eyebrows and eyes.

B. Nursing diagnosis associated with eye disorders include those that alter satisfaction of human needs at every level from physiological to self-actualization needs.

C. Planning.

1. Specific outcome objectives are written for each individual nursing diagnosis.

2. The nurse must plan extra time to assist patients who have a vision loss.

D. Implementation.

1. Give support and encouragement to patient adjusting to loss of eyesight.

2. Guidelines for helping a blind person.

   a. Do not shout.

   b. Speak to the patient as you enter the room so he will know you are there. Notify him when you are leaving.

   c. Remove hazards from environment so patient will not accidentally fall or injure himself.

   d. Assess amount of assistance patient will need with self-care activities.

   e. Orient patient thoroughly to room at time of admission.

   f. Use "clock method" to tell patient about arrangement of food on his plate. Set up tray for him. Feed the patient if necessary.

   g. Allow patient to maintain his dignity while his needs are being met.

3. Nursing care of the patient having eye surgery; most eye surgery is done on a short-stay basis.

   a. Preoperative care: nursing care planned according to individual needs.

   b. Orient patient to short-stay surgery area and preoperative routine and procedures.

   c. Emphasis on teaching for home care.

   d. Verify that preoperative eye drops are placed in the correct eye: OD for right eye; OS for left eye; OU for both eyes.

4. Postoperative care: gentleness is very important.

   a. No jarring of head when transferring patient.

   b. Speak before touching patient who cannot see.

   c. Medicate for nausea and vomiting immediately to prevent increased IOP from vomiting.

   d. Report sudden pain in eye immediately as it may indicate hemorrhage.

   e. Use cold compresses to reduce swelling.

   f. Teach activity restrictions and positioning while in bed (i.e., which side the patient can lie on).

   g. Avoid straining, lifting, bending from the waist, and other activities that elevate IOP.

   h. Follow-up care with physician is essential.

5. Care of an artificial eye.

   a. Handle it very carefully.

   b. Care is similar to that for dentures; cleanse and reinsert.

   c. Remove carefully, wash with mild soap and water, store in container of water or contact lens solution. Wet prosthesis before reinserting.

E. Evaluation.

1. Based on reassessment data and determining whether outcomes have been met.

2. Assessments are made to evaluate vision improvement.

V. **Eye Disorders**

A. Common errors of refraction.

1. Refraction: light rays are bent so that they are not properly focused on the retina.

   a. Myopia (nearsightedness): light rays converge and focus in front of the retina. Person has difficulty seeing distant objects.

   b. Hyperopia (farsightedness): light rays converge behind the retina; person has difficulty seeing objects close at hand.

   c. Presbyopia: visual defect of old age; improper accommodation of the ciliary muscles and ligaments when switching between distant and near vision.

   d. Astigmatism: results from a warped lens or irregular curvature of the cornea.

B. Cataract: opacity of the lens.

1. Symptoms and medical diagnosis: complaint of distortion of vision, floaters, photosensitivity.

2. Diagnosis by examination under slit lamp; lens appears opaque.

3. Surgical treatment: removal of affected lens and implant of intraocular lens, or prescription of contact lens or eyeglasses for aphakic eye.

4. Nursing intervention.

   a. Preoperative nursing care: explain expected outcome of surgery. Orient patient to room. Implement safety measures. Administer eyedrops precisely as ordered.

   b. Postoperative nursing care.

      (1) Observe patient for sudden and severe pain in eye, bleeding, and signs of infection.

      (2) Warn patient not to cough, sneeze violently, squeeze eyelids, or make sudden movements of head.

      (3) Ambulation and other physical activity usually are not restricted unless otherwise ordered by surgeon.

      (4) Discharge planning should include instruction of patient about limitations on physical activities, instillation of eyedrops, and application and removal of eye dressings and shield.

      (5) Patient warned that adjustment to artificial lens will take time.

         (a) Contact lenses provide better vision than cataract glasses but require manual dexterity to remove, care for, and reinsert.

         (b) Intraocular lens implanted during surgery. Should not cause discomfort or inconvenience. There is risk of damage to eye.

C. Glaucoma: a complex group of disorders that have in common an increase in intraocular pressure.

   1. Due to either excessive production or inadequate drainage of aqueous from the chamber of the eye. Increased pressure of accumulating fluid damages optic disc.

   2. Two major types: acute, or angle-closure, glaucoma, and chronic, or open-angle, glaucoma.

      a. Acute, angle-closure glaucoma.

         (1) Characterized by sudden and severe pain in eye, blurred vision, and regional headache.

         (2) Medical and surgical treatment:

            (a) Treated as an emergency. Effort is made to reduce pressure immediately by administration of drugs.

            (b) As soon as inflammation subsides, surgery is done (periph-

eral iridectomy) before vision is destroyed.

      b. Chronic, open-angle glaucoma more insidious and more common. Can lead to blindness without ever producing an acute attack.

         (1) Symptoms and medical diagnosis:

            (a) Symptoms relatively mild: blurred vision, trouble adjusting to dark, narrowing of vision, seeing halos around objects and light.

            (b) Persons most at risk for glaucoma are diabetics, those with recently controlled hypertension, blacks, those with family history of glaucoma, those with facial hemangioma or nevi, children with large eyes, and victims of eye injury.

            (c) Diagnosis confirmed by applanation tonometry.

         (2) Medical and surgical treatment:

            (a) Chronic glaucoma treated by drugs to enhance the outflow of aqueous and decrease its production. Diuretics also may be used. Patients with glaucoma being treated in a hospital for unrelated illnesses must continue to receive their eye medication.

            (b) Surgical treatment: trabeculoplasty or filtering procedure by laser beam to facilitate drainage of aqueous.

         (3) Nursing intervention:

            (a) Patient education of utmost importance. Failure to follow prescribed treatment can mean loss of vision.

               (i) Nature of disorder and how it affects the eye.
               (ii) Treatments available.
               (iii) Expected result of currently prescribed treatment.
               (iv) Possible outcome of not following prescribed treatment.

D. Retinal detachment.

   1. A separation of the sensory layers from the pigmented epithelial layer due to holes or tears in the retina.

   2. Incidence increases dramatically after age 40, most common in 50- and 60-year-olds.

   3. Symptoms and diagnosis: flashes of light, floaters, cloudy vision, sometimes sudden loss of vision. Diagnosis confirmed by direct ophthalmoscopy.

4. Surgical treatment:
   a. Repair of holes and tears by photocoagulation or cryosurgery. More extensive surgery may be required to position retinal breaks in contact with epithelial layer.
   b. Vitrectomy: removal of opaque vitreous and stabilization of retina against choroid.
5. Nursing intervention: preoperative and postoperative care require specialized skills and knowledge. Instructions for Home care (Table 30-11).

E. Retinopathy: two causes are diabetes mellitus and hypertension.
1. Diabetic retinopathy: two types, proliferative and nonproliferative.
   a. Nonproliferative retinopathy: vessels develop microaneurysms, which tend to rupture and hemorrhage into the vitreous.
   b. Proliferative retinopathy: neovascularization with fragile vessels that rupture and hemorrhage into the vitreous or between layers of the retina.
2. Diabetic retinopathy controlled by laser photocoagulation treatments.

F. Corneal disorders.
1. Keratitis: inflammation of the cornea from irritation or infection.
2. Corneal ulceration: from foreign body, trauma, or infection with bacteria, fungi, or protozoa.
3. Treatment to erradicate infection and decrease inflammation.
4. Scarring of cornea may cause visual impairment.
5. Corneal transplant (keratoplasty) done to replace cornea damaged by trauma, ulcers, or disease and restore vision.
   a. Two types: full-thickness and lamellar keratoplasty.
   b. Cornea is not vascular and heals very slowly; takes up to 1 year for complete healing.

G. Macular degeneration occurs with aging and affects color vision, acute vision, and central vision.
1. Cigarette smokers more likely to develop macular degeneration.
2. Wearing protective sunglasses may help prevent the disorder.
3. Two types of macular degeneration: atrophic (most common) and exudative.
4. Visual loss is bilateral and progressive.
5. Peripheral vision is retained, but central vision is lost; the person can walk around and perform many functions but cannot read.
6. Low-vision aids can be used to enhance vision.

H. Eye trauma.
1. Corneal abrasion is very painful; infection is a danger.
2. Removing a foreign body from surface of cornea is best done by irrigation.
3. Foreign body penetrating the cornea should be removed by physician.
4. Chemical burns require extensive irrigation.
5. Foreign body is removed by everting the lid and using cotton swab.
6. Deeply embedded objects must be removed by an ophthalmologist.

VI. Causes and Prevention of Hearing Loss
A. Table 30-12 presents some causes of hearing loss.
B. Measures to prevent hearing loss:
1. Refrain from putting sharp instruments into the ear to clean or relieve tickling in the canal: hairpins, pencils, etc.
2. Keep the ear canal clean by removing cerumen with irrigation or drops as necessary.
3. Avoid loud noise; continual exposure to music amplified to more than 104 to 111 decibels may damage hearing.
4. Avoid drugs that are ototoxic; monitor hearing when ototoxic drugs are prescribed.

VII. Diagnostic Tests and Examinations (Table 30-13)
A. Visual examination with otoscope.
B. Whisper test for simple evaluation of hearing ability.
C. Test for nystagmus by having patient follow finger with eyes while observing for oscillation of eyeballs.
D. Rhomberg test for balance.

VIII. Nursing Management of Ear Disorders
A. Assessment.
1. History taking (Table 30-14).
2. Physical examination.
   a. Outer ear inspected for developmental anomalies, encrustations, and lesions.
   b. Note enlargement of lymph nodes in front of ear and over mastoid process.
   c. Patient reports tinnitus, pain, dizziness, or vertigo.
B. Common nursing diagnoses:
1. Activity intolerance.
2. Pain.
3. Impaired verbal communication.
4. Risk for injury.
5. Knowledge deficit.
6. Social isolation.
C. Planning.
1. Expected outcomes are written for each nursing diagnosis chosen.

2. Planning of care is a collaborative process and may involve the nurse, physician, audiologist, and speech pathologist.

3. When hearing is impaired, communication may take longer, and the nurse should plan sufficient time into the schedule to work with a hearing-impaired patient.

D. Implementation (Table 30-16).

1. Instill ear drops; position the patient supine with the affected ear up; pull the pinna slightly up and back.

2. Warm ear drops to room temperature before instilling.

3. Interventions for communicating with the hearing impaired (Table 30-17).

4. Nursing care of the patient having ear surgery.

   a. Preoperative care: physical preparaion and administration of eardrops, if ordered.

   b. Postoperative care: varies according to surgical procedure:.

      (1) Patient usually kept flat in bed with head kept still for several hours for major surgery.

      (2) Watch for signs of injury to facial nerve.

      (3) Assist when up until all dizziness has passed.

      (4) Instruct in home care (Table 30-18).

E. Evaluation.

1. Reassess to determine whether outcomes are being met.

2. Determine if hearing is improving.

IX. Common Ear Disorders

A. Hearing impairment: types of hearing loss.

1. Conductive: external and middle ear unable to conduct sound waves.

2. Sensorineural: dysfunction located in inner ear of the eighth cranial nerve; not due to malfunction of outer or middle ear.

3. Central hearing loss: pathology above junction of eighth cranial nerve and brain stem.

B. Otitis media: inflammation of the middle ear:

1. Acute serous otitis media: usually follows upper respiratory infection or trauma.

2. Secretory otitis media: due to primary allergic response and increased secretions.

   a. Treatment: antihistamines, decongestants, myringotomy with insertion of ventilating tubes.

3. Suppurative otitis media: caused by bacterial infection, usually from an upper respiratory tract infection. Treatment: systemic antibiotics, eardrops, tympanoplasty to repair ruptured eardrum, and sometimes mastoidectomy.

C. Otosclerosis: a hereditary disease of the bone in the middle ear.

1. Symptoms and medical diagnosis.

   a. Progressive hearing loss begins in late teens or early twenties. Patient complains that the voices of others are muffled but can hear his own voice very well.

   b. Treatment: some cases respond to a hearing aid; others require stapedectomy and the insertion of a prosthetic device.

2. Nursing intervention: postoperative care.

   a. Position patient properly for first 48 hours.

   b. Help patient avoid sudden, violent movements.

   c. Instruct in self-care before discharge.

D. Labyrinthitis: inflammation of labyrinth of inner ear:

1. Symptoms: loss of hearing, dizziness, nausea and vomiting, nystagmus.

2. Treatment: antibiotics, bedrest, drugs to control motion sickness, possibly mastoidectomy if that bone is involved.

E. Menière's syndrome: group of symptoms due to an increase of fluid in labyrinthine spaces, with swelling and congestion of cochlear mucosa.

1. Symptoms: tinnitus, headache, poor coordination, hearing loss. Vertigo and nausea and vomiting when head is moved.

2. Treatment: bedrest during attacks of vertigo, drugs to control nausea and motion sickness, restriction of fluid intake, and surgical destruction of the eighth cranial nerve.

F. Dizziness and vertigo.

1. Caution patient to avoid sudden movements.

2. Assist patient to get up, go to bathroom, ambulate, etc.

3. Administer medication to minimize motion sickness before symptoms become severe.

4. Encourage patient to limit fluid intake if this is recommended.

5. Encourage patient to not smoke.

6. Teach patient coping mechanisms to deal with stress.

G. Tinnitus: noise in the ear, "head noise."

1. Common to many disorders of the ear, cardiovascular disease, neurological disorders, and thyroid disease.

2. Biofeedback training and masking techniques are sometimes successful when all other treatments fail.

X. Rehabilitation

A. Speech reading.

1. Not a panacea. Experienced speech readers understand fewer than half the words spoken.

2. Enhanced by nonverbal cues.

3. Requires special abilities.
4. Hearing aids.
   a. Can improve hearing for various kinds of hearing loss.
   b. Must receive special care to avoid damage. Clean ear mold with soap and water. Other parts should not be wet. Avoid hair spray on hearing aid.
5. Cochlear implants now available; success is variable among patients.
6. Hearing assistive devices.
   a. Aids for amplification of telephone and sound systems in churches and theaters.
   b. Closed-captioning on T.V.
   c. Hearing dog to provide safety when out-of-doors.
   d. Devices around house such as flashing light attached to doorbell.

XI. Elder Care Points

A. Older persons often suffer from dry eyes; this is treated by instillation of replacement tears, an artificial tear solution.
B. Elderly persons undergoing eye surgery often have other chronic diseases. These must be considered when planning care. Instructions and information should be given both verbally and in written form.
C. Hearing loss is very common in those over 75 years of age; nurses should pay close attention to communication with senior adults. Be certain you have the person's attention, speak distinctly, and validate communication by asking for feedback.
D. Arteriosclerosis may contribute to hearing loss in the elderly by decreasing blood flow to the 8th cranial nerve.
E. The elderly person with arthritis may have difficulty in changing a battery in a hearing aid; offer assistance.

XII. Community Care

A. Nurses should constantly teach about eye and ear safety.
B. All nurses assess for vision and hearing problems.
C. Home care and long-term care nurses should regularly assess all patients for vision deterioration and for hearing loss.
D. Encouraging those with vision loss or hearing loss to have a thorough evaluation may help improve the quality of life of these patients.
E. Frequently assess the function of a hearing aid for patients; batteries may run down and need replacing; elderly often forget when the battery was last replaced.
F. Resources for the visually impaired and hearing impaired.
   1. Vision services, information, and support available to patients and their families.
   2. Services and aids available for the hearing impaired.

CHAPTER 31

Medical–Surgical Nursing in Emergency and Disaster

PREVENTION OF ACCIDENTS

◆ Home Safety

According to statistics compiled by the National Safety Council, accidents in the home account for one fourth of all fatal accidents. People under 5 and over 65 years of age are the principal victims of fatal mishaps occurring in the home. Because these individuals spend a large majority of their time inside the house, safety hazards must be identified and removed if accidental deaths are to be avoided.

Nurses, physicians, and others concerned with safety and welfare must take an active part in educating the public about ways to prevent home accidents. The two most dangerous rooms in the house are the kitchen and the bathroom. Table 31-1 shows some of the most common home hazards and how they can be eliminated.

Think about . . . Can you find three ways to increase safety in your own home?

◆ Highway Safety

Motor vehicle accidents are the leading cause of accidental death in the United States. Every year, thousands of Americans are killed in motor vehicle accidents and millions are disabled by some kind of injury sustained in a traffic accident.

The two principal causes of motor vehicle accidents are human failure and mechanical failure. Human failure is by far the greater danger. Improper driving, which is responsible for almost 90% of all accidents, can be caused by the influence of alcohol and/or drugs, fatigue, excessive speed, or emotional instability. Mechanical failure often is not detected as the cause of an accident; however, there has been much interest recently in built-in safety devices and inspection for safety hazards in new automobiles. The use of seat belts and air bags, lowering the speed limit on major highways, and better enforcement of laws against drunk driving have made a significant impact on vehicular deaths. The effect of again raising the speed limit on major highways is yet to be seen. The decrease in the number of vehicular deaths also reflects improvements in emergency medical

TABLE 31-1 ◆ Home Safety Chart

Kitchen

For gas, coal, or wood-burning stove, have vents or flues; keep windows open a crack. Never light stove with kerosene or gasoline. Turn off all flames after cooking. Repair any gas leakage.

Use potholders. Keep handles of pots and pans turned away from edge of stove.

Keep knives, sharp instruments, and poisons, such as bleach and household cleansers, out of children's reach. Keep matches out of reach of children. Place child safety locks on all cupboard doors within reach where dangerous substances are stored.

Wipe up spills on floor.

Keep electric appliances in good working order.

Place broken glass in heavy paper sack to prevent cuts through plastic bags.

Storage areas

Always keep cellars, attics, garages neat.

Clean and disinfect area where garbage is kept, and dispose of it frequently.

Never place poisonous substances in drinking glasses, cold drink bottles, or other containers that have been used for food or drink.

Always label poisonous compounds; read labels of poisons you have purchased and store out of reach.

Living room

Be sure floors are not slippery. Use rubber mats under rugs to prevent slipping.

Replace frayed or torn carpets.

Cover electric sockets.

Replace frayed electric cords. Keep electric cords off floor where people walk.

Place heaters a safe distance from walls. Use screens around fireplace. Keep fireplace matches out of reach of children.

Pad sharp edges on furniture as necessary.

Check ashtrays for lit matches or cigarettes when going to bed or leaving house.

Furnace

Have furnace checked every year, especially for leaks in tank of oil-burning furnaces.

Never light furnace with gasoline or kerosene.

Change filters monthly.

Bathroom

Use rubber mat in tub.

Store medicines out of children's reach. Keep all medicines capped and labeled. Throw out old medicines. Keep phone number of poison center close to telephone.

Install child safety locks on cupboards where dangerous substances or medicines are stored.

Dispose of razor blades immediately after use.

Keep hot water heater set at 120° F or lower.

Bedrooms

Do not smoke in bed.

Use rubber mats under scatter rugs.

Stairways

Cover with carpeting or rubber safety treads.

Replace torn or frayed carpeting. Keep stairs cleared of toys and cleaning equipment.

Install handrails, proper lighting.

Use gates at top and bottom if there are young children.

General areas

Install smoke alarms throughout the house.

Install carbon monoxide alarms.

---

services, which provide prompt and effective first aid and emergency care of accident victims.

◆ Water Safety

Weekends and vacations are an opportunity for Americans to enjoy water sports. With increased participation has come a proportionate increase in accidental deaths and injuries in or on the water. Many water accidents involve jet skis or wave riders. People who use these recreational items should take a safety test before unsupervised use. Many of these accidents could have been prevented if the simple rules of water safety had been observed. **These rules include using good judgment about the choice of swimming area, ensuring proper supervision of children and adults who are not strong swimmers, diving only in areas where the water is sufficiently deep and is free of rocks or other obstacles, never swimming alone, and avoiding overexertion or swimming distances beyond one's ability.** A life jacket and appropriate rescue equipment should be available for each occupant of a boat. Life jackets should be worn by all water skiers and jet ski users.

Above all, one should know how to handle an emergency should it arise. Panic frequently increases the danger for both the victim and the would-be rescuer.

The victim of a diving injury should not be removed from the water until emergency medical personnel are in attendance. The chance of a neck and spinal cord injury is considerable. The victim is placed on a flat surface and moved as a unit taking care to rigidly stabilize the neck.

Rescue of a drowning person requires clear thinking and deliberate action. First, the rescuer should call for help. If possible, he should try to reach the victim without going in water over his head. It is often possible to reach him by extending an arm, towel, rope, pole, or any long and sturdy object that is available. When the victim has grasped the object, he can be pulled slowly to safety. If a boat is available, it should be used to rescue the person who is beyond reach by other methods.

A swimming rescue is very difficult, even for the most experienced swimmer. Because the victim is frightened, he may demonstrate abnormal strength and be quite capable of drowning both himself and his rescuer. After the rescued person is brought out of the water, he must be given cardiopulmonary resuscitation (CPR) if he is not breathing. If he is breathing, he should be placed in a reclining position and covered with a blanket or coat. His head should be turned to one side so that if he vomits, he will not aspirate the vomitus into his lungs.

Because near-drowning victims usually aspirate water, pulmonary edema may occur and the victim should be transported to a medical facility promptly for evaluation and treatment. Bacterial or fungal pneumonia may follow aspiration of fresh water. There is danger of delayed cardiac irregularities in all persons who have been rescued from drowning, no matter how short a time they might have been struggling in the water.

GENERAL PRINCIPLES OF FIRST AID

The following guidelines explain specific actions to take when called upon to provide first aid.

◆ *Try to keep calm and think before acting. Concentrate on what should be done first and the manner in which to proceed step by step.* Move slowly and deliberately so that you can gain time to think things through and at the same time instill confidence in those you are trying to help. Identify yourself as a nurse. This will serve to reassure the victim and the onlookers.

◆ *Before attending to the victim or victims of an accident, quickly survey the accident scene to determine whether there are further hazards to yourself and the victims.* For example, spillage of gasoline after a motor vehicle accident can cause a fire or explosion, or there may be danger to the victim, yourself, and onlookers from oncoming traffic and secondary collisions. In both highway and home accidents, live electric wires may be in the vicinity. Whenever there is a high risk of death from hazardous conditions in the immediate environment, the victims should be moved at once, regardless of the nature of their injuries. One factor that often is overlooked is the heat of the pavement in the summertime. Victims may receive severe burns from lying on a sun-baked street or sidewalk while waiting for the ambulance. Although it may not be safe to move the victim to a shaded area, it is advisable to place clothing, newspaper, or some other protective covering between his skin and the hot pavement.

◆ *If there are several victims of the accident, make a quick check of each one before beginning treatment.* The most serious and life-threatening injuries must be treated first; those who do not seem to be in immediate danger can be attended to by someone else who is capable of watching the victim and reporting to you any change in his condition.

◆ Assess the victim as soon as possible after you are sure that there is no further danger in the immediate environment.

◆ Look for a Medic-Alert bracelet or necklace. If the victim is wearing one or has some other identification showing specific medical needs, bring this to the attention of the ambulance or hospital personnel.

◆ Try to determine the kind of instrument that caused the injury; for example, the column of the steering wheel, a drug or poison, or electric current. This will give clues about the type of injury sustained and the treatment required. **When evaluating the victim, begin at the head and work downward to the toes.** Refer to the evaluation checklist in Table 31-2.

◆ *Do not move the victim unless, as explained, he is in immediate danger or until you have immobilized injured parts.* This is particularly true if spinal injury is suspected.

◆ *Do not remove an object that has penetrated a part of the body and is still in place.* For example, a knife, piece of metal, or sliver of wood that is protruding from the chest or abdomen should be left as is. Bandages are applied around the object to stabilize it and control bleeding as necessary.

◆ *Do not try to give anything by mouth to a person who is unconscious;* he may aspirate the material into his air passage.

◆ *Explain to the victim in a calm and positive tone of voice what you are doing for him and why.* Give honest answers, but do not alarm him unduly. You must sound as if you are in control of yourself and the situation.

◆ *Remember that most states have adopted "good Samaritan" laws that protect medical personnel from malpractice suits in the case of emergency medical care for victims of accidental injury.* These laws prevent litigation for malpractice as long as medically trained individuals act in good faith and to the best of their ability.

Even in states where there are no such protective laws, malpractice suits of this kind very rarely occur. For many people, the advantages derived from knowing that they have used their skills and experience to help someone in need outweigh the risk of a lawsuit.

Think about . . . If you came upon an automobile accident in which several people were involved and stopped to render aid, how would you assess the situation for safety of yourself and the victims? How would you act to ensure as safe a scene as possible for evaluation of the victims?

TABLE 31-2 ◆ *Checklist for Evaluating Accident and Emergency Patients*

Area of Assessment	Mode of Assessment	Possible Causes
ABCs		
A—airway	Look and listen for signs of respiratory distress: gasping, wheezing, stridor, choking, restlessness. Check mouth for easily removable foreign body. Do *not* tilt head and hyperextend neck if spinal injury is suspected.	Airway obstruction, acute allergic reaction.
B—breathing	Put ear close to nose and mouth and listen for breathing. Watch chest and abdomen for rhythmic rise and fall. Note rate and quality of respirations.	*Absence of respirations:* cardiac arrest, airway obstruction. *Rapid, shallow respirations:* hyperventilation, pain, fear.
C—circulation	Feel for pulse in carotid or femoral artery; note rate and quality. Check for bleeding.	*Absence of pulse:* cardiac arrest. *Rapid, bounding pulse:* hemorrhage, fright, hypertension. *Rapid, weak pulse:* hemorrhage, shock.
Head-to-toe examination		
1. General appearance and level of consciousness	Note if alert, oriented to time, place, person. Note response to verbal stimuli. Check for MedicAlert ID.	*Momentarily unconscious:* fainting, mild concussion. *Disoriented, confused, combative:* substance abuse, head injury, cerebral ischemia, insulin reaction, diabetic ketoacidosis. *Comatose:* severe brain damage, poisoning, diabetic ketoacidosis.
2. Pupils	Lift eyelid and check pupils for equality in size and shape and response to light.	*Dilated, fixed:* brain damage, drug overdose, shock, cardiac arrest. *Constricted:* CNS disorder, drug overdose. *Unequal:* intracranial lesion, stroke. *No response to light:* cerebral ischemia, brain damage.
3. Ability to move	Ask conscious victim to move extremities	*Paralysis on one side:* stroke, head injury with brain damage, hemorrhage. *Inability to move extremities:* spinal cord injury.
4. Ears, nose	Look for drainage, note character.	Facial trauma, skull fracture.
5. Skin color and temperature	Note circumoral pallor. In dark-skinned victims evaluate skin changes in conjunctiva, soles of feet, and palms of hands.	*Pallor:* shock, heart attack. *Bright red lips and skin:* carbon monoxide poisoning. *Cyanosis:* asphyxia, electrocution, cold, shallow respirations. *Hot, dry skin:* heatstroke. *Cool, dry skin:* hypothermia. *Cold, clammy skin:* shock.
6. Head, mouth, and neck	Check for lacerations, soft depressed area of skull, avulsed tissue. Note breath odor. Check for loose or missing teeth, lacerations inside mouth. Check for pulsating, distended, or collapsed jugular vein.	Skull fracture, hematoma. Alcohol. *Fruity odor:* diabetic ketosis. Facial trauma. Cardiopulmonary pathology, injury.
7. Chest	Check lung sounds, change in position of trachea. Palpate for crepitus. Note skin integrity, open wounds. Check symmetry of chest movement during respirations. Splinting due to pain. Shoulder pain on left side.	Pneumothorax. Hemothorax. Fractured ribs. Possible ruptured spleen.

TABLE 31-2 ◆ *Checklist for Evaluating Accident and Emergency Patients (Continued)*

Area of Assessment	Mode of Assessment	Possible Causes
8. Abdomen	Palpate for hard, distended abdomen. Listen for bowel sounds *before* palpation. Check for wounds, drainage. Assess pain.	Abdominal trauma.
9. Genitalia	Look for lacerations, trauma, discharge, bloody urine. Assess pain.	Trauma to genitalia, bladder, or kidney.
10. Extremities	Look for deformities, lacerations, missing fingers and toes. Check for ability to move, abnormal sensations. Assess pain.	Trauma, fractures, nerve damage.

EMERGENCY CARE

Emergency care may be provided in the emergency room, a clinic, or out in the community (Figure 31-1). Those emergencies affecting the heart, thorax and lungs, musculoskeletal system, head and spine, eye and ear, skin (burns), gastrointestinal (abdominal injuries), and genitourinary systems are discussed within the chapters related to the specific body system. Acute alcohol or drug intoxication is discussed in Chapter 33 on substance use disorders. General emergency nursing, disorders that affect the entire body, and disaster nursing are presented in this chapter.

◆ Cardiopulmonary Resuscitation (CPR)

The first priority in administering emergency medical care is to assess the airway, then check for signs of breathing, as listed in Table 31-2. The second priority is to determine whether the heart is beating by assessing circulation. When neither breathing nor circulation is present, cardiopulmonary resuscitation, usually abbreviated CPR, is indicated.

Many phenomena cause sudden cessation of breathing and circulation, from electric shock to drowning to heart attack and cardiac arrest. The technique for CPR is complex and requires special knowledge and skills that can be mastered only by diligent study and practice. The following text gives the basic facts about CPR, for review of the procedure. **Supervised practice is recommended at least once a year to maintain previously learned skills.**

Prompt action is vitally important to the success of CPR. When a person stops breathing spontaneously and his heart stops beating, "clinical death" has occurred. Within 4 to 6 minutes, the cells of the brain, which are most sensitive to lack of oxygen, begin to deteriorate. If the oxygen supply is not restored immediately, the patient suffers irreversible brain damage and "biological death" occurs.

Cardiopulmonary resuscitation is indicated when the person shows signs of cardiac arrest. **These signs include (1) absence of response to stimuli, (2) absent respirations, and (3) absence of a carotid pulse.** Failure of the pupils to react to light eventually will occur as the brain is deprived of its oxygen supply.

To make the steps in CPR easier to remember, the American Heart Association suggests using the *ABC's*. The letter *A* reminds one of "airway," *B* of "breathing," and *C* of "circulation" (Figure 31-2). Resuscitation for the infant and child is somewhat different. See Table 31-3.

Steps for Cardiopulmonary Resuscitation   Follow these steps to administer CPR:

◆ *Call for help.* Do this as you start to check the person. Activate the emergency medical system (call "911").

◆ *Establish unresponsiveness.* Gently shake and shout "Are you okay?" Unless he answers immediately, call loudly for help again.

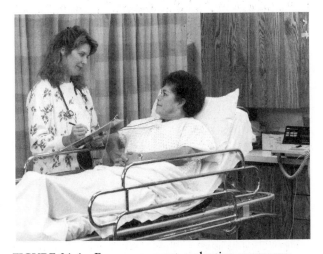

FIGURE 31-1   Emergency nurse evaluating emergency room patient. (Photo by Glen Derbyshire; courtesy of Goleta Valley Cottage Hospital, Goleta, CA.)

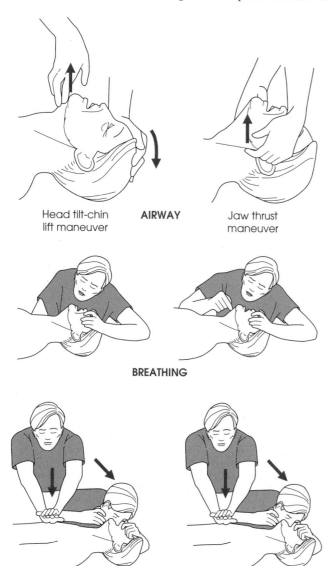

Head tilt-chin   **AIRWAY**   Jaw thrust
lift maneuver   maneuver

BREATHING

CIRCULATION

FIGURE 31-2   Cardiopulmonary resuscitation. (*Source:* Modified from Lammon, C. B., et al. [1995]. *Clinical Nursing Skills.* Philadelphia: Saunders, p. 37.)

◆ *Check for airflow and establish an airway.* Kneel close to the victim's body, turn him as a unit onto his back, and place the heel of one hand on the forehead and two fingers of your other hand on the bony prominence of his chin; lift the chin to open the airway. Be careful not to put the fingers on the soft tissue under the chin. **If neck injury is suspected, use the jaw-thrust maneuver.** Grasp the angles of the patient's lower jaw and lift with both hands, displacing the jawbone forward while tilting the head backward (Figure 31-2).

◆ *Assess for absence of airflow.* Tilt your head down with your ear over the victim's nose and mouth area, and listen and feel for his breath while looking at

the chest to see if it rises and falls with respiratory movements. Do this for 3 to 5 seconds.

◆ *Supply rescue breathing.* If the victim is not breathing, maintain the head tilt/chin lift with the hand on the forehead, and pinch the nose shut. Take a deep breath, and, forming a seal around his mouth, deliver two full breaths watching to see whether the chest rises. If the first breath did not go into the victim, the airway may have become obstructed; reposition with head tilt/chin lift, and try to deliver the breaths again. If the air still cannot be delivered, the Heimlich maneuver will have to be used to open the airway before further intervention can be done. (See description of Heimlich maneuver.) If the two breaths have been delivered successfully, continue with the following steps.

◆ *Assess for presence of pulse.* Locate the victim's larynx with two fingers and then slide them slightly laterally with gentle pressure to locate the carotid pulse. If the pulse is present, but the patient is not breathing, continue rescue breathing at a rate of 12 per minute (one every 5 seconds) and be certain the emergency medical system (EMS) is activated. If there is no pulse detected after 5 to 10 seconds, begin chest compressions by placing the heel of the hand closest to the victim's head on the sternum two fingerbreadths above the xiphoid process. Placing the heel of the other hand over the first hand and

TABLE 31-3 ◆ *Differences in CPR Between Infants and Children*	
Infants	**Children**
Use "puff" breaths to make the chest gently rise.	Use sufficient breath to just make the chest rise for each of the two breaths delivered.
Check for a brachial pulse in the arm between the shoulder and the elbow.	Check the carotid pulse.
Locate chest compression position with fingers in center of chest over sternum.	Locate chest compression position from tip of sternum, placing hand over sternum.
Using two fingers, compress chest five times, no more than ½ inch deep, at a rate of 100 per minute.	Use one hand and align shoulders over your hand.
Tilt head back and cover infant's mouth and nose with your mouth; give one breath at end of each five compressions.	Deliver five compressions, ½ to 1 inch deep, at a rate of 100 per minute.
	Pinch off nose, cover mouth with your mouth, and give one slow breath between sets of five compressions.
Check pulse and breathing at end of four cycles; continue CPR if no pulse or breathing are detected.	Check pulse and breathing at end of four cycles; continue CPR if no pulse or breathing are detected.

keeping the fingers up off the chest, locking your elbows to keep arms straight, and keeping your body aligned directly over the hands, depress 1½–2 inches. Give 15 compressions at a rate of at 80 to 100 per minute. Stop compressions; perform head tilt/chin lift and give 2 breaths; begin another cycle of compressions. Check the carotid pulse every minute (after 4 cycles of 15 compressions and 2 breaths). If the pulse resumes, continue breathing for the patient if he is not breathing on his own. Obtain transport to a medical facility as soon as possible.

In the hospital, initiate CPR and call for help. Have someone alert the full medical emergency team—physician, respiratory therapist, or pharmacist—as soon as possible.

The most common cause of airway obstruction in the unconscious person is the tongue. The head tilt/chin lift maneuver repositions the trachea and tongue so that the airway is open. Because this maneuver also repositions the cervical spine, the jaw thrust method of opening the airway should be used if a spinal injury in the neck area is suspected. For this, kneel at the head of the victim with your elbows on the ground, and place your thumbs on his lower jaw near the corners of the mouth and pointing toward his feet; place your fingertips around the bone of the lower jaw, and lift.

Although transmission of the human immunodeficiency virus (HIV) is highly unlikely via saliva, many health professionals are hesitant to give mouth-to-mouth rescue breathing to strangers. A pocket mask that can be carried in a purse, pocket, or car is available can be used to provide a barrier while giving rescue breathing.

It is essential to have the victim on a firm surface when giving chest compressions. A board or other firm, flat surface can be placed under the upper back of the victim, or he must be moved to the ground or floor. Otherwise the heart will not be compressed between the sternum and the spine.

Hand and body position is very important while giving chest compressions. Improper hand positioning can cause broken ribs which can lacerate the liver or damage the lung. The rhythm of compressions should be regular and steady.

Two-Person CPR The compression-to-ventilation ratio is 5 to 1 with a pause for ventilation of 1½ seconds. Exhalation occurs during chest compressions. As a nurse, you may assist another rescuer by positioning yourself opposite the person performing CPR and offering to help. When CPR is stopped at the end of a cycle and the first rescuer is checking the pulse for 5 seconds, find your hand position for compressions. If the first

rescuer says, "No pulse; continue CPR," wait for him to give a breath and then begin compressions. He will then give one breath during your fifth compression. When you tire (after a minimum of 10 cycles), call out, "Switch on five," and count with your compressions, "one–and–two–and–three–and–four–and–switch," as you give the five compressions and then move to the patient's head; check the carotid, indicate the result, and continue CPR by giving a breath.

◆ Choking Emergencies

Obstructed airway is the sixth leading cause of accidental death. Adults as well as children can become choking victims and need immediate intervention to prevent death from asphyxiation. Both partial and complete airway obstruction should be treated, especially if there is evidence of poor air exchange with the partial obstruction. **If the person is conscious and able to cough or speak, he may not need assistance in expelling the object from his throat.** In this situation it is best to simply encourage him to cough and breathe as deeply as he can.

A weak and ineffective cough indicates poor air exchange and the need for assistance. The person may make snoring sounds if the airway is obstructed by the tongue. Crowing sounds are indicative of spasm of the larynx, and gurgling sounds indicate foreign matter in the air passages. The victim also may start to become cyanotic, or he may clutch his throat in the universal sign for choking (Figure 31-3).

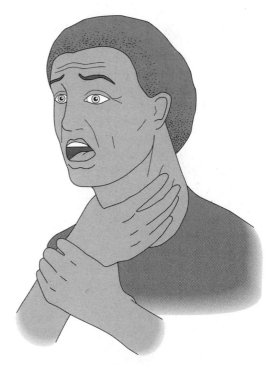

FIGURE 31-3 Universal distress signal for choking.

When the choking victim cannot speak or cough and is unable to remove the obstructing foreign object in his throat on his own, an attempt must be made to help him expel it.

The Heimlich Maneuver   If the victim is standing, the rescuer positions herself beside or slightly behind him. Tell the victim you can help him, and place your arms around his waist. Make a fist with one hand and place the thumb toward victim just above the umbilicus. Grasp your fist with your other hand and deliver five thrusts upward into the abdomen. This is the *Heimlich maneuver* (Figure 31-4). Each squeeze-thrust should be strong enough to dislodge a stuck foreign body in the airway. These thrusts create an artificial cough, making the diaphragm move and forcing air out of the lungs. Keep a good grip on the victim, as he may lose consciousness and will have to be lowered to the ground.

Heimlich Maneuver for an Unconscious Victim
When you are administering CPR to an unconscious victim and cannot get a breath into the victim because of an obstructed airway, first let go of the head and then reposition with the head tilt/chin lift to clear any tongue obstruction. If you still cannot get a breath in, kneel straddling the victim's body. Place the heel of one hand

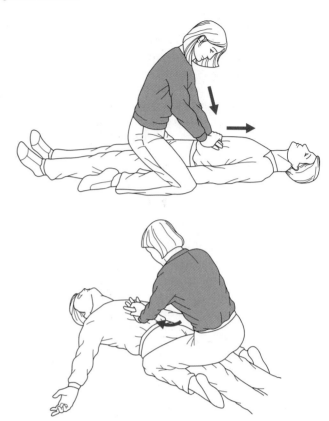

FIGURE 31-5   Abdominal thrust for an unconscious victim.

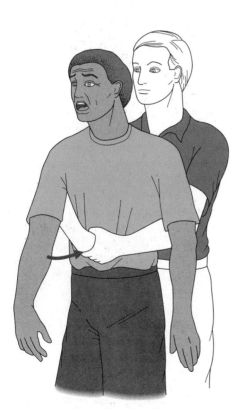

FIGURE 31-4   Abdominal thrust, standing.

on top of the other with the hands positioned between the umbilicus and the tip of the xiphoid process at the midline of the body (Figure 31-5). Push up five times forcefully enough to dislodge an obstruction. Then open the airway by grasping the tongue and lower jaw between your thumb and fingers and lifting the jaw. Look into the mouth, and if you see an object, sweep it out with the index finger of your other hand, using a hooking motion to remove the obstruction. (The finger sweep is not done for children.) Now try to ventilate again. If the airway is still obstructed, give five more abdominal thrusts, open the airway, check the mouth with a sweep, and start the process again. **This maneuver should only be used in an unconscious victim, never in a seizure victim.**

The initial maneuver alone may dislodge the foreign object so that it can be coughed out by the victim. At this point the rescuer should encourage the victim to persist with coughing until the foreign body is removed. No effort should be made to interfere with the victim's efforts as long as he has good air exchange and his color is good.

An alternative to the abdominal thrust is the chest thrust (Figure 31-6). This maneuver can be used for pregnant women and others in whom an abdominal thrust is contraindicated, such as very obese people.

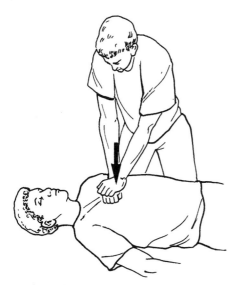

FIGURE 31-6   Chest thrust for an unconscious victim.
(*Source:* Lammon, C. B., et al. [1995]. *Clinical Nursing Skills.*
Philadelphia: Saunders, p. 50.)

Think about . . . If you are dining in a restaurant and observe someone at another table apparently choking, can you describe the exact steps you would take to assist?

◆ Control of Bleeding

The only emergency conditions that have priority over control of hemorrhage are cessation of breathing and a sucking wound of the chest. Severe bleeding can rapidly lead to irreversible hypovolemic shock from loss of intravascular fluid and to circulatory collapse.

Blood issuing from an artery is bright red and will gush forth in spurts at regular intervals. Blood loss from an artery is more rapid than from a vein. Blood from a severed or punctured vein leaks slowly and steadily and is dark red. **Apply pressure to the wound or compress the artery above the wound** (see Chapter 17).

Applying Pressure   Even major bleeding can usually be stopped by applying pressure directly over the wound. The palm of the hand is used, preferably after a clean cloth or sterile dressing has been placed over the open wound. However, if no dressing is available and the victim's life is in danger from blood loss, trying to avoid contamination of the wound is not as important as controlling the hemorrhage.

Once the bleeding has stopped, a compression dressing and bulky bandage are gently but snugly tied in place. Do not wrap the body part so tightly as to constrict circulation completely.

The amount of blood leaking from a wound can be minimized somewhat by elevating the injured part and immobilizing it so that clots are not disturbed and the pumping action of neighboring vessels is decreased.

Once the bleeding has been controlled, the pressure dressing is left in place so as not to disturb clots and renew the bleeding. If blood soaks through the original dressing, additional dressings are applied over the soaked ones, but none of the dressings should be removed until medical help is available.

If bleeding is copious and cannot be stopped with a pressure bandage and immobilization, the artery leading to the wound can be compressed to decrease or perhaps stop altogether the flow of blood from the wound. Pressure points for control of arterial bleeding are shown in Figure 17-6. If the pressure point has been covered properly, there should be no pulse below the point of pressure and the victim should notice tingling and numbness in the area. Pressure points in the neck and head must be used with caution, because there is danger of interrupting blood supply to the brain or of blocking the intake of air.

◆ Shock

The term *shock* means inadequate tissue perfusion. In emergency nursing shock usually is *neurogenic* (caused by psychological factors, such as pain, fright, or trauma); *hypovolemic* or *hemorrhagic* (caused by decreased blood volume, as in severe bleeding, loss of fluid from nausea and vomiting of gastroenteritis, or loss of plasma, as in burns); *septic* (caused by infection), or *cardiogenic* (caused by decreased cardiac output and collapse of the peripheral vascular system).

Symptoms   Shock symptoms result from complex pathological and psychological mechanisms. These involve inadequate blood volume, reduction of the cardiac output, loss of tone in and collapse of the blood vessels near the surface of the body, increased permeability of the capillaries with a shift of the body fluids from one compartment to another, and alterations in the chemical characteristics of the blood.

Not all the signs and symptoms of shock need be present in every patient; they can occur in varying combinations and in different degrees of severity, depending on the cause of shock and the patient's response to it.

The classic symptoms and signs of shock include cold, moist skin, especially in the extremities; pallor, especially of the lips and fingers; and rapid and weak pulse, decreased blood pressure, listlessness, thirst, and oliguria.

Management of Shock   Whenever possible in an emergency situation, the nurse must attempt to prevent shock or at least to lessen its severity. **This is done by acting quickly to control bleeding, relieving pain through proper splinting or positioning, keeping the victim warm, and treating the wound.** The body has several defense mechanisms that are automatically called into action as soon as injury occurs. By supporting these mechanisms through simple nursing measures, the nurse can reduce the severity of shock and mitigate its effects on an accident victim. Management of hemorrhagic shock is discussed in Chapter 17.

◆ Chemical Burns

Strong chemicals capable of burning the skin and mucous membranes will continue to destroy tissue unless they are diluted and removed immediately. **For this reason one must act quickly to irrigate any area burned by chemicals with large amounts of water until all traces of the chemical have been removed.** Once this has been done, the burned area is covered with a dressing, and the patient is transported to a hospital.

However, water is not used for burns caused by dry lime or phenol. Dry lime should be brushed from the skin and clothing unless there is enough water to remove *all* traces of the powder. The nurse should use gloves to protect the hands. Small amounts of water will only react chemically with the lime to produce a highly **corrosive** (destroys gradually) substance. Phenol (carbolic acid) is not water-soluble. The phenol is first removed by alcohol and the burned area is then rinsed with water.

If a corrosive chemical has been ingested, the poison control center should be contacted for instructions and proper dosage of an antidote. Vomiting should **not** be induced or encouraged by overloading the stomach. No attempt should be made to neutralize a chemical substance, as this can cause further damage to the esophagus and stomach.

◆ Poisoning

Poisoning from gases, chemicals, drugs, and other toxic substances accounts for many deaths in the United States every year. The death rate for accidental poisoning has not dramatically changed since 1965.

Prevention of accidental poisoning begins with a realization that there are literally hundreds of thousands of poisonous substances in our environment. Every home has a variety of poisons sitting on the shelves of the medicine cabinet, under the kitchen sink, or in the laundry room, utility room, and garage. **Children are the most frequent victims of poisoning, and medicines account for half of all accidental poisonings of children under the age of 5.** Aspirin has consistently been the leading cause of death in accidental poisoning in children of this age. Other poisons frequently ingested by children include bleaches, soaps and detergents, insecticides, and vitamin and iron preparations. In the past decade, there has been an increase of poisoning in children who have ingested a parent's prescribed medications.

Since the government began requiring "child-proof" caps on all medications and many poisonous substances ordinarily found in households, the incidence of poisoning in children has decreased somewhat, but carelessness on the part of adults continues to be a major factor in the accidental poisoning of children.

> Despite this progress in prevention of accidental poisoning in children, acute poisoning still is the most frequently encountered pediatric emergency in this country.

Prevention   As a member of the health team, the nurse must do all she can to educate the public in the ways in which accidental poisoning can be prevented. She should remember the following simple rules and use every opportunity to teach them to her friends and neighbors:

* *Destroy all medicines that are no longer being used.* An overdose can be fatal, especially to a child. In some instances, drugs undergo chemical changes with age and become toxic compounds.
* *Store poisons and inedible products separately from edible foods.*
* *Do not transfer poisonous substances from their original container to an unmarked one.* NEVER place a poison in a container (such as a soft drink bottle) that is normally used for edible solids or liquids.
* *Never tell a child that the medicine he is being given is candy.* Tell him it is a drug to make him feel better and that it must be taken only as the doctor has directed.
* *Always read the labels of chemical products before using them.*

Symptoms of Poisoning   The symptoms of poisoning vary according to the substance ingested and the time that has elapsed since it first entered the body. Poisoning should be suspected if the victim becomes ill very suddenly and there is an open poison or drug container nearby. In children, one should be alert to the possibility of poisoning when there is a peculiar odor to the breath or when there is evidence that the child has eaten leaves or wild berries. Always remember that children are naturally very curious and that a substance need not taste good for a child to place it in his mouth and swallow it.

Other symptoms of poisoning include pain or burning sensation in the mouth and throat, nausea, vomiting, disorientation, visual disturbances, loss of consciousness, or a deep, unnatural sleep.

General Principles of First Aid for Poisoning   Call the local poison control center first. All cases of poisoning demand immediate action. The longer the delay before treatment, the greater the chance of the poison being absorbed in the body and permanently damaging body tissues.

Always save the container and any of its contents that may help in identifying the poison. If the container cannot be found and the type of poison is not known, try to save a sample of vomitus for analysis and identification.

Swallowed Poisons   Generally, the first step is *dilution* of the poison, immediately followed by *removal* of the stomach contents. In the absence of a stomach pump, vomiting can be induced, but this is contraindicated for certain kinds of poisons, such as corrosive chemicals and petroleum products. A liquid such as water or milk can usually serve to dilute the poison.

Vomiting is induced by placing a spoon or an index finger down the back of the throat to stimulate the gag reflex. An emetic such as 2 tablespoons of salt in a glass of warm water or 15 to 30 mL of syrup of ipecac diluted in a glass of water can be used, but gastric lavage in the emergency room is more effective. The smaller amount is given to children, and the larger amount is for adults. Be sure that during the vomiting episode, the victim is positioned so that the vomitus will not be aspirated into the lungs.

Antidotes to specific poisons often are printed on the labels of the containers. A phone call to the nearest hospital emergency department can provide specific instructions on what to do until the patient can reach the emergency department and be treated by a physician. If possible, the specific antidote should be given as soon as the stomach has been emptied of the poison. In the emergency department, activated charcoal is given to absorb any poison remaining in the stomach and the stomach is evacuated.

When a patient has swallowed a corrosive poison, such as a strong acid or alkali, vomiting is contraindicated, because there is the danger of further irritating and damaging the upper intestinal tract. In addition, the corrosive substance also may be aspirated into the respiratory tract during vomiting.

Corrosive substances should be diluted with milk or water given orally. Never induce vomiting if the victim is unconscious.

Inhaled Poisons   When a patient has inhaled a poisonous substance, he should be transported out into fresh air immediately. Carry him out and loosen any tight clothing. Alert the emergency medical system and obtain transport to a medical facility immediately. Give CPR as needed. If carbon monoxide has been inhaled, the mucous membranes will be cherry red.

When the patient is stable, the nurse should gently try to find out whether the poisoning was accidental or if a suicide attempt has occurred. If suicide was attempted, the patient needs further counseling.

Food Poisoning   This type of poisoning is produced by the toxins of bacteria present in contaminated food. The term *ptomaine poisoning,* so frequently associated with food poisoning, is actually misleading. Ptomaines are substances formed by the decomposition, or "spoilage," of protein foods. The digestive system is able to cope with these substances, and they do not necessarily cause illness. Decomposing food is not of itself necessarily harmful, but because foods in the process of decomposition frequently harbor pathogenic organisms and serve as excellent media for their growth, they should be avoided.

Prevention. Cleanliness, good personal hygiene, and proper preparation and handling of foods are essential to prevent food poisoning.

Symptoms and treatment. Food poisoning should be suspected when more than one person in a group, family, or community is affected by an acute febrile gastrointestinal disturbance. The onset is sudden, with nausea, vomiting, diarrhea, and abdominal cramps. Food is withheld, drugs are administered to control diarrhea, and sedation and parenteral fluids are given.

Types. Food poisoning may be bacterial or chemical. The chemical types, however, are not true food poisonings, but toxic conditions caused by poisonous mushrooms, toxic berries, or foods that have not been cleansed of insecticides or other chemicals.

Staphylococcus aureus frequently grows in creamed foods that have not been refrigerated adequately. Custards, cream pies, mayonnaise, and processed foods commonly used for picnics often are the source of this type of food poisoning. The illness rarely is fatal, and symptoms are usually limited to nausea, vomiting, diarrhea, and abdominal cramps. The patient should be kept quiet and given sedation and parenteral fluids as necessary.

◆ Neck and Spine Injuries

In emergency or accident situations, it is not uncommon for severe bleeding, absence of respirations, or other life-threatening conditions to distract the rescuer and cause her to overlook the possibility that the victim also might have a spinal cord injury. If this happens, and the rescuer proceeds to treat the more obvious injuries and moves the victim before properly immobilizing the neck and back, permanent damage and paralysis may result.

Types of accidents in which spinal injury should be suspected are motor vehicle, diving, biking, and sledding mishaps. A person who has been injured by diving into shallow water must be moved by rescuers, because he may be in danger of drowning. Efforts to remove him from the water and to resuscitate him must be gentle and undertaken only after the neck and back have been properly supported to avoid further damage to the spinal cord. The victim of a sledding or skiing accident may not show signs of injury because of bulky clothing, but he should be moved only after careful evaluation and immobilization, as indicated.

Evaluation of a victim for a spinal cord injury is described in Table 31-2. **If an injury to the neck is a possibility, a cervical collar is applied before the person is moved to a stretcher.** This should be done only by trained personnel familiar with the techniques of applying and maintaining traction on the head while the collar is being applied. When a cervical collar is not available and the victim must be moved to safety, the neck may be immobilized with any material handy, such as a coat, shirt, or towel, rolled in the shape of a collar. The purpose of the collar is to keep the neck as straight as possible, preventing it from flexing or hyperextending. Treatment for neck and spinal cord injuries is covered in Chapter 14.

♦ Electric Shock

When an electric current passes through the body, it can cause severe shock to the entire body, cessation of breathing, circulatory failure, and serious burns. The current travels along the path of least resistance and may be conducted through the heart.

Emergency treatment of electric shock involves CPR if breathing has ceased or the heart has stopped, general measures to treat shock, and emergency treatment of a major burn if one has been sustained. The proper procedure for separating a victim from a live conductor of electricity is shown in Figure 31-7. Remember that water serves as a conductor of electricity **and wet objects can transmit a fatal electric current to a person trying to rescue the victim of electric shock.** A person who is struck by lightning suffers from electric shock. All electrical shock victims must be observed for cardiac dysrhythmias after the injury.

♦ Animal Bites

Family pets, especially dogs and cats, are the most common source of animal bites. When a wild animal, such as a squirrel or fox, attacks and bites a human

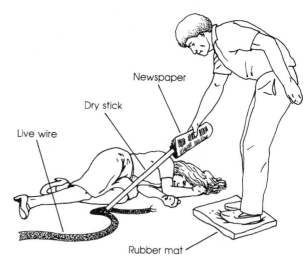

The rescuer stands on a rubber mat or dry board and wears rubber-soled shoes. The rescuer does not touch the victim until certain that wire contact has been broken.

FIGURE 31-7 Separating a victim from a live electric wire while avoiding similar shock.

being without provocation, one should always suspect rabies as the cause of the animal's unusual behavior. All animal and human bites should be treated as potentially dangerous because of the presence of pathogenic microorganisms in the mouth that can cause a serious infection.

Treatment. **Wounds from animal bites should be rinsed immediately with soap and hot running water for 5 to 10 minutes.** The affected area is then treated with antibiotic ointment, covered with a clean bandage and immobilized. Medical attention should be given to the wound as soon as possible.

Because the possibility of rabies must always be considered in an animal bite, the animal must be confined and observed for signs of the disease. The Animal Control Agency should be contacted to catch the animal if necessary. If it has been killed, its head should be sent to a laboratory for examination. If a diagnosis of rabies in the animal has been confirmed or if there is no proof that the animal has been immunized against rabies, the victim is given a series of injections to build up antibodies against the virus. Newer vaccines require fewer injections and are more effective in stimulating antibody production than the traditional Pasteur treatment.

♦ Snakebite

Although bites from poisonous snakes are rare in the United States, they do occur and can be fatal if not treated promptly and effectively. There are four kinds of poisonous snakes in this country: copperheads, rattlesnakes, and cottonmouths (or water moccasins) are all called pit vipers because they have pits or depressions behind their nostrils; coral snakes are small snakes with characteristic red, black, and yellow bands. Coral snakes do not have fangs; they inject their venom by a chewing motion.

A venomous snakebite usually can be distinguished by two fang marks (though there may be only one on a small surface, such as the toe or finger), severe pain and swelling in the area, discoloration at the site of injection of venom, nausea and vomiting, respiratory distress, and shock. Nonpoisonous snakebites usually appear as either small scratches or lacerations.

Treatment. Nonpoisonous snakebites are treated as simple wounds and require only a cleansing of the wound with soap and water and the application of a mild antiseptic. Venomous snakebites should receive medical attention as quickly as possible.

> The victim of a poisonous snakebite should be kept as quiet and calm as possible while being transported. Under no condition should he be given an alcoholic beverage or stimulant.

Current treatment for poisonous snakebite consists of washing the wound, lowering the extremity or area and immobilizing it, keeping the victim calm and seeking medical attention as quickly as possible. **Tourniquets, incision, and sucking the area to extract venom are no longer recommended.**

Once the snakebite victim reaches a hospital or clinic, the wound is debrided and irrigated to remove the venom and damaged tissues. Skin grafting may be required later. The victim is given antivenin, medications to counteract the specific pharmacological action of the venom, and other drugs to avoid complications and provide relief.

◆ Insect Bites and Stings

Systemic reactions to the bites and stings of insects and bees account for more deaths each year in the United States than do snakebites. A systemic reaction is caused by hypersensitivity to the venom of bees, wasps, hornets, fire ants, or harvester ants.

Symptoms of a systemic reaction include hives, swelling, general weakness, tightness in the chest, abdominal cramps, constriction of the throat, loss of consciousness, and possibly death from severe **anaphylaxis.** Whenever a person suffers from any of these symptoms after a sting or insect bite, treatment must be started immediately. The shorter the interval between the time of the sting or bite and the development of symptoms, the more likely the possibility that death will result. Ice packs may be applied to the area of the bite or sting while medical help is being sought.

Treatment. First aid treatment for a systemic reaction is to inject aqueous epinephrine (1/1,000 solution) in dosages of 0.3 to 0.4 mL for adults and 0.15 to 0.3 mL for children. An antihistamine, such as Benadryl, also is given.

The female worker honeybee injects a venom sac that may remain embedded in the victim's skin. This sac may be removed by gently scraping the site with a fingernail or knife blade, being careful not to squeeze the sac and force the venom into the tissues. **The "stinger" should be removed as quickly as possible.**

An ice pack may be applied to reduce swelling and relieve pain. Patients who appear to be in shock should be kept warm and should remain lying down with the legs elevated and the head flat. If symptoms persist after 20 minutes and the patient has not yet reached a medical facility, a second injection of epinephrine should be given.

An emergency kit that contains the drugs, syringe, constricting band, towelette, and tweezers needed for prompt treatment of a systemic reaction to stings and bites is available by prescription. Individuals known to be hypersensitive to insect and bee venom should keep such a kit with them at all times and be thoroughly familiar with its use *before* the need for it arises. These people also should wear some kind of medical identification that indicates their hypersensitivity. Any person who has had a systemic reaction or even a severe local reaction with swelling beyond two joints should receive hyposensitization therapy to increase his tolerance to insect and bee stings.

Less serious stings of bees, wasps, yellow jackets, and hornets are treated by applying a paste of baking soda and water or household ammonia and a cold compress. Meat tenderizer also has been found effective in relieving the symptoms of minor insect sting reactions. Bites from venomous spiders, scorpions, and other poisonous insects are treated in the same manner as poisonous snakebites.

Ticks, which can carry diseases such as Rocky Mountain spotted fever or Lyme disease, are removed by grasping the tick as close to the skin as possible with tweezers and pulling it straight out without twisting. Some people feel that placing a drop of turpentine, mineral oil, or petroleum jelly on its body makes it let go before pulling it out.

After the tick is removed, wash the area with soap and water and apply a mild disinfectant. If there is some question as to whether or not the tick may be carrying an infectious disease, a physician should be consulted.

◆ Injuries Due to Extreme Heat and Cold

Heatstroke   Heatstroke, a rare condition also called *sunstroke,* is the result of a serious disturbance of the heat-regulating center in the brain. Normally, the body responds to higher environmental temperatures by increasing perspiration and by using other internal mechanisms that keep the body temperature within normal limits. In heatstroke, these mechanisms fail to function properly and the patient's temperature rises, the skin becomes dry and hot, and there may be convulsions and collapse. Other symptoms include visual disturbances, dizziness, nausea, and a weak, rapid, irregular pulse. Because the body temperature may go as high as 108° F to 110° F (42.2° C to 43.3° C), the patient is likely to die if his condition is not treated.

A person suffering from heatstroke should be placed in the shade and cooled immediately by being sprinkled with water and fanned. He should be immersed in cold water or have ice packs applied to his body as soon as possible to lower his temperature. Ice water enemas and gastric lavage may be utilized to speed cooling. Chlorpromazine (Thorazine) may be given to relieve muscle spasms.

If the body's heat-regulating mechanism is impaired, the person may experience heatstroke any time he is exposed to extremely high temperatures, and he may need to adjust his life so that he can avoid repeated episodes of heatstroke.

Heat Exhaustion (Heat Prostration)   Heat exhaustion is caused by excessive sweating, which removes large quantities of salt and water from the body. **The patient appears to be in shock with cool, damp skin, pallor, increased pulse and heart beat, dizziness, or stupor.** He may also have muscle cramps and poor coordination. Treatment is aimed at replacing the essential salts and fluids. A person suffering from heat exhaustion should be placed in a cool area and kept quiet. As much salt and water (¼ teaspoon of salt to an 8-oz glass of liquid), tomato juice, or Gatorade as he can drink is administered. If he is unable to swallow the salt solution, replacement fluids are administered IV. Muscular cramps may be relieved by gently massaging the affected muscles. Dorsiflexing the toes helps decrease calf pain.

Sunburn   Immediate treatment of a minor sunburn involves the application of cool compresses soaked with a solution of magnesium sulfate (Epsom salts) or sodium bicarbonate (baking soda) to relieve the discomfort. If chills, fever, swelling, or gastrointestinal disturbances occur, the patient should receive medical attention. Nonsteroidal antiinflammatory drugs (NSAIDs) may be taken to alleviate pain.

Hypothermia   Hypothermia is a serious lowering of the total body temperature caused by prolonged exposure to cold. Persons most at risk for hypothermia are the elderly, very young and thin children, the mentally ill or deficient, alcoholics, the homeless, and drug addicts.

Hypothermia is a chilling of the entire body, but the extremities can withstand lower temperatures (20° F to 30° F lower) than the torso, where vital organs are located. When the core (central) temperature drops even 2° F or 3° F, physiological changes that can lead to fatal cardiac arrhythmias and respiratory failure occur.

Symptoms of hypothermia range from mild shivering and complaints of feeling cold to loss of consciousness and a death-like appearance. Indeed, persons in profound hypothermia may be presumed dead, because the body's protective mechanisms have drastically slowed its metabolic processes. The body uses less than half its normal requirement for oxygen in severe hypothermia. Pulse and respiration are barely detected, reflexes are absent, and the person is unconscious.

Prevention.   **Prevention of hypothermia includes eating high-energy foods, exercising, wearing layers of clothing, and covering the head.** From one-half to two-thirds of the body's heat is lost through the head. Elderly persons particularly need protection against the effects of extreme cold (Table 31-4). Hypothermia in these persons can easily be misdiagnosed because its symptoms resemble those of so many diseases to which the elderly and weak are most susceptible.

Another reason for failing to diagnose profound hypothermia is improper procedure and equipment for measuring body temperature. In profound hypothermia the core temperature can be as low as 86° F (30° C), but clinical thermometers used in hospitals and clinics rarely register temperatures below 94° F (34.5° C), and

---

TABLE 31-4 ◆ *Suggestions for Helping the Elderly Prevent Accidental Hypothermia*

◆ Room temperature should not be lower than 65° F. An indoor thermometer should be kept in the house and checked daily during the cool seasons.

◆ An energy audit by the utility company can identify ways to prevent heat loss from the home. Check with the gas or electric company.

◆ If heating the entire house presents economic problems, suggest heating one or two rooms adequately and closing off the other rooms of the house.

◆ Suggest aids, such as throw or quilted snuggle bag (a quilt with snaps or zipper that becomes a bag), extra socks, and warm hats to be worn indoors.

◆ Recommend wearing several loose layers of clothing to retain body heat.

◆ Head covering should be worn even while sleeping, as two-thirds of the body's heat is lost through the head.

◆ Advise against using fireplaces in extremely cold weather, unless no other heat source is available; much heat is lost through the flue. If a fireplace is used, close the damper as soon as the fire is completely extinguished.

◆ Arrange for someone to check in daily with elderly persons who live alone.

many times the temperature is taken orally rather than rectally.

Treatment. Once hypothermia is diagnosed, rewarming is begun. The method varies according to the age and physical condition of the patient. The core must be rewarmed first to prevent lactic acid in the extremities from being rapidly shunted to the heart, which can cause ventricular fibrillation. **The heart is extremely sensitive when cold, and the patient must be handled carefully to prevent dysrhythmias.** If rewarming is done in an emergency care facility, monitoring equipment must be readily at hand. Rewarming outside a health care facility probably should be more gradual. This must be done properly to avoid sending cold blood that has pooled in the extremities back to the heart, where it can cause deadly arrhythmias. The body is warmed by wrapping it in a blanket or submerging it in a tepid bath.

Frostbite   Frostbite is a localized injury to tissue caused by freezing. Exposure of the tissues to extreme cold constricts the blood vessels, damages vessel walls and tissue cells, and leads to the formation of blood clots. Frostbite occurs most often in the fingers, toes, cheeks, and nose, where exposure usually is greatest and blood supply is most easily impeded.

Symptoms of frostbite include numbness and a prickling sensation in the affected area. The skin appears dull and opaque and may have a yellowish cast. Eventually, edema occurs as fluid escapes from the damaged vessel walls.

Prevention. Like hypothermia, frostbite can be prevented by wearing protective clothing and avoiding exposure to extreme cold. Sometimes this is not possible if a person is caught unaware or unprepared. Those who are intoxicated or under the influence of drugs may not realize they are suffering from frostbite. If the person also is suffering from hypothermia, he cannot think clearly and does not realize that his skin is being exposed to severe cold.

Treatment. Once the patient is removed from the cold, the affected area should be warmed by immersion for about 10 minutes in water heated to between 100° F and 110° F (38° C to 43° C). Do not try to hasten the process by using water that is hotter, as this can only add to the damage. Handle the frostbitten part gently. *Never* rub or massage skin that has been frozen. The practice of rubbing snow or ice on the part is dangerous and completely without benefit. Rubbing or rough handling can cause further damage to the fragile tissues.

Wrap the affected area in bulky clean or sterile bandages, being sure to separate skin areas, as between the fingers. Give the person hot tea or coffee to drink. Elevate the affected area. Later on, after emergency treatment has been given, debridement of dead tissue and skin grafting will be necessary if the deeper tissues are destroyed by gangrene resulting from impaired circulation.

◆ The Combative Patient

The use of tranquilizing drugs has greatly reduced the occurrence of violent behavior in people who are temporarily unable to control their emotions because of a psychological disorder. This does not mean, however, that psychiatric emergencies no longer occur or that the nurse will never need to know how to handle such patients. When a person becomes greatly agitated and experiences an uncontrollable urge to act violently, he may be extremely frightened and usually welcomes help in regaining control if it is offered in the correct way.

Success in dealing with an unruly patient is more easily achieved if help is offered on a one-to-one basis. Several people trying to talk to him or subdue him at once may only add to his fright and disorientation. However, if physical restraint becomes necessary, one should be sure that enough people are on hand to control the patient.

When the nurse is talking to a person who is combative, it is best that she use his name frequently, tell him who she is, and what she is trying to do, and express genuine concern about his feelings and the situation he is in.

Patients who are not diagnosed as mentally ill or psychotic also can become "violent" when nurses and other health care personnel fail to respect their rights and needs. **Everyone has a right to privacy and to know what is happening to him.** Patients should be told what procedures are planned and why they are necessary. When an emergency patient seems to be out of control and combative, it might be that he perceives himself to be in danger from the emergency staff as well as from his injuries.

When a patient gives verbal and nonverbal clues that he is agitated, fearful, and likely to assault a nurse or other staff member, measures should be taken to calm him. This is done by cautiously approaching the patient in a nonthreatening manner, establishing eye contact with him, and in a soft voice explaining what is being done for him and why it is necessary. Taking time to listen as well as talk to the patient can help the nurse understand why a potentially violent or combative patient feels the need to defend himself and regain control over what is happening to him.

It may be necessary to help the patient by exerting some outside controls. These may be verbal or physical, but physical force should be used only after it is apparent that talking with the patient is not going to calm him. One may simply tell him to stop screaming, to sit down, or to put down an object that he apparently intends to use as a weapon. If verbal control does not work, it may be necessary to restrain the overwrought patient. If restraints are used, the patient should not be left alone immediately after he has been restrained, as this action will give him the impression that he is being punished for wrongdoing rather than being assisted in controlling himself.

It is strongly suggested that any nurse who works regularly in an emergency department, psychiatric unit, or other setting where she will have occasion to deal with violent patients obtain additional information and training in handling such situations. Lack of knowledge and experience in emergency psychiatric situations can be detrimental to the patient as well as to those who are trying to help him.

◆ Domestic Violence

Sometimes the emergency department patient is a victim of abuse. Signs of battering include bruises, swellings, lacerations, fractures, hematomas, blackened eyes, abdominal injuries (especially during pregnancy), burns, and open wounds. Bruises or fractures in various stages of healing and signs of old lacerations and wounds in the presence of new ones indicate a need for a thorough assessment for battering. Often the victim may explain all of the injuries as the result of logical accidents rather than disclose that battering by an intimate partner has occurred. Psychologically the person may display signs of depression, low self-esteem, anxiety, and stress. Asking the following questions after establishing rapport with the patient may encourage honest sharing of thoughts and feelings:

- ◆ Have you been hit or hurt in any way in the past year?
- ◆ Who injured you? Has it occurred before?
- ◆ Are you afraid of anyone?
- ◆ Do you feel safe at home?
- ◆ Does your partner use drugs or alcohol? How does his or her behavior change after using them?

Although many more women are battered by their intimate partners, men sometimes also suffer from battering. If battering is revealed, the person is referred to an appropriate shelter.

Any time a child is brought into the emergency department with unexplained or questionably explained injuries, a thorough physical assessment is performed for signs of physical abuse. If such signs are found, the case is referred to the proper authorities. **Child abuse or suspicion of child abuse must be reported by law.**

Unfortunately elder abuse is common. Elderly patients also should be assessed for signs of abuse. The attitude of the elderly patient toward the caregiver should be assessed to determine whether there is any element of fear. The same signs of physical abuse should be searched for, as well as signs of malnutrition, uncleanliness, or severe depression. **The law requires that signs of elder abuse be reported.**

DISASTER NURSING

A disaster may be defined as *any catastrophe in which numbers of people are plunged into helplessness and suffering*. Natural disasters include epidemics, earthquakes, explosions, hurricanes, tornadoes, fires, floods, and transportation accidents. War-caused disasters may result from enemy attacks with chemical, biological, nuclear, psychological, and conventional weapons. Terrorist bombings also are classified as disasters.

Whether the disaster is natural or war-caused, it will involve physical injuries, loss of property, and interruption of the normal activities of daily living. Victims often will need food, clothing, shelter, medical and nursing or hospital care, and other basic necessities of life.

The nurse has a definite role in helping to relieve the suffering inflicted by such tragedies, and she should actively participate in community planning and civil defense programs so that, in time of disaster, she will be prepared to function effectively as a member of the health team.

◆ Disaster Planning

The governmental agencies for disaster planning are the Office of Civil Defense and the U.S. Public Health Service. The American Red Cross is a voluntary organization that traditionally provides nursing care and the basic essentials of shelter and food during a natural disaster. In most communities, the local civil defense agency and the Red Cross work together to formulate disaster plans to coordinate their services with each other and with other agencies planning for essential services, such as transportation, communication, and welfare.

Special courses in civil defense and disaster nursing are usually offered by the Office of Civil Defense, the Red Cross, and professional organizations. These courses help the nurses and volunteer workers in the community understand the function of each agency in a particular type of disaster and serve to coordinate the planning for each kind of emergency nursing.

◆ Psychological Responses to Disaster

Since the 1940s many studies have been conducted to determine the needs and problems of persons trying to cope with a major disaster. Typical responses are not unlike those of any person who is overwhelmed with sudden and profound change, death, or destruction of a former way of life.

One would expect people to panic when they are caught up in a major disaster, but this is not a common reaction, except when there is life-threatening danger that occurs in a matter of moments and without warning. More typical of psychological responses to a major disaster are the three states described in the following section.

- Stage I is the *impact stage.* Survivors are stunned, apathetic, and disorganized. For several hours after the initial blow they may have difficulty following directions and will need strong support and firm guidance.
- Stage II is the *recoil stage.* During this stage individuals are very compliant, want to be helpful, and may minimize or ignore their own injuries. At this stage some persons may need to be protected from themselves if they are indeed injured or physically and emotionally exhausted.
- In Stage III, called the *posttrauma stage,* some survivors become elated, grateful that they are still alive. Others might feel guilty when they realize they did not suffer as much as their friends and neighbors. At this stage the attention of the survivors turns toward rebuilding, and they have a strong sense of brotherhood and community spirit.

Later on, victims of a disaster probably will begin to complain about the help provided by various agencies, governmental and private. If the disaster could have been avoided or at least mitigated by an efficient civil defense or similar agency, the psychological effects may be more severe and psychological recovery will take longer.

◆ Nursing Intervention

After a disaster care of victims is prioritized according to a triage system. Those with life-threatening conditions and a good chance of survival are cared for first. These are Class I or life-threatened patients. Class II patients are treated next and have conditions that are urgent and require treatment within a 2-hour time frame. Class III patients come last and are considered nonurgent; treatment can be delayed for 4 to 6 hours. **When there are more victims of a disaster than medical personnel to treat them, those that are mortally wounded and not expected to survive are not treated until those more likely to survive are treated.** This is a difficult choice for most nurses, but in a disaster instance, the good of the most must prevail over that of the few.

The focus of assessment during triage is assessing for level of acuity. Many emergency department nurses use the mnemonic OLD CART to obtain sufficient details from the patient to classify their acuity.

O = Onset of symptoms

L = Location of problem

D = Duration of symptoms

C = Characteristics the patient uses to describe the symptoms

A = Aggravating factors

R = Relieving factors

T = Treatment administered before arrival

These assessment techniques are useful both in the ER and out in the field.

A booklet published under the direction of the U.S. Department of Health and Human Services includes the following list of nursing responsibilities in case of a disaster. All nurses should:

- Be prepared for self-survival and for performing emergency nursing measures.
- Know the community disaster plans and organized community health resources.
- Know the meaning of warning signals and the action to be taken.
- Know measures for protection from radioactive fallout.
- Know measures for prevention and control of environmental health hazards.
- Be prepared to interpret health laws and regulations.
- Know and interpret community resources for citizen preparedness, such as first aid and medical self-help courses.

In many types of disaster, the nurse may need to improvise because of lack of equipment. She must always bear in mind the basic principles of nursing that she has been taught and has practiced in the hospital environment. If there is a great disparity between need and availability of medical and nursing personnel, she may be called upon to exercise leadership and judgment in determining the condition of each victim, using supplies and equipment, and detecting changes in the environment that might be hazardous.

The U.S. Department of Health and Human Services recommends that the nurse be skilled in the following areas if she is to be involved in disaster health care. The nurse participates in planning and providing care for large groups of people under extreme duress in various types of disaster situations. Developing and revising nursing procedures aimed at providing comfort and safety during and after a disaster helps the nurse to deal more efficiently with the actual crisis situation.

The emotional and physical comfort and safety of large numbers of disaster victims must be attended to with limited supplies, equipment, utilities, and personnel. The nurse must understand the emotional stress caused by personal fear, problems of displacement and separation of families, increasing anxiety, and continuing danger. She helps people of different cultural backgrounds and religious beliefs accept and adapt to temporary living conditions in crowded and often adverse situations.

Recognizing and understanding the effect of disrupted social and economic patterns, such as personal and material losses, emotional trauma, and crowded living conditions, helps the nurse deal with the victims more effectively. It is helpful to encourage patients to verbalize their concerns and fears and to guide them in performing certain tasks.

Providing basic instruction to disaster victims in the aspects of appropriate self-care and encouraging them to further provide for their own needs and the needs of others are essential responsibilities of the nurse in any disaster situation.

Water Purification   When the normal water supply is disrupted, water may be purified by bringing it to a rolling boil for 3 to 5 minutes. Let the water cool before drinking. Household liquid bleach containing 5.25% sodium hypochlorite may be used to disinfect water. Add 16 drops of bleach to a gallon of water and let stand for 30 minutes. Distillation is the third method of preparing safe water from a possibly contaminated supply. To distill, fill a pot halfway with water. Tie a cup to the handle on the pot's lid so that the cup will hang right side up when the lid is upside down (the cup should not dangle in the water). Boil the water for 20 minutes. The water that drips from the lid into the cup is distilled. This method frees water of microbes that may remain after bleach treatment.

Major Chemical Emergency   When a chemical emergency has occurred in your neighborhood, you should do the following:

- Close all windows and doors to the dwelling.
- Turn off all fans, heaters, and air conditioning systems.
- Close the fireplace damper.
- Go to an above-ground room with the fewest windows and doors.
- Take your emergency kit and a portable radio with you.
- Wet some towels and jam them in the crack under the doors. Tape around doors, windows, exhaust fans or vents. Use plastic garbage bags to cover windows, outlets and heat registers.
- Stay put until you are told all is safe or you are asked to evacuate.

In the Event of an Earthquake   Each household should have earthquake supplies in readiness. If an earthquake strikes and you are indoors, stay there. Get under a desk, table, or stand in a corner or door frame. Cover your head with your arms. If outdoors, get into an open area away from trees, buildings, walls, and power lines. If driving, pull over to the side of the road and stop away from trees, buildings, and power lines. Stay inside the vehicle. If you are in a crowded public place, do not rush for the doors. Move away from display shelves containing objects that could fall. If you are in a high-rise building, stay away from windows and outside walls. Avoid using the elevators. Get under a table or desk.

After the quake, assist those injured, applying first aid as needed. Do not use the telephone unless there is a life-threatening injury or fire. If uninjured, check for gas leaks. If you find any, turn off the utility at once. Turn off water if water pipes are broken. Turn on the portable radio for instructions and news reports.

In Case of Fire   If the smoke detector goes off, don't wait to dress or gather belongings, get out of the dwelling. If fire or smoke is evident, drop to the floor and crawl to the exit. Feel any door before opening it. If it is hot, find another way out. If clothes catch on fire, drop to the ground and roll to suffocate the fire. Keep rolling until flames are out.

♦ Further Intervention

Observing, recording, and reporting information to appropriate people must be carried out in an organized manner. General physical and mental conditions of patients and signs and symptoms that may be indicative of changes in their conditions must be accurately observed. Stresses in relationships between patients, their families, visitors, and personnel must be kept to a minimum.

Performing nursing procedures in a disaster situation demands skill and judgment to provide for the good of the greatest number of people. The nurse must administer medications and treatments as directed and improvise supplies, equipment, and techniques as necessary. She also must carry out precautionary measures, including maintaining a safe and sanitary environment and separating patients with communicable diseases. Instituting emergency first aid measures also is a duty of the nurse, and usually she is forced to use improvised supplies and to observe aseptic techniques under very chaotic conditions.

Working toward restoring community and family life according to available resources once the disaster has occurred also involves the nurse and other members of the health care team. Individual self-help and work therapy are encouraged, as are activities of family living, with adaptations designed to attain and maintain a sanitary and healthy environment. Existing community facilities and resources must be used as much as possible for continued patient care.

The nurse can promote the effectiveness of the health service agency in disaster preparedness by knowing and interpreting the agency's disaster plan. She must understand the relationship between the agency plan, the local government plan, and the local Red Cross plan. Trying to maintain and restore community health by controlling environmental health hazards also is an important responsibility for any nurse.

Think about ... Are you and your family prepared for a disaster? Do you have a disaster kit on hand? If you have children, do you have measures in place for their care by others if you are unable to reach them?

CRITICAL THINKING EXERCISES

Clinical Case Problems

Read each clinical situation and discuss the questions with your classmates.

1. While driving home from work one afternoon, you come upon the scene of an accident. There are two victims inside a wrecked automobile and one lying on the side of the road. The two in the car are bleeding moderately from small lacerations. One is unconscious and has a large bruised and swollen area on his forehead. The other person is hysterical and cannot move his leg without great pain. The victim lying on the side of the road has no visible signs of injury, but he is not breathing.
   a. Which victim is treated first? How is he treated?
   b. If help is available, what should be done for the apparent fracture?
   c. If help is not available, what would you say to the victim with the fracture?
   d. How would you control moderate bleeding?

2. While working as a student nurse in the hospital's emergency unit, you notice that patients who have been injured or are very ill sometimes become hostile and combative. Some try to assault members of the emergency team and others use abusive and threatening language.
   a. Discuss with your classmates some reasons why patients may behave in these ways when they are injured or very ill.
   b. What are some ways in which so-called violent patients who are not mentally ill can be handled so as to calm them and prevent assault on and encourage cooperation with the emergency staff?

3. Your community has been hit by a hurricane. There are many people injured, several fatalities, and widespread destruction of property.
   a. What kinds of psychological responses would you expect to see in the people who have survived the hurricane but have minor injuries, even though many have lost their homes?
   b. What kinds of nursing intervention would be helpful to people in each of the stages of response to a major disaster?
   c. What are your responsibilities as a nurse for planning and implementing health care in the case of a disaster?

BIBLIOGRAPHY

American Heart Association. (1994). *Textbook of Advanced Cardiac Life Support*. Dallas: Author.

Antai-Otong, D. (1995). *Psychiatric Nursing: Biological and Behavioral Concepts*. Philadelphia: Saunders.

Babb, D., Jenkins, B. (1990). Action Stat! Alcohol withdrawal syndrome. *Nursing 90*. 20(10):33.

Bailey, M. M. (1996). Emergencies handbook: You can't afford to waste time during a code. *Nursing 96*. 26(3):61–64.

Beachley, M., Farrar, J. Abdominal trauma: putting the pieces together. *American Journal of Nursing*. 93(11):26–34.

Braun, A. E. (1993). Emergency cardiac care: the new drug protocols. *RN*. 56(11):52–58.

Cardona, V. D. (1994). *Trauma Nursing*, 2nd ed. Philadelphia: Saunders.

Clunn, P. A. (1996). The nurse's kit for survivors. *Reflections*. 22(1):8–9.

deWit, S. C. (1994). *Rambo's Nursing Skills for Clinical Practice*, 4th ed. Philadelphia: Saunders.

Emergency Nurses Association (1993). *Emergency Nursing Core Curriculum*, 4th ed. Philadelphia: Saunders.

Huston, C. J. (1993). Action Stat! Assessing a spider bite. *Nursing 93*. 23(2):33.

Huston, C. J. (1993). Action Stat! Treating a jellyfish sting. *Nursing 93*. 23(8):33.

Jackson, L. (1995). Quick response to hypothermia and frostbite. *American Journal of Nursing*. 95(3):52.

Keep, N. B., Glibert, C. P. (1995). How safe is your ED? *American Journal of Nursing*. 95(9):45–50.

Kitt,. S., et al. (1995). *Emergency Nursing: A Physiologic and Clinical Perspective*, 2nd ed. Philadelphia: Saunders.

Kohl, J. (1996). Heat stroke. *American Journal of Nursing*. 96(7):51.

Lammon, C. B., et al. (1995). *Clinical Nursing Skills*. Philadelphia: Saunders.

Laskowski-Jones, L. (1995). First-line emergency care: what every nurse should know. *Nursing 95*. 25(1):34–43.

Maher, A. B., Salmond, S. W., Pellino, T. A. (1994). *Orthopaedic Nursing*. Philadelphia: Saunders.

Mattice, C. (1996). Consult stat: it's not always obvious when a patient's in shock. *RN*. 59(3):61–62.

Pezzella, D. (1994). Responding to the hypothermic patient. *Nursing 94.* 24(2):50–51.

Soloway, R. A. G. (1993). Emergency nursing: street-smart advice on treating drug overdoses. *American Journal of Nursing.* 93(9):65–72.

Sommers, M. S. (1996). The shattering consequences of CPR. *C. E. Test Handbook.* Vol. 7:3–7.

Sullivan, S. A. (1993). Derm detective: how severe is this frostbite? *American Journal of Nursing.* 93(2):59, 61–62, 64.

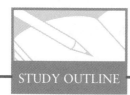

STUDY OUTLINE

I. Prevention of Accidents

A. Home safety.

  1. More than one-fourth of accidental deaths occur in the home.

  2. Principal victims are children and elderly.

  3. Education of the public will help prevent accidents.

B. Highway safety.

  1. Motor vehicle accidents are the leading cause of accidental death in this country.

  2. Major causes of such accidents are human and mechanical failure.

C. Water safety.

  1. Observing the common-sense rules of water safety helps prevent accidents.

  2. Rescue methods vary; attempt a swimming rescue only if you are experienced.

  3. Cardiopulmonary resuscitation may be necessary.

  4. Have victim lie down, and treat him for shock.

  5. Transport near-drowning victim to medical facility for evaluation of fluid and electrolyte status and cardiac irregularities.

II. General Principles of First Aid

A. Think before acting. Move slowly and deliberately; act with confidence.

B. Survey scene to determine hazards to victims, onlookers, and rescuers.

C. Check each victim quickly, treat the most serious injuries first.

D. Evaluate injuries and summon help.

E. Do not move victim unless necessary.

F. Do not remove an impaled object unless it is in the cheek and bleeding must be controlled.

G. Do not try to give anything by mouth to an unconscious person.

H. Explain in a calm voice what you are doing for the victim; be honest.

I. Good Samaritan laws in many states protect medical personnel giving first aid at the scene of an accident.

III. Cardiopulmonary Resuscitation (CPR)

A. Reestablishment of heart and lung action.

B. Indicated when there is no breathing and no heart beat in people who have suffered near-drowning, electric shock, or cardiac arrest.

C. Prompt action essential to prevent biological death.

D. Should be administered only by trained personnel because of possible complications.

E. Indications for CPR.

  1. Absence of carotid pulse.

  2. Absence of response to stimuli.

  3. Absent respiration.

F. Artificial breathing given by mouth-to-mouth technique.

  1. Open airway.

  2. Breathe into victim's mouth about 12 times per minute.

G. Cardiac compression: applied to lower half of sternum.

  1. Press downward to squeeze heart between sternum and spinal column.

  2. Press without interruption 80 to 100 times per minute.

IV. Choking Emergencies

A. Obstructed airway is the sixth leading cause of accidental death.

B. Victim may give universal signal for choking, be unable to speak or cough, and begin to turn cyanotic.

C. If victim is able to cough and expel the foreign object on his own, this should be encouraged.

D. Abdominal thrust and chest thrust used.

V. Control of Bleeding

A. Place clean or sterile dressing over wound.

B. Apply firm, steady pressure with hand.

C. When bleeding has decreased, apply bandage. Do not wrap wound so tightly as to constrict circulation.

D. Elevate and immobilize injured part.

E. If pressure to wound does not decrease blood loss from wound, apply pressure to pressure point above the artery serving the wounded area.

VI. **Shock**

A. There are four types of shock: neurogenic, hypovolemic, septic, and cardiogenic.

B. Shock is the inadequate perfusion of body tissues or perfusion failure.

C. Symptoms are due to inadequate blood volume, loss of tone and then collapse of peripheral vessels, and shift of body fluids.

D. Symptoms are pallor, weak pulse, clammy skin, and thirst.

E. Management of shock.

1. Reassure and comfort patient.

2. Maintain body heat.

3. Place patient flat.

4. Restore circulating blood volume, relieve respiratory embarrassment, and control pain.

VII. **Burns**

A. Two dangers are shock and infection.

B. Minor burns should be immersed in cold water or covered with cold compresses.

C. Major burns.

1. Cover with clean, dry dressing and transport victim to hospital or clinic.

2. Give victim fluids to drink only if transport to hospital will be delayed for several hours.

3. Never apply ointments or disturb blisters.

D. Chemical burns.

1. Flush with water; exceptions are burns from dry lime and phenol (carbolic acid).

2. Cover with a dressing and transport victim to hospital.

3. For ingestion of corrosive poison, give victim milk or water to drink. Do not induce or encourage vomiting or try to chemically neutralize the poison.

VIII. **Poisoning**

A. Education can help prevent accidental poisoning.

B. Poisoning should be suspected if the victim suddenly becomes ill, if there is a peculiar odor to the breath, and if an open drug or poison container is found nearby. Save container or vomitus for identification.

C. Swallowed poisons.

1. Induce vomiting, except for corrosive poisons or petroleum products or if patient is unconscious.

2. Give specific antidote if it is known; contact poison control center.

3. Give activated charcoal.

D. Inhaled poisons.

1. Transport victim to source of fresh air.

2. Give CPR as necessary.

3. Keep victim warm and quiet; do not give alcohol or stimulants.

E. Food poisoning due to toxins produced by bacteria in contaminated foods.

1. Prevented by proper preparation, storage, and handling of food.

2. Onset is acute with severe gastrointestinal disturbances.

3. Treatment: begin supportive measures.

IX. **Electric Shock**

A. Give CPR; treat burns as needed.

B. Use caution in separating victim from source of electric current.

X. **Animal Bites**

A. Treat wound immediately.

B. Vaccinations necessary if examination of the animal reveals the possibility of rabies.

C. Snakebite.

1. Nonpoisonous snakebite is treated as minor wound.

2. Poisonous snakebite is treated by keeping the patient calm, placing the bitten part in a dependent position, and transporting the patient to medical facility.

D. Insect bites or stings.

1. Serious stings require immediate attention.

a. Give aqueous epinephrine and Benadryl.

b. Keep victim calm and treat for shock.

2. Apply paste of baking soda and water or meat tenderizer and cold compresses to less serious stings.

3. Apply a drop of turpentine or mineral oil to ticks and remove; wash area with soap and water and apply an antiseptic.

XI. **Injuries Due to Extreme Heat and Cold**

A. Heatstroke (sunstroke): a disturbance in the heat-regulating mechanism in the brain allows patient's body temperature to become extremely high.

1. Cool with cool water.

2. Transport to a medical facility.

B. Heat exhaustion (heat prostration): caused by excessive loss of salt and water through perspiration. Treated by replacing these substances.

C. Sunburn: treat minor burn with application of solution of baking soda or Epsom salts and water.

D. Hypothermia: drastic lowering of body temperature.

1. Symptoms: mild shivering and complaints of cold to unconsciousness.

2. Prevention (Table 31-4).

3. Treatment.

    a. Depends on age and physical condition of patient.

    b. Rewarm body.

    c. Submerge in tepid bath or wrap in blanket.

    d. Improper warming can cause cardiac arrhythmias and respiratory and cardiac arrest.

E. Frostbite: local condition associated with constriction of blood vessels and damage to tissue and vessel walls.

    1. Rewarm quickly by immersion in warm water.

    2. Do not rub; handle very gently.

XII. The Combative Patient

A. Patient who is violent may be terribly afraid.

B. Identify yourself; speak to the patient, using his name frequently.

C. Try simple commands to help patient gain control of himself.

D. If physical restraint is used, be sure enough people are available to subdue patient.

E. Do not leave him alone immediately after he is restrained.

XIII. Disaster Nursing

A. A disaster involves loss of property, physical injuries, and interruption in activities of daily living on a large scale.

B. Agencies involved in planning disaster nursing are the Office of Civil Defense, Red Cross, and other local voluntary organizations.

C. Psychological responses.

    1. Impact stage: survivors and victims need firm guidance and support.

    2. Recoil stage: persons may overextend themselves.

    3. Posttrauma stage: survivors are compliant and want to be helpful.

D. Nursing Intervention.

    1. Know community disaster plans.

    2. Provide leadership and nursing care.

    3. Provide for emotional and physical comfort and safety of victims.

    4. Work to increase effectiveness of local disaster planning agency.

    5. Use mnemonic OLD CART for data gathering.

    6. Water purification by chlorination with bleach, boiling, or distillation.

    7. Care for major chemical emergency: seal off dwelling.

    8. Earthquake safety: seek shelter under sturdy object; if outside go away from trees, buildings, and power lines.

    9. Fire safety: if smoke alarm sounds, go outside immediately; if smoke or fire is detected, fall to the floor and crawl to exit.

    10. Further interventions.

        a. Assess victims' physical and mental condition.

        b. Improvise supplies and procedures for treatment as necessary.

UNIT FOUR

Mental Health Nursing of the Adult

The four chapters in this unit present the basic information needed by the nurse to assist patients with mental health problems. Chapter 32 covers disorders of anxiety and mood and presents assessment and interventions for depression and to prevent suicide. Chapter 33 discusses nursing care for patients with substance use disorders. Chapter 34 talks about cogitive disorders, such as confusion, delirium, and dementia. Care of the Alzheimer's patient is a large part of this chapter. Chapter 35 presents characteristics of personality and thought disorders and the modalities used to treat them.

The student will find considerable information in this unit that will be applicable to the care and concerns of patients that also are being treated for a medical–surgical disorder. Depression and anxiety often accompany chronic illness. Substance use may become apparent when a patient is admitted after an accident of some sort. Confusion and delirium are frequently seen in patients after anesthesia or with serious infections. Many disruptions of homeostasis can cause confusion to occur in elderly patients. Often times patients with personality and thought disorders are hospitalized or being treated in clinics for other medical–surgical problems. The nurse needs to understand these disorders adequately to plan care for such patients.

These chapters also present a solid foundation for the LPN who wishes to pursue further study to work in a psychiatric facility.

CHAPTER 32

Care of Patients with Anxiety and Mood Disorders

In this chapter disorders of anxiety and mood are discussed. Disorders of anxiety affect 3% to 8% of the general population and up to 15% of the elderly population. Anxiety is considered normal and healthy unless it becomes debilitating and prevents a person from functioning in everyday life. Abnormal or debilitating anxiety is intense and feels life-threatening to the individual. Intervention by health care professionals is necessary to prevent potential harm toward self or aggression toward others.

The incidence of mood disorders is very high. Unfortunately these disorders are frequently inaccurately diagnosed and treated. A term used to describe normal mood (a feeling state) is **euthymia. Dysthymia** refers to a disturbance in mood that may manifest in either depression or elation (**mania**). An individual experiencing clinical depression is more than just sad. Depressed or dysthymic individuals feel a sense of hopelessness and despair that cannot be alleviated by usual means. This hopelessness can lead to thoughts of suicide.

Mania, on the other hand, is an elevation in mood that is characterized by feelings of elation, excitement, or extreme irritability. Manic individuals may not sleep or eat for days and intervention is necessary to prevent complete physical and mental exhaustion and aggressive behavior. Sometimes individuals switch from being extremely depressed to becoming manic. This condition is called bipolar disorder. It often is initially diagnosed in young adults, but it may be diagnosed at anytime during the life span.

NURSING MANAGEMENT

◆ Assessment

A thorough assessment of anxiety and mood is necessary to prevent inaccurate diagnosis and inadequate treatment. Anxiety and depression are self-limiting conditions and often are alleviated without specific medical or nursing interventions. However, because both conditions usually recur, often in greater levels of severity, early intervention is important.

Severe levels of anxiety affect one's ability to think rationally. Exaggeration of normal feelings and specific physical symptoms are apparent. The physical signs include dry mouth, elevated blood pressure, heart rate and respirations, increased perspiration, nausea, irritability, diarrhea, increased urination, and insomnia. Patients often describe feelings of fear, impending doom, helplessness, low self-esteem, guilt, and anger. See Table 32-1 for assessment and nursing management of anxiety.

Elder Care Point... The elderly population often present anxiety as somatic complaints rather than openly verbalize emotional distress. The nurse may observe the anxious elder complaining of an upset stomach, inability to sleep, fatigue, or increased need to urinate. Medications that the elder is taking may increase feelings of anxiety. Certain medical conditions, such as problems with the thyroid gland, the cardiac system, and altered blood sugar, also can mimic anxiety disorders.

TABLE 32-1 ◆ *Assessment and Nursing Management of Anxiety*

Assessment of Anxiety

Physiological	Psychological
Tachycardia	Restlessness
Elevated blood pressure	Agitation
Increased perspiration	Tremors (fine to gross shaking of the body)
Dilated pupils	Startle reaction
Hyperventilation with difficulty breathing	Rapid speech
Cold, clammy skin	Lack of coordination
Dry mouth	Withdrawal
Constipation	Impaired attention
Urinary frequency	Poor concentration
Diarrhea	Forgetfulness
	Decreased perceptual field
	Decreased productivity
	Confusion

Nursing Management of Anxiety

Level of Anxiety	Assessment	Goal	Nursing Management
Mild	Increased alertness, motivation, and attentiveness.	To assist client to tolerate some anxiety.	Help client identify and describe feelings Help client develop the capacity to tolerate mild anxiety, take deep breaths, focus on pleasant thoughts.
Moderate	Perception narrowed, selective inattention, physical discomforts.	To reduce anxiety; LTG: directed toward helping client understand cause of anxiety and new ways of controlling it.	Provide outlet for tension such as walking, crying, working at simple, concrete tasks. Encourage client to discuss feelings.
Severe	Behavior becomes automatic; connections between details are not seen; senses are drastically reduced.	To assist in channeling anxiety.	Recognize own level of anxiety. Encourage use of coping mechanisms. *Report escalating anxiety to RN.*
Panic	Overwhelmed; inability to function or communicate; possible bodily harm to self and others; loss of rational thought.	To be supportive and protective.	Provide nonstimulating, structured environment. Avoid touching. Stay with client. Medicate client with tranquilizers if necessary.

Source: Zerwekh, J., Claborn, J. (1992). *NCLEX-PN: A Study Guide for Practical Nursing.* Dallas, TX: Nursing Education Consultants. Reprinted with permission.

Assessing for mood disorders involves observing not only mood and affect, but also physical signs and symptoms. The nurse assesses mood by both asking the patient questions and observing facial expressions and verbalizations. **Affect** is a term used to describe a person's feelings. A person with a flat or blunted affect may tell you she is feeling fine, but you notice by her facial expression and overall demeanor that she appears sad. The sadness described by depressed individuals is intense and renders them hopeless and feeling worthless. The mood of a manic patient, on the other hand, is one of grandiosity and general well-being. In the midst of a manic episode the manic patient will tell the nurse that anything is possible.

Many physical signs and symptoms are classic for mood disorders. An initial question concerns sleep. A depressed patient may say that she sleeps all the time (**hypersomnia**) or that she falls asleep easily, but wakes up after 2 to 3 hours and is unable to get back to sleep (**insomnia**). Manic patients are unable to sleep, and it is not unusual for them to tell you they have not slept for days.

Think about... How would you differentiate an individual who is agitated from sleep deprivation from an individual who is in the manic phase of bipolar disorder?

Appetite also must be assessed. Assess for recent weight loss or gain and patterns of eating. A person who is depressed also may have many somatic complaints, such as headache, stomachache, dizziness, nausea, indigestion, and change in sexual responsiveness. The inability to concentrate and indecisiveness also are hallmarks of mood disorders.

The depressed patient often presents with psychomotor retardation. Speech is slowed, as are movements and thought processes. However, it is not uncommon to see agitation and irritability in a depressed person. **The agitation and irritability seen in manic patients can often lead to aggressive behavior.**

♦ Nursing Diagnoses

Nursing diagnoses for anxiety and mood disorders are listed in Table 32-2.

♦ Planning

Planning care for a patient with an anxiety or mood disorder involves promoting safety; reducing symptoms of anxiety, depression, and mania; and providing adequate nutrition and sleep. Once the patient is able to concentrate, nursing goals focus on teaching about the illness and medications the patient will be taking. Medication compliance is very important because it is

not unusual for the patient to stop taking medications once the symptoms subside.

Nursing goals include:

- Promoting safety
- Providing for rest
- Correcting nutritional deficiency
- Reducing external stimuli
- Educating patient about the illness
- Educating patient about medications

♦ Implementation

Nurses can be very instrumental in helping a patient recover from a panic level of anxiety. Remaining calm and supportive provides a safety net for the patient. Patients with anxiety need teaching about how to prevent further attacks. They need to be taught how to relax and should attempt to determine the underlying cause of their anxiety.

Protecting a suicidal patient from self-harm is a priority nursing intervention. If the patient is hospitalized, suicide precautions must be initiated. For individuals not hospitalized, a suicide contract, preferably written, should be initiated until the patient can seek further help. Active listening and a caring attitude are necessary to build a trusting relationship with a severely depressed, suicidal patient. Even if the patient is unwilling to talk to you, you must indicate to the patient both verbally and nonverbally that you care.

Think about... Describe at least three ways in which a nurse shows caring and empathy.

Patients in a manic state can be a source of danger to others on the unit. The moods of manic patients can escalate quickly from good-natured humor into active aggression. Decreasing stimuli and/or removing the manic patient may be necessary.

Manic patients often come into the hospital malnourished. Provide small frequent, high-calorie meals. Finger foods often are necessary because the manic patient will not sit down long enough to eat. Knowledge about medications and the need for long-term use of medications is another very important intervention. Appropriate interventions for patients experiencing anxiety and mood disorders are listed in Table 32-2.

♦ Evaluation

Evaluating patients with anxiety, depression, or mania is necessary not only immediately, but also upon discharge from the hospital or emergency room. The nurse must determine whether the outcome criteria initiated for the patient were met. Assessing whether the symp-

TABLE 32-2 ◆ *Common Nursing Diagnoses and Interventions for Patients with Anxiety and Mood Disorders*

Nursing Diagnosis	Goals/Expected Outcomes	Interventions
Anxiety, related to lack of knowledge, real or perceived threat to self-concept, unmet needs.	Vital signs will return to normal limits. Patient will be able to verbalize reasons for anxiety. Patient will be able to verbalize at least three anxiety-reduction methods.	Maintain a calm, nonthreatening manner. Reassure patient that she is safe. Keep immediate surroundings low in stimuli. Administer anxiolytics as ordered by the physician. When anxiety is sufficiently reduced, explore possible reasons for the anxiety with the patient. Teach signs and symptoms of escalating anxiety and ways to prevent it.
Ineffective individual coping, related to situational crisis, maturational crisis, inadequate support systems.	Patient will be able to describe two new coping methods by discharge. Patient will identify a supportive network by discharge.	Support the patient's efforts to explore the meaning and purpose of behavior. Encourage the patient to verbalize the significance of the current crisis in her life. Encourage the patient to develop a supportive network.
Social isolation related to panic level of anxiety, repressed fears.	Anxiety will be relieved within 30 minutes of taking medication. Patient will be able to verbalize fears. Patient will practice at least one method of relaxation while in the hospital.	Monitor level of anxiety on a frequent basis. Foster a therapeutic nurse–patient relationship by staying with the patient during social interactions and keeping all promises. Administer anxiolytics as ordered by the physician. Monitor effectiveness of medication and side effects. Teach the patient how to recognize increasing levels of anxiety and ways to interrupt the response (relaxation techniques). Encourage patient to express fears.
Spiritual distress related to sense of despair and feelings of abandoment by God.	Patient will verbalize hope for the future within 1 week.	Engage in active listening and convey a caring, genuine attitude. Encourage the patient to remember a time in her life when she felt nurtured, loved and accepted. Encourage and accept verbalization of all feelings.
Risk for violence: Self-directed, related to severely depressed mood, feelings of hopelessness, anger turned inward, statements and cues indicating a desire to commit suicide.	Patient will verbalize a desire to live. Patient will sign a no-suicide contract. Patient will not harm self.	Determine appropriate level of suicide precautions and initiate them. Monitor closely for any change in mood and temperament. Initiate a 24-hour verbal or written contract with the patient stating that she will not harm herself.
Risk for violence: directed toward others, related to manic state, delusions of grandeur.	Patient and others on unit will remain free from harm. Patient will show evidence of decreased aggression within 20 minutes of medicine administration.	Maintain low stimuli in environment. Observe patient's behavior frequently (every 15 minutes). Try to redirect or distract patient. Administer tranquilizing medications as ordered and as indicated. Monitor effectiveness of medications.
Altered nutrition, more or less than body requirements, related to inability to sit still long enough to eat, lack of appetite, low energy level.	Patient will assume regular eating habits within 1 week. Patient will verbalize the essentials of a healthy diet within 1 week. Patient will be weight/height proportionate within 6 months.	Weigh daily. Record intake and output. Determine food likes and dislikes. Offer small frequent, high-calorie meals and finger foods. Stay with the patient during meals. Administer vitamin and mineral supplements.
Sleep pattern disturbance: related to erratic sleeping patterns, too much sleep, too little sleep.	Patient will report a restful sleep pattern within 3 days.	Provide a quiet environment with low stimuli that is conducive to rest. Monitor and record sleeping patterns. Prior to bedtime provide comfort nursing measures, such as a backrub, warm bath, and relaxing music. Prohibit intake of caffeine foods in the evening hours. Administer sedative medications as ordered to assist the patient in establishing a normal sleep pattern.

toms of anxiety, depression, or mania are relieved is essential. Part of this overall assessment will include determining the effectiveness of medications. Sometimes it takes several different trials of a combination of drugs to achieve the desired effect. In addition, many of the medications take 2 to 3 weeks to become effective and the initial side effects of drowsiness and nausea may discourage long-term compliance.

Think about ... What type of approach would a nurse follow to help a patient who is fearful agree to take antidepressant medication? The patient tells you that medication would not be necessary if she tried harder. In addition the patient is concerned that the medication is addictive.

DISORDERS OF ANXIETY AND MOOD

◆ Generalized Anxiety Disorder

A persistent, unrealistic, or excessive worry about two or more life circumstances characterizes a person who exhibits symptoms associated with generalized anxiety disorder. Physical symptoms include trembling, feeling shaky, increased muscle tension, muscle soreness, easy fatiguability, and restlessness. In addition, an automatic nervous system response causes an increase in vital signs, dyspnea, palpitations, dry mouth, dizziness, and nausea. **The person experiencing this disorder is hypervigilant, has difficulty sleeping, and can be irritable.** Worry over children, finances, employment, and health are typical concerns that keep these individuals chronically worried.

Diagnosis To help clinicians define and diagnose behavioral disorders more consistently, the American Psychiatric Association publishes the Diagnostic and Statistical Manual, which establishes guidelines for how diagnoses are made. According to the DSM-IV, the diagnosis of generalized anxiety disorder can be made only when the anxiety has been present for at least 6 months.

Treatment Persons with this disorder respond very well to supportive therapy and anxiolytic (antianxiety) medications. Supportive therapy may include individual therapy, education about relaxation techniques, and stress management. These patients need much reassurance and a nurse who is a good listener.

The major category of drugs used to treat anxiety disorders are benzodiazepines. Some of the more commonly prescribed drugs prescribed from this category are alprazolam (Xanax), chlordiazepoxide (Librium), oxazepam (Serax), lorazepam (Ativan), and diazepem (Valium). Patients taking these drugs must be advised to

use them with caution because of their highly addictive nature. It is very easy to become physically and psychologically dependent on these medications. However, anxiolytics are very effective in reducing the symptoms of anxiety.

A newer anxiolytic currently being prescribed that is not a benzodiazepene is buspirone (Buspar). Although anti-anxiety effects take longer to become therapeutic (4–6 weeks), the advantage is that patients are not as prone to becoming dependent. See Table 32-3 for a list of common medications used to treat anxiety.

Nursing Intervention **When intervening with a patient who is experiencing extreme levels of anxiety, the most helpful response by the nurse is a calm, reassuring attitude.** Stay with the patient and attend to physical needs as necessary. Attempt to make the immediate surrounding environment less stimulating. For example, dim the lights, turn off the television or radio, and limit the number of people in the area. Be sure to use clear simple statements and repeat as necessary. Assess the patient's need for a short-acting anxiolytic and medicate as necessary. When the anxiety is under control, help the patient determine root causes for the anxiety and assist in problem-solving behaviors that worked to alleviate anxiety in the past.

Think about ... What behavior would indicate to the nurse that a short-acting anxiolytic is indicated for a patient who is extremely anxious?

TABLE 32-3 ◆ *Medications Used to Treat Anxiety*

Category of Medication	Nursing Implications
Benzodiazepines	
Alpraolam (Xanax)	Can cause drowsiness and lethargy.
Chlorodiazepoxide (Librium)	Do not stop taking these medications abruptly.
Diazepam (Valium)	Potentially addictive. Use cautiously.
Lorazepam (Ativan)	Do not take any other CNS depressants, including alcohol, while taking
Oxazepam (Serax)	these medications.
	Watch patient for signs of orthostatic hypotension.
	May cause paradoxical excitement, especially in the elderly. Report to physician.
Nonbenzodiazepine	
Buspirone (BuSpar)	Takes 7 to 10 days for symptoms to subside.
	No evidence of tolerance or physical dependence.
	Does not cause as much lethargy or drowsiness as benzodiazepines.

◆ Bipolar Disorder

Signs and Symptoms   When a patient experiences episodes of extreme sadness, hopelessness, and helplessness interspersed with periods of extreme elation and hyperactivity, bipolar disorder is suspected. According to the DSM IV, two types of bipolar disorder are recognized. Bipolar I disorder is characterized by episodes of major depression with at least one episode of manic or hypomanic behavior. Bipolar II disorder is characterized by one or more depressive episodes with at least one episode of hypomania. See Table 32-4 for descriptions of depressive, manic, and hypomanic episodes.

Treatment   Lithium carbonate is the drug of choice used to stabilize manic behavior. See Table 32-5 for nursing implications for lithium. As it may take 2 to 3 weeks for Lithium to become effective, antipsychotics such as chlorpromazine (Thorazine) or haloperidol (Haldol) are given to decrease the level of hyperactivity. In addition to stabilizing the patient with medication, it is sometimes necessary to hospitalize patients with manic symptoms, particularly if they are of danger to themselves or others, or are suffering from exhaustion caused by extreme hyperactivity.

Nursing Intervention   Nursing interventions for a hospitalized manic patient involve keeping the patient safe, providing, a high-calorie intake, administering

TABLE 32-5 ◆ *Nursing Implications for the Administration of Lithium*
◆ Inform patient that it takes 7 to 14 days to reach therapeutic levels of this medication.
◆ This drug does not cure bipolar disorder. Initially it helps decrease the manic behavior, but may need to be taken on an ongoing basis.
◆ There is a small margin between therapeutic levels and toxic levels. A therapeutic level is 1.0 to 1.5 meq/L. It is necessary for the patient to have blood levels drawn biweekly to monthly until a maintenance level is maintained.
◆ Lithium can cause sodium depletion. A low-sodium diet could cause toxicity. Maintain normal salt intake and drink adequate fluids.
◆ Take Lithium with meals to prevent gastric distress.
◆ Do not take diuretics while taking Lithium.
◆ Monitor the patient closely during any type of dehydration. A decrease in fluid volume can lead to toxicity.
◆ Monitor renal and thyroid function periodically.

antimanic medications, and providing for a restful sleep. It may be necessary to place a manic patient in a quiet area to decrease environmental stimulation. Often it is necessary to assign a nurse or nurse assistant to stay with the manic patient until the medications have reduced agitation and hyperactivity.

Behavior in manic patients can escalate rapidly from a mood of frivolity and joking to agitation and extreme paranoia. Close observation and documentation of mood, verbalizations, and behavior are very important. **When communicating with a manic patient, it is essential that the nurse maintain a calm demeanor.**

Until the medications are effective, therapeutic communication consists of setting limits. When setting limits it is necessary that you initially clearly state your expectation of the patient's behavior. State the consequences for the patient's not complying with the request, and always follow through with the stated consequence. To avoid being manipulated by the patient it is important that all staff members be consistent. Sometimes, because of the severity of the mania, the manic patient is unable to comply with simple requests. In these instances it is necessary to distract the patient rather than attempt to use reason.

◆ Major Depressive Disorder

Signs and Symptoms   Major depressive disorder is diagnosed when at least five symptoms characteristic of depression have been present for at least 2 weeks. **These symptoms include an overwhelming feeling of sadness, inability to feel pleasure or interest in daily activities, weight gain or loss not attributed to dieting, sleep disturbances, fatigue or loss of energy, feelings of worthlessness, difficulty in making decisions or concen-**

TABLE 32-4 ◆ *Characteristics of Depressive, Manic and Hypomanic*	
Episodes	
Depressive	Overwhelming sadness and loss of interest in most activities. Symptoms must be present for at least 2 weeks. Change in appetite, hypersomnia or insomnia, inability to concentrate or make decisions, feeling hopeless, guilt-ridden and worthless. Suicidal ideation also may be present.
Manic	Change in mood that includes increased grandiosity or irritability that is present for at least 1 week. Manic person may exhibit pressured speech and flight of ideas, inability to concentrate, decreased need for sleep or nutrients, increase in goal-directed activity, psychomotor retardation, impulsive spending and hypersexuality. May require hospitalization.
Hypomanic	Inflated or irritable mood for at least 4 days. May experience loud and rapid speech, decreased need for sleep, distractibility and increase in goal-directed activity. Hospitalization is not indicated because it does not involve psychotic behavior.

trating, and suicidal thoughts. These symptoms may be subjective (described by the patient) or observable by significant others.

Prior to making a diagnosis of depression, the physician must be certain that there are no medical conditions present that could mimic depression. Patients who have suffered a stroke, have cancer, a myocardial infarction, or are newly diagnosed with diabetes all need to be screened for depression. Moreover, many classifications of medications may induce a pharmacological type of depression. Examples are antihypertensives, sedatives, and antianxiety agents, antipsychotic drugs, and steroids and hormones.

In addition, abuse of alcohol often produces symptoms that mimic depressive symptoms. In some instances a person drinks alcohol to alleviate the symptoms of depression—drinking to drown sorrows. In other cases, drinking large amounts of alcohol will actually cause a person to feel depressed because alcohol is a central nervous system depressant. In either instance a diagnosis of alcohol dependence needs to be considered when the symptoms associated with depression are present.

Elder Care Point... There is a high incidence of depression among the elderly, and it often is misdiagnosed. Elders and their caretakers frequently attribute the depression to the increasing number of losses that is part of the aging process. These losses include decreases in bodily function and loss of friends and family. Symptoms of major depression are not a normal part of the aging process, and a differential diagnosis needs to be made. The cause may be due to a general medical condition or a pharmacological intervention.

There is increasing evidence that major depressive disorder is caused by a biochemical imbalance. However, most scientists today agree that most major illnesses are the result of a combination of heredity and environment. What is not understood is how these two elements interact to precipitate an episode of major mental illness. More research needs to be done in this area. Remember, however, that, regardless of the cause, depression needs to be treated and not ignored. The signs and symptoms of depression will eventually subside. However, research findings indicate that an attack of major depression is very likely to recur at a later time, with even greater severity.

Treatment   Patients who are depressed respond best to a combination of antidepressant medication and psychotherapy. Hospitalization may be necessary if there is a high potential of suicide. In that instance it would be necessary to protect the patient from impulses over which he or she has little control. See assessment for suicide in Table 32-6.

TABLE 32-6 ◆ *Questions to Ask a Potentially Suicidal Patient*
◆ Are you feeling suicidal? If yes, ask question number 2.
◆ Do you have a plan? If the patient answers, Yes, ask patient to describe the plan: How do you plan to take your life?
◆ Can you think of any event that may have caused you to feel this way?
◆ Do you have a lethal weapon in your possession?
◆ Who comprises your support system?
◆ Do you drink or use drugs on a regular basis?
◆ Has anyone in your family history made a previous suicide attempt?
◆ Are you currently taking any antidepressants?
◆ Have you experienced a major loss within the last year?
◆ What is your history with past close relationships?
◆ Have you given away any of your possessions recently?
◆ Have you been having difficulty remembering things lately?

Since the 1960s medications have made a great difference in the lives of people who are depressed. The three main categories of medications used to treat depression are the monamine inhibitors (MAOIs), tricyclics, and selective serotonin reuptake inhibitors (SSRIs). Tricyclics and MAOIs are very effective in treating depressive symptoms. However, they can cause some very serious side effects that are unpleasant for the patient and cause noncompliance. The SSRIs cause fewer side effects, but are much more expensive and therefore not as readily prescribed for patients on limited incomes or without insurance coverage. For a list of nursing implications of commonly prescribed antidepressant medications, see Table 32-7.

Electroconvulsive therapy (ECT) also is a treatment for severe depression. Before ECT is considered, several regimens of medication are given. If the depression is not relieved, ECT is considered. Basically, ECT consists of electric shock to the brain waves via electrodes applied to the temples. This shock artificially induces a grand mal seizure. How this mechanism actually relieves depression is not understood. The patient typically receives two to three treatments a week for several weeks.

Nursing Intervention   The priority nursing intervention for a depressed patient is to protect the patient from acting on impulses and harm him/herself. This is especially true once the antidepressant medications begin to take effect. Prior to that time, the patient may not have adequate energy to commit suicide. Once the patient begins to feel somewhat better, but has not recovered completely, there is sufficient energy to complete the act. Monitoring the patient closely at this time is very important. Genuine caring and concern for the patient who is depressed is essential. Depressed patients can

TABLE 32-7 ◆ *Nursing Implicatins for Antidepressant Drugs*

Category of Medication	Nursing Implications
Tricyclics	
Amitriptyline (Elavil)	Mood elevation may take from 7 to 28 days. Full recovery from major depression may take 6 to 8 weeks. Encourage patient to keep taking the medication.
Imipramine (Tofranil)	
Nortriptyline (Pamelor)	Inform patient that side effects of drowsiness, dizziness, and hypotension will subside after the first few weeks.
Amoxapine (Ascendin)	
Maprotyline (Ludiomil)	Inform patient to avoid taking alcohol and working around machines and heavy equipment.
Clomipramine (Anafranil)	Anticholinergic side effects, such as dry mouth, blurred vision, tachycardia, postural hypotension, constipation, urinary retention, and esophageal reflux, are common.
	Tricyclics are usually taken at bedtime.
	Inform the patient not to stop taking these medications suddenly.
	Monitor patient for suicidal ideation. An overdose of these medications could be fatal.
MAO Inhibitors	
Isocarboxazid (Marplan)	Certain foods, medications, and beverages can cause a hypertensive episode that can be life-threatening. Tell the patient to avoid foods high in tyramine, such as aged cheeses, red wine, sherry and beer, pickled or smoked fish, fermented meats, and artificial sweeteners. Also inform the patient not to take any medications that increase the heart rate, such as ephedrine, stimulants, alcohol, narcotics, tricyclic antidepressants, or antihypertensives.
Phenelzine (Nardil)	
Tranylcypromine (Parnate)	
	Common side effects are weight gain, postural hypotension, edema, change in cardiac rate and rhythm, urinary retention, constipation, insomnia, weakness, and fatigue.
	Monitor blood pressure very closely during the first few weeks of treatment.
	Inform the patient to go to the emergency room immediately if a headache begins.
	If the medication is discontinued for any reason, inform the patient to continue the dietary restrictions for at least 14 days.
Selective serotonin reuptake inhibitors (SSRIs)	
Fluoxetine (Prozac)	These medications effect an elevation in mood faster than the TCAs or MAOs. In addition, they are not as sedating and do not have the anticholinergic side effects of TCAs or MAOs.
Sertaline (Zoloft)	
Paroxetine (Paxil)	Common side effects include nausea, nervousness, insomnia, anxiety, and sexual dysfunction.
Nefazodone (Serzone)	These medications work by blocking the reuptake of a chemical in the brain, serotonin, allowing increased levels of serotonin to be available. Serotonin is involved in the transmission of stimuli between cells in the brain; higher levels affect a person's mood positively.
Mirtazapine (Remeron)	
Atypical antidepressants	
Trazodone (Desyrel)	These medications act similarly to the SSRIs. Trazadone not only blocks the reuptake of serotonin, but also stimulates serotonin receptors.
Bupropion (Wellbutrin)	
	Side effects are similar to the SSRIs with the exception that Trazadone is known to cause priapism, a painful, prolonged erection of the penis.
	Bupropion, in doses above 450 mg/day, is known to cause seizures. It should be used cautiously in patients with any type of previous head trauma or seizure disorder.

be difficult to be with because of their self-defeating thoughts and verbalizations.

In addition to being supportive, the nurse needs to help the patient begin to set some goals. Begin with small goals, such as grooming, and work toward the greater goals of reentry into the work force. Goal setting and problem solving require mental energy and concentration that are not available to a person who is still in the depths of depression.

Think about . . . What types of goals would be suitable for a 25-year-old female nursing student who is depressed? She is taking Prozac, an SSRI, and feeling better, but continues to feel overwhelmed.

Most depressed persons complain of some type of sleep deprivation. Providing the patient with restful sleep is very important. Many of the antidepressant medications have a sedative effect. However, the nurse should provide the patient with an environment that is conducive to sleep and needs to educate the patient and family about the importance of regular sleep.

Intervention for a patient receiving ECT involves basic preoperative preparation, including obtaining a signed consent, removing dentures, keeping the patient NPO for at least 6 hours, and administering a preoperative medication such as Atropine sulfate. The patient will receive a short-acting general anesthesia.

After the seizure is completed, monitor vital signs, reorient the patient, and prepare for discharge. Electroconvulsive therapy frequently is done on an outpatient basis in the early morning. Prior to discharge the patient is given breakfast. Short-term memory loss is expected, and this fact should be explained to the patient and family prior to treatment.

♦ Assessment of the Suicidal Patient

One of the outcomes of untreated depression is suicide.

> Persons at risk for suicide are as follows: family history of suicide, history of a previous attempt, terminally ill patients, people addicted to drugs or alcohol, patients diagnosed with major depressive disorder or bipolar disorder, and persons under considerable stress.

Suicide assessment includes determining the level of lethality (low, moderate, or high), the presence of a distinct plan, and collecting a family history. It is important that your questions be direct and concise. See Table 32-6 for examples of questions to ask potentially suicidal patients.

All suicide threats and gestures should be taken seriously. Feeling suicidal is extremely painful, and your caring and concern may help the patient find a better way to cope with the stressors that everyday living brings.

Medications to treat an underlying depression often are indicated, and the nurse must help the patient understand that depression is a real illness for which sometimes pharmacological intervention is necessary. Too many people who are depressed and suicidal are told by well-intentioned friends or uninformed medical personnel that they just need to get on with their life and think happy thoughts. **This type of advice reinforces the hopelessness that a suicidal patient feels.**

Nursing Intervention   Interventions for suicidal patients can be divided into two major categories: first the nurse must make the initial assessment and determine the degree of probability of suicide. The probability of a completed attempt (lethality) increases when there is a weapon available (guns or knives), when there is a poor support system, with social isolation, with persons under the influence of mood-altering chemicals, and with males. Statistically, men are more likely to complete a suicide.

Second, some type of suicide precautions must be initiated. Suicide precautions could consist of placing the patient in a seclusion room for 24-hour observation. When assessment indicates that the actual suicide intent is not as lethal, maintaining close observation and contracting with the patient to refrain from taking action will suffice. In addition, all items that the patient might use for self-harm must be removed, such as razor blades, belts, ropes, or pills.

Think about . . . What contact have you had in your own life with someone who attempted or actually committed suicide? How might this affect your nursing care of others?

It is important for the nurse to connect with the suicidal patient and build a trusting relationship. The patient must know that the nurse cares. Active listening and spending time with your patient is very important. Showing a willingness to listen to your patient's pain and your calm presence indicate to the patient that you will provide a safe environment.

COMMUNITY CARE

As hospital stays are becoming shorter, many patients with disorders of anxiety or mood will be hospitalized only long enough to stabilize the life-threatening symptoms. They will then be seen in outpatient clinics, long-term care, at home, or in day hospitals. Medication compliance is a major nursing responsibility. Once they feel better and the crisis that impelled them to seek help is over, patients may decide that medications are no longer needed. Regular visits to the clinic or physician are as important, as is some type of continued support system.

CRITICAL THINKING EXERCISES

Clinical Case Problems

Read each clinical case problem and discuss the questions with your classmates.

1. You are working in an emergency room and the mother of an adolescent who was in an automobile accident becomes hysterical. You assess her briefly and find she is in a panic level of anxiety.
   - What nursing actions will you take to decrease the anxiety level of this mother?
   - When might it be appropriate for you to let this mother see her son?

2. You are caring for an elderly couple in their home 6 months after the husband had a stroke. One day the wife takes you aside and tells you that she is concerned about her husband. She says that he is not sleeping well and that his appetite is poor. Upon further questioning, you find that he is verbalizing a desire to "end it all."
   - What initial priority nursing action should be taken at this time?
   - How would you assess the level of caregiver stress the wife is experiencing?
   - What type of community supports might be available for this couple?

3. Mrs. Gonzalez, an elderly female you are caring for in the nursing home is being treated for generalized anxiety disorder. The anxiolytic medications seem to be working in relieving the overall anxiety. She is sleeping better and feels calmer. However Mrs. Gonzalez tells you that she continues to be fearful of going on outings with the other residents.

   ◆ What types of nursing interventions would be necessary in this situation?

   ◆ What needs to be included on the overall care plan for the staff to follow?

4. Mr. Bill Jones, a 35-year-old male, comes into the emergency room after a high speed chase with the police. He is using vulgar, profane language and is unable to sit down even for a few minutes. Bill switches rapidly from being fun loving and humorous to angry and aggressive. The psychiatrist tells you that Bill has bipolar disorder and orders Thorazine to be given intramuscularly.

   ◆ What would be the best way to approach Bill safely to give him the injection?

   ◆ What are your major safety concerns regarding this patient in the emergency room?

   ◆ What other nursing interventions are necessary at this time?

BIBLIOGRAPHY

American Psychiatric Association. (1994). *Diagnostic and Statistical Manual of Mental Disorders—IV*. Washington, D.C.: American Psychiatric Association.

Badger, J. (1995). Reaching out to the suicidal patient. *American Journal of Nursing*. 95(3):24–32.

Bihm, B. (1996). Psychotropic medications and the elderly. *MEDSURG Nursing*. 5(3):191–194.

Carson, V., Arnold, E. (1996). *Mental Health Nursing: The Nurse Patient Journey*. Philadelphia: Saunders.

Chez, N. (1994). Helping the victim of domestic violence. *American Journal of Nursing*. 94(7):33–37.

Dossey, B. (1996). Help your patient break free from anxiety. *Nursing 96*. 26(10):52–54.

Ferdinand, R. (1995). I'd rather die than live this way. *American Journal of Nursing*. 95(12):42–48.

Fortinash, K., Holoday-Worret, P. (1995). *Psychiatric Nursing Care Plans*. St. Louis, MO: Mosby-Year Book.

Kotin, B. (1993). Shock therapy: facts, not myths. *R.N.* 56(7):26–30.

Lynch, S. H. (1997). Elder abuse: what to look for, how to intervene. *American Journal of Nursing*. 97(1):27–32.

Mayo, T. L. (1997). Menatl health services in the home: a balance of sophistication and caring. *Home Healthcare Nurse*. 15(4):271–274.

McCullough, P. K. (1992). Evaluation and management of anxiety in the older adult. *Geriatrics*. 47(4):35.

Mellick, E. (1992). Suicide among elderly white men: development of a profile. *Journal of Psychosocial Nursing*. 30(2):29–34.

Spear, H. L. (1996). Anxiety: when to worry, what to do. *RN*. 59(7):40–45.

Valente, S. (1994). Recognizing depression in elderly patients. *American Journal of Nursing*. 94(12):18–25.

Zerwekh J., Claborn, J. (1992). *NCLEX-PN: A Study Guide for Practical Nursing*. Dallas, TX: Nursing Education Consultants.

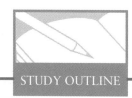

STUDY OUTLINE

I. **Significance of Anxiety and Mood Disorders**
   A. Incidence high for both disorders, especially depression.
   B. Both often go undiagnosed and untreated.

II. **Normal Anxiety Versus Anxiety Disorders**
   A. Levels of anxiety.
      1. Mild.
      2. Moderate.
      3. Severe.
      4. Panic.
   B. See Table 32-1 for descriptions of levels of anxiety and interventions.

III. **Normal Mood versus Mood Disorders**
   A. Descriptors of mood or affect.
      1. Euthymia: normal mood.
      2. Dysthymia: disturbance in mood.
      3. Mania: elevation in mood (elation).
   B. Extremes require intervention.

IV. **Nursing Assessment of Anxiety and Mood Disorders**
   A. Early intervention is important.
   B. Severe levels of anxiety affect ability to think rationally.

C. Signs and symptoms of increasing levels of anxiety.

    1. Increased blood pressure and pulse.

    2. Dry mouth.

    3. Increased respirations.

    4. Nausea.

    5. Irritability.

    6. Diarrhea.

    7. Increased urination.

    8. Insomnia.

    9. Feelings of impending doom.

    10. Fear, guilt, anger, and helplessness.

    11. Low self-esteem.

D. Observation of affect is important.

    1. Descriptions of affect: flat or blunted.

    2. Descriptions of mood: depressed or manic.

E. Physical indicators of mood disorders.

    1. Hypersomnia or insomnia.

    2. Change in appetite: overeating versus undereating.

    3. Somatic complaints: headache, stomachache, dizziness, nausea, indigestion, and change in sexual responsiveness.

    4. Indecisiveness and inability to concentrate.

    5. Psychomotor retardation.

    6. Agitation and irritability that can lead to aggressive behavior.

F. Planning: nursing goals include:

    1. Promoting safety.

    2. Providing for rest.

    3. Correcting nutritional deficiency.

    4. Reducing external stimuli.

    5. Educating patient about the illness and medications.

G. General interventions for anxiety and mood disorders.

    1. Remain calm.

    2. Develop trusting relationship.

    3. Teach methods of relaxation.

    4. Use active listening.

    5. Initiate suicide contract.

    6. Decrease environmental stimuli.

    7. Monitor food intake.

    8. Medicate as necessary.

H. Evaluation: expected outcomes.

    1. Symptoms of anxiety, mania, or depression will be relieved.

    2. Patient demonstrates understanding of medications.

    3. Patient compliant with medication regimen.

V. Common Nursing Diagnoses, Expected Outcomes, and Interventions (Table 32-2)

VI. Disorders of Anxiety and Mood

A. Generalized anxiety disorder.

    1. Persistent, unrealistic, or excessive worry about two or more life circumstances for 6 months.

    2. Physical symptoms include:

        a. Trembling, feeling shaky.

        b. Increased muscle tension.

        c. Muscle soreness.

        d. Easily fatiguability.

        e. Restlessness.

        f. Increase in vital signs.

        g. Dyspnea.

        h. Palpitations.

        i. Dry mouth.

        j. Dizziness and nausea.

        k. Hypervigilance.

        l. Insomnia.

        m. Irritability.

B. Bipolar disorder: episodes of extreme sadness, hopelessness, and helplessness alternating with periods of extreme elation and hyperactivity.

    1. Bipolar I: characterized by episodes of major depression with at least one episode of manic or hypomanic behavior.

    2. Bipolar II: characterized by one or more depressive episodes with at least one episode of hypomania.

    3. For descriptions of manic, hypomanic, and depressive episodes, see Table 32-4.

C. Major depressive disorder: diagnosed when at least five symptoms characteristic of depression have been present for at least 2 weeks.

    1. Symptoms (subjective and objective) include:

        a. Overwhelming feeling of sadness.

        b. Inability to feel pleasure or interest in daily activities.

        c. Weight gain or loss not attributed to dieting.

        d. Sleep disturbances.

        e. Fatigue or loss aof energy.

        f. Feelings of worthlessness.

        g. Difficulty in making decisions or concentrating.

        h. Suicidal thoughts.

VII. Treatment for Anxiety Disorders

A. Psychotherapy.

    1. Supportive.

    2. Individual.

    3. Relaxation techniques.

    4. Stress management.

B. Anxiolytic therapy (Table 32-3).

C. Nursing interventions.
1. Stay calm.
2. Stay with patient.
3. Attend to physical needs.
4. Decrease environmental stimulation.
5. Medicate with anxiolytics as necessary.
6. Evaluate effectiveness of medications.
7. Determine root causes of anxiety if indicated.

VIII. Treatment for Mood Disorders
A. Bipolar disorder.
1. Hospitalization may be necessary.
2. Lithium carbonate: drug of choice to stabilize manic behavior (Table 32-5).
3. Nursing interventions.
   a. Provide for safety for patient and others.
   b. Provide high-calorie diet (finger foods).
   c. Administer antimanic medications.
   d. Monitor effectiveness of medications.
   e. Encourage rest and sleep.
   f. Maintain calm demeanor.
   g. Set limits on behavior.
B. Major depressive disorder.
1. Hospitalization may be necessary if patient is suicidal.
2. Psychotherapy: individual and group.
3. Antidepressant medications (Table 32-7).
4. Electroconvulsive therapy (ECT): indicated for severe depression.
   a. ECT is the delivery of electric shock to brain waves via electrodes.
   b. Used as treatment modality when others failed.
   c. Consist of two to three treatments per week for several weeks.
5. Nursing interventions.
   a. Protect patient from self-harm.
   b. Monitor closely.
   c. Assist patient in setting goals.
   d. Provide for restful sleep.
   e. Administer antidepressant medications.
   f. Monitor effectiveness of medications.
   g. For ECT, routine preoperative preparation.
   h. After ECT, routine postoperative recovery.
   i. Short-term memory loss is expected.

IX. Assessment and Intervention for a Suicidal Patient
A. Assessment: see Table 32-6 for questions to ask.
1. Persons at risk.
   a. Family history of suicide.
   b. History of a previous attempt.
   c. Terminally ill patients.
   d. Drug addiction and alcoholism.
   e. Diagnosis of major depressive disorder or bipolar disorder.
   f. Considerable stress.
2. Level of lethality: low, moderate, or high.
   a. Increases when the following are present:
      (1) A distinct plan.
      (2) Weapons present (guns, knives).
      (3) Poor support system.
      (4) Influence of mood-altering chemicals.
      (5) Being male.
3. Take all threats seriously: initiate written or verbal contract.
4. Encourage treatment of underlying mental disorder, such as depression.
5. Nursing interventions for suicide.
   a. Determine lethality.
   b. Institute suicide precautions if necessary.
      (1) Place in seclusion.
      (2) One-to-one observation.
      (3) Remove all sharp objects.
   c. Build trusting relationship.
   d. Demonstrate caring.
   e. Use active listening.
   f. Provide safety.

X. Elder Care Points
A. Elders often present anxiety as somatic complaints. Certain medications produce symptoms that mimic those of anxiety.
B. Incidence of depression in the elderly is high and often is misdiagnosed or discounted.

XI. Community care
A. Decrease in hospital stays.
B. Patients treated in outpatient clinics, long-term care, in the home, and in day hospitals.
C. Once symptoms are relieved, continued treatment is necessary.

CHAPTER 33

Care of Patients with Substance Use Disorders

O B J E C T I V E S

Upon completing this chapter, the student should be able to:

1. Discuss the significance of substance use disorders in the general adult population.
2. Explain the difference between abuse of mood-altering substances versus dependence on mood-altering substances.
3. Discuss methods of withdrawal from mood-altering substances.
4. Outline the factors to be considered when performing an assessment of a patient who abuses substances.
5. From a list of NANDA nursing diagnoses, identify at least four nursing diagnoses that would be appropriate for a patient with a substance use disorder.
6. From the nursing diagnoses identified, choose appropriate nursing interventions and expected outcomes.
7. Describe the signs and symptoms of alcoholism and of abuse of stimulants, central nervous system depressants, opiates, nicotine, cannabis, hallucinogens, and inhalants.
8. Discuss the nursing interventions for each of these disorders, including the major teaching implications.
9. Describe the effects of substance use disorders on the family and friends of the abuser.

Substance abuse is a major problem throughout the world. Not only does drug abuse have the potential for causing death and medical problems for the abuser, but also it causes many emotional and physical problems for the immediate family, coworkers, and friends of the abuser. In 1956 alcoholism was recognized by the American Medical Association as a medical disease rather than a moral weakness. Change in attitude takes time, and there are still many stigmas associated with alcoholism and use of other drugs that have potential for abuse. Even though research since the mid-1980s tells us that there is a genetic predisposition to alcoholism, society continues to blame families and individuals for the problem. This attitude frequently keeps addicted individuals from seeking treatment.

The term currently used to describe problems with alcoholism and drug abuse is **substance use disorder.** This term implies that a recognizable set of signs and symptoms become apparent when a person ingests a psychoactive substance. **Psychoactive substances** are any mind-altering agents capable of changing a person's mood, behavior, cognition, arousal level, level of consciousness, and perceptions.

In this chapter the following categories of drugs will be studied: central nervous system depressants, including alcohol; central nervous system stimulants, including cocaine, amphetamines, and nicotine; and opiates (narcotic analgesics). Other types of drugs that have potential for abuse are cannabis (marijuana), hallucinogens (LSD), and inhalants.

TERMINOLOGY

Several terms are used to describe substance use disorders. Abuse of substances is different from dependence on substances.

Dependence on substances implies that there are physical and psychological symptoms of addiction and that when the drug or chemical is stopped for any reason, the individual experiences symptoms of withdrawal. Abuse of substances implies that an individual is using a psychoactive drug in a nontherapeutic manner or is illicitly using prescription drugs.

See Table 33-1 for a list of additional terms commonly used in understanding substance use disorders.

For most of the categories of drugs discussed in this chapter there are a certain group of symptoms that will be present when the patient attempts to stop using a drug. This phenomenon is called **withdrawal,** and in some instances it can be fatal. **An easy way to remember withdrawal symptoms is that they are the opposite of the symptoms caused by the ingestion of the chemical.** For example, withdrawal symptoms for a substance that depresses the central nervous system, such as alcohol, are elevation in pulse and blood pressure, nervousness, and heightened anxiety. Persons who are withdrawing from stimulants will experience drowsiness, headache, lethargy, nausea, alterations in eating and sleeping patterns, and sometimes craving.

Think about... How would you recognize the symptoms of withdrawal in a alcoholic hospitalized for another condition?

> **TABLE 33-1 ♦ *Terms Associated with Substance Use Disorders***
>
> * **Addiction:** Symptoms of withdrawal are present when a drug is no longer taken. Usually accompanied by tolerance. Specific withdrawal symptoms vary depending on the particular drug.
> * **Delusion:** A false, fixed belief that cannot be changed with rational explanation.
> * **Detoxification:** The process of eliminating the drug from the body with medical supervision.
> * **Hallucination:** A sensory perception (touching, tasting, feeling, hearing, seeing) that occurs without external stimulation.
> * **Illusion:** A misperception of an actual sensory perception.
> * **Physical dependence:** Same as addiction. May or may not be accompanied by craving or psychological dependence.
> * **Psychological dependence:** Implies the craving or compulsion to take a drug to feel good.
> * **Tolerance:** The need for increased amounts of substances to receive the desired effect.
> * **Withdrawal:** Specific symptoms that are apparent when a drug is no longer taken.

NURSING MANAGEMENT

✦Assessment

Physical Signs and Symptoms   **Symptoms of substance abuse vary greatly depending on the drug and also on how long a person has been abusing the substance.** For example, symptoms in the early stages of alcoholism are vastly different from symptoms in chronic, end-stage alcoholism. Results also vary depending on when the assessment was done. For example, is the individual acutely intoxicated or in the early stages of withdrawal?

A general body systems check, including vital signs, is necessary to determine whether the individual is abusing or dependent on a certain drug. Blood pressure, pulse, and respiration may be decreased or increased. The temperature may be elevated. Impaired coordination may be apparent when the individual is asked to walk or attempt to complete a task that requires fine motor control.

Pupils may be dilated or constricted, and there may be little or no direct eye contact. The eyes may be bloodshot. Observe the skin for needle tracks, bruises, excess perspiration, and excoriation. The nurse also might observe rhinorrhea and a congested, red nose. Grooming could vary from extreme neatness to being unkempt. Try to detect any type of odor that would indicate heavy alcohol use.

Behavioral Indicators   Speech may be slurred, incoherent, or loud and boisterous. Mood or affect will vary from calm and relaxed to extremely agitated and hostile. It would not be unusual to observe some paranoid ideation, particularly if the drug used is illegal. Is the person oriented to time, place, and person?

Do not overlook the possibility of suicide. Certain drugs decrease inhibitions. If suicidal feelings are present prior to the ingestion of the drug, taking the drug may precipitate action. Moreover, determine whether altered perceptions, such as **delusions, hallucinations, or illusions,** are present. See Table 33-1 for descriptions of these terms.

Psychological Indicators of Abuse   **Denial** and **rationalization** are the main two defense mechanisms used by substance abusers. A typical example of the use of denial is characterized by the following statement: "I never drink more than two beers at a time, and I never drink before noon." "If you had my problems, you would drink, too" is a classic example of rationalization. To be effective in treating substance abusers, nurses must remember that substance abusers usually do not seek help voluntarily. Denial and rationalization become very entrenched behaviors and are difficult to eradicate.

History   Obtaining a drug history is an essential part of the assessment for drug abuse and alcoholism. Remember to take into account, however, that denial is a primary defense mechanism used by substance abusers. Therefore, it often is equally necessary to take a family history. An alcoholic may tell you that he is only a social drinker, but his wife or children may say that he drinks to the point of intoxication at least three times a week.

Think about . . . How would you confront a discrepancy in what the client and the family report about the amount of alcohol or drugs taken? What would you say to the family and what would you say to the addict?

In taking a history the nurse needs to find out the type of substance used, the amount taken, and the pattern of use. Examples of questions to ask either the individual or the family member are listed in Table 33-2.

◆ Nursing Diagnoses

Common nursing diagnoses, expected outcomes, and interventions for persons with substance use disorders are included in Table 33-3.

TABLE 33-2 ◆ *Guide to History Taking: Questions to Determine Past and Present Drug and Alcohol Use*

- What is your drug of choice?
- What other types of drugs do you routinely take?
- How much do you drink or how much do you use?
- How often do you drink or use substances?
- Have you ever tried to cut down or control your drug use or drinking?
- When did you last drink or use drugs of any kind?
- Have you noticed that now it takes more of the drug or drink to get the same effect you got several months ago?
- Have you noticed any withdrawal symptoms?
- Have you ever been treated for liver disease, hepatitis, heart disease, anemia, or drug overdose?
- Have you had any recent falls, accidents, or injuries?
- Have you ever stopped drinking or using drugs for a period of time?
- Have you ever been in treatment for substance abuse?
- Is there a family history of alcoholism or drug abuse?
- What is your marital status? If married, are you happily married?
- Have you ever been in trouble with the law?
- What is your occupation? Are you experiencing any difficulties at work?

◆ Planning

Collaborative goal setting is very important when working with an individual who is addicted to a substance. In addition to working with the patient, it is necessary that the nurse collaborate with the family. All addicts have one or several friends or family members who enable their behavior. Setting goals with the patient and excluding the family or friends often leads to failure or relapse. Planning care for a patient with a substance use disorder includes promoting safety (physical and psychological); providing a safe withdrawal from the substance; and ensuring adequate nutrition and sleep.

To prevent relapse, considerable education regarding substance abuse becomes a priority goal. The education may be started in a treatment center, but needs to be continued after discharge for at least 1 year. Persons who abuse substances need to learn new coping skills, and practicing these new skills in a supportive environment is necessary.

Nursing goals include:

- Promoting safety.
- Ensuring adequate rest.
- Correcting nutritional deficiencies.
- Educating the patient and family about substance abuse.
- Providing safe detoxification.
- Teaching the family about enabling behaviors.
- Encouraging long-term follow-up care.

◆ Implementation

A genuine, caring, nonjudgmental nurse can be very helpful in the recovery process, not only for the person who is abusing substances, but also for the family. Often by the time medical treatment is sought, there have been many instances of crisis in the family. For example, the legal system may be involved if the person is abusing illegal drugs or if there was an arrest for driving while intoxicated. Also, because there is stigma associated with the abuse of alcohol and other chemicals, the patient and the family feel shame and guilt. Many individuals consider substance abuse a moral weakness, rather than a disease. **To be effective in working with substance abusers nurses must examine their own attitudes and make certain the patients and families are treated with respect.**

Think about . . . What personal experiences have you had with substance abuse, and how might this experience affect your care of the abuser and the family?

TABLE 33-3 ◆ *Common Nursing Diagnoses, Expected Outcomes, and Interventions for Substance Use Disorders*		
Nursing Diagnoses	**Goals/Expected Outcomes**	**Interventions**
Risk for injury related to effects of drug, complications of withdrawal.	Patient will remain free from any injury. Patient will withdraw from drugs or alcohol without any undue effects.	Assess the patient for symptoms of withdrawal as early as 8 hours after the ingestion of alcohol. Administer medications at the first sign of withdrawal symptoms. Remain with the patient during times of confusion and disorientation. Restrain and/or place in seclusion if the patient becomes a danger to self or others. Monitor the withdrawal process closely.
Alteration in nutrition, less than body requirements, related to poor food intake, inadequate absorption of nutrients, poor appetite.	Within 1 week patient will self-select a nutritious diet. Patient will gain 5 lb within 1 month. Signs of peripheral neuropathy (numbness and tingling) will disappear.	Document intake and outut and food intake. Collaborate with patient to determine food preferences. Encourage small, frequent meals. Administer multivitamins, especially thiamin (vitamin B_1) and niacin.
Sensory-perceptual alterations related to withdrawal from drug.	Vital signs will remain within normal limits. Patient will experience no harmful side effects from withdrawal. Within 48 hours patient will be oriented to time, place, and person.	Call the patient by name, and demonstrate respect and caring. Monitor vital signs, and administer medications for withdrawal as indicated. Assess and record mental status and reality orientation. Reorient the patient on a regular basis. Reduce environmental stimuli. Encourage restful sleep. Administer medications as necessary.
Altered family process: Alcoholism, related to altered family roles, unexpressed feelings, family history of alcoholism.	Family will be able to identify and share feelings. Family will role-play at least one situation of potential enabling. Family will agree to attend at least six 12-step meetings.	Educate the family about the altered roles present in addictive families. Assess family members for presence of denial, shame, or guilt. Encourage expression of genuine feelings. Teach family members how to recognize feelings and safe ways to express them. Encourage family members to attend a 12-step support meeting. Define the term *enabling* for the family members. Encourage family members to state at least one time when they engaged in enabling behavior. Offer family members alternative choices to enabling behavior. Have family members practice what they will say and do when a situation arises that might lead to enabling behavior.
Thought process, altered, related to cognitive impairment, intoxication.	Patient will become oriented to time, place, and person within 48 hours. Patient will be free from injury. Patient will be able to participate in ADL. Patient will be able to distinguish between reality and nonreality.	Approach the patient in a calm, slow manner. Continuously assess mental status and orientation. Use simple explanations and repeat as necessary. Protect the patient from injury. Assist the patient with ADLs until ability to think and problem-solve returns. Use reality orientation to help the patient distinguish between what is real and what might be illusions, hallucinations, or delusions. If the patient is experiencing altered perceptions, present reality in a caring, noncritical manner.
Denial, ineffective, related to minimization of the symptoms of addiction, knowledge deficit regarding the negative effects of alcohol.	Patient will acknowledge the abuse of substances and the subsequent unmanageability of his life to the staff, peers, and the immediate family. Patient will openly acknowledge the need for substance abuse treatment. Patient will agree to attend ninety 12-step meetings in 90 days.	Approach the patient in a nonjudgmental manner. Gently confront the denial as you gain the trust of the patient. Help the patient see the need for treatment and abstinence. Inform the patient about the negative aspects of addictive processes. Encourage patient to make a list of harmful effects of drugs that he has experienced and to share them with you. Encourage attendance at a 12-step program to help break through the denial.

Another priority intervention is to ensure that the patient does not suffer ill consequences from a poorly managed detoxification. **Detoxification refers to the process of ridding the body of the drug without causing harmful ill effects.** At one time it was thought that allowing alcoholics to experience a painful withdrawal would frighten them so much they would never drink again. Today we know that is not true; **withdrawal can be life-threatening,** especially from alcohol and certain anxiolytics, such as benzodiazepines.

Other general nursing interventions include orienting the patient to reality if the patient is intoxicated or cognitively impaired. Potentially fatal effects of drugs and/or alcohol, such as cardiac arrythmias, hypotension, and respiratory depression, must receive priority attention. Seeing that the patient gets adequate sleep and a balanced diet high in proteins and multivitamins also is part of early intervention.

The use of drugs to medicate symptoms of depression or other underlying mental illnesses is common. Schizophrenics often use drugs and alcohol in an attempt to stop the voices (auditory hallucinations) that torment them. Once a patient stops using chemicals, it is very important to assess for underlying mental disorders. Failing to assess and treat these conditions often results in relapse.

Patients who are in the early recovery process from substance abuse benefit greatly from therapeutic conversations with the nurse. Patients must grieve the loss of the substance, and they also feel guilt and shame for acts that were committed while under the influence. To help the patient "work through" these feelings, the nurse needs to be an excellent active listener, offering support and validation as necessary.

◆ Evaluation

Recovery from a substance use disorder is a lengthy process. Ridding the drug from the body can take weeks, particularly if there is coexisting liver damage. Often the patient is malnourished, physically exhausted, and in poor general health. Return to an optimum healthy state may take 6 months to 1 year. Recovery of psychological or emotional health takes even longer. If the patient started abusing drugs at a very young age, emotional development was arrested. Coping mechanisms to deal with anxiety or emotional pain were never developed; the addict used the drug(s) instead.

Consequently nurses working in the hospital may see only a very small part of the recovery process—early physical recovery. Evaluating overall effectiveness of substance abuse treatment is measured in years rather than weeks. Admitting a patient to a hospital and guiding him safely though detoxification is a very necessary, but small, beginning step in the overall process.

DISORDERS ASSOCIATED WITH SUBSTANCE ABUSE

◆ Alcohol Abuse and Dependence

Alcohol is a central nervous system (CNS) depressant and is the most commonly abused substance. It is widely available, legally sanctioned, and relatively inexpensive. A 12-oz bottle of beer, a 6-oz glass of wine and a 1.5-oz single shot of whiskey contain the same amount of alcohol. It takes approximately 1 hour for the body to metabolize one standard drink.

Because of the widespread availability of alcohol, abuse of this substance is found in all socioeconomic levels. Coexisting abuse of other substances (polydrug abuse) is frequent. Until alcoholism reaches advanced stages, it is often easy to conceal the problem from the general community. Family members also participate in the denial and often feel helpless to effect any change.

Nurses who work in emergency rooms and busy outpatient clinics often see alcoholics who are admitted for medical problems related to alcohol abuse. **Some of the types of medical conditions seen are liver damage, cardiomyopathy, hypertension, stroke, sleep disturbances, malnutrition, peripheral neuropathies, cognitive impairment, and chronic infection.** Often these patients are treated only for their presenting medical problem. In these instances the medical treatment team is reinforcing the patient's denial system.

It also is not uncommon for a patient to return from surgery to a busy surgical unit and develop symptoms of alcohol withdrawal. An event of this type complicates postoperative recovery and can be fatal. Taking a thorough preoperative history is absolutely essential. Medications and IV fluids can be given to prevent severe withdrawal.

Alcoholism is a major health problem in the United States and is a factor in many other instances of death and morbidity. For instance, use of alcohol is frequently associated with traffic accidents, murder, spousal abuse, child abuse, rape, and suicide. See Table 33-4 for the symptoms of intoxication and withdrawal.

Elder Care Point... The elderly are at very great risk for alcohol abuse. Drinking is an attempt to alleviate depression or loneliness. Remember that the function of vital organs, especially the liver and kidneys, is diminished with increasing age. Therefore, the by-products of alcohol are not cleared from the body as efficiently, and many medical problems occur.

TABLE 33-4 ◆ *Characteristics of Commonly Abused Substances*

Drug	Usual Methods of Administration	Effects on Body	Effects of Overdose	Withdrawal Syndrome
Alcohol	Oral.	Drowsiness, ataxia, initial euphoria and aggressive or belligerent behavior, muscular incoordination. At higher alcohol levels, slurred speech, marked ataxia and muscular incoordination, marked cognitive impairment.	Amnesia, tremors, hypothermia, seizures, respiratory failure, coma, death.	Nausea, vomiting, anorexia, agitation, hallucinations, seizures, increased body temperature, increased blood pressure and heart and respiratory rate, possible death.
Opiates (narcotic analgesics)	Oral, inhalation, IV.	Euphoria, drowsiness, decreased respiration, constricted pupils.	Decreased respirations, shallow breathing, clammy skin, seizures, possible death.	Watery eyes, runny nose, yawning, anorexia, irritability, tremors, panic, cramps, nausea, chills and sweating.
CNS stimulants (cocaine, amphetamines)	Inhalation, oral, IV, smoked.	Increased alertness, excitation, euphoria, increased pulse and blood pressure, insomnia, anorexia.	Agitation, hyperthermia, hallucinations, convulsions, possible death.	Apathy, long periods of sleep, irritability depression, disorientation.
CNS depressants (anxiolytics and barbiturates)	Oral.	Slurred speech, disorientation, drunken behavior without odor of alcohol.	Shallow respiration, clammy skin, dilated pupils, weak, rapid pulse, coma, possible death.	Anxiety, insomnia, tremors, delirium, convulsions, possible death.
Cannabis (marijuana)	Inhaled, oral.	Euphoria, relaxed inhibitions, increased appetite, disoriented behavior.	Fatigue, paranoia, psychosis.	None.
Hallucinogens (LSD, PCP)	Oral.	Illusions, hallucinations, impaired perception.	Effects are increased and intensified, psychosis, flashbacks, and possible death.	None.

Diagnosis

To establish a diagnosis of alcohol dependence the following criteria must be met: presence of withdrawal, and significant impairment in family relationships and occupational productivity; blackouts (a temporary loss of recent memory that occurs while drinking); drinking in spite of serious consequences to health or occupation; and evidence of tolerance.

Making the diagnosis of alcohol dependence is not necessarily difficult. The difficulty lies in getting the alcoholic to admit that there is a problem. Unless there is *self-diagnosis* ("I am an alcoholic"), treatment will be for the benefit of the treatment team and the family, but will not foster long-term recovery for the alcoholic.

Treatment   Treatment consists of two phases. Initial priorities consist of detoxifying and stabilizing the patient. Librium (chlordiazepoxide HCL) is the drug of choice for this process. **Once the patient is stable and able to participate in a treatment program, therapy consists of confronting the patient's denial and encouraging self-diagnosis.** Sometimes it is necessary to have the family and coworkers assist in this process.

Group and behavioral therapy are part of the treatment plan for the alcoholic. Group therapy helps break through denial and also gives the alcoholic a new sense of belonging and identity. Behavioral therapy helps the patient with self-discipline and discourages impulsive behavior. Limit-setting is one of the hallmarks of behavioral therapy. It is essential that all members of the team participate and completely agree about the limits.

Referral to a 12-step program, such as Alcoholics Anonymous (AA), also is integral to most treatment plans. Alcoholics Anonymous has been in existence for over 50 years and has helped millions of alcoholics throughout the world get and stay sober. See Table 33-5 for a description of 12-step programs.

Think about... Consider visiting an Alcoholics Anonymous meeting while you are studying about the disorder. What do you think it might feel like to walk through the doors? Would you want to remain anonymous?

Complications of Alcoholism   A serious effect of chronic alcohol abuse is damage to brain cells. A condition that is reversible with treatment is **Wernicke's encephalopathy**. This condition precedes **Korsakoff's syndrome (substance-induced persisting dementia)**, which is irreversible. The alcoholic presenting with Wernicke's encephalopathy is confused, ataxic, and has significant memory loss. Treatment involves giving large doses of thiamin (vitamin B_1) and abstaining from alcohol. Thiamin acts as a nerve insulator in the body and is absent in the diets of most chronic alcoholics.

The alcoholic presenting with Korsakoff's syndrome has grossly impaired memory and gait disturbance. **Confabulation** (making up stories) frequently is seen as an attempt to communicate. A brain scan will show brain atrophy. No treatment to reverse this condition is available.

Nursing Intervention   Interventions for the alcohol abuser must include the family. Families need to learn in what manner they might have been enabling the alcoholic, and they need time to practice new behaviors that will require the alcoholic to be responsible for himself or herself.

Initial interventions for the alcoholic focus on physical recovery. Orienting the patient to time, place, and person is necessary, as is providing for physical safety.

Detoxification is managed medically by giving antianxiety agents, such as Librium. Close monitoring of vital signs is important, because signs of alcohol withdrawal include an increase in blood pressure and heart rate. Preventing the patient from experiencing a seizure (delirium tremens, DT) is an essential part of the detoxification process.

Once the alcohol is cleared from the body, intervention for psychological homeostasis is begun. The patient needs to be educated about the disease process and needs to learn new coping methods. See Table 33-3 for additional interventions.

◆ Abuse of Other Central Nervous System Depressants

Other CNS depressants subject to abuse and dependence are barbiturates and anxiolytics, including benzodiazepines. Drugs in this category may be purchased illegally, or initially they may be prescribed by a physician. It is not uncommon to use these drugs in conjunction with alcohol, but it can be fatal because of the synergistic effects. Drugs in this category are frequently prescribed by physicians for insomnia or to ease anxiety. Patient education is very important in preventing addiction to this category of drugs.

TABLE 33-5 ◆ *Description of 12-Step Programs*

◆ What do you mean by a 12-step program?
A 12-step program is a fellowship of men and women who have a common problem (alcoholism, substance abuse, relationships, overeating, gambling, etc.). The only requirement for membership is the desire to stop a behavior that has become unmanageable. Twelve-step programs are not allied with any sect, denomination, political affiliation, religious institution, or organization. These programs will not endorse or oppose any causes and are completely based on voluntary membership and totally self-supporting.

◆ Where did 12-step programs originate?
In 1935 Bill W. and Dr. Bob founded the original 12-step support group for alcoholics. Shortly thereafter, Alanon was founded by Lois Wilson, the wife of Bill W. Since that time, there have been hundreds of 12-step support groups that follow the model of Alcoholics Anonymous.

◆ How are 12-step programs helpful?
Twelve-step programs provide an anonymous setting where people with similar problems can share experience, strength, and hope. People who attend these meetings on a regular basis find a sense of community and are able to find acceptance and unconditional love and support. The 12 steps are "worked through" with the help of the members and/or a sponsor. The essence of the steps entails admitting that you have a problem, acknowledging that you are in need of a power greater than yourself to stop the behavior, admitting strengths and weaknesses, making amends to others you have offended as a result of the problem, and helping others through the same process. Twelve-step members do not actively solicit members, but are always available when a potential member asks for help.

◆ Isn't it necessary to have professional help when you have a substance abuse disorder?
To help an addicted person with the potentially harmful symptoms of withdrawal, medical attention is often necessary because death can be a complication of improperly managed withdrawal. Also in some cases where there is a dual diagnosis (an addictive process and a mental illness) present, professional help is indicated. Otherwise, programs such as Alcoholics Anonymous have helped millions of people worldwide.

Source: Carson, V., Arnold, E. (1996). The Journey Anesthetizied by Substance Abuse. In *Mental Health Nursing: The Nurse–Patient Journey*, ed. V. Carson and E. Arnold. Philadelphia: Saunders, pp. 793–839. Reprinted with permission.

Insomnia is not an uncommon event in the elderly population. Great care must be taken when prescribing sedatives and hypnotics for the elderly. Decreased liver and renal function can lead to toxicity and dependence quickly. Benzodiazepines, in particular, have a long half-life and are not excreted readily by the body. Therefore patients with poor liver and renal function are subject to a cumulative effect and may experience toxic side effects.

Treatment   **Because withdrawal from this category of drug can be fatal, it is considered best to have the patient hospitalized and closely monitored when withdrawing the drug.** As with detoxification from alcohol, the patient is given a drug from a similar category in titrated doses. The amounts depend on the severity of the addiction. With the long half-life of benzodiazepines, the initial symptoms of drug withdrawal may not appear for 3 to 5 days. See Table 33-4 for symptoms of intoxication and withdrawal from CNS depressants.

Long-term treatment consists of referral to a 12-step program and perhaps individual and/or group psychotherapy. Patients need to be taught different ways to induce sleep and relieve anxiety.

Nursing Intervention   Again, considering the potential lethality of withdrawal, astute assessment is of prime importance. Frequent monitoring of vital signs, mood, and general functioning are necessary to avert a seizure. See Table 33-3 for general nursing interventions.

◆ Abuse of Opiates

Opiate analgesics also can be obtained both legally and illegally. Many addicts begin the process of addiction with a prescription drug for severe pain. If these individuals rely totally on narcotics to relieve chronic pain and have a tendency to abuse drugs, addiction may occur. On the other hand, if a variety of measures are used to alleviate the pain, and narcotics are necessary, there may be some increased tolerance and physical dependence. Both tolerance and physical dependence can be treated by slowly decreasing dosages of the opiates.

Addiction implies the presence of psychological craving and of withdrawal symptoms. When addiction occurs, the addict needs the drug to prevent symptoms of withdrawal, not to sustain the feeling of euphoria that was present with early use of the drug.

Treatment   Treatment involves helping the patient withdraw from the drug. Withdrawal from opiates is not life-threatening, but there can be considerable

discomfort experienced. The greatest danger with opiates is an overdose. Prompt medical intervention is essential. Treatment for an overdose usually consists of administration of a narcotic antagonist, such as Naltrexone.

If heroin, which is a street drug, is the drug of choice, success of rehabilitation is poor unless the environment also is changed. It is not unusual for a heroin addict to require up to 2 years in some type of supervised alternative living program. Group, individual, and behavioral therapy also are essential to success.

Why is it usually necessary to have a different approach for addicts who obtain their drugs legally versus addicts who obtain their drugs illegally on the street?

Nursing Intervention   Nursing intervention depends on the severity of the addictive process. If the patient overdoses, emergency measures are indicated. In other instances, nursing intervention is aimed at alleviating the symptoms and confronting denial. If the patient is addicted to heroin, the recovery process will be lengthy because of the lifestyle changes that are necessary. Typically, with heroin addiction, there has been considerable legal involvement and maladaptive coping. Each situation must be considered individually. See Table 33-3 for specific interventions.

◆ Abuse of Stimulants

The two common categories of CNS stimulants are cocaine and amphetamines. Both categories of drugs have legitimate medical uses, but have become widely abused. Amphetamines cause an increase in pulse rate, blood pressure, general excitation, anorexia, and hyperactive reflexes. Misuse can range from small amounts used infrequently to ingestion of large amounts, causing sleeplessness and anorexia for days. **Sleep deprivation of this magnitude can lead to extreme agitation and hostility, a transient psychosis, and can eventually be fatal.**

Cocaine use has increased dramatically. It is highly addictive and also can cause death, even in small doses. **Cocaine is a short-acting drug and is more commonly used as a binge drug rather than a maintenance drug.** The powder is either "snorted" (intranasal administration) or dissolved and administered IV.

Crack, a purified form of cocaine, is smoked by placing it in a pipe or smoking it with marijuana or tobacco. Freebasing cocaine reduces it to its purest form. This type of administration gets the chemical into the lungs and into the bloodstream much faster and produces a more immediate rush. It also is the most dangerous method and accounts for many overdoses and lethal reactions.

Cocaine produces euphoria, increased energy, and a sense of well-being. The stimulating effects are very fast-acting and energizing. However, the effects after the "high" are equally intense, and individuals are subject to severe emotional lows.

Treatment   Treatment for abuse of CNS stimulants is similar to treatment for alcohol abuse. Initially the treatment protocol is symptom specific and managed by medications. Expected symptoms are agitation, depression, cardiac arrythmias, seizures, or hyperthermia. Anxiolytics or antipsychotics may be used for agitation, and antidepressants may be used for the depressive symptoms.

An issue in the long-term recovery for abuse of stimulants is how to treat depression, which is inevitable. A combination of behavioral and group therapy and referral to a 12-step program is necessary. Addicts also must be taught ways to cope with the psychological craving that often leads to relapse.

Nursing Intervention   In the initial phase of recovery from stimulants, assessment skills are critical. **Patients can and do die from cardiac arrythmias associated with stimulant abuse.** Once the drug has cleared the body, which can be relatively fast, the nurse must observe the patient for signs of suicide. Patients often feel they cannot live without the intense highs experienced by cocaine use. It also is very possible that abuse of stimulants has caused the addict legal and financial problems. A caring, concerned attitude by the nurse is very important. For further interventions see Table 33-3.

◆ Abuse of Nicotine

Abuse of nicotine is an increasingly common problem and has great potential for mortality and morbidity. Nicotine is inhaled in the form of cigarettes or cigars or chewed as chewing tobacco. **Nicotine is very addictive and causes increased respiration, decreased pulmonary function, and a chronic cough.** The danger of this drug is not only to the user of the substance, but also to others who are in close proximity to the smoker. Effects of passive smoke have received much attention in the literature since the mid-1980s.

The development of lung cancer and other lung diseases, such as emphysema, poses the greatest danger for the user. In addition, pipe smokers and persons who chew tobacco are more prone to oral cancer.

Withdrawal symptoms include irritability, tension, decreased heart rate, and insomnia. Withdrawal can begin as soon as 24 hours after the cessation of smoking. **Craving is especially intense with nicotine addiction and continues long after the patient quit smoking.**

Treatment   **Nicotine patches, self-help groups, hypnosis, and acupuncture are among the treatments available for nicotine addiction.** Because cigarettes are both legal and accessible and the withdrawal symptoms are uncomfortable, most smokers stay in denial about the effects of nicotine. Frequently it is not until later years that the devastating effects are apparent.

Nursing Intervention   Mandating a person to stop smoking or shaming a person who smokes usually is not an effective intervention. **Basically, the decision to stop smoking rests with the individual.** The appropriate intervention at that time is to support the decision to stop. A reminder that the physical symptoms of withdrawal will not last forever is important. The craving will last longer than withdrawal symptoms, but is manageable if a change toward a healthy lifestyle is desirable. As with other addictions, new, more adaptive coping styles need to be learned.

◆ Abuse of Cannabis

Cannabis salvia (marijuana) is a plant grown in many parts of the world. The leaves and flowering tops of the plant are dried and loosely rolled in cigarette paper and smoked. It is a commonly used substance, both as a gateway drug for teenagers and as a recreational drug for adults. Cannabis is currently illegal in the United States; however there is active discussion of legalizing marijuana for medical purposes. The active ingredient in marijuana is effective in controlling nausea in patients who are receiving chemotherapy, and studies also indicate that it lowers intraocular pressure in patients who have glaucoma.

Marijuana is typically smoked, but it also can be ingested. It acts quickly (15 minutes), and the effects last for up to 4 hours. General effects are a mild euphoria, increased appetite, and increased sensitivity to sound, colors, and other environmental elements. Impaired coordination, mental concentration, and altered judgment also are present. In large doses the person may experience psychotic symptoms. Marijuana often is one of the first drugs that teenagers try, and this experimentation often leads to use of stronger drugs. Long-term effects for adult users are a lack of motivation and ambition. Marijuana is not physically addictive, but it may lead to psychological dependence.

Treatment   There is no particular withdrawal syndrome for cannabis, so treatment must focus on issues related to the dangers of substance abuse in general.

Nursing Intervention Nursing intervention is directed toward helping the patient lead a life that is drug free. However, in some instances a person who is intoxicated may need to be placed in a protected environment until judgment and coordination return. A thorough assessment of concomitant drug use also must be done. It would not be unusual for the person to be taking more than one drug.

◆ Abuse of Hallucinogens and Inhalants

Two common drugs that cause hallucinations are lysergic acid diethylamide (LSD) and phencyclidine hydrochloride (PCP, or angel dust). These drugs are not physiologically addictive, but have extremely unpredictable effects. Hallucinogens cause distortion of the senses, an inability to separate fact from fantasy, impaired sense of time, and severely impaired judgment. Users never know whether they will have a good "trip" or a bad one. Flashbacks are common and often very distressing. This group of drugs is very dangerous because use is known to cause panic, paranoia, and death from extremely impaired judgment.

Commonly abused inhalants include glue, nail polish remover, aerosol-packaged products, paint thinner, and other types of solvents. Symptoms of use are acute confusion, excitability, and sometimes hallucinations. Prolonged use of inhalants causes permanent damage to all body organs and a psychological dependence. Inhalants are most frequently used by the younger population because they are inexpensive and easily accessible.

Medical treatment and intervention for both hallucinogens and inhalants may include provision of safety for the individual who may be experiencing a bad "trip." Emergency measures may be necessary to provide respiratory support for an individual who acquires permanent lung damage as a result of inhalants.

EFFECTS OF SUBSTANCE ABUSE ON FAMILY AND FRIENDS

Anyone living in close proximity to a substance-dependent person will be affected. Persons who are abusing substances are unavailable for emotional intimacy because life becomes centered around the drug of choice rather than family or friends. **Family members experience a multitude of feelings, which include anger, rage, embarrassment, guilt, shame, and hopelessness. Denial and rationalization are as common in the family of the addict as they are in the substance abuser.**

Two terms commonly associated with the family and friends of a substance abuser are *enabling* and *co-dependency*. **Enabling basically entails doing some-**thing for people that they could do themselves. In maintaining their own denial about the situation, enablers cover up for the addict and attempt to maintain a status quo. Calling in sick for the abuser is one common example of enabling behavior. This behavior keeps the substance-dependent person from facing consequences and ultimately breaking through denial.

Think about . . . In which ways might a family enable? Is enabling ever helpful?

Co-dependency is another term that describes enabling behavior. **The co-dependent is any family member or friend who attempts to control the behaviors of the dependent person. Co-dependents typically overfunction in an attempt to stabilize the out-of-control substance abuser.** Because overfunctioning does not work, co-dependents feel powerless and attempt to control even more. A vicious, self-destructive cycle is established and is difficult to break. The overfunctioning keeps the substance abuser from facing objective reality.

Enablers often have a difficult time understanding that their behavior is counterproductive to the overall health and well-being of the substance abuser and the family. Self-righteousness is a typical attitude observed in enablers and is difficult to confront.

Nursing Intervention Intervening with the family of the co-dependent can be quite difficult because the enabling behaviors are so entrenched. **Initially family members must be allowed to express their anger, frustration, and shame.** It is imperative that the nurse remain caring and nonjudgmental at this time. Confrontation should be gentle, not forceful. A trusting relationship needs to be developed with the family or they may continue to focus on the addict rather than focus on their own recovery.

Referral to a 12-step program is equally important for family members. Alanon, Alateen, and Alatot have been in existence for years and can be very helpful. See Table 33-5 for information on 12-step programs. For specific nursing interventions for the family, see Table 33-3.

COMMUNITY CARE

As is the case with the general patient population, in-patient hospital stays for individuals who are addicted are usually short. If the patient has some type of insurance, it is not unusual for the insurance company to pay only for medical detoxification. Any further treatment that is necessary would be performed on an outpatient basis.

Making a decision to become sober and/or drug free often requires lifestyle changes. Changes of this magnitude are not made overnight. Addicted individuals often need ongoing medical support as well as support from the recovery community. Nurses must encourage persons who are attempting recovery to seek out necessary help and make the recovery process a number-one priority.

Because treatment for substance abuse is costly, the better response from society should be prevention. Increased public awareness is crucial, as is education of youth about the responsible use, and ultimate hazards, of mood-altering substances.

CRITICAL THINKING EXERCISES

Clinical Case Problems

Read each clinical case study and discuss the questions with your classmates.

1. Mr. Samm is a 65-year-old white male who was recently widowed. He misses his wife very much. When he comes to the doctor's office where you work today, he appears to be under the influence of alcohol. He is stumbling, his speech is slurred, and his breath has an alcohol-like odor.

   ◆ What should be your immediate action?

   ◆ If you were going to confront Mr. Samm, how would you go about it?

   ◆ What type of help is available for the elderly with a drinking problem?

2. You are working the evening shift and Mr. Martinez, a 32-year-old construction worker begins yelling profanity and tries to get out of bed. He is confused and can't remember why he came to the hospital. He went to surgery for repair of a broken femur this morning. You take his vital signs and find his blood pressure is 170/90. One hour ago it was 120/80. His wife says he forgot to tell the doctor that Mr. Martinez drinks twelve beers every night.

   ◆ What should your initial action be at this time?

   ◆ What is wrong with Mr. Martinez?

   ◆ What might happen to this patient if you don't act on the information you have?

   ◆ After his blood pressure returns to normal, list the necessary interventions.

3. You are a home health nurse and, when you arrive at the home of Mr. and Mrs. Brown, Mrs. Brown confides in you that she is concerned that her husband, age 29, is abusing alcohol and drugs. You are visiting the couple because they have a 7-year-old son with severe cerebral palsy. You have been visiting them for 2 years on a monthly basis and you are surprised when Mrs. Brown approaches you.

   ◆ How would you respond to Mrs. Brown?

   ◆ Why did Mrs. Brown wait this long to tell you about her husband?

   ◆ What resources are available for Mrs. Brown?

   ◆ What might your feelings toward Mr. Brown be, now that she has confided in you?

BIBLIOGRAPHY

Alcoholics Anonymous. (1995). *Twelve Steps.* New York: AA World Services.

American Psychiatric Association. (1994). *Diagnostic and Statistical Manual of Mental Disorders–IV.* Washington, D.C.: American Psychiatric Association.

Antai-Otong, D. (1995). Helping the alcoholic patient recover. *American Journal of Nursing.* 95(8):22–26.

Babb, D. (1990). Action stat! Alcohol withdrawal syndrome. *Nursing 90.* 20(10):83–84.

Belcaster, A. (1994). Caring for the alcohol abuser. *Nursing 94.* 24(2):56–59.

Brown, R. L. (1992). Identification and office management of alcohol and drug disorders. In *Addictive Disorders,* ed. M. F. Flemming, K. L. Barry. St. Louis, MO: Mosby.

Carson, V., Arnold, E. (1996). The journey anesthetized by substance abuse. In *Mental Health Nursing: The Nurse–Patient Journey,* ed. V. Carson and E. Arnold. Philadelphia: Saunders.

Dubiel, D. (1990). Cocaine overdose. *Nursing 90.* 20(3):33.

Fortinash, K., Holoday-Worret, P. (1995). *Psychiatric Nursing Care Plans.* St. Louis, MO: Mosby-Year Book.

Gorman, M. (1996). Alcoholic patients: keeping hope alive. *American Journal of Nursing.* 96(1):20.

Gorman, M. (1996). Substance abuse: culture clash: working with a difficult patient. *American Journal of Nursing.* 96(11):58.

Gorman, M. (1997). Substance abuse: treating acute alcohol withdrawal. *American Journal of Nursing.* 97(1):22–23.

Haack, M., Hughes, T. (1989). *Addiction in the Nursing Profession.* New York: Springer.

House, M. (1990). Cocaine. *American Journal of Nursing.* 90(4):41–45.

Montgomery, P., Johnson, B. (1992). The stress of marriage to an alcoholic. *Journal of Psychosocial Nursing.* 32(10):12–16.

Navarra, T. (1995). Enabling behavior: the tender trap. *American Journal of Nursing.* 95(1):50–52.

Patch, P. B., Phelps, G. L., Cowan, G. (1997). Alcohol withdrawal in a medical-surgical setting: the 'too little, too late' phenomenon. *MEDSURG Nursing.* 6(2):79–89.

Sajo, E. (1996). Nurses can intervene to stop abuse of methamphetamine. *Nurseweek.* 9(8):8–9.

Sullivan, E. (1995). *Nursing Care of Clients with Substance Abuse.* St. Louis, MO: Mosby-Year Book.

Wilson, S. (1994). Can you spot an alcoholic patient? *R.N.* 57(1):46–51.

Wing, D., Hammer-Higgins, P. (1993). Determinants of denial: a study of alcoholics. *Journal of Psychosocial Nursing.* 31(2):13–17.

Yates, J., McDaniel, J. (1994). Are you losing yourself in co-dependency? *American Journal of Nursing.* 94(3): 32–36.

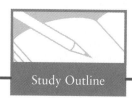

Study Outline

I. Significance of Substance Use Disorders

A. Major problem throughout the world.

B. Problems for both the abuser and family and friends.

C. Alcoholism recognized as disease in 1956 by American Medical Association.

D. Substance use disorder.

   1. Recognizable signs and symptoms after the ingestion of psychoactive substance.

   2. Psychoactive substances: any mind-altering agents capable of changing or altering a person's mood, behavior, cognition, arousal level, level of consciousness, and perceptions.

   3. Terminology.

      a. Abuse: implies use of a psychoactive drug in a nontherapeutic manner or the illicit use of prescription drugs.

      b. Dependence: implies the presence of physical or psychological symptoms of addiction; when the drug is stopped, withdrawal symptoms appear.

      c. Withdrawal: a certain group of symptoms that appear when there is an attempt to stop using a substance.

         (1) Withdrawal from CNS depressants: increased BP, pulse, nervousness, heightened anxiety.

         (2) Withdrawal from CNS stimulants: drowsiness, headache, lethargy, nausea, alterations in eating and sleeping patterns, and craving.

II. Nursing Assessment

A. Physical signs and symptoms vary according to length of use.

   1. Change in vital signs.

   2. Impaired coordination.

   3. Pupillary changes.

   4. Bloodshot eyes.

   5. Needle tracks, bruises.

   6. Congestion.

   7. Variations in grooming.

   8. Odor of alcohol.

B. Behavioral indicators.

   1. Slurred speech.

   2. Incoherent or loud and boisterous.

   3. Variation in mood.

   4. Altered orientation to time, place, and person.

   5. Suicidal ideation.

   6. Illusions, hallucinations, or delusions.

C. Psychological indicators.

   1. Denial and rationalization.

   2. Both are entrenched behaviors.

D. History.

   1. Take history from family as well as patient.

   2. Determine type of substance used, the amount taken, and the pattern of use.

   3. See Table 33-2 for examples of questions to ask.

III. Planning

A. Collaborative goal setting very important.

B. Educating about substance abuse is a priority goal.

C. Goals include:

   1. Promoting safety.

   2. Ensuring adequate rest.

   3. Correcting nutritional deficiencies.

   4. Educating patient and family.

   5. Providing for safe detoxification.

   6. Teaching family about enabling behaviors.

   7. Encourage long-term follow-up care.

IV. Implementation

A. Use gentle, caring nonjudgmental approach.

B. Safely manage detoxification (ridding the body of the drug without causing harmful ill effects).

C. Implement reality orientation.

D. Foster adequate sleep.

E. Provide balanced diet high in protein and multivitamins, especially thiamin.

F. Once detoxification is complete, observe for underlying mental disorders.

G. Assist in grieving process.

V. **Evaluation—Expected Outcomes**
  A. Has completed safe detoxification.
  B. Admits problem: self-diagnosis.
  C. Experiences restful sleep.
  D. Eats well-balanced diet.
  E. Learns new coping mechanisms.
  F. Interacts appropriately with family.
  G. Maintains abstinence.

VI. **Common Nursing Diagnoses, Expected Outcomes, and Interventions (Table 33-3)**

VII. **Disorders Associated with Abuse and Dependence**
  A. Alcohol abuse and dependence: CNS depressants.
    1. Widely available and legal.
    2. Twelve-oz beer, 6-oz wine and 1.5-oz single shot contain same amount of alcohol.
    3. Takes 1 hour for body to metabolize one standard drink.
    4. Many medical conditions related to alcohol abuse.
      a. Liver damage.
      b. Cardiomyopathy.
      c. Hypertension.
      d. Stroke.
      e. Sleep disturbances.
      f. Malnutrition.
      g. Peripheral neuropathies.
      h. Cognitive impairment.
      i. Chronic infection.
    5. Diagnosis of alcohol dependence.
      a. Presence of withdrawal and significant impairment in family relationships and occupational productivity.
      b. Blackouts: temporary loss of memory.
      c. Drinking in spite of serious consequences.
      d. Evidence of tolerance.
    6. For successful treatment, alcoholic must admit to alcoholism: self-diagnosis.
    7. Treatment: two phases:
      a. First phase: detoxify and stabilize the patient. Librium used for detoxification.
      b. Second phase: confront the patient's denial and encourage recovery.
        (1) Group and behavioral therapy.
        (2) Referral to Alcoholics Anonymous.
        (3) Limit-setting.
    8. Complications.
      a. Wernicke's encephalopathy: treated with thiamin (reversible).
      b. Korsakoff's syndrome (irreversible).
    9. Nursing interventions.
      a. Must include the family.
      b. Educate families about enabling.
      c. Provide safe environment for detoxification.
      d. Administer medications to assist in detoxification.
      e. Monitor vital signs.
      f. Observe for possible seizure.
      g. Educate the patient about substance abuse.
      h. Teach new coping methods.
  B. Abuse of other CNS depressants: anxiolytics and barbiturates.
    1. May be purchased legally and illegally.
    2. Often used in conjunction with alcohol and can be fatal due to synergistic effect.
    3. Withdrawal also can be fatal.
    4. Need to be hospitalized for detoxification.
    5. Benzodiazepines have long half-life. Withdrawal may not appear for 3 to 5 days.
    6. Long-term treatment includes referral to support group and sometimes psychotherapy.
    7. Nursing interventions.
      a. Monitor safe withdrawal.
      b. Teach patients different ways to induce sleep and relieve anxiety.
  C. Abuse of opiates: narcotic analgesics.
    1. Can be obtained both legally and illegally.
    2. Addiction often begins with a prescription for severe pain.
    3. Tolerance occurs with increased use, but addiction occurs when there are craving and withdrawal symptoms.
    4. Treatment involves assisting the patient in the withdrawal process.
      a. Withdrawal from opiates is not life-threatening.
    5. Greatest danger with opiates is from an overdose.
    6. With heroin addiction long-term rehabilitation is necessary—up to 2 years.
    7. Nursing interventions.
      a. Initiate emergency measures if overdose occurs.
      b. Alleviate symptoms of withdrawal.
      c. Confront denial.
  D. Abuse of CNS: cocaine and amphetamines.
    1. Both drugs have legitimate medical uses, but have become widely abused.
    2. Symptoms of amphetamine abuse.
      a. Increased pulse, blood pressure.
      b. General excitation.
      c. Anorexia.
      d. Hyperactive reflexes.

e. Large amounts can cause sleep deprivation, which leads to extreme agitation and hostility and a transient psychosis.

3. Symptoms of cocaine abuse.

   a. Used as binge drug.

   b. Very short-acting.

   c. Can be taken intranasally, inhaled, or injected.

   d. Produces euphoria.

   e. Increased energy.

   f. Sense of well-being.

   g. Subject to severe "lows" after the "highs."

4. Treatment: similar to treatment for alcohol abuse.

   a. Management is symptom specific and achieved with medications.

   b. Patient may experience agitation, depression, cardiac arrythmias, seizures, or hyperthermia.

   c. Behavioral therapy and support group referral are necessary.

5. Nursing interventions.

   a. Assessment skills are critical.

   b. Death is possible because of cardiac involvement.

   c. Assess for suicidal ideation.

E. Abuse of nicotine.

1. Great potential for morbidity and mortality.

2. Inhaled, smoked, or chewed.

3. Symptoms of addiction.

   a. Increased respirations.

   b. Decreased pulmonary function.

   c. Chronic cough.

   d. Craving.

4. Passive smoke dangerous to family and friends.

5. Withdrawal symptoms.

   a. Irritability.

   b. Tension.

   c. Decreased heart rate.

   d. Insomnia.

   e. Craving.

6. Treatment.

   a. Nicotine patches.

   b. Self-help groups.

   c. Hypnosis.

   d. Acupuncture.

e. Denial remains intact until serious physical symptoms appear.

7. Nursing interventions.

   a. Patient must have desire to stop smoking.

   b. Support the patient's decision.

VIII. Effects of Substance Abuse on Family and Friends

A. Impossible for family to escape the effects of substance abuse.

B. Family members experience wide range of feelings.

1. Anger and rage.

2. Embarrassment.

3. Guilt.

4. Shame.

5. Hopelessness.

C. Denial and rationalization are equally common in the family.

D. Enabling behaviors: doing things for others they could or should do for themselves.

E. Co-dependent: a family member or friend who attempts to control the behaviors of the substance abuser.

1. Becomes a vicious circle.

2. Leads to frustration and anger.

F. Nursing interventions with the family.

1. Allows family members to express feelings.

2. Nurse must remain caring and nonjudgmental.

3. Nurse must develop trusting relationship.

4. Refer to 12-step program for family members.

IX. Elder Care Points

A. Elderly are at great risk for alcohol abuse.

1. Drink to alleviate depression and loneliness.

2. Decreased liver function leads to decreased clearance of by-products of alcohol.

B. Care must be taken when prescribing sedatives and hypnotics for the elderly.

1. Insomnia is common with advanced age.

2. Decreased liver and renal function can lead to toxicity and dependence quickly.

3. Benzodiazepines have long half-life.

   a. Not excreted rapidly from the body.

   b. Increased danger with the elderly.

X. Community Care

A. Shorter hospital stays are inevitable.

B. Majority of treatment is outpatient.

C. Prevention of substance needs to be a focus.

CHAPTER 34

Care of Patients with Cognitive Disorders

OBJECTIVES

Upon completing this chapter the student should be able to:
1. Discuss the incidence and significance of cognitive disorders in the aged population.
2. Differentiate between delirium (acute cognitive disorder) and dementia (chronic cognitive disorder).
3. Discuss the assessment skills necessary accurately to document a cognitive disorder.
4. From a list of NANDA nursing diagnoses, identify at least four nursing diagnoses that would be appropriate for a patient with delirium or dementia.
5. From the diagnoses listed, choose appropriate nursing interventions and expected outcomes.
6. Describe the signs and symptoms and treatment of drug-induced delirium, Alzheimer's disease, and vascular dementia.
7. Describe the nursing interventions for drug-induced delirium, Alzheimer's disease, and vascular dementia.
8. Discuss the nursing measures necessary to care for a patient who is confused and disoriented.

Cognitive disorders are especially troubling conditions both to those persons affected by them and to family and friends. Cognitive disorders are very common, especially with the increase in the elderly population since the mid-1980s. Although these disorders do occur across the life span, they are very common with the neurobiological changes that accompany aging.

Cognition refers to mental processes of perception, memory, judgment, and reasoning. **A cognitive disorder is diagnosed when there is a significant change in cognition from a previous level of functioning.**

Disorders of cognition include both delirium and dementia. **Delirium (acute confusion) is characterized by a change in overall cognition and level of consciousness over a short time. Dementia, on the other hand, is characterized by several cognitive deficits, memory in particular, and tends to be more chronic. Both conditions are classified according to etiology.** Possible etiologies for delirium are substance-induced delirium or delirium caused by the ingestion of a substance that for some reason is toxic to the patient. Alzheimer's disease is an example of dementia. A simple way to remember the difference between the two conditions is that **delirium is an acute condition that requires immediate treatment and dementia is a chronic one.**

Reversing the symptoms of delirium depends on timely diagnosis and treatment. It also is important to note that **delirium can coexist with dementia.** If delirium is recognized and promptly treated, the patient with preexisting dementia should be restored to a previous level of functioning.

Elder Care Point... In hospitalized elders with preexisting dementia, it is not unusual to see the patient who was previously fully conscious become drowsy, disoriented, combative, and unable to recognize family and friends. The astute nurse suspects delirium or acute confusion. One of the first interventions is to note what type of medications the patient is receiving. Anticholinergic medications have potent central nervous system (CNS) effects and can cause a sudden episode of confusion. Is the dose too high for age and physiological functioning? Is there a cumulative effect? Are the medications synergistic? Nurses need to be careful not to dismiss situations of this type when evaluating dementia. Delirium and dementia can coexist, and the acute condition needs to be recognized and treated, not merely dismissed as part of the overall dementia.

NURSING MANAGEMENT

◆ Assessment

Differentiating between delirium (acute confusion) and dementia can be very difficult for the nurse because often the patient is not a reliable historian. A mood disorder, such as depression, also may be present and further complicate the picture. Accurate recognition of these three conditions requires excellent assessment skills. For a review of the symptoms of depression, see Chapter 32.

The onset of acute delirium is sudden and often appears at sundown. The patient may be either very alert or lethargic, depending on the cause of the delirium. The attention span changes, and overall awareness of the environment is lower. Orientation to time, place, and person is impaired, as well as recent and immediate memory. Speech may be incoherent and overall thinking is disorganized and distorted. The patient will not be able to communicate his thoughts to the nurse in a meaningful way. **Delusions, hallucinations, and illusions** also may be present, as well as a disturbed sleep cycle, which is usually reversed. The patient appears very confused, and the nurse may question the need for physical or chemical restraints.

The onset for dementia is slow and may progress over a long time (months to years). The patient is generally alert and has a normal attention span. Orientation to time, place, and person may be impaired, as well as recent memory. In later stages of dementia, patients lose remote memory as well. The nurse would observe that the patient has both difficulty with abstracting thoughts and a poverty of thoughts. **Confabulation** (making up conversation to fill in gaps) is common. Impaired judgment also is common. Hallucinations, delusions, and illusions usually are not present. These patients experience fragmented sleep rather than a reversed cycle. There also often is a notable change in personality.

An effective way to assess whether a patient has delirium or dementia is to note the following five areas: **judgment, affect, memory, cognition, and orientation (JAMCO).** What is the status of the patient's judgment? Did the patient say he would stay in bed if you left the rails down and when you checked 15 minutes later, he was walking the hall? This connotes poor judgment and the nurse must provide for the patient's safety at this time.

Assessing and documenting affect also are important. Has there been a sudden change in mood from the previous assessment. Often the family will say that they note a difference in mood when they visit the patient. Always pay attention to what family members tell you. They know the patient much better than you do.

When assessing memory it is important to note both recent and remote memory. In some types of dementia, a patient may not be able to remember what was on the breakfast tray, but may be able to talk at great length about events in their younger years. When assessing delirium the nurse may find that both recent memory (a few hours before) and immediate memory (a few minutes before) are absent.

Think about... Think of one or two ways you can assess immediate, recent and remote memory. How does the nurse know whether the patient's memory is accurate?

Cognition refers to the ability, based on previous knowledge, to perceive information and make sense of it. In delirium a patient may experience **illusions** (misinterpretations of reality). Intravenous tubing might be perceived as a snake. Patients also may see or hear things that are not there (**hallucinations**) or believe that something is true that is not (**delusions**).

Problem-solving ability and judgment often are diminished, but not completely absent. Consequently the patient may not only be able to make good decisions, but also become combative or hostile if the nurse or family member attempts to intervene.

Finally, is the patient oriented to time, place, and person? Are there times when the patient is oriented? It is not unusual for a patient to be completely oriented during the daytime hours and become confused and disoriented at night. This phenomenon is known as **sundowning** and needs to be documented by the nurse. See Table 34-1 for a list of questions to ask using the JAMCO assessment guide.

TABLE 34-1 ◆ *Quick Assessment Guide for Delirium and Dementia*

Use the mnemonic JAMCO (*J*udgment, *A*ffect, *M*emory, *C*ognition, *O*rientation).

Judgment
  Does patient have insight into his behavior? Is the patient aware of danger or safety issues?

Affect
  Is affect blunt, flat, inappropriate, suddenly changed, or variable?

Memory
  Is memory intact? Does patient have remote memory, but not recent or immediate? Is memory better during the day?

Cognition
  Is the patient able to process abstract thoughts? Are thoughts fragmented or disorganized? Does the patient make up answers to questions *(confabulate)* to hide deficits?

Orientation
  Is the patient oriented to time, place, and person? Does the patient recognize family and friends?

Think about . . . How would a nurse know the difference between sundowning and a sudden onset of delirium?

A mental status assessment of this type needs to be completed at least once a shift, so that any change can be detected promptly and appropriate interventions taken. When abrupt changes are noted, a more detailed assessment should follow, in addition to notifying the physician. In cases of delirium or acute confusion the nurse must assess the patient's medication history, look for any signs of infection and assess current fluid and electrolyte balance.

◆ Nursing Diagnoses

Nursing diagnoses for patients with disorders of cognition are listed in Table 34-2.

TABLE 34-2 ◆ *Nursing Diagnosis, Expected Outcomes and Nursing Interventions for Cognition Disorders*		
Nursing Diagnosis	**Goals/Expected Outcomes**	**Nursing Interventions**
Acute confusion related to overdose of medication, electrolyte imbalance, drug withdrawal, infections, vascular insufficiency or cerebral vascular accident.	Vital signs and level of consciousness will return to normal within 24 h. Patient will return to previous state of neurological functioning. Patient will demonstrate socially acceptable behavior.	Approach patient gently with relaxed manner. Assess judgment, affect, memory, cognition, and orientation. Monitor vital signs. Check level of consciousness as patient's condition indicates. Notify physician of your findings. Administer medications as ordered. Decrease environmental stimuli. Provide for reality orientation, especially time. Identify usual patterns of behavior. Refrain from using restraints. Identify comfort strategies used by the caregiver at home. Limit visitors.
Chronic confusion related to memory loss, altered perceptions.	The patient will function at an optimal level for the degree of cognitive losses at this time. The patient will be able to communicate with others. The patient will participate in group activities within 1 week.	Speak slowly and calmly. Use simple phrases and words. Face the patient directly when you talk. Be consistent in approach to patient. Assign the same staff to work with the patient. Maintain daily structure and routine. Encourage reminiscing about the past. Provide group activities that are simple, such as singing or simple crafts. Monitor closely for behavioral indicators of pain or discomfort. Use pictures to communicate with the patient. Break down all tasks into simple steps. Encourage patient to complete one step at a time.
Altered thought process related to inability to retrieve and process information, impaired abstract thinking, loss of judgment, insight, cognition, and problem-solving ability.	Patient will remain free from harm. Patient will respond coherently to simple statements. Patient will participate in ADLs with assistance from caregivers.	In a caring and gentle manner, frequently orient patient to the surroundings. Use both verbal and visual reminders. Encourage other caregivers to do the same. Provide for safety, and make a safe environment a number-one priority. Observe the patient closely for any behavioral cues that indicate pain or discomfort. Place familiar objects in the patient's room. Avoid argument or confrontation about the patient's misperceptions. Educate the family about the patient's cognitive deficits. Promote interactions between the patient and family.
Impaired social interaction related to anxiety and depression, apathy, confused state.	The patient will demonstrate increased comfort in social situations. The patient will be able to sit through an activity without an increase in agitation.	Use a calm, caring approach when approaching patient. Use therapeutic, gentle touch as indicated. Encourage patient to wear or use any prostheses or ambulatory aids as needed. Adhere to routine care. Be certain that all structured activities are brief. Do not force a client who is becoming agitated to participate in any social activity. Teach family members the importance of reminiscing with the patient rather than focusing on events of the day. Assess the patient's ability to perform tasks that were familiar in earlier years.

(Table 34-2 continued)

TABLE 34-2 ◆ *Nursing Diagnosis, Expected Outcomes and Nursing Interventions for Cognition Disorders* (Continued)

Nursing Diagnosis	Goals/Expected Outcomes	Nursing Interventions
Risk for caregiver stress, related to high emotional and physical demands placed on the caregiver, safety concerns for the relative, caregiver isolation.	Caregiver will verbalize ways to facilitate the caregiver role without becoming exhausted. Caregiver will openly express feelings. Caregiver will demonstrate adaptive coping skills to regain equilibrium.	Assess caregiver's ability to meet the needs of the patient. Make caregiver aware of community resources. Actively listen to caregiver's fears and concerns. Educate the caregiver about cognitive disorders. Help caregivers be realistic about the prognosis for their loved one. Encourage participation in support groups for families who have similar problems. Support caregiver in taking steps to maintain own health
Bathing/self-care deficit related to cognitive and perceptual impairment.	The patient will feed self without assistance. The patient will groom self daily without assistance.	Encourage patient to perform ADLs within current ability. Have patient wear own clothes. Use clothing with zippers and fastening tape (Velcro). If client is resistant to self-care, offer to come back later. Encourage as much independence as possible. Praise patient for any and all accomplishments. Use simple, direct explanations when demonstrating the specific behavior you want the patient to complete. Encourage the use of finger foods. Maintain toileting schedule.
High risk for injury related to poor judgment, impaired cognition, poor memory.	The patient will remain free from physical harm.	Put mattress on the floor. Place patient in a limited-access unit. Put complex locks on the doors. Use identification bracelets. Label all rooms and doors. Install safety bars in the bathroom. Supervise smoking. Encourage activity during the day.

◆ Planning

In planning care for a patient with a cognitive disorder safety is a number-one priority. Patients in the early stages of Alzheimer's disease, for example, may attempt to hide their condition and may be experiencing difficulties with activities of daily living (ADLs). Forgetting to turn off the stove or to lock the doors is not uncommon.

Planning care for a patient with delirium involves accurately assessing the acute condition, stabilizing the patient, reducing environmental stimuli, providing reality orientation, and assisting the physician in determining the cause. Planning care for a patient with dementia is long term and frequently involves the caregivers. Because the loss of cognition is so devastating, it is important to maintain the patient's dignity, provide for safety and optimal level of functioning, and promote quality of life.

Nursing goals for patients with cognitive disorders include:

- Providing safety.
- Reducing environmental stimuli.
- Assessing frequently.
- Providing reality orientation.
- Eliminating causative factors.
- Promoting dignity and self-worth.
- Maintaining optimal functioning.
- Educating family about dementia.

◆ Implementation

When caring for a patient whose sudden change in behavior may be due to delirium, time is of the essence. Assess the patient frequently, document your findings, and be certain the physician is notified. Because the level of consciousness for this type of patient is clouded, reduce any and all distractions in the environment. It may be necessary to medicate patients if their anxiety is great or if the misinterpretation of the environment causes them to be aggressive. Anxiolytics are given for anxiety and antipsychotics are given for aggressive behavior.

Repeated orientation to the environment also is an essential intervention. Patients may be able to remember their own name, but may be confused about place and time. It is not adequate to repeat this information once or twice. It must be repeated frequently and in a calm, soothing manner. The calm attitude of the nurse is very important in reducing the anxiety that is inevitably present for the patient.

A patient who is experiencing acute confusion or delirium will benefit from repeated orientation to time, place, and person. An individual with chronic confusion in the late stages of dementia will not benefit from this type of intervention. If **global amnesia** is present, the patient will not be able to remember family, friends, or events, regardless of how many times you repeat the information. Moreover, expecting the patient to re-member leads to frustration for both the nurse and the patient. Orienting this type of patient to the location, day, and time with verbal reminders and pictures or symbols can be helpful. See Table 34-3 for guidelines for the use of reality orientation for confused patients.

Think about . . . Is it always necessary to encourage a patient to see reality as the nurse sees it? What about elderly patients who have severe dementia and believe they are living in their own homes, even though they are in a nursing home?

TABLE 34-3 ◆ *Guidelines for the Use of Reality Orientation*

What is reality orientation?
Reality orientation is a therapeutic program implemented **consistently** by all nursing staff to orient a patient to time, place, and person. This method includes the use of verbal communication techniques, as well as written signs indicating the current date, month, or room iden-tification. Clocks with large letters also are included to help the patient know the correct time.

   Special group sessions also are used to orient patients. These sessions focus on time, place, and person, as well as certain holiday events. These groups not only improve orientation, but also break social isolation.

When to use reality orientation
◆ The use of reality orientation is appropriate when a patient is experiencing acute confusion or delirium. A sudden episode of confusion is very frightening, and orienting the patient is a way to allay fear and anxiety.
◆ Patients experiencing dementia or chronic confusion often have global amnesia and do not benefit from repeated verbal reality orientation. Gentle reminders of the day or time is helpful, but need to be repeated often and without the expectation that the patient will remember something that was said 5 minutes before.
◆ All of the aspects of reality orientation mentioned are helpful for all patients with cognitive disorders. However, in patients experiencing acute confusion, the ultimate expectation is that the patient will become completely oriented and return to a previous level of functioning. With chronic confusion the goal is to preserve dignity and maintain optimum function.

Examples of ways to implement reality orientation and reduce confusion
◆ Under no circumstances should nurses ever chastise or become frustrated with a patient for not remembering. This has no therapeutic value.
◆ Verbalize to patients in a consistent and caring manner who you are, where they are, and the date and time: "Hi, Mr. Jones. I am your nurse, Betty, at the Davis Nursing Care Center. It is 8 A.M. on Wednesday, October 25, and it is time for breakfast."
◆ Look directly at the patient when you are speaking.
◆ Ask only one question at a time.
◆ Ask questions where the patient can respond with a yes or no answer: "Would you like to eat in the dining room?" Too many options will frustrate the patient.
◆ Eliminate environmental distractions when talking to a patient.
◆ Break down tasks such as dressing into simple one-step tasks.
◆ Ask the client to do only one task at a time.
◆ Gently touch the patient to convey acceptance.
◆ If possible, provide caregivers who are familiar to the patient.
◆ Provide general orientation of the year by using holiday decorations.
◆ Decrease the noise level in the environment by avoiding paging systems and call lights that ring or buzz.
◆ Label photos of people familiar to the patient with the names of the people who are in the photos.
◆ Limit visitors to one or two at a time.
◆ Place the patient's name in large block letters in his or her room and on clothing.
◆ Use symbols rather than words on signs indicating location of dining room or bathroom.
◆ When misperceptions are present, clarify them for the patient. "No Mr. Jones, I am not your daughter; I am your nurse, Betty. Your daugh-ter will be here after you eat your lunch."
◆ When units specifically designed for patients with chronic confusion (low-stimulus units) are not available, use yellow tape to mark spe-cific boundaries for the patient.
◆ Give frequent reassurances.
◆ Keep the patient's room well lit.
◆ Encourage the use of hearing aids and prescription glasses.
◆ Have clocks, calendars, and personal items in clear view of the patient.
◆ Encourage reminiscing about happy times in life.

A patient experiencing acute confusion may become combative or attempt to crawl out of bed. In 1992 the Food and Drug Administration issued a warning stating that restraints should no longer be considered as first-line management of patient's behavioral problems. As reported by J. Stolley, (1995), "Restraints worsen confusion and foster depression, anger, and humiliation." It is recommended that institutions have in place policies and procedures that address the safe use of restraints when they are necessary and encourage informed consent for the patient and family. See Table 34-4 for guidelines on the use of restraints and alternatives to restraints.

Interventions to provide safety and minimize anxiety for patients with dementia and delirium are similar.

However, nurses who care for patients with dementia need to be aware of the importance of maintaining the dignity of the patient and family. In the later stages of dementia there are numerous deficits in self-care, such as grooming and toileting. It is very important to treat both patients and families with respect. **Call the patient by name, provide for privacy, and individualize your care for this patient based on culture and history.** It is a well-documented fact in the nursing literature that when patients are seen as people or human beings, nurses are likely to be more compassionate and caring .

Patients with dementia will respond much better if there are daily routines and the environment is structured. If the patient lives at home, the family will need to receive both education and support in this effort.

TABLE 34-4 ◆ *Alternatives and Guidelines for the Use of Restraints*

Alternatives to restraints

Acute cate settings

- Encourage family members and friends to stay with the patient.
- Encourage oral feedings instead of intravenous or nasogastric feedings. Avoid inserting tubes that can be pulled out.)
- Remove catheters and drains as soon as possible.
- Decrease environmental stimulation. Decrease glaring lighting, reduce noise, and minimize stimulation.
- Keep patient close to the nurse's station.
- Be certain patient has a call button within easy reach.
- Place the bed in the lowest setting, and use half-siderails to keep patient from rolling out.

Long-term care facilities

- Place mattress on the floor to prevent patient from falling out of bed.
- Talk to the patient, even when the patient is not responding to you or is responding in an inappropriate way.
- Incorporate relaxation techniques into the care plan, such as back massage and hydrotherapy.
- Gently touch the patient to convey acceptance.
- Use therapeutic communication techniques to encourage the patient to verbalize feelings.
- Encourage ambulation whenever feasible.
- Encourage the patient to participate in recreational, physical, and occupational therapy.
- Encourage the patient to participate in as many ADLs as possible.
- Initiate diversional activities, such as listening to radio, television, and music.
- Keep the patient on a schedule for toileting.

Guidelines for the safe use of restraints

- Use the least restrictive type of restraint that will accomplish the objective.
- Obtain informed consent from the patient or the patient's relatives before using restraints.
- Have an institutional policy on restraints written and available for the patient and family.
- Make certain that all staff have adequate in-service training on the use of restraints.
- Use hand mitts for patients who are receiving IV therapy or have catheters or nasogastric tubes.
- If hand mitts do not work, consider wrist restraints.
- Use a belt, jacket, or vest restraint for patients who are confused and prone to wandering.
- All restraints must have a doctor's order.
- Restraints must not be used to punish or control the patient.
- Apply restraints snugly, but not so tight that they impede circulation in any manner.
- Check the area distal to the restraint every 2 hours (or according to the hospital policy) for circulation and function.
- Remove the restraints, and change the patient's position at least every 2 hours.
- Apply active or passive range of motion (ROM) to the affected joints and muscles.
- Secure restraints to the bedframes, not siderails.
- Tie with knots that can be quickly released.
- Consider restraints as only temporary solutions.
- Clearly document in the patient record the reason for the restraint, the type selected, and the time frame for use.
- Document care given to the patient while in restraints.

Family members often are exhausted from the daily requirements of round-the-clock care. Nurses can encourage caregivers to consider day care or respite care. Both of these types of care give the family members a much-needed psychological and physical rest.

Families also need to be encouraged to talk openly and frankly about quality of life and advance directives. Preferably these talks should be completed prior to the diagnosis of dementia when the patient still has cognitive functioning. If not, the family caregiver becomes the spokesperson and needs to be encouraged to get a power of attorney and a living will for the patient. Families need considerable support in these matters. **Observing someone you love deteriorate neurologically is very difficult.**

Think about... How might a nurse approach the family of an elder who is approaching the end stages of dementia? What are some creative ways to introduce the subject of advance directives?

◆ Evaluation

Evaluating the care for a patient with cognitive disorders is accomplished by determining whether the stated expected outcomes were met. Returning the patient to a previous level of cognitive and psychomotor functioning whenever possible is essential. Because confusion is present in all cognitive disorders, regardless of the cause, keeping the patient free of injury is of primary importance. Eliminating or determining the cause of acute delirium is a main priority for nurses during the process of assessment.

An additional expected outcome, particularly with patients with dementia, is that the family will be able to verbalize the stages of illness and maintain realistic expectations for their loved one. Maintaining the dignity and self-respect of both the patient and the family is very important.

COGNITIVE DISORDERS

◆ Delirium

Many conditions or physiological alterations can cause delirium. **Some examples are cerebrovascular accident, drug overdose, toxicity or withdrawal, tumors, systemic infections, fluid and electrolyte imbalances, and malnutrition.** The general features of delirium are the same for all the causes, and nursing care is basically the same; the main difference is in diagnosis and treatment of the underlying cause. In this chapter the prototype condition of substance-induced delirium will be discussed.

Substance-Induced Delirium **Substance-induced delirium can be caused by withdrawal from a substance, intoxication with a substance, or side effects from a medication.** For a review on intoxication and withdrawal delirium, see Chapter 33. Many classes of medications can produce symptoms of delirium. Some common examples are anesthetics, analgesics, sedative-hypnotics, any product with anticholinergic activity (tricyclic antidepressants, antihistamines, theophylline derivatives, and antipsychotics), histamine$_2$-blocking agents (cimetidine and ranitidine). Commonly prescribed beta-blockers and nonsteroidal antiinflammatory drugs (NSAIDs) also can cause symptoms of delirium. Diagnosis and treatment depend on thorough history taking. It is not unusual for a person to be taking large amounts of over-the-counter medication and forget to mention that fact because the medications were not prescribed by a physician.

Nursing Intervention **Always monitor the effects of medications.** Take a thorough medication history. If the patient is unable to give you a history, elicit help from the family. Pay attention to drug interactions and incompatibilities. Never be hesitant to consult with the pharmacist. Encourage patients to take medications only when medically indicated. Also report any unusual effects of medications promptly. Early recognition can assist in a faster recovery. If the medication accumulates over several days, elimination of the substance from the body takes much longer and places the patient in even greater danger. See Table 34-2 for specific nursing interventions for patients with cognitive disorders.

Elder Care Point... The elderly are at a particularly high risk for substance-induced delirium because of overall decreased metabolism and reduction in liver and kidney function. A general principle to use in prescribing medications to elders is to give the smallest amount possible and increase the amount only as symptoms indicate.

◆ Dementia

There are several different types of dementia, and these conditions also are classified according to the underlying cause. **Examples of illnesses classified as dementia are Alzheimer's a disease, Pick's disease, Huntingdon's chorea, Korsakoff's syndrome, vascular dementia, acquired immune deficiency syndrome (AIDS) dementia complex, and Parkinson's disease.** The two most common prototypes, Alzheimer's disease and vascular dementia, are discussed in this chapter.

Alzheimer's disease. Alzheimer's disease (AD) is the most common degenerative disease of the brain.

Approximately four million Americans have AD, and there is no known cause or cure. Alzheimer's disease typically affects people over the age of 65, but can strike younger people, too. The incidence increases as age advances, and it is estimated that 20% of people over 85 have the disease. The average age of onset of symptoms to the time of death is 8 to 10 years.

Signs and Symptoms   Behavioral patterns and symptoms associated with AD are typically divided into four stages: mild, moderate, moderate to severe, and late. See Table 34-5 for common behavioral manifestations associated with stages of AD.

Alzheimer's disease is difficult to diagnose and is frequently diagnosed only when other types of dementia are excluded or ruled out. Basically, there is a loss of neurons in the frontal and temporal lobes. The atrophy in these areas accounts for the patient's inability to process and integrate new information and to retrieve memory. The use of tropicamide solution is a potential diagnostic aid for Alzheimer's disease. A research study was conducted using a 0.01% solution as eye drops. Pupils dilated consistently in all but one subject with Alzheimer's disease and pupils did not dilate in the control group. Further studies are underway.

Treatment   Treatment is primarily symptomatic. A new medication, Tarcine HCl (Cognex), is used to improve memory and reasoning ability. This medication works by elevating the levels of acetylcholine in the cerebral cortex. During use of this drug, liver functions need to monitored closely. This drug has had modest effects, but even minor improvement in reasoning and memory is helpful for both the patient and caregivers.

Nursing Intervention   General nursing interventions for patients with AD depend on the stage of illness the patient is experiencing. In the early stages general measures for intervening with a confused patient are necessary. In progressive stages, supportive care is indicated. Working with the family is of utmost importance, as family members are most often the primary caregivers until the later stages. At that time nursing home placement is common. See Table 34-2 for specific nursing interventions for patients with cognitive disorders.

Vascular dementia.   Prior to the publication of DSM–IV vascular dementia was called multi-infarct dementia. It is the second most common type of chronic cognitive disorder. **Vascular dementia is a broad term used to describe any type of dementia caused by vessel disease.** Persons who are predisposed to this type of dementia have a history of hypertension, hyperlipidemia, diabetes mellitus, and abuse of nicotine and alcohol.

Any type of vessel disease in the brain will cause brain damage. Lack of oxygen to the brain tissue because of ministrokes (clots or hemorrhage) can cause death of brain tissue in a short time. The parts of the brain originally affected with cell death will be permanently damaged.

Signs and Symptoms   The onset is rather abrupt, and the neurological impairment is localized rather than global. The progression of symptoms is more rapid than with AD, which tends to progress more slowly. Neurological deficits are present in whatever part of the brain has been destroyed. Prompt treatment of hypertension and vascular disease is necessary to prevent long-term complications.

Nursing Intervention   Nursing interventions are basically supportive and will depend on which part of the brain suffered damage. See Table 34-2 for specific nursing interventions for patients with dementia.

TABLE 34-5 ◆ Behavioral Patterns Found in Mild, Moderate, Moderate to Severe and Late Stages of Alzheimer's Disease

Early stage
Slow, progressive loss of intellectual ability.
Difficulty in learning new things.
Mild depression.
Personality and social interactions remain intact.

Middle stage
Increase in memory loss.
Decreased ability to perform usual ADLs.
Variable mood.
Noticeable personality change (e.g., easy-going person can become angry and paranoid).
Social withdrawal.
Monitor for safety.
Should not drive.

Middle to late stage
Unable to recognize familiar objects and family (agnosia).
Needs repeated instructions for simple tasks.
Needs total care—can be very burdensome for the family.
Wanders away.
Incontinent.
Outbursts of anger, hostility, paranoia.

Late stage
Unable to speak or ambulate.
Profound memory loss.
Difficulty swallowing.
Weight loss.
Bedridden.
Fetal position.
End-stage consequences of poor nutritional state and bedridden status: pressure sores, respiratory failure, contractures, pneumonia.

TABLE 34-6 ◆ *Patient Education: Suggestions for Families Caring for a Patient with Alzheimer's Disease*

Family members should be advised to do the following.

- Protect the patient from various forms of stress, such as changes in caregiver, routine, or environment.
- Keep the daily routine the same.
- Establish bedtime rituals.
- Make and keep a copy of the daily schedule, and stick to the schedule as closely as possible.
- Orient the patient to time, place, and person as necessary to maintain safety and promote maximum functioning.
- Simplify the environment to minimize illusions and confusion; keep decorative items to a minimum.
- Keep the environment as quiet as possible.
- Schedule rest breaks throughout the day for both yourself and the patient.
- Lower your expectations of the patient; forcing the patient to think too much causes frustration.
- Offer help when needed, and distract as necessary.
- Always supervise the patient when taking medications.
- Use sense of touch. Visual and auditory perceptions are distorted; therefore patients have an increased need for touch.
- Always approach the patient from the front prior to touching.
- Use distraction if patient becomes agitated. Walking, gardening, rocking in a rocking chair, sanding wood, or folding laundry are good examples of distraction.
- Remove all potential safety hazards.
- Use many of the safeguards used for young children, such as storing all cleaning solutions, pesticides, medications, and nonedible items in locked cabinets.
- Put protective caps on all unused electrical outlets.
- Remove all sharp objects.
- Lower temperature of water heater.
- Remove all throw rugs, and keep hallways and stairs free of clutter.
- Provide a low bed for the patient.
- Keep the house well-lit.
- If patient wanders, alert local police and neighbors.
- Attach safety rails in the bathroom.
- Provide an identification bracelet for the patient.
- Allow the patient to smoke only under very close supervision.
- Protect windows and door with Plexiglas.
- Rather than restrict a patient with dementia from wandering, provide them with some safe areas in which to wander. For example, gates could be installed in a fenced backyard.
- As the illness progresses, gradually restrict car use.

COMMUNITY CARE

If patients with dementia or delirium are hospitalized, the inpatient stay will typically be for a short time. For a variety of reasons, financial and personal, many families are choosing to keep their elders at home. Nurses who make home visits will often encounter families attempting to care for a relative who is experiencing either of these conditions. Considerable teaching must be done about the causes and stages of these illnesses. In addition, families are eager for practical knowledge that will make the living arrangement more acceptable. See Table 34-6 for some tips on caring for a patient with dementia at home.

In the later stages of dementia, nursing home placement sometimes is necessary. Many nursing homes have special units set aside for AD patients. In these units safety precautions are a primary concern. Entrance and exit doors have special codes so that patients cannot wander off the unit. Nurses in these units spend considerable time educating families about the stages of AD and help families with the inevitable grieving process.

In addition to observing patients with delirium in the acute hospital setting, nurses often interact with these patients in outpatient clinics, emergency rooms, or doctor's offices. Excellent assessment skills are necessary to prevent any further decline.

CRITICAL THINKING EXERCISES

Clinical Case Problems

Read each clinical case problem and discuss the questions with your classmates.

1. You are a nurse working in a nursing home and Mr. Dixon, a 75-year-old patient you have been caring for over the past 6 months suddenly becomes combative when the nurse's aide attempts to give him his morning bath. You have never

observed Mr. Dixon exhibit this type of behavior before.

- ◆ What would your initial nursing intervention be?
- ◆ How might you explain Mr. Dixon's sudden change in behavior?

2. You are newly assigned to work on the Alzheimer's unit in the nursing home where you work. Mrs. Oneida Lampert, 82 years old, is admitted during the afternoon. Her daughter tells you her mother has Alzheimer's disease and she can no longer care for her at her home because she is incontinent and wanders off. She says she feels guilty about leaving her mother at the nursing home, but knows it is the best thing for everyone.

- ◆ How would you initially respond to Mrs. Lampert's daughter?
- ◆ What could you say to the daughter that would allay some of her feelings of guilt?
- ◆ What type of behavior might you expect from Mrs. Lampert during her initial adjustment to the nursing home?

3. John Miller, Jr., a 40-year-old school teacher, accompanies his father, John Miller, Sr., to the doctor's office where you are working. The elder Mr. Miller, currently 62 years old, was diagnosed with vascular dementia 3 years before. His condition is progressively deteriorating, and the younger Mr. Miller, tells you that he is fearful that this type of dementia could happen to him.

- ◆ How would you respond to the younger Mr. Miller?
- ◆ What type of preventive education might be helpful for Mr. Miller, Jr.?

BIBLIOGRAPHY

Allen, T. (1994). Understanding Alzheimer's disease: an overview. *Nurseweek.* 25(7):8–9.

American Psychiatric Association. (1994). *Diagnostic and Statistical Manual of Mental Disorders–IV.* Washington, D.C.: American Psychiatric Association.

Cummings, J. (Interview). (1995). Alzheimer's disease: a look at disease characteristics and etiology. *Current Approaches to Geriatric Psychiatry.* 1(1):5–6.

Foreman, M., Zane, D. (1996). Comparing acute confusion, dementia and depression. *American Journal of Nursing.* 96(4):49.

Fortinash, K., Holoday-Worret. (1995). *Psychiatric Nursing Care Plans.* St. Louis, MO: Mosby-Yearbook.

Fraser, C. (1996). This dementia patient can be helped. *RN.* 59(1):38–44.

Gray, G. E. (Interview). (1996). Maintaining adequate nutrition in patients with Alzheimer's disease. *Current Approaches to Geriatric Psychiatry.* 2(4):7–8.

Hall, G. R., Wakefield, B. (1996). Acute confusion in the elderly. *Nursing 96.* 26(7):33–37.

Jones, C. P. (1994). In Sam's shop. *American Journal of Nursing.* 94(3):50–52.

Lyons, J. S. (Interview). (1995). Administering the behavioral syndromes scale for dementia. *Current Approaches to Geriatric Psychiatry.* 1(1):8–9.

McCracken, A. (1994). Special care units: meeting the needs of cognitively impaired patients. *Journal of Gerontological Nursing.* 20(4):41–44.

Miller, J. (1996). A clinical project to reduce confusion in hospitalized older adults. *MEDSURG Nursing.* 5(6):436–444.

Neal, L. (1996). The home care client with Alzheimer's disease. Part I. *Home Health Care Nurse.* 14(2):175–178.

Nelson, D. (1995). Massaging victims of Alzheimer's disease: communication and caring through touch. *Massage.* 53(2):24–31.

Perlaky, D. (1994). A bearable solution: responding creatively to dementia. *Nursing 94.* 24(1):60–62.

Powell, L. S., Courtice, K. (1993). *Alzheimer's Disease: A Guide for Families.* Reading, MA: Addison-Wesley.

Rabins, P. (Interview). (1995). Antipsychotic therapy in elderly patients with dementia: factoring in sedation potential. *Current Approaches to Geriatric Psychiatry.* 1(1):7–8.

Reisberg, B. (Interview). (1995). Functional assessment staging (FAST) in Alzheimer's disease: a practical approach to diagnosis. *Current Approaches to Geriatric Psychiatry.* 1(1):10–11.

Roca, R. (Interview). (1996). Alternative care settings: the homebound patient with Alzheimer's disease. *Current Approaches to Geriatric Psychiatry.* 3(2):10–11.

Shelden, L. J. (Interview). (1996). Management of aggressive behavior in the patient with dementia. *Current Approaches to Geriatric Psychitry.* 2(2):1–2.

Stolley, J. (1995). Freeing your patient from restraints. *American Journal of Nursing.* 95(2):26–31.

Sultzer, D. L. (Interview). (1996). Treatment of delusional and agitated behavior in elderly patients. *Current Approaches to Geriatric Psychiatry.* 2(4):1–3.

Varacolis, E. (1995). *Foundations of Psychiatric Mental Health Nursing.* Philadelphia, PA: Saunders.

Weiler, K. (1994). Legal aspects of nursing documentation for the Alzheimer's patient. *Journal of Gerontological Nursing.* 20(4):31–40.

Williams, L. (Interview). (1996). Polypharmacy and the elderly patient with dementia. *Current Approaches to Geriatric Psychiatry.* 3(2):1–4.

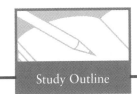

I. **Incidence and Significance of Cognitive Disorders**

   A. Very common, especially among the elderly population.

   B. Increasing with the increase in the elderly population.

   C. Cognition: mental processes of perception, memory, judgment, and reasoning.

   D. Disorders of cognition occur when there is a significant change in cognition from a previous level of functioning.

II. **Delirium versus Dementia**

   A. Delirium: change in overall cognition and level of consciousness over a short time (acute confusion).

   B. Dementia: presence of several cognitive deficits, memory in particular (chronic).

   C. Both conditions are classified according to etiology.

   D. Delirium and dementia can coexist in the same patient.

III. **Nursing Assessment of Delirium and Dementia**

   A. Patient is usually not a good historian.

   B. Need to differentiate between delirium, dementia, and depression.

   C. Depression: see Chapter 32.

   D. Delirium.

     1. Onset is sudden and often appears at sundown.

     2. Patient may be either very alert or lethargic, depending on cause.

     3. Change in attention span and reduction in overall awareness of environment.

     4. Disoriented.

     5. Impaired recent and remote memory.

     6. Incoherent speech.

     7. Thinking disorganized and distorted.

     8. Presence of delusions, hallucinations, and illusions.

     9. Disturbed, possibly reversed sleep cycle.

     10. Patient appears very confused.

   E. Dementia.

     1. Slow onset (months to years).

     2. Generally alert and normal attention span.

     3. May be disoriented and lose recent memory.

     4. In later stages, global amnesia present.

     5. Unable to abstract thoughts.

     6. Poverty of thoughts.

     7. Uses confabulation to fill gaps in conversation.

     8. Impaired judgment.

     9. Fragmented sleep.

     10. Usually do not experience hallucinations, delusions, or illusions.

     11. Notable change in personality.

   F. Necessary to assess *j*udgment, *a*ffect, *m*emory, *c*ognition, and *o*rientation (JAMCO).

     1. Judgment: presence of judgment and insight.

     2. Affect: description of change in mood and affect.

     3. Memory: difference between recent, remote, and immediate memory.

     4. Cognition: presence of illusions, hallucinations, and delusions.

     5. Orientation: time, place, and person.

   G. Sundowning: tendency to be oriented during the daytime hours and become confused and disoriented during the evening hours.

   H. Complete physical and mental status assessment at least once per shift.

   I. Planning.

     1. Delirium.

       a. Provide for safety.

       b. Reduce environmental safety.

       c. Assess frequently.

       d. Provide reality orientation.

       e. Eliminate causative factors.

     2. Dementia.

       a. Provide for safety.

       b. Promote dignity and self-worth.

       c. Maintain optimal functioning.

       d. Educate family about dementia.

   J. General nursing interventions.

     1. Assess patient frequently.

     2. Notify physician if findings change.

     3. Medicate for anxiety and aggression.

     4. Orient to time, place, and person, if appropriate (Table 34-3).

     5. Follow appropriate guidelines for use of restraints (Table 34-4).

     6. Maintain calm, soothing manner.

     7. Maintain dignity of patient and family.

8. Encourage respite care or day care.

9. Encourage family members to talk about advance directives.

K. Evaluation.

1. Return to previous level of functioning.

2. Freedom from injury.

3. Elimination of the cause of acute delirium.

4. Increased knowledge base of family (caregivers).

IV. **Common Nursing Diagnoses, Expected Outcomes and Interventions for Patients with Cognition Disorders (Table 34-2)**

V. **Disorders of Cognition**

A. Causes of delirium (acute confusion).

1. Cerebrovascular accident.

2. Drug overdose.

3. Toxicity or withdrawal.

4. Tumors.

5. Systemic infections.

6. Fluid and electrolyte imbalances.

7. Malnutrition.

B. Causes of dementia.

1. Alzheimer's disease.

2. Pick's disease.

3. Huntington's chorea.

4. Korsakoff's syndrome.

5. Vascular dementia.

6. Acquired immune deficiency syndrome (AIDS).

7. Parkinson's disease.

C. Substance-induced delirium.

1. Caused by withdrawal from substance, intoxication, or side effects from a substance.

2. See Chapter 33 for information on delirium due to intoxication or withdrawal.

3. Examples of medications that can cause delirium.

a. Anesthetics.

b. Analgesics.

c. Sedative-hypnotics.

d. Tricyclic antidepressants.

e. Antihistamines.

f. Theophylline derivatives.

g. Antipsychotics.

h. Histamine$_2$ blocking agents.

i. Beta-blockers.

j. Nonsteroidal antiinflammatory drugs (NSAIDs).

k. Various over-the-counter medications.

4. Nursing interventions.

a. Always monitor the effects of medications.

b. Take thorough medication history.

c. Look for interactions and incompatibilities.

d. Consult with pharmacist as necessary.

D. Alzheimer's disease: the most common degenerative disease of the brain.

1. No known cause or cure.

2. Usually affects people over the age of 65.

3. Incidence increases as age advances.

4. Signs and symptoms: vary according to stages of disease. (Table 34-5 for common signs and symptoms of Alzheimer's disease.)

5. Diagnosed when other types of chronic dementias are ruled out.

6. Treatment is primarily symptomatic.

7. New medication (Tarcine) is being used with some success to improve memory and reasoning ability.

a. Elevates acetylcholine levels in the brain.

b. Carefully monitor liver function.

8. Nursing interventions.

a. Depends on the stage of illness the patient is experiencing.

b. Use general measures for working with a confused patient.

c. Include family.

d. May require nursing home placement in the later stages.

E. Vascular dementia: second most common type of dementia.

1. Describes any type of dementia caused by vessel disease, which causes brain damage.

2. Onset usually is abrupt.

3. Neurological impairment is localized rather than global.

4. More rapid progression than Alzheimer's disease.

5. Nursing interventions.

a. Prompt recognition of symptoms of hypertension and vascular problems.

b. Supportive depending on the part of the brain affected.

VI. **Elder Care Points**

A. Elders who have a preexisting dementia also can have a sudden episode of delirium.

B. Consider cumulative effects of medications.

C. The correct etiology for acute delirium needs to be recognized and treated.

D. Elders are sensitive to the cumulative effects of medications because of decreased metabolic and liver function.

E. Elders should be prescribed the smallest amount of medication possible, and doses should be increased only when symptoms indicate.

VII. **Community Care**

A. Shorter inpatient stays.

B. Often cared for in the home.

C. Family needs considerable teaching (Table 34-6).

D. Nursing home placement may be necessary in the later stages of dementia.

E. May also see patients with disorders of cognition in outpatient clinics, emergency rooms, or doctor's offices.

F. Excellent assessment skills are necessary.

CHAPTER 35

Care of Patients with Thought and Personality Disorders

OBJECTIVES

Upon completing this chapter, the student should be able to:

1. Discuss the incidence of thought and personality disorders in the general population.
2. Differentiate between thought and personality disorders.
3. Outline the facts to be considered when performing a nursing assessment of a patient with either a thought or a personality disorder.
4. From a list of NANDA nursing diagnoses, identify at least four nursing diagnoses that would be appropriate for a patient with either a personality or a thought disorder.
5. From the nursing diagnoses identified, choose appropriate nursing interventions and expected outcomes.
6. Describe appropriate nursing interventions for a patient who is angry, manipulative, hostile, paranoid, or aggressive.
7. Describe the signs and symptoms of schizophrenia and borderline personality disorder.
8. Describe the major nursing interventions for schizophrenia and borderline personality disorder.

This chapter focuses on patients who are experiencing a disorder of thought or personality. Diagnosis of a thought disorder (e.g., schizophrenia) is made when a person is unable to think in an organized way and has serious misperceptions of reality (**hallucinations** and **delusions**). The hallucinations often are frightening and tormenting. Affect or mood also is affected, as are interpersonal relationships.

The incidence of thought disorders is not as high as that of mood disorders, but they tend to be more chronic and debilitating. It is estimated that between 0.5% and 1% of the general population is affected with schizophrenia.

Disorders of personality are long-term conditions. Prevalence varies, according to the type and population studied. Borderline personality disorder is diagnosed most frequently and is seen in 2% of the general population, 10% among mental health clinic patients, and about 20% among psychiatric inpatients. *(American Psychiatric Association, 1994)*

Symptoms of personality disorders are first observed in late adolescence and early adulthood. An actual diagnosis may not be made until the person reaches the late twenties or thirties. By this time the entrenched behaviors are quite evident. It is not uncommon to note failed marriages, poor work histories, and considerable difficulty with interpersonal relationships. Four characteristics of personality disorders are:

1. Inflexible and maladaptive response to life events.
2. Serious difficulty in areas of personal and work relationships.
3. Tendency to evoke interpersonal conflict.
4. Tendency to evoke a negative empathic response from others.

The main difference between thought disorders and personality disorders is that individuals with thought disorders experience an altered reality and impaired ego

functioning (sense of self). Individuals with personality disorders do not experience a break with reality, and their ego remains intact.

Another difference is that some of the symptoms of thought disorders can be relieved with antipsychotic medications. Medications are not indicated for personality disorders, although they are sometimes prescribed when there is a concurrent mood disorder. Individuals with symptoms of either thought or personality disorders will benefit from various types of psychotherapies.

NURSING MANAGEMENT

◆ Assessment

Assessment of a thought disorder involves observing the person's ability to think in a logical manner and the presence of **psychotic features (hallucinations, delusions, and grossly disorganized behavior). An individual with a thought disorder will act and look bizarre.** Voices (auditory hallucinations) will be telling the person what to do, and delusions (false, fixed beliefs) develop as the disorder progresses. Delusions can be either grandiose or persecutory. An example of *delusions of grandeur* would be to believe that you are from royalty. Individuals with *delusions of persecution* believe that they are being persecuted by agencies or other people.

Ideas of reference also are common among individuals with thought disorders. In this instance the person with the thought disorder believes that he or she is being specifically targeted for a message from an important person. A common manifestation is to believe that the news anchor on the television is sending special messages telepathically.

When assessing thought disorders, the interview must be brief. Because there is a problem with logical thought processing, it is difficult for the individual to remain focused for very long. Also the thinking process is very concrete, and the ability to abstract information is not present. See Table 35-1 for definition of terms associated with assessment of a thought disorder.

Personality disorders are enduring patterns of behavior where there is no loss of contact with reality or impaired cognition. These individuals do not look or act bizarre or different. The nurse needs to assess how the individual views self and others, how feelings are typically expressed, and obtain a history of former relationships.

It is important not to make a hasty assessment and label a person with a personality disorder. An individual may have some traits of a particular disorder, but not exhibit enough of the criteria for a DSM–IV

TABLE 35-1 ◆ *Definition of Terms Used in Assessing a Thought Disorder*

- **Delusions:** grandeur (inflated notion of self-importance); persecution (belief that one is being persecuted). Patient has false, fixed beliefs that cannot be changed by logical reasoning. Delusions can be fleeting or fixed.
- **Echolalia:** involves involuntary repetition of words spoken by others. Seen in catatonic schizophrenia.
- **Echopraxia:** involves imitating the motions of others. Seen in catatonic schizophrenia.
- **Emotional blunting or flat affect:** type of affect seen in schizophrenia where there is a reduction in intensity of affect or absence or near absence of emotional expression.
- **Hallucinations:** auditory (hearing); visual (seeing); gustatory (tasting); olfactory (smelling); tactile (feeling or touching). Patient experiences various sensory perceptions without a corresponding stimuli in the environment. Auditory hallucinations are common in schizophrenia.
- **Ideas of reference:** a type of delusion where the theme is that events, objects, or other persons in the patient's immediate environment have a particular and unusual significance for them only. For example, a schizophrenic may believe that the anchorman on a television news show is speaking directly to him.
- **Illusions:** patient misinterprets reality. For example, patient may perceive IV tubing as a snake.
- **Neologisms:** involves making up new words to express confused thoughts. Seen in schizophrenics with a serious thought disturbance.
- **Waxy flexibility:** a state seen in catatonic schizophrenia where the person maintains a limb in one position for a long time. Movement of limbs appears to be "waxlike."
- **Word salad:** a disorganized mix of words, phrases, and fragments that lack comprehension. Seen in severe schizophrenia.

---

diagnosis. If a hasty unconfirmed assessment is made and a patient is labeled a "borderline," nurses may view the patient as "hopeless" or "chronic." This type of labeling is counterproductive for both the patient and nursing staff. See Table 35-2 for examples of

---

TABLE 35-2 ◆ *Guide for Assessing Patients with Personality Disorders*

Observe and assess the patient for the following behaviors:

- Low self-esteem.
- Constant seeking of praise and admiration.
- Self-centeredness.
- Extreme envy of others.
- Anger and possible rage when others do not share the same point of view.
- Acts without thinking; impulsivity.
- Consistent poor judgment in making decisions.
- Unreliable.
- Evidence of self-destructive behavior.
- Treatment of others as objects, not people.
- Expression of a need to control others.
- Excessive use of manipulation to get needs met.

behaviors nurses might observe when assessing a personality disorder.

◆ Nursing Diagnoses

See Table 35-3 for nursing diagnoses, expected outcomes, and nursing interventions for individuals with thought and personality disorders.

◆ Planning

Planning care for a patient with a personality or thought disorder involves promoting safety, monitoring medications intended to relieve symptoms of agitation or psychosis (thought disorders), and ensuring adequate nutrition and sleep. Care for both of these types of disorders will be long term with intermittent treatment

---

TABLE 35-3 ◆ *Common Nursing Diagnoses, Expected Outcomes, and Nursing Interventions for Patients with Disorders of Thought and Personality*

Nursing Diagnoses	Goals/Expected Outcomes	Nursing Intervention
Thought Disorders		
Altered thought process related to delusional thinking, loosening of associations.	Patient will be able to distinguish between reality and nonreality. Absence of delusional thinking.	Approach the patient in a calm, matter-of-fact manner. Avoid challenging the patient's delusional system. Assess for evidence of situations that trigger anxiety for the patient, and determine whether these situations also trigger increased delusions. Administer antipsychotic medications as ordered. Monitor medications for effectiveness and side effects.
Self-care deficit related to alteration in thought processes, social withdrawal.	Patient will provide self-care without nurse's prompting. Patient will dress appropriately and maintain appropriate hygiene.	Encourage the patient to perform normal activities according to level of ability. Make available only the clothes the patient is to wear. Minimize environmental stimuli. Intervene as necessary if patient is unable to complete daily care. Offer positive reinforcement when patient does complete ADLs.
Sensory-perceptual alteration: hallucinations: auditory, and visual related to psychotic features of formal thought disorder, heightened level of anxiety.	Patient is able to make association between increased anxiety and increase in hallucinations. Patient is able to recognize states of increased anxiety. Patient is able to hold conversations without hallucinating.	Observe and assess for hallucinations. Once it is established that the content of the hallucinations will not cause harm to the patient or others, distract or redirect the patient when hallucinations occur. Help patient recognize the feeling states that are present prior to the hallucination rather than focusing on the content. State your reality about the patient's hallucinogenic experience ("I understand that you hear voices telling you are a bad person; I do not hear those voices"). Administer antipsychotic medications and monitor effectiveness and side effects.
Social isolation related to interpersonal withdrawal associated with psychotic disturbance, altered thought process.	Patient will engage in social interaction with others on the psychiatric unit (meals, outings, groups). Patient will express pleasure in social interactions with others.	When interacting with the patient, convey a warm, accepting attitude. Spend some structured time with the patient everyday to promote trust. Keep all appointments with the patient. Determine patient's interests. Encourage the patient to interact with other patients on the unit, even if for a brief time.
Personality Disorders		
Ineffective individual coping related to loss of a relationship, real and perceived stressors, loss of structure.	The patient will verbalize a desire to stop being manipulative to get needs met. The patient will neither idealize nor devalue staff members. The patient will verbalize a plan to reduce stressors.	Convey an accepting attitude to the patient. Set firm limits as necessary. Support the patient in the use of clear, direct communication. Assist the patient to attempt to redirect angry feelings in constructive activities, such as crafts, games, or exercises. Assist the patient in developing a realistic plan to minimize stressors.

TABLE 35-3 ◆ *Common Nursing Diagnoses, Expected Outcomes, and Nursing Interventions for Patients with Disorders of Thought and Personality* (Continued)		
Nursing Diagnoses	**Expected Outcomes**	**Nursing Intervention**
Personality Disorders (Continued)		
Risk for violence, self-directed, related to history of suicidal gestures, history of self-mutilating behavior.	The patient will stop self-mutilating behaviors. The patient will sign a no-suicide contract. The patient will not commit suicide.	Encourage the patient to identify, label, and express feelings. Assist patient to become aware of escalating levels of anxiety and the desire to self-mutilate. Encourage the use of diversional activities, such as journal writing or crafts, when the desire to self-mutilate is present. If the patient does engage in any self-mutilating behavior, care for the wound in a matter-of-fact manner, so that the nurse does not overtly encourage maladaptive coping. Assess degree of suicidality. Implement suicide precautions. Formulate a short-term, no-harm contract with the patient. Renew contract as necessary.
Self-esteem disturbance related to unmet dependency needs, perceived abandonment/rejection.	The patient will consistently verbalize positive comments about self and realistic comments about others. The patient will not manipulate others.	Assist the patient in setting goals that are realistic. Encourage patient to set goals and monitor progress. Assist the patient in becoming aware of manipulative behavior. Set limits on manipulative behavior. Explain consequences of manipulative behavior in a calm, rational manner. Teach the patient basic assertive techniques.
Impaired social interaction related to disturbance of self-concept, inability to maintain a healthy relationship.	The patient will be able to have a healthy relationship. The patient will be able to identify and set personal boundaries.	Teach the patient the essential components of a healthy relationship, such as trust or honesty. Make patient aware that intensity of emotions is not an essential part of healthy relationships. Teach the patient the necessity of personal boundaries and how to maintain them. Role-model boundaries for the patient by being consistent and congruent in your interactions. Observe patient setting boundaries and give appropriate feedback as necessary.

for acute episodes. Patients need to be educated about the medications and coping skills necessary to function outside of a hospital setting. For individuals with thought disorders, medication is very important. It is not unusual for a patient to stop taking medications because the voices returned with a warning that all medications are poison.

Nursing goals for thought disorders include:

◆ Promoting safety and trust.
◆ Educating about medication.
◆ Monitoring medication compliance and effectiveness.
◆ Ensuring adequate sleep and nutrition.
◆ Minimizing social withdrawal.

Nursing goals for personality disorders include:

◆ Setting limits.
◆ Teaching coping skills.
◆ Promoting safety.

◆ Encouraging insight into behavior.
◆ Monitoring behavior changes.

◆ Implementation

When caring for a patient with a thought disorder, an attitude of acceptance is necessary to promote trust. Individuals with thought disorders often have *paranoid delusions* and live within the confines of their own reality. Unless trust is established, interventions will be difficult to accomplish.

Administering medications and teaching the patient and family about antipsychotic medications are two additional nursing interventions. In addition, the side effects of the medications must be monitored. Antipsychotic medications can cause serious, irreversible adverse effects. See Table 35-3 for specific nursing interventions for individuals with thought disorders.

For individuals with personality disorders, setting limits is a priority intervention. Patients must be taught ways to get their needs met that are not manipulative. Often it is necessary to implement suicide precautions and help the patient stop self-mutilating behaviors. See Table 35-3 for specific nursing interventions for individuals with personality disorders.

Patients with disorders of thought and personality can sometimes be angry, manipulative, hostile, paranoid, or aggressive. These behaviors can be difficult and require thoughtful interventions by nurses. See Table 35-4 for specific ways to intervene with each of these behaviors.

◆ Evaluation

To evaluate the effectiveness of nursing interventions, it is necessary to determine appropriate expected outcomes and then monitor the patient's progress. Hospitalization may be necessary to protect the patient from harm to self or others or to ensure the patient will maintain compliance on a medication regime. In these instances the focus of the outcome is on ensuring safety and alleviating the symptoms of psychosis.

Expected outcomes for the positive symptoms of schizophrenia are easier to achieve than the outcomes for the negative symptoms. **Compliance with antipsychotic medications will improve sleep and decrease hallucinations and delusions (positive symptoms). Outcomes for the negative symptoms would include a decrease in psychomotor retardation, increase in self-care, improved affect, and an increase in motivation. In addition, the patient would exhibit a trusting attitude toward others and a decrease in social withdrawal.** Achieving expected outcomes for the negative symptoms of schizophrenia is a much longer process than for the positive symptoms.

Long-term outcomes for patients with personality disorders include demonstrating new coping strategies for handling stressors, verbalizing anger without acting

---

TABLE 35-4 ◆ *Specific Nursing Interventions for Patients Who Are Angry, Hostile, Aggressive, Manipulative, or Paranoid*

Angry, hostile, and aggressive behavior

- Continuously assess for nonverbal cues (pacing, fidgeting, increase in verbalizations) that the patient's anger is increasing.
- Recognize that in some situations anger can rapidly escalate to hostility and aggression toward others.
- Encourage the patient to find a quiet, safe place.
- Offer PRN medications if they are ordered and if it is appropriate.
- Listen to the patient, and acknowledge that you care and want to help.
- Maintain a calm, self-assured attitude, even if you are frightened.
- Allow the patient adequate personal space.
- If the patient is using abusive language, know that this is the only way that the patient can express feelings.
- Honestly verbalize the patient's options. For example, say, "You can stay in the dayroom if you can remain calm; otherwise it will be necessary for you to go to the quiet (seclusion) room."
- Always ask the patient's permission before touching. Touching can be soothing, but only if the patient feels okay with it.
- Set a time frame for verbal de-escalation and stand by it. If the patient is making progress within 15 minutes, continue. If not, remind the patient of the limits that were initially set.
- Maintain your own safety—have adequate staff backup. However, only one person should attempt verbal de-escalation.
- If the patient continues to escalate and the behavior becomes aggressive, physical restraints may be necessary.
- Application of physical restraints in a psychiatric setting always is a team approach by trained staff.
- The patient must always be made aware of the staff's intentions and actions, and the entire episode must be accurately documented.
- A guiding principle is that less restrictive measures must always be tried before physically restraining a patient.

Manipulative behavior

- Set clear and realistic limits on specific behaviors.
- Establish realistic and enforceable consequences.
- Make certain that all staff are informed of the limits and are in agreement.
- Specific limits on the plan of care need to be documented.
- The decision to discontinue limits should be made by the entire staff and should be made only when the patient has demonstrated consistent behavior.

Paranoid behavior

- Attempt to assign only one or two nurses to the patient.
- Initially make brief contact with the patient, and do not make unnecessary demands.
- Increase credibility by being honest, adhering to a stated schedule and following through on commitments.
- Do not touch a patient who is paranoid.
- Do not mix medications with food.

out, increasing independent decision making, and decreasing manipulative behaviors to get needs met. It is expected that in times of stress the patient will revert to previously learned behaviors and at times will need to be encouraged to continue implementing new behaviors. **Recovery from a personality disorder is a long-term process.**

DISORDERS OF THOUGHT

The DSM–IV describes disorders of thought as disorders where there are psychotic symptoms present. **Examples of psychotic features associated with thought disorders are hallucinations, delusions, or disorganized speech and/or behavior.** Schizophrenia is the most common thought disorder and consequently, is discussed in this chapter. Other types of thought disorders are brief psychotic disorder, schizoaffective disorder, delusional disorder, schizophreniform disorder, shared psychotic disorder, psychotic disorder due to a medical condition, and substance-induced psychotic disorder. In addition there is a category that includes psychotic disorder N.O.S. (not otherwise specified). In this instance the patient does not meet enough of the criteria to be diagnosed with any of the thought disorders listed.

◆ Schizophrenia

Schizophrenia is a serious medical illness that, when left untreated, causes people to have unusual, bizarre behavior (hallucinations and delusions). The illness usually develops in late adolescence or the early twenties. Because these behaviors are so inappropriate and out of the norm, **individuals with schizophrenia are shunned and stigmatized.** They are then particularly vulnerable to poverty, homelessness, drug abuse, and suicide. New methods of treatment are available to help schizophrenics maintain independent, productive lives outside of an institution.

Diagnosis   The exact cause of schizophrenia is unknown. However, current research indicates that there may be a biological basis. It is known that schizophrenia is more likely to occur among the poor and unemployed and when there is an increase in environmental stressors.

The signs and symptoms of schizophrenia are divided into negative (absent) and positive (present) symptoms. **Positive symptoms include the presence of hallucinations, delusions, and disordered thinking or loose associations between thoughts. Negative symptoms include apathy, social isolation, poverty of thoughts, psychomotor retardation, blunted affect, and lack of motivation.** See Table 35-5 for a description of the different types of schizophrenia.

TABLE 35-5 ◆ *Types of Schizophrenia*	
Type	**Behavioral Manifestations**
◆ **Paranoid:** exhibits extreme suspiciousness, **delusions of grandeur,** and **delusions of persecution.** Can be hostile and aggressive. Auditory hallucinations are common.	
◆ **Catatonic:** exhibits a stuporous condition associated with rigidity, unusual posturing and **waxy flexibility.** Also demonstrates **echopraxia** and **echolalia.** Exhibits unpredictable behavior because behavior is controlled by delusions and hallucinations.	
◆ **Disorganized:** exhibits flat affect, silliness, and incoherence. Has gross thought disturbances, including **word salad** and **neologisms.** Delusions and hallucinations are common.	
◆ **Undifferentiated:** exhibits symptoms found in more than one type, but does not meet adequate criteria for paranoid, catatonic, or disorganized types.	
◆ **Residual:** exhibits negative symptoms of schizophrenia, with no evidence of hallucinations, delusions, or disorganized thoughts.	

Treatment   **Antipsychotic medications (neuroleptics) treat the positive symptoms of schizophrenia.** These medications are very effective in stopping the voices (auditory hallucinations), enabling the patient to connect thoughts in a logical manner (loose associations), and eliminating the delusional system. **Because antipsychotics do cause some serious and unpleasant side effects, patients often are noncompliant.** Moreover, once patients are on medications for a while, they begin to feel better and stop taking the medications. In time, the hallucinations, delusions, and disorganized thought and behavior return.

Negative symptoms are treated with a therapeutic environment, including a therapeutic relationship with the nurse, and education regarding basic living skills. These symptoms are notoriously more difficult to treat because treatment is long and the symptoms, in and of themselves, inhibit the schizophrenic from seeking help.

Think about... Noncompliance with medications often leads to a rehospitalization for schizophrenics. Can you think of some ways that nurses could devise to help schizophrenics comply with the medication regimen?

Nursing Intervention   **A priority intervention in working with schizophrenics is to administer antipsychotic medications.** As with any medication, nursing responsibility includes not only giving the medication, but also monitoring the effectiveness of the medications and any adverse effects. Antipsychotics have many serious side effects, some of which can be life-threatening. See Table 35-6 for the nursing implications of antipsychotic medications, including adverse reactions.

TABLE 35-6 ◆ *Nursing Implications for Antipsychotic Medications Used to Treat Schizophrenia*

Medications commonly used to treat schizophrenia

Chlorpromazine (Thorazine)
Thioridazine (Mellaril)
Mesoridazine (Trilafon)
Trifluoperazine (Stelazine)
Fluphenazine (Prolixin)

Thiothixene (Navane)
Haloperidol (Haldol)
Loxapine (Loxitane)
Molindone (Moban)

Recent medication used to treat schizophrenia

Clozaril (Clozapine) is a relatively new drug for the treatment of schizophrenia. Mild extrapyramidal symptoms do occur, but at much lower rates than with traditional antipsychotics. A major adverse side effect is agranulocytosis. Weekly monitoring of the white blood count is necessary. In spite of the potentially serious side effects, Clozaril is very effective in obliterating the positive symptoms of schizophrenia. This drug is reserved for patients with severe schizophrenia who have not responded to traditional antipsychotics.

Common anticholinergic side effects seen with antipsychotics

◆ Dry mouth.
◆ Constipation.
◆ Nasal congestion.
◆ Sexual dysfunction.

◆ Urinary retention and hesitancy.
◆ Blurred vision.
◆ Photophobia.

Nursing implications
◆ Provide adequate fluids.
◆ Monitor voiding and elimination patterns.
◆ Administer stool softener.
◆ Remind patient that blurred vision and nasal congestion will cease once the body becomes accustomed to the drug.
◆ Remind patient to wear sunglasses when in the sun.
◆ Remind patient to alert treatment team if sexual difficulties continue.

Common extrapyramidal side effects seen with antipsychotics

◆ Pseudo-Parkinsonism.
◆ Akathisia and tardive dyskinesia.

◆ Acute dystonic reactions.

Pseudo-Parkinsonism: Masklike facies, stiff and stooped posture, shuffling gait, drooling, fine tremors, and pill-rolling movement.

Nursing implications
◆ May need to switch to a different antipsychotic.
◆ Administer anticholinergic medications such as Artane (trihexyphenidyl) or Cogentin (benztropine).

Dystonic reactions: Acute contractures of tongue, face, neck, and back.

Nursing implications
◆ Administer Benadryl (diphenhydramine hydrochloride) 25–50 μg stat. Relief is usually immediate.
◆ Experience is very frightening for the patient.
◆ Stay with the patient.

Akathisia: characterized by pacing, inner restlessness, and leg aches relieved by moving.

Nursing implications
◆ Notify physician.
◆ Antipsychotic may need to be changed or an anticholinergic added to the drug regimen.
◆ Symptoms disappear when the drug is discontinued.

Tardive dyskinesia: tongue protrusion, lip-smacking, sucking, chewing, blinking, lateral jaw movements, grimacing, rapid, purposeless and irregular movements, shoulder shrugging, pelvic thrusting, wrist and ankle flexion or rotation, foot tapping and toe movements.

Nursing implications
◆ Discontinuing the drug does not always relieve the symptoms.
◆ No specific treatment other than discontinuing the drug.
◆ Give soft foods.
◆ Have patient wear soft shoes or slippers.
◆ Encourage patients to be screened for tardive dyskinesia every 3 months.

TABLE 35-6 ◆ *Nursing Implications for Antipsychotic Medications Used to Treat Schizophrenia (Continued)*

Cardiovascular side effects

◆ Orthostatic hypotension.

◆ Tachycardia.

Nursing implications
◆ Check blood pressure before giving medications.
◆ Inform patient to dangle feet prior to getting out of bed to prevent falls.
◆ Inform patient that tolerance will develop in several weeks.
◆ Make certain there is no underlying cardiac disease prior to starting the drug.
◆ Increase fluid intake to expand vascular volume.

Miscellaneous side effects

◆ Sleepiness and fatigue.

◆ Weight gain.

◆ Photosensitivity.

◆ Hives and contact dermatitis.

Nursing implications
◆ Administer medication at bedtime.
◆ Inform patient that tolerance to the dosage will develop in 1 to 2 weeks.
◆ Avoid direct sunlight.
◆ Wear protective clothing and sunscreen when outside.
◆ Notify physician if there is a rash; may need to discontinue or change the drug.
◆ Monitor food intake.

Neuroleptic malignant syndrome

◆ High fever.

◆ Muscle rigidity.

◆ Incontinence.

◆ Hyperkalemia.

◆ Diaphoresis.

◆ Increased pulse.

◆ Stupor.

◆ Elevated white blood count.

◆ Renal failure.

Nursing implications
◆ Stop all medications.
◆ Give supportive, symptomatic care.
◆ Hydrate (oral and IV).
◆ Renal dialysis for renal failure.
◆ Correct electrolyte imbalance.
◆ Decrease body temperature.
◆ Medicate for arrythmias.
◆ Early detection increases survival rate.

Elder Care Point . . . Elders who are taking antipsychotic medications are at a higher-than-usual risk for developing serious side effects. Baseline cardiac, renal, hepatic, and hematological studies need to be done before initiating psychotropic drugs. The beginning dosages should be one-half to one-third of the normal adult dose. Elders need to be watched very closely for difficulty swallowing, constipation and fecal impactions, weight gain, memory impairment, and orthostatic hypotension.

General nursing interventions for the negative symptoms include teaching the patient and family about the illness and how to manage the signs and symptoms. Because social withdrawal is a common symptom, helping the schizophrenic learn to trust others is a major

consideration. See Table 35-3 for additional nursing interventions for patients with schizophrenia.

Think about . . . If you were caring for a patient who did not trust you, what would your approach be?

DISORDERS OF PERSONALITY

The DSM–IV describes 10 different personality disorders. Depending on the descriptive characteristics, these disorders are clustered into three separate categories. Cluster A includes behaviors that are considered **odd** or **eccentric** (schizotypal, schizoid, and paranoid). Cluster B describes behaviors that are considered **dramatic, emotional, and erratic** (antisocial, borderline, histrionic, and narcissistic). Individuals with Cluster C behaviors appear **anxious and fearful** (avoidant, dependent, and obsessive-compulsive). The tenth personality disorder described is personality disorder N.O.S. (not otherwise specified). An individual with this disorder could display characteristics from several of the 10 disorders listed. However, there would not be enough defining traits from any one category to diagnose that specific disorder. See Table 35-7 for a brief description of each of these personality disorders.

Think about... After reviewing the table on personality disorders, try to match each of the disorders to someone you know or a patient you may have cared for.

The focus for this chapter will be borderline personality disorder because it is one of the more commonly diagnosed disorders. Moreover, this particular disorder presents nurses with many challenges in the process of providing nursing care.

◆ Borderline Personality Disorder

Diagnosis   Borderline personality disorder is defined by the DSM–IV as "a pattern of instability in interpersonal relationships, self-image and affects, and marked impulsivity" (American Psychiatric Association, 1994: 629). Patients with this disorder attach quickly and easily to others and fear **real or imagined abandonment.** Emotions and relationships are very intense. In response

---

TABLE 35-7 ◆ *Description of Personality Disorders*

Cluster A (odd and eccentric)
Schizotypal: exhibits difficulty with close relationships, distortions in thinking and feeling, and odd or eccentric behavior.
Schizoid: exhibits withdrawal from social relationships and a restricted affect.
Paranoid: exhibits distrust and suspiciousness of others and feels others wish them harm or evil.

Cluster B (dramatic and emotional and erratic)
Antisocial: exhibits disregard for, and violation of, the rights of others; lack empathy.
Borderline: exhibits instability in interpersonal relationships, self-concept, labile emotions, and marked impulsivity.
Histrionic: exhibits pattern of extreme emotionality and attention-seeking behavior.
Narcissistic: exhibits grandiose behavior, intense need for admiration, and lack of empathy.

Cluster C (anxious and fearful)
Avoidant: exhibits social inhibition, feelings of inadequacy, and fear of rejection.
Dependent: exhibits behavior that is submissive and clinging; needy.
Obsessive-compulsive: exhibits behavior that is concerned with excessive orderliness, perfectionism, and need for control.

---

to potential abandonment from caregivers or significant others, it is not unusual to see **self-mutilating behavior** (cutting on hands and wrists, cigarette burns) or **suicidal gestures.**

Splitting is a common trait seen in borderline patients. This trait involves the initial idealization of a caregiver or friend, followed, sometimes very quickly, by a devaluing of that same person. For example, it is common for a patient with borderline traits to tell the nurse, "You are the best nurse I have ever had. No one else understands me like you do." When the nurse returns after 2 days off, the patient would say, "I can't believe you didn't call me when you were off. I felt horrible and began cutting on my wrists, and it is your fault."

The patient with borderline personality disorder also may idealize one or two team members and devalue others. It is very important that the staff decide on an approach to use with a particular patient. To implement the plan properly, all team members must be consistent with the approach.

Impulsivity in at least two of the following areas also is characteristic of Borderline Personality Disorder: **gambling, overeating, spending impulsively, abusing substances, engaging in unsafe sex, or driving recklessly.** Engaging in one or more of these impulsive behaviors often is the reason for admission to a hospital.

Treatment   Treatment first depends on accurate diagnosis. Adolescents who are impulsively acting out with substances and have identity problems may appear to have borderline personality disorder, but these traits often disappear with increased maturity.

Treatment for persons with this disorder involves long-term psychotherapy and sometimes a structured environment. Medications can be used to treat symptoms as they occur, such as depression or anxiety, but do not actually treat the disorder.

Nursing Intervention   To work effectively with borderline personality disorder patients, nurses need to maintain good boundaries without being controlling, rigid, and inflexible. Patients with this disorder often ask nurses to "bend the rules" or grant special privileges. **The nurse needs to set limits and offer a rationale, and should not be open to negotiation. Limit setting must be done with caring and empathy.** If the patient views the limit setting as punitive, the behavior is certain to recur at a later time.

This does not mean that the patient will always gladly accept the limit setting and be grateful for your concern. It does mean that the nurse is assisting the patient in developing some internal boundaries and subsequent changes in behavior.

It is necessary for the nurse to maintain a safe environment for patients with borderline disorder because these patients are impulsive and do not have the internal controls available to do this for themselves. It may be necessary to initiate suicide precautions. See Chapter 32 for information on suicide precautions.

Patients with personality disorders have an ability to "get under the skin" of caretakers. If you note a particularly intense reaction to a patient (excessive sympathy, empathy, anger, or frustration), it is important to talk about these feelings with a more experienced nurse or a peer whom you trust. **Keep the focus on the feelings that were evoked in yourself.** If you are able to find the origin of these feelings, subsequent reactions of a similar kind may be averted with other patients. See Table 35-3 for common nursing interventions for patients with borderline personality disorder.

COMMUNITY CARE

At one time patients with thought disorders were hospitalized indefinitely. With the introduction of antipsychotic medications, these patients are much more likely to be hospitalized for medication stabilization and released to a less restrictive type of care. Therefore, it would not be unusual for nurses to care for patients with thought disorders in a variety of settings, such as nursing homes, clinics, or home care.

Elder Care Point... Although elderly schizophrenics are few in number, they can present unique challenges for nurses who work in long-term care. Because of the negative symptoms of social withdrawal, apathy, and sometimes paranoia, schizophrenic elders are not as likely to seek out nurses for help. They may ignore physical problems and often will not seek help for pain associated with physical disabilities.

Patients with personality disorders are not hospitalized unless there is imminent danger to themselves via self-mutilation or suicidal gestures. Again, nurses come into contact with patients with personality disorders in a variety of settings outside the hospital. Setting limits and appropriate boundaries for these patients continue to be effective interventions, regardless of the setting.

CRITICAL THINKING EXERCISES

Clinical Case Problems

Read each clinical case and discuss the questions with your classmates.

1. You are a nurse working for a home health agency. Your supervisor assigns you to visit Mr. John Hammer, a 42-year-old man who just returned from an extended stay at a psychiatric facility. He was diagnosed schizophrenic at age 25 and currently lives with his parents. He had abdominal surgery for an intestinal obstruction a week ago and you need to change the dressing. He is taking two different antipsychotic medications and has a history of noncompliance with medications.

    ◆ What type of initial approach would you use with Mr. Hammer?
    ◆ How might this approach differ from how you would deal with other patients?
    ◆ What type of teaching needs does Mr. Hammer have?
    ◆ How might you include his family in the teaching plan?

2. You are a nurse working in a psychiatric facility and care for a 65-year-old woman, Anna Leiber, who was placed in the nursing home by her daughter. The daughter is an attorney, but the mother's current psychotic state prevents her from recognizing her daughter. Anna has a fixed delusional system with many religious overtones. She is unable to carry on a conversation for more than a few minutes without preaching about God and salvation. Anna began antipsychotic medications 3 days ago. You observe that she is attempting to talk with her daughter who is visiting. You notice that she is becoming increasingly agitated and is pacing. She begins talking in a loud voice and yelling at her daughter about not being saved.

    ◆ How might you approach Anna and her daughter at this time?
    ◆ What needs to be included in a teaching plan for the daughter?

3. A 32-year-old female patient, Betsy Jones, arrives at the clinic where you work and proceeds to remove a towel from around her right arm. You observe a superficial wound on the wrist, approximately one-half inch in length, that is bleeding, but not profusely. Betsy tells you that she cut herself because she just broke up with her boyfriend and her psychiatrist is out of town. Her breath smells of alcohol. The physician on duty tells you that he has seen Betsy several times and that she is a "psych" patient.

    ◆ What type of psychiatric diagnosis might be applicable for Betsy?
    ◆ How would you approach this patient to care for the wound?
    ◆ Why do you think the doctor called Betsy a "psych" patient?
    ◆ How would you respond to the doctor's comment?
    ◆ What type of referral might be appropriate for Betsy?

4. While at work in a busy doctor's office, you notice that a male patient suddenly begins to talk very loudly and says if he isn't seen soon, he is going to punch somebody. His wife is trying to calm him down, but it is not helping. One of the other patients in the waiting room comes and tells you to please do something.

◆ How would you approach this male patient?

◆ Outline a plan to de-escalate his anger.

BIBLIOGRAPHY

American Psychiatric Association. (1994). *Diagnostic and Statistical Manual of Mental Disorders–IV*. Washington, D.C.: American Psychiatric Association.

Banez, M. E. (1996). Responding effectively to the angry patient. *MEDSURG Nursing*. 5(6):461–463.

Barstow, D. (1995). Self-injury and self-mutilation: nursing approaches. *Journal of Psychosocial Nursing and Mental Health Services*. 33(2):19–22.

Bihm, B. (1996). Psychotropic medications and the elderly. *Medsurg Nursing*. 5(3):191–194.

Fortinash, K., Holoday-Worret, P. (1995). *Psychiatric Nursing Care Plans*. St. Louis, MO: Mosby-Yearbook.

Lee, Mary. (1996). Drugs and the elderly: do you know the risks? *American Journal of Nursing*. 96(7):25–32.

Lucas, M. (1990). Understanding schizophrenia. *R.N.* 53(10): 52–56.

Piccinino, S. (1990). The nursing care challenge: borderline patients. *Journal of Psychosocial Nursing*. 28(4): 22–27.

Stuart, G., Sundeen, S. (1995). *Principles and Practice of Psychiatric Nursing*. St. Louis, MO: Mosby-Yearbook.

Torrey, E. F. (1988). *Surviving Schizophrenia: A Family Manual*. New York: Harper & Row.

Valente, S. (1991). Deliberate self-injury: management in a psychiatric setting. *Journal of Psychosocial Nursing*. 29(12):19–24.

Vallone, D. C., Stephanos, M. J. (1990). Minimizing drug reactions. *R.N.* 53(11):36–42.

Varacolis, E. (1994). *Foundations of Psychiatric Mental Health Nursing*. Philadelphia: Saunders.

Winter, D. (1990). Questions and answers about schizophrenia. *Journal of Psychosocial Nursing*. 29(8):7.

Zollo, M. B., Derse, A. (1997). The abusive patient: Where do you draw the line? *American Journal of Nursing*. 97(2): 31–35.

Zook, R. (1997). Handling inappropriate sexual behavior with confidence. *Nursing 97*. 27(4):65.

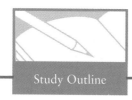

Study Outline

I. **Introduction**

A. Thought disorder: disorganized thought, behavior, hallucinations, and delusions are present.

1. Mood is altered, as are interpersonal relationships.

2. Incidence lower than mood disorders, but tends to be more debilitating and chronic.

3. Population affected is 1%.

B. Personality disorders: long-term conditions.

1. Borderline personality disorder most prevalent.

2. Diagnosis made in early adulthood.

3. Typical to see failed marriages, poor work histories, and difficulty with interpersonal relationships.

4. Four hallmarks of personality disorders.

a. Inflexible and maladaptive response to life events.

b. Serious difficulty in areas of personal and work relationships.

c. Tendency to evoke interpersonal conflict.

d. Tendency to evoke a negative empathic response from others.

C. Comparisons between thought and personality disorders.

1. Persons with thought disorders experience an altered reality and impaired ego functioning.

2. Thought disorders can be treated with medications.

3. Both benefit from psychotherapy.

II. **Nursing Assessment**

A. Thought disorders.

1. Presence of psychotic features (hallucinations, delusions, and grossly disorganized behavior and thinking).

2. Individuals look and act bizarre.

3. Ideas of reference present.

4. Delusions of grandeur and persecution.

5. Keep interview brief.

B. Personality disorders: enduring patterns of behavior where there is no loss of reality or impaired cognition.

   1. Patients do not look or act in bizarre or different ways.
   2. Assess view of self and others.
   3. Assess expression of feelings.
   4. Determine history of relationships.
   5. Determine history of impulsive behaviors.
   6. Do not make hasty diagnosis; leads to "labeling" behavior and can be counterproductive for both patient and staff.

III. Planning

A. Care for both of these disorders will be long term with intermittent treatment for acute episodes.

B. Goals for patients with thought disorders.
   1. Promote safety and trust.
   2. Educate about medication.
   3. Monitor medication compliance and effectiveness.
   4. Ensure adequate sleep and nutrition.
   5. Minimize social withdrawal.

C. Goals for patients with personality disorders.
   1. Set limits.
   2. Teach coping skills.
   3. Promote safety.
   4. Encourage insight into behavior.
   5. Monitor behavior changes.

IV. General Nursing Interventions

A. Thought disorders.
   1. Attitude of acceptance is important to promote trust.
   2. Administer antipsychotic medications.
   3. Encourage patient compliance with medications.
   4. Observe for toxic side effects of antipsychotic medications (Table 35-6).

B. Personality disorders.
   1. Set limits.
   2. Confront manipulative behavior.
   3. Monitor for self-mutilation.
   4. Implement suicide precautions, if necessary.

C. For specific interventions for patients with angry, hostile, aggressive, manipulative, or paranoid behavior, see Table 35-4.

V. Evaluation

A. Expected outcomes: thought disorders.
   1. Medication compliance.
   2. Relief of symptoms, positive and negative.
   3. Improved sleep and thinking.
   4. Decrease in psychomotor retardation.
   5. Improved affect.
   6. Improved trust.
   7. Improved motivation.

B. Expected outcomes: personality disorders.
   1. Demonstration of new coping strategies for handling stressors.
   2. Verbalization of anger without acting out.
   3. Increase in independent decision making.
   4. Decrease in manipulative behaviors.

VI. Common Nursing Diagnoses, Expected Outcomes and Nursing Interventions for Disorders of Thought and Personality (Table 35-3)

VII. Disorders of Thought

A. Include brief psychotic disorder, schizoaffective disorder, delusional disorder, schizophreniform disorder, shared psychotic disorder, psychotic disorder due to medical condition, substance-induced psychotic disorder, and psychotic disorder N.O.S.

B. Schizophrenia.
   1. Develops in late twenties.
   2. Schizophrenics are shunned and stigmatized because of their bizarre behavior.
   3. Are vulnerable to poverty, homelessness, substance abuse, and suicide.
   4. Cause.
      a. Biological basis probable.
      b. Increase in incidence when poverty, unemployment, and many environmental stressors are present.
   5. Signs and symptoms.
      a. Positive symptoms: hallucinations, delusions, and loose associations.
         (1) Easier to treat.
         (2) Treated with antipsychotic medications (Table 35-6).
      b. Negative symptoms: apathy, social isolation, poverty of thoughts, psychomotor retardation, blunted affect, and lack of motivation.
         (1) More difficult to treat.
         (2) Treated with therapeutic relationships and therapeutic environment.
   6. Treatment medications and therapeutic environment.
   7. Nursing interventions.
      a. Monitor medication compliance.
      b. Monitor side effects of antipsychotics.
      c. Promote trust.
      d. See Table 35-3.

VIII. Disorders of Personality

A. See Table 35-7 for description of personality disorders.

B. Borderline personality disorder.

1. Pattern of instability in relationships, affect, and self-image, and impulsive behavior.

2. Attach to others quickly and fear abandonment by others.

3. Engage in self-mutilation and suicidal gestures.

4. Use splitting behaviors: idealize a person and then devalue or idealize one and devalue another group.

5. Marked impulsivity: gambling, drinking, eating, sex, spending, or driving recklessly.

6. Treatment: long-term psychotherapy and medications to treat the symptoms of anxiety and depression.

7. Nursing interventions.

   a. Set limits without being rigid, controlling, and inflexible.

   b. Maintain good personal boundaries.

   c. Maintain safe environment.

   d. Initiate suicide precautions if necessary.

   e. Be aware of your own feelings.

IX. **Elder Care Points**

A. Elders who are taking antipsychotics are at a greater risk for developing extrapyramidal symptoms, tardive dyskinesia, and neuroleptic malignant syndrome.

B. Beginning doses should be one-half to one-third of the normal adult dose.

C. Elderly schizophrenics who are in nursing homes need particular attention paid to their physical health because they are less likely to seek attention because of social isolation and paranoia.

X. **Community Care**

A. Less frequent hospitalization noted.

B. See patients with thought and personality disorders in hospitals, nursing homes, clinics, and in the home.

Managing Medical–Surgical Issues

The two chapters in this unit deal with issues that every medical–surgical nurse must face in practice. Chapter 36 presents information on leadership and management skills. The realities of working with unlicensed assistive personnel (UAPs) is dealt with at length. Learning to delegate appropriately is part of learning to work efficiently. It also is necessary to conform to the boundaries of legal nursing practice. Chapter 37 discusses finding employment, becoming a good employee, broadening career goals, maintaining current knowledge and skills, and terminating employment gracefully. These chapters will assist the practical nurse graduate to make the transition more easily from student to employed nurse.

Leadership in Medical–Surgical Nursing

With the current changes in health care delivery, the licensed practical nurse (LPN) is taking on more and more leadership functions. Leadership is a comprehensive process that includes guiding staff, matching talent to task, and using resources to meet patient needs efficiently. Leadership requires a good grasp of basic management techniques. This chapter discusses the management skills and leadership qualities that the LPN needs *to be effective as a new nurse the first year after graduation.* More extensive leadership-management positions require considerable experience and advanced management skills.

THE CHAIN OF COMMAND

Once you are hired, it is important that you become familiar with the organizational structure of the health facility for which you work. This information is generally provided during your formal orientation to the facility. Be certain you know the chain of command for the area in which you are employed. Who is your immediate supervisor? From whom do you take orders? To whom does your supervisor report? To whom should you report changes in patient condition, signs of complications, and so on? To whom do you go with concerns or complaints? Who is in charge of scheduling your hours? Whom should you call if you are ill and cannot make it to work?

LEADERSHIP STYLES

Most leaders employ a blend of leadership styles. A permissive, or *"laissez-faire,"* leader does not attempt to control the team and offers little, if any, direction. This leader assumes that the members of the team are competent and self-directed and will do what needs to be done correctly and efficiently. This leader often needs to be liked by everyone and therefore avoids any blame for things that go wrong by allowing members to function completely independently.

The *authoritarian* or *autocratic* leader tightly controls team members. Staff are rarely consulted when decisions are to be made. Rules are set without input from the staff and directives, and orders are given out constantly. **This leader closely supervises the work of each staff member.** When mistakes are made, they are quickly pointed out. The goal of this leader is to accomplish tasks without regard to the effect on the people.

The *democratic* leader frequently consults with staff members and seeks staff participation in decision making. The skills and knowledge of the team members are readily used to ensure that the team functions

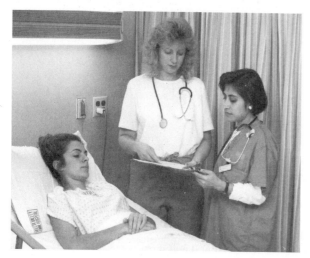

FIGURE 36-1.   Licensed practical nurse delegating a task to a nursing assistant.

efficiently. Team members are respected as individuals, and there is an open and trusting attitude overall. The democratic leader is part of the team, not sitting above it, and accepts responsibility for the actions of the team.

There is no one set of qualities that make a good leader. Table 36-1 lists responses that nurses have given when asked what they think makes a good leader. Such a leader instills confidence, trust, and spirit into the team. Appropriate leadership fosters growth among the team members.

***Think about* . . .** With what type of leader do you prefer to work? Why? Is there a situation in which an autocratic leader is needed? Can you explain why?

KEYS TO EFFECTIVE LEADERSHIP

As an LPN you will be expected to work with other members of the health care team. **Collaboration is essential for cost-effective patient care.** Part of your collaborative practice will be to learn to work effectively

TABLE 36-1 ♦ *Attributes That Make a Good Leader*	
♦ Ability to teach	♦ Flexible
♦ Active listener	♦ Good role model
♦ Articulate	♦ Good sense of humor
♦ Assertive	♦ Objective
♦ Calm	♦ Open-minded
♦ Considerate	♦ Organized
♦ Consistent	♦ Responsible
♦ Decisive	♦ Sensitive
♦ Excellent clinical skills	♦ Strong character
♦ Excellent problem solver	♦ Tactful
♦ Fair	

with unlicensed assistive personnel (UAPs), which include unit secretaries, nursing assistants, homemaking aids, housekeeping personnel, and various types of technicians. To be effective in this role, you must learn to delegate tasks appropriately and effectively.

♦ Effective Communication

Leaders use good communication skills. Communicating in direct, concise terms in a tactful, friendly, nonthreatening way is essential to create a supportive work environment. Obtaining feedback about directions given and listening actively to reports, suggestions, and complaints establishes a pattern for two-way communication. This helps the leader stay in tune with the atmosphere, attitudes, and problems of others on the health care team.

Communicating effectively includes taking the time to attend to the person by stopping what you are doing, establishing eye contact with the other person, remembering to be polite by saying "Please" and "Thank you," and using a warm tone of voice. Saying "I would like you to take vital signs on the right side of the hall please," rather than "Go and take vital signs on that side of the hall," usually enlists better cooperation and a more pleasant attitude toward the task. **Treat others in the manner you prefer to be treated.**

When assigning tasks, be certain to be very specific about what is to be done, how it is to be done, and when the task is to be completed. Inquire if there are questions before ending the interaction. Many a conflict can be avoided by being thorough when giving directions, making a request, or assigning a task.

If a conflict does arise, try to remain calm and open, and actively listen to the problem. Accept responsibility for any part you played in the development of the conflict. Focus on the issue rather than on the feelings of those involved. Mediate by communicating openly. Sort out the issues involved by identifying key themes in the discussion. Consider the options, and weigh the consequences of each option. Choose the option for conflict resolution that offers the best outcome.

♦ Clinical Competence and Confidence

As a nurse leader you must demonstrate competence in the skills of the profession. Confidence in the ability to perform those skills well is essential if you are to have the respect of the other members of the team. Along with this competence and confidence should be sufficient self-esteem to readily admit when a mistake has been made or when you don't know something. Announcing "I don't know, but I will find out," is the best way to handle such a situation. Others will respect you more if you openly admit that you don't know everything. The ability to admit such a thing shows your human side and provides an atmosphere in which others can admit what they don't know and can ask for help.

◆ Organization

Being a leader requires good organization. Organizing the work of a unit requires time-management skills. Each day should be carefully planned, but the plan should have some built-in flexibility for unforeseen events and needs. Knowing the strengths of each member of the health care team helps the leader divide the workload more effectively. Decision-making ability is needed quickly to divide up patients and assign tasks to various personnel. Problem-solving skills enable difficult decisions to be made. The good problem solver first defines the problem, then looks at the alternatives. The outcomes of using each of the alternatives is estimated, and then one of the alternatives is chosen. If the alternative chosen does not work to solve the problem, then the whole process is repeated.

◆ Delegation

You are accountable for the tasks you delegate. Legally, as a licensed nurse, you are responsible and accountable for the outcome of any task you delegate to another. Delegating appropriately means that you must (1) know the capabilities and competencies of the person to whom you are delegating a specific task; (2) know whether or not the task falls within the domain of tasks that can legally be delegated by you; (3) communicate effectively with the person to whom you are delegating; and (4) understand the patient's needs.

Before any tasks are delegated to a UAP, the person should be thoroughly oriented to the facility and the unit on which he or she is employed. **Competencies of unlicensed personnel must be documented before tasks are delegated to them.** This requires evidence of a training program and *written evidence by a qualified nurse or instructor that the person has demonstrated competence in the task or skill.* If you do not have access to such written documentation, it is best to observe the UAP perform the task or skill the first time you delegate it to verify that a level of competence has been reached. If the task has not been a part of formal training program for the UAP, then you should demonstrate how the task should be done and ask for a return demonstration.

Think about . . . How would you tactfully tell UAPs that you would like to see a particular task performed before assigning them to do it on their own?

Be familiar with your nurse practice act so that you know what tasks and skills fall within your legal domain. This tells you what you must not delegate. Your agency should have a job description that spells out what the UAPs can and cannot do. Be certain that you are familiar with the UAP job description before you delegate a task. *It is up to you to know what the UAP cannot do.* The policies and procedures of the agency and the standards of practice for your area of nursing help define what the UAP is allowed to do. **Do not delegate assessment or aspects of the analysis, planning, or evaluation phases of the nursing process. These must be performed by the licensed nurse.** The majority of tasks that are to be delegated to UAPs are technical, repetitive skills. **Interventions that require professional judgment should not be delegated.** Within the area of general competencies, the UAP should be assessed for competence in patient safety issues such as infection control and moving and positioning patients.

Effective communication to the UAP means sending clear, concise messages and listening carefully to feedback. It is better to say, "Please take Mrs. Jones's temperature at 2:00 P.M. and let me know right away what it is so that I can let her doctor know," than to just say "Mrs. Jones's temperature needs to be taken at 2:00 P.M." "Tell me immediately if Mr. Hoskin's temperature is above 101.2° F.," is better than "Let me know if Mr. Hoskin's temperature is high." Delegating effectively means including the result desired and the timeline for completion. Ask the UAP whether there are any questions about what is to be done, and ask for a summary of what he or she understands is to be done. Asking the person to share with you what you have just said, or for their understanding of what you have requested will verify that your request has been received as intended. Tell the UAP where you will be if a problem or question arises during performance of the task. Be certain that delegation of the task has been accepted by the delegatee, and then give up responsibility for that task to that person. **Remember that when you delegate you do not give up your responsibility for overall patient care.** You must follow through by verifying that the task has been completed in a timely manner.

Effective delegation includes giving feedback on how the task was performed. Give praise where it is due; share favorable comments from patients about the UAPs' work and interactions. If things did not go well, communicate exactly what went wrong in a supportive manner. **Be certain that privacy is provided before giving criticism.** Be tactful. You might share that the patient was upset that it took three tries for the UAP to obtain an accurate blood pressure. Asking "do you think you need some more supervised practice and suggestions on how to take blood pressures smoothly? Would you like me to demonstrate it again?" allows the UAP a face-saving way to admit that more instruction is needed. Ask what might help the UAP perform better the next time.

When giving constructive criticism begin by tactfully acknowledging feelings or expressing empathy. Statements such as "I understand that we are one aide short today," begin the interaction on a less threatening note. Next describe the behavior. An example would be: "I've noticed that it has been 9:30 three mornings this week before vital signs you took were posted." Then state the expectation for future compliance, such as: "It is necessary for the vital signs to be posted no later than 8:30 A.M. from now on." Last state the consequences if the expected action does not occur. This can be done by stating something like "the physicians and medication nurses have to track you down when the vital signs are not posted on time. If posting is late again, I will have to document your inability to complete the task on time." When delegating a variety of tasks you also will probably need to help the UAP prioritize the order in which they should be done. It takes many months for most UAPs to be able to discern which tasks take priority over others. **When performance by a UAP has been poor, documentation of the specific facts (not your opinions) must be done.** The unit manager should also be made aware of the performance problem.

The patient must be told when an unlicensed person will be performing some tasks that were formerly performed only by nurses. This is within the domain of patient's rights. Simply tell the patient that you, the nurse, have primary responsibility for the care given, but that the UAP is your assistant and will be doing certain tasks (Table 36-2).

TABLE 36-2 ♦ *Delegatable Tasks for Unlicensed Assistive Personnel (UAPs)* *

♦ Applying cold packs	♦ Give a vaginal douche
♦ Applying a condom catheter	♦ Hair care
♦ Applying elastic stockings	♦ Measuring weight and
♦ Applying a hearing aid	height
♦ Applying warm compresses	♦ Oral hygiene
♦ Assisting to deep-breathe	♦ Performing ROM exercises
and cough	♦ Providing skin care
♦ Assisting with ambulation	♦ Removing a foley catheter
♦ Baths	♦ Recording intake and output
♦ Bed making	♦ Repositioning patients
♦ Blood glucose monitoring	♦ Stocking supplies
♦ Collection of specimens	♦ Taking specimens to the
♦ Emptying drainage	laboratory
containers	♦ Toileting patients
♦ Feeding patients	♦ Transfering to a chair
♦ Filling water pitchers	or bed
♦ Giving an enema	♦ Turning patients
♦ Give a sitz bath	♦ Vital signs

*May vary from state to state and from facility to facility.

♦ Beginning Leadership Roles

Initially the new LPN will be performing leadership functions in working with UAPs. This requires appropriate delegation of tasks and supervision of the UAPs' work. Later on, when the new graduate is thoroughly oriented to the facility and its policies and is functioning competently, team leading may be required. A team leader coordinates and assigns other personnel, assists with patient care, helps resolve conflicts, assists with the writing of policies and procedures, contributes information for evaluation of UAPs, and collaborates with physicians and other health team members.

When working in a medical clinic, the LPN team leader often is responsible for overseeing the scheduling of patients, performing quality assurance audits, training other staff, evaluating other staff, coordinating the members of the team to accomplish the daily work, assisting with the writing of policies and procedures, attending staff meetings, and resolving staff conflicts.

An LPN working in home care may be asked to assign and supervise nursing assistants and home health aides, in which case she or he will make patient care assignments, assist with orientation and evaluation, verify that paperwork ensuring reimbursement is correctly completed, and give and receive report on assigned patients.

Think about . . . What leadership functions do LPNs perform in the facility in which you are assigned for clinical experience?

ADVANCED LEADERSHIP ROLES

Eventually the LPN may become a charge nurse or a supervisor of UAPs in settings such as home care or outpatient clinics. **A charge nurse must have some training and experience in nursing administration and supervision and additional preparation in a specialized area.** At least one year's experience as a staff nurse is required before taking on charge nurse duties.

The ability to recognize significant changes in patient condition and to take necessary action is a primary quality in a charge nurse. **This person is responsible for the total nursing care of the patients on the unit during the shift.**

In a long-term care facility, the charge nurse receives reports from the previous shift, makes patient assignments, makes rounds and assesses all patients, directs the administration of medications and treatments, confers with team members throughout the shift, and reports to the oncoming shift on patient status. Charge nurses also may be responsible for overseeing training of UAPs and for evaluating members of the unit's health care team.

MANAGEMENT SKILLS FOR THE LICENSED PRACTICAL NURSE

All nurses are expected to be able to manage time, use a computer, order supplies, transcribe physician's orders, place phone calls for needed orders, process verbal orders, and document care appropriately for reimbursement of patient costs.

◆ Time Management

Leaders need to use time efficiently. Some techniques can be learned to assist with time management. Each work day should begin by making a "to-do" list before the shift starts. This just provides a loose structure for the day. One or two general goals for the day should be formulated. The goal for the home care nurse might be to complete four visits by lunchtime. Work organization for this nurse involves determining the most efficient order for the visits scheduled for the day, gathering all needed supplies, notifying patients of the approximate time of the visit, organizing the paperwork to be completed, and making certain there is gas in the car.

Organizing for the work day in a medical clinic varies depending on the type of clinic and the assigned duties of the nurse. Treatment rooms may need to be stocked and set up for scheduled treatments, charts pulled for patients scheduled to be seen, or supplies in examining rooms replenished.

For the staff nurse in the hospital, the shift's goal might be "to ensure that all assigned patients be kept comfortable and safe and that all scheduled treatments and medications are given." This is a measurable goal. After receiving report and obtaining the patient assignment, priorities should be set. To do this, identify the patients with the most significant or life-threatening problems. Which patients are physically unstable and need to be checked frequently? Which patients have frequently scheduled assessments or treatments? Which patients are most at risk for complications? Which patients are a safety risk because they are confused? Priorities are set according to patient need. Unstable patients take precedence over stable patients. Scheduled medications and treatments must be done before tasks that are ordered t.i.d.

The goal for the long-term care nurse might be to delegate and coordinate care of assigned patients and finish all scheduled tasks on time and keep the patients safe and comfortable. Take a few minutes before making rounds to devise a time schedule for the work of the shift. Use a grid that shows each hour of the shift and each patient and room number. Note times you will delegate tasks, assess patients, check IVs, give treatments, turn patients, document care, perform teaching, and prepare for report. **Documentation is a critical task in all settings and must be considered a priority when organizing to accomplish the daily workload.**

Use a separate grid to note when medications are due for each patient. Use this sheet to note when you give PRN medications. That way you have a quick refresher for charting the PRN medications in the progress notes. As you work throughout the day, you can make small notes on your work organization sheet that will provide data and a guide for charting.

Next, consider what has to be done sometime during the shift. Checking the "crash" cart would be such a task. Note on your work schedule when you feel you will have time to do that. Finally consider things that you would like to do if time permits, such as spending time talking with a lonely patient, giving a backrub, or making a phone call to a patient's family. Jot these at the bottom of the worksheet.

Once the work is organized, begin your patient assessment rounds. This should be done early in the shift. Patient status can sometimes change dramatically during the change-of-shift time. Quickly assess each patient's area of greatest problem (usually the one for which they were admitted). Check all tubes and equipment attached to the patient. You will be able to do more in-depth assessments later in the shift. Right now you just need to determine whether there are any emergencies, get a feel for the patient's status and needs, and determine what equipment and supplies you will need for each patient during the shift. Inquire about the need for pain medication or other PRN medication while initially in the room. These then can be brought back during early-morning medication rounds unless the medication is a badly needed analgesic; this should be administered immediately.

At the end of the day you should evaluate the effectiveness of your time management. Did your schedule help? Did it work pretty well, as you had it planned? Did you need more time to complete a task than you thought it would take? This analysis helps you create a more workable plan the next time. Keep in mind that work plans must be flexible. Even the best plans can get destroyed if one patient's status deteriorates markedly. This happens to all nurses from time to time.

Think about . . . Can you design a shift time management sheet for yourself that suits your work style and needs?

◆ Using Computers

Computers are used in all health care facilities. The nurse must become proficient in using them to perform everyday functions for patient care and unit administration. The computer is used to place orders to the various departments for supplies, medications, diets, laboratory and diagnostic tests, and engineering and housekeeping needs. Surgery is scheduled by computer. Staffing patterns may be scheduled by computer. Nursing care plans are constructed on the computer and are updated and revised as needed every 24 hours by the nurse. Acuity levels for patients are tracked. Agency census is compiled on the computer. Laboratory results often are sent to the unit via computer.

It is evident that each nurse must quickly learn to use the agency's computers efficiently to perform all necessary tasks for the job. Some agencies are now requiring nurses to chart actions completed and to write progress notes on the computer. It may not be long before paper charts will be a thing of the past.

◆ Transcription of Orders

When handling newly written orders, first read all the orders. Then transcribe the *"stat"* (do immediately) orders first. Transfer the orders to the Kardex, computer "care plan," medication and treatment cards (if used), and the medication administration record (MAR). Each medication order must include the patient's name and room number, the name of the medication (preferably both generic and trade name), ordered dosage, route of administration, the times the doses are to be given, the date the order was written, and the date it is to be discontinued and/or renewed. **Check off each order as it is transcribed.** Narcotics, anticoagulants, hypnotics, and antibiotics must be renewed every 48 to 72 hours depending on agency policy and state laws. Sign off the order with a red line across the page under the physician's signature and your first initial, last name, and official designation. Include the date and the time. Notify the person who will be giving the medication of the new order. The order is transmitted to the pharmacy by phone or computer and a copy of it is sent to the pharmacy.

Dietary orders are transmitted to the dietary department and entered on the Kardex or computer "care plan" along with notations for any fluid restrictions or requirements for intake and output recording. If intake and output records are required, a recording sheet is placed in the patient's room or on the door to the room.

Unclear orders should be clarified directly with the physician who wrote them. When medications arrive on the unit from the pharmacy, they should be checked with the physician's orders before placing them in the patient's drawer or bin. This may be completed by a pharmacy technician. Because of frequent changes in orders, all medication orders on the MAR or Kardex should be verified with the chart orders once every 24 hours.

Positioning, intake and output, treatment requirements, and use of special equipment are noted on the Kardex or on the computer "care plan" for each patient. **Allergies are noted on the MAR sheet and on the front of the chart to alert all personnel.**

When a medication is discontinued, cross out the item on the MAR/Kardex by using a highlighter over it and write "DC" with the date and time. Notify the nurse giving the medications for the shift. Alert the pharmacy of the discontinuation order and return leftover doses of the medication to the pharmacy for proper crediting to the patient's account. Sign off the discontinue order on the physician's order sheet.

Orders for laboratory and diagnostic tests require that the order be transmitted to the appropriate department by phone or computer and the correct requisition slip filled out. The forms and labels for specimen containers are stamped with the patient's addressograph plate. If blood samples are to be drawn when the patient is in a "fasting" state, then an "NPO" status must be transmitted to dietary, to the nurses, and to the patient. An "NPO" sign is posted on the door to the patient's room. The test must be ordered to be drawn before the breakfast hour. A barium enema (BE) and upper gastrointestinal (GI) series are scheduled with the BE before the upper GI series to prevent swallowed barium from interfering with the BE. Laboratory and diagnostic test orders are recorded on the Kardex or computer "care plan" along with dietary restrictions and pretest medications.

Preoperative orders should include diet/NPO status desired, necessary preoperative treatments, a notation regarding the operative consent and the exact procedure to be performed, laboratory and diagnostic tests to be completed, patient education required, and orders for sedatives or preoperative medications. There also may be orders for the type of surgical preparation to be performed and when, insertion of an IV cannula and what solution is to be started, insertion of a Foley catheter, or application of elastic hose. **All preoperative orders are considered canceled at the time the patient enters surgery.**

Postoperative orders should include a schedule for vital sign measurement; directions for care of tubes, suction, and dressings; IV solutions to be infused; medications to be administered; diet permitted; measurement of intake and output; directions for positioning, activity, turning, coughing and deep-breathing; and time to catheterize if the patient is unable to void and does not have an indwelling catheter. Additional orders may request circulation checks or monitoring of neurological status.

◆ Taking Verbal Orders

Orders by physicians should be written, but at times verbal orders or telephone orders are given, with the expectation that the nurse will write the orders in the chart for the physician to sign later. If a physician asks a nurse to write a verbal order on a chart while they are together on the unit, the nurse should have the physician verify and sign the order before leaving the unit.

The legal ability of the LPN to take verbal orders from a physician depends on the laws of the state and the written policies of the agency in which he or she is employed. **Verbal orders can be taken only by licensed nurses and in some states only by an RN.**

If your state and agency allow you to take a verbal or telephone order, follow the guidelines in Table 36-3. After verifying that the order is correct, the nurse enters it on the physician's order sheet and marks it "V.O." (verbal order) or "T.O." (telephone order) with the date, time, first initial, last name, and professional designation (RN or LPN). **The physician must sign the written form of the verbal order as soon as possible.**

◆ Documentation for Reimbursement

All nurses must document care delivered. Each type of agency has guidelines about the details of care that must be documented and how often each must be noted. **Any time equipment is in use that is being billed to the patient's account, a note must be in the chart that explains why the equipment is being used as well as objective statements that show that the equipment is still needed.** When a patient is receiving specific treatments, the reason the treatment is needed and each time a treatment is given must be documented. An example would be a home visit for wound care. The nurse must document objectively the appearance of the wound, how it is cleaned and dressed, and an assessment of whether it is improving or not. Specific objective information, such as actual wound dimensions, color, and characteristics, is included. **For a home care patient, the nurse also must document evidence that the patient still needs to be treated at home rather than at the doctor's office.** Orientation at the employing agency should include specifics of the type of documentation necessary for reimbursement.

Leadership and management skills develop with practice and continued learning. Professional growth is an important aspect of an evolving career in nursing. Each nurse should seek his or her own direction and pursue growth opportunities. Once the nurse has solid clinical skills and at least a year of experience, there is the confidence necessary to take on greater responsibility. It is at this point that the opportunity to accept a greater leadership role should be considered.

CRITICAL THINKING EXERCISES

Situations

1. You are assigned 10 patients on the day shift. You have one nursing assistant who can help you but who also is helping another nurse.
   - ◆ What tasks should you consider delegating to this UAP?
   - ◆ How would you verify that tasks you have delegated have been done and done correctly? Would this method help build team spirit?

2. Within your patient care assignment you have a gentleman with pneumonia, a woman with heart failure, a postoperative colectomy patient, a diabetic with an infected leg ulcer, and a man with pancreatitis. When organizing your work for the day, in what order of priority would you place each patient?
   - ◆ If within your assignment are patients that have scheduled neurological checks, glucose monitoring, and wound care, in which order would you handle these tasks?
   - ◆ If you have a patient with nausea and vomiting, one with postoperative pain, and one with chest pain, whose needs would you try to meet first?

3. You are team-leading. Two of your staff begin to bicker about who should be answering the call light that keeps coming on. How would you handle the situation?

4. Mrs. Horton needs to have her blood sugar checked before lunch. You want the nursing assistant to perform this task and she was trained to do it. Mrs.

TABLE 36-3 ◆ Guidelines for Taking Telephone Orders

- ◆ Write the order down on a piece of paper.
- ◆ Read it back to the physician; verify spelling of medications or diagnostic tests. Do this every time with every physician.
- ◆ Write the order on the physician's order sheet, note the date and time, and indicate "TO" for telephone order with your first initial, last name, LVN or LPN.
- ◆ See that the physician signs off on the order when making rounds; this must be done within 48 hours in most agencies.
- ◆ If a telephone order is requested from midnight to 6:00 A.M., have another person, preferably a nurse, on an extension to verify the order. Physicians awakened from a sound sleep sometimes do not recall the exact order. Have the other nurse initial the order; or have the other person document the order as they heard it given and sign it.
- ◆ Make an entry in the nurse's notes describing the circumstances that prompted a telephone order. Include the statement that the orders were read back to the physician and that they were confirmed to be accurate by the physician when read back.

Horton is fussy and dislikes having her finger stuck for this procedure.

- ◆ Describe the phrases you would use to delegate this task and to prepare the UAP to interact with this patient.
- ◆ Mrs. Horton later complains to you that the UAP didn't wash her hands before performing the procedure. How would you handle this breach of procedure with the UAP?

BIBLIOGRAPHY

Arnold, E., Boggs, K. (1995). *Interpersonal Relationships: Professional Communication Skills for Nurses,* 2nd ed. Philadelphia: W. B. Saunders.

Canavan, K. (1997). Combating dangerous delegation. *American Journal of Nursing.* 97(5):57–58.

Douglass, M. E., Douglass, D. N. (1994). Handling change effectively: ten tips for weathering the storm. *Nursing 94.* 24(9):92, 95.

Grensing-Pophal, L. (1997). How to become a master juggler. (1997). *Nursing 97.* 27(3):79.

Grensing-Pophal, L. (1997). Improving your leadership skills. *Nursing 97.* 27(4):41.

Grippando, G. M., Mitchell, P. R. (1993). *Nursing Perspectives and Issues,* 5th ed. Albany, NY: Delmar.

Hansten, R. I., Washburn, M. (1992). Working with people: what do you say when you delegate work to others? *American Journal of Nursing.* 92(7):48, 50.

Hansten, R. I., Washburn, M. (1992). Working with people: what's your feedback style? *American Journal of Nursing.* 92(8):56–61.

Hawke, M. (1995). Are you management material? *Nursing 95.* 25(11):82–83.

Hill, S. S., Howlett, H. A. (1997). *Success in Practical Nursing,* 3rd ed. Philadelphia: Saunders.

Huston, C. J., Marquis, B. L. (1995). Seven steps to successful decision-making. *American Journal of Nursing.* 95(5):65–67.

Kroll, B. N. (1993). Taking charge: decisions: A good manager has to delegate. *RN.* 56(2):23–23, 26.

Kurzen, C. R. (1993). *Contemporary Practical/Vocational Nursing,* 3rd ed. Philadelphia: Lippincott.

Manion, J. (1995). Understanding the seven stages of change. *American Journal of Nursing.* 95(4):41–43.

Osborn, E. (1997). Organizational skills: Half the battle. *Home Healthcare Nurse.* 15(1):1997.

Osguthorpe, S. G. (1997). Managing a shift effectively: The role of the charge nurse. *Critical Care Nurse.* 17(2):64–69.

Parkman, C. A. (1996). Delegation: are you doing it right? *American Journal of Nursing.* 96(9):43–47.

Rich, P. L. (1995). Becoming a team: working with nursing assistants. *Nursing 95.* 25(5):100–103.

Sheehan, J. (1996). Safeguard your license: Avoid these pitfalls. *RN.* 59(12):59–62.

Sullivan, E. J., Decker, P. J. (1992). *Effective Management in Nursing,* 3rd ed. Redwood City, CA: Addison-Wesley.

Sullivan, G. H. (1995). Legally speaking: when assignments don't match skills. *RN.* 58(4):57–58, 60.

Tappen, R. M. (1994). *Nursing Leadership and Management: Concepts and Practice,* 3rd ed. Philadelphia: Davis.

Walton, J. C., Waszkiewicz, M. (1997). Managing unlicensed assistive personnel: Tips for improving quality outcomes. *MEDSURG Nursing.* 6(1):24–28.

Zerwekh, J., Claborn J. C. (1997). *Nursing Today: Transition and Trends,* 2nd ed. Philadelphia: Saunders.

Zimmerman, P. G. (1997). Delegating to unlicensed assistive personnel. *Nursing 97.* 27(5):71.

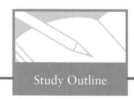

Study Outline

I. **Introduction**
   A. More and more LPNs have to assume increasing leadership functions with the changes in the health care system.
   B. Leadership requires a good grasp of management techniques.

II. **The Chain of Command**
   A. To be an effective leader you must understand the organizational structure of the agency for whom you work.
   B. Know the chain of command within the agency.

III. **Leadership Styles**
   A. Most leaders use a blend of leadership styles.
   B. A *laissez-faire* leader offers little, if any, direction.
   C. The *authoritarian* or *autocratic* leader tightly controls team members.
   D. The *democratic* leader frequently consults other staff members and seeks participation in decision making.
   E. No one set of qualities makes a good leader (Table 36-1).

IV. Keys to Effective Leadership

A. Collaboration is essential for cost-effective patient care.

B. The LPN must learn to work effectively with UAPs.

C. Effective communication is one key to good leadership.

   1. Communicate in direct, concise terms in a tactful, friendly, nonthreatening way.

   2. Obtain feedback about directions given to a UAP.

   3. Listen actively to reports, suggestions, and complaints.

   4. Attend to the person with whom you are communicating by stopping what you are doing and establishing eye contact (unless this is culturally unacceptable to the other person).

   5. Phrase requests politely instead of issuing commands to do tasks.

   6. Treat others as you would prefer to be treated.

   7. When assigning tasks, be specific about what is to be done, how it is to be done, and when the task is to be completed.

   8. When a conflict arises, remain calm and open and actively listen to the problem. Focus on the issue rather than on the feelings involved.

D. Clinical competence and confidence are necessary for a leader.

   1. Display expert skills.

   2. Admit a mistake or when you don't know something.

E. Organization of work tasks for the unit is essential.

   1. Allow some flexibility in work schedules.

   2. Become a good problem solver: define the problem; look at the alternatives; estimate the outcome for each alternative; choose the best alternative to solve the problem.

F. Delegation is essential to accomplish the workload.

   1. You are accountable for the tasks you delegate.

   2. To delegate appropriately you must:

      a. Know the capabilities and competencies of the person to whom you are delegating a specific task.

      b. Understand which tasks you can legally delegate.

      c. Communicate effectively with the person to whom you are delegating.

      d. Understand the needs of the patient for whom the task is delegated.

      e. The competencies of UAPs must be documented before tasks are delegated to them.

      f. Most tasks that can be delegated are technical, repetitive skills; **interventions that require professional judgment should not be delegated.**

      g. Be certain that the task has been accepted by the UAP and then give up the responsibility for the task; follow up to see that the task was completed satisfactorily.

      h. Provide feedback on how the task was performed.

      i. Be certain privacy is provided if criticism of performance is necessary.

      j. Document unsafe behaviors or poor performance factually and report it to your supervisor.

V. Beginning Leadership Roles

A. Delegation of tasks to UAPs is a beginning leadership function.

B. Team leading may follow at a later date after thorough orientation and adjustment to the facility.

C. In a medical clinic, the team leader may oversee scheduling of patients, perform quality assurance audits, train other staff, evaluate other staff, coordinate the team, and perform other duties.

D. In home care, the LPN may be asked to assign and supervise certified nurse aids (CNAs) and home health aides by making assignments, assisting with orientation and evaluation, completing paperwork for reimbursement of agency services, and receiving report on assigned patients.

VI. Advanced Leadership Roles

A. Eventually the LPN may become a charge nurse in a long-term care facility or a supervisor of UAPs in home care or outpatient settings.

B. A charge nurse must have some training and experience in nursing administration and supervision and additional preparation in a specialized area. At least 1 year's experience as a staff nurse is required.

C. The charge nurse is responsible for the total nursing care of the patients on the unit during the shift.

VII. Management Skills for the Licensed Practical Nurse

A. Time management must be efficient.

   1. To-do lists help organize tasks.

   2. Goals should be set.

   3. A work organization plan for the day should be made.

   4. Time for documentation should be inserted into the work schedule.

B. Patient rounds should be made early in the shift.

   1. Develop the ability to perform a quick head-to-toe initial assessment.

   2. Assess what supplies and equipment will be needed in that room or place for the day's work.

C. At the end of the day evaluate the effectiveness of the day's work plan.

D. Using computers.

1. The computer must be used to place orders to various departments, obtain data, schedule surgery, update acuity levels and census, and in some institutions, to chart.

2. Computer expertise is essential for work efficiency.

E. Transcription of orders.

1. Do "stat" orders first.

2. Transfer orders to the Kardex, computer "care plan," medication, and treatment cards or medication administration record (MAR).

3. Check off each order as it is transcribed.

4. Sign off orders correctly.

5. Clarify unclear orders with the physician who wrote them.

6. Verbal orders should be signed by the physician as soon as possible.

7. The legality of an LPN taking telephone or verbal orders varies from state to state. **Know your state's laws.**

8. Follow guidelines in Table 36-3 for taking telephone orders.

F. Documentation for reimbursement.

1. All care must be documented.

2. Each agency will have guidelines for the type of documentation that must be done to obtain reimbursement for services rendered.

3. Any time special equipment is in use, there must be notes in the chart indicating that there is still a need for the equipment.

4. Documentation of a home care visit must include evidence that the patient is still homebound and could not be treated elsewhere.

CHAPTER 37

Professional Issues

O B J E C T I V E S

Upon completing of this chapter the student should be able to:
1. Apply for a nursing position by filling out the application and submitting a résumé.
2. Participate appropriately in a job interview.
3. State methods to maintain a current knowledge base in nursing.
4. Identify three reasons to belong to professional organizations.
5. Discuss ways to contribute to the community as a nurse.

The completion of nursing school brings the challenge of finding appropriate employment as a nurse. To become employed, the nurse must fill out job applications, prepare and submit a résumé, and participate in job interviews. This chapter prepares you for these tasks.

Nursing licensure in many states requires a certain number of hours of continuing education for renewal. Legally a nurse must meet current standards of practice in carrying out duties and responsibilities. To do this, the nurse needs to be up-to-date on procedures and knowledge of disease conditions, treatments, and medications. A lifelong commitment to continuing education is the only way to achieve the knowledge needed. There are various ways to obtain this knowledge, and they are discussed in this chapter.

Belonging to a professional organization also is part of being a professional. Such membership brings many benefits and offers ways in which the nurse can contribute to nursing as a profession.

The nurse's role as a teacher of preventive health care and self-care requires that there be involvement with the community. Through participation in community activities, membership in community organizations, and using teaching skills regarding health wherever possible, the nurse can truly contribute to the community.

PREPARING TO APPLY FOR A JOB

Networking with others you meet who are employed as nurses or who have positions in health care agencies is a good way to establish a base of contacts for possible leads to open nursing positions. **Networking** means getting out and meeting people, exchanging phone numbers, expressing interest in other persons and what they are doing, and establishing a business relationship that might be mutually beneficial. Performing volunteer work or working as a patient care assistant during nursing school can put you in a position to meet other members of the health care professions. These contacts are valuable when it comes time to look for employment.

Think about... How many people do you have in your professional network? How can you add network contacts?

The first step in applying for employment is to determine what type of position you desire and in what geographical location you are willing to work. Factors such as transportation to and from work, cost of commuting, and time spent commuting should be taken into consideration. No matter how desirable the job, if it is going to cause extra stress for you to reach the location where children need to be dropped off in the morning and picked up at the appointed hour, perhaps a position closer to that location would be better. Search out the availability of the type of position that is best for you first; if no such position is available in your chosen geographical area, then you have the option of looking for a different position or of widening the area of search.

Newspaper ads, journal advertisements, community or school job fairs, the local state nurse's association office, peers, instructors, and friends may all provide news of job openings. Calling the personnel office of any agency in which you wish to work to find out whether a position is open is another avenue. Once a position vacancy is located, then an appointment for an interview can be made. This can be done either by phoning the agency or by writing a query letter inquiring about the availability of a position. When you send a query letter you also should include your résumé. Figure 37-1 shows an example of a cover letter.

Usually an application for the position is filled out by the applicant before a job interview takes place. Some agencies may do a preliminary interview first. To fill out a job application you will need the following:

- Your social security number.
- Dates of graduation from high school and nursing school.

- Other dates of attendance and degrees obtained from any college.
- Dates of previous employment (starting and ending) and name of supervisor.
- Names, addresses, and telephone numbers of three references. At least two of these should be "professional" references. You should ask your teachers if they will act as a reference for you before their names are submitted.

The application should be filled out legibly in ink or typed if you fill it out at home. **Neatness and accuracy are very important.** You should take a résumé with you to the interview in case the interviewer asks for it. Place it in a folder so that it stays clean and neat.

Nancy S. Crebs
8746 Old Springs Road
Dallas, Texas 75218
(214) 348-0186

March 30, 1996

Ms. JoAnn Normandy
Nurse Recruiter
Oakhaven Medical Center
21215 Audelia Rd.
Dallas, Texas 75238

Dear Ms. Normandy:

I will be graduating from my Vocational Nursing program in May. I will take my licensure examination the last week of May. I'm writing to inquire if your institution will have an LVN opening in June? I completed a semester of my clinical experience in your facility and really liked the type of nursing that is practiced there and the upbeat attitude of all the staff.

I have worked for three years as a Certified Nursing Assistant and am well organized in my work. I relate well to elderly clients and enjoy working with them and their families.

I am available after 3:30 p.m. Monday, Wednesday, and Friday, and during Spring Break week, April 3 -7, for an interview.

I am enclosing my resume and hope to hear from you regarding a possible position in the near future.

Sincerely,

Nancy S. Crebs
Enc.

FIGURE 37-1   Example of a cover letter.

It is important to start job hunting well in advance of graduation. There will be lots of other graduates out there looking for positions. "The early bird gets the worm" often applies in these situations. A good time to start is one month after the beginning of your last semester of nursing school, assuming you plan to begin work shortly after graduation.

Think about . . . How many ads are there in the Sunday edition of the local paper for LPN positions? Would you be interested in applying for any of them?

PREPARING YOUR RÉSUMÉ

A résumé may be the employer's first introduction to you. It is your first opportunity to sell yourself by presenting your strengths. It must be neat and presentable. Table 37-1 lists the guidelines for résumé preparation. It is very important that the résumé be neatly typed and that all grammar and spelling errors be eliminated. Ask someone knowledgeable about such things to "proofread" it before you submit it.

The demographic data should include a daytime telephone number. The professional objective may be short term, such as "staff nurse position on a general medical unit," or it may include a long-term objective such as "obtain R.N. within 5 years."

The Experience data are an overview of your work history and may display any special skills or talents you possess. It is written in chronological order with the most current employment first. Include the job title, place in which you worked, and the dates during which you were employed. Beneath that information you may want to include particular responsibilities or skills used in that position ("interacted with the public, counseled

with clients, ordered all supplies, developed teaching materials, supervised other staff, etc.").

The Education section includes date and place of high school graduation, any colleges attended, and nursing school. It should include:

◆ Name of school or college and city and state in which it is located.
◆ Degree obtained: major and minor (for college).
◆ Date completed or date of graduation.
◆ Certification courses or specialized training or education programs. (Continuing education courses relevant to your profession or skills used in your profession are appropriate.)

Include the state in which you are licensed, or where you will be seeking licensure, and the date you will take the NCLEX-PN examination.

If you are a new graduate and have received honors, scholarships, or special relevant awards, you may include a section that lists them on your résumé. This may help you be more competitive for a position that has several applicants. Volunteer work may also be listed here. If this section does not apply to you, do not include it on the résumé.

If you belong to any professional or community organizations, and/or have held an office, you may wish to include such a section on your résumé. This section is optional.

Under references, put "available upon request," but have your references chosen and listed on a separate sheet. Each person whose name you submit should have your prior permission to do so. This way they know that they may be called and asked questions about you. If they know this ahead of time, they will be better prepared to give answers that display you in the most positive light. Figure 37-2 presents a sample résumé. A cover letter should accompany any résumé sent in by mail. The cover letter should be only about a half-page long and is very similar to a query letter. It should state why you wish to work at this particular place. It is best to find out the name of the person who will be doing the hiring, but, if this is not possible, address the letter to "Nurse Recruiter" or the "Director of Nursing." Calling the nursing office of the agency and asking the name of the individual who hires nurses is acceptable. The letter may end with a request for an interview. State the time period during which you are available (i.e., hours after classes and clinical, or during a vacation break).

Persons reviewing résumés generally spend only 2 to 3 minutes on each. Therefore, having your résumé correctly formatted and one page long will give you an advantage over applicants submitting a lengthy, multi-page document.

TABLE 37-1 ◆ *Guidelines for Résumé Preparation*

◆ Use high-quality bond paper that is white, off-white, light blue, or light grey.
◆ Type the résumé in easy-to-read type.
◆ Be certain there are no abbreviations, spelling errors, or grammatical errors in the résumé; there should be no typing errors, and no correction fluid should be used.
◆ Use underlining, bold face, or capital letters for headings.
◆ Do not include more than two pages of information.
◆ Items that must be included are name and address, phone number for daytime hours, education completed, licensure held, previous experience, and references.
◆ Items that are optional are career/professional objective, honors and awards, professional organizations, community service.

Nancy S. Crebs
8746 Old Springs Road
Dallas, Texas 75218
(214) 348-0186

Licensure	Will take NCLEX-PN on May 15, 1996
Experience	Certified Nursing Assistant Oakgrove Care Center Oak Cliff, Texas 9/91 - present Responsibilities: taking vital signs, weighing patients, bathing, bedmaking, personal care, feeding, I & O, assisting with ambulation, social interaction.
Education	Vocational Nursing Program El Centro College Dallas, Texas Completion May, 1996 Lake Highlands High School 1986 - 1989 Intravenous Therapy Certification El Centro College Continuing Education March 1996
Community Service	Volunteer Los Amigos Medical Clinic 1991 - 1995; assisted with examinations and performed client teaching.
References	Available upon request

FIGURE 37-2   Example of a résumé.

Think about . . . If you do not own a typewriter or a computer with a printer, how will you go about securing a service to type your résumé and cover letters?

THE JOB INTERVIEW

After making an appointment for an interview, it is wise to plan ahead. Prepare to dress appropriately for the interview. Neat, clean, and pressed business or professional attire is best. Table 37-2 presents the do's and don'ts of what to wear.

The next step is to consider the answers to the questions you may be asked. Table 37-3 shows often-asked questions. Answer every question you are asked honestly. Be careful not to criticize past employers or

instructors, and don't dwell on your shortcomings. Turn them into an area for future improvement: "I need to improve my time-management and organizational skills. Working regularly on one unit full-time will provide me with the opportunity to do that."

If you have little experience with interviews, you may wish to role-play an interview situation with a friend to help you feel more at ease on the actual day of your appointment. Knowing exactly where you are going, where to park, and how to locate the interviewer's office before you set out also helps decrease tension. Allow sufficient time to arrive calm, cool, and collected before the appointment.

Try to find out as much as you can about the agency in which you are applying for a position. What is their philosophy of nursing? How many beds do they have? What patient services do they offer? Are they full

TABLE 37-2 ◆ *Do's and Don'ts of What to Wear to an Interview*	
Do's	**Don'ts***
Clothes	
Ladies: suit, skirt with coordinated top or jacket, business-type dress. *Don't buy an outfit for interviewing that you will never wear again.* Hose should be worn with dress shoes that are polished. *Gentlemen:* suit, dress slacks and sport jacket with shirt and tie; dress slacks with shirt and pullover sweater; dressy pants with shirt and tie (hot weather attire). Appropriate dark socks to be worn with polished dress shoes.	Flashy clothes, unpressed clothes, clothes with spots or that fit very poorly and consequently appear "sloppy." No T-shirts, shorts, short skirts, jeans, tennis, or athletic shoes, or sandals. Shoes that hurt your feet.
Grooming	
Nails should be clean, manicured, and with subdued polish, if any.	No vivid red polish or odd colors of nail polish; no decals or ornaments on nails.
Hair should be clean and neatly combed or styled.	Men with long hair should wear it tied back. No unshaven face or untrimmed beard.
Jewelry should be minimal and appropriate to a business outfit.	No more than one pair of earrings for women. Men should forego wearing any earring; if one is worn, it should be small. No nose rings.
Makeup for women should be minimal and subdued.	No heavy eye shadow, vivid lipstick, or blush.

*Some of the don't items may reflect the "real you," but this is not the place to display this part of your personality.

service, or do they just treat medical–surgical problems of adults? Do they use patient care assistants? Unlicensed assistive personnel? What is the average patient-to-nurse ratio? How many patients are usually assigned to a licensed practical nurse (LPN) per shift? What other responsibilities does a staff nurse undertake at this agency? If committee participation is part of the job, is it done during work hours, or is it expected that meetings are attended outside of work hours? What is the procedure for promotion?

As you are called in for the interview, establish eye contact with the interviewer, and maintain reasonable eye contact during the interaction. Try not to display any nervous mannerisms, such as rhythmic movements of leg, hands, or feet. If you wish to take notes, ask the interviewer if he or she minds if you do.

Should you be offered a position at the end of the interview, avoid being pressured to say "Yes" if you are not certain about committing to the job at this point. Request a few days to consider the position. If you have other interviews scheduled, say so, and tell the interviewer when you will be able to make a decision regarding the position. If you know that you definitely do not want the position, decline it graciously, and express appreciation for the interviewer's time and interest in you. If you are interested, simply ask, "When will a decision be made about filling this position?" Not every applicant will develop rapport with every interviewer. If things seemed "cool" and the position desired is not offered, try elsewhere.

Once a position is offered, you will want to know what the salary will be and what other benefits you will receive as an employee. Table 37-4 presents areas of

benefits that might be available and that you might want to compare between institutions if you are offered more than one position. Inquiring about opportunities for advancement is wise; just be certain to word your questions politely so that you don't present a "what's in this for me" attitude. **Your whole demeanor during an interview should be based on the attitude of looking at what you might be able to contribute to the institution or business.**

After the interview, take a few minutes to write a note of thanks to the interviewer expressing appreciation for the interest and time spent with you. Mention any special effort extended to you, such as a lunch or personal tour of the facilities or unit. Close with an expression of continued interest in the position for which you are applying if it is one you really desire. Notes also should be written for interviews that do not develop into positions that you want. You may want to apply for a different position at that agency sometime in the future.

If you do not hear from the interviewer by the date that was indicated, a follow-up phone call is appropriate. A position offered may be declined by phone, but be sure to speak personally with the individual and not just leave a message on the voice mail system.

RETAINING THE POSITION

Once you obtain a position, effort must be extended to keep it. Most new graduates have a 6-month probation period before employment is considered permanent. Showing interest in duties, patients, and other staff

TABLE 37-3 ◆ *Often Asked Interview Questions*

Interviewers rarely ask all of these questions; these are just some that you should be prepared to answer. Sit down and write out your answers before the interview; don't memorize your answers. This exercise just prepares you by having you "prethink," which will decrease your tension during the actual interview.

◆ What is your professional goal at this time?
◆ What was your favorite unit of study in nursing school?
◆ What area of nursing interests you the most?
◆ Which clinical rotations did you enjoy the most? Why?
◆ Which did you like the least? Why?
◆ What do you feel are the strengths that you could contribute here?
◆ What do you see as your weaknesses?
◆ What particular qualifications do you have that make you feel you will be successful in such a staff position?
◆ What skills from past work experiences do you feel would be useful in this position?
◆ How would others describe you?
◆ How do you feel about "collaborative care"?
◆ How would you describe your communication skills?
◆ How do you feel about working with computers?
◆ How do you plan to update your nursing knowledge?
◆ What are your future career goals? Where do you want to be a year from now? Three years from now? Five years from now?
◆ How are your time-management skills?
◆ What types of situations cause you to feel considerable stress?
◆ If you find yourself in a situation that you don't know how to handle or are assigned a task in which you are not competent, what would you do?
◆ What is your philosophy of nursing?
◆ Why do you wish to work for this organization?
◆ Do you want full-time or part-time work?
◆ What are your salary expectations?
◆ Which shift do you prefer to work? Which shifts can you work?
◆ Do you have any questions?

members is important. Using good communication techniques, courtesy, and tact in dealing with patients, families, and staff, maintaining patient confidentiality, and treating others respectfully shows others that you are a valuable staff member.

Arriving to work on time, clean and neat, and ready to begin your duties calmly and in an organized manner provides the best opportunity to shine each day. Remember to sign in or report on and off duty as required. If duties are not completed by the end of the day, notify the charge nurse or supervisor of tasks undone. If illness prevents you from reporting to work, notify the proper person **as soon as you know you will not be able to work.**

◆ Confidentiality

Patient confidentiality is vitally important; it is a legal and ethical issue with many possible consequences if violated. Patients should not be discussed with unit colleagues in areas off the unit. Refrain from talking about patients or family members in elevators or stairways where others not involved in their care or family members may hear you. The particulars about patient situations should not be discussed with friends or at home. Patients' names should not be attached to any anecdotes shared with other people. **Maintaining patient confidentiality is a professional responsibility.**

Think about . . . Can you think of three instances during your clinical experiences in which you have heard nurses break the rule about patient confidentiality? How could the nurse(s) in question have handled the situation more professionally?

TABLE 37-4 ◆ *Benefit Package Options to Consider and Compare*

The following are some of the fringe benefits available with many health care employers. Each benefit represents a money outlay for the benefit of the employee and should be considered as part of the total "salary" being offered. A lower salary with more benefits may be the best bet in the long run, if the benefits are of interest to you, for example, child care availability or subsidy does you no good if you do not have eligible children.

◆ Health insurance with choices of providers
◆ Dental and vision insurance
◆ Paid sick days
◆ Vacation days
◆ Disability insurance
◆ Life insurance or accidental death or dismemberment coverage
◆ Credit union membership
◆ Free parking
◆ Bus passes
◆ Retirement plan
◆ Profit sharing
◆ Tuition reimbursement/scholarship program
◆ Loan program
◆ Day care program
◆ Health and wellness program
◆ Uniforms (scrubs)
◆ Free meals
◆ Cafeteria or snack shop
◆ Medical library
◆ Nursing learning center with resources available
◆ Nursing education department
◆ Discount on health services
◆ Career ladder program
◆ Available counseling services
◆ Scholarship program for continuing education offerings
◆ Discount/wholesale club membership
◆ Fitness center for employee use

◆ Terminating Employment

Do not consider resigning hastily. Any new position takes a considerable period of adjustment to reach an "ideal" working situation. It is very costly to hire and train nursing personnel. It takes many months before a new employee really is integrated and can work efficiently within the system. A position someplace else may not be better, only different.

Before terminating employment, it is always best to have a new job. However, it is courteous to let your employer know that you are considering changing jobs in case word gets back that you are out looking. If dissatisfaction is the main reason for a desired change, sometimes things will improve if you sit down with your supervisor and express your concerns. **This works best if you can manage to phrase each point as a "concern" rather than a criticism or complaint.** This is another area in which role-play works well to prepare for the actual interaction.

Once you have decided to leave your position, you must follow the agency's policy for termination. Give 4 weeks' notice whenever possible. If 2 weeks' notice is required by your contract, allow time for that. Submit your resignation in writing *after* notifying your supervisor verbally that you are resigning. You may need to submit a resignation letter to the director of nurses or personnel department with a copy to your supervisor. Check to see what the proper protocol is. The letter should be brief. If you are leaving with bad feelings, do not mention that in the letter. You may take up grievances with the personnel or human resources department. Figure 37-3 is an example of a letter of resignation.

MAINTAINING CURRENT NURSING KNOWLEDGE

Now that you are employed, you need a plan to maintain and improve your knowledge base and skills. In-service programs at the place of employment are one way that nurses learn about new equipment and procedures. Subscribing to and regularly reading one or more professional nursing journals is a very good way to learn about advances in medicine and nursing care, new drugs, new diagnostic tests, and new ways to care for

Nancy S. Crebs
8746 Old Springs Road
Dallas, Texas 75218
(214) 348-0186

March 15, 2002

Ms. Joan Stenz, R.N., M.S.N.
Assistant Vice President
Oakhaven Medical Center
21215 Audelia Rd.
Dallas, Texas 75238

Dear Ms. Stenz:

It is with regret that I submit my resignation. My husband has been transferred out of state. My period of employment at Oakhaven Medical Center has been very rewarding. I have gained a wealth of experience that will be of great benefit to me in my career. My last day of work will be April 30, 2002.

Thank you for the opportunity you have provided for me at your institution and for your kindness to me.

Sincerely,

Nancy S. Crebs

FIGURE 37-3   Example of a letter of resignation.

patients. Attending seminars and workshops on timely topics in nursing is very beneficial as well. Many times the employing institution has a program that will provide "scholarship" money for nurses to attend these offerings.

Many states now require mandatory continuing education for renewal of the nursing license. Be certain to check with the State Board of Licensed Practical Nursing to see what, if any, requirements there are in your state. Units to meet these continuing education requirements (CEs) can be obtained by attending approved seminars and workshops and by completing continuing education materials offered in journals or by mail. Many companies offer short correspondence courses. Once you are licensed as a nurse, you will begin to receive brochures.

Even if your state does not require continuing education units, the prudent nurse will work at keeping his or her knowledge base current. Legal determinations are made on what a "prudent" nurse would do in any given situation. A "prudent" nurse always is one who has kept up with current information and skills. A word to the wise should be sufficient.

MEMBERSHIP IN PROFESSIONAL AND COMMUNITY ORGANIZATIONS

Licensed practical nurses are eligible for membership in the National Association for Practical Nurse Education and Service (NAPNES). The NAPNES was founded in 1941 to promote national understanding of the purpose of practical nursing schools and continuing education for the LPN. The group has defined ethical conduct and published standards of practice. Members receive the *Journal of Practical Nursing,* published by NAPNES. The address is 1400 Spring Street, Suite 310, Silver Springs, MD 20910.

The National Federation of Licensed Practical Nurses (NFLPN), founded in 1949, informs members of current issues and also makes available malpractice, personal liability, health, and accident insurance to members. This group lobbies on state and national levels for issues of interest and concern to members. It publishes a journal, *The Licensed Practical Nurse.* The address is P.O. Box 11039, Durham, NC 27703.

The National League of Nursing has a Council of Practical Nursing Programs to which LPNs may belong. This body accredits and provides continuing education for LPN faculty. The NLN publishes *Nursing and Health Care,* a journal. The NLN provides professional testing services and studies and surveys aspects of nursing education.

Community organizations in which nurses may be interested in becoming members are the American

Heart Association, the American Lung Association, the American Red Cross, the American Cancer Society, the Diabetes Association, and any number of smaller groups related to Alzheimer's disease, Multiple sclerosis, cystic fibrosis, and other disorders. Community organizations greatly depend on volunteer help to provide services to citizens who need them. Nurses can be very instrumental in the success of such organizations in their community. Belonging to any community organization provides an opportunity for the nurse to interact with the public and provide health education. Community service is an excellent way for the nurse to share expertise and service, practice skills, contribute to the community, and—network.

CRITICAL THINKING EXERCISES

Situations

1. What type of nursing position would be best for you considering your abilities, preferences, skills, family situation, and salary needs?
2. How would you respond if an interviewer asked you whether you are married? If you have small children? Are these appropriate questions during an employment interview?
3. Pretend you have landed the job you want. What will you do if your car breaks down just before you are ready to leave for work?
4. You often share experiences with other members of your household at dinner time. How will you protect patient confidentiality in these situations?

BIBLIOGRAPHY

Editors of *Nursing 95.* (1996). Dispelling the myths about job security. *Nursing 96 Career Directory.* Springhouse, PA: Springhouse.

Engram, B. (1991). Yes, you can land the job you really want! *Nursing 91.* 21(2):116–120.

Hanger, T. I. (1991). Presenting yourself successfully. *Nursing 91.* 21(6):87–88.

Hunt, B. H., James, M. K. (1997). Tomorrow's LPN understanding the role. *Nursing 97.* 27(3):52–53.

Kurzen, C. R. (1993). *Contemporary Practical/Vocational Nursing,* 2nd ed. Philadelphia: Lippincott.

Mitchell, P. R., Grippando, G. M. (1993). *Nursing Perspectives and Issues,* 5th ed. Albany, NY: Delmar.

Rutkowski, B. L. (1989). Six steps to building your confidence. *Nursing 89.* 19(9):124–130.

Shuman, J. (1994). Six ways to take this job . . . and love it! *American Journal of Nursing.* 94(6):59–62.

Smith, C. E. (1990). Changing jobs, making the right move. *Nursing 90.* 20(9):107–110.

Trudeau, S. E. (1992). Job hunting: will your references help? *RN.* 55(11):65–68.

Weis, D. (1990). Ten questions recruiters will ask. *Nursing 90.* 20(3):116–118.

Welton, R. H., Morton, P. G. (1995). Strategies for writing an effective resume. *Critical Care Nurse.* 15(6):118–126.

Zerwekh, J., Claborn, J. C. (1997). *Nursing Today: Transition and Trends,* 2nd ed. Philadelphia: Saunders.

Zimmermann, P. G. (1995). Ten tips for a top interview. *Nursing 95.* 25(9):83–87.

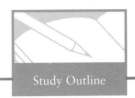

Study Outline

I. Introduction

A. The next step after nursing school is to seek employment.

B. Continuing education often is required for license renewal and is a professional responsibility.

C. The nurse contributes to the community and to nursing by becoming an active member of a professional organization.

D. Involvement in the community and community organizations provides opportunities for teaching preventative health and self-care practices.

II. Preparing to Apply for a Job

A. Networking provides valuable contacts for locating job openings.

B. Determining the type of job desired and the geographical location in which you wish to work is the first step.

C. Gathering data about possible nursing positions is the next step.

D. Compiling the data and dates necessary to fill out a job application should be done ahead of time.

E. Job hunting should begin well in advance of graduation.

III. Preparing Your Résumé

A. A résumé must be typed on good-quality paper and be neat and without spelling or grammatical errors.

B. A résumé includes sections on personal demographic data, education history, past work experience, licensure, and references. Optional sections are honors and awards, volunteer activities, and professional goals.

C. Include a cover letter with any résumé sent by mail.

IV. The Job Interview

A. Plan ahead. Prepare clothes and rehearse.

B. Consider answers to questions most frequently asked.

C. Role-playing helps reduce tension during the actual interview.

D. Make an appointment for an interview.

E. Know exactly where you are going and where you will park.

F. Allow sufficient time to get there, so you will be calm and not hurried.

G. Find out as much about the agency/institution as possible before the interview.

H. Establish eye contact with the interviewer, and maintain reasonable eye contact throughout the interview.

I. Write a follow-up note after the interview thanking the person for his or her time and interest in you.

V. Retaining the Position

A. A probation period is usual.

B. Showing interest and enthusiasm is a plus.

C. Be on time; report on and off duty.

D. Report any undone tasks at the end of the shift.

E. Use good communication skills.

F. Show respect for and interest in others.

G. When ill, call in to the appropriate person as soon as possible.

VI. Confidentiality

A. Patient confidentiality is vitally important.

B. Do not discuss patients or their families anywhere off of the unit or with others not directly involved in their care.

VII. Terminating Employment

A. Do not consider resigning hastily.

B. A great deal of time and money is spent on orienting and integrating a new employee; give it a chance.

C. Obtain a new position before quitting an old one.

D. Follow the agency's personnel policy and terms of your contract for resignation.

E. Submit the resignation in writing after verbally notifying your immediate supervisor.

VIII. Maintaining Current Nursing Knowledge

A. Make a plan to keep your knowledge up-to-date.

B. Take advantage of in-service offerings at your place of employment.

C. Subscribe to at least one professional nursing journal.

D. Attend nursing seminars or workshops on a regular basis.

E. Complete continuing education offerings in journals or from correspondence companies as needed to increase your knowledge and to maintain licensure.

IX. **Membership in Professional and Community Organizations**

A. LPNs are eligible for membership in NAPNES, NFLPN, and the NLN.

B. Community organizations such as the American Heart Association, American Lung Association, Diabetes Association, American Cancer Society, and the American Red Cross need volunteers; nurses can be valuable to these organizations.

C. Community service is a good way to network and to share expertise, skills, and teaching with people in the community.

Table of Most Common Laboratory Test Values

The following tables list normal values, now termed *reference values,* for the most commonly performed laboratory tests. Clinical laboratories use various forms of tests to derive the needed information, and therefore each laboratory has its own set of reference values.* The International System of Units designated by "S.I. units" has been adopted by clinical laboratories in many countries and represents a modification of the metric system.†

---

*The reference values in the Tables of Diagnostic Tests within individual chapters may differ depending on the laboratory used and type of testing procedure.

†The tables are adapted from Conn, R. B.: Laboratory values of clinical importance. In Rakel, R. E. ed. (1997). *Conn's Current Therapy.* Philadelphia: Saunders, pp. 1242–1249.

TABLES OF REFERENCE VALUES

Some of the values included in the tables have been established by the Clinical Laboratories at Thomas Jefferson University Hospital in Philadelphia and have not been published elsewhere. Other values have been compiled from the sources cited herein. These tables are provided for information and educational purposes only. They are intended to complement data derived from other sources, including the medical history and physical examination. Users must exercise individual judgment when employing the information provided in this Appendix.

Reference Values for Hematology

	Conventional Units	SI Units
Acid hemolysis (Ham test)	No hemolysis	No hemolysis
Alkaline phosphatase, leukocyte	Total score 14–100	Total score 14–100
Cell counts		
Erythrocytes		
Males	4.6–6.2 million/mm^3	$4.6–6.2 \times 10^{12}$/L
Females	4.2–5.4 million/mm^3	$4.2–5.4 \times 10^{12}$/L
Children (varies with age)	4.5–5.1 million/mm^3	$4.5–5.1 \times 10^{12}$/L
Leukocytes, total	4,500–11,000/mm^3	$4.5–11.0 \times 10^9$/L
Leukocytes, differential counts*		
Myelocytes	0%	0/L
Band neutrophils	3%–5%	$150–400 \times 10^6$/L
Segmented neutrophiils	54%–62%	$3,000–5,800 \times 10^6$/L
Lymphocytes	25%–33%	$1,500–3,000 \times 10^6$/L
Monocytes	3%–7%	$300–500 \times 10^6$/L
Eosinophils	1%–3%	$50–250 \times 10^6$/L
Basophils	0%–1%	$15–50 \times 10^6$/L
Platelets	150,000–400,000/mm^3	$150–400 \times 10^9$/L
Reticulocytes	25,000–75,000/mm^3 (0.5%–1.5% of erythrocytes)	$25–75 \times 10^9$/L
Coagulation tests		
Bleeding time (template)	2.75–8.0 min	2.75–8.0 min
Coagulation time (glass tube)	5–15 min	5–15 min
D–Dimer	<0.5 μg/mL	<0.5 mg/L
Factor VIII and other coagulation factors	50%–150% of normal	0.5–1.5 of normal
Fibrin split products (thrombo-Welco test)	<10 μg/mL	<10 mg/L
Fibrinogen	200–400 mg/dL	2.0–4.0 g/L
Partial thromboplastin time (PTT)	20–35 s	20–35 s
Prothrombin time (PT)	12.0–14.0 s	12.0–14.0 s
Coombs' test		
Direct	Negative	Negative
Indirect	Negative	Negative
Corpuscular values of erythrocytes		
Mean corpuscular hemoglobin (MCH)	26–34 pg/cell	26–34 pg/cell
Mean corpuscular volume (MCV)	80–96 μm^3	80–96 fL
Mean corpuscular hemoglobin concentration (MCHC)	32–36 g/dL	320–360 g/L
Erythrocyte sedimentation rate (ESR)		
Wintrobe		
Males	0–5 mm/h	0–5 mm/h
Females	0–15 mm/h	0–15 mm/h
Westergren		
Males	0–15 mm/h	0–15 mm/h
Females	0–20 mm/h	0–20 mm/h
Haptoglobin	20–165 mg/dL	0.20–1.65 g/L
Hematocrit		
Males	40–54 mL/dL	0.40–0.54
Females	37–47 mL/dL	0.37–0.47
Newborns	49–54 mL/dL	0.49–0.54
Children (varies with age)	34–49 mL/dL	0.35–0.49
Hemoglobin		
Males	13.0–18.0 g/dL	8.1–11.2 mmol/L
Females	12.0–16.0 g/dL	7.4–9.9 mmol/L
Newborns	16.5–19.5 g/dL	10.2–12.1 mmol/L
Children (varies with age)	11.2–16.5 g/dL	7.0–10.2 mmol/L
Hemoglobin, fetal	<1.0% of total	<0.01 of total
Hemoglobin A$_{1C}$	3%–5% of total	0.03–0.05 of total
Hemoglobin A$_2$	1.5%–3.0% of total	0.015–0.03 of total
Hemoglobin, plasma	0.0–5.0 mg/dL	0.0–3.2 μmol/L
Methemoglobin	30–130 mg/dL	19–80 μmol/L

*Conventional units are percentages; SI units are absolute counts.

Reference Values for Clinical Chemistry (Blood, Serum, and Plasma)*

	Conventional Units	SI Units
Acetoacetate plus acetone		
Qualitative	Negative	Negative
Quantitative	0.3–2.0 mg/dL	30–200 µmol/L
Acid phosphatase, serum (thymolphthalein monophosphate substrate)	0.1–0.6 U/L	0.1–0.6 U/L
ACTH (see corticotropin)		
Alanine aminotransferase (ALT, SGPT), serum	1–45 U/L	1–45 U/L
Albumin, serum	3.3–5.2 g/dL	33–52 g/L
Aldolase, serum	0.0–7.0 U/L	0.0–7.0 U/L
Aldosterone, plasma		
Standing	5–30 ng/dL	140–830 pmol/L
Recumbent	3–10 ng/dL	80–275 pmol/L
Alkaline phosphatase (ALP), serum		
Adult	35–150 U/L	35–150 U/L
Adolescent	100–500 U/L	100–500 U/L
Child	100–350 U/L	100–350 U/L
Ammonia nitrogen, plasma	10–50 µmol/L	10–50 µmol/L
Amylase, serum	25–125 U/L	15–250 U/L
Anion gap, serum, calculated	8–16 mEq/L	8–16 mmol/L
Ascorbic acid, blood	0.4–1.5 mg/dL	23–85 µmol/L
Aspartate aminotransferase (AST, SGOT), serum	1–36 U/L	1–36 U/L
Base excess, arterial blood, calculated	0 ± 2 mEq/L	0 ± 2 mmol/L
β-carotene, serum	60–260 µg/dL	1.1–8.6 µmol/L
Bicarbonate		
Venous plasma	23–29 mEq/L	23–29 mmol/L
Arterial blood	21–27 mEq/L	21–27 mmol/L
Bile acids, serum	0.3–3.0 mg/dL	0.8–7.6 µmol/L
Bilirubin, serum		
Conjugated	0.1–0.4 mg/dL	1.7–6.8 µmol/L
Total	0.3–1.1 mg/dL	5.1–19.0 µmol/L
Calcium, serum	8.4–10.6 mg/dL	2.10–2.65 mmol/L
Calcium, ionized, serum	4.25–5.25 mg/dL	1.05–1.30 mmol/L
Carbon dioxide, total, serum or plasma	24–31 mEq/L	24–31 mmol/L
Carbon dioxide tension (P_{CO_2}), blood	35–45 mmHg	35–45 mmHg
Ceruloplasmin, serum	23–44 mg/dL	230–440 mg/dL
Chloride, serum or plasma	96–106 mEq/L	96–106 mmol/L
Cholesterol, serum or EDTA plasma		
Desirable range	<200 mg/dL	<5.20 mmol/L
LDL cholesterol	60–180 mg/dL	1.55–4.65 mmol/L
HDL cholesterol	30–80 mg/dL	0.80–2.05 mmol/L
Copper	70–140 µg/dL	11–22 µmol/L
Corticotropin (ACTH), plasma, 8 A.M.	10–80 pg/mL	2–18 pmol/L
Cortisol, plasma		
8 A.M.	6–23 µg/dL	170–630 nmol/L
4 P.M.	3–15 µg/dL	80–410 nmol/L
10 P.M.	<50% of 8 A.M. value	<50% of 8:00 A.M. value
Creatine, serum		
Males	0.2–0.5 mg/dL	15–40 µmol/L
Females	0.3–0.9 mg/dL	25–70 µmol/L
Creatine kinase (CK), serum		
Males	55–170 U/L	55–170 U/L
Females	30–135 U/L	30–135 U/L
Creatine kinase MB isoenzyme, serum	<5% of total CK activity	<5% of total CK activity
	<5% ng/mL by immunoassay	<5% ng/mL by immunoassay

(Table continued on following page)

Reference Values for Clinical Chemistry (Blood, Serum, and Plasma)* (Continued)

	Conventional Units	SI Units
Creatinine, serum	0.6–1.2 mg/dL	50–110 μmol/L
Estradiol–17β, adult		
Males	10–65 pg/mL	35–240 pmol/L
Females		
Follicular phase	30–100 pg/mL	110–370 pmol/L
Ovulatory phase	200–400 pg/mL	730–1470 pmol/L
Luteal phase	50–140 pg/mL	180–510 pmol/L
Ferritin, serum	20–200 ng/mL	20–200 μg/L
Fibrinogen, plasma	200–400 mg/dL	2.0–4.0 g/L
Folate, serum erythrocytes	2.0–9.0 ng/mL	4.5–20.4 nmol/L
	170–700 ng/mL	385–1590 nmol/L
Follicle-stimulating hormone (FSH), plasma		
Males	4–25 mU/mL	4–25 U/L
Females, premenopausal	4–30 mU/mL	4–30 U/L
Females, postmenopausal	40–250 mU/mL	40–250 U/L
γ-glutamyltransferase (GGT), serum	5–40 U/L	5–40 U/L
Gastrin, fasting, serum	0–110 pg/mL	0–110 mg/L
Glucose, fasting, plasma or serum	70–115 mg/dL	3.9–6.4 nmol/L
Growth hormone (hGH), plasma, adult, fasting	0–6 ng/mL	0–6 μg/L
Haptoglobin, serum	20–165 mg/dL	0.20–1.65 g/L
Immunoglobulins, serum (see reference values for immunological procedures)		
Insulin, fasting, plasma	5–25 μU/mL	36–179 pmol/L
Iron, serum	75–175 μg/dL	13–31 μmol/L
Iron binding capacity, serum		
Total	250–410 μg/dL	45–73 μmol/L
Saturation	20%–55%	0.20–0.55
Lactate		
Venous whole blood	5.0–20.0 mg/dL	0.6–2.2 mmol/L
Arterial whole blood	5.0–15.0 mg/dL	0.6–1.7 mmol/L
Lactate dehydrogenase (LD), serum	110–220 U/L	110–220 U/L
Lipase, serum	10–140 U/L	10–140 U/L
Lutropin (LH), serum		
Males	1–9 U/L	1–9 U/L
Females		
Follicular phase	2–10 U/L	2–10 U/L
Midcycle peak	15–65 U/L	15–65 U/L
Luteal phase	1–12 U/L	1–12 U/L
Postmenopausal	12–65 U/L	12–65 U/L
Magnesium, serum	1.3–2.1 mg/dL	0.65–1.05 mmol/L
Osmolality	275–295 mOsm/kg water	275–295 mOsm/kg water
Oxygen, blood, arterial, room air		
Partial pressure (Pa_{o2})	80–100 mm Hg	80–100 mm Hg
Saturation (Sa_{o2})	95%–98%	95%–98%
pH, arterial blood	7.35–7.45	7.35–7.45
Phosphate, inorganic, serum		
Adult	3.0–4.5 mg/dL	1.0–1.5 mmol/L
Child	4.0–7.0 mg/dL	1.3–2.3 mmol/L
Potassium		
Serum	3.5–5.0 mEq/L	3.5–5.0 mmol/L
Plasma	3.5–4.5 mEq/L	3.5–4.5 mmol/L
Progesterone, serum, adult		
Males	0.0–0.4 ng/mL	0.0–1.3 mmol/L
Females		
Follicular phase	0.1–1.5 ng/mL	0.3–4.8 mmol/L
Luteal phase	2.5–28.0 ng/mL	8.0–89.0 mmol/L

Reference Values for Clinical Chemistry (Blood, Serum, and Plasma)* (Continued)

	Conventional Units	SI Units
Prolactin, serum		
Males	1.0–15.0 ng/mL	1.0–15.0 µg/L
Females	1.0–20.0 ng/mL	1.0–20.0 µg/L
Protein, serum, electrophoresis		
Total	6.0–8.0 g/dL	60–80 g/L
Albumin	3.5–5.5 g/dL	35–55 g/L
Globulins		
Alpha$_1$	0.2–0.4 g/dL	2.0–4.0 g/L
Alpha$_2$	0.5–0.9 g/dL	5.0–9.0 g/L
Beta	0.6–1.1 g/dL	6.0–11.0 g/L
Gamma	0.7–1.7 g/dL	7.0–17.0 g/L
Pyruvate, blood	0.3–0.9 mg/dL	0.03–0.10 mmol/L
Rheumatoid factor	0.0–30.0 IU/mL	0.0–30.0 kIU/L
Sodium, serum or plasma	135–145 mEq/L	135–145 mmol/L
Testosterone, plasma		
Males, adult	300–1200 ng/dL	10.4–41.6 nmol/L
Females, adult	20–75 ng/dL	0.7–2.6 nmol/L
Pregnant females	40–200 ng/dL	1.4–6.9 nmol/L
Thyroglobulin	3–42 ng/mL	3–42 µg/L
Thyrotropin (hTSH), serum	0.4–4.8 µIU/mL	0.4–4.8 mIU/L
Thyrotropin-releasing hormone (TRH)	5–60 pg/mL	5–60 ng/L
Thyroxine (FT$_4$), free, serum	0.9–2.1 ng/dL	12–27 pmol/L
Thyroxine (T$_4$), serum	4.5–12.0 µg/dL	58–154 nmol/L
Thyroxine–binding globulin (TBG)	15.0–34.0 µg/mL	15.0–34.0 mg/L
Transferrin	250–430 mg/dL	2.5–4.3 g/L
Triglycerides, serum, after 12-hour fast	40–150 mg/dL	0.4–1.5 g/L
Triiodothyronine (T$_3$), serum	70–190 ng/dL	1.1–2.9 nmol/L
Triiodothyronine uptake, resin (T$_3$RU)	25%–38%	0.25–0.38
Urate		
Males	2.5–8.0 mg/dL	150–480 µmol/L
Females	2.2–7.0 mg/dL	130–420 µmol/L
Urea, serum or plasma	24–49 mg/dL	4.0–8.2 nmol/L
Urea nitrogen, serum or plasma	11–23 mg/dL	8.0–16.4 nmol/L
Viscosity, serum	1.4–1.8 × water	1.4–1.8 × water
Vitamin A, serum	20–80 µg/dL	0.70–2.80 µmol/L
Vitamin B$_{12}$, serum	180–900 pg/mL	133–664 pmol/L

*Reference values may vary depending on the method and sample source used.

Reference Values for Therapeutic Drug Monitoring (Serum)

	Therapeutic Range	Toxic Concentrations	Proprietary Names
Analgesics			
Acetaminophen	10–20 µg/mL	>250 µg/mL	Tylenol Datril
Salicylate	100–250 µg/mL	>300 µg/mL	Aspirin Bufferin
Antibiotics			
Amikacin	25–30 µg/mL	Peak >35 µg/mL Trough >10 µg/mL	Amikin

(Table continued on following page)

Reference Values for Therapeutic Drug Monitoring (Serum)

	Therapeutic Range	Toxic Concentrations	Proprietary Names
Chloramphenicol	10–20 µg/mL	>25 µg/mL	Chloromycetin
Gentamicin	5–10 µg/mL	Peak >10 µg/mL Trough >2 µg/mL	Garamycin
Tobramycin	5–10 µg/mL	Peak >10 µg/mL Trough >2 µg/mL	Nebcin
Vancomycin	5–10 µg/mL	Peak >40 µg/mL Trough >10 µg/mL	Vancocin
Anticonvulsants			
Carbamazepine	5–12 µg/mL	>15 µg/mL	Tegretol
Ethosuximide	40–100 µg/mL	>150 µg/mL	Zarontin
Phenobarbital	15–40 µg/mL	40–100 ng/mL (varies widely)	Luminal
Phenytoin	10–20 µg/mL	>20 µg/mL	Dilantin
Primidone	5–12 µg/mL	>15 µg/mL	Mysoline
Valproic acid	50–100 µg/mL	>100 µg/mL	Depakene
Antineoplastics and immunosuppressives			
Cyclosporine	50–400 ng/mL	>400 ng/mL	Sandimmune
Methotrexate, high dose, 48 hours	Variable	>1 µmol/L 48 hours after dose	Mexate Folex
Tacrolimus (FK-506), whole blood	3–10 µg/L	>15 µg/L	Prograf
Bronchodilators and respiratory stimulants			
Caffeine	3–15 ng/mL	>30 ng/mL	
Theophylline (Aminophylline)	10–20 µg/mL	>20 µg/mL	Elixophyllin Quibron
Cardiovascular drugs			
Amiodarone (Obtain specimen more than 8 hours after last dose)	1.0–2.0 µg/mL	>2.0 µg/mL	Cordarone
Digitoxin (Obtain specimen 12–24 hours after last dose)	15–25 ng/mL	>35 ng/mL	Crystodigin
Digoxin (Obtain specimen more than 6 hours after last dose)	0.8–2.0 ng/mL	>2.4 ng/mL	Lanoxin
Disopyramide	2–5 µg/mL	>7 µg/mL	Norpace
Flecainīde	0.2–1.0 ng/mL	>1 ng/mL	Tambocor
Lidocaine	1.5–5.0 µg/mL	>6 µg/mL	Xylocaine
Mexiletine	0.7–2.0 ng/mL	>2 ng/mL	Mexitil
Procainamide	4–10 µg/mL	>12 µg/mL	Pronestyl
Procainamide plus NAPA	8–30 µg/mL	>30 µg/mL	
Propranolol	50–100 ng/mL	Variable	Inderal
Quinidine	2–5 µg/mL	>6 µg/mL	Cardioquin, Quinaglute
Tocainide	4–10 ng/mL	>10 ng/mL	Tonocard
Psychopharmacologic drugs			
Amitriptyline	120–150 ng/mL	>500 ng/mL	Elavil
Bupropion	25–100 ng/mL	Not applicable	Triavil Wellbutrin
Desipramine	150–300 ng/mL	>500 ng/mL	Norpramin Pertofrane Tofranil
Imipramine	125–250 ng/mL	>400 ng/mL	Janimine
Lithium (Obtain specimen 12 hours after last dose)	0.6–1.5 mEq/L	>1.5 mEq/L	Lithobid
Notriptyline	50–150 ng/mL	>500 ng/mL	Aventyl Pamelor

Reference Values for Clinical Chemistry (Urine)

	Conventional Units	SI Units
Acetone and acetoacetate, qualitative	Negative	Negative
Albumin		
Qualitative	Negative	Negative
Quantitative	10–100 mg/24 hours	0.15–1.5 μmol/day
Aldosterone	3–20 μg/24 hours	8.3–55 nmol/day
δ-Aminolevulinic acid (δ-ALA)	1.3–7.0 mg/24 hours	10–53 μmol/day
Amylase	<17 U/hour	<17 U/hour
Amylase/creatinine clearance ratio	0.01–0.04	0.01–0.04
Bilirubin, qualitative	Negative	Negative
Calcium (regular diet)	<250 mg/24 hours	<6.3 nmol/day
Catecholamines		
Epinephrine	<10 μg/24 hours	<55 nmol/day
Norepinephrine	<100 μg/24 hours	<590 nmol/day
Total free catecholamines	4–126 μg/24 hours	24–745 nmol/day
Total metanephrines	0.1–1.6 mg/24 hours	0.5–8.1 μmol/day
Chloride (varies with intake)	110–250 mEq/24 hours	110–250 mmol/day
Copper	0–50 μg/24 hours	0.0–0.80 μmol/day
Cortisol, free	10–100 μg/24 hours	27.6–276 nmol/day
Creatine		
Males	0–40 mg/24 hours	0.0–0.30 mmol/day
Females	0–80 mg/24 hours	0.0–0.60 mmol/day
Creatinine	15–25 mg/kg/24 hours	0.13–0.22 mmol/kg/day
Creatinine clearance (endogenous)		
Males	110–150 mL/min/1.73 m^2	110–150 mL/min/1.73 m^2
Females	105–132 mL/min/1.73 m^2	105–132 mL/min/1.73 m^2
Cystine or cysteine	Negative	Negative
Dehydroepiandrosterone		
Males	0.2–2.0 mg/24 hours	0.7–6.9 μmol/day
Females	0.2–1.8 mg/24 hours	0.7–6.2 μmol/day
Estrogens, total		
Males	4–25 μg/24 hours	14–90 nmol/day
Females	5–100 μg/24 hours	18–360 nmol/day
Glucose (as reducing substance)	<250 mg/24 hours	<250 mg/day
Hemoglobin and myoglobin, qualitative	Negative	Negative
Homogentisic acid, qualitative	Negative	Negative
17–Hydroxycorticosteroids		
Males	3–9 mg/24 hours	8.3–25 μmol/day
Females	2–8 mg/24 hours	5.5–22 μmol/day
5–Hydroxyindoleacetic acid		
Qualitative	Negative	Negative
Quantitative	2–6 mg/24 hours	10–31 μmol/day
17–Ketogenic steroids		
Males	5–23 mg/24 hours	17–80 μmol/day
Females	3–15 mg/24 hours	10–52 μmol/day
17–Ketosteroids		
Males	8–22 mg/24 hours	28–76 μmol/day
Females	6–15 mg/24 hours	21–52 μmol/day
Magnesium	6–10 mEq/24 hours	3–5 mmol/day
Metanephrines	0.05–1.2 ng/mg creatinine	0.03–0.70 mmol/mmol creatinine
Osmolality	38–1400 mOsm/kg water	38–1,400 mOsm/kg water
pH	4.6–8.0	4.6–8.0
Phenylpyruvic acid, qualitative	Negative	Negative
Phosphate	0.4–1.3 g/24 hours	13–42 mmol/day

(Table continued on following page)

Reference Values for Clinical Chemistry (Urine) *(Continued)*

	Conventional Units	SI Units
Porphobilinogen		
Qualitative	Negative	Negative
Quantitative	<2 mg/24 hours	<9 µmol/day
Porphyrins		
Coproporphyrin	50–250 µg/24 hours	77–380 nmol/day
Uroporphyrin	10–30 µg/24 hours	12–36 nmol/day
Potassium	25–125 mEq/24 hours	25–125 mmol/day
Pregnanediol		
Males	0.0–1.9 mg/24 hours	0.0–6.0 µmol/day
Females		
Proliferative phase	0.0–2.6 mg/24 hours	0.0–8.0 µmol/day
Luteal phase	2.6–10.6 mg/24 hours	8–33 µmol/day
Postmenopausal	0.2–1.0 mg/24 hours	0.6–3.1 µmol/day
Pregnanetriol	0.0–2.5 mg/24 hours	0.0–7.4 µmol/day
Protein, total		
Qualitative	Negative	Negative
Quantitative	10–150 mg/24 hours	10–150 mg/day
Protein/creatinine ratio	<0.2	<0.2
Sodium (regular diet)	60–260 mEq/24 hours	60–260 mmol/day
Specific gravity		
Random specimen	1.003–1.030	1.003–1.030
24-hours collection	1.015–1.025	1.015–1.025
Urate (regular diet)	250–750 mg/24 hours	1.5–4.4 mmol/day
Urobilinogen	0.5–4.0 mg/24 hours	0.6–6.8 µmol/day
Vanillylmandelic acid (VMA)	1.0–8.0 mg/24 hours	5–40 µmol/day

Reference Values for Toxic Substances

	Conventional Units	SI Units
Arsenic, urine	<130 µg/24 hours	<1.7 µmol/day
Bromides, serum, inorganic	<100 mg/dL	<10 mmol/L
Toxic symptoms	140–1,000 mg/dL	14–100 mmol/L
Carboxyhemoglobin, blood	% Saturation	Saturation
Urban environment	<5%	<0.05
Smokers	<12%	<0.12
Symptoms		
Headache	>15%	>0.15
Nausea and vomiting	>25%	>0.25
Potentially lethal	>50%	>0.50
Ethanol, blood	<0.05 mg/dL	<1.0 mmol/L
	<0.005%	
Intoxication	>100 mg/dL	>22 mmol/L
	>0.1%	
Marked intoxication	300–400 mg/dL	65–87 mmol/L
	0.3%–0.4%	
Alcoholic stupor	400–500 mg/dL	87–109 mmol/L
	0.4%–0.5%	
Coma	>500 mg/dL	>109 mmol/L
	>0.5%	
Lead, blood		
Adults	<25 µg/dL	<1.2 µmol/L
Children	<15 µg/dL	<0.7 µmol/L
Lead, urine	<80 µg/24 hours	<0.4 µmol/day
Mercury, urine	<30 µg/24 hours	<150 nmol/day

Reference Values for Cerebrospinal Fluid

	Conventional Units	SI Units
Cells	<5/mm³, all mononuclear	$<5 \times 10^6$ L, all mononuclear
Glucose	50–75 mg/dL (20 mg/dL less than in serum)	2.8–4.2 mmol/L (1.1 mmol less than in serum)
IgG		
Children under 14	<8% of total protein	<0.08% of total protein
Adults	<14% of total protein	<0.14% of total protein
IgG index $\left(\frac{\text{CSF/serum IgG ratio}}{\text{CSF/serum albumin ratio}} \right)$	0.3–0.6	0.6–0.6
Oligoclonal banding on electrophoresis	Absent	Absent
Pressure, opening	70–180 mmH₂O	70–180 mmH₂O
Protein, total	15–45 mg/dL	150–450 mg/L
Protein electrophoresis	Albumin predominant	Albumin predominant

Reference Values for Tests of Gastrointestinal Function

	Conventional Units		Conventional Units
Bentiromide	6–hour urinary arylamine excretion greater than 57% excludes pancreatic insufficiency	Maximum (after histamine or pentagastrin)	
		Males	9.0–48.0 mmol/hour
β-Carotene, serum	60–250 ng/dL	Females	6.0–31.0 mmol/hour
Fecal fat estimation		Ratio: basal/maximum	
Qualitative	No fat globules seen by high-power microscope	Males	0.0–0.31
Quantitative	<6 g/24 hours (>95% coefficient of fat absorption)	Females	0.0–0.29
		Secretin test, pancreatic fluid	
Gastric acid output		Volume	>1.8 mL/kg/hr
Basal		Bicarbonate	>80 mEq/L
Males	0.0–10.5 mmol/hour		
Females	0.0–5.6 mmol/hour	D-Xylose absorption test, urine	>20% of ingested dose excreted in 5 hours

Reference Values for Immunologic Procedures

	Conventional Units	SI Units
Complement, serum		
C3	85–175 mg/dL	0.85–1.75 g/L
C4	15–45 mg/dL	150–450 mg/L
Total hemolytic (CH₅₀)	150–250 U/mL	150–250 U/mL
Immunoglobulins, serum, adult		
IgG	640–1350 mg/dL	6.4–13.5 g/L
IgA	70–310 mg/dL	0.70–3.1 gL
IgM	90–350 mg/dL	0.90–3.5 g/L
IgD	0.0–6.0 mg/dL	0.0–60 mg/L
IgE	0.0–430 ng/dL	0.0–430 μg/L

Lymphocyte Subsets, Whole Blood, Heparinized

Antigen	Cell Type	Percentage	Absolute
CD3	Total T-cells	56–77	860–1880
CD19	Total B-cells	7–17	140–370
CD3 and CD4	Helper-inducer cells	32–54	550–1190
CD3 and CD8	Suppressor-cytotoxic cells	24–37	430–1060
CD3 and DR	Activated T-cells	5–14	70–310
CD2	E rosette T-cells	73–87	1,040–2,160
CD16 and CD56	Natural killer (NK) cells	8–22	130–500

Helper/suppressor ratio: 0.8 to 1.8.

Reference Values for Semen Analysis

	Conventional Units	SI Units
Volume	2–5 mL	2–5 mL
Liquefaction	Complete in 15 minutes	Complete in 15 minutes
pH	7.2–8.0	7.2–8.0
Leukocytes	Occasional or absent	Occasional or absent
Spermatoza		
Count	$60–150 \times 10^6$ mL	$60–150 \times 10^6$ mL
Motility	>80% motile	>0.80 motile
Morphology	80%–90% normal forms	>0.80–0.90 normal forms
Fructose	>150 mg/dL	>8.33 mmol/L

BIBLIOGRAPHY

AMA Drug Evaluations, Annual. (1994). Chicago: American Medical Association.

Bick, R. L. ed. (1993). *Hematology—Clinical and Laboratory Practice.* St. Louis, MO: Mosby-Year Book.

Borer, W. Z. (1992). Selection and use of laboratory tests. In Tietz, N. W., Conn, R. B. Pruden, E. L. *Applied Laboratory Medicine,* ed. Philadelphia: Saunders, pp. 1–5.

Campion, E. W. (1992). A retreat from SI units. *New England Journal of Medicine.* 327:49.

Friedman, R. B., Young, D. S. (1989). *Effects of Disease on Clinical Laboratory Tests,* 2nd ed. Washington, DC: AACC Press.

Henry, J. B. (1991). *Clinical Diagnosis and Management by Laboratory Methods,* 18th ed. Philadelphia: Saunders.

Hicks, J. M., Young, D. S. (1992). *DORA 1992–1993: Directory of Rare Analyses.* Washington, DC: AACC press.

Jacobs, D. S., Kasten, B. L., Demott, W. R. Wolfson, W. L. (1990). *Laboratory Test Handbook,* 2nd ed. Baltimore: Williams & Wilkins.

Kaplan, L. A., Pesce, A. J. (1989). *Clinical Chemistry—Theory, Analysis, and Correlation,* 2nd ed. St. Louis, MO: Mosby.

Kjeldsberg, C. R., Knight, J. A. (1993). *Body Fluids—Laboratory Examination of Amniotic, Cerebrospinal, Seminal, Serous, and Synovial Fluids,* 3rd ed. Chicago: ASCP Press.

Laposata, M. (1992). *SI Unit Conversion Guide.* Boston: New England Journal of Medicine Books.

Scully, R. E., McNeely, W. F., Mark E. J., McNeely, B. U. (1992). Normal reference laboratory values. *New England Journal of Medicine,* 327:718–724.

Speicher, C. E. (1993). *The Right Test—A Physician's Guide to Laboratory Medicine,* 2nd ed. Philadelphia: Saunders.

Tietz, N. W., ed. (1990). *Clinical Guide to Laboratory Tests,* 2nd ed. Philadelphia, Saunders.

Wallach, J. (1992). *Interpretation of Diagnostic Tests—A Synopsis of Laboratory Medicine,* 5th ed. Boston: Little, Brown.

Young, D. S. (1992). Determination and validation of reference intervals. *Archives of Pathologic and Laboratory Medicine.* 116:704–709.

Young, D. S. (1990). *Effects of Drugs on Clinical Laboratory Tests,* 3rd ed. Washington, DC: AACC Press.

Young, D. S. (1987). Implementation of SI units for clinical laboratory data. *Annals of Internal Medicine.* 106: 114–129.

Diet Therapy

THE NORMAL DIET

The normal diet consists of foods chosen from the food pyramid (Figure A-1). The base of the diet is 6 to 11 servings of breads, cereals, rice, or pasta. To this is added 3 to 5 servings of vegetables and 2 to 4 servings of fruit. Meat, poultry, fish, dry beans, eggs, and nuts are limited to 2 to 3 servings per day. An additional 2 to 3 servings of milk, yogurt, or cheese round out the diet. Fats and sweets are used sparingly. Examples of one serving are:

- **Breads, cereals, rice, and pasta**
  1 slice of bread
  ½ cup of cooked rice or pasta
  ½ cup of cooked cereal
  1 ounce of ready-to-eat cereal
- **Vegetables**
  ½ cup of chopped raw vegetables
  ½ cup of cooked vegetables
  1 cup of leafy raw vegetables
- **Fruits**
  1 piece of fruit or melon wedge
  ¾ cup of juice
  ½ cup of canned fruit
  ½ cup of dried fruit
- **Milk, yogurt, and cheese**
  1 cup of milk or yogurt
  1½ to 2 oz of cheese
- **Meat, poultry, fish, dry beans, eggs, and nuts**
  2½ to 3 oz of cooked lean meat, poultry, or fish.
  Count ½ cup of cooked beans, 1 egg, 2 tablespoons of peanut butter as 1 oz of lean meat (about ⅓ of a serving).

Each part of a meal may consist of more than one serving. For example a dinner portion of spaghetti would consist of 2 to 3 servings of pasta. Table A-1 shows daily calorie requirements.

THERAPEUTIC DIETS*

◆ Clear Liquid Diet

Purpose: Provides an oral source of calories and electrolytes as a means of preventing dehydration and reducing colonic residue to a minimum.

Indications: The immediate postoperative period, acute debilitation, acute gastroenteritis, upper gastrointestinal lesions; also to reduce the amount of residue in the colon in preparation for bowel surgery, barium enema, or after colon surgery (Table A-2).

◆ Full Liquid Diet

Indications: Oral surgery, mandibular fracture, plastic surgery to the face, esophageal strictures; also for acutely ill client for whom chewing may be difficult, or other postoperative states in transition between a clear liquid and other diet; three to six small feedings a day are recommended (Table A-3).

Contraindications: Nausea, vomiting, distension, or diarrhea when advanced to this diet postoperatively, lactose intolerance.

◆ Prudent Diet (Low Cholesterol and Sodium)

This diet is aimed at lowering low-density lipoprotein (LDL) cholesterol levels and sodium intake.

High-sodium foods include pickles, olives, salted nuts, soy sauce, frankfurters, bacon, sausage or

*The pages that follow are reprinted from Melonakos, K. (1991). *Saunders Pocket Reference for Nurses.* Philadelphia: Saunders, pp. 316–321. Reprinted with permission.

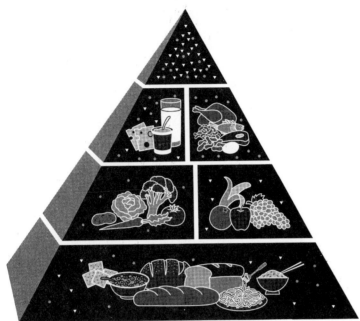

FIGURE A-1 The Food Pyramid. (*Source:* U.S. Government. Reprinted in Monahan, F., Drake, T., Neighbors, M. [1994]. *Nursing Care of Adults.* Philadelphia: Saunders, inside back cover.)

TABLE A-1 ◆ *Servings Needed per Calorie Requirements*

	Women, Some Older Adults	Children, Teen Girls, Active Women, Most Men	Teen Boys and Active Men
Calorie level*	About 1,600	About 2,200	About 2,800
Bread group	6	9	11
Vegetable group	3	4	5
Fruit group	2	3	4
Milk group	2–3†	2–3†	2–3†
Meat group	2, for a total of 5 oz	2, for a total of 6 oz	3, for a total of 7 oz

*These are the calorie levels if you choose low-fat, lean foods from the five major food groups and use foods from the fats, oils, and sweets group sparingly.
†Women who are pregnant or breastfeeding, teenagers, and young adults to age 24 need three servings.
Source: U.S. Government. Reprinted in Monahan, F., Drake, T., Neighbors, M. (1994). *Nursing Care of Adults.* Philadelphia: Saunders, inside back cover. Reprinted with permission.

TABLE A-2 ◆ *Clear Liquid Diet*

Type of Food	Foods Included	Foods Excluded
Beverage	Carbonated beverages, tea, coffee, strained fruit juice (apple, cranberry, cranapple, grape, punch, powdered fruit beverage mixes)	Milk, milk drinks
Soup	Fat-free bouillon or broth	Any other
Dessert	Plain gelatin, popsicles, sherbert sometimes allowed	Any other
Condiments	Sugar, honey, plain hard candy	Any other

TABLE A-3 ◆ *Full Liquid Diet*

Type of Food	Foods Included	Foods Excluded
Beverage	Carbonated beverages, coffee, tea, fruit juices, milk, milk drinks	None
Bread	None	All
Cereal	Soft cooked cereals	Any other
Fat	Butter, cream, margarine	Any other
Vegetables	Tomato juice, vegetable puree in soup	Any other
Meat, egg, cheese	Raw pasteurized eggs.* Soft cooked egg sometimes allowed	Any other
Soup	Broth, strained cream soups, yogurt	Any other
Dessert	Yogurt, custard, ice cream, plain pudding, tapioca	Any other
Condiments	Pepper, salt, sugar, honey, hard candy	Any other

*Raw, unpasteurized eggs should not be used because of the danger of *Salmonella* infection. In addition, the avidin in the egg white prevents the absorption of biotin.

scrapple, processed cheese, canned soups, potato chips and other snack chips, canned fish and meats, luncheon meats, ham, mustard, and ketchup (Table A-4).

Indications: Heart disease, atherosclerosis, hyperlipidemia.

◆ Sodium-Restricted Diet

Along with foods, the sodium content of medications and local water should be considered. Potent oral diuretics have lessened the need for severe limitation of sodium in the diet (Table A-5).

Indications: chronic heart failure, hypertension, atherosclerosis, edema, cirrhosis of the liver, or chronic kidney disease

◆ High-Fiber Diet

Fiber increases fecal bulk, holds water, and binds calcium, magnesium, and other needed nutrients. The

TABLE A-4 ◆ *Low-Cholesterol Diet*

Type of Food	Foods Allowed	Foods Excluded
Beverage	Herb tea, carbonated beverages, fruit drinks, skim milk, coffee,* wine,* beer,* low-fat milk*	Whole milk, chocolate milk, nondairy creamers, canned evaporated whole milk, hard liquor
Bread	Whole-grain breads, white enriched breads, rolls, muffins, melba toast, biscuits, water bagels, oatmeal, oat bran	Egg bread, cheese bread, commercial biscuits, muffins, donuts, sweet rolls, snack crackers
Cereals	Whole-grain or enriched cereals, hot or cold	Commercial granola
Fats	Polyunsaturated vegetable oils, such as corn, cottonseed, safflower, sesame seed, soybean, sunflower; margarines or salad dressings made with allowed oils; Monounsaturated fats, such as olive oil, peanut oil, canola oil	Solid fats, shortenings, butter, lard, cream, hard margarines, salt pork, meat fat, coconut oils, palm oil, mayonnaise, hydrogenated fat
Fruits and vegetables	All fruits and vegetables may be used unless prepared with restricted ingredients	Vegetables in cream, butter or cheese sauce; vegetables fried in saturated fat
Meat, eggs, cheese	Chicken, turkey, veal, fish, shellfish, dried peas, beans, lentils (prepared with allowed ingredients); natural-style peanut butter, egg substitutes, and egg whites if desired; very lean beef, lamb, pork, or ham once or twice a week; cheeses made from skim milk, low-fat cottage cheese, baker's cheese, farmer's cheese, baker's cheese; part-skim-milk mozzarella; fatty fish such as bluefish, salmon, mackerel—three to four times a week	Duck, goose, fatty meats (spareribs, frankfurters, sausages, ham, bacon, bologna, lunch meats, regular hamburger); egg, yolks except 3 per week; cheeses made from whole milk or cream, processed cheese
Soups	Broth, vegetable soup (not creamed)	Creamed soups, or those made with fatty meats
Desserts	Cocoa powder, fruit whip, gelatin, puddings made with skim milk, ice milk, sherbet, homemade baked goods made with allowed ingredients, hard candies, angel food cake	Chocolate, whole-milk puddings, ice cream, candies, caramels, butterscotch, coconut, macadamia nuts, cashews, commercial cakes, pies, cookies mixes
Condiments	Jelly, jams, honey, sugar, salt, pepper, herbs, spices, vinegar, mustard, ketchup, soy sauce	Potato chips and other commercial fried snacks

*With approval of physician

TABLE A-5 ◆ *Low-Sodium Diet*

Type of Diet	Sodium per Day Allowed	Foods Excluded
Mild	2.4–4 g	Added salt, salty foods, such as salted nuts, potato chips, pretzels, smoked meats, bouillon, frozen entrees, salted or smoked meat and fish, luncheon meats, processed cheese, regular peanut butter, sauerkraut, olives, pickles, salted chips or popcorn, salted nuts, canned soups, commercial bouillon, instant cocoa or hot cereals, cooking wine, celery salt, garlic salt, onion salt, commercial salad dressings or meat extracts, meat tenderizers, soy sauce, Worcestershire sauce
Moderate	1,000 mg	All foods restricted in "mild" sodium restriction. Low-sodium products are to be used. No salt added to food; preservatives or flavor enhancers that contain sodium (e.g., monosodium glutamate [MSG] or disodium phosphate); commercial baked products unless prepared without salt, salted margarine or butter, breakfast cereals containing salt, cheese containing salt, any canned or frozen vegetables with salt; other vegetables found to be high in sodium content in any form* **Meal Pattern** Milk limited to 2 cups; meat, fish, and poultry to 4 servings (1 oz); bread (salted), 2 servings; salted margarine or butter, 2 teaspoons; fruits/vegetables, 4 servings per allowed lists (1½ cups total)
Strict low sodium	500 mg	All foods excluded in mild and moderate lists. Only salt-free bread is allowed* **Meal Pattern** Milk limited to 2 cups; meat to 4 servings (1 oz); no salted margarine or butter, no salted breads, no salted fats; fruits, 4 servings; vegetables 1½ cups total from allowed lists*
Severe	250 mg	All foods excluded in restrictions above* Only salt-free bread **Meal Pattern** No salted milk; meat, 4 servings (1 oz); vegetables 1½ cups total from allowed lists;* fruits, 4 servings; no salted bread, no salted fats

*Note: These vegetables should be avoided for moderate, strict, or severe sodium-restrictive diets; artichokes, beets, carrots, celery, Swiss chard, dandelion greens, beet greens, collard greens, mustard greens, kale, spinach, turnip greens or white turnips, sauerkraut, hominy.

TABLE A-6 ◆ *Low-Fiber Diet*

Type of Food	Foods Included	Foods Excluded
Beverage	Carbonated beverages, coffee, tea, milk, milk drinks, fruit juices	None
Bread	White or fine rye bread or rolls, soda crackers	Whole-grain products, any breads with nuts or dried fruits
Cereal	Refined wheat, rice, or corn cereals	Whole-grain cereals, bran, cereals cooked with nuts and fruits, hard or firm dry cereal
Fats	Butter, cream, margarine	Fried foods
Fruit	Fruit juices, ripe avocado, banana, cooked or canned apples, apricots, cherries, pears, all above without skin or seeds, dried fruit puree	Raw fruits, skins, or seeds
Vegetables	Cooked, pureed vegetables, vegetable juices	Raw vegetables, skins
Meat, eggs, cheese	Ground or tender meat, fish, or chicken, eggs, cottage cheese, cheddar or American cheese, yogurt, tofu, and smooth peanut butter	Fried meat, chicken, fish, strong cheeses
Soup	Puree from food allowed, all cream and broth soups	Whole vegetable or meat soups unless adjusted in consistency for patient
Dessert	Custard, gelatin, angel food cake, tapioca, puddings, ice cream, cake, plain cookies	Rich desserts, nuts, raisins, coconut
Condiments	Salt, pepper, sugar, vinegar, sauces, gravy, catsup	Olives, pickles, popcorn, relishes, strong spices

inclusion of high-fiber foods in the diet is recommended for patients on a general diet and those with constipation, and it may be helpful in the treatment of diverticular disease. High-fiber foods include whole-wheat breads and cereals, bran, oatmeal, wheat germ, millet, brown rice, cornmeal, legumes (dried beans), nuts, seeds, and fresh fruits and vegetables with skins (e.g., apples, grapes, apricots, raw cauliflower, carrots, celery, cabbage, lettuce). Bananas, prunes, dates, figs, and rhubarb are good laxatives as well as being high in fiber.

◆ Soft Low-Fiber Diet

Indications: Gastrointestinal disturbances, general physical weakness, or poor chewing ability (Table A-6).

Note: Soft diet contains whole pieces of food that are not chopped or pureed. Some elements of this soft diet may need to be adjusted in consistency to fit the needs of the particular client (e.g., pureed meats and fruits).

◆ High-Calorie, -Protein, -Vitamin Diet

This diet is indicated for underweight or malnourished clients. The normal diet is supplemented with foods high in protein, vitamins, and calories. Small, frequent feedings are best (six to eight per day). The caloric value can be 25% to 50% above normal, and the protein increased to 90 to 100 g/day for adults (Table A-7).

Cheeses, sauces, cream soups, potatoes, ice creams, puddings, and milk shakes may be used liberally. Prepared nutritional supplements such as Ensure, Ensure plus, Sustacal, or Carnation Instant Breakfast may be used at meals or between meals. Supplementary vitamins may be indicated.

TABLE A-7 ◆ *High-Calorie, -Protein, and -Vitamin Diet*	
Group	Number of Servings
Milk	4 or more
Meat or meat substitutes	3 or 4
Breads and cereals	4 to 8
Fruits and vegetables	4 or more

*The pages that follow are reprinted from Melonakos, K. (1991). *Saunders Pocket Reference for Nurses.* Philadelphia: Saunders, pp. 316–321. Reprinted with permission.

Glossary

Abduction: Movement away from the midline of the body.

Ablation: Removal of a part, as by incision; eradication.

Abrasion: A wound caused by rubbing or scraping the skin or mucous membrane.

Absorption: The passage of liquids or other substances through a body surface and into its tissues and fluids, as in absorption of the end products of digestion into the intestinal villi.

Abuse: Misuse; excessive or improper use.

Acceptance: Admission of reality, as in the reality of death; the final stage in the process of dealing with dying and death.

Accommodation: Adjustment, especially of the ocular lens for seeing objects at varying distances.

Acid: A substance that yields hydrogen ions in solution.

Acid–base balance: A normal condition in which the narrow range of normal pH and the normal ratio of carbonic acid to bicarbonate ions are maintained.

Acidosis: A condition in which the pH of body fluids is below normal range because of either a loss of base bicarbonate or an accumulation of acid.

Acquired: Occurring from factors outside the organism, as in response to the environment.

Acquired immunodeficiency syndrome (AIDS): A group of symptoms believed to be caused by a virus (HIV) that infects and destroys T-lymphocytes.

Acupressure: Application of digital pressure on a part of the body to relieve pain or produce anesthesia.

Acupuncture: Technique for treating certain painful conditions and for producing regional anesthesia by passing long, thin needles through the skin to specific points.

Acute myocardial infarction: Ischemic necrosis of an area of the heart muscle resulting from sudden occlusion of blood flow through one or more branches of the coronary arteries.

Acute pain: Sharp, severe pain.

Addiction: A psychological craving for alcohol or drugs with the presence of withdrawal symptoms if the substance cannot be obtained.

Adduction: Movement toward the midline of the body.

Adhesion: A fibrous band that binds two parts together that are normally separated; often occurs after surgery in the abdomen.

Adjuvant: That which assists, such as a drug added to a prescription that enhances the principal ingredient.

Adrenergic: Action that mimics that of the sympathetic nervous system.

Adrenocortical: Indicating the cortex of the adrenal gland.

Adulthood: A stage of life at which the individual has reached biological maturity, usually at age 20.

Advance directive: a document prepared for future health care while an individual is alive and competent.

Adventitious: Acquired; arising sporadically.

Aerobe: A microorganism that requires oxygen for survival.

Aerobic: Term for an organism that requires oxygen to live.

Aerosol: A suspension of a drug or other substance that is dispensed in a cloud or mist.

Affect: The external expression; mood.

Ageism: Prejudice against aging and aged persons.

Agglutination: One type of antigen–antibody reaction in which a solid antigen clumps together with a soluble antibody.

Agranulocytosis: Condition of deficiency, or absolute lack, of granulocytic white blood cells.

Airway: The passage by which air enters and leaves the lungs; also, a device used to secure unobstructed respiration.

Albumin, serum: A plasma protein formed principally in the liver and constituting about 60% of the protein concentration in the plasma.

Alkalosis: A condition in which the pH of body fluids is above normal because of either a loss of acid or an accumulation of base bicarbonate.

Allergen(s): Any substance capable of triggering an exaggerated immune response.

Allergy (allergies): An abnormal and individual hypersensitivity to a particular allergen; acquired by exposure to the allergen and manifested after reexposure.

Alleviate: Relieve; to make easier to bear.

Allogeneic: Having a different genetic constitution but belonging to the same species.

Allograft: Transplant tissue obtained from the same species.

Alopecia: Baldness or loss of hair.

Amenorrhea: Absence of menstruation.

Anabolism: The building up of the body substance; the constructive phase of metabolism.

Anaerobic: Term for an organism that lives in an oxygen-free environment.

Analgesia: Absence of normal sense of pain.

Analgesic(s): Pain reliever.

Anaphylaxis: An unusual or exaggerated allergic reaction.

Anastomosis: Communication between two tubular organs; also surgical, traumatic, or pathological formation of a connection between two normally distinct structures.

Androgen(s): Any steroid hormone that promotes male characteristics.

Anemia(s): A condition in which there are too few functioning red blood cells to meet the oxygen needs of tissues.

Anesthesia: Loss of feeling or sensation.

Aneurysm: Sac formed by localized dilatation of the wall of a blood vessel or the heart.

Anger: A feeling of hostility and bitterness against a situation or person; a second stage in acceptance of death.

Angina pectoris: Exertional chest pain caused by ischemia of heart muscle and increased demand for oxygen.

Angiography: X-ray studies of the arteries, veins, or lymph vessels of the body.

Animate: Alive.

Anion: A negatively charged atomic particle.

Ankylosis: Abnormal immobility and consolidation and obliteration of a joint.

Anorexia: Lack or loss of appetite for food.

Anorexia nervosa: An eating disorder in which there is an aberration of eating patterns, severe weight loss, and malnutrition.

Antiarrhythmic agents: Substances that help return the heart rate and rhythm to more normal values and restore the origin of the heart's electrical activity to its natural pacemaker.

Antibiotic: An agent that is capable of either killing or inhibiting the growth of microorganisms.

Antibody (antibodies): An immunoglobulin molecule that is capable of adhering to and interacting only with the antigen that induced its synthesis.

Anticoagulants: Substances that suppress, delay, or nullify the coagulation of blood.

Antiemetic: An agent that prevents or relieves nausea and vomiting.

Antigen(s): Any substance that can produce an antagonist.

Antifungal(s): Agents destructive to or inhibitive of the growth of fungi.

Antigen–antibody reaction: An immune response that occurs when an antibody comes in contact with the specific antigen for which it was formed. In a transfusion reaction the response is a clumping together, or agglutination, of the red blood cells carrying the antigens.

Antihistamine: An agent that counteracts the effects of histamine; used to relieve the symptoms of an allergic reaction.

Antihypertensive: A medication to prevent or control high blood pressure.

Antimicrobial agent: Substance capable of either killing or suppressing the multiplication and growth of microorganisms.

Antineoplastic agent: Substance that inhibits the maturation and proliferation of malignant cells.

Antiseptic(s): Any substance that inhibits the growth of bacteria outside the body; in contrast, a germicide kills the bacteria outright.

Antitoxin: A specific kind of antibody produced in response to the presence of a toxin.

Antitussive: An agent that inhibits the cough reflex in the cough center in the brain.

Antivenin: A substance used to neutralize the venom of a poisonous animal.

Anuria: Diminished or absent production of urine by the kidney.

Aphakic eye: Eye without a lens, as after a cataract extraction.

Aphasia: A defect in or loss of the power of expression by speech, writing, or signs or in the comprehension of spoken or written language.

Apical: Pertaining to the apex of a structure; particularly the heart.

Aplastic: Having deficient or arrested development.

Apnea: Temporary cessation of breathing.

Apraxia: Loss or impairment of acquired motor skills.

Arrhythmia: Variation from the normal rhythm, especially of the heartbeat.

Arteriosclerosis: A group of diseases characterized by thickening and loss of elasticity of the arterial walls.

Arthritis: Inflammation of a joint.

Arthrocentesis: Surgical puncture of a joint cavity for aspiration of synovial fluid.

Arthroplasty: Surgery of a joint to increase mobility or decrease pain.

Arthroscopy: Endoscopic examination of the interior of a joint.

Ascites: Accumulation of edematous fluid within the peritoneal cavity.

Asepsis, medical: Destruction and containment of infectious agents after they leave the body of a patient with an infectious disease.

Assessment, nursing: Data-gathering activities for the purpose of collecting a complete, relevant data base from which a nursing diagnosis can be made.

Astigmatism: Error of refraction in which light rays are not sharply focused on the retina, because of abnormal curvature of the cornea or lens.

Ataxia: Uncoordinated motor movements.

Atelectasis: The collapsed or airless state of the lung.

Atherosclerosis: A disease process in which fibrinous plaques are laid down on the inner walls of the arteries, thus narrowing the lumens of the vessels and predisposing them to the development of intravascular clots.

Atrial fibrillation: Rapid, irregular, and ineffective contractions of the atria.

Atrophy: Wasting or a decrease in size from lack of use.

Audiometry: Measurement of sound perception.

Audit: An official examination of the record of all aspects of patient care.

Aura: A peculiar sensation preceding the appearance of more definite symptoms, especially a sensation, that occurs immediately before an epileptic seizure.

Aural: Pertaining to the ear.

Autograft: A graft transferred from one part of a patient's body to another.

Autoimmune disease: One caused by the body's failure to recognize its own cells, thus rejecting them as it would a foreign substance.

Autologous: Indicating something that has its origin within an individual, as in transfusing with one's own blood.

Autonomic dysreflexia: Hyperreflexia, an uninhibited and exaggerated reflex response of the autonomic nervous system to some type of stimulation.

Avulsion: The tearing away of part or all of an organ or structure.

Axon: The process of a neuron that transmits impulses away from the cell body.

Azotemia: Retention in the blood of urea, creatinine, and other nitrogenous protein metabolites that are normally eliminated in the urine.

B-lymphocyte: A sensitized lymphocyte that is responsible for antibody formation and the development of humoral immunity.

Babinski's reflex: A reflex action elicited by stimulating the sole of the foot and characterized by dorsiflexion of the great toe and flaring of the smaller toes. A positive Babinski indicates an abnormality in the motor control pathways of the nervous system.

Bacteria: Microscopically small organisms belonging to the plant kingdom, some of which are capable of producing disease in humans.

Bactericidal: Able to kill bacteria.

Bacteriophage: A virus that destroys bacteria by lysis. The virus is usually of a type specific for the particular kind of bacteria it attacks.

Bacteriostatic: Able to slow duplication of bacteria.

Bargaining: An attempt to make an arrangement whereby one gives something in order to gain something in return; the third stage in acceptance of death.

Base: A substance that combines with acids to form salts.

Behavior: The manner in which one conducts oneself in response to social stimuli, an inner need, or a combination of the two.

Belief: Currently held idea or value derived from culture and experience.

Benign: Not very harmful; nonmalignant.

Bereaved: Experiencing the reaction of grief and sadness upon learning of the loss of a loved one.

Biliary: Pertaining to bile, the bile ducts, or the gallbladder.

Biliary colic: Acute pain resulting from obstruction of a bile duct, usually caused by cholelithiasis.

Binder: A broad bandage most commonly used as an encircling support of abdomen or chest.

Biofeedback: A training program designed to develop one's ability to control the autonomic (involuntary) nervous system.

Biological response modifier (BRM): An agent that manipulates the immune system in hopes of controlling or curing a malignancy.

Biopsy: Removal of living cells for the purpose of examining them microscopically.

Bisexual: An individual who is sexually attracted to others of either sex.

Bladder, cord: Dysfunction of the urinary bladder caused by damage to the spinal cord.

Bladder, neurogenic: A dysfunction of the urinary bladder caused by a lesion of the central or peripheral nervous system and characterized by lack of awareness of the need to void.

Blepharitis: Infection of glands and lash follicles along the margin of the eyelid.

Blood gases, arterial (ABGs): The partial pressure exerted by oxygen and carbon dioxide in the arterial blood. ABGs reflect the ability of the lungs to exchange these gases, the effectiveness of the kidneys to retain and eliminate bicarbonate, and the efficiency of the heart as a pump.

Borborygmi: Gurgling, splashing sounds normally heard over the large intestine; rumbling in the bowels.

Botulism: Food poisoning caused by a neurotoxin produced by *Clostridium botulinum*, sometimes found in improperly canned or preserved foods.

Bradycardia: Slowness of the heart beat, as evidenced by slowing of the pulse rate to less than 60 per minute.

Bradypnea: Abnormally slow breathing.

Bronchodilator: A drug that acts directly on the smooth muscles of the bronchi to relax them and relieve bronchospasm.

Bronchogram: An x-ray of the bronchial tree using a radiopaque substance that is introduced into the trachea.

Bronchoscopy: Insertion of an endoscope for diagnosis and treatment of disorders of the bronchi.

Bruit: An abnormal sound of venous or arterial origin heard on auscultation.

Bulla (bullae): A blister; a round, fluid-filled lesion of the skin, usually more than 5 mm in diameter.

Burns, full-thickness: One in which all of the epithelializing elements and those lining the sweat glands, hair follicles, and sebaceous glands are destroyed.

Burns, partial-thickness: One in which the epithelializing elements remain intact.

Cachexia: A profound state of general ill health and malnutrition.

Calculus (calculi): An abnormal concretion, usually of mineral salts, occurring mainly in hollow organs or their passages (e.g., renal calculus, or kidney stone).

Callus: A thickened area of the epidermis caused by pressure or friction.

Carcinogen: Any substance or agent that produces or increases the risk of developing cancer in humans or lower animals.

Carcinoma: A malignant growth made up of epithelial cells.

Cardiac glycosides: A group of compounds containing a carbohydrate molecule (for example, digitalis) that affect the contractile force of the heart muscle.

Cardiac tamponade: Compression of the heart caused by collection of fluid in the pericardial sac.

Cardiogenic shock: Shock state caused by pump failure of the heart.

Cardiomyopathy: Disease of the myocardium, especially due to primary disease of the heart muscle.

Cardiopulmonary resuscitation: Reestablishment of heart and lung action after they have suddenly stopped.

Cardiotonic(s): Agent having the effect of strengthening contractions of heart muscle.

Carriers: Persons who harbor infectious organisms within their bodies without manifesting any outward symptoms of the infection.

Catabolic: The destructive phase of metabolism, the opposite of anabolism.

Catabolism: The phase of metabolism in which larger molecules are broken down and energy is released.

Cataract(s): Opacity of the lens of the eye.

Category-specific precautions: A system of precautionary measures organized according to types of diseases (for example, respiratory or enteric) and employed to prevent the spread of disease.

Cations: Positively charged atomic particles.

Cauterize: To burn with a cautery, or to apply one.

CD lymphocyte: A type of lymphocyte that is the master regulator of the human immune system. It is the primary site of replication for HIV.

Cell(s): The basic structural unit of living organisms.

Cell-mediated immunity: Immunity resulting from activation of sensitized lymphocytes.

Cellulitis: Inflammation of cellular or connective tissue.

Central hearing loss: Impaired perception of sound caused by pathology above the junction of the eighth cranial nerve and the brain stem (in the brain).

Cerumen: Earwax.

Chalazion: Infection of the Meibomian gland of the eye; internal stye.

Chemonucleolysis: Treatment of a herniated intervertebral disk by dissolution of a portion of the nucleus pulposus by injection of a chemolytic agent.

Chemotherapy: Use of chemicals, especially drugs, in the treatment of such diseases as cancer, infection, and some mental illnesses.

Cholecystitis: Inflammation of the gallbladder.

Cholelithiasis: Presence of stones within the gallbladder or biliary tract.

Cholinergic: Agent that produces the effect of acetyl-choline.

Chorea: Involuntary muscle twitching.

Chronic pain: Pain of long duration showing little change or slow progressive pain.

Chronological: Occurring in natural time sequence.

Chyme: The mixture of partly digested food and digestive secretions found in the stomach and small intestine during digestion of a meal.

Cirrhosis of liver: A condition characterized by destruction of normal hepatic structures and their replacement with necrotic tissue and scarring.

Claudication, intermittent: A syndrome characterized by intensification of limb pain as exercise is increased; related to occlusion of arteries in the legs.

Climacteric: Endocrine, somatic, and psychic changes occurring at the end of the female reproductive period (menopause); also normal diminution of testicular activity in the male.

Clinical pathway: Tool used to track patient progress along a set path in a managed care system.

Clonic: Alternating contraction and relaxation of muscles.

Code of ethics: A set of rules governing one's conduct.

Cognition: Refers to mental processes of perception, memory, judgment, and reasoning.

Coitus: Sexual intercourse.

Colic: Spasm causing pain; may be biliary, renal, intestinal, or uterine.

Collaboration: The act of working or cooperating with another.

Collaborator: One who works cooperatively with another.

Collagen: Fibrous protein found in skin, bone, cartilage, and ligaments.

Colonization: The process of a group of organisms living together, especially bacteria.

Colostomy (colostomies): Surgical creation of an opening in the colon to allow fecal material to pass outside.

Colposcopy: Visual examination of the vagina and cervix with a specially designed endoscope that allows the detection of malignant growths in their early stages.

Comedo (comedones): A plug of keratin and sebum in an enlarged pore; a blackhead.

Communicable disease: A disease that may be transmitted directly or indirectly from one individual to another.

Complement system: A complex series of enzymatic proteins that interact to combine with the antigen–antibody complex, producing lysis of intact antigen cells.

Complete blood count (CBC): The number of each kind of cell in a sample of blood.

Compliance: Expression of ability of lung tissue to distend when filled with air.

Computed tomography (CT) scan: A computer-aided technique in which small sections of tissue within an organ can be visualized by radiograph.

Concept(s): An idea, thought, or notion derived from experiences and information acquired from one's external environment.

Conductive hearing loss: Impaired perception of sound caused by a dysfunction of either the external or the middle ear.

Confabulation: A behavioral reaction to memory loss in which the patient fills in memory gaps with inappropriate words.

Confusion: Not being aware of or oriented to time, place, or self.

Congenital: Present at birth.

Congestive heart failure: Exhaustion of heart muscle and a resultant engorgement of the heart's chambers and the blood vessels. Eventually, sluggish blood flow leads to retention of fluid and edema in lungs and elsewhere in the body.

Conjugate: Working in union; equally coupled.

Conjunctivitis: Inflammation of the membrane covering the eyeball and lining the eyelids.

Consciousness: Responsiveness of the mind to impressions made by the senses.

Contactant: A substance that produces an allergic or sensitivity response when in direct contact with the skin.

Contamination: Presence of a noxious agent, such as bacteria or radiation, in a place where it is not wanted.

Contracture: Adaptive shortening of skeletal muscle tissue that is not subjected to normal stretching and contraction.

Convulsion: State of involuntary muscle contractions and relaxations.

COPD: Chronic obstructive pulmonary disease.

Coronary occlusion: Closing off of a coronary artery and interruption of its blood flow.

Corrosive: Containing a destructive agent that produces disintegration or wearing away.

Creatinine: A nonprotein substance that is formed in muscle in relatively small and constant amounts, passes into the bloodstream, and is eliminated by the kidney. Urine creatinine levels are diminished when glomerular filtration is impaired.

Crede technique: Downward pressure with the open hand over the suprapubic area to facilitate emptying of the urinary bladder.

Crepitation: A sound like that of hair rubbed between the fingers; occurs when bone fragments rub together.

Cretinism: A congenital condition due to lack of thyroid secretion, characterized by arrested physical and mental development, dystrophy of the bones and soft parts, and lowered basal metabolism.

Criterion: A standard for judging a condition or establishing a diagnosis.

Crust: An outer layer of solid matter formed by dried exudate or secretion.

Cryoprecipitate: Any precipitate that forms as a result of cooling.

Cryosurgery: Destruction of tissue by application of extreme cold, as in removal of cataracts.

Cryotherapy: The therapeutic use of cold or freezing.

Cryptorchidism (cryptorchism): Failure of one or both of the testes to descend into the scrotum during fetal life.

Culdoscopy: Direct inspection of the female viscera through an endoscope introduced into the pelvic cavity through the posterior vaginal fornix.

Culture: Propagation of microorganisms or living tissue cells in media conducive to their growth.

Curettage: Cleansing of a surface of an organ with a spoon-shaped instrument (curet).

Cyanosis: A bluish tinge to the skin caused by lack of oxygen and accumulation of carbon dioxide in the blood.

Cystitis: Inflammation of the urinary bladder.

Cystogram: Radiograph of the urinary bladder using a contrast medium.

Cystoscopy: Endoscopic examination of the interior of the bladder.

Cytology: The study of cells, their origin, structure, function, and pathology.

Cytotoxic: Destructive to cells.

Dactylitis: An inflammation of a finger or toe.

Data base: A collection of facts and figures for analysis from which conclusions may be drawn.

Deaf: Partially or completely lacking the sense of hearing.

Death(s): The cessation of all physical and chemical processes that invariably occurs in all living organisms. See also *Dying.*

Debridement: Removal of all foreign material and dead tissues from or adjacent to a traumatic or infected lesion until healthy tissue is exposed.

Decubitus ulcer(s): A breakdown in the skin and underlying tissues caused by long-standing pressure, ischemia, and damage to the underlying tissue.

Defecate: To evacuate the bowels; to have a bowel movement.

Defibrillation: To stop fibrillation of the heart with electrical current.

Dehiscence: Separation of all layers of a surgical wound.

Delegate: To authorize and send another as one's representative (to carry out a task).

Delirium: An altered state of consciousness that is usually acute and of short duration.

Delusion: A false, fixed belief that cannot be changed with rational explanation.

Dementia: A broad impairment of intellectual function that usually is progressive.

Demyelinization: Destruction of the myelin sheath of nerve tissue.

Dendrite: Any of the thread-like extensions of the cytoplasm of a neuron.

Denial: Defense mechanism in which existence of intolerable conditions are unconsciously rejected; first stage in the acceptance of death.

Denuded: Removal of the protective layer or covering through surgery, trauma, or pathological change.

Depression: A morbid sadness, dejection, or melancholy; a stage in the acceptance of death.

Dermabrasion: Planing of the skin done by mechanical means to smooth the skin and remove scars.

Dermatitis: Inflammation of the skin.

Dermatology: The medical specialty concerned with the diagnosing and treating skin disorders.

Dermatome: Nerve tract.

Developmental task(s): One that should be completed during a specific life period to ensure continuing psychosocial growth and maturity.

Deviation: Departure from normal.

Diabetic neuropathy: A disorder of the peripheral nerves that is associated with diabetes mellitus and is characterized by sexual impotence in the male, neurogenic bladder, and pain or loss of feeling in the lower extremities.

Diabetogenic: Causing diabetes.

Diagnosis, nursing: A concise statement of a patient's actual or potential health problems that nurses, by virtue of their education and experience, are capable and licensed to treat.

Dialysis: The diffusion of solute molecules through a semipermeable membrane, the molecules passing from the more concentrated solution to the less concentrated one.

Dialysis, peritoneal: Use of the peritoneum as a dialyzing membrane to remove waste products that have accumulated in the body as a result of renal failure.

Diaphoresis: Excessive perspiration.

Diastole: The phase of the cardiac cycle in which the heart muscle relaxes between contractions; during this phase the two ventricles are dilated by blood flowing through them. Diastolic blood pressure is recorded as the bottom number in the pressure measurement.

Diastolic blood pressure: Arterial pressure during diastole.

Diffusion: The spontaneous mixing of the molecules or ions of two or more substances; the result of random thermal motion.

Digital: Pertaining to or resembling a finger or toe.

Digitalization: Initial administration of digitalis to build up a therapeutic blood level of the drug.

Diplopia: Double vision; seeing two images.

Disability: Difficulty in performing certain tasks because of impairment.

Disease-specific precautions: A system of precautionary measures organized according to the specific infectious disease presented by the patient.

Disinfectant(s): An agent that destroys infection-producing organisms.

Dislocation: Stretching or tearing of ligaments around a joint with complete displacement of a bone.

Disseminated: Widespread.

Distal: In a position farthest from the point of reference.

Distraction: Having attention diverted from present experience (i.e., pain).

Diuresis: Excretion of excess fluid in the urine.

Diuretic(s): Agents that promote secretion of urine.

Diurnal: Happening during daylight hours.

Diverticulum (diverticula): Small blind pouches resulting from a protrusion of the mucosa of a hollow organ through weakened areas in the organ's muscle wall.

Documentation: The recording of significant information on a patient's chart.

Down's syndrome: A congenital disorder characterized by physical malformations and some degree of mental retardation; also called trisomy 21 syndrome because there is a defect in chromosome 21.

DRGs: Diagnostic-related groups.

Dumping syndrome: A group of symptoms caused by too rapid a passage of food through the upper gastrointestinal tract.

Dying: A stage of life; a process that from a medical point of view begins when a person has a disease that is untreatable and inevitably ends in death; or the final stages of a fatal disease. See also *Death(s)*.

Dynamic: Having vital force or inherent power.

Dysarthria: Slurring or indistinct speech articulation; difficulty speaking.

Dyscrasia: An imbalance of formed elements, as in blood dyscrasia.

Dysfunctional uterine bleeding: Uterine bleeding at times other than during normal menstruation.

Dysmenorrhea: Painful or difficult menstruation.

Dyspareunia: Difficult or painful coitus in women.

Dysphagia: Difficulty in swallowing.

Dysphasia: Difficulty speaking; usually caused by a brain lesion.

Dyspnea: Labored or difficult breathing.

Dysrythmia: Variation from the normal rhythm, especially of the heartbeat.

Dysthymia: A disturbance in mood that may manifest in either depression or elation.

Dysuria: Painful urination.

Eccentric: Departing from conventional custom or practice; differing conspicuously in behavior, appearance, or opinions.

Ecchymosis: An irregularly shaped, blue-black skin discoloration caused by bleeding beneath the skin.

ECG: The record produced by amplification of the electrical impulses normally generated by the heart.

Ectopic: Located away from normal position, as in ectopic pregnancy.

Ectropion: Outward turning of the eyelid.

Edema: An accumulation of fluid surrounding the cell.

Edematous: Pertaining to, or affected with, edema (abnormal fluid in the tissue).

EEG: A recording of changes in electrical potentials in the brain.

Effluent: A flowing out (i.e., out of ileostomy, colostomy).

Ejaculation: Ejection of the seminal fluid from the male urethra.

EKG: The record produced by amplification of the electrical impulses normally generated by the heart.

Elastance: The extent to which the lungs are able to return to their original position after being barely distended.

Electrocardiogram: The record produced by amplification of the electrical impulses normally generated by the heart.

Electroencephalogram: A recording of changes in electric potentials in various areas of the brain.

Electrolyte(s): A chemical substance that, when dissolved in water, dissociates into ions and thus is capable of conducting an electric current.

Electromyography: The recording and study of intrinsic electrical properties of skeletal muscle; useful in diagnosing neuromuscular disorders.

Elimination: Discharge from the body of indigestible materials and waste products of metabolism.

Embolism: Sudden obstruction of arterial blood flow by a blood clot or a mass that has been brought to the site in the bloodstream.

Embolus: A clot or plug of material (usually from a thrombus) carried by blood flow that lodges in a vessel and obstructs blood flow.

Emesis: Substance produced by vomiting.

Emphysema: A chronic pulmonary disease characterized by increase beyond normal in the size of air spaces distal to the terminal bronchiole with destructive changes in their walls.

Empyema: The presence of infected and purulent exudate within the pleural cavity.

Encephalopathy: Any dysfunction of the brain.

Endarterectomy: Surgical removal of thickened atheromatous areas of the innermost coat of an artery.

Endemic: Present in a community at all times.

Endocarditis: Inflammation of the membrane lining the cavities of the heart and of the connective tissue bed on which it lies.

Endocrine: Secreting internally; refers to glandular function.

Endogenous: Coming from within.

Endometriosis: The presence of endometrial tissue in locations outside the uterus.

Endorphin: One of a group of opiate-like peptides naturally produced by the body.

Endoscopy: Examination with an endoscope that allows for direct visual inspection of the interior of hollow organs and body cavities.

Endotoxin(s): Heat-stable toxin that is present in the intact bacterial cell wall, is pyrogenic, and is capable of increasing capillary permeability.

Engraftment: Successful establishment of the graft in bone marrow transplantation.

Enteral feeding: Feeding a patient by means of a tube passed into the stomach from the nasal passage.

Enterostomal: Refers to an abdominal stoma opening of the intestine.

Entropion: Inversion of the eyelid margin.

Enucleation: Removal of an organ or other mass intact, as of the eyeball from the orbit.

Enzyme: Any protein that acts as a catalyst, increasing the rate at which chemical reaction occurs.

Epidemic(s): Disease that simultaneously attacks many people in a geographic area, is widely diffused, and spreads rapidly.

Epidermophytosis: A fungal infection that most often affects the feet, especially between the toes; also called *athlete's foot* or *dermophytosis*.

Epididymis: A small oblong body resting upon and beside the posterior surface of the testes that constitutes the first part of the excretory duct of each testis.

Epidural: Situated upon or outside of the dura mater.

Epigastric: Pertaining to the region over the pit of the stomach.

Epistaxis: Nosebleed.

Equilibrium: Balance.

Erection: The state of swelling, hardness, and stiffness observed in the penis of the male and to a lesser extent in the clitoris of the female.

Erythema: Redness of the skin.

Erythrasma: A chronic bacterial infection of the major skin folds, marked by red or brownish patches on the skin.

Erythrocyte sedimentation rate: The rate at which red blood cells settle out of unclotted blood in 1 hour.

Erythropoiesis: Formation of red blood cells, erythrocytes.

Eschar: A castout of dead tissue, as from a burn, corrosive application, or gangrene.

Esophageal varices: Varicosities of branches of the azygous vein that connects with the portal vein in the lower esophagus; related to portal hypertension and cirrhosis of the liver.

Estrogens: The female sex hormones, including estradiol, estriol, and estrone.

Etiology: Study of the cause of disease; origin.

Euthanasia: An easy or painless death; active euthanasia, or mercy killing, is the deliberate ending of the life of a person who is incurably and terminally ill; passive euthanasia is the withholding of "heroic" measures and allowing the person to die.

Euthymia: A normal mood or feeling state.

Evaluation,
   of outcome: Appraisal of the patient's progress toward achievement of the goals and objectives stated in the nursing care plan.
   of process: Appraisal of nursing activities and what has been done to assess, plan, and implement nursing care.
   of structure: Appraisal of the physical facilities, equipment, staffing, and other characteristics of an agency that affect the quality of nursing care.

Evisceration: (1) extrusion of internal organs; (2) removal of the contents of the eyeball, leaving the sclera intact.

Excess: An amount beyond what is usual or necessary.

Excoriation: Any superficial loss of substance, such as that produced by scratching the skin.

Exercises, isometric: Active exercise performed against stable resistance, without change in the length of the muscle.

Excursion: Range of movement (of the lungs).

Exfoliate: To separate or peel off in scales, layers, or flakes.

Exocrine: Secreting externally via a duct.

Exogenous: Coming from outside.

Exophthalmia: Abnormal protrusion of the eyeball.

Exotoxin: A potent toxin formed and excreted by the bacterial cell.

Expectorate: To spit out saliva or cough up materials from the air passageways leading to the lungs.

Extension: A movement that brings a limb into or toward a straight condition. Opposite of flexion.

Extracellular fluids: Body fluids outside the cell walls that constitute the environment of each cell.

Extracorporeal: Outside the body.

Exudate: Fluid that contains dead cells, serum, phagocytes, bacteria, or pus.

Fecal impaction: Accumulation of puttylike or hardened feces in the rectum or sigmoid colon.

Feedback: The process of providing a system information about its output.
   negative: A corrective action in which a system is informed that its output is not satisfactory and a change is needed.
   positive: Information that tells a system its output is satisfactory.

Fibroid: A thickened vascular mass in the uterus.

Fibroma: A fibrous, encapsulated connective tissue tumor.

Fibrosis: Fibrous tissue formation.

Fistula(s): Any abnormal, tube-like passage within the body between two internal organs or leading from an internal organ to the body surface.

Flaccid: Limp, weak, or relaxed.

Flatus: Gas in the digestive tract.

Flexion: To decrease the angle between the bones forming a joint; opposite of extension.

Flora: Plant life as distinguished from animal life.

Fluid(s): The water and substances dissolved in it that form the internal environment.
   transcellular: Body fluids that pass through cellular structures and eventually are eliminated from the body.

Fluid balance: Equilibrium between the amount of fluid taken into the body and that lost through urine, feces, the lungs, skin, and possibly vomiting and fistulas.

Fluid deficit(s): Fluid imbalance in which there is not enough fluid in one or more of the body's fluid compartments as a result of either inadequate intake or excessive loss.

Fluid excess: Imbalance in which too much fluid accumulates in one or more of the body's fluid compartments. See also *Edema.*

Fracture(s): Interruption in the continuity of a bone.

Fulguration: Destruction by electric cautery.

Functional disorder: A disorder that affects function but not the structure of the body or body part.

Fungus (fungi): A member of a group of organisms (mushrooms, yeasts, molds, etc.) that thrive in a warm, moist climate and can cause infections difficult to eradicate because they tend to reproduce by means of spores that are resistant to ordinary disinfectants and antiseptics.

Galactosemia: A genetic disorder in which there is a lack of the enzyme necessary for proper metabolism of galactose.

Gangrene: A necrosis, or death, of tissue, usually due to deficient or absent blood supply.

Gastritis: An inflammation of the mucous membrane lining the stomach.

Gastrostomy: Surgical creation of an opening into the stomach to administer food and liquids.

Gate control theory: The proposal that synapses in the dorsal horn of the spinal cord act as gates and that pain signals compete with those of other kinds of stimuli for passage through the gate and transmission to the brain.

Gene: One of the self-reproducing biological units of heredity that make up segments of the DNA molecule that controls cellular reproduction and function.

Genital: Pertaining to the genitals (reproductive organs).

Geriatrics: Medical treatment of diseases commonly associated with aging and aged persons.

Gerontology: Study of the problems of aging in all its aspects.

Glaucoma: A group of diseases of the eye, characterized by increased intraocular pressure, that can produce blindness if not managed successfully.

Global amnesia: Irretrievable total loss of memory.

Globulin(s): General term for proteins; separated into five fractions by serum protein electrophoresis and classified in order of decreasing electrophoretic mobility. The fractions are alpha$_1$-, alpha$_2$-, beta$_1$-, and beta$_2$-globulins and the gamma globulins.

Glucocorticoid: Any hormone released from the adrenal cortex that increases glucogenesis and thus raises the level of liver glycogen and blood glucose.

Glucogenesis: Formation of glucose from glycogen.

Glycosuria: Glucose in the urine.

Glycosylated hemoglobin (HGB A$_{1C}$): Hemoglobin with glucose attached to it; periodic measurements of hemoglobin A$_{1C}$ can help determine a diabetic patient's average blood glucose level over a period of 3 to 4 months.

Goal(s): A broad statement describing what is to be accomplished over a specified period.

Goiter: An enlargement of the thyroid gland.

Goniometry: Measurement of range of motion in a joint.

Graft: Implant or transplant of tissue or an organ.

Granulocyte: Leukocyte containing abundant granules in its cytoplasm; granulocytes include neutrophils, eosinophils, and basophils.

Gynecomastia: Development of abnormally large mammary gland in the male.

Hallucination: A sensory perception (touching, tasting, feeling, hearing, seeing) that occurs without external stimulation.

Handicap: Social disadvantage that exists because of a disability.

Health: The ability to function well physically and mentally and to express the full range of one's potentialities.

Hearing loss: Impaired perception of sound.

Heat exhaustion: A disorder resulting from overexposure to heat or to the sun; also called *heat prostration*. It is caused by excessive perspiration and loss of body water and salt.

Heatstroke: A life-threatening condition resulting from prolonged exposure to environmental heat; also called *sunstroke*.

Helping relationship: One in which at least one of the parties intends to promote growth, development, maturity, improved functioning, and improved coping in the life of the other.

Hemarthrosis: Collection of blood in the joint space.

Hematemesis: Vomiting of blood.

Hematocrit: The volume percentage of red blood cells in whole blood.

Hematoma (hematomas): A localized collection of blood, usually clotted, that has leaked from adjacent blood vessels into an organ, space, or tissue.

Hematuria: Blood in the urine.

Hemiparesis: Weakness affecting only one side of the body.

Hemiplegia: Paralysis of one half, or one side, of the body.

Hemodialysis: Removal of nitrogenous wastes from the blood by circulating arterial blood through a dialysate and returning it to venous circulation.

Hemodynamics: Study of the movements of blood and the pressures being exerted in the blood vessels and the chambers of the heart.

Hemoglobin: The protein found in red blood cells that transports molecular oxygen in the blood; oxygenated hemoglobin (oxyhemoglobin) is bright red in color; unoxygenated hemoglobin is darker.

Hemolysis: Rupture of red blood cells with release of hemoglobin into the plasma.

Hemolytic: Pertaining to the breakdown of red blood cells.

Hemophilia: An inherited disorder in which there is deficiency of one or more specific clotting factors in the blood.

Hemoptysis: Coughing and spitting of blood that can originate in the lungs, larynx, or trachea.

Hemothorax: Collection of blood in the pleural cavity.

Hepatic encephalopathy: Degenerative changes in the brain associated with liver failure.

Hepatitis: Inflammation of the liver.

Hernia: Protrusion or projection of an organ or a part of an organ through the wall of the cavity that normally contains it.

Herpesvirus: Any of a large group of DNA viruses found in many animal species. Type 1 herpes simplex virus (HSV) produces lesions that are primarily nongenital. Type 2 HSV lesions most often are genital.

Heterosexual: A person who is sexually attracted to a person of the opposite sex.

Hiatus hernia: Protrusion of a portion of the stomach through the opening in the diaphragm through which the esophagus passes.

Hierarchy: The arrangement of objects, elements, or values in a graduated series.

Hirsutism: Excessive growth of hair on the body.

HIV: Human immunodeficiency virus. The causative agent for AIDS.

HLA: Human leukocyte antigen.

HMO: Health maintenance organization.

Holism: The belief that each person is a unified whole.

Holistic health care: Attention to the mental, social, spiritual, and physical aspects of health and illness.

Homeopathy: A practice based on the theory that large doses of drugs that produce symptoms of a disease in healthy people will cure the same symptoms when administered in small amounts.

Homeostasis: A tendency of biological systems to maintain stability in the internal environment while continually adjusting to changes necessary for survival.

Homosexual: Person who is sexually attracted to a person of the same sex.

Homozygous: Gene inherited from both parents.

Hordeolum: An external stye.

Hormone: A chemical produced by the cells of the body and transported by the bloodstream to target cells and organs on which it has a regulatory effect.

Hospice: A program that provides a continuum of home and inpatient care for the terminally ill and their family.

Human needs: Basic needs for survival and personal growth shared by all humans.

Human needs theory: The proposal that basic human needs act as stimuli to human behavior; Maslow postulated five levels of human needs: physiological, safety and security, love and belonging, esteem, and self-actualization.

Humoral: Pertaining to body fluids or substances contained in them.

Humoral immunity: Antibody-mediated immunity, the result of B-cell action and the production of antibodies.

Hydrocephalus: Increased cerebrospinal fluid in the ventricles of the brain.

Hydronephrosis: Distention of the renal pelvis and calices with urine that cannot flow through obstructed ureters.

Hydrostatic pressure: The pressure or force due to the presence of a fluid.

Hyperalimentation: Total parenteral nutrition.

Hypercalcemia: An above-normal level of calcium in the blood (i.e., more than 5.5 mEq/L or 11 mg/dL).

Hypercapnia: Increased amount of carbon dioxide in the blood.

Hyperglycemia: Increase of blood sugar as in diabetes.

Hyperkalemia: Excessive amount of potassium in the blood.

Hyperlipidemia: Excessive lipids in the blood.

Hypernatremia: Excess of sodium in the blood.

Hyperopia: A visual defect in which parallel light rays reaching the eye focus behind the retina; farsightedness.

Hyperplasia: Increase in the number of cells of an organ; extra cell growth.

Hypersensitivity: An exaggerated immune response to an agent perceived by the body to be foreign. See also *Allergy (allergies)*.

Hypersomnia: Sleeping for long periods.

Hypertension: Persistently high blood pressure; in adults, a systolic pressure equal to or greater than 140 mm Hg and a diastolic pressure equal to or greater than 90 mm Hg.

Hypertonic solution: One in which the osmotic pressure (concentration) is greater than that of body fluids.

Hyperthermia: Unusually high fever.

Hypertrophy: Increase in size of a structure or organ.

Hyperuricemia: Excessive uric acid in the urine.

Hyperventilation: An abnormal breathing pattern in which an above-normal amount of air is inhaled into the lungs.

Hypervolemia: Abnormal increase in the volume of circulating blood.

Hypnosis: A subconscious condition, usually artificially induced, in which there is a response to suggestions and commands made by the hypnotist.

Hypoalbuminemia: Decreased albumin in the blood.

Hypocalcemia: A below-normal level of calcium in the blood (i.e., less than 4.5 mEq/L or 8.5 mg/dL).

Hypocapnia: A deficit of carbon dioxide in the blood resulting from hyperventilation.

Hypochromic: Pertaining to a condition of the blood in which the red blood cells have a reduced hemoglobin content.

Hypogammaglobulinemia: An immune deficiency characterized by abnormally low levels of generally all classes of serum gammaglobulins with increased susceptibility to infectious diseases.

Hypoglycemia: Deficiency of sugar in the blood.

Hypoglycemic agents: Those that lower the blood glucose level (i.e., oral medications that are used to treat some forms of diabetes mellitus).

Hypokalemia: Extreme potassium depletion in the circulating blood.

Hyponatremia: Decreased concentration of sodium in the blood.

Hypophysectomy: Excision of the hypophysis cerebri.

Hyposensitization: A treatment used in managing hypersensitivity to a known allergen; the program involves regular injections of minute quantities of selected antigens over an extended period.

Hypothalamus: That portion of the diencephalon that lies beneath the thalamus at the base of the cerebrum; it activates, controls, and integrates many of the body's vital functions (e.g., regulation of metabolism, volume of body fluids, electrolyte content, and release of hormones).

Hypothermia: A serious loss of body heat caused by prolonged exposure to cold.

Hypotonic solution: One in which the osmotic pressure (concentration) is less than that of body fluids.

Hypotonic state: Pertaining to abnormally decreased muscular tone or tension.

Hypoventilation: An abnormal breathing pattern in which insufficient amounts of air are inhaled into the lungs.

Hypovolemia: Diminished blood volume.

Hypoxemia: Insufficient oxygenation of the blood.

Hypoxia: Deficiency of oxygen.

Iatrogenic disorder: An adverse condition induced by effects of treatment by a physician or surgeon.

Icterus: Bile pigmentation of the tissues, membranes, and secretions.

Idiopathic: Of unknown cause.

Idiosyncrasy: Special characteristic by which persons differ from each other.

Ileal conduit: Surgically created passageway that uses a portion of the ileum to direct the flow of urine from the ureters to the outside.

Ileostomy (ileostomies): An artificial opening in the ileum, created surgically to drain fecal material from the small intestine.

Ileus: Intestinal obstruction, especially failure of peristalsis.

Illusion: A misperception of an actual sensory perception; misinterpretation of reality.

Imagery: Imagination; the calling up of mental pictures or events.

Immune deficiency: A lack of immune bodies and resultant impairment of the immune response to foreign agents.

Immunity: Resistance to a specific disease.

    active: That acquired by producing one's own antibody.

    passive: That acquired by receiving antibody from a source other than one's own body.

Immunization: The process of rendering an individual immune by passive immunity or of becoming immune by active immunity.

Immunocompetence: The capacity to develop an immune response after exposure to antigen.

Immunoglobulin(s): A protein of animal origin with known antibody activity and a major component of humoral immunity. See also *Antibody (antibodies)*.

Immunosuppression: Deliberate inhibition of antibody formation; used in transplantation to prevent rejection of the donor organ.

Immunotherapy: Passive immunity of a person by administration of preformed antibody; also the administration of immunopotentiators and immunocompetent lymphoid tissue for cancer treatment.

Impairment: Dysfunction of a specific organ or body system.

Impetigo: An infection of the skin, usually by streptococci or staphylococci.

Impotence: Inability of the male to achieve or maintain an erection.

Impulsive: Acting in response to an impulse because the action brings emotional release or pleasure even though the action may be harmful to the self or socially unacceptable.

Inanimate: Not alive; dull, lifeless.

Incontinence: An alteration in the control of bowel or urinary elimination, or both.

Incubation: The interval between exposure to infection and the appearance of the first symptom.

Infarct: Localized area of necrosis produced by ischemia caused by obstructed arterial supply or inadequate venous drainage.

Infarction: Occurrence of localized area of dead tissue produced by inadequate blood flow.

Infection: Invasion and multiplication of pathogenic microorganisms in body tissue.

Inference: A deduction or conclusion.

Inflammation: An immediate cellular response to any kind of injury to the cells and tissues.

Ingestants: Any substances taken orally, such as food or drink.

Ingestion: The taking of any substance, such as food, drugs, water, chemicals, by mouth or through the digestive system.

Inhalants: Medication or compounds suitable for inhaling.

Initial: The beginning of a thing or process; the first.

Injectables: Appropriate fluids capable of being injected.

Innate: Belonging to the essential nature of something; existing in or belonging at birth.

Insensible: Unconscious; without feeling or consciousness.

Insomnia: A sleep disorder; an inability to sleep.

Insufficiency: The condition of being inadequate for a given purpose.

Insulin-dependent diabetes mellitus: Type I diabetes; a form of the disease that requires replacement of endogenous insulin with regular injections of exogenous insulin.

Intention tremor: Tremor that occurs upon attempt at voluntary movement.

Interstitial: Placed or lying between.

Interstitial fluids: Body fluids that are located in the tissue spaces around the cells. See also *Edema*.

Intervention: Nursing activities performed by the nurse to meet the specified goals of a nursing care plan.

Intracellular: Within cells.

Intracellular fluids: Body fluids that are within cell walls.

Intraocular: Within the eye.

Intrathecal: Injection into the subarachnoid space of the spinal cord via lumbar puncture.

Intravascular fluids: Body fluids within the blood vessels; they are composed of plasma and the substances it transports.

Intravenous therapy: The administration of fluids through a vein.

Intussusception: Telescoping of one part of the bowel into another.

Ion: A particle carrying an electric charge, consisting of an atom or group of atoms into which the molecules of an electrolyte are divided or one of the electrified particles into which the molecules of a gas are divided by ultraviolet rays, gamma rays, or x-rays, or by other ionizing agents.

Iridectomy: Excision of part of the iris.

Ischemia: Deficiency of blood supply to a part as a result of functional constriction of a blood vessel or of actual obstruction, as by a clot.

Isolation technique: Special precautionary procedures used to set apart patients with communicable diseases; the purpose is to prevent the spread of infectious agents from the patient to others.

Isometric: Having equal dimensions; maintaining the same length.

Isotonic contraction: Occurs when tension is developed in a muscle.

Isotonic solution: A solution in which the osmotic pressure is the same as that of intracellular fluid (e.g., normal saline [0.9% concentration]).

Isotope: One of a series of chemical elements that have nearly identical chemical properties but differ in their atomic weight and electric charge. Many isotopes are radioactive.

Jaundice: A yellowing of the skin and mucous membranes that reflects excessively high blood levels of bilirubin (bile pigment).

Keloid: Excessive, abnormal scar formation in the skin following trauma or surgical incision.

Keratitis: Inflammation of the cornea.

Ketoacidosis: Accumulation of ketone bodies in the blood because of incomplete metabolism of fats, resulting in metabolic acidosis.

Ketonuria: Acetone bodies in the urine.

Ketosis: The accumulation in the body of the ketone bodies: acetone, beta-hydroxybutyric acid, and acetoacetic acid.

Kinetic motion: The motion of material bodies and the forces and energy associated with it.

Korsakoff's syndrome: Substance-induced persisting dementia.

Kupffer's cells: Large, highly phagocytic cells in the liver; they form part of the reticuloendothelial system.

Kyphosis: Abnormally increased curvature of the thoracic spine, which gives a "hunchback" appearance.

Labile: Unsteady, not fixed; easily disarranged.

Labyrinthitis: Inflammation of the internal ear, including the vestibule, cochlea, and semicircular canal.

Laparoscopy: Examination of the peritoneal cavity with a fiber-optic instrument inserted through a small abdominal incision.

Laryngectomy: Partial or total removal of the larynx by surgical excision; the person who has had a laryngectomy is called a *laryngectomee*.

Laryngoscopy: Direct or indirect visual examination of the larynx.

Laser: Stands for *l*ight *a*mplification by *s*timulated *e*mission of *r*adiation; converts light wavelengths into one small, intense unified beam of one wavelength radiation; used for diagnosis and surgery.

Latent: Not obvious; hidden.

Lesion: A circumscribed area of pathologically altered tissue.

Leukapheresis: Separation of leukocytes from blood that is then transfused back into the patient.

Leukemia: Malignant disease of the blood-forming organs, marked by abnormal proliferation and development of leukocytes and their precursors in the blood and bone marrow.

Leukocyte: A colorless blood cell whose chief function is to protect the body against pathogenic microorganisms.

Leukocytosis: An increase in the number of white blood cells, leukocytes, in the blood.

Leukopenia: Reduction in the number of leukocytes in the blood to 5,000 or less.

Leukoplakia: Patches of thickened, white tissue on mucous membrane; considered a precursor to cancer.

Level of consciousness (LOC): A standardized system to describe the state of consciousness (i.e., alert wakefulness, drowsiness, stupor, or coma).

Lhermitte's sign: An electric shock–like sensation felt along the spine when the neck is flexed.

Libido: Conscious or unconscious sexual drive.

Lifestyle habits: Entrenched practices related to work, recreation, diet, exercise, and other activities of daily living.

Ligate: To tie or bind.

Lipodystrophy: Disturbance or defectiveness of fat metabolism.

Lipoma: A fatty tumor.

Lipoprotein: Any of the macromolecular complexes that are transported in the blood.

Lithiasis: Formation of stones.

Lithotripsy: Crushing of a calculus in the kidney, bladder, urethra or gallbladder.

Lordosis: Abnormal forward curvature of the spine.

Lucid: Clear, especially applied to clarity of the mind.

Lymphadenitis: Inflammation of the lymph nodes.

Lymphadenopathy: Disease of the lymph nodes, often producing enlargement.

Lymphangiography: Radiograph of lymphatic vessels after injection of a contrast medium.

Lymphangitis: Inflammation of the lymph vessels.

Lymphatic system: An accessory system by which fluids can flow from tissue spaces into the blood.

Lymphedema: Swelling of tissues drained by the lymphatic system.

Lymph nodes: Small bundles of lymphatic tissue containing lymphocytes, the functions of which are filtration and phagocytosis.

Lymphocyte: A mononuclear, nongranulous leukocyte that is chiefly a product of lymphoid tissue and is important in the development of immunity.

  sensitized: A nongranular lymphocyte that has been processed either by the thymus (T-lymphocyte) or an unknown processing area (B-lymphocyte) and is responsible for either cellular or humoral immunity.

Lymphocyte-transforming factor: A protein mediator that causes transformation and clonal expansion of nonsensitized lymphocytes that produce a toxin destructive to antigen.

Lymphoma: Any neoplastic disorder of lymphoid tissue.

Lysis: The gradual decline of a fever or disease; the opposite of crisis.

Macrophage: Large, mononuclear phagocytes derived from monocytes; they are components of the reticuloendothelial system.

Macrophage-activating factor: A mediator released by sensitized lymphocytes on contact with an antigen, the function of which is to induce in macrophages an increased content of lysosomal enzymes, more aggressive phagocytosis, and increased mitosis.

Macrophage chemotaxis factor: A protein mediator released by sensitized lymphocytes on contact with antigen, the function of which is to attract macrophages to the antigen site.

Macule (macula): A discolored spot on the skin that is not raised above the surface.

Malignancy: See *Cancer.*

Malignant: Becoming progressively worse; resisting treatment and resulting in death; having the properties of anaplasia, invasiveness, and metastasis.

Mammography: X-ray examination of the soft tissues of the breast.

Mammoplasty: Plastic surgery of the breast.

Managed care: Organization of health care delivery that coordinates care delivery by various health team members in a timely, cost-effective, manner.

Mania: An elevation in mood characterized by feelings of elation, excitement, or extreme irritability.

Mastication: Chewing.

Mean, mathematical: An average (e.g., mean corpuscular hemoglobin concentration, which is the concentration of hemoglobin in the average erythrocyte).

Mediastinum: The mass of tissues and organs separating the sternum in front and the vertebral column behind.

Mediate: Accomplished by indirect means; act between two parties or sides.

Meditation: The act of contemplative thinking.

Melanoma: A malignant, darkly pigmented mole or tumor of the skin.

Melena: Black, tarry stools.

Menarche: Onset of menstruation.

Menière's syndrome: A group of symptoms produced by an increase in fluid in the labyrinthine spaces with swelling and congestion of the mucosa of the cochlea.

Menopause: The span of time during which the menstrual cycle wanes and gradually stops; see *climacteric.*

Menorrhagia: Excessive menstruation.

Menses: The onset of the menstrual cycle.

Menstruation: Shedding of the uterine lining.

Mentate: To think.

Metabolic acidosis: A condition in which the pH of body fluids is below 7.4 because of either an excessive production of carbonic acid through the oxidation of fats or because of a loss of bicarbonate.

Metabolic alkalosis: A condition in which the pH of body fluids is above 7.4 because of an excessive loss of acid, above-normal intake or retention of base, or a low level of potassium in the blood.

Metabolism: The sum of the physical and chemical processes by which living tissue is formed and maintained and by which large molecules are disassembled to provide energy.

Metastasis: The movement of disease from one organ or body part to a distant location; for example, the migration of microorganisms and of malignant cells.

Metrorrhagia: Uterine bleeding occurring at irregular intervals and sometimes for prolonged periods.

Microcytic: Smaller-than-normal blood cells.

Micron: Unit of linear measure; equal to 0.001 mm.

Micturition: The voiding of urine.

Milliequivalent: One-thousandth of a chemical equivalent, expressed as mEq; the concentration of electrolytes in a certain volume of solution is usually expressed as milliequivalents per liter (mEq/L).

Mineralocorticoids: A group of hormones elaborated by the adrenal cortex that have an effect on sodium, chloride, and potassium levels in extracellular fluid.

Miotic: Drug that constricts the pupil.

Mitosis: Type of cell division of somatic cells in which each daughter cell contains the same number of chromosomes as the parent cell. It is the process by which the body grows and by which somatic cells are replaced.

Monocytes: Mononuclear phagocytic leukocytes.

Morphological: Science of structures and forms without regard to function.

Mucolytic: Dissolving or destroying mucus.

Mucositis: Inflammation of a mucous membrane.

Muscle tone: Readiness of a muscle to contract and relax normally.

Mycosis (mycoses): Any disease caused by a fungus.

Mydriatic: Dilating the pupil.

Myocarditis: Inflammation of the heart muscle.

Myopia: The error of refraction in which parallel light rays focus in front of the retina; nearsightedness.

Myringotomy: Incision into the eardrum.

Myxedema: Condition in the adult in which there are low thyroid levels.

Nebulizer: An atomizer; a device for delivering drugs or water to the respiratory tract by forcing air or oxygen through a solution.

Necrotic: Pertaining to death of a portion of tissue.

Necrosis: The changes that occur as a result of death of cells; caused by enzymatic degradation.

Neoplasm: Tumor; any new and abnormal growth.

Nephron: The structural and functional unit of the kidney, which consists of the renal corpuscle, the proximal convoluted tubule, limbs of the loop of Henle, the distal convoluted tubule, and the collecting tubule; thus each nephron is able to form urine independently.

Nephrosclerosis: Atherosclerotic disease of the small renal arteries related to hypertension and eventual destruction of renal cells.

Nephrostomy: Formation of an artificial fistula into the renal pelvis of the kidney.

Nephrostomy tubes: Tubes inserted to drain the renal pelvis.

Networking: Meeting people, exchanging phone numbers, expressing interest in other persons and what they are doing, and establishing a business relationship that might be mutually beneficial.

Neuron: Any of the conducting cells of the nervous system; consists of a cell body containing the nucleus and cytoplasm and the axon and dendrites.

Neuropathy: Any disease of the nerves.

Neutrophilia: Increase in the number of neutrophils in the blood.

Neutrophils: Granular leukocytes; also called *polymorphonuclear leukocytes.*

Nocturia: Excessive urination during the night.

Nodules: Small masses of tissue that can be detected by touch.

Noncommunicable Cannot be carried from one person to another.

Non-insulin-dependent diabetes mellitus (type II): A form of diabetes in which levels of endogenous insulin are adequate and control can be managed by diet and exercise and perhaps by an oral hypoglycemic agent.

Normo-: A combining form indicating normal or usual.

Nosocomial: Pertaining to or originating in a hospital.

Nuchal rigidity: Stiffness and pain in the neck from inflammation of the meninges.

Nursing: The diagnosis and treatment of human responses to actual or potential health problems. See also *Nursing process.*

Nursing care plans: Written plans of care that serve to communicate to the nursing staff and others the specific nursing diagnoses and prescribed nursing orders for directing and evaluating the effectiveness of the care given.

Nursing process: A goal-directed series of activities whereby the practice of nursing accomplishes its goal of alleviating, minimizing, or preventing real or potential health problems.

Nystagmus: Involuntary, rapid rhythmic movement of the eyeball.

Objective data: Information obtained through the senses or measured by instruments.

Objectives: Well-defined steps toward the accomplishment of a goal; they should be realistic, be stated in measurable terms, and include the conditions under which they will be accomplished.

Obsessive: Having ideas, thoughts, or impulses that are persistent to an excessive degree.

Occult: Obscure, concealed, hidden.

Oliguria: Diminished amount of urine formation.

Oncogene: A gene in a virus that has the ability to induce a cell to become malignant.

Oncology: The study of tumors.

Oophoritis: Inflammation of an ovary; ovaritis.

Ophthalmologist: A physician who specializes in treating eye disorders.

Ophthalmoscope: An instrument for examining the eye; the direct ophthalmoscope is used to inspect the back portion of the interior of the eyeball; the indirect ophthalmoscope permits stereoscopic inspection of the interior of the eye.

Opportunistic pathogen: Fungi or bacteria, usually harmless, that cause infection in a person with a depressed immune system.

Optician: A specialist in the making of optical apparatus.

Optometrist: A professional person trained to examine the eyes and prescribe eyeglasses to correct irregularities of vision.

Orchiectomy: Excision of one or both testes.

Orchitis: Inflammation of the testes.

Orthopedic: Referring to the correction of deformities of the musculoskeletal system.

Orthopnea: Ability to breathe easily only in the upright position.

Orthostatic hypotension: A fall in blood pressure that occurs when standing up from a sitting or lying position or when standing in a fixed position; it is characterized by dizziness, syncope, and blurred vision.

Oscilloscope: An instrument that makes visible on a screen the nature of an electrical current.

Osmosis: The passage of solvent from a solution of lesser concentration to one of greater concentration through a selectively permeable membrane.

Osmotic pressure: Pressure that develops when two solutions of different concentrations are separated by a semipermeable membrane.

Ossification: Formation of or conversion into bone or a bony substance.

Osteoporosis: A porous condition of bone due to demineralization associated with aging.

Otalgia: Pain in the ear.

OTC: Over the counter.

Otitis media: Inflammation of the middle ear.

Otorrhea: Inflammation of the ear with purulent discharge.

Otoscope: Instrument for examining the ear canal and eardrum.

Outcome: The result of an action.

Ovulation: The periodic ripening and rupture of the mature Graafian follicle and the discharge of the ovum from the cortex of the ovary.

Oxidation: The process of a substance combining with oxygen.

Pacemaker: A mechanical device that provides electrical stimulation when an anatomic pacemaker fails; a cardiac pacemaker provides electrical stimulation when there is heart block.

Pain: A feeling of distress or suffering caused by stimulation of specialized nerve cells; considered to occur whenever a person says it is present.

Palliative: Relief of symptoms when a disease cannot be cured.

Palpitation: Rapid, violent, or throbbing pulsation, as an abnormally rapid throbbing or fluttering of the heart.

Pancreatitis: Inflamed condition of the pancreas.

Panhysterectomy: Surgical removal of the entire uterus.

Papule: A small, round, solid, elevated lesion of the skin.

Paracentesis: Surgical puncture of a cavity to aspirate fluid.

Paradoxical respirations: Those in which, upon inhalation, the traumatized portion of the chest wall moves inward rather than outward.

Paralytic ileus: Absence of peristalsis; paralysis of the intestines.

Paranoia: A disorder that exhibits delusions of persecution or of grandeur or a combination of both.

Paraplegia: Paralysis of the lower extremities.

Parenteral: Route other than the digestive tract.

Paresthesia: Feeling of tingling or numbness.

Patent: Wide open.

Pathogen: A microorganism or substance capable of producing a disease.

Pathological: Caused by a disease.

PCA: Patient-controlled analgesia.

Pediculosis: Infestation with lice.

Pelvic inflammatory disease: Any inflammation in the pelvis that occurs outside the uterus, uterine tubes, and ovaries.

Peptic ulcer: Loss of tissue lining the esophagus, stomach, or duodenum.

Percutaneous: Through the skin.

Perforation: A hole or break in the retaining walls or membranes of an organ, as in perforated ulcer and perforated eardrum.

Perfusion: Supplying tissues and organs nutrients and oxygen by blood flow through the arteries.

Pericarditis: Inflammation of the sac that encloses the heart and the roots of the great vessels.

Periodontal: Located around a tooth.

Periorbital: Surrounding the socket of the eye.

Periostomal: The area around the stoma.

Peripheral: Pertaining to the area outside the central region or structure.

Peristalsis: Involuntary wavelike contraction of organs with both longitudinal and circular muscle fibers that passes along the organ and propels its contents, as in peristalsis of the digestive tract.

Peritonitis: Inflammation of the serous sac that lines the abdominal cavity and encloses the abdominal organs.

Permeable: Permitting passage of a substance.

Pessary: A hard rubber ring inserted in the vagina to help keep the abdominal organs in place.

Petechiae: Very small, nonraised, round, purplish spots caused by intradermal or submucosal bleeding that later turn blue or yellow.

pH: The concentration of hydrogen (H) in a solution; the higher the concentration of hydrogen ions, the lower the pH of the solution.

Phacoemulsification: A technique of cataract extraction in which high-frequency vibrations are used to fragment the lens.

Phagocytosis: The engulfing of microorganisms and other foreign matter by phagocytes.

Phenylketonuria: A genetic disorder in which there is a defect in the metabolism of phenylalanine resulting in the presence of this amino acid in the urine.

Phlebitis: Inflammation of a vein.

Phlebotomy: Surgical opening of a vein to draw blood, often done with a needle.

Photocoagulation: Alteration of proteins in tissue by the use of light energy in the form of ordinary light rays or a laser beam.

Photophobia: Difficulty tolerating light.

Pilonidal sinus: A lesion located at the cleft of the buttocks in the sacrococcygeal region; also called pilonidal cyst.

Placebo(s): A supposedly inactive substance or procedure that can have either positive or negative effects on the relief of symptoms and that is usually given under the guise of effective treatment or in clinical trials of new drugs.

Planning: A phase of the nursing process in which a plan is developed with the patient, family, or significant other to provide a blueprint for nursing intervention to achieve specified goals. See also *Nursing care plans.*

Plaque: A patch or flat area.

Plasma: The liquid portion of blood in which formed elements are suspended; it contains plasma proteins, inorganic salts, nutrients, gases, wastes from the cells, and various hormones and enzymes.

Plasma cell: A spherical or ellipsoidal cell involved in the synthesis, storage, and release of antibody.

Plasmapheresis: Separation of the cells and components of the blood.

Platelets: The smallest formed elements in the blood; important in coagulation and blood clotting.

Plethora: A general term denoting a red florid complexion or an excess of blood.

Pneumocystis carinii: An opportunistic protozoan infection of the lung associated with acquired immunodeficiency syndrome (AIDS).

Pneumothorax: Accumulation of air or gas in the pleural cavity, resulting in collapse of the lung on the affected side.

Polyarteritis: Multiple sites of inflammatory and destructive lesions in the arterial system.

Polycythemia: An elevation in the total number of blood cells.

Polydipsia: Excessive thirst that results in drinking large quantities of water.

Polymorphonuclear leukocytes: The fully developed cells of the granulocyte series, especially neutrophils of which the nuclei contain three or more lobes.

Polyuria: Production of an excessive amount of urine.

Postictal state: Condition of a person right after a seizure.

PPO: Preferred provider organization.

Precancerous: Said of a growth that is not yet, but probably will become, cancerous.

Precipitate: A deposit separated from a suspension or solution by precipitation; the reaction of a reagent that causes the deposit to fall to the bottom or float near the top.

Premenstrual syndrome: A group of symptoms experienced by some women for several days before the onset of the menstrual period.

Prepuce: The foreskin or fold of skin over the glans penis in the male.

Presbycusis: Impairment of hearing in old age.

Presbyopia: Farsightedness that occurs normally with aging.

Pressure ulcer: A sore caused by pressure from a splint or other appliance or from the body itself when it has remained immobile in bed for extended periods.

Preventive: Hindering the occurrence of something, especially disease.

Primary union of wounds: The joining of two edges of a wound that are close together, resulting in a thin scar after healing; also called *healing by first intention.*

Priority: A first right established on emergency or need.

Problem-oriented medical records (POMR): A system of documentation in which the information is arranged according to specific problems presented by the patient at the time of seeking health care. The four components are data base, problem list, initial plan, and follow-up. See also *Progress notes.*

Process: A series of actions that move from one point to another on the way to completing a goal.

Prodromal stage: Early or very beginning stage of an illness.

Prognosis: Predicted outcome of the course of a disease.

Progress notes: Entries in the medical record describing what has been done in the care of the patient and his response to the intervention.

Prolapse: The falling down or displacement of a part or all of an organ, as in prolapse of a stoma and prolapse of the uterus.

Prophylactic: Something done or used to prevent infection or disease.

Prostaglandins: A group of naturally occurring fatty acids that stimulate contraction of the uterine and other smooth-muscle tissue.

Prosthesis: An artificial substitute for a missing part, such as an eye, limb, or tooth, used for functional or cosmetic reasons, or both.

Protective isolation: Special precautionary procedures to minimize exposure to infectious agents in a patient who has an immune deficiency or who is otherwise susceptible to infection.

Proteinuria: An excess of serum proteins in the urine.

Protocol: The plan for a course of medical treatment.

Protozoa: A phylum comprising the unicellular organisms; most are free-living, but some lead commensalistic, mutualistic, or parasitic existences.

Proximal: Closest to a point of reference.

Pruritus: Itching.

Psychoactive substances: Mind-altering agents capable of changing or altering a person's mood, behavior, cognition, arousal level, level of consciousness, and perceptions.

Psychotic features: Hallucinations, delusions, and grossly disorganized behavior.

Ptomaines: Toxic substances produced by the action of putrefactive bacteria on proteins and amino acids.

Ptosis: The dropping of an organ below its usual position, for example, lowering of the eyelid so that it partially or completely covers the cornea.

Pulmonary edema: Diffuse accumulation of fluid in the tissues and air spaces of the lung.

Pulse deficit: The difference between the radial and apical pulse rates.

Purpura: Purplish areas caused by bleeding into the skin or mucous membranes.

Purulent: Full of pus.

Pus: Liquid product of inflammation composed of albuminous substances, a thin fluid, and leukocytes; generally yellow in color.

Pustule: A small, round, pus-filled lesion of the skin.

Pyelogram: X-ray film of the kidney and ureters after injection of a contrast medium that may be administered intravenously (IV pyelogram) or by way of the ureters (retrograde pyelogram).

Pyelonephritis: Inflammation of the kidney and renal pelvis.

Pyrogen: Any agent that causes fever.

Pyuria: Pus in the urine.

Quadriplegia: Paralysis of all four extremities.

Rad: Radiation absorbed dose; the unit used for measuring doses of radiation.

Radiation therapy: The use of radiant energy from radioactive materials or high-voltage x-ray to treat disease.

Radioimmunoassay: A laboratory method for measuring minute quantities of specific antibodies or any antigen, such as a hormone or drug, against which antibodies have been produced.

Radionuclide: A radioactive substance given to the patient prior to the X-ray filming or scan.

Radiopaque: Not penetrable by x-ray; appears white.

Rales: Abnormal respiratory sounds heard in auscultation with a stethoscope indicating some pathological condition.

Range of motion: The extent, measured in degrees of a circle, through which a joint can be extended and flexed.

Rationalization: A defense mechanism in which a patient finds logical reasons (justification) for his behavior while ignoring the real reasons.

Recurrent: Returning at intervals.

Referred pain: Pain felt in a part away from its point of origin.

Reflex (reflexes): The sum of any particular autonomic (automatic) response mediated by the nervous system and not requiring conscious movement.

Refraction: Determination of refractive errors (inability to focus light rays on the retina) and their correction with eyeglasses.

Regeneration: The natural renewal of a structure.

Regimen: A prescribed scheme of diet, exercise, or activity to achieve certain ends.

Rehabilitation: The processes of treatment and education that helps the disabled individual attain maximum function, a sense of well-being, and a personally satisfying level of independence.

Remittent: Alternation of abating and returning, such as a fever that comes and goes.

Replication: The process of duplicating or reproducing.

Reservoir: A passive host or carrier that harbors pathogenic organisms without harm to itself and is a source from which others can be infected.

Residual urine: Urine that remains in the bladder immediately after urination.

Resorption: Taking in or absorbing again.

Respiration: The taking in of oxygen, its utilization in the tissues, and the giving off of carbon dioxide.

Respiratory acidosis: A condition in which the pH of body fluids is below 7.4 because of failure of the lungs to remove sufficient amounts of carbon dioxide.

Respiratory alkalosis: A condition in which the pH of body fluids is above 7.4 because of excessive removal of carbon dioxide by the lungs, as in hyperventilation.

Resuscitation: Revival after apparent death.

Reticuloendothelial system: A network of cells and tissues found throughout the body, especially in the blood, connective tissue, spleen, liver, lungs, bone marrow, and lymph vessels; these cells play a role in blood cell formation and destruction and in inflammation and immunity.

Retinopathy: A pathological condition of the retina associated with diabetes mellitus.

Retrograde: Moving backward; degenerating from a better to a worse state.

Retrospective: Dealing with the past.

Retrovirus: A type of virus that contains RNA.

Rhonchi: Coarse rattling sounds in the bronchial tubes caused by a partial obstruction.

Rickettsia: A genus of small, rod-shaped to round microorganisms found in tissue cells of lice, fleas, ticks, and mites and transmitted to humans by their bites.

Rigor mortis: The stiffness that occurs in dead bodies.

Safer sex: Any sexual practice that is performed with the use of a barrier to prevent the exchange of body fluids.

Salpingitis: Inflammation of a uterine tube.

Sarcoma: A tumor, often highly malignant, composed of cells derived from connective tissue.

Scabies: Infestation with the mange mite.

Scaling: Shedding of small, thin, dry layers of skin.

Scarring: Replacement of damaged tissue with fibrous tissue.

Schizophrenia: An illness that causes unusual, bizarre behavior (hallucinations and delusions).

Scleropathy: Injection of a solution that causes the vessel to dry up and disintegrate.

Scoliosis: Lateral curvature of the spine.

Scotoma: An area of lost vision in the visual field.

Sebaceous: Containing, or pertaining to sebum, an oily, fatty matter secreted by the sebaceous glands.

Secondary union: Healing of a wound in which the edges are far apart and cannot be brought together; the wound fills with granulation tissue and heals from the edges inward.

Sedative(s): An agent that calms nervousness, irritability, and excitement.

Seizure(s): An attack of uncontrollable muscular contractions; a convulsion.

Self-care: The process whereby one initiates and carries out certain health practices to maintain life, health, and personal well-being.

Semen: A thick, opalescent, viscid secretion discharged from the urethra of the male at the climax of sexual excitement (orgasm).

Seminal: Concerning the semen or seed.

Sensitivity reaction: An exaggerated response to agents perceived by the body as foreign.

Sensorineural hearing loss: Impaired perception of sound caused by a dysfunction in the inner ear or the eighth cranial nerve.

Sensory loss: Impairment of acuity of sight, hearing , taste, touch, and smell.

Septicemia: Invasion of the bloodstream by infective microorganisms.

Sequela: Condition resulting from a disease that follows the disease.

Seroconversion: The point at which antibodies to specific antigens are detectable in the blood.

Seroma: A collection of serum forming a tumor-like mass.

Serosanguinous: Containing both serum and blood.

Serum (sera): The clear, liquid portion of blood that does not contain fibrinogen or blood cells. Immune serum is blood serum from the bodies of persons or animals that have produced antibody; inoculation with such serum produces passive immunity.

Serum sickness: A hypersensitivity reaction to a foreign serum or other antigen.

Shock: Acute peripheral circulatory failure due to derangement of circulatory control or loss of circulating fluid.

Shunting: Physiologically bypassing, as when blood flows past the alveoli but the membrane is thickened and gases cannot cross into or out of the blood.

Sickle cell disease: All those genetic disorders in which sickle hemoglobin is found in the red cells.

Slit lamp: An instrument for examining the surface of the eye through a biomicroscopic lens.

Smear: A specimen for microscopic and cytological study; the material is spread thinly and evenly across a slide with a swab or loop.

SOAP: Acronym for *S*ubjective and *O*bjective data, *A*ssessment, and *P*lanning

Solute: The substance that is dissolved in a solution.

Somogyi effect: A rebound phenomenon due to overtreatment with insulin.

Source-oriented record keeping: A system of documentation in which information is arranged according to the person, department, or other source of information.

Specific gravity: The weight of a substance compared with the weight of an equal amount of another substance taken as a standard; for liquids the standard usually is water (specific gravity of 1).

Spermatozoa: The mature male sex or germ cells formed within the seminiferous tubules of the testes.

Spirochete: Any organism that is a member of the order *Spirochaetales*.

Spirometer: Instrument for measuring air taken into and expelled from the lungs.

Splenomegaly: Enlargement of the spleen.

Splitting: A trait that involves initial idealization of a care-giver or friend, followed by a devaluing of that same person.

Spores: Reproductive cells, usually unicellular, produced by plants and some protozoa.

Sprain: Wrenching or twisting of a joint with partial or complete tearing of the ligaments.

Sputum: Substance expelled by coughing or clearing the throat.

Stapedectomy: Surgical removal of the stirrup of the middle ear and replacement with a prosthetic device.

Stasis: Standing still; stagnation; usually refers to fluid.

STD: Sexually transmitted disease.

Stem cells: Generalized mother cells the descendants of which specialize, often in different functions; an example is an undifferentiated mesenchymal cell that is the progenitor of the blood and fixed-tissue cells of the bone marrow.

Stenosis: Narrowing or contraction of a passageway or opening.

Stent: Tubular device to give support to the interior of a vessel or tube, preventing its collapse.

Stereotaxis: Method of precisely locating areas in the brain.

Sterilization, microbe: The process of rendering an article free of microorganisms and their pathogenic products.

Steri-strips: Small, reinforced, adhesive strips placed over a healing incision to hold it together after sutures are removed.

Stoma (stomas): A mouth-like opening, especially one that is created surgically for the elimination of urine or fecal material.

Stomatitis: Generalized inflammation of the oral mucosa.

Strabismus: Deviation of the eye that cannot be controlled voluntarily.

Strain: Pulling or tearing of either muscle or tendon, or both.

Stye: Infected swelling near the margin of the eyelid.

Subcutaneous: Beneath or to be introduced beneath the skin.

Subluxation: Partial or incomplete dislocation of a bone from its place in a joint.

Substance use disorder: Problems with alcoholism or drug abuse.

Subsystem: A system within a larger system.

"Sucking" chest wound: One in which the pleural cavity has been penetrated, allowing air and gas to enter the cavity and produce pneumothorax.

Suicidal gestures: Things done or said that indicate a patient is contemplating committing suicide.

Sundowning: The phenomenon of becoming confused and disoriented at night.

Suprasystem: A highly complex system.

Sympathectomy: Surgical excision or interruption in some portion of the sympathetic nerve pathways.

Syncope: Fainting.

Syndrome: Combination of signs and symptoms associated with a pathological process or disease.

Synovial fluid: The transparent viscid fluid found in joint cavities, bursae, and tendon sheaths.

Synthesis: The process or processes involved in the formation of a complex substance from simpler elements or compounds; opposite of decomposition.

Synthesize: Put together (data) into a logical whole.

System: An organized whole composed of interacting parts.

Systole: The phase of the cardiac cycle in which the ventricles contract and force blood into the aorta and pulmonary arteries; the systolic pressure is recorded as the top number in a blood pressure reading.

Systolic (BP): Arterial pressure during systole.

Tachycardia: Abnormally rapid heart rate, usually to be over 100 beats per minute.

Tachypnea: Abnormal rapidity of respiration.

TENS: *T*ranscutaneous *e*lectrical *n*erve *s*timulator.

Tertiary: Third in order or stage.

Testis: The male gonad. One of two reproductive glands located in the scrotum that produce the male reproductive cells and the male hormone, testosterone.

Tetany: Continuous tonic spasm of a muscle; associated with calcium deficit, vitamin D deficiency, and alkalosis.

Thalamus: Either of two large structures composed of gray matter and situated at the base of the cerebrum and acting as a relay station for impulses traveling from the spinal cord and brain stem to the cerebral cortex.

Thanatologist: One who studies death.

Thanatology: The medicolegal study of the dying process and death.

Theory (theories): A belief, policy, or principle proposed or followed as the basis of action.

Therapeutic: Having medicinal or healing properties.

Thermal: Pertaining to heat.

Thoracentesis: Surgical puncture and drainage of the thoracic cavity.

Thrombocytopenia: Decreased number of platelets.

Thrombophlebitis: Inflammation of a vein related to formation of a blood clot within the vessel.

Thrombosis: Formation, development, or presence of a blood clot within a blood vessel.

Thrombus: A blood clot that obstructs a blood vessel or a cavity of the heart.

Thymus: An endocrine gland that lies in the upper chest beneath the sternum and which, during fetal life, sensitizes certain stem cells that eventually become T-lymphocytes.

Thyroid crisis: Sudden increase in the output of thyroxine and resultant extreme elevation of all body processes.

Thyroid storm: See *thyroid crisis*.

Thyrotoxicosis: Toxic condition due to hyperactivity of the thyroid gland.

Tinea: Ringworm; a name applied to many different kinds of fungal infections of the skin; the specific type usually is designated by a modifying term (e.g., tinea capitis, or ringworm of the scalp).

Tinnitus: Ringing, buzzing, or other continuous noise in the ear.

T-lymphocytes: Those white cells destined to provide cellular immunity that have passed through the thymus and migrated to the lymph nodes.

Tonic: State of rigid contraction of the muscles.

Tonometer: An instrument for measuring tension or pressure, especially intraocular pressure.

Tophus (tophi): Deposit of sodium biurate in tissues near a joint, in the ear, or in bone, as occurs in gout.

Topical: Pertaining to a particular area, as in topical medications applied to an area of the skin.

Torsion: Act of twisting or condition of being twisted.

Total parenteral nutrition: Intravenous feeding to provide all nutritional needs over time.

Tourniquet: A device for compressing an artery or vein; its use as an emergency measure to relieve hemorrhage is generally recommended only if the victim's life is threatened and other measures fail to stop massive blood loss.

Toxin: Poisonous substance.

Tracheostomy: A surgical incision into the trachea to insert a tube through which the patient can breathe.

Traction: Exertion of a pulling force, as that applied to a fractured bone or dislocated joint, to maintain proper positioning.

Tranquilizers: A group of agents that provide calm and relief from anxiety.

Transcellular fluid: Secretions and excretions that move through cell membranes and eventually leave the body.

Transfer factor: A factor occurring in sensitized lymphocytes that recruits additional lymphocytes and transfers to them the ability to confer cell-mediated immunity.

Transfusion: The administration of whole blood or blood components directly into the bloodstream.

Tuberculin test: An evaluation of sensitivity to the tubercle bacillus; the most common method is intradermal injection of a purified protein derivative of tuberculin (the Mantoux test); a positive reaction indicates the need for further diagnostic procedures.

Tumor node metastasis, staging system for: A system for classifying cancers according to the extent to which the malignancy has spread.

Turgor: Normal tension of a cell; swelling, distention.

Ultrasonography: A radiological technique in which deep anatomic structures are recorded by depicting the echoes of ultrasonic waves that have been directed into the tissues; the echoes (reflections) returning from the structures are converted into electrical impulses that are displayed on a screen, thus presenting a "picture" of the tissues being examined.

Unlicensed assistive personnel (UAP): Nursing assistants, technicians, unit secretaries, and aides who do not hold a professional license to perform some aspects of health care delivery and are hired to perform specific repetitive tasks.

Urea nitrogen: A major protein metabolite that is not recycled by the body but is excreted in the urine; blood urea nitrogen levels indicate the ability of the kidney to filtrate and excrete waste products.

Uremia: Retention in the blood of urea, creatinine, and other nitrogenous wastes normally eliminated in the urine; more correctly called *azotemia*.

Ureterostomy (ureterostomies): Surgical creation of a stoma to divert urine to the outside.

Urinalysis: Analysis of a sample of urine, most often done to detect protein, glucose, acetone, blood, pus, and casts.

Urticaria: Hives.

Vaccination: Injection of a vaccine into the body to produce immunity to a specific disease.

Vagotomy: Interruption of impulses carried by the vagus nerve or nerves; may be done to reduce the production of gastric secretions and to inhibit gastric motility, as part of the treatment for peptic ulcer.

Valsalva maneuver: Increase of thoracic pressure by forcible exhalation against the closed glottis, as in straining at stool.

Value: Something that is cherished or held dear.

Varices: Twisted and swollen veins.

Varicose veins: Enlarged and tortuous veins in which the distorted shape is the result of accumulations of pooled blood.

Vasectomy: Excision of the vas (ductus) deferens, or a portion of it; bilateral vasectomy results in sterility.

Venereal: Pertaining to or resulting from intercourse.

Ventilation: The movement of air from the external environment to the gas exchange units of the lung.

Vertigo: A sensation of movement of one's self or of one's surroundings.

Vesicant: Blistering; causing or forming blisters.

Vesicle: A small sac containing a serous liquid; a small blister.

Vesicostomy: Formation of an opening into the urinary bladder.

Viable: Capable of living.

Virulence: Degree of ability of an organism to cause disease.

Viscera: Internal organs contained within a cavity.

Viscous: Sticky, gummy, gelatinous; thicker than usual.

Vitrectomy: Removal of the contents of the vitreous chamber, and replacing them with a sterile physiological saline solution.

Volvulus: A twisting of the bowel upon itself, causing obstruction.

Wart: Epidermal growth of viral origin.
Wernicke's encephalopathy: Damage to brain cells caused by chronic alcohol abuse.
Wheal: Localized area or edema on the body surface.
Withdrawal: Symptoms that are the opposite of the symptoms caused by the ingestion of chemicals or drugs.

Xanthoma: Lipid deposit in the skin.
Xenograft: Surgical graft of tissue from one species to an individual of a different species.
Xerostomia: Lack of saliva; dry mouth.

Yeast: Term for fungi that reproduce by budding.

Zygomatic: Pertaining to zygomatic bone.

Index